THE HISTORY OF
OBSTETRICS &
GYNAECOLOGY

MICHAEL J. O'DOWD & ELLIOT E. PHILIPP

With a foreword by
J. J. SCIARRA

informa
healthcare

New York   London

First published in 2000 by the Parthenon Publishing Group Inc.

This edition published in 2011 by Informa Healthcare, Telephone House, 69-77 Paul Street, London EC2A 4LQ, UK.

Simultaneously published in the USA by Informa Healthcare, 52 Vanderbilt Avenue, 7th Floor, New York, NY 10017, USA.

Informa Healthcare is a trading division of Informa UK Ltd. Registered Office: 37–41 Mortimer Street, London W1T 3JH, UK. Registered in England and Wales number 1072954.

A CIP record for this book is available from the British Library.

Library of Congress Cataloging-in-Publication Data available on application

ISBN-13: 9781850700401

Orders may be sent to: Informa Healthcare, Sheepen Place, Colchester, Essex CO3 3LP, UK
Telephone: +44 (0)20 7017 5540
Email: CSDhealthcarebooks@informa.com
Website: http://informahealthcarebooks.com/

For corporate sales please contact: CorporateBooksIHC@informa.com
For foreign rights please contact: RightsIHC@informa.com
For reprint permissions please contact: PermissionsIHC@informa.com
Printed and bound in the United Kingdom.

THE HISTORY OF
OBSTETRICS &
GYNAECOLOGY

Dedication

This book is dedicated to our loved ones

Contents

Acknowledgements

We would like to acknowledge the very great help given to us by many friends and colleagues in the medical profession, and above all by librarians and curators of museums. It would have been quite impossible to research the history without their unfailing help always given most willingly and constructively. We are immensely grateful. The names are not written in any particular order, but much of the work was done in the libraries of The Royal College of Obstetricians and Gynaecologists, The Royal Society of Medicine, The Wellcome Institute, Cambridge University and two universities in Los Angeles.

In particular we single out the help given to us by Miss Patricia Want and her team at The Royal College of Obstetricians and Gynaecologists; Mr John Ayres, Deputy Librarian at The Royal Society of Medicine and his team; Mr Stephen Johnson, the Systems Librarian at The British Institute of Radiology in London; and the librarians at the Mercer's Library in Dublin.

We are particularly grateful to Dr Richard Smith and Professor Geoffrey Chamberlain for permission to reproduce statistical tables from *The ABC of Antenatal Care*, published originally in the *British Medical Journal* and later in book form by the *British Medical Journal*; to the President and Council of the Royal College of Surgeons of England for permission to reproduce the portraits of John Hunter and William Hunter in their council room; to Dr Stefan Reif of Cambridge University Library; to Dr Stephen Carstairs, Consulting Radiologist at the Royal Northern Hospital and archivist to the Royal College of Radiology; to Dr Jordan Phillips of Los Angeles for much information about American and Chinese gynaecological history; to Dr Felip Cid Rafael, Curator of the Barcelona Museum of the History of Medicine; to Dr Yvonne Hackenbroch, FSA, for much information about art and for

obtaining photographs of ivory models for us; to Dr Barbara Watterson of Liverpool for much help and for information about Egyptian medicine; to Mr E. L. Holland, FRCOG, for information about Egyptian medicine; to Mr Nigel Phillips and Mr Peter Young for help in obtaining books and booklets from which many of the reproductions were taken; to Dr Catherine James and to Miss Mary-Lou Nesbitt of the Medical Defence Union; as well as to the late Dr Clifford Hawkins for help with information about medico-legal matters; to the curator of the special collections in the Hunterian Museum in Glasgow for permission to reproduce the plates prepared originally for William Hunter's *Gravid Uterus*; to Dr Edith Gilchrist and to Dame Josephine Barnes for much information and for many helpful suggestions; to Ms Rochelle Clary, librarian at the University of California, Irvine; to Professor Edwin Malcolm Symonds, the University of Nottingham, Department of Obstetrics and Gynaecology; to Mr Martin Powell, the University of Nottingham, Department of Obstetrics and Gynaecology for slides of magnetic resonance imaging; to Mr Mervyn Griffiths the Registrar at the Medical Society of London for the photograph of the Medical Society of London; to Mrs Christine O'Dowd for her support and word processing. Thanks also to Margaret Mannion and Florence Grenham.

There are two people who have alas passed on who were the original inspiration for this book. The first was the late Dr Robert Greenblatt, the pioneer in gynaecological endocrinology who was the original person to suggest that this book should be written and who had already himself written the outlines of gynaecological history, and the late Lucie Ruth Philipp who was the real inspiration and who helped greatly in the early days of its preparation.

Foreword

Once or twice in a generation, a book is published that seems destined to become a classic. This is such a volume. It is a monumental achievement of scholarship and research – clearly a labour of love by the authors, whose interest in the history of obstetrics and gynaecology is long and illustrious. At the approach of a new millennium, Michael J. O'Dowd and Elliot E. Philipp have compiled *The History of Obstetrics and Gynaecology* to serve as an appropriate reference point: '. . . in the last decade of this twentieth century, during which more progress has been made in medicine than in the whole of the previous thousand and more years'.

The authors have produced a masterpiece. The text is completely original and contains a large number of illustrations, many searched out by the authors over many years. The narrative engages and draws the reader along, page after page. The work contains several special features – in particular, a detailed chronological table at the end of each section, and a large number of short biographies in a separate section, at the end of the book, of individuals who have made significant contributions – physicians and non-physicians, obstetricians and gynaecologists, as well as leaders in other fields. The extensive reference lists will greatly benefit those many readers inspired by this volume to further their study of medical history.

This remarkable history book recounts the events and changes – admittedly not always improvements – that have taken place over many centuries in society, changes in scientific knowledge and the way it is communicated, in technology, and in the lives and times of those persons who have dedicated their efforts to the health of women and their progeny. Of particular interest are those developments in seemingly unrelated fields that were vital to advances in gynaecology and obstetrics. This multi-faceted approach, which considers a topic not only in the appropriate biographies, but also in narratives, chronological tables, and reviews of related subjects and technologies, provides a far richer and more comprehensive treatment than would be possible if the authors had written from a century by century perspective.

In some 700 pages, the authors achieve the seemingly impossible – an account of history that is both meticulous and fascinating. Every aspect of obstetrics and gynaecology is here: prehistory and the early communications in writing; the discovery of the Rosetta Stone, which allowed modern scholars to decipher the mysteries of ancient Egyptian medicine; the earliest contraceptive practices and those only now being developed; the achievements of the Middle Ages, the Renaissance, and of more recent centuries, in Europe and Asia and the Americas. The authors have also included discussions of the contributions of such American pioneers as Oliver Wendell Holmes, Kermit Edward Krantz, Ephraim McDowell, Ralph Hayward Pomeroy, Isidor Clinton Rubin, and James Marion Sims because their work had widespread international implications.

At a time when major universities are removing to remote locations all scientific journals published before 1975 and authors are instructed to cite only articles published within the past 20 years, and when medical information is captured in the media in sound bites of 15 or 30 seconds' duration, this book is an indispensable addition, not only to every medical library throughout the world, but to the personal collections of books read again and again over many years by physicians, graduating medical students – indeed by anyone who is interested in the history of obstetrics and gynaecology.

J. J. Sciarra, MD, PhD
President of the International Federation
of Gynecology and Obstetrics
and
Thomas J. Watkins Professor and Chairman
Department of Obstetrics and Gynecology,
Northwestern University Medical School,
Chicago, Illinois, USA

The Authors

MICHAEL J. O'DOWD, MD, FRCOG, DCH, DA

*Consulting Obstetrician/Gynaecologist
Portiuncula Hospital, Ballinasloe
County Galway, Ireland*

ELLIOT E. PHILIPP, MA, FRCS, FRCOG

*Consulting Gynaecologist
Royal Northern and Whittington Hospitals
London, UK*

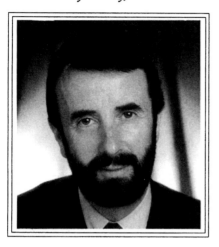

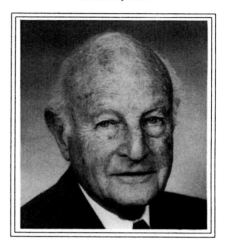

Following his qualification in medicine from University College Galway, Michael O'Dowd entered the postgraduate training programme in Belfast, Northern Ireland. After working in Canada and Zambia he settled as a specialist in a Franciscan hospital.

Due to a singular disinterest in history he dropped the subject during second level education and shifted to biology which led to a medical career. However, because of an interest in art he discovered the anatomical works of Leonardo da Vinci and thus began an embryonic interest in the past. Influenced by a set of prints depicting famous scenes in medical history he entered the fetal stage of development; the discovery of Harold Speert's *'Iconographia Gyniatrica'* led to the delivery of a 'neophyte' medical historian.

Michael O'Dowd's early development was 'nurtured' by the works of Harvey Graham and the other leading historians of obstetrics and gynaecology.

The mythology and archaeology of civilization prior to AD 500; the evolution of Celtic society; historical aspects of art, and music, and aspects of investigative journalism all fascinate him – as do libraries and book shops. He has written for stage, radio and television and also shares a deep interest in music with his wife Christine and their four children.

On completion of his medical studies at Cambridge University and in London and Switzerland, Elliot Philipp served as a doctor in the Royal Air Force. He then completed his specialist gynaecology training at teaching hospitals in London and Cambridge.

As a hospital consultant he researched, particularly into all forms of pain relief in childbirth, and into rare blood diseases in pregnancy; he pioneered 'key-hole' surgery and micro-operations, especially on infertile women.

He has been President of the Hunterian Society (1989–1990) and of the Medical Society of London (1993–1994). He serves on an Ethics Committee dealing with complicated problems that arise from new *in vitro* fertilization techniques.

He has published some 30 books, and edits a postgraduate text book on Obstetrics and Gynaecology. He has been an invited speaker in many Universities in the United States, Europe and the Middle and Far East.

In 1971 the French Government made him Chevalier de la Legion d'Honneur. He continues to write, adding to the 300 articles and papers already published.

His family is the most important thing in his life.

The photograph was kindly supplied by Elliot Philipp's grandson, Mr Guy Hills.

Introduction

It is appropriate in the last decade of this twentieth century, during which more progress has been made in medicine than in the whole of the previous thousand and more years, to review the history of the important specialty of obstetrics and gynaecology. Its edifice has been built on foundations laid by the great discoverers of the past working within our subject, and by wonderful polymaths, such as William Harvey who wrote with great originality about the human organs of generation after he had discovered and described the circulation of the blood.

Recently, many advances in obstetrics and gynaecology have resulted mainly because of discoveries by scientists working in totally different fields, which may have been only indirectly or even not at all related to the specialty. To give examples: the art of imaging the uterus and pelvis has been based on the discovery of X-rays by Roentgen, to which more recently has been added the use of ultrasonic machines that have been developed from apparatus invented to detect the presence of submerged submarines on the sea bed, and flaws in steel beams. Magnetic resonance imaging was initially used in medicine for the detection of lesions in the brain, and only later in the lower abdomen and pelvis.

In the 1990s no gynaecologist in the developed world can work without using the special skills and machinery of colleagues working in pathology, anaesthetics, imaging and in radiotherapy. The story of how the subjects developed side by side and of how gynaecologists came to use the various new tools is described in this book.

There have, of course, been previous histories of our own subject; and we have not hesitated to refer to them and especially to Fasbender's *History of Obstetrics* and Ricci's monumental works on gynaecological surgery. Harvey Graham's *Eternal Eve* written for a broader public is a splendid history, and in the first edition had many good references. There are also Harold Speert's and other outstanding gynaecological history books. Sherwin B. Nuland has added a splendid set of biographies of medical heroes.

We have told ourselves occasionally that we are plagiarizing as we refer to the books mentioned and to other works; but there is no other way of writing history except for 'inventing it'! We are only too aware that some previously written histories are mythical inventions and may be completely untrue, such as the claim that John Hunter inoculated himself with syphilis and gonorrhoea, repeated so often in the history books but now proved by careful examination of his notebooks to be a complete forgery (Woolf, 1986). Michael Holroyd a most eminent modern biographer recently said that history will look totally different in 50 years time, but that he hopes his books will still be useful as references. We hope ours will too.

The planning and structure was shared by us with the inspired encouragement of Mr David Bloomer, our publisher. His company has already published a series on the history of medical specialties.

We have tended to keep the narrative in each chapter a little short, but we add a 'chronology' to some, as well as a large list of references for the most modern elements.

The last section of the book is devoted to short biographies of outstanding masters from all of whose works in obstetrics and gynaecology and in other medical subjects new developments in ours have occurred. Such a man is Lord Lister, who is remembered because his discoveries, together with those of Pasteur, indirectly made possible much modern gynaecological surgery as well as improvements in obstetrics.

A few maps show how the knowledge of the art spread initially in the Eastern Mediterranean countries and then, in the sixteenth to nineteenth centuries, world-wide by travel. Now information is relayed instantaneously to all countries of the world. Yet, for all this, mortality in childbirth remains catastrophically high in the so-called 'developing' countries because of their weak economies and because of national catastrophes as well as man-made wars which make it impossible for them to acquire the new, mostly expensive, technologies which have so markedly lowered mortality from childbirth and operations in the developed world. It would be wrong by describing great changes to be insensitive to the restrictions placed for the major part of the world's population on acquiring the benefits of these changes.

We think that this book can be used in many different ways; as a work of reference by referring to the index, and by reading the appropriate biographies which should give an impression of the characters and accomplishments of the various men and women who have made discoveries in obstetrics and gynaecology. For example, if knowledge is sought about the subject of 'extended hysterectomy' reference to the index will show the pages in which there is a main essay on this subject. This happens to be in the section on the development of surgery. Hysterectomy is also touched on in the Narrative chapter. In the main essay the name of Ernst Wertheim features as the chief exponent of the operation in its early development. His life is described in the Biographies chapter. But the prospects for success in the operation improved greatly, as mentioned in the text, because of the advent of safe blood transfusions, asepsis, antisepsis and antibiotics. The subject of blood transfusion appears in a separate chapter on the blood and in the biography of Landsteiner, the discoverer of the blood groups. Information about asepsis can be found in the Narrative chapter and in the section dealing with the control of sepsis where the names of Lister, Pasteur, Fleming and Colebrook, appear. Details of these masters' work will also be found in the Biographies chapter under their names.

This form of construction makes it possible to give detailed information about how the extended hysterectomy operation developed and how difficulties and dangers were overcome without making the main essay very long, or duplicating information in different parts of the book. If the book were written era by era it would not be possible to trace so effectively the development of a subject. The book therefore does not give a century by century overview of all the advances occurring in, say, the eighteenth century, although what was happening in the eighteenth century is sketched out in the Narrative chapter. Furthermore, if the chronological tables to be found at the end of most chapters are referred to, a further idea about what was happening century by century can be obtained.

The Narrative chapter is written mainly to provide an overview of what happened in different eras. Much that has been described at length in the main body of the book is mentioned briefly in the Narrative; but when something like the fight against sepsis is described, that description can be found at length in the Narrative and in the Biographies. We have tried to make the work as authentic as history can be and to cover most of the obstetric and gynaecological changes made since the earliest times.

REFERENCES

Fasbender, H. (1906). *Geschichte der Geburtshulfe.* (Jena: Gustav Fischer)

Graham, H. (1950). *Eternal Eve.* (London: W. Heinemann)

Harvey, W. (1651). *Exercitationes de Generatione Animalium, quibus accendunt quaedam De Partu: de Membranis ac humoribus Uteri: a de conceptione.* (London & Amsterdam)

Nuland, S. B. (1988). *Doctors.* (New York: Alfred A. Knopf)

Ricci, J. V. (1945). *One Hundred Years of Gynaecology.* (Philadelphia: Blakiston Co.)

Ricci, J. V. (1949). *Development of Gynaecological Surgery and Instruments.* (Philadelphia: Blakiston Co.)

Ricci, J. V. (1950). *The Genealogy of Gynaecology.* (Philadelphia: Blakiston Co.)

Speert, H. (1973). *Iconographia Gyniatrica.* (Philadelphia: F. A. Davis)

Woolf, D. (1986). *Hunterian Society Transactions,* **XLIV**, 59–60

Narrative – historical overview

A man who has been concerned in a transaction will not write it fairly; and a man who has not cannot. But not withstanding all this uncertainty, history is not the less necessary to be known . . .
Letters written by Earl Chesterfield to his son.
Letter CXLIX, 26 April 1748

INTRODUCTION

The purpose of this history book is to record the changes that have taken place in obstetrics and gynaecology over many centuries. The key word is 'changes', not 'progress' because that word implies betterment and it is questionable whether all the changes that have occurred are beneficial. Also, saving lives by preventing or curing diseases, can eventually lead to overpopulation and starvation.

Changes in society are reflected in changes in obstetrics and gynaecology and are influenced by many features in scientific discovery and reasoning occurring at the time those changes are made. Such a time for instance was the industrial revolution which altered all aspects of life, including medicine. The study of history soon reveals that nearly all medical endeavours are accompanied by struggles – like those against the unknown, such as the agents that cause sepsis, or those struggles between feminists and their opponents, or perceived opponents, for domination in maternity care. This particular struggle was a direct result of the increasing mechanization in the seventeenth and eighteenth centuries; that mechanization itself being a male-dominated movement. Struggles do not have to be bitter, but some in our subject have been and that lends interest to this history.

COMMUNICATION

'In the beginning was the word' says the Gospel of St. John 1:1. The ability to communicate in writing was the first great change leading to the spread of knowledge, to the wide interchange of ideas and to the communication of new discoveries. The early teaching of obstetrics and gynaecology was written in hieroglyphics which were followed by the earliest form of the alphabet – the North Semitic alphabet – which, according to most evidence, originated in the lands on the eastern shores of the Mediterranean. It is not absolutely certain whether hieroglyphics were the forerunners of the alphabet, but it is certain that the first writings on clay tablets were in a cuneiform alphabet and later writings were on papyri, then on parchment and, much later, on paper.

Handwriting was followed by printing. The earliest forms of printing originated in China in the second century. A wood block was inked with a paint brush, a sheet of paper was spread on it and its back rubbed with a brush. The first movable type seems to have been thought out by a Chinese alchemist in the eleventh century. By the fourteenth century in China some form of printing seems to have been well established (Duhalde, 1763). Paper also originated in China and the secret of how to produce it was transmitted by the Chinese to the Arabs, who not only lived and worked in the eastern Mediterranean countries but also in Spain which they dominated during the thirteenth century. Slowly the process moved to western Europe where Gutenberg probably invented typographic printing and also the printing press in the middle of the fifteenth century, probably about AD 1450.

Old Egyptian stone and clayware, early manuscripts and, from the fifteenth century onwards, the printed word in books and articles, and still more recently recordings on film, sound and videotapes, have therefore formed the bricks from which the edifice of history is made. Writing has also fomented struggles between different and highly important schools of thought. To give an example: the followers of Galen (c. AD 131–201) (q.v.), whose writing was thought to be almost holy script, battled against those who first appreciated the remarkable changes brought

1

about by Vesalius (1514–1564) (q.v.), who inaugurated scientific dissection of the human body in the sixteenth century.

The great founding teachers of our subject, Hippocrates and Galen, spread the word by personal travel, although their journeys were far more limited than any undertaken after the fifteenth century, when travellers discovered new continents.

TOOLS OF THE TRADE

Men have designed tools for every trade since prehistoric times. Most notable for our subject have been tools of iron to make operating instruments, specula and obstetric forceps, and in the twentieth century monitoring and imaging instruments. Mauriceau (1637–1709) (q.v.) initiated operative obstetrics and with it the decline of the birthing stools. Some changes came about with dramatic suddenness over just a few decades. These included the discovery of the microscope and the ability to use it to identify organisms that could not be seen with the naked eye. Slowly developing discoveries have been those leading to birth control in all its various forms from, in

ancient Egypt, plugs made of grass to be put into the vagina, leading to those of sponge and rubber and finally in the late twentieth century, to the synthetic hormones used in the contraceptive pill.

General anaesthesia was developed to make major operations, such as amputation, painless, but was quickly applied to midwifery and some of the new volatile substances were used first by obstetricians such as James Young Simpson of Edinburgh (q.v.). Knowledge of molecular biology is the latest great 'change' and it can be applied to another recent change, namely the spin off from *in vitro* fertilization techniques. This chapter records in outline the story of the changes as a whole, and the rest of the book records the changes in specific subjects.

PREHISTORY

The development of obstetrics and gynaecology possibly started in the Indus valley where civilization was flourishing 5 millennia ago (Thomas, 1964). A map illustrating how the knowledge of medicine spread from the Indus Valley, west to the Middle East and eastwards across India, is shown in Figure 1. This was followed

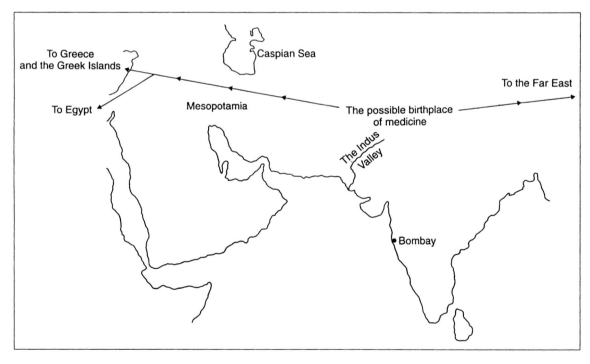

Figure 1 A map showing how the knowledge of medicine spread from the Indus Valley, west to the Middle East and eastwards across India

about 1500 years later by the Maurian Empire named after Chan Dragupta Mauria. From his name were derived the names of the island of Mauritius and the country in the most north-western part of Africa, Mauritania; but not a great deal is known about medicine in the Maurian Empire.

Even though obstetrics may have started in the Indus valley, Aurignacian art, which is represented by paintings of animals and by statues and is the earliest phase of Paleolithic art, was carried out in Europe between south-west Russia and Spain and depicted drawings and statues of interest to gynaecology (Speert, 1973). Art and obstetrics and gynaecology have always been linked from the days of those who drew the earliest illustrations depicting pregnant women and fertility goddesses to those who today design videographics and computer diagrams.

The most famous of all female statues of antiquity is the 'Venus of Willendorf'. It is one of the earliest statuettes of the female figure. It was found in the loess of the middle Aurignacian period which was about 22 000–24 000 BC. A loess is a light-coloured, fine-grained accumulation of clay and silt particles deposited by the wind. These findings were made in 1908 in western Europe, not in the Middle or Far East. The 'Venus of Willendorf' is thought to have been a fertility figure and is now in the Natural History Museum in Vienna (Lyons and Petrucelli, 1987).

Paintings are the earliest form of wall decoration in the caves which were inhabited by peoples in antiquity. There is a picture on a cave wall in Spain of a pregnant woman carrying a fetus in her abdomen, and of a baby emerging from the womb at birth. There is similarly a chalk figure of a female from the Neolithic Bronze Age about 2000 BC which was found in a pit at the flint-mining site of Grimes Graves in Norfolk, England. This figure is now in the British Museum.

Figures of women giving birth are extremely old. There is a seated female figure (c. 6500–5700 BC) found in excavations of Catal Huyak in central Turkey. The figure is thought to be that of a fertility goddess giving birth in a sitting position, with the baby between her legs.

Jacques von Siebold, or according to the French de Siebold, pointed out that the origins of obstetrics differ from those of medicine because obstetrics deals with normal states of affairs, whereas medicine deals with abnormality. Obstetrics is as old as humanity but that is not true of medicine. In old texts there is no mention of male obstetricians although there are references to midwives. In ancient mythology the goddesses were present at deliveries, but not the gods. There was a problem in the harems of the ancient Middle East because most of the women in them were young and as it was important to have old women to help with the deliveries, particularly if something was going wrong, they had to recruit these women from outside. No matter how bad things were, no man was ever called.

Although it is almost certain that there were inhabitants long ago in the Americas, and particularly in the south, the centre of all so-called civilized existence was in the Mediterranean basin and particularly the eastern Mediterranean countries. There was already a map showing some of the world 500 years BC. Europe was somewhat amorphous although the coastline of Italy had been charted. Libya occupied most of the southern shore of the Mediterranean. The Atlantic coasts of Europe had however, not been explored until the fourth century BC. Since it was possible to travel overland from the Mediterranean to India, intrepid voyagers knew the 1800-mile Indus River – one of the longest in the world – which rises in Tibet, flows through the Karakoram range across the Kashmir border into Pakistan, and ends in the Arabian sea. It was in the valley of this great river that the art of obstetrics seems to have started. The Indus had been explored by the officers of Darius I, King of Persia (550–486 BC) in about 510 BC. Roman power was fed by some of the luxuries of the Indus valley but from the second century onwards its influence was gradually taken over by that of the Abyssinians and Arabs, who dominated science and the eastern sea routes.

In Abyssinia women were delivered kneeling and in Kamschatka (in the north-east of the former Soviet Union) not only delivered kneeling, but in the presence of all the inhabitants of the village (Ludolf, 1681). We may infer what went on 2000 years ago from the behaviour of so-called 'primitive' tribes today; we know that in some primitive places, when a woman was going to have a baby they built a small hut for her so that she could stay modestly concealed from view. No man was present but the woman's mother or other female relative was. A male was allowed by some communities to cut the cord with a stone and then to tie a knot in the cord. That particularly happened in Sandwich Island, in the New Hebrides (now called Etate).

The writings of G.H. de Langsdorff, published in Frankfurt in 1812, describe how a cloth was placed on the ground and another one on the woman who was in labour. Once the parturient was delivered her husband came to cut the cord. The husband still does this in Brazil, where they use the shell of a shellfish to cut the cord. This was also done until recently in Kamschatka in the Khabarovsk territory in the extreme north-east of the former Soviet state, a very mountainous district.

ANTIQUITY

Egypt (6000–1200 BC)

We have chosen to concentrate in some detail on the role of gynaecology in Egypt because of information gained from the discoveries of ancient papyri by German and English explorers. Joachim translated the Ebers Papyrus (Figure 2), named after George Maurice Ebers, a German egyptologist who obtained the papyrus during a stay in Egypt in the winter 1872–1873 from a citizen of Luxor (Ebers, 1875). It contains, amongst its other medical compendia, treatments for various gynaecological matters. These include prolapse of the uterus, the preparation of various lotions, honey, petroleum and so on and the use of the fumes of wax and hot charcoal to help a prolapse go back!

On page 171 of Joachim's German translation (1890) are instructions on how to carry out an abortion, on page 173 the beginning of a remedy to prevent both breasts from shrinking, on page 174 a remedy against corrosion of the vulva, and on page 175 a remedy to prevent disease starting in the labia and against shooting pains in the vulva. On page 176 is a remedy to cool the vulva and uterus and to disperse inflammation of these parts. This consisted of a diet of palm fruit and cypress blended with oil and was probably an astringent remedy. At that time peppermint water was already being used for vaginal douching. There were remedies for pruritus, and there is a phrase in the book (on page 173) which makes it appear as though the ancient Egyptians knew of the existence of the ovaries, possibly from the rites preceding the embalming process and from vaginal examinations. They almost certainly knew the difference between the vulva, the vagina and the uterus and made pessaries from lint impregnated with various drugs which were rolled into a rod-shaped body and applied to the vagina.

In most Moslem countries and in ancient Egypt before the advent of Islam women were attended only by women and men were excluded from

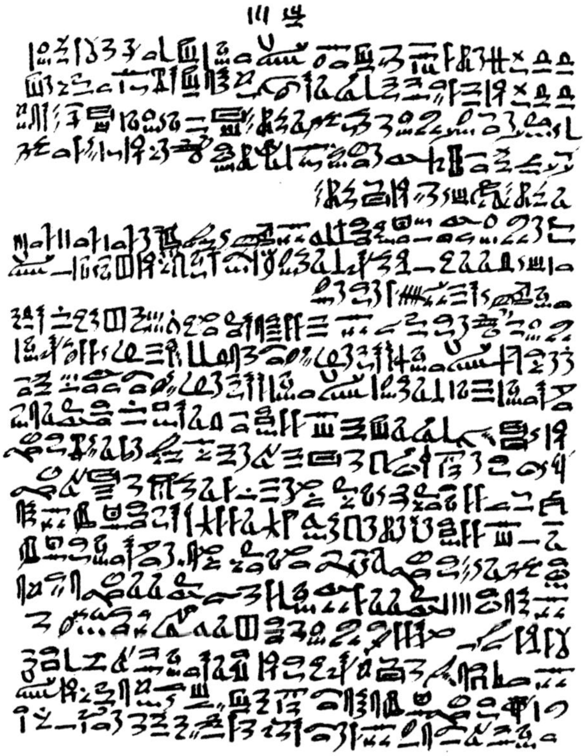

Figure 2 The Ebers Papyrus. Dated from circa 1550 BC this contains the first known reference to the use of a spermicidal chemical. Reproduced with kind permission from the International Planned Parenthood Federation (IPPF)

places where women were labouring. This is still so in many Middle-Eastern and eastern areas of the world. Women squatted either on the ground or on bricks to deliver. There has been a return to the squatting position in the second half of the twentieth century. (In fact, delivery with the patient lying on her back may only have come into fashion in the era of Louis XIV who is said to have wanted to look at one of his mistresses giving birth.)

Labour stimulants were used and these are recorded in the Ebers Papyrus. They consisted of salt, onions, oil, mint, incense, wine and even ground-up scarabs and tortoise shells. Once the child was born attention was paid to the way it gave its first cry and this was supposed to be prognostic of its future health. The cord was cut only after the midwife had washed the baby, according to the Westcar Papyrus. If the mother could not breast-feed then a 'wet-nurse', whose breasts would continue to lactate after she had finished suckling her own child providing that a new baby was placed on them, was engaged. In Thailand today women breast-feed squatting on the floor or on their beds with the babies supported by being held on or over their thighs. This seems to have been the state of affairs in ancient Egypt, too. (Breast-feeding, is still almost universal in the Far East except in those places where the baby food formula manufacturers have invaded.) In the Egyptian Middle Kingdom ivory wand amulets carried representations of Thoeris, a goddess shown as a pregnant female hippopotamus standing on its hind legs. This deity was at all periods much revered by all levels of society as the protectress of women in childbirth. (The Middle Kingdom covered the eleventh and twelfth dynasties, about 2050–1750 BC.) There was another domestic god, Bes, a dwarf-deity with leonine features, protector against snakes and various terrors and helper of women in childbirth. Heqet, a frog goddess of Antinopolis where she was associated with Khnum (a ram-headed god of elephantine appearance), was also a helper of women in childbirth.

In the Old and Middle Kingdoms there existed crude female figures of bound captives, the most likely purpose of which was for use in magical practices designed to secure fertility, safe child delivery and power over personal enemies and malignant forces. The god Bes is represented as an oil lamp with two wickholders on a stand with a central opening for filling with oil and a nozzle with a hole for a wick of twisted flax or papyrus. There were also predynastic potteries with painted designs carrying representations of a large female figure which has similarly been identified as a fertility goddess.

Pregnancy was diagnosed by a woman urinating over a mixture of wheat and barley seeds combined with dates and sand. If the grains sprouted the woman was sure to give birth! If only wheat then a boy would be born. If only barley, then a girl. The hormones in the urine could possibly have made a difference.

Mesopotamia (4000–331 BC)

The practice of medicine in Mesopotamia began either simultaneously with that in Egypt or soon thereafter. The history of the area is complex and is divided into the various eras of Sumerian, Semitic, Babylonian, Assyrian, Chaldean and Persian. The code of Hammurabi (c.1700 BC), the famous ruler of the old Babylonian Dynasty, was one of the first codes to regulate the practice of medicine. It is probable that the ancient Hebrews inherited many of their beliefs and codes, especially in medicine, from the old Mesopotamian cultures. The old Hebrew codes, many of which are still observed by orthodox Jews today, concerned among other things the frequency and timing of sexual intercourse (mid-cycle after about 12 days of abstinence) and the avoidance of intercourse after childbirth (longer after delivering a girl than after delivering a boy).

India (1500 BC – AD 500)

The enlightened one, Buddha – the Prince Gautama Siddhãrtha born c.563 BC and brought up as a Hindu – started his own 'religion and philosophy' which greatly altered and raised the status of women. Buddhism dominated religious worship in India from the time of Asoka until about the eighth century AD and it still has an enormous influence. Buddhism stood for the individual rights of women and secular conceptions of marriage. It checked the spread of purdah which led to seclusion of females, and was most beneficial as compared to Braminism by giving far greater attention to women. It gradually declined from the fifth to the sixth century AD onwards, but in his time, Buddha, was a great liberating influence.

The Buddha did not consider marriage as an inviable sacrament. He married Yasodhara and gave her his own ring, but he also gave presents to a very large number of other ladies. He and Yasodhara were probably both 16 years old when they married, but he left her and their son after some time to retreat and lead an ascetic life while he did his thinking and philosophizing. There is good reason to believe that before his death, at the age of 80, he consorted with the famous courtesan A. M. Ambapala. Courtesans in ancient India held a very high position and the Indian race had most sophisticated ideas about sexual activity, the rights of women and the maintenance of their health. When women were highly esteemed their physical health was treated as being as important as that of men.

Greece and Rome (500 BC – AD 500)

Our knowledge of pre-Hippocratic Greece depends on the findings of those archaeologists who excavated in Troy and Crete. The excavations carried out by Sir Arthur Evans (1851–1941), especially those of the ruins of Knossos in Crete, uncovered evidence of a sophisticated Bronze Age civilization which he called Minoan. Among the artefacts which he dug up and which are on exhibition on Knossos are 3000 clay tablets inscribed with a form of Minoan writing, the linear B script. Although this has been very difficult to decipher there are illustrations in the museum which show that the Minoans certainly knew the results of sexual congress and there are hints at their use of birth stools. Crete is probably the starting point of European civilization because it is one of the places, as is Turkey, where East meets West.

Greek medicine was dominated first by the Greek gods such as Apollo, Diana, Mercury and so on, and then by the writings of the great Hippocrates (q.v.). Asclepius (q.v.) has been enormously important in the culture of medicine. It is possible to see that if obstetrics and gynaecology started near India, their practice gradually moved westward so that it reached the Greek islands and then mainland Greece before arriving in Italy, and then specifically in Rome. In the main text and also in the Biographies section we discuss the work of some of the important Greek and Roman doctors but it is worth mentioning the great Soranus of Ephesus, a prolific writer of some 20 important works. Ephesus is, appropriately, a city in Asia Minor and so east of Greece, and west of India. Soranus studied in Alexandria, the great coastal city in the north of Egypt and eventually went to Rome where he practised medicine in the reigns of Trajan (98–117) and Hadrian (117–138). He died at about the time Galen (q.v.) was born (Temkin, 1956).

Soranus, whom Temkin said was one of most learned, critical and lucid authors of antiquity, wrote his *Gynaecology* in Greek. He also wrote about bandages, fractures and surgery but most important was his biographical *Life of Hippocrates*. Soranus's gynecology was paraphrased in part by Muscio (or Mustio) around AD 300–500. Muscio wrote mainly from the shorter catechism which Soranus had written for midwives and Muscio's translation or adaptation was used by Rösslin (q.v.) in his famous Rosegarden book of 1513. Soranus mentioned a Greek author Moschion who formulated prescriptions for gynaecological treatment. He is not to be confused with Muscio.

The various illustrated positions of the fetus in Temkin's edition of Soranus's Gynaecology, may

have been added after Soranus's original text had been written; but Soranus knew that the fetus could take up various positions in the uterus and described them. It seems likely that Paulus Aeginetta also taught that feet presentation could be natural. Soranus described the qualities needed by a good midwife: she had to have a good memory, love her work, be respectable, be sound of limb, robust and 'endowed with long slim fingers and short nails to be able to touch a deep-lying inflammation without causing too much pain'.

Soranus when speaking about the attitude of midwives said 'she will not change her methods when the symptoms change, but will give her advice in accordance with the course of the disease'. He usually advised bland treatment especially during the initial stage or attack of the disease (epitasis), but he advocated 'cyclic treatment' consisting first of a 'restorative treatment' to build up the patient's strength, and then of a 'metasyncritic treatment' in which diet was carefully directed to include acrid and pungent substances and local treatment was with cupping, with or without scarification or metasyncritic drugs. Vomiting may have been provoked by inserting the fingers far into the mouth, and infusions prepared with honey, wine and vinegar were also given.

Soranus was not a great believer in dissection saying 'and since dissection, although useless, is nevertheless studied for the sake of profound learning, we shall also teach what has been discovered by it'. He went on to write that he would not be believed that dissection was useless unless he showed that he knew all about it. Soranus gave one of the earliest full descriptions of the uterus, with its narrow neck, and with a 'didymus' on each corner.

It may be that Soranus's rejection of dissection because it was useless, helped to perpetuate Galen's anatomy which was based on the dissection of lower animals, particularly the Barbary apes found in North Africa. Galen had done quite extensive dissection on lower animals but his greatest fault was to imagine that what he found in these non-primates could apply to the anatomy of the human female. It may be that Soranus's views on dissection which upheld Galen held obstetrics and gynaecology back until the time of Vesalius.

Soranus's writings were translated into Latin by Caelius Aurelianus in the fifth or sixth century. Caelius Aurelianus should not be confused with Aurelius Cornelius Celsus, the compiler of scientific and medical knowledge who lived in the reign of Tiberius Caesar (Garrison,1921). Manuscripts of antiquity were written for the layperson as well as for professionals, unlike present day books. Most of course were written by physicians, but Celsus was a lay-man of the noble family of Cornelii (Morton, 1983).

Galen's authority predominated in Alexandria from the fourth century onwards, and by the sixth century had reached the dominating position which it held for another thousand years. Soranus's teachings were reasonably dominant until then, and were also accepted by a large number of people for quite a long time afterwards. He had written not only a description of the female genital organs, but also a discussion on fertilization and embryology quoted in Oribasius's medical encyclopaedia 200 years later. In talking about midwives, Soranus demanded that 'she should be free from superstition': He wrote about a 'natural sympathy' between the uterus and the breasts in his Book 1 page 15. Galen and Soranus were preceded by Celsus who lived from 25 BC to AD 50 in the reigns of Augustus and Tiberius and who had made observations on the anatomy of the uterus and had described some gynaecological operations. Pliny (AD 23–79), who lived soon after Celsus, described various therapeutic agents in the treatment of diseases of women, and he was followed by two other teachers, Aylen born in AD 170 and Oribasius (AD 325–403). The latter compiled a vast encyclopaedia of 70 volumes, some of which concerned gynaecology.

Galen who had been born in 131 in Pergamum, a city in Mysia, now part of Turkey, was influenced by the fact that his birthplace was a shrine of the healing god Asclepius to which many distinguished persons from the Roman empire came for cures, and by the teaching in the city's medical school at which Galen first studied, before moving to Smyrna (Ismir today), then Corinth in Greece and Alexandria in Egypt. Inevitably he travelled to Rome returning 5 years later to Pergamum.

The Bible

The Hebrew Bible in Leviticus 15:2 described a discharge that was probably gonorrhoeal in men. The same chapter, verse 9 deals with menstruation; and verse 33 seems to hint at the sexual transmission of discharges (Siebold, 1891; Stewart-McKay, 1901).

The *mshnt* was a type of confinement chair made of brick and there were also birthing stools recorded in the Old Testament. These were made of wood and were sometimes highly decorated. The front of the seat was hollowed out into a semicircle and two upright wooden rods were affixed to each corner of the front so the women could grasp them when pushing in the second stage of labour. It is recorded that there was often a midwife in front as well as behind the mother, the role of the one behind being to support her.

Siebold in his history quotes Rachel's delivery in Genesis 35:17–18, to show that she had a difficult delivery; and in fact it must indeed have been very difficult because she died after Benjamin had been born, and she was apparently on her own when she was delivering him. She had a long labour but according to some authorities quoted by Siebold she was already around 50 years of age, and she had of course long been infertile.

In Genesis 38: 27–30 when Thamar was delivering, the first twin put out its hand and the midwife tied a red thread on its wrist, but then it went back in and his brother came out! This story shows according to Siebold, that spontaneous version could occur. The reason why the midwife put the thread around the first child's hand was to give it precedence for legal purposes. The midwife was very surprised by the outcome and the mother was very badly torn!

The Hebrew Texts

In antiquity Rabbis were teaching the Talmud which was studied intensively. It consisted of the Mishna and its lengthy commentary the Gemara, slowly compiled over several centuries in Palestine and Babylonia. In the university centres there, thousands of students studied in the Academies and often moved from one to another and even from country to country. The Talmud deals with many medical matters. It is diverse and complicated and it required new Rabbis to codify the laws contained in it. These laws contain among other matters much about menstruation, religious purification, discharges from the penis and the vagina, laws appertaining to childbirth and divorce as well as to fertility and infertility. One of the great commentators who codified the Talmud was Maimonides (1135–1204) (q.v.). The Jewish philosophers were much influenced by Greek philosophical concepts, particularly by the writings of Plato and Aristotle.

In 1896–1897 100 000 fragments of documents relevant to medieval history were discovered in the Genizah of the old Ben Ezra Synagogue of

Old Cairo. A Genizah is a room in a synagogue into which material that should not be destroyed because it contains the name of God or a reference to him, is stored. The discovery of the Cairo Genizah was made by two very learned Scottish Presbyterian ladies from Ayrshire, a Mrs Lewis and a Miss Gibson who had some knowledge of Hebrew. They obtained a rare fragment of a Hebrew manuscript which was identified by Rabbi Dr Solomon Schechter, Professor in Rabbinics at Cambridge University, as a part of 'Ecclesiasticus' a book of the Apocrypha. Dr Charles Taylor, Master of St John's College, Cambridge, helped Dr Schechter to bring all the contents of the Genizah to Cambridge where they are now being studied in the Cambridge University library. Among these are some fragments related to excessive uterine bleeding and its treatment (T-Sar 43/21), to the early diagnosis of pregnancy (T-Sn 90/36) and for inducing abortion (T-Sar 45/30). (T-S stands for Taylor-Schechter the names under which the fragments are classified) (Price and Wigham Price,1964).

THE DARK AND MIDDLE AGES (AD 500–1450)

It does seem as though there were real 'Dark Ages' from the years AD 400 to AD 1000. It seems extraordinary that after the burgeoning of art, culture and medicine in the Middle East and in the countries under the influence of Greece and Rome everything should have come to a standstill for a lengthy period of 600 or more years. The so-called Dark or early Middle Ages followed the collapse of the Roman Empire in the fifth century. However, the monks in their monasteries, the Rabbis in their schools of learning and the stonemasons who started to build the great cathedrals and churches travelled from country to country and ensured that neither art not science died away completely. One of the great glories of the ninth century is the Irish Books of Kells, still to be seen in Trinity College, Dublin.

Paulus Aegineta (Paul of Aegina) (AD 625–690) summarized much ancient medicine in his manuscript *An Epitome*, later printed in 1528. In it he described amputation of the breast. His compilations of Graeco-Roman medicine extended to seven books.

The Middle Ages stretched in time from the decline of the Roman Empire to the beginnings of the Renaissance in the mid-fifteenth century. As the Roman Empire came to an end, its capital moved to Byzantium on the shores of the Bosphorus. The study of medicine also moved to Byzantium close to its site of origin in Greece. In the sixth century the medical schools of Alexandria and Athens were shut down. Interest in medicine waned as the concern with scholasticism became all consuming. Human dissection was forbidden and all aspects of medicine went into decline. Fortunately the art of obstetrics and gynaecology as practiced in antiquity was recorded and compiled for posterity.

Oribasius (c. AD 325–403) of Pergamum had a high reputation as an obstetrician in Byzantium. He also produced an encyclopaedia of medicine which promulgated the ideas of Galen. Another compiler in Byzantium was Aetius of Amida (AD 502–575) whose obstetrics and gynaecology was based on that of Soranus. His compilations on gynaecology were abstracted by other workers and were translated into Arabic. These translated texts formed the basic knowledge by which Arabian physicians understood gynaecology between the ninth and twelfth centuries. The Arabian texts were later translated and adopted by the Byzantine physicians in the fourteenth century and eventually formed the basis of Caspar Wolff's *Harmonia Gynaeciorum* in the sixteenth century.

Arabian medicine which was based on Graeco-Roman precepts, came to the forefront from the middle of the of the eighth century, and its main school was in Baghdad. The Arabians collected all available manuscripts and translated the works into Arabic. Among those compilers of importance in obstetrics and gynaecology was Rhazes (AD 850–923) who studied and worked in Baghdad. In one of his books, called the *Continens*, there are references to gynaecology, while a further book the *Liber Helchavy* was devoted mainly to midwifery. Another physician of the era who was held in very high esteem was Avicenna (980–1037) and although his writings were not original, he kept alive the teachings of the ancients, which were to form the basis of some of the best European medical books of the sixteenth century. Also of importance was Albucasis (936–1013) who gains the credit for the introduction of the cautery, and also Moses Maimonides (1135–1204) the Jewish scholar and physician.

Over the next few centuries European medicine gradually re-emerged. Universities were founded in Paris, Bologna, Oxford, Cambridge, Padua, Montpellier and Naples during the course of the twelfth and thirteenth centuries. Knowledge of anatomy was based on that of the pig until 1316 when Mundinus at Bologna wrote a book on human dissection. Mundinus perpetuated the concept that the uterus contained seven cells, but disagreed with the concept of the wandering uterus as proposed in ancient Greece.

In Salerno near Monte Cassino in southern Italy a medical school was founded in about the sixth century and was of importance until the twelfth century. In the eleventh century Trotula wrote a book in Salerno known as *de Passionibus Mulierum Curandarum, De Aegritudinibus Mulierum De Curis Mulierum*, also known as just *Trotula*. She was possibly a woman doctor of Salerno and she may have practised midwifery. The book most probably was translated from Latin into English in the early fifteenth century (Rowland, 1981). In this book different positions and malpresentations of the child are described and illustrated. (Another book which shows abnormal fetal positions is Jane Sharp's (q.v.) *The Compleat Midwive's Companion* in 1671.) In 1566 Caspar Wolff wrote an essay denying that Trotula was a woman. In the essay he not only wrote about the original Trotula, but about 'old Trots', who at the end of the Middle Ages were considered to be procuresses and women who still wished to have sexual pleasures. William Shakespeare (1564–1616) wrote in *The Taming of the Shrew* 'an old Trot, with ne'er tooth in her head although she may have as many diseases as two and fifty horses', commemorating the name of Trotula (Rowland, 1981). Another physician surgeon of the thirteenth century Italian school was Richard of Salerno. His book the *Anatomia Vivorum* contained some gynaecological anatomy and is said to have been the first text to show the importance of the subject in the understanding of women's diseases.

Medicine in the twelfth and thirteenth centuries was dominated by the Islamic and Arabic influences. Their principles were: not to dissect because it was against their religion, for men not to deal with gynaecological or obstetrical matters because these were for midwives to deal with, for operations to be carried out by wandering specialists and to argue about fees! There were great teaching hospitals in Baghdad, Damascus and Cairo of which the Hall of Wisdom in Cairo was the most famous (Garrison, 1921).

The earliest printed book in the library of the Royal College of Obstetricians and Gynaecologists in London is a work of Albertus Magnus (q.v.), a Dominican monk born Albert von Volstadt and educated at Padua, who lived from about AD 1193 to 1280. It took until the third quarter of the fifteenth century before his book, which had been handed down in manuscript, became printed and for its information to be widely spread. The work

is important because it is the first printed work concerning gynaecology in a section entitled *A Comment on the Secrets of Women*. This incidentally contains one of the first printed endocrinological prescriptions; for Albertus advocated using the powdered testis of a hog in wine for men of poor sexual power, and the powdered womb of a hare in wine to make women fertile. (A similar prescription is to be found in a manuscript in the British Library. This manuscript has recently been printed in a Middle English text together with a translation into modern English by Beryl Rowland. The manuscript dates from the early fifteenth century.) The Albertus text was probably printed first in Venice in 1478 and then again in Venice in 1509 and in Amsterdam, and more than a century later in 1643 and 1648.

THE RENAISSANCE (c. 1450–1600)

After the long doze of the Middle Ages came the Renaissance when, (according to Jacob Burckhardt, a Swiss historian in 1860) in Italy particularly there was an awakening from the 'sleep of the dead of all cultural life in the Middle Ages'. It was characterized according to Burckhardt by 'the development of the individual which made possible the discovery of the world and the discovery of man'. This was achieved by extraordinary developments in the fifteenth, sixteenth and part of the seventeenth centuries.

In 1492 Christopher Columbus discovered America and in the same year the Jews were expelled from Spain. Ten years later the Muslims and some Spanish Protestants became victims of the inquisition. To escape its edicts Moslems, Jews and Protestants started to migrate to other countries and in their migration took with them their medical knowledge and helped it spread throughout the rest of Europe.

The great stars of the new science that overruled Galen's medicine and Ptolomy's astronomy were Copernicus followed by Galileo, William Harvey and Isaac Newton, who were leaders in the scientific revolution of the seventeenth century. The great Leonardo da Vinci who illustrated among other anatomical structures both the female and the male genital organs and in the famous *De Coitu* drawing showed the two joined together, lived at a time when mathematics was advancing rapidly.

Dissection was performed particularly by such men as Gabrielis Falloppio (1523–1562) whose first anatomical works were published 2 years before he died (Figure 3). Falloppius or Falloppio was an Italian who described the Fallopian tubes connecting the ovaries to the the uterus, as well as the semicircular canals of the inner ear. He was a friend of the great anatomist Vesalius. Although Italian was his spoken language his monumental three-volume collected works (1050 pages plus index), published in Venice in 1606 after his death, were written in Latin. They contained not only a considerable amount of anatomy, but also a great deal of theory as to the causation of tumours and medication for almost all conditions known in those days.

In the sixteenth century the other great anatomists were Aranzo and Eustachius. They dissected and made marvellous illustrations in textbooks and atlases. Another of the very early atlases of gynaecological interest was written by John Johannes Ketham and published in Venice in 1513. It is one of the oldest printed illustrated atlas folios, notable for its beautiful line drawing and engravings of the human body that are admirably clear.

One of the most colourful personalities of the sixteenth century was Paracelsus. Philippus Aureolus Theophrastus Bombast von Hohenheim (1493–1541), who called himself Paracelsus signifying above or beyond Celsus, qualified as a doctor probably at the University of Ferrara where the medicine of Galen and of the Arab teachers of the Middle Ages was already being loudly criticized. 'Bombastic' is named after him and not vice versa. He has been described as a genius and as a vitriolic scathing caustic critic. His great ability for upsetting people turned him inevitably into a traveller visiting England, Ireland, Scotland, most European countries and Russia. One of his great claims to fame in his day was that he burnt the books of Avicenna and of Galen in front of the University of Basle to which he had been appointed a lecturer in medicine. He probably was the first man to use any form of chemotherapy and probably anticipated homeopathy and the works of Ehrlich because he prescribed mercury by mouth for syphilis, the great scourge. The illness was said to have been brought by Columbus's sailors back from America, but while there is little good evidence to support this, it is certain it spread like a plague and was one of the biggest killer diseases until, first Ehrlich and then Fleming, Chain and Florey discovered how to use arsenic, sulphonamides and later penicillin in the twentieth century. Paracelsus's great book on surgery, published in 1536, remade his reputation

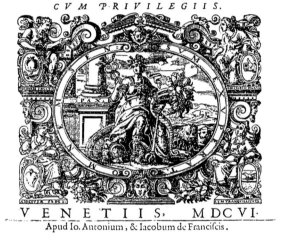

Figure 3 The Frontispiece of Gabrielis Falloppio's book

after he had had to leave Basle following disputes with his colleagues there.

Eucharius Rösslin who died in 1526 produced a book in 1513 entitled *Der Schwangern Frawen und Hebammen Roszgarten* (The Rose Garden for Pregnant Women and Midwives) much of which was derived from the works of Moschion of the sixth century AD and Soranus of Ephesus of the second century. The 'Rosegarden' was eventually translated from the German into Latin in the early 1530s. An English translation by Richard Jonas was published by Thomas Raynold as *The Byrth of Mankynde* in 1540. This was to remain the most popular textbook of midwifery until late in the seventeenth century. *The Byrth of Mankynde* devotes a whole chapter to ailments in pregnancy but does not advocate any kind of regular antenatal care. Antique book collectors have long treasured *The Byrth of Mankynde* as one of the most desirable of old obstetric books to possess.

The great names of the end of the Renaissance include those of midwives such as Louise Bourgeois (q.v.) and her French contemporaries. Ambroise Paré (1510–1590) (q.v.) a great teacher of midwives at the Hotel Dieu in Paris was not only a very great surgeon, but also greatly advanced obstetrics and its teachings. Paré revitalized the idea of podalic version. This involves turning the baby by 'inserting the hand into the uterus, clasping one or two feet (hence podalic) of the unborn child and turning it (i.e. version) into such a position that it could be born'. Although it seems to have been a very obvious procedure to carry out, it had not been done apparently between Soranus's time and Paré's time.

The Hotel Dieu in Paris was from the fifteenth century onwards the most famous maternity unit in Europe and therefore in the world. It still functions today. While the Hotel Dieu and the school for midwives, probably the first founded in Europe under the direction of Ambroise Paré, helped to spread the knowledge of midwifery widely because people came from many countries to learn there, the main centres for the propagation of knowledge were the universities founded from the eleventh century onwards, and such institutions as the Royal Society with its publications.

In England the first formal arrangement for the control of midwives was made under Henry VIII by an Act of 1512 and was incorporated into the Act which dealt with the regulation of physicians and surgeons. This arrangement continued until 1902 when the Central Midwives Board began to issue licences. Most of the licences contained about two full pages of conditions under which the licence was granted and the oath which the midwife took on being granted her licence.

Also of importance during the Renaissance were the naming of the venereal disease 'syphilis'; the putting to death of Agnes Sampson of Edinburgh in 1591 apparently for attempting to alleviate labour pains; the performance of Caesarean section in 1500 by a Swiss sow gelder called Jacob Nufer; the publication of Scipione Mercurio's *La Commare O Riccoglitrice* in 1596, the first authorative obstetric text published in Italy; and the institution and retention of Records of Christenings, Marriages and Deaths c.1538 in the reign of King Henry VIII.

SEVENTEENTH CENTURY

The obstetric forceps were developed, but kept secret, by the Chamberlen family. Major advances were made in our understanding of embryology, and knowledge of reproductive anatomy was enhanced with the advent of microscopic examination.

The development of the obstetric forceps was the major advance in the seventeenth century. Instruments to assist delivery had been in use for centuries, but were mainly for extracting dead infants. There were various forms of hooks which were used to grasp the fetal buttocks or head. Also fillets or bandages of soft leather, linen, muslin or whale bone were used which could be passed around the limbs in breech presentation and traction applied. The vectis (tractor or lever), was a long narrow instrument which was slightly similar to the single blade of a forceps in appearance. However, it was inefficient and also likely to cause gross injury to both the infant and mother. The only methods used to extract a living infant were by version and breech extraction or by delivery with unaided hands.

The possibility of constructing an obstetric forceps which could be used with safety was probably suggested by Jacob Rueff about 1554, although a bas relief from Rome c. second century AD illustrated what appeared to be a pair of obstetric forceps. However, the Chamberlen family are usually credited with the invention and development of the instrument which was to save the lives of countless numbers of infants and mothers. Peter Chamberlen the elder (1575–1628) was born in Paris but emigrated to England in the mid-sixteenth century. He invented the forceps about 1598. The instruments were kept secret by the Chamberlen family for almost 150 years. The forceps were of clever design and the two halves could be separated at the point at which they crossed over one another. This allowed for separate insertion of each blade into the pelvis. The cross-over point could then be stabilized, allowing the fetal head to be gripped and extracted from the pelvis. Jean Palfyne (1650–1730) of Ghent devised instruments known as the Palfyne or Douglas forceps in 1723 and many other varieties of obstetric forceps were introduced thereafter.

William Harvey (1578–1657) (q.v.) was born in Folkestone and educated at Cambridge (Figure 4). From there he went to Padua in Italy where he studied under Fabricius and was influenced by Galileo. In 1628 his pioneering work on the

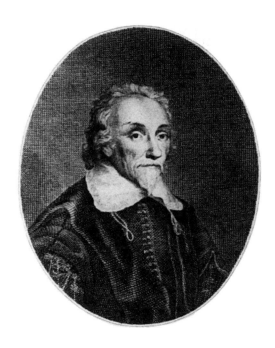

Figure 4 William Harvey (1578–1657). The discoverer of the circulation of blood and a founder of the science of embryology. Reproduced with kind permission from the Wellcome Institute Library, London

circulation of the blood was published in his *De Motu Cordis et Sanguinis in Animalibus* (On the Motion of the Heart and Blood in Animals). Harvey was also renowned as one of the founders of embryology. In 1651 his *De Generatione Animalium* (On the Generation of Animals) was published. In it he maintained that the embryo developed by differentiation and growth, and was not entirely preformed in the egg as was thought at that time. He thus helped to establish the theory of epigenesis. Harvey studied the development of the chick embryo in detail and also dissected human embryos. In his writing on labour, *De Partu*, he recommended patience and advised against unnecessary interference. Harvey's *De Generatione Animalium* with its chapter *De Partu* was the first original English book on obstetrics to replace translations of German and French publications.

Robert Hooke (1635–1703) studied both astronomy and microscopy and in his work *Micrographia* of 1665, was the first to name the cell as seen by him in a sample of cork. With the aid of microscopic magnification, Marcello Malpighi (1628–1694) discovered the capillary circulation and thus completed Harvey's earlier work.

Malpighi studied embryology and also documented microscopic investigations of the endometrium, myometrium, ovary and hydatidiform degeneration of placental tissue. Further anatomical observations were made by Johann van Horne (1621–1678) of Leiden who accurately described the round ligament and ovary.

One of the most important anatomical descriptions in gynaecology was that by Regnier de Graaf (1641–1673) (q.v.) who, whilst still a young man, first published his book in 1668 from Leiden in Holland where he lived, describing the structure of the testis and the sections of the female genital organs including the ovaries with follicles in them. Regnier de Graaf's findings were quickly recognized as of great interest throughout the world because not only were there two editions of his book published in Holland in 1668 and 1677 but there was also a French edition in 1678 and many subsequent editions in other countries.

De Graaf's work was in part dependent on the discovery of the microscope. Who actually invented the microscope is not certain, but improvements were definitely made to it by Galileo. It is likely that the microscope had been invented by Hans Lippershey at the end of the sixteenth or perhaps even at the beginning of the seventeenth century. Galileo was not only a very great astronomer, but understood well how to make use of optical lenses to magnify the very-near-by with a microscope and very-far-away with a telescope. It was from these very early discoveries that such marvels as the radio telescope and the electron microscope – the latter most important in modern gynaecological research – have developed.

François Mauriceau (1637–1709) of Paris was a renowned obstetrician of the time, who investigated the mechanism of labour and devised a method of delivery for the aftercoming head in breech presentations. He described brow presentation; difficult labours due to pelvic contraction; and may have been the first to advocate delivery in bed rather than on a birth stool. Mauriceau is known to have used the crotchet to expedite delivery but was against the use of Caesarean section. The forceps had not yet arrived in France, so in a difficult labour he could only help to deliver a baby by a destructive operation or breech extraction in an effort to save the life of the mother. In his *Traité des Maladies des Femmes Grosses et Accouchées* (Treatise on the Illnesses of Pregnant Women) of 1668 he disagreed with the theory that the pelvic bones separated during labour. Mauriceau described and named the fourchette and fossa navicularis. His book, which went into many editions, had 80 pages on hygiene and diseases of pregnancy, including the advice to pregnant women not to live in narrow streets with rubbish in them because 'there are women so delicate that the odour of a badly snuffed candle can bring about premature labour'.

Great authors such as Mauriceau, Levret and later Smellie and William Hunter with their Atlases and Notebooks were a potent force for the spread of information, but the journals describing transactions of learned societies, were able to have a wider, quicker distribution than large books. The foundation of the Royal Society in 1660 was followed before very long, by the publication of its journal (*The Philosophical Transactions*) which still continues today. This is a strong vehicle for the distribution of knowledge between scientists of many disciplines who would otherwise not know in an era of specialization, what was being done in other fields. Since modern obstetrics and gynaecology feed on the discoveries of scientists working in chemistry, physics and other fields, journals such as those of the Royal Society and *Nature* which similarly covers most of science are of immense value.

The seventeenth and eighteenth centuries were known as the 'Age of Enlightenment' because it was an age which spawned a philosophical movement characterized by the belief in the power of human reason and by changes and innovations in political, religious and educational doctrines. It was an age in which philosophical and religious thought found freedom of expression. James II (1633–1701) reigned only from 1685 to 1688 when he was deposed to be succeeded by William and Mary. The Act of Settlement in the year 1688 allowed only Protestants to succeed to the British throne. Queen Mary, William of Orange's wife, in 1694 commissioned Sir Christopher Wren to rebuild the Royal Hospital for old and disabled seamen, now known as the Royal Naval College, Greenwich.

Some of the first descriptions of the microscopic appearances of bacteria were made by Antony van Leeuwenhoek (1632–1723) (q.v.) Figure 5). Leeuwenhoek was one of the first to describe 'the little animals of the sperm' in the early 1670s, as well as bacteria. He described the spermatozoa among other of his discoveries in the 300 letters that he wrote to the British Royal

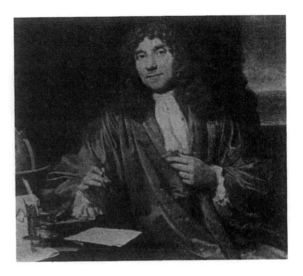

Figure 5 Antony van Leeuwenhoek – pioneer microscopist

Society in the mid-1670s. It took a century or two more before the great importance of the discovery by Leeuwenhoek of bacteria was appreciated. Leeuwenhoek was not a doctor and had had no scientific training. He was a draper who lived in Delft (The Netherlands). His contemporary was Jan Swammerdam (1637–1680) of Amsterdam who produced in 1669 his *Bible of Nature* which dealt mainly with the microscopic examination of insects.

Hendrik van Deventer (1651–1727) of the Hague wrote about obstructed labour and deformities of the pelvis. He became an accepted authority on pelvic shapes and architecture. Deventer's book *The Art of Midwifery Improved* was translated into English in the early eighteenth century. Around the same time, another Dutchman, Hendrik van Roonhuyze (1622–1672) of Amsterdam, described vesico-vaginal fistula. He advocated the use of Caesarean section in cases of obstructed labour, but the procedure was outlawed in Paris because of its associated high mortality.

Other discoveries of note included Caspar Bartholin's description of the glands in the vulva which bear his name, and Wharton's dissection findings of the umbilical cord. Louise Bourgeois, a Paris midwife, published her work on obstetrics in 1609. A pupil of Ambroise Paré, her work was translated into English as the *Compleat Midwifes Practice Enlarged* in 1659. Following experiments in which scientific obstetrics began. A number of obstetricians achieved fame for their outstanding contributions to the art of obstetrics and gynaecology.

The eighteenth century was not only a time of enlightenment, but also if one had enough money, a time of elegance. It was possible for a clever obstetrician such as William Hunter to amass a great fortune. That did not stop him from working and his, as well as his contemporary William Smellie's Atlas, bear witness not only to their immense industry but also their ability to call on the finest artists to illustrate their dissections.

William Smellie (1697–1763) (q.v.), born in Lanarkshire Scotland, studied at Glasgow but then moved to London. He eventually became known as the 'Master' of British midwifery (Figure 7) Smellie introduced variations of the obstetric forceps while at the same time advocating reduced interference in the labour process. He recognized the adverse effect of rickets on the pelvis and also investigated the pelvic soft tissues (Smellie, 1752). Another Lanarkshire man, William Hunter

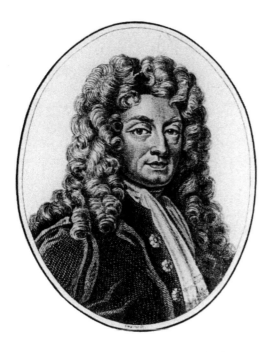

Figure 6 Sir Christopher Wren was the first man to give an intravenous injection into a mammal – a dog in 1656. Reproduced with kind permission from the Wellcome Institute Library, London

made by Sir Christopher Wren (Figure 6), Richard Lower of Oxford attempted blood transfusions in 1665, laying the foundations for twentieth century interest in this area. It was in the seventeenth century also that the idea of the wandering uterus was finally dispelled. In 1618 Chales le Pois showed that hysteria occurred in both men and women, and thus dispensed with the notion that hysterical attacks resulted from the wandering uterus – an erroneous ancient belief that had ben disputed by Rhazes (AD 850–923) and also by Mondinus de Luzzi in the fourteenth century.

EIGHTEENTH CENTURY

The eighteenth century was known as the 'Age of Reason'. The beliefs and ideas which had been accepted for centuries were questioned and new solutions sought. Also called The 'Age of Humanitarianism' it was an era in which the medical profession was known for its caring attitude and charitable works. This was the century

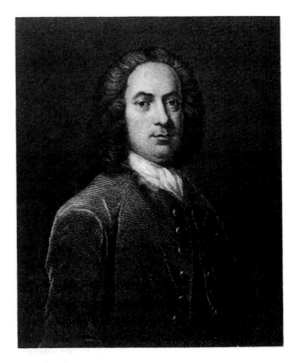

Figure 7 William Smellie (1697–1763). The 'Master' of British midwifery

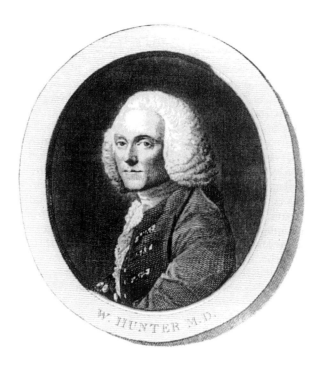

Figure 8 William Hunter (1718–1783). Great anatomist and Royal Obstetrician. Author of *The Anatomy of the Human Gravid Uterus Exhibited in Figures* (1774); one of the finest anatomical atlases ever; printed by the famous Baskerville Press. Reproduced with kind permission from the Wellcome Institute Library, London

(1718–1783) (Figure 8), carried out detailed investigations into the anatomy of the pregnant and non-pregnant uterus and the embryo. Smellie and Hunter established the scientific basis for obstetrics and gynaecology in Britain.

Another obstetrician of note was Charles White (1728–1813) of Manchester who in 1773 stressed the need for cleanliness to avoid the onset of puerperal sepsis. While White proclaimed the need for aseptic obstetrics, Alexander Gordon (1750–1799) of Aberdeen was the first to demonstrate with clarity the infective nature of puerperal sepsis in 1795. Jean Astruc (1684–1766) of Montpellier wrote a six volume *Treatise on the Diseases of Women* which was published in 1761–1765. He described the difference between gonorrhoea and syphilis and espoused medical rather than surgical gynaecology. Other Frenchmen of importance were André Levret (1703–1780) of Paris who designed forceps and also carried out important work on the pelvic architecture, and Jean Louis Baudelocque

(1748–1810) who developed techniques for pelvic mensuration.

Bartholomew Mosse (1712–1759) founded the Rotunda Hospital Dublin in 1745. His successor Fielding Ould (1710–1789) introduced the left lateral position for delivery and was known as the first important teacher of midwifery in Ireland. In America much thought was given to the building of hospitals and while there were several firsts recorded it is said that the Pennsylvania hospital founded in 1751 by Benjamin Franklin and Dr Thomas Bond is the oldest in the United States. William Shippen Jr (1736–1808) taught anatomy and some obstetrics from 1762 onwards in Philadelphia. Meanwhile in Europe hospitals were also founded, some with lying-in wards. In London St George's Maternity Hospital was built in 1733 and later became Queen Charlotte's in 1739. The Middlesex Hospital of 1745 was the first to incorporate lying-in beds in a general hospital, and the City of London Maternity Hospital was founded in 1750 (Chamberlain and Turnbull, 1989).

The pathological basis of many disease processes was founded on the work of Battista Morgagni (1682–1771) who described various forms of gynaecological pathology, and also by Marie François Xavier Bichat (1771–1802) who claimed that organic changes in the composition of tissues caused disease (Ricci, 1950).

Medical treatment, which in ancient times consisted mainly of the use of herbs, grasses, leaves, the barks of trees and alcohol, developed slowly. But, even in the late Middle Ages discoveries and inventions in one country soon became known in other countries. Until then international communication had been very slow indeed. One example of how knowledge spread in the eighteenth century is illustrated by a Japanese textbook containing woodcuts which were surprisingly like those copper engravings that had appeared in Mauriceau's famous book printed in 1668 (Figure 9). Apparently, the way this had happened was that van Deventer initially translated Mauriceau's book into Dutch. The Dutch occupied and had influence on the island of Java, which later came under Japanese domination. The Dutch influence in the island began in 1610 soon after the Japanese had started commerce with the island, and the Japanese had probably found van Deventer's translation of Mauriceau's book there. They took copies of the book to Japan, and since the Japanese could not reproduce the steel or copper plate illustrations in Deventer's edition of

15

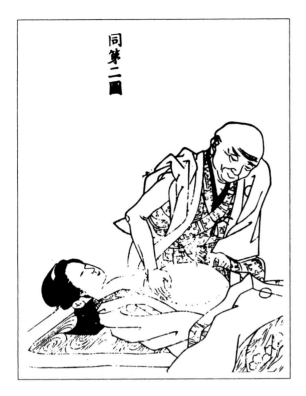

Figure 9 Woodcut from an eighteenth century Japanese text-book based on a French illustration of 1668

Mauriceau's book onto metal engravings, they did so onto woodcuts in the eighteenth century. Other adaptations of the woodcuts followed.

NINETEENTH CENTURY

In this century there were notable advances in the development of gynaecological surgery, in anaesthetics and in the fight against puerperal sepsis. Gynaecology developed separately from midwifery; and the female reproductive tract was subjected to much unnecessary, but some beneficial, surgical assault.

The development of gynaecological surgery

Ephraim McDowell (1771–1830) (q.v.) was born in Rockbridge County, Virginia, and moved to Danville, Kentucky in his early teens. In 1809 he performed an ovariotomy on a Mrs Crawford of Green County, Kentucky. He first removed 15 lb of gelatinous substance from the tumour and then extracted an ovarian sac with remaining

material which weighed 7.5lb. The operation lasted 25 minutes and the patient recovered. McDowell's success led to an upsurge of interest in gynaecological surgery, mainly aimed at the removal of apparently diseased ovaries. Over the centuries, numerous attempts were made to repair vesico-vaginal fistulae. However it was James Marion Sims (1813–1883) (q.v.) who carried out the first successful repair of a fistula in 1849 (Figure 10). He is remembered also for his double-ended speculum, the introduction of a sharp curette with a flexible blade in 1866 and the introduction of the Sim's position for gynaecological examination. In 1855 he established a hospital for women in New York. Osiander of Gottingen, Germany, amputated a cancerous cervix in 1801 and this is said to have stimulated an interest in vaginal hysterectomy. The operation was perfected in the nineteenth century. However, the technique had been attempted as early as the second century AD, when Soranus of Ephesus amputated a prolapsed uterus. It was Vincent Czerny (1842–1916) of Heidelburg who systematized the operation in 1879 and brought it into general use. The first abdominal hysterectomies were carried out by A.M. Heath and Charles Clay of

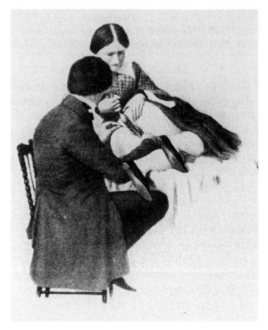

Figure 10 Sims operating on a vesico-vaginal fistula. The patient is in the semiprone position, and the correct use of his retractor is clearly shown. The original of this picure was prepared under Sims' supervision for Savage's *Female Pelvic Organs*

Manchester in 1843 and 1844. Walter Burnham of Massachusetts is credited with first performing abdominal hysterectomy in a case of malignancy. Freund of Strassburg improved the technique in 1878, and popularized the operation. It was Wertheim who performed the first really radical hysterectomy in 1898.

Caesarean section was modified and mortality rates improved towards the end of the nineteenth century. In 1876 the introduction of the Porro technique, in which subtotal hysterectomy was performed after the child had been extracted, dramatically improved survival rates. In 1882 Adolph Kehrer, and also Sanger, closed the uterine wound and thus laid the foundations for the modern Caesarean section operation.

Symphyseotomy, which is division of the symphysis pubis, had been practised for many years. Percival Willughby (q.v.) reported that the operation was known in Ireland. Jean Rene Sigault is said to have performed the first symphyseotomy on a living woman in Paris in 1777. The end result for this patient who had had four previous stillborn babies was that she had a live child, but she suffered from a vesico-vaginal fistula for the rest of her life (van Roosmalen, 1991).

In 1842–1846 approximately, Recamier invented the uterine curette, or rather rediscovered it, thus making it possible to explore the cavity of the uterus. In 1870 there were descriptions of how prolapse could be treated by applying leeches to the vulva as well as solutions containing hyocyamus. At that time dysmenorrhoea was considered to be a very serious although common condition. It was in this century that psychosomatic gynaecology was beginning to be taught by Charles Mansfield Clark.

No surgical inventions are accepted easily, as Judge T. J. Mackey of Washington, who wrote a memorable introduction to Sims' autobiography, said 'of all professions the medical is slowest to welcome reform. It has always stood in the rear ward of reform. The reason is obvious, its theories are translated into action on the living human body, and, as it deals with vital problems, it accepts with caution that novelty and theory that might prove mortal in practice'. Mackey quotes the fate of the great Cullen, William Hunter's teacher, as a reproach because his novel views of obstetrics were only slowly accepted. The great John Hunter had no audience for his first lectures on comparative anatomy, so that he asked his servant to take down the male skeleton from the wall and place it in a chair beside the servant so that he could start his lecture with the word 'Gentlemen' Jenner had a rough passage when he introduced vaccination. Harvey 'encountered trenchant criticism over many years', and James Y. Simpson, when he introduced obstetric anaesthesia was 'anathematized from the pulpit as opposing the revealed will of God, declared in the primal curse upon women'.

The introduction of anaesthetics had a major impact on both gynaecological surgery and analgesia in obstetrics. Dental extraction under nitrous oxide was carried out on Horace Wells by a Dr Riggs in 1844. Two years later James Young Simpson (1811–1870) of Edinburgh used ether successfully on an obstetric patient. In the following year he used chloroform as an analgesic in labour. However, it was not until John Snow of London administered chloroform to Queen Victoria in 1853, that anaesthesia and analgesia in labour became socially acceptable. Prior to that the lay public and many of the medical profession actively campaigned against its use.

Maternity care

Throughout the period between the sixteenth and the twentieth centuries, and continuing still, there have been disputes about the relative roles of men and women in obstetrics and gynaecology. Certainly midwives carried out almost all normal deliveries whether their patients came from the poor peasants in the villages, or from the Queens in Royal courts. For instance in his Day Book of Attendance on Queen Charlotte, William Hunter points out that Mrs Draper the midwife, delivered the Queen's first two children and kept Hunter out of the room by various false descriptions of the progress of her labour.

In the nineteenth century Thomas Bull wrote the first book that was devoted solely to antenatal care. The book was entitled *Hints to Mothers for the Management of Health During the Period of Pregnancy and in the Lying-in Room* with an exposure of common errors in connection with these subjects. The book was so immensely successful that it sold 25 editions between 1837 and 1877. Although there was plenty of advice to the mother on what she should do, there was little evidence that either doctors or midwives were involved much, actively, in her care during pregnancy.

It seems that Dr A. Pinard of France was one of the first to advocate antenatal examination of the abdomen. The reason for this was, he said, to try to avoid malpresentations of the fetus. Pinard was

17

also an advocate of induction of labour prematurely in order to avoid disproportion. He reported that Madame Becquet of Vienne (France) had established a refuge for unsupported pregnant women in Paris in 1892, so this may have been one of the first antenatal inpatient hostels. Although Sir Richard (Dick) Whittington seems already to have opened a refuge for the unwed women of St Thomas in Southwark in 1423, commanding that 'all the things that occurred in that room should be kept entirely secret under the pain of loss of livelihood'. Pinard was an assiduous and inventive obstetrician and his name was long remembered in French maternity units for his design of a fetal stethoscope (Pinard, 1895). Madame Becquet and Pinard opened a hostel for pregnant women who were abandoned and without means. They were admitted to the hostel and then delivered in Dr Pinard's department in the Baudeloque hospital. They fared better and had heavier babies than those mothers admitted from their own homes.

It was Madame Becquet's example, published in a journal, that was followed by Dr Haig Ferguson who opened a hostel similar to hers in Edinburgh for antenatal patients in 1899, next door to the Royal Maternity Hospital in that city. The Hotel Dieu in Paris has played, as can be seen throughout this book, an enormous role in obstetrics. First of all it admitted antenatal patients if they had reached 'the end of the 9th month'. Before that, those who wished to keep their pregnancies secret could find admission to a neighbouring hospital in Paris, the Hôpital de la Salpetriere where there was an antenatal ward. In the Hotel Dieu patients before the end of the 9th month who were not well could be admitted, but they may have had to share a double bed with another patient, even if they had itching disorders or venereal diseases. The spread of infection was thus facilitated.

The conquest of puerperal fever

In 1662 Thomas Willis described a condition which he termed *puerperarum febris*. It was in 1716 that Edward Strother introduced the term 'puerperal fever'. The conquest of this condition that killed thousands of women who had delivered in maternity hospitals all over the world, is a history of the control of infection initially, and later the treatment of infection by killing the organisms causing it. The fight against infection which had started in the latter part of the eighteenth century through the work of Charles White (Figure 11)

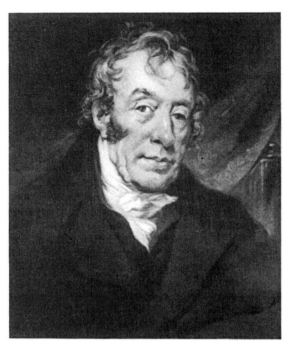

Figure 11 Charles White (1728–1813). Pioneer Obstetrician who first suggested aseptic midwifery. Author of *A Treatise on the Management of Pregnant and Lying-in Women* (1773)

and also Alexander Gordon of Aberdeen was expanded in the nineteenth century. Robert Collins (1801–1896) of Dublin began his system of chlorine disinfection during 1826–1833 and thus reduced deaths from puerperal fever. In America, Oliver Wendell Holmes (1809–1894) published his essay on puerperal fever in 1843, pointing out that the disease was carried to the patient by her physician or nurse. Meanwhile in Vienna, Ignaz Philipp Semmelweis (1818–1865) (q.v.) noted that women who were attended by medical students were much more likely to develop puerperal sepsis. From the 1840s, he ordered that all students who attended the dissecting room should wash their hands with 'chlorina liquida' before entering the wards to examine obstetric patients. This method of management led to a major reduction in mortality rates from sepsis. The streptococcus, which was the main cause of puerperal sepsis, was first isolated in 1860 by Louis Pasteur (1822–1895).

Five years later Joseph Lister (1827–1912) introduced antiseptic techniques using a carbolic spray to eliminate bacteria from the air and from patients' wounds. In spite of their wonderful work and in spite of the hand washing and aseptic and antiseptic measures taken, puerperal fever was not fully conquered, and even in 1987 sepsis caused 4.3% of all maternal deaths in the UK (HMSO, 1991).

In the second half of the nineteenth century the maternal mortality rate in hospitals was very high indeed and this was in great measure due to infection. For instance at Queen Charlotte's Hospital, London as Sir John Dewhurst (1989) writes 'the causation of puerperal fever was at the time not understood, but the design of lying-in hospitals and the failure adequately to isolate women were clearly involved'. Florence Nightingale (1820–1910) in her *Introductory Notes on Lying-in Institutions* was critical of the design of several establishments including Queen Charlotte's which she castigated in these terms 'it would be seen that the rooms are placed on the opposite sides of a main corridor running the length ways of the building; the corridors of the different floors communicate with the stairs; the ventilation of each room communicates with the ventilation of every other room through the corridors; but none of the rooms have windows on opposite sides, and there are water closets having their ventilation in common to that of the building. Now every one of these structural arrangements is objectionable and would be considered so at any hospital, and nobody nowadays would venture to include all of them in a general hospital plan. They are hence *a fortiore*, altogether inadmissible in a building for lying-in women' (Nightingale, 1861).

Florence Nightingale recognized that one had to have a very good ventilation system in order to keep the number of infections down. The figures of women dying in 1868 were 84.4 per 1000 deliveries. Not all deaths were due to infection, because such measures as forceps deliveries and Caesarean section for disproportion were not yet in vogue and women died of obstructed labours and other obstetric complications. In spite of improvements in the ventilation system at Queen Charlotte's the maternal mortality remained very high. In 1876 the figure was 45.7 per 1000, so it was necessary to close the wards for many weeks in order to disinfect them. Part of the trouble was overcrowding and the very poor ventilation system. Windows were closed so that the patients should 'not catch cold'. Both midwives and pupil midwives went from ward to ward without washing their hands while the patients wandered about the corridors freely.

There were other obstetric problems such as eclampsia and babies lying the wrong way, haemorrhage before and after delivery, and single women 'many poor deserted homeless girls' who suffered malnutrition. There were more of these than married women at Queen Charlotte's. In the years 1857–1879, 5269 were single, 3632 married and 133 widowed. These latter suffered the greatest mortality, one in 20 of them dying at the hospital, whereas one in 48 who were married died. It is revealing that the figures were much better for home deliveries where infection was less likely to occur, and these high figures were present even though Semmelweis had, since the early 1850s at least, been teaching about antiseptic precautions; but handling patients with antiseptics was not enough. Ventilation, then as now, had to be good and no risk from sewage and its gases entering the ward could be allowed. Fortunately, maternal mortality dropped in the first and second decades of the twentieth century, the best figures for these years being reported for 1912 when it was 2.6 per 1000 deliveries, but it rose again in 1916 to 9.1 per 1000 deliveries. It was not only mothers who were dying from infection but babies too. The discoveries of antibiotics as described in Chapter 17 dramatically reduced deaths and morbidity from infections (Colebrook, 1954).

Other events

The art of auscultation was markedly advanced by the invention of the stethoscope in 1819 by René Laennec (1781–1826). Laennec's student, Kergaradec, applied a stethoscope to the maternal abdomen in 1822 and was the first to hear the fetal heart beat by mediate auscultation. Progress in scientific obstetrics and gynaecology occurred over a wide front. Albert Neisser (1855–1916) discovered the cause of gonorrhoea in 1879. The development of the knowledge of pathology and bacteriology was mainly due to the efforts of Rudolf Virchow (1821–1902), Louis Pasteur (1822–1895), and Robert Koch (1843–1910). Karl Ernst von Baer (1792–1876) visualized the ovum for the first time in 1827. Gregor Johann Mendel (1822–1884), a monk of Czechoslovakia, enunciated the laws of inheritance in 1866. Five years before the end of the century Wilhelm Conrad Röntgen (1845–1923) discovered X-rays, and soon afterwards, in 1896, radioactivity was discovered by Antoine Henri Becquerel (1852–1908). The Curies isolated radium in 1898.

Further names of note in this century were Friedrich Trendelenburg (1844–1925) of Berlin who introduced the head-down position for surgery with which he is eponymously related; James Mathews Duncan (1826–1886) of Aberdeen who made notable contributions to the debate on managing placenta praevia and antepartum haemorrhage; Gustav A. Michaelis (1798–1848) who discovered that a true conjugate measurement of less than 8.75 cm indicated a contracted pelvis; Alexander J.C. Skene (1838–1900) of Brooklyn, discoveror of the glands at the external urethral orifice; Howard A. Kelly (1858–1943) who developed an interest in female urology; Karl S.F. Crede (1819–1892) of Leipzig who introduced his method of placental delivery and prophylactic management for ophthalmia neonatorum; and John Braxton Hicks (1825–1897) who, among his other observations, noted that rhythmical uterine contractions occurred during pregnancy.

The menstrual cycle was studied by a number of investigators and many erroneous theories were propounded on the relationship between ovulation and the menstrual flow. In 1839 Augustin Nicolas Gendrin was first to suggest that menstruation was controlled by ovulation. Kundrat and Engelmann in 1873, Williams in 1876, Moricke in 1882, Leopold in 1885, and Westphalen in 1896 carried out valuable investigations on the endometrium, initially from autopsy material but later from curettings taken at various stages of the cycle in living women. Prenant in 1898 suggested a secretory role for the corpus luteum and set the scene for the many advances in our knowledge of hormones during the following century.

The Voltaire chair, hysterometry, and wax models

There is, in the Barcelona museum of the History of Medicine in Spain, a padded Voltaire Chair, made by Maison Dupont in Paris, France, in the middle of the nineteenth century. It is a little difficult to know why the chair was called a Voltaire Chair, probably after Francois-Marie Arouet Voltaire (1694–1778), the great French eighteenth century philosopher, playwright and wit, although Voltaire certainly had nothing to do with gynaecology and lived a century before the chair was designed (Figure 12). The chair is somewhat similar to those now used in all gynaecological departments for colposcopic examinations, where the patient is placed in the lithotomy position, and since she is often awake, the back has to be hinged. The word lithotomy derived from the

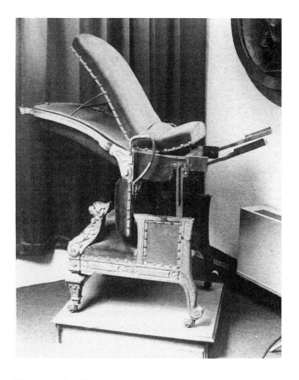

Figure 12 The Voltaire Chair in the Barcelona museum of the History of Medicine – mid-nineteenth Century (*see* text). Reproduced with kind permission from The Museum of the History of Medicine, Barcelona

Greek 'lithos' for stone, is used for this position because perineal lithotomy was often practised, to remove stones from the bladder particularly following the perineal incisions originally designed by Mariano Santo Di Barletta in the sixteenth century and others earlier.

The beautiful chair in Barcelona is covered in a light yellow velvet of the highest quality. It is still in pristine condition; and it may be that it was never used for any surgical procedure. In order for the patient to sit comfortably the hinged back is raised and the feet are supported on movable foot-rests jutting out from the front of the chair. Underneath the chair is a flat square upholstered platform which when the chair is flattened can be raised up to convert the whole apparatus into an elegant chaise-longue suitable, as the inscription states, to grace any elegant Parisian salon. The chaise is supported on four legs under which are casters so that it can be moved about in any direction. The director of the museum Dr Felip Cid I Rafael believes that the chair was designed for hysterometry or the practice of sounding the uterus with a uterine sound, called in French a hysterometer. In the same museum there is a small collection of hysterometers. One, most interestingly, has a curved intrauterine end with five hinges on it. The instrument, made in France between 1850 and 1860, has a serrated inner edge and was bought in Paris by a Catalan doctor who took it to Barcelona for his own use. When introduced into the uterus it was not only used to measure the size of the cavity, but also hopefully to remove small polyps and even to decapitate a dead fetus for easier removal.

In the same museum, dating from the beginning of the twentieth century, there is a series of wax models to teach students embryology. These models show the intrauterine appearance of early embryos up to 6–8 weeks' gestation.

The nineteenth century was the era of modesty, as exemplified by the famous illustration in Maygrier's Atlas describing how he conducted vaginal examination of a patient lying or standing, but covered in both postures by a long flowing skirt (Figure 13).

TWENTIETH CENTURY

The advances in society, scientific medicine and obstetrics and gynaecology during this century have surpassed those of all previous eras. J.P. Greenhill, Professor of Gynecology, Cooke County Graduate School of Medicine, Chicago and editor of the *Year Book of Obstetrics and Gynecology* bade farewell to that journal in 1975 by summarizing a personal experience of 55 years of change in obstetric practice from 1921 to 1975. Greenhill was a resident house officer in gynaecology at Johns Hopkins Hospital during 1919–1920. He became the first resident at the Chicago Lying-In Hospital in 1921 at a time when ... 'the practice of obstetrics was rather primitive. We did not even have a test for pregnancy other than bimanual vaginal examination. Aschheim and Zondek did not describe their test until 1927'. It was Voge who first introduced a flocculation test for pregnancy in 1926. The earliest pregnancy tests were carried out on animals and results could take up to 6 weeks to materialize. In 1930 the Hogben test was introduced and results were available within 48 hours. The Kupperman test was introduced in 1943, and pregnancy was detectable within 2 hours.

Regarding the care of the pregnant woman, Greenhill recalled that 'Relatively few pregnant

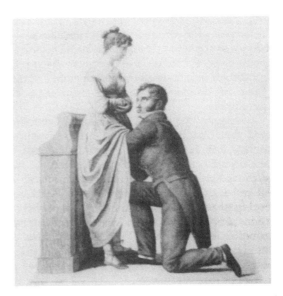

Figure 13 Illustration from Jacques Pierre Maygrier's Atlas – *Nouvelles Demonstrations d'Accouche-ments*, Paris, Bechet (1822)

women were given good prenatal care ... Our office routine was to take the patient's blood pressure, examine her urine and weigh her. We made vaginal examinations, listened to the fetal heart tones if the gestation was advanced and answered many questions'. Weight restriction was a common method of management, with only 15 lb gain being allowed throughout pregnancy. Salt was severely restricted. The routine laboratory tests were blood counts, blood tests for gonorrhoea and syphilis and urinalysis. There were no specialized clinics and the term 'high-risk patient' did not exist. With regards to delivery 'Most ... were spontaneous ... we performed many low and mid-forceps deliveries and even high forceps operations ... we delivered nearly all breeches from below and we became extremely skilful in this art ... we did extremely few Caesarean sections for placenta praevia ... In the early days we made the diagnosis by vaginal examination, a practice that can be dangerous. For treatment we used rubber bags of various types and sizes and we also packed the vagina with gauze. Because we delivered most of the babies from below, we lost most of them in cases of total placenta praevia. A few mothers died also'. Greenhill went on to say that blood transfusion was unusual and the rhesus factor was only discovered about 1940 by Landsteiner and Wiener. No antibiotics were available and many patients died, particularly from criminal abortions or puerperal sepsis. Many cases of eclampsia were referred by midwives. Caesarean section was not often performed until Dr De Lee improved the technique of the cervical operation. Most women with chorionepithelioma died within a year of diagnosis despite curettage or hysterectomy.

Turning to the fate of the infants, Greenhill noted that 'Another disease in which fantastic progress has been made is erythroblastosis, a disease which caused innumerable deaths . . . we saw many babies with congenital deformities . . . we knew nothing about amniocentesis'. With the development of the new subspecialty, Neonatology, there was a reduction in fetal morbidity and mortality. The introduction of 'ultrasound or sonar in obstetrics has been a great boon . . . Many years ago we had a large number of cases of postpartum haemorrhage . . . we had no available pituitary extract until a few years later even though it had been advocated by Hofbauer as early as 1918. We also gave hot intrauterine douches for the treatment of uterine haemorrhage. Every labour room had a sterilized can with a rubber tubing and hot water'. Greenhill wondered whether the 'young men and women practising obstetrics today realize how easy and gratifying is the practice of this specialty as compared with our difficulties and lack of essential knowledge 50 years ago'.

Turning his attention to gynaecology, Greenhill paid tribute to the work of Papanicolaou who introduced the cervical smear test. Knowledge of the test spread world-wide after the publication of Papanicolaou and Traut's book *Diagnosis of Uterine Cancer by the Vaginal Smear* in 1943. The use of Lugol's iodine by Schiller, and also the use of colposcopy as described by Hinselmann, were major advances in the diagnosis of cervical abnormalities. Gynaecological surgery was improved and operations were simplified. Culdoscopy and laparoscopy were introduced. Studies and tests for infertility resulted in the births of thousands of healthy infants. Rubin introduced and popularized tests for tubal patency, treatments of gonorrhoea, artificial insemination and plastic operations of the tubes. Fertilization *in vitro* 'popularly called "genetic engineering" is creating serious problems and debates . . . the field of endocrinology has become awesome . . . a great contribution, to mention only one, is the induction of ovulation in women who do not produce ova spontaneously'. *In vitro* fertilization is, of course, not 'genetic engineering'; although

research into the former may facilitate the latter. As such, *in vitro* fertilization does not interfere in any way with the embryo's genetic inheritance. Greenhill also recalled the advances in the surgery of genetic malformations, and in the treatment of cancer. This personal insight into 55 years of obstetric practice highlights not only the progress but also the rapid pace of change in our specialty during this century.

Obstetrics

Maternal mortality

Maternal mortality rates have long been used as an index of the effectiveness of maternity care. At the beginning of this century the rates in Europe and America were in the region of five deaths per 1000 maternities. Between 1901 and 1905 the rate for the UK was 5.6, similar to that in Australia. In the USA after 1915, the rate fluctuated between seven and nine per 1000 about as high as those of the nineteenth century. Various Ministries of Health investigated the high maternal mortality rates and it became apparent that well-fed, parous, rural women were the least likely to die as a result of pregnancy, whereas city dwellers, those who delivered in institutions and particularly primigravidae and mothers of large families were at high risk. Up to two-thirds of the deaths were preventable. Failure of obstetricians, general practitioners and midwives to provide adequate antenatal care and proper supervision and management of women in labour were indicted as major reasons for the high death rates. From the 1930s on there was a major drive to ensure better education of the health professionals involved in maternity care, while mothers were encouraged to attend for antenatal care, and hospital delivery was recommended (Figure 14).

Tackling a number of factors influenced the maternal mortality rates, and advances on many fronts, medical and social, gradually effected a large reduction in maternal mortality over the years.

The many scientific discoveries which were put into practice, were complemented by the improvement in living standards slowly achieved from the time of the First World War onwards, and helped the trend to fewer deaths.

Antenatal care The introduction of antenatal care, which is generally attributed to J.W. Ballantyne, a lecturer in Antenatal Pathology at the University

Perinatal mortality rate (per thousand births)

Maternal mortality rate (per million births)

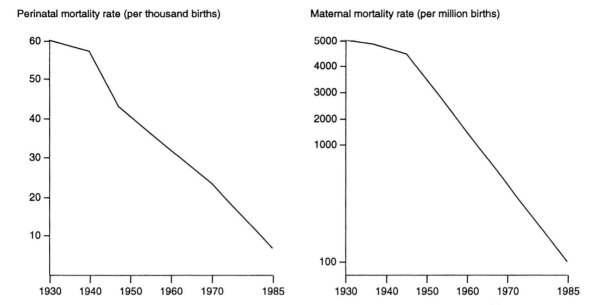

Figure 14   Decline in perinatal mortality and maternal mortality from 1930–1985

of Edinburgh, gave health professionals the possibility to assess the general health and welfare of pregnant women. Ballantyne's first antenatal bed was endowed at the Royal Maternity and Simpson Memorial Hospital in 1901. In the same year in Boston, USA, home visits to antenatal patients began and the first antenatal clinic was opened there in 1911. In Australia the first antenatal clinic opened in 1912 in Sydney.

Pre-eclampsia   The recognition of antenatal pathology and particularly the early diagnosis of pre-eclampsia had a major impact on maternal mortality. Although eclampsia had been recognized for centuries it was John Charles Weaver Lever in 1811 who discovered that proteinuria was associated with eclampsia. Alexandre Henri Pilliet, a French pathologist, showed the relationship between eclampsia and liver changes late in the nineteenth century. The sphygmomanometer was perfected in 1896 by Scipione Riva-Rocci, so that the relationship of hypertension, proteinuria and oedema with pre-eclampsia and eclampsia was recognized at the beginning of the twentieth century. However, even by 1915 blood pressure readings were seldom taken so that the toxaemia of pregnancy was usually well established before it was recognized. Mortality from eclampsia was as high as 40%. When

Stroganoff introduced antieclamptic therapy in 1909 it led to a remarkable fall in death rates from the disease. The combination of anticonvulsant with antihypertensive treatment that was introduced in the 1960s, lowered the death rates still further.

Antepartum haemorrhage   This was a leading cause of maternal mortality. There were two main categories, one in which the patient was 'toxic' and the other in which the placenta was abnormally sited. Maternal mortality due to haemorrhage from placenta praevia was 6 or 7% while its perinatal mortality was in the order of 50%. The treatment in 1900 was by tamponade of the cervix and vagina to try to control the bleeding. When and if the bleeding was under control the pack was removed and the cervix was manually dilated. Internal version and fetal extraction were then performed. Expectant management was introduced by Macafee of the Royal Maternity Hospital, Belfast, who reduced maternal mortality to 0.57% and perinatal mortality to less than 25% during the years 1932–1944. During the same years Caesarean section, which had been considered a dangerous operation until about 1912, became more commonly used in the management of the low-implanted placenta. By 1931 Arthur H. Bill showed that cases treated by

Caesarean section were likely to have a maternal mortality of less than 2%. Also of benefit was the introduction of the Obstetric Flying Squad, to attend to women in danger in their own homes, instituted by Farquahar Murray in Newcastle in about 1937, and soon established in most areas of the country.

Expectant treatment for antepartum haemorrhage, particularly if placenta praevia was suspected, continued to be the method of management achieving the best results. Until the 1970s it was routine that expectant treatment was followed by an examination under anaesthesia at 38 weeks' gestation; and Caesarean section was performed if the digital examination revealed a placenta praevia. Various methods were used to diagnose placental location, including soft tissue X-ray, amniography and radioisotope estimation. In the 1970s however, ultrasound techniques became available and replaced all other methods in the diagnosis of placenta praevia. Blood transfusions became a real possibility after Landsteiner had shown in 1900 that there were different blood groups and that reactions did not occur when group-compatible blood was transfused. From 1914 blood banks were introduced with citrate being used to inhibit blood coagulation. Karl Landsteiner and Alexander Wiener discovered the rhesus factor in 1940. This had a major impact on the blood transfusion services; and particularly for rhesus factor disease.

Anaesthesia Although the development of anaesthesia was to have a major impact on obstetrics and gynaecology, many maternal deaths were caused by poor anaesthetic techniques. Some volatile agents were not suitable for use during Caesarean section. There was the ever present danger of regurgitation of stomach contents as highlighted by Mendelson in 1946 and again by Sellick in 1961. The institution of proper training and supervision for junior staff, the introduction of adequate premedication and good anaesthetic techniques, and the use of epidural or caudal analgesia were of importance in reducing maternal mortality.

Sepsis The introduction of antibiotics had a major role to play in combating all forms of infection. It was estimated that in the USA in 1914 almost 5000 women died of puerperal sepsis. Tuberculosis, pelvic inflammatory disease and syphilis were also major causes of mortality and morbidity. The introduction of sulphonamides in the 1930s and of penicillin from 1941, combined with adequate aseptic techniques, dramatically reduced but did not eliminate mortality and morbidity from sepsis. The general improvement of the care of women in labour; of the patient with miscarriage or ectopic pregnancy, the recognition of causes of pulmonary embolism and their adequate treatment, the treatment of heart disease, anaemia and undercurrent illness have all played their part in reducing maternal mortality.

Confidential enquiries into maternal mortality and morbidity were stimulated by the investigations of Dr Janet Campbell in 1924. Unfortunately despite the great strides made in the battle against maternal mortality in the West, the rates in developing countries remain at least a hundred times greater than those of the USA or Britain.

Perinatal mortality

The registration of live births in England and Wales began in 1837 and became compulsory from 1874 on. Stillbirths only became registrable in 1928. Towards the end of the last century the emphasis was on the health of the mother rather than that of her fetus. Many perinatal deaths resulted from deliberate sacrifice of the infant, particularly in difficult deliveries. However, as the birth rate declined from 1920 onwards infant mortality became a major issue, and attention was focused on the prevention of perinatal death.

Infant mortality was about 156 per 1000 live births at the turn of the century, having remained at that level since the early nineteenth century. The rate dropped slowly to 36 per 1000 over the subsequent 50 years. From 1906 infant mortality was categorized as early neonatal (1 week postdelivery), late neonatal (2-4 weeks postdelivery), and postneonatal (over 4 weeks from delivery). The early neonatal death rate stayed static until the 1940s. The recorded stillbirth rate of 1928 was about 41 per 1000 (live and stillbirths) and did not alter until the 1940s. At that time, the principal causes of perinatal mortality were documented as maternal toxaemia, antepartum haemorrhage, difficult labours, congenital malformations and premature birth. It was later recognized that other factors such as rhesus isoimmunization and teratogenic drugs were also involved (Hibbard, 1988).

In the 1940s Dugald Baird, Professor of Midwifery at Aberdeen University in Scotland, noted the association of low social class and poor nutrition with high obstetric and perinatal mortality. He assembled data on stillbirths and early neonatal deaths which he categorized into 'obstetrical' and 'environmental' groups. He discovered that perinatal deaths due to asphyxia, possibly from placental insufficiency, increased when the duration of gestation exceeded 40 weeks, particularly in older mothers. This led to the concept of induction of labour for 'postmaturity' and a liberal policy of Caesarean section to avoid hypoxia in labour. In 1949 the perinatal mortality rate in England and Wales was 38.1 per 1000 and by 1991 about eight per 1000 total births – a remarkable drop.

Perinatal mortality surveys were carried out in Britain on a number of occasions between 1958 and 1982. Perinatal deaths were found to be highest in consultant-staffed units, lowest in home deliveries and intermediate for general practitioner units. It was suggested that the differences arose partly because of the transfer of difficult cases in late pregnancy and labour and also to the booking of high-risk patients into hospital units.

Birth trauma was reduced by better training of obstetric personnel, by the abandonment of high forceps and difficult vaginal breech deliveries and by the introduction of new methods of labour management. Hypoxia in labour was sought after more diligently, with scanty liquor or meconium-staining signalling the need for more intensive monitoring, or urgent interference. However, the hypoxic stillbirth remained difficult to eliminate as a problem. Prematurity rates fell in response to better nutrition and increased standards of living. Heavy sedation was employed in an effort to halt premature labour and in the 1970s β-sympathomimetic agents were introduced for the same purpose. The neonatal care of the premature infant had little to offer until the 1950s. High concentration oxygen therapy was introduced, but this led to infant blindness from retrolental fibroplasia. The iatrogenic prematurity due to induction of labour in women supposedly at term but with incorrect dates was eventually curtailed by the introduction of ultrasound technology with more accurate pregnancy dating in the 1980s. Although first introduced in the 1960s, ultrasound pregnancy dating only became widely available in the 1980s. Rhesus isoimmunization was tackled after the discovery of the rhesus factor by Levine and Stetson and independently by Landsteiner and Wiener in 1940,

by replacement transfusions of blood in the affected newborn babies and subsequently by the development of anti-D immunoglobulin by C.A. Clarke of Liverpool in 1966. The legalization of therapeutic abortion in many countries reduced the perinatal rates of severe fetal congenital malformation from approximately 6% to to less than 2%.

As antenatal care developed, mothers were placed in high- or low-risk categories. It gradually became apparent that the fetus could also be categorized in this way. As large- or small-for-dates infants posed a special threat so intrauterine fetal measurement became of importance. Biochemical assessment of the fetoplacental unit was born with the discovery of a gonad-stimulating substance in the urine of pregnant women by Aschheim and Zondek in 1927. Soon called 'chorionic gonadotropin', this was the first of many substances isolated from the placenta. In the mid-1950s, Arnold Klopper and Jim Brown of Edinburgh developed methods for measurement of progesterone and oestrogens in urine. This led to the concept of hormonal tests for fetoplacental function. Ito and Higashi reported their detection of human placental lactogen in 1961, and soon after assays of human placental lactogen and oestriol production were commonly used to test fetoplacental function. Biochemical assessment of the placenta and fetus remained popular until the early 1980s. Meanwhile biophysical assessment of the fetus evolved. The method based on ultrasound examination and cardiotocography, was introduced by Frank Manning and Larry Platt in the early 1980s. Fetal kick counting was introduced by Sadovsky et al. in Israel in 1976.

Labour and delivery

Profound changes occurred in the understanding and management of induction of labour, of delivery and of the third stage in the twentieth century. There was also a gradual trend towards delivery in hospital. By the 1990s almost 100% of women attended hospitals for childbirth in many developed countries. In the Netherlands, however, 35% of births occurred at home. A Commons Health Committee in the UK advised in 1992 that for low-risk mothers there should be a return to births at home, in general practitioner or in midwifery units. In response, the Royal College of Obstetricians and Gynaecologists pointed to a 51.7 per 1000 perinatal mortality from such a system in the Netherlands.

Induction of labour The concept of induction of labour to effect preterm delivery in cases of contracted pelvis was introduced in the mid-eighteenth century. Ergot, derived from a fungal growth on rye grain, had been known to traditional midwives for centuries. Stearns of the USA 'discovered' the drug in about 1808 and reported its use in 100 cases of augmentation of labour, but its general use led to a high number of stillbirths and the drug fell into disuse for speeding up the first two stages of labour. Ergot continues to be very useful for management of the third stage. Throughout the nineteenth century a large number of strategies for inducing labour were tried. A favourite method was that of 'bougie induction', and although maternal and perinatal mortality were reported from their use, these and other mechanical methods of induction were used until the 1950s. Towards the end of the nineteenth century induction by artificial rupture of the membranes became popular in Britain. Around the same time the use of quinine for induction was described by Porak in 1878. This method remained popular until the 1930s although it too was associated with poor maternal and neonatal outcome. Sparteine sulphate, an alkaloid of ergot, was introduced in the 1940s and was quite commonly used until the mid-1960s. At the same time the O.B.E. (oil, bath, enema) routine was used for most labour inductions, and for many women in spontaneous labour, to empty the lower bowel in an attempt to facilitate their labours.

'Pitocin induction' was initiated by Theobald of Bradford in 1952, who advocated the physiological use of intravenous pitocin. He later worked at University College Hospital with Nixon. The drug was first extracted from the posterior pituitary gland by Henry Dale in 1906. Blair Bell described its application to the pregnant uterus in 1909 and in the following year a pituitary extract was administered in cases of uterine inertia during labour, but maternal deaths from shock were reported after the intramuscular pitocin injections.

That the pituitary extract contained both vasopressin and oxytocin was determined by Vincent du Vigneaud who isolated purified oxytocin in 1954 from pituitary extracts and then manufactured synthetic oxytocin or Syntocinon. Its use was reported by Boissonnas *et al.* in 1955. Transbuccal induction using 'linguets' of pituitary extract was quite commonly used in the 1960s.

A pelvic scoring system was devised by Bishop in 1964 who found that the ripe cervix was more likely to respond to induction. The cervical ripening agent prostaglandin was introduced by Karim *et al.* in 1968. At the same time Turnbull and Anderson introduced their method of titrated oxytocin infusion via an electric pump. By the 1980s two main methods of induction had evolved. Artificial rupture of the membranes with Syntocinon infusion if labour did not ensue within 12 hours was the first method. Cervical ripening with prostaglandin followed by artificial rupture of the membranes 4–5 hours later, with the addition of Syntocinon soon afterwards if labour had not supervened, the second method, became a standard practice in many obstetric units.

In the mid-1950s about 13% of births in Britain were induced. This figure reached 26% in 1970 and almost 40% in 1974. Most cases of induction were for maternal toxaemia and for 'postmaturity'. After many women had complained about this active intervention, induction rates fell to about 20% in the late 1980s.

Duration of labour The uterus and its contractions were actively investigated in the first half of the century. This followed earlier work by Kristeller of Germany who had reported on the characteristics of uterine action in 1861. Different methods of tocodynamometry (measurement of uterine muscle activity) were invented by Schatz in 1872, Poullet in 1880, Podleschka in 1932, Alvarez and Caldeyro-Barcia in 1950 and others. The measurement of the activity of various drugs on uterine contractility was established by the mid-1960s. It was in the same era that incompetence of the cervix was investigated by Lash and Lash in 1950, Rubovits in 1953, Palmer and Shirodkar in 1953 and McDonald in 1957. The duration of spontaneous labours was assessed in the 1958 and 1970 Perinatal Surveys in the UK; and it was found that the perinatal mortality rates rose if the duration of labour was less than 3 hours or more than 48 hours. Mortality rates were lowest when the first stage lasted between 12 and 24 hours in primigravidae or between 3 and 24 hours in multiparae. The optimum duration of the second stage was between 30 minutes and 4 hours for primigravidae. From the early 1970s intervention to speed up the first stage of labour, by artificial rupture of membranes and intravenous infusion of oxytocin, became more commonplace even when labour had not been induced artificially. During that decade, O'Driscoll and Meagher of the National Maternity Hospital, Dublin, introduced their 'active management of labour', which provided low rates of obstetrical intervention combined with a high level of support in labour. Philpott of Rhodesia introduced the 'partographic control of labour', a method by which uterine hypotonus or disproportion could be recognized and appropriate action taken before the mother or fetus became exhausted.

Analgesia Although extracts of mandrake, poppy and other methods were used for pain relief over many centuries, it was not until Queen Victoria accepted chloroform analgesia in 1853 for the birth of her eighth child Leopold, that pain relief for the labouring woman became socially acceptable and known as *Chloroform a la Reine.* Although morphine and scopolamine were used from 1902, it was not until 1932 that R.J. Minnitt of Liverpool designed a portable gas and air analgesic system and so introduced the use of volatile gases in obstetric analgesia. By 1946 gas/air analgesia was commonly used. Trilene was also used. Pethidine (meperidine or demerol in the USA and Dolantine in other parts of the world) was introduced as an alternative to heroin and morphine in 1940 and was first used as an 'antispasmodic' to relieve uterine pain. However, it soon became the most commonly used analgesic in labour. The drug had adverse effects on the fetus so pethilorphan, a mixture of pethidine with a narcotic antagonist was introduced, and was used in almost a quarter of labours during the early 1970s. Various forms of tranquillizers, including promazine and diazepam, were used, as were the phenothiazine derivatives perphenazine and promethazine.

Regional analgesia in the form of caudal anaesthesia which was first described by Sicard and Catheline in 1901 was applied to obstetrics by Edwards and Hingson in 1942. Lumbar epidural analgesia became more popular and gradually replaced caudal analgesia from the mid-1970s onwards. Pudendal block enjoyed a vogue during the 1960s and 1970s although already advocated in the 1940s.

The 'natural methods' of pain relief in labour failed to achieve popularity until their use was demanded by some women's groups in the mid-1980s

Assisted delivery Caesarean section delivery was performed in less than 2% of labours at the beginning of the twentieth century, but by 1990 was carried out in 12% of deliveries in the UK and rates of over 25% were recorded in some centres in the USA and even higher in the upper social

classes there. While forceps delivery was uncommon in the early 1900s, approximately 5% of all deliveries were effected by this means in 1958. The figure rose to 12–16% in 1990. The ventouse or vacuum extractor was introduced in the 1950s and replaced the use of forceps somewhat, but did not achieve the same popularity in the Anglo-Saxon world as in French-speaking countries. The practice of episiotomy with or without instrumental delivery became common after 1950. At that time about 15% of deliveries were accompanied by this practice, but by the mid-1980s anything up to 50% of labouring women had the procedure carried out. Women's groups then actively campaigned against the unnecessary performance of episiotomy.

Electronic fetal monitoring Auscultation of the fetal heart in labour was first performed in the mid-nineteenth century. Towards the end of that century it was recognized that variations of the fetal heart rate were related to the fetal condition at birth. In the 1960s the science of electronics was applied to the monitoring of the woman and fetus in labour. Due to the work of Hon and Caldeyro-Barcia, Guttmacher and others, certain changes in fetal heart traces were found to predict fetal hypoxia. Electronic fetal monitoring gradually appeared to be essential for the proper supervision of the fetus in labour. However, MacDonald's study and other studies in the mid-1980s showed that electronic monitoring as compared to intermittent auscultation had probably not improved the outcome for the fetus; yet electronic monitoring in high-risk cases, combined with Saling's technique of fetal scalp pH monitoring was still considered valuable. The condition of the newborn infant was affected not only by hypoxia but also by the use of drugs in labour. Virginia Apgar, an American anaesthetist, introduced a scoring system which allowed definitive evaluation of the newborn's condition in 1953.

The third stage In the 1930s the use of ergot was again revived, and ergometrine was developed in Britain. Syntocinon, which was produced in 1954, was later combined with ergometrine to form the compound syntometrine, which came into general use in the 1960s.

Hospital delivery During the 1920s in the UK approximately one-fifth of mothers were delivered in hospital. By 1954 this figure had reached almost

27

64%. By 1972 that figure was almost 92% and by 1991 approximately 99% of women were delivered in maternity institutions. Trends in the introduction of 'user-friendly' domiciliary-type birthing rooms in hospital contrasted sharply with the regimented authoritarian attitudes of the 1970s. The humanization of labour suites and lying-in wards reflected changing attitudes among health professionals who gradually understood that a caring approach to labouring women and their partners could rate as highly as technological intervention. The admission of fathers and other supporters to the labour wards was one of the major advances starting in British hospitals in 1962.

The role of midwives

In the early twentieth century Ballantyne initiated routine antenatal care and with the encouragement of Dr Janet Campbell of the Ministry of Health, antenatal clinics were set up throughout the UK. Midwives ran the clinics with the help of doctors who were mainly junior residents.

The changes in midwifery care in the years from 1960 onwards were enormous, so that the term 'Childbirth Revolution' was no exaggeration. Although theoretically independent most midwives considered themselves to be assistants to the doctors who had an ever increasing role in running the maternity units, especially in hospitals. The result of technological changes was to be far reaching. Partograms became widely used by obstetricians, and to a certain extent replaced the verbal descriptions of the progress of each labour, as midwives on one shift handed over to the next. Cardiotocographs became increasingly used in labour wards that were sited away from the antenatal and postnatal wards and resembled operating theatres.

The pattern of labour changed in the 1980s; chiefly because of the increasing use of Syntocinon, it became more painful so epidural analgesia was more often used, leading to more forceps deliveries. The higher forceps rates, the greater intervention rates and the higher Caesarean section rates, all diminished the role of the midwife. By 1974 the Central Midwives Board (CMB) in a statement of policy stressed that pupil midwives should receive instruction in the management of natural birth in addition to the new techniques of 'active labour' (Central Midwives Board, 1974). Some obstetricians stimulated by requests from mothers for a more

'natural' process to be reintroduced managed to lower the induction and the Caesarean section rates. The role of the midwives *vis à vis* doctors has changed throughout the ages and will continue constantly to change. This relationship and the seeking for a greater say in delivering women on the part of both doctors and of midwives has been a constant and continuing theme throughout the history of midwifery.

Womens' groups

As the century advanced the medical profession became much more involved in womens' health care. Some women felt they had lost control of their natural body functions, and were frightened by the ever advancing tide of medical interventions. By the mid-1970s a major confrontation between womens' groups and obstetricians developed. As a result obstetricians re-evaluated their role as health professionals and came to involve the woman in making decisions to a much larger extent. Women writers made a major contribution to our understanding of the woman's point of view. Their publications include valuable works by Sally Inch (1982), Ann Oakley (1984), Marjorie Tew (1990) and Ann Dally (1991).

Neonatal paediatrics

Neonatology was pioneered by the work of the French physician Charles Michel Billard during the 1820s when he worked at the Hospice des Enfants in Paris. It is claimed however that the first neonatal paediatrician was August Ritter von Reuss who was appointed to the New Born Department of the University Women's Clinic in Vienna in 1911.

Incubators were introduced at that time. The Rotch model became available in 1903 and the Hess water-jacketed incubator was designed in 1914. An important advance in 1935 was the work of Gibberd and Blaikley of Guy's Hospital, London who pioneered infant resuscitation in this century. Hyaline membrane disease or respiratory distress syndrome previously known as congenital atalectasis, was described in 1953. Six years later Avery and Meade discovered that deficiency of surfactant led to the syndrome. Surfactant replacement therapy began in the 1960s and is still being developed in the 1990s.

Aggressive oxygen therapy was instituted in the 1940s in a bid to prevent or ameliorate the syndrome. However, Theodore Terry soon described blindness caused by retrolental fibroplasia which itself was due to the high concentration oxygen therapy. Modern neonatology began in the 1960s with the advent of umbilical catheterization and controlled oxygen therapy and the measurement of blood gases.

Erythroblastosis This was recognized by Diamond, Blackfan and Batty in 1932 as a major cause of perinatal mortality. The discovery of the main blood groups in 1900, and the rhesus system in 1940, and the application of umbilical vein catheterization for exchange transfusion in 1951 only partially contained the problem. It was the introduction of anti-D immunoglobulin in 1966 which eventually brought rhesus isoimmunization under a great measure of control.

Grief counselling

One of the greatest advances in neonatal care was the introduction of grief or bereavement counselling from the mid-1970s. From that time onwards counselling skills were applied to parents who had suffered stillbirths, neonatal deaths and miscarriages and were also introduced to other areas of obstetrics and gynaecology.

Genetics, congenital defects and teratology

Although infants with genetic malformations had been recognized from antiquity it was Mendel's publication of 1866 which had a major bearing on the development of genetic investigations. Watson and Crick in 1953 described the double helix molecular model for DNA. Amniocentesis was reported by Menees *et al.* in 1930 and Bevis in 1953, while Liley in 1961 further refined the technique. Brock and Sutcliffe in 1972 discovered that high α-fetoprotein levels in the amniotic fluid were associated with neural tube defects thus paving the way for the antenatal assessment of some congenital malformations. New techniques included fetoscopy, introduced by Westin in 1954; ultrasound by Ian Donald in 1958; chorionic villus biopsy by Evans *et al.* in 1972 and gene probe analysis by E.M. Southern in 1975. By these methods many congenital malformations could be diagnosed antenatally with termination of pregnancy being offered in some appropriate cases and intrauterine surgery on the fetus in a few others (Pauerstein, 1987).

As with so many other subjects in obstetrics it was Paré in the sixteenth century who was the first to use the word 'teratology'. It is taken from the Greek word for 'wonderful or monstrous' but in modern terms it signifies a whole variety of aberrations of development. It has only recently been realized that there are many agents that can cause abnormalities in the fetus and newborn infant. This is despite the fact that old wives' tales have abounded for centuries about the effects of antenatal happenings on fetal development. For instance, strawberry marks or naevi were said to have been the result of mothers walking or falling in a field of strawberries, or seeing abnormal children, and hare-lip (cleft palate) was firmly thought to be due to a mother being frightened by a hare running across her path at night. In fact about 2–4% of liveborn children do suffer from serious structural abnormalities (Butler and Alberman, 1969). A most dramatic event was the recognition by McBride (1961) that Thalidomide could cause abnormalities in newborn babies. Twenty years passed before Herbst and others discovered in 1971 that diethylstilboestrol taken in pregnancy can cause adenocarcinoma of the vagina of girls born to the mothers who took the drug (Herbst *et al.*, 1971) and it took still longer to realize that males born to women who had taken this drug could be sterile.

It did not take long for research to show that a whole series of exposures in pregnancy to such different factors as radiation, infections, hormone abnormalities of the mother and drugs could cause serious congenital defects in newborn children. In 1973 Wilson published an important work in which among other things he pointed out the most susceptible times in pregnancy for the fetus to be affected by teratogens; and he showed that the time of laying down of specific organs was an important feature in the action of noxious elements on the fetus when they were most vulnerable (Wilson, 1973).

It had long been realized that alcohol could have an adverse effect on newborn babies. For instance in the Bible (Judges 13:7) it says 'Behold thou shalt conceive and bear a son; and drink no wine or strong drink'. In 1726 a report to the British Parliament said 'Parental drinking causes weak, feeble and distempered children'. In more recent times French observers realized that there was a condition that they termed the 'fetal alcohol syndrome' (Lemoine *et al.*, 1968). The children are usually small and have short palpebral fissures, a low nasal bridge, a short nose, indistinct philtrum and a narrow upper lip, together with a small chin and a flat mid-face. They are mentally handicapped, too. A very large percentage of chronically alcoholic mothers have babies who suffer from the fetal alcohol syndrome.

It is now known that there is a very large variety of metals and drugs that can cause abnormalities in babies, as well as such abnormalities being caused by vitamin and other food deficiencies. Because of the risks of possible ill-effects from X-rays and radiotherapy as well as radiography there has been increasing caution in protecting the fetus from being exposed to such rays.

In 1941 Gregg, an Australian doctor, noted that infection with the rubella virus, hitherto thought to be quite innocuous, was associated with a large number of congenital cataracts, deafness and cardiovascular defects in Australia (Gregg, 1941).

Had Gregor Mendel not founded genetics and the laws of heredity in 1864 while working in his monastery, knowledge of the science of teratology, could not have been advanced so quickly (Wilson, 1973). As a result of this explosion of information about teratogenic agents, all drugs now placed on the market that can possibly be given to pregnant women are assessed for their teratogenic effects. Sometimes it is difficult to decide whether to take the risk of an abnormal baby in order to treat the mother, and this is particularly so when the mother has to receive anti-cancer drugs.

Imaging

Radiology became available through the work of Wilhelm Conrad von Röntgen who in 1895 discovered 'a new kind of ray' which he called X-rays. He received the first Nobel Prize in 1901. X-ray techniques became widely used in the early part of the century, and as early as 1908 X-rays were used from the 7th week of pregnancy onwards. X-ray dating in late pregnancy became common place but was inaccurate. Spalding documented the overlapping of skull bones found on X-ray in intrauterine death in 1922. The bony and soft pelvis were investigated in great detail. Herbert Thoms improved the technique of X-ray pelvimetry and on his findings based his Thoms' Classification of Pelvic Types. For a time 'routine radiography' was common. In the mid-1920s however, came warnings that exposure to X-rays could have a damaging effect on both infant and mother. Despite that, radiology remained widely used until 1956, when Alice Stewart and her associates in Oxford reported that childhood cancer was more common in infants who had

been subjected to radiation *in utero*. At that time, over 60% of expectant mothers were subjected to radiology in some 'centres of excellence'.

Ultrasound was introduced by Ian Donald, J. MacVicar and T.G. Brown in 1958. They originally investigated abdominal masses with pulsed ultrasound. A-mode, or one-dimensional scanning, and B-mode or two-dimensional scanning were later developed. The third technique of Doppler ultrasound was found useful in detection of the fetal heart beat. Ultrasound techniques were soon applied to obstetrics and the first scanner for use in obstetric care was completed in 1960. Magnetic resonance imaging was described independently in 1946 by Purcell and also by Bloch. Eric Odeblat used the technique to examine the uterine musculature and cervical mucus during the 1950s and 1960s and Mansfield and Maudesley obtained the first human *in vivo* images in 1977.

Termination of pregnancy

The first liberal abortion law was passed in the Soviet Union in 1920 but was later repealed by Stalin in 1936. However, Iceland in 1935 and most other East and West European countries liberalized abortion legislation over the following 40 years.

In Britain restrictive abortion laws were passed in 1861 and such legislation rapidly spread through the British Empire. These laws were repealed in 1967. Under the 'code Napoleon' of France abortion became a capital offence in French law, but attitudes changed in the second half of the century due to the power of 'Pro-Choice' Groups in particular 'Choisir'. In the USA restrictive abortion State Laws were repealed from the mid-1970s in most but not in all States.

Litigation

Malpractice claims became of increasing importance from the 1950s. The first laws which mentioned malpractice appeared in the Code of Hammurabi in ancient Babylon where stringent penalties were outlined against physicians for failure of treatments. In ancient Greece the concept of peer review was introduced and Plato advocated that putative physician malpractice should be judged only by other physicians. Civil liability for the actions of physicians and surgeons was recorded in England in the fourteenth and fifteenth centuries and in America in 1794. The

Medical Defence Union of the UK came into being in 1885 and the Medical Protection Society was formed 7 years later. By the 1990s medical malpractice claims had become a multi-million pound 'industry'. One response of the profession was to engage in defensive medicine. The realization that obstetrics and gynaecology was a high-risk area forced many practitioners to abandon established positions or promising careers in the profession (Varian, 1991).

Gynaecology

Cancer

Cervix The earliest form of cervical cancer was described by Rudolph Virchow in 1858 and John Williams in 1886 (Ricci, 1945). These superficial lesions were again described in the 1900s by Cullen and other investigators. The so-called 'surface carcinoma' or 'intraepithelial carcinoma' was later termed 'carcinoma *in situ*' by Broders in 1932. In 1962 Reagan *et al.* introduced the term 'dysplasia'. A further change occurred when Richart introduced cervical intraepithelial neoplasia terminology in 1964. Cells from the abnormal cervix were subjected to microscopy by Daniel and Babes and also O. Viana who reported tumour cells in vaginal fluids in 1927. The work of Papanicolaou and Traut in 1943 stimulated cervical cytology screening which was first introduced in 1948.

Examination of the cervix under magnification was introduced by Hans Hinselmann in 1925. He first used acetic acid to coagulate cervical mucus, and this later led to the 'acetic acid test'. Three years later Schiller advocated the use of Lugol's iodine to stain the cervix. Various classifications were introduced to describe the colposcopically detected cervical abnormalities and their relationship to cancer. Initially the treatment of premalignancy was by biopsy or cone biopsy, but these methods were complemented by laser therapy from the mid-1960s and by cryocautery from 1970. Electrocautery techniques introduced in the late 1940s were again revived in the 1970s. The cold coagulator was first brought to attention by Kurt Semm in 1966. Diathermy loop excision was pioneered by Cartier in 1981 and popularized by Prendiville in 1989.

Invasive cervical cancer was being treated by radical abdominal hysterectomy by Ernst Wertheim in 1900; and his technique was continuously modified by Schauta, Victor Bonney and others over the years. Radiotherapy was first used in 1903 by Cleaves and also by Danysz. In the same year Abbe started to use radium to treat cervical cancer in the USA. At first it was thought that radiation would replace surgery but it has not done so entirely, and they are complementary treatments.

Ovary The Pfannenstiel Classification of ovarian tumours of 1898 was replaced by Robert Meyer's Classification in 1915. Although various forms of ovarian tumour had been described prior to this century, much of our knowledge is due to observations made between 1900 and 1940. The mainstay of treatment has been surgery but chemotherapy was introduced in the form of alkylating agents in 1952 by Rundels and Burton. Early ovarian cancer has proved notoriously difficult to detect. Because of this there developed an interest in tumour markers particularly following Witebsky and his associates' isolation of antisera to mucinous cancers in 1956. Perhaps in the future a simple blood test will be able to be used as a screening device. Early detection and treatment would drastically improve the high mortality rates of 75% within 10 years of first diagnosis.

Vagina Cruveilhier of Paris first described carcinoma of the vagina in 1827. The condition was rare, but in 1971 Herbst *et al.* described the association between stilboestrol treatment of pregnant women and the onset of vaginal adenocarcinoma in their daughters.

Vulva In 1912, Basset and also Kehrer devised their radical operations for cancer of the vulva.

Uterus In 1900 Pusey and Pfahler used X-ray therapy for endometrial carcinoma. Radiotherapy was gradually introduced as a treatment in the 1920s. Surgery however became the more popular form of treatment so that by the end of the 1940s, a cure rate of almost 70% was claimed for surgery. Rita Kelley and William Baker introduced progesterone therapy in 1950 and cytotoxic treatment was used from the 1970s onwards to supplement surgery.

Cytotoxics In the fight against cancer, surgery and radiotherapy were, until 1946, the main modes of treatment. In that year the first publications appeared suggesting that drugs could be used to combat certain forms of neoplasia. These drugs were called cytotoxic, the word being derived from the Greek word for cell and the Greek word *toxicon* or the Latin word *toxicum* for poison. The Greeks had used the word *toxicon* for the poison they used on arrows.

The first clinical use of a cytotoxic drug was followed by its report by Gilman and Frederick Phillips (1946). The drug urethane, was used in the treatment of leukaemia by Patterson (1946). Nitrogen mustard was also used in the same year and induced remission in patients with lymphoma. Nearly all cytotoxic drugs were, and most still are, difficult for patients to tolerate because of their side-effects.

Other substances with cytotoxic properties were developed. They included low molecular weight chemicals, hormones, enzymes, naturally occurring antibiotics, plant alkaloids and cytokines. Choriocarcinoma was the first dangerously malignant disease to yield to chemotherapy. The drugs being used by 1970 were amethopterine (methotrexate), mercaptopurine, actinomycin D, and vinblastine. They had all been used separately, in combination or sequentially. The drugs were dangerous because they depressed bone marrow function, causing a fall in leukocyte and platelet counts and sometimes also diminished erythrocyte formation. They also, because of this, tended to lower resistance to infection.

Much of the work was carried out by Professor Kenneth Bagshawe, at the Charing Cross Hospital in London, where he treated the first cases in the UK. Choriocarcinoma or chorionepithelioma is not a very common condition in the UK so it was decided to limit treatment to three centres in Edinburgh, Sheffield and London. Because of the principle of freedom of choice, consultants could treat their own cases; but only in those three centres could the very rigid hormone assays needed for assessing whether the condition was responding be carried out. Between the years 1946 when the first drugs were given and 1991, there were great improvements, particularly in lessening the toxic side-effects by changing the drug regimens.

In 1965 Skipper first advanced the 'fractional cell kill' hypothesis. He based his experiments on transplantable murine leukaemia cell lines and studied them *in vivo*. He found that a given dose of drug killed a fixed proportion of tumour cells irrespective of the initial number rather than a fixed number of tumour cells. He thus postulated that the cytotoxic killing of cells followed first order kinetics.

The next gynaecological malignancy to respond to the cytotoxic drugs was probably carcinoma of the ovary. Not all ovarian cancers respond, but some do, particularly dysgerminomas, which may respond to chemotherapy with a single agent. Teratomas also respond well. Combinations of substances derived not only from moulds but also from heavy metals were used so that platinum was combined with vinblastine and bleomycin, or etoposide. Dennis Talbot and Maurice Slevin (1991) were able to report that it was likely that major advances would be made in optimizing the scheduling of cytotoxic drugs by using them with other forms of treatment and by changing and better planning the schedules for treatment.

None of this cytotoxic chemotherapy would have been developed if it had not been for the work of Peyton Rous (1879–1970) showing that it was possible for sarcoma to be transmitted in normal fowls (1910; 1913). Alexis Carell (1873–1944) and Montrose Burrows (1884–1947) were the first to grow the sarcoma *in vitro*. It may well be that it is logical that cytotoxic drugs, which bear in many ways a similarity to antibiotics, should be used against tumours (Carell and Burrows, 1910). The virus transmission of tumours has not been proved except for a few tumours and even these are the cause of some debate so that Albert Singer and David Jenkins (1991) in a review editorial in the *British Medical Journal* pointed out that although the human papillomavirus has been implicated as a transmitting virus for cervical cancer it is possible that other viral agencies could be responsible and in particular the herpes simplex virus type 2.

Benign pathology

Endometriosis Although discovered by Karl von Rokitansky the pathologist in 1860 and described by other workers in the 1800s, it was Sampson in 1921 who first wrote of 'chocolate cysts' of the ovary; terming the condition 'endometriosis'. In 1922 Blair Bell coined the term 'endometrioma'. Fraser in 1925 suggested surgical treatment for the condition and Karnaky introduced high-dose oestrogen treatment in 1948 and thus laid the foundations for hormonal and biochemical treatments for the condition.

Family planning

In the early twentieth century the American champion of birth control was Margaret Higgins Sanger. She resolved to change 'the destiny' of mothers, having observed the mortal effects of criminal abortion. Her first birth control clinic opened in Brownsville, Brooklyn in 1916. Marie Stopes of England met Margaret Sanger in 1915 and later developed a commitment to the birth control movement. Stopes' first clinic was opened in 1921 in the Holloway district of London (Figure 15).

Natural family planning methods were boosted by the introduction of the 'calendar method' based on the work of Ogino of Japan and Knaus of Austria in the early 1930s. They worked out the dates of ovulation in the menstrual cycle. Also at that time Van de Velde noted the relationship between the basal body temperature rise in the second half of the cycle and ovulation, and so the temperature control method came into use. Seguy and Simonnet related increased cervical mucus production to ovulation in 1933. By 1972 John and Evelyn Billings and co-workers in Australia had perfected their Billing's mucus technique.

Barrier methods of contraception were in use for centuries but the process of vulcanization only became available in 1834. In the early 1900s rubber condoms had a shelf life of 3 months, but by the 1930s the latex process improved the shelf life, quality and efficacy of the sheath. Diaphragms, cervical caps and spermicides were all available prior to 1900, but were improved and became more reliable from the 1950s onwards.

Intrauterine contraceptive devices became available from 1909 when Dr Richter of Waldenburg described the method. Ernest Graefenberg, Jack Lippes, Jaime Zipper and others are eponymously related to various forms of the device also named after flowers in China and the Far East.

Hormonal contraception was based on the discovery of oestrogen by Edgar Allen and Edward Doisey in 1923 and of progesterone by George Corner, Willard Allen and Walter Bluer in 1928. In the 1940s Russel Marker was responsible for a major breakthrough when he isolated progesterone from the Mexican yam and thus found a cheap method of obtaining the hormone. In 1956 Pincus, Chang, Rock and Garcia used norethisterone to inhibit ovulation. Enovid, the first commercially available contraceptive pill, was marketed in the USA in 1960, to be followed by many others with diminishing quantities of hormones.

Various *sterilization* procedures were described by Madlener in 1910 and by Irving, Pomeroy and Kroener in the subsequent 20 years. Laparoscopic sterilization was first used by Power and Barnes in

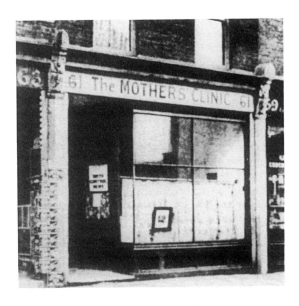

Figure 15 One of the first Family Planning Clinics to be established – Marie Stopes' clinic in the Holloway district of London, established in 1921. Reproduced with kind permission from the IPPF

1941 and Fallopian tube occlusion devices became available in the early 1970s. Common types included the Hulka–Clemens clip, the Fallope–Yoon ring, and the Filshie clip. Vasectomy was first used at the end of the nineteenth century and became commonplace from 1960 onwards.

Hormones

The various hormones involved in the female and male reproductive tracts were all isolated in the twentieth century. Allen and Doisey isolated a potent oestrogen from the follicular fluid of sows' ovaries in 1923. Corner and Allen (1929) developed a bioassay which enabled them to isolate progesterone. They used the term 'progestin' but Butenandt in 1930 suggested the suffix 'sterone' and thus the term 'progesterone' arose. In 1931 Butenandt isolated a male hormone from urine which he called androsterone. The pituitary gland was the subject of intensive study from the late nineteenth century and Oliver and Schafer in 1895 obtained extracts with pressor and oxytocic effects. Du Vigneaud *et al.* eventually had isolated, analysed and synthesized vasopressin and oxytocin in 1954. It was Fevold, Hisaw and Leonard who discovered that two different pituitary hormones influenced the ovarian cycle. Three years later the separation of follicle stimulating and luteinizing hormones was described and the pituitary gland was named the 'leader of the endocrine orchestra', the 'conductor' being the hypothalamus.

Stricker and Grueter of France in 1928 described secretion of milk following administration of a pituitary extract. Their discovery led to the isolation of prolactin and led to important work being carried out on hyperprolactinaemia in the 1930s by Krestein, Ahumada and del Castillo. In 1972 Meites *et al.* discovered that inhibitory control was exerted by secretions from the hypothalamus; and from this Besser *et al.* were able to report that bromo-criptine was effective in lowering high prolactin levels. The portal system between the hypothalamus and the pituitary was described by Popa and Fielding in the early 1930s. Harris, Professor of Anatomy in Oxford, carried out important work in evoking ovulation by stimulating the tuber cinereum and preoptic areas of the hypothalamus. Saffran and Schally after extracting substances from many tons of pigs' hypothalamic tissues identified the decapeptides in them and named them the hormone releasing factors in 1955. For this Andrew Schally received the Nobel Prize in 1977.

An endocrine function of the placenta was first described by Aschheim and Zondek (Figure 16) in 1927 although it had been first suggested by Halban in 1904. Chorionic gonadotrophin production was tracked down to the syncytium in 1963. Ovulation induction techniques employing placental hormones had been introduced by Davis and Koff as early as 1938 using an extract of pregnant mare's serum.

Polycystic ovaries, first described by J. Lisfranc in 1830, came under scrutiny from Irving Stein (Figure 17) and Michael Leventhal (Figure 18) of Chicago in 1935. They described women with amenorrhoea and cystic ovaries whose menstruation returned following bilateral ovarian wedge resection. Initially diagnosed at laparotomy, the large pearly ovaries of the condition could also be seen at laparoscopy, and later the typical ultrasound findings were fully described and illustrated in the 1980s, by Judy Adams working in the Middlesex Hospital, London.

Prostaglandins were discovered by Kurzrok and Lieb in 1930 and became of great importance for the induction of labour and abortion from the 1970s.

It is of interest that stilboestrol the first synthetic oestrogen, widely used in the late 1940s and early 1950s after its synthesis by Dodds and by Cooke and Hewitt, proved not only to be ineffective in treating toxaemia and diabetic pregnancies, but also to be teratogenic, as shown in 1971 by Herbst who discovered that there were disastrous changes

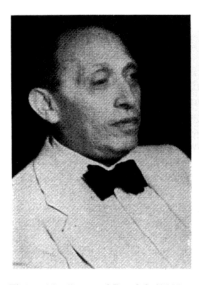

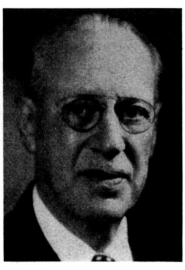

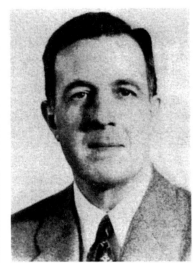

Figure 16 Bernard Zondek (1891–1967). Obstetrician and endocrinologist. The inventor with Selmar Aschheim of a test for pregnancy

Figure 17 Irving Freiler Stein

Figure 18 Michael Leo Leventhal

in the genitalia of women whose mothers had been given the substance in their pregnancies. It was later realized that their sons, too, might be infertile.

Infertility

The investigation of infertility became more scientific for the first time with the description by Rindfleisch in 1910 of hysterosalpingography. Better known, however, in history, was Isidor Rubin, who is remembered for the introduction in 1920 of 'Rubin's test' which first involved tubal insufflation with oxygen and later with carbon dioxide. The endometrium was investigated by Hitschmann and Adler in 1908 and by others, but it was not until 1950 that Noyes, Hertig and Rock demonstrated that the endometrium could be dated accurately histologically. Semen analysis was introduced in the late 1920s and in 1931 Moench and Holt analysed sperm morphology. A large number of workers evaluated semen and the World Health Organization and the American Fertility Society issued guidelines to standardize the reporting of sperm morphology. Hormone profiles only became readily available from the 1970s onwards.

The concept of the induction of ovulation was introduced in the 1930s but suitable agents did not become available until the 1960s. Tubal surgery played an important role, later supplemented by the advent of *in vitro* fertilization and gamete intrafallopian transfer technology, which became widely available after the birth of Louise Brown in 1978, the first baby resulting from the *in vitro* fertilization work of Robert Edwards (q.v.) and Patrick Steptoe (q.v.). Artificial insemination with donor semen was extensively used in the 1970s but received a set-back with the realization that donor semen could transmit the human immunodeficiency virus.

Venereal disease

Syphilis and gonorrhoea were the main forms of venereal disease in the 1900s when no successful method of treatment was available. Millions of people world-wide died from the ravages of syphilis. The Lock (venereal disease) Hospitals provided care for some of the sexually infected. The introduction of the arsenicals in the first third of the century was instrumental in altering the course of syphilis. The sulphonamides and penicillin followed and the latter could treat both syphilis and gonorrhoea.

Paul Ehrlich had patented Salvarsan (arsphenamine or 606) in 1907. He also produced neoarsphenamine which was more soluble and which was found to cure syphilis in humans in 1910. This drug became known as the 'magic bullet' or therapeutica magnans. The spirochaete had been discovered in 1905, and the Wassermann reaction to diagnose the disease from blood samples was described in the following year. During the First World War, one venereal disease officer was employed for every 10 000 troops. By the 1930s blood tests for syphilis were required premaritally in some states in USA and soon after this, antenatal screening for syphilis was introduced as a routine. Penicillin was found to be an effective treatment in 1943 but syphilis still existed in epidemic proportions until the 1970s.

The acquired immune deficiency syndrome (AIDS) was first reported in the USA in 1981, although the first cases had been seen but not recognized for what they were in 1978. AIDS had replaced syphilis as the major killer venereal disease world-wide by 1985.

In 1975 it seemed as though the major epidemics had been eliminated. There was no recurrence of the plague that had occurred in the fourteenth century, the endemic syphilis that could be found all over the world from the sixteenth century onwards was at least under control, if not eliminated, and smallpox had been completely eliminated. Then there arose the new scourge, the human immunodeficiency virus (HIV), that led on in very many cases to AIDS. Once the first signs of this disease have started, death is almost inevitable within 10 years or so of the first symptoms. Many women were infected by heterosexual intercourse and their babies were subsequently infected either *in utero* or postnatally through breast-feeding.

In January 1983 Professor Luc Montagnier of the Pasteur Institute in Paris isolated the virus for the first time. In May 1983 Dr Ann-Marie Casteret wrote an article in *Le Quotidien du Medecin* pointing out that the USA was about 2 years ahead of France in its experience of the disease.

In January 1985 Robert Gallo taking part as the head of a group in the USA in the race with the French to identify the virus and delineate its characteristics, published an article in *Nature* describing the complete nucleotide sequence of HIV. It required the work of several extremely well-funded laboratories to produce this article of great complexity. In fact the article had 19 named authors and received help from many other individuals; but Gallo's priority has been disputed.

Another multi-author article in the *British Medical Journal* in 1991 underlined the fact that very heavy investment and the work of many individuals and teams are required not only for the successful performance of this kind of research; but also for research into molecular biology, and that teams of trained researchers were continuing to probe towards the complete mapping of the human genome.

At first it seemed as though AIDS, which appears after a lengthy incubation of HIV in the human body, occurred particularly in homosexual communities in California and later in New York. However, by the late 1980s it was quite clear that world-wide the most common cause of infection was unprotected vaginal intercourse, and that increasingly large numbers of women were being infected and were infecting their casual or permanent partners as well as the fetuses in their wombs with this deadly virus. *Pneumocystis carinii* pneumonia outbreaks occur as the great final killer of people with AIDS who have insufficient immunological protection, not only for the virus causing the disease, but for the other opportunistic infections which eventually kill them.

Many of these infections are acquired before the appearance of AIDS and several such as salmonellosis, herpes simplex and cytomegalovirus (CMV colitis) were recognized in the 1970s and 1980s not only in homosexuals but also in their partners appearing in gynaecological clinics.

The presence of HIV in obstetrics, with the birth of congenitally infected children, has been a very serious development.

Gynaecologists were being infected by hepatitis B virus and developing viral hepatitis after acquiring small, almost subclinical, injuries while operating or giving injections in the 1980s. This meant that many gynaecological patients undergoing major surgery were tested for the antigens of hepatitis. It also became recognized that gynaecologists themselves *could* pass their viral infections (hepatitis and HIV) on to patients when they operated on them.

The menstrual cycle

The physiological changes of the menstrual cycle were the subject of intense scientific scrutiny from the late 1900s. The introduction of the uterine curette by Recamier in the 1840s provided the means by which endometrial tissue could be sampled. Hitschmann and Adler of Vienna first clearly illustrated the changing endometrial histological appearances throughout the cycle in 1907–1908. The mechanism of menstrual haemostasis was investigated by Schickele in 1912. Calendar records of thousands of menstrual cycles were investigated by Arey in 1939 who discovered the average interval of 28.4 days. Markee in 1940, by extremely skilful experiments, investigated the role of the endometrial vasculature in menstruation.

Excess menstrual loss was correlated with abnormal histological characteristics of the endometrium by Cullen in 1900, Schroder in 1914 and Novak in 1927. Hormone therapy for menorrhagia was given first by Albright in 1938, while cyclical oestrogen and progesterone therapy was suggested by Hamblen and colleagues 3 years later. Dilatation and curettage were also advocated as a treatment as well as for diagnosis. A large number of drugs were evaluated, but hysterectomy was the mainstay in treatment of women who had completed their families until the advent of endometrial ablation in the 1980s. The menopause came under intense scrutiny from 1966 when Wilson's publication *Feminine Forever* brought hormone replacement therapy to the public's attention. The premenstrual tension syndrome became a popular target for medical treatment in the 1980s.

Endoscopy

Both laparoscopy and hysteroscopy date from the development of the cystoscope in the nineteenth century. George Kelling described 'coelioscopic' examinations in 1901 and Jacobaeus of Stockholm introduced the term 'laparoscopy' in 1910; the term 'peritoneoscopy' being coined by Orndoff in 1920. During the 1940s culdoscopy was popularized by the work of Albert Decker and became more commonly used than laparoscopy in the USA. However, the introduction of modified instrumentation and cold light illumination sources in Europe, following the work of Hopkins of Reading in the UK, led to a second surge of popularity for laparoscopy from the 1960s. Names associated with the laparoscopic technique in Europe were Raoul Palmer of Paris who taught Patrick Steptoe of the UK and Kurt Semm of Germany.

Pantaleoni described successful hysteroscopy in 1869. Clado in 1898 and David in 1907 refined the technique and there were further improvements and popularization in the 1930s and 1940s, but it was not until the 1970s and 1980s that hysteroscopy became more widely used after techniques were improved by Hamou, Parent, Baggish and Barbot. Endometrial ablation techniques, which were first reported by Droegemueller and his associates in 1971, became an alternative to hysterectomy in cases of menorrhagia.

Urology

In the early part of the century much of the scientific activity in this area was based on the treatment of vesico-vaginal fistulae following Sims' example. However, 'stress incontinence', first named as such by Eardley Holland in 1922, and the 'unstable bladder' became relatively more important as cases of vesico-vaginal fistula were less frequently seen in the developed countries. Various forms of vaginal and abdominal operations to cure stress incontinence were perfected from the 1920s. New procedures are still being reported in the 1990s.

The unstable bladder became suitable for investigation after the introduction of the cystometric technique by Mosso and Pellacani in 1882. Drug therapies for the condition first began when belladonna was used by Langworthy in 1936. Gradually more sophisticated pharmaceuticals were used to relieve this unsocial condition.

DNA manipulation

It was in the 1970s that precise cutting and joining of DNA molecules in the test tube first came about, leading to the possibility of constructing new combinations of DNA segments. Recombinant techniques were used first in plant cultures but later with the aid of *in vitro* fertilization to obtain embryos for culture it became possible to mix cells from different embryos and produce chimeras.

By putting DNA into a newly fertilized egg adult animals can be bred so that transgenic progeny lines are produced. This has been performed successfully in mice and in farm animals. In this way, due to the development of transgenic technology based on *in vitro* fertilization, new animal models can be produced to test for possible treatments for genetic disorders. This is achieved by inactivating targeted genes and culturing different types of cells which can be introduced into small animal embryos (Benz, 1989). This is now leading to very difficult ethical situations.

DNA sequences and recombinant technology It was the *in vitro* fertilization techniques developed in the 1960s that made it possible to make transgenic animal technology an almost daily event in farm animals. One of the off shoots of the *in vitro* fertilization procedures has been the production of monoclonal antibodies by cell fusion. The antibody molecule is obtained by fusing E lymphocytes (the antibody-secreting cells of the immune system) with 'immortal', malignant myeloma cells obtained from mice. While these techniques may not be considered to be pure gynaecology they certainly will in the future help gynaecologists to deal with various abnormalities and even perhaps with cancers. The public however, tends to be very suspicious of recombinant technology.

RECENT DEVELOPMENTS IN CHINA

Until the 1970s the Eastern system of barefoot doctors had prevailed, providing most medical treatment. Barefoot doctors were, and are, mainly trained in County and Commune Hospitals. In the 1990s there are 1.5 million barefoot doctors for the population of China, which is over 1000 million.

The Peking Union Medical College was in existence by the 1920s and trained women gynaecologists from then onwards. The most famous of these was Doctor Lin Qiaozhi, born in 1901, and a gynaecologist from the age of 30 onwards, most of the time at the Peking Union Medical College. There had been no women resident doctors in Chinese hospitals before her; and she was certainly the first woman to hold the post of Chief of Gynaecology in any University Hospital.

The medical educational system in the 1990s includes medical colleges and very advanced medical technology and in particular microsurgery; but together with this modern surgery, traditional Chinese medicine, Chinese herbal medicine and pharmacology are still taught.

Until the 1940s there were very few fully trained doctors in China. Most of these were medical missionaries from European countries; but the traditional doctors in China had been using drugs which were discovered only much later by Western doctors. For instance, some cardiac patients were being treated for hundreds of years with *Rauwolfia* which grows well in some parts of China.

China started to catch up very quickly from the 1940s onwards, and such techniques as Caesarean section and forceps became more commonly used than previously. All the same it has not been easy to reduce the stillbirth and 1st year death rate from 50% of all deliveries to something resembling Western figures.

Maternal mortality is still very high in China. In 1950 it was about 1500 per 100 000 deliveries and in 1990 it had dropped to 94.7 per 100 000 deliveries. This is to be compared to a figure of less than 10 per 100 000 deliveries in Western Europe. The rate in China is far worse in the remote rural and mountainous areas than it is in the urban areas where it has dropped to under 50 per 100 000 deliveries. China still needs programmes of antenatal care and health examinations and now Chinese medical services are beginning to make contact with the World Health Organization, United Nations International Children's Emergency Fund (UNICEF) and United Nations Family Planning Association (UNFPA).

Population and birth planning in the People's Republic of China

China had its first census in 1953 and it was then realized that there was a population of almost 600 million, growing at about 2% annually. The Chinese leaders tried to start family planning programmes. These were interrupted in the late 1950s by the Great Leap Forward, and again in the 1960s by the Cultural Revolution, but since 1971 birth planning has been given consistently high priority by the ruling Communist Party leadership.

Medical schools in China all closed in 1966 and only re-opened in December 1970 when their administration was placed under the control of revolutionary committees, the chairman of which was always an army officer. They set up a campaign in 1971 with 'later, longer, fewer' as the reproductive norms or goals for China. Later meant later marriages, women first being recommended not to marry before their mid-twenties, and then the late twenties. Longer, stood for longer intervals between births with 3 or 4 years recommended, and fewer meant fewer children. In the early 1970s this meant two children per family but it has now been reduced to one child per family. This is now considered to be 'better'.

The campaign to introduce intrauterine devices has been successful and about 100 million were said to have been inserted between 1971 and 1978. Some of these have shapes that appear unusual to Western eyes such as the 'Canton flower'. About 30% of couples are sterilized – either the husband or the wife.

The Communist regimen was only established in China in 1949. Before that there had been Emperors who had not apparently encouraged any systematic method of training gynaecologists and obstetricians.

China is a huge country. Most of its population is concentrated along the eastern coast of the country, with only 15% of the country's population inland. It was only during the cultural revolution that doctors became dispersed throughout the country, so that for the first time, rural populations had medical attention. The barefoot doctors brought contraception to the masses of the population. They, in turn, were supervised by higher trained doctors, insufficient in numbers. Female sterilization is mainly carried out by tubectomies, with the removal of most of the Fallopian tube on each side. There are two tubectomies for every vasectomy; and 20 million tubectomies were done between the years 1971 and 1978. It was in that decade that the American doctor Jordan Phillips introduced laparoscopy and laparoscopic sterilization into China. His teachings and techniques became disseminated from the 1970s onwards.

This may have an effect on the number of induced abortions in China, where in 1978 in Beijing there were 940 induced abortions for every 1000 live births. In the countryside there were about 300 per 1000 live births. Vacuum aspiration, pioneered by the Chinese, is the main method of abortion; and has spread throughout the world.

At one time, Chinese women were not allowed by law to marry younger than the age of 20; but this law became unworkable. Although young couples are still encouraged to marry later in life, penalties for early marriage are not so great in the 1990s as they were 20 years earlier.

THE FUTURE

The conditions in time to come cannot be foreseen, but it is likely that progress will continue. Societies, governments and health professionals must together determine methods by which the unnecessary mortality and morbidity in the developed and developing nations are reduced to a minimum. Purported advances in diagnostic methods and treatments should be subjected to rigorous trials before their introduction to clinical practice. The mistakes of the past may be repeated unless we heed the admonition *Primum Non Nocere.* It is hoped that the increasing interest of obstetricians and gynaecologists in medical audit and consumer satisfaction will convince the public of the underlying humanity, high ideals and caring attitudes of all who espouse this most noble profession.

REFERENCES

Many of the references in this chapter, particularly those relating to the twentieth century may be found in the appropriate sections of the book

Benz, E.J. (1989). *Molecular Genetics,* pp. v–20. (Edinburgh: Churchill Livingstone)

Butler, N.R. and Alberman, E.D. (1969). *Perinatal Problems,* pp. 283–320. (Edinburgh: E. & S. Livingstone)

Carell, A. and Burrows, M.T. (1910). Culture de sarcoma en dehors de l'organism. *C. R. Soc. Biol. (Paris),* **69**, 332–4

Central Midwives Board (1974). *Active Management of Labour,* Statement to Training Schools. (London: Central Midwives Board)

Chamberlain, G. and Turnbull, A. (1989). The continuum of obstetrics. In Turnbull, A. and Chamberlain, G. (eds.) *Obstetrics,* pp. 3–8. (Edinburgh, London, Melbourne, New York: Churchill Livingstone)

Colebrook, L. (1954). Puerperal infection. In Munro Kerr, J.M., Johnston, R.W. and Phillips, M.H. (eds.) *Historical Review of Obstetrics and Gynaecology 1800–1950,* pp. 202–25. (London: E. & S. Livingstone)

Corner, G.W. and Allen, W.M. (1929). Physiology of the corpus luteum (II) Production of a special reaction: progestational proliferation: by extracts of corpus luteum. *Am. J. Physiol.,* **88**, 326–39

Dally, A. (1991). *Women Under the Knife, A History of Surgery.* (London, Sydney: Hutchinson Radius)

Dewhurst, Sir J. (1989). *Queen Charlotte's – The Story of a Hospital,* p. 68. Private Publication

Duhalde, J.B. (1763). *Description de l'Empire de chine et de la Tartarie Chinoise,* published in the Hague.

Ebers, G. (1875). *Papyros Ebers: das hermetische Buch über die Arzeneimittel der altem. Ägypter in hieratischer Schrift,* 2 vols. (Leipzig)

Garrison, F.H. (1921). *An Introduction to the History of Medicine,* 3rd edn. pp. 96–105. (Philadelphia London: W.B. Saunders & Co.)

Gilman, A. and Phillips, F.S. (1946). The biological actions and therapeutic applications of the beta chloroethyl amines and sulphides. *Science,* **103**, 409–15

Greenhill, J.P. (ed.) (1975). Progress in Obstetrics and Gynaecology– 1921–75. In *Year Book of Obstetrics and Gynecology,* pp. 9–15. (Chicago: Year Book Medical Publishers Inc.)

Gregg, N. McA. (1941). Congenital cataract following german measles in the mother. *Trans. Ophthalmol. Soc. Aust.,* **3**, 35

Herbst, A.L., Ulfeder, H. and Poskanzer, D.C. (1971). Adenocarcinoma of the vagina. Association of maternal diethylstilboestrol therapy with tumour appearance in young women. *N. Engl. J. Med.,* **284**, 878–81

Her Majesty's Stationery Office (1991). *Report on Confidential Enquiries into Maternal Deaths in the United Kingdom 1985–1987.* (London: Her Majesty's Stationery Office)

Hibbard, B.M. (1988). *Principles of Obstetrics,* pp. 1–18. (London, Boston: Butterworths)

Inch, S. (1982). *Birthrights. A Parents Guide to Modern Childbirth.* (London, Melbourne: Hutchinson and Co. Publishers Ltd)

Joachim, H. (1890). Papyros Ebers: das älteste Buch über Heilkunde. Aus dem Aegyptischen zum erstemal Vollstandig ubersetz von H. Joachim (Berlin: G. Reimer)

Lemoyne, P. *et al.* (1968). Les enfants de parents alcoholoques: anomalies observés, a propos de 127 cas. *Arch. F. Pediatr.,* **25**, 830

Ludolf, A. (1681). *Historia Aethiopica Sile Brevis et Succincta Descriptio Regni Habessinorum,* Frankfurt

Lyons, A.C. and Petrucelli, J. (1987). *Medicine: An Illustrated History,* p.24. (New York: Harrier & Abrahams)

McBride, W.G. (1961). Thalidomide and congenital abnormalities. *Lancet,* **2**, 1358

Morton, L.T. (1983). *Medical Bibliography,* 4th edn. (London: Gower Medical Press)

Nightingale, F. (1861). *Introductory Notes on Lying-in Institutions.* (London: Longmans)

Oakley, A. (1984). *The Captured Womb. A History of the Medical Care of Pregnant Women.* (Oxford, Glasgow: Blackwell Scientific Publishers)

Patterson, E. (1946). Leukaemia treated with urethane compared to deep X-ray therapy. *Lancet,* **46**, 677

Pauerstein, C.J. (1987). *Clinical Teratology in Clinical Obstetrics,* pp. 317–26. (New York: Wiley Medical)

Pinard, A. (1895). *Bull. de L'Academie de Med.,* **3**, 33–34, p. 593–7

Price, W. and Wigham Price, A. (1964). *Ladies of Castlerae: The Life of A.S. Lewis and M.D. Gibson,* (Durham: Presbyterian Historical Society of England)

Ricci, J.V. (1945). *One Hundred Years of Gynecology, 1800–1900.* (Philadelphia: Blakiston Co.)

Ricci, J.V (1950). *The Genealogy of Gynecology.* (Philadelphia: Blakiston Co.)

Rous, F.P. (1910 and 1913). A transmissible avian neoplasm (sarcoma of the common fowl). *J. Exp. Med.,* **12**, 696–705, **13**, 397–411

Rowland, B. (1981). *Medieval Woman's Guide to Health.* (London: Croom Helm)

Siebold, B.C.J. (1891). *History of Obstetrics, Essai d'un Histoire de l'obstetrique,* translated from the German by F.J. Herrgot. (Paris: G. Steinheil)

Singer, A. and Jenkins, D. (1991). Viruses and cervical cancer. *Br. Med. J.,* **302**, 251 and 659

Smellie, W. (1752). *Treatise on the Theory and Practice of Midwifery,* 2nd edn. (London: Wilson & Durham)

Speert, H. (1973). *Iconographia Gyniatrica. A Pictorial History of Gynecology and Obstetrics.* (Philadelphia: F.A. Davis Co.)

Stewart-McKay, W.J. (1901). *The History of Ancient Gynaecology.* (London: Bailliere Tindall & Cox)

Talbot, D.C. and Slevin, M.L. (1991). Cytotoxic drugs. In Philipp, E.E. and Setchell, M.E. (eds.) *Scientific Foundation of Obstetrics and Gynaecology,* 4th edn. (Oxford: Butterworth-Heinemann Ltd)

Temkin, O. (1956). *Soranus' Gynaecology,* (Baltimore: Johns Hopkins Press)

Tew, M. (1990). *Safer Childbirth? A Critical History of Maternity Care,* pp. 147–79. (London, New York: Chapman & Hall)

Thomas, P. (1964). *The Indus Valley Civilisation.* (London: Asia Publishing House)

van Roosmalen, J. (1991). Symphyseotomy – a re-appraisal for the developing world. *Prog. Obstet. Gynaecol.,* **9**, 149–62

Varian, J.P.W. (ed.) (1991). *Handbook of Medicolegal Practice.* (Oxford: Butterworth-Heinemann Ltd)

Willughby, P. (1863). *Observations in Midwivery; the Country Midwife's Opusculum,* manuscript in Royal Society of Medicine, c.1670: also (1863) edited from the original by Henry Blenkinsop Warwick: also (1972) re-edited by Wakefield, S.R.

Wilson, J.R. (1973). *Environment and Birth Defects.* (New York, London: Academic Press)

FURTHER READING

Brown, W.G. (1799). *Travels in Africa Egypt and Syria in the Years 1792–98.* (London)

Rother, M.C. (1970) *The Medieval Hospital of England*

Antiquity

MESOPOTAMIA

About 6000 years ago the flat coastal clay and marshlands of what is now Iran and southern Iraq became populated with tribes who migrated from the surrounding areas. The land which became known as Mesopotamia lay between the twin rivers, the Tigris and the Euphrates, which originated in the mountains of Asia Minor and merged to flow into the Persian Gulf. The region became known as 'the cradle of civilization'.

The first recognizable civilization in the area was that of the Sumerians who populated the southern part of Mesopotamia c. 4000–2400 BC. Several cities were established, the best known of which was Ur. Although the city may have lain on the coast the ruins now stand 160 km inland. The Sumerians developed the world's oldest written language. Cuneiform script was committed to soft clay using a hard reed with wedge-shaped end. The clay tablet was allowed to dry in the sun or was baked in an oven. The Sumerians also used cylindrical seals for official documents. When rolled over a clay tablet, an impression of the cuneiform script or pictograph remained on the clay. Over 30 000 cuneiform tablets detailing the life in ancient Mesopotamia survive, 800 of which deal with the practice of medicine.

The Sumerians were overrun by the Akkadians, a Semitic warrior people from the north. Their leader, Sargon the Great, was supposedly found as a baby, floating on the river, in a basket made of reeds. The Semites ruled from 2400 to 1900 BC. The Babylonian era (1900–1100 BC) began when Amorite tribes conquered the small town of Babylon. This era's most famous ruler was the lawyer–king Hammurabi (c.1700 BC). He built a city at that site in Babylonia. Hammurabi is remembered for his code of laws which governed the rights of citizens, and which contained a number of directives for the medical profession. The laws not only governed the economic relationship between doctor and patient but also laid down punishment for those who were negligent. A thousand years after Hammurabi,

Babylon became known for its hanging gardens. The Assyrian peoples in the north-east of Mesopotamia slowly developed power from 1900 BC and were the dominant group in Mesopotamia from 1100 to 606 BC. Two further eras occurred, those of the Chaldeans (c.606–539 BC) and the Persians (539–331 BC).

Although symptoms were elicited, doctors depended on divination to discover what sin committed against the gods had caused the patient's illness. Hepatoscopy was practised, in which the liver or entrails of sacrificed animals were examined. The patient's prognosis depended on the findings, and physicians referred for guidance to clay models of a sheep's liver on which diagnostic inscriptions were written. Cosmology was important and diagnosis and prognosis were deduced from the alignment of the stars. Another prognostic aid came from the observation of birds in flight. The direction of flight was important. If the bird veered left, the outcome was pessimistic, and this may have been the origin of the belief that the left was sinister.

The medicine practised in Mesopotamia was mainly of mystical or magical nature but the medical 'texts' contained almost 250 drugs of vegetable origin, 120 of mineral origin and 180 which came from other sources. Very little was written on obstetrics or gynaecology. However, it is known that women gave birth while squatting on a birth chair, or on bricks. The occurrence of miscarriage was sometimes ascribed to injury. Infants judged to be of poor quality were exposed and allowed to die. Menstruating women were considered unclean and were isolated. This practice of isolation was also used for many forms of disease. Adultery was a serious crime.

The peoples of Mesopotamia understood the principles of scientific agriculture and were also interested in mathematics. Their numbered systems were based on units of 60 but a decimal system was also in use. The 60-minute hour and 360-degree circle was passed on by them to the present day.

EGYPT

The ancient Egyptians began farming along the valley and delta of the Nile about 6000 years ago. Egypt's small states were united by King Menes to form one long narrow kingdom extending about 900 km along the river. The city of Memphis, which was situated near the Nile delta, became the capital soon after 3000 BC. The first calendar was invented, and hieroglyphic writing came into use, around the same time.

The Kings, or Pharaohs, were recognized as gods in their own right. The Pharaohs divided Egypt into 'nomes' or regions, each of which had a Governor. Due to its geographical position, being surrounded by sea and desert, Egypt remained relatively isolated over a long period of time and this insularity allowed the development of a strong and unadulterated culture. Historians have divided Egypt's history between 3100 BC and 332 BC into 31 Royal Periods or Dynasties. Three eras, or Kingdoms, were also recognized within that timespan. The ancient Egyptians wrote prolifically but their hieroglyphic script was undecipherable. Our knowledge of their culture was therefore based on archaeological evidence, their 'oral' tradition, and the observations of the Greeks and Romans who wrote hundreds of years later.

Hieroglyphic (Greek: Hieros–sacred, Glyphein – to carve) writing was developed from pictographs where objects were represented by their images. The ancient Egyptians learned to write on papyrus (obtained from papyrus reed, by cutting its pith into thin strips and pressing these together as a writing material) using ink made of gum or soot. The hieroglyphics were difficult and time consuming to inscribe. A simple and quicker form called 'demotic hieroglyphics' – from democratic, or available to all – was developed, along with an alphabet of 24 letters.

The translation of these sources became possible after the discovery of the Rosetta Stone. During Napoleon's conquest of Egypt in August 1799, a squad of French soldiers carried out repairs to an outpost named Fort St Julien at Rosetta near Alexandria. An officer called Bouchard (Boussard) discovered a flat slab of black basalt stone measuring roughly 114 x 71 cm which was divided into three horizontal registers each of which contained an inscription in a different script. The inscriptions were in hieroglyphics (sacred writing), the abbreviated demotic script (the language of the common people), and Greek. Many attempts were made to decipher the hieroglyphics. Dr T. Younge of England and Rosellini of Pisa were partially successful.

Eventually the Frenchman, Jean-Francois Champollion translated the hieroglyphics in 1822. Thus the Rosetta Stone, attributed to Ptolemy the Fifth (c. 196 BC), became the key which unlocked the vast storehouse of Egyptian knowledge. Our main sources of knowledge of Egyptian medicine came from the hieroglyphic inscriptions on temple and tomb walls, from examination of embalmed mummified remains, and also from a series of papyri which were discovered in the last century.

The papyri, supplemented by the archaeological evidence, described Egyptian medical practice relatively well. The reputed founder of medicine was Thoth who presided at the Temple of Hermopolis. He is said to have written the Hermetic books, a collection of 42 sacred books which contained the available knowledge of the time, covering a wide range of subjects. Six of these books were devoted to medicine and the Ebers Papyrus may have been one of the them. There were a number of goddesses of fertility, pregnant women, and childbirth. Imhotep (c. 2900 BC) was a famous physician who was later venerated as a god.

Women's diseases were adequately represented in the papyri. The ancient Egyptians evolved over a hundred anatomical terms and described the external, but not internal, female genitalia. They documented menstrual problems and leukorrhoea and were the first to describe uterine prolapse. Male and female circumcision was practised. The Arabic word for this mutilation is *Chafadh*. A medical school was founded in the city of Sais and women physicians taught obstetrics and gynaecology. The birth stool was used and vaginal fumigation was an important method of administering medications.

Contraceptive methods were described, including the application of dung, honey and carbonate salt. Acacia leaf tips, which produced lactic acid, were also used. Surgery was limited to the repair of fractures and of various injuries. However, abcesses, boils and superficial growths were also treated. The copper salts contained in their eye paints had an antiseptic effect, and wound dressings of honey combined with grease or resin promoted healing. The ancient Egyptians gained their limited anatomical knowledge from their observation of injuries, preparation of animals for food, and the embalming of the dead. As their knowledge was limited they developed an almost entirely speculative approach to anatomy and physiology.

Papyri are writings made on special sheets made out of reeds. The reeds are grown on the banks of the River Nile. They are still harvested today between the months of June and September most years. The outer rind of the reed is cut off, then the pith is cut into thin strips which are laid horizontally and vertically. The criss-cross pattern of the reeds is pressed and it thus makes a sheet of papyrus. The standard sheet of the 5th Persian period was 15 x 30 cm. There is still a papyrus institute on the banks of the Nile, near Cairo.

The Kahun Papyrus dates from about 1850 BC and was discovered by Flinders Petrie, an English archaeologist, at Kahun, south-west of Cairo in 1899. It is a copy of a much older text. The papyrus was translated by F.L. Griffith in 1893, and its contents related to gynaecology and veterinary medicine. The first two pages contain 17 gynaecological prescriptions and instructions; surgical methods are not included in the instructions. On the third page are 17 prescriptions for the assessment of sterility and pregnancy and for ascertaining the sex of the unborn child. There is much about magic spells in the Kahun Papyrus. It is probably the first textbook on gynaecology in medical history. There are references to vulval pruritus, for which oil and incense, or asses' urine, were applied. Uterine prolapse was treated with a concoction containing grain, fruit and cows' milk, which was cooked and then taken as a gruel. Putrefaction of the womb, due to infection or neoplasia is mentioned. Lower abdominal pain with swelling, and also urinary discomfort are alluded to, and treatments offered. There are various methods used to determine whether a woman is fertile. Crocodile dung is advocated as a contraceptive. Crocodile dung does have sponge-like properties and peasant women in Egypt still use sponges soaked in vinegar, placed in the vagina as 'barrier' contraceptives.

The Ebers Papyrus is called after the German Egyptologist, George Ebers, and was bought by him in 1873 from an Arab in Luxor and translated into German by Joachim. The writing, in black and red ink, dates to about 1550 BC and is apparently a copy of an older papyrus. Its text contains a pharmacopoeia. There are prescriptions to regulate menstruation, to prevent leukorrhoea, correct uterine displacement, induce labour, increase lactation, and to remedy breast disease. Treatments were administered orally, by vaginal fumigation or irrigation, or by insertion of linen pessaries impregnated with medication.

The Ebers Papyrus recommends a mixture of Acacia tips, bitter apples and dates, bound together with honey and placed in the vulva. These give off lactic acid, which is not a bad spermicide. The Ebers Papyrus, which is over 65 feet long, contains 108 pages. It dates from the reign of Amenhotep 1 (1526–1505 BC). Although it deals with 'the preparation of medicine for all parts of the human body', it has a special section of gynaecology, including prolapse (found in several Egyptian mummies), gonorrhoea, contraception, assistance in childbirth, and possibly cancer of the womb.

The Edwin Smith Papyrus was discovered in a grave near Luxor in 1862 and dates from c.1700 BC. It is a copy of a document devoted to surgery which probably dated back to 3000 BC. It contains the oldest known Egyptian prescription, is over 15 feet long, and was translated by James Henry Breasted, the doyen of American Egyptology.

The Hearst Papyrus c.1550 BC was acquired during an expedition by Hearst in 1901. It contains 204 sections, and refers to genitourinary diseases in women. Most of the content is similar to the Ebers papyrus.

The Greater Berlin Papyrus also known as the Bruge Papyrus, deals with 25 medical conditions including breast disease and fertility. The Berlin Papyrus gives a prescription for a mixture of fat, also mandrake and sweet ale, boiled together and swallowed by the woman, to be taken every morning for four mornings after intercourse. This presumably increases fertility.

The Lesser Berlin Papyrus c.1300–1600 BC, contains incantations for mothers and sick children, the contents being mainly of a mystical or magical nature.

The London Papyrus c.1350–1600 BC, consists mainly of mystical prose.

The Chester Beatty Papyrus deals mainly with diseases of the anus. It dates from Dynasty XIX (1315–1200 BC). It is now in the British Museum, and the most important part, number VI, has a section on gynaecological problems, whilst number X concerns aphrodisiacs.

It seems likely that gonorrhoea existed in ancient Egypt. It also seems likely that infertility was common and was known as 'want in her womb' which meant an overwhelming desire to bear a child. It is of interest that nomadic traders of Arabia brought plants to be used as medicines in Egypt, from India and China. Cinnamon was one of these plants.

Although childbirth was attended by a high mortality, both of mothers and infants, it was regarded in Egypt as a natural event and not as an illness. It was 'women's business' with no men in attendance. The mummy of the XIth Dynasty Princess Hehenit shows that she had a narrow pelvis and died shortly after delivery with a vesico-vaginal fistula. It is not possible to calculate the maternal and infant mortality at this distance in time. Women squatted to deliver.

'Fertility figurines' made of faience or clay have been found in old Egyptian tombs (Figure 1). They are nearly always naked women. Little attention has been paid to the modelling of breasts or faces, but hips and buttocks are exaggerated in size and the genitalia are emphasized. Quite often the pubic triangle is picked out with paint on faience figurines or pricked with dots on figures made with clay. If they were put into graves containing male bodies then they were probably to ensure that the man's sexual potency would carry through to the afterlife.

In 1896–97 100 000 fragments of documents relevant to ancient history were discovered in the geniza of the old Ben Ezra Synagogue of Old Cairo. A geniza is a room in a synagogue into which material that should not be destroyed because it contains the name of God or a reference to him, is stored. The discovery of the Cairo geniza was made by two very learned Victorian ladies, a Mrs Lewis and a Miss Gibson who had some knowledge of Hebrew. They obtained a rare fragment of a Hebrew manuscript which was identified by Rabbi Dr Solomon Schechter, Professor in Rabbinics at Cambridge University, as a part of Ecclesiasticus, a book of the Apocrypha. Dr Charles Taylor, Master of St John's College, Cambridge, helped Dr Schechter to go to Cairo to bring back all the contents of the geniza, which are now being studied in the Cambridge University Library. Among these are some fragments related to excessive uterine bleeding and its treatment (T-Sar 43/21), the early diagnosis of pregnancy (T-Sn 90/36) and for the induction of abortion (T–Sar 45/30). (T–S stands for Taylor-Schechter the names under which the fragments are classified).

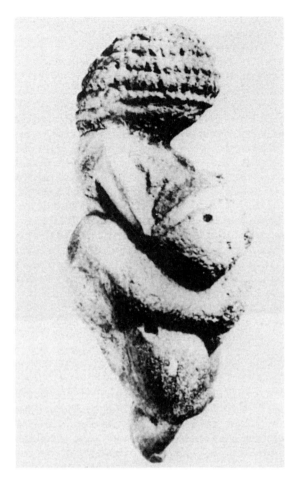

Figure 1 An early fertility symbol emphasizing the importance of fertility in society. Reproduced with kind permission from Gunn, A.D.G. (1987). *Oral Contraception in Perspective*, p. 14. (Carnforth UK : Parthenon Publishing)

Pregnancy tests in ancient Egypt

The Berlin and the Carlsberg Papyri deal with pregnancy tests. A woman who thought she may be pregnant was asked to urinate daily on two cloth bags, one containing wheat and the other barley mixed with sand and dates. If both germinated she was said to be pregnant. If neither did then she was not. It may be possible that hormones contained in the urine did cause germination. The experiment has been repeated today and sometimes found to work!

Not only in ancient Egypt but until the beginning of the twentieth century, male doctors had nothing to do with pregnant women. Hieroglyphs described the *Mshnt* which was used sometime before 2500 BC. It was a sort of confinement chair made of brick, later replaced by wooden ones.

The placenta and the umbilical cord seem to have a special place in Egypt, especially those emanating from Royal Princesses, and even today in Egypt, a peasant woman who wishes to have another child may bury her placenta and cord under the threshold of her house, considering it to be 'the other or second child'.

GREECE

The legendary Greek physician Asclepius (Figure 2) became deified as God of the Healing Arts. In mythological terms, he was the son of Apollo the Sun God (who was also God of Music, Fine Arts, Poetry, Eloquence, and Medicine), and a mortal woman, the legendary Thessalian Princess, Coronis. Coronis was killed for her unfaithfulness to Apollo but he snatched the unborn Asclepius from her as she became engulfed by the flames of

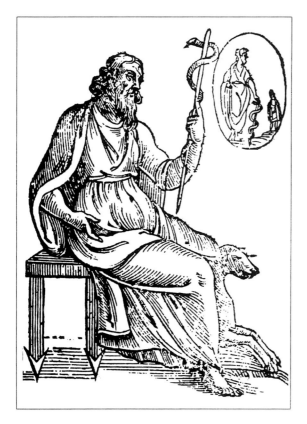

Figure 2 Asclepius, Greek God of Medicine. Reproduced with kind permission of Akademische Druck-u. Verlagsanstalt, Graz, Austria

her funeral pyre. Apollo's son was raised by the centaur Chiron, who instructed him in the healing arts. (Apollo may have delivered his son by Caesarean section and the funeral pyre may have referred to the burning fever of puerperal sepsis from which Coronis died.)

Whether mythological or not, Asclepius was said to be a tribal chief who was skilled in the art of healing. His sons followed in his footsteps. Asclepius trained them and they were known as Asclepiads and Physicians. Asclepius became a figure of such central importance that temples were built in his honour. The priests of the temples were also called Asclepiads and were clinicians who practised conservative medicine.

The first Asclepian Temple was erected about 1200 BC, at Titane. At least 200 other Asclepian Temple sites have been discovered in Greece and the Mediterranean basin. The best known were at Epidaurus and Cos. The temples were usually built in sites of natural beauty. The sick underwent a process of 'incubation' or 'temple sleep' and their dreams were interpreted by the priests or Asclepiads. Bathing, massage and the application of soothing ointments were all practised, but surgery was less frequently attempted. Sacred serpents played an important role in healing and the typical Asclepian staff was entwined by a snake (the serpent symbolism originated with the Minoans). Recreational activities and fresh air were encouraged so that the patient left the temple refreshed, strengthened in faith, and in harmony with nature.

The causation of disease was pondered by the philosophers. Their teachings were combined with clinical medicine about 500 BC and culminated in a new breed of medical scientists. Greek medicine was influenced and enriched by contact with Babylonia, Egypt and the East. However, the Greeks were the first to separate medicine from sorcery and magic. This new attitude began during the Trojan Wars which ended with the destruction of Troy in 1193 BC. Greek physicians of the time removed arrow heads, stopped the bleeding, applied medications, and cared for the sick and wounded without the use of magic. The doctors were practical men whose chief function was the care of war wounds.

In the pre-Hippocratic era, animal experimentation formed the basis of much of the available knowledge on anatomy and physiology. Alcmaeon of Crotona (c. 500 BC) was a famous physician who held the view that illness was brought about as a result of imbalance between the different components of the body. He also theorized that the fetus nourished itself through its body in a sponge-like fashion. His contemporary, Anaxagoras, believed however that the fetus was fed through the umbilical vessels.

The medical writers and philosophers began to show a deeper interest in the reproductive process from about the fifth century BC. In the Hippocratic corpus, ten treatises dealt with gynaecology or embryology. Hippocrates (Figure 3) advanced a theory of 'pangenesis' or 'preformation'. This theory held that sperm were produced by both partners and contained elements from all parts of their bodies. It was assumed that simultaneous orgasm must occur for conception to take place. Aristotle replaced the theory of preformation with that of 'epigenesis' which was based on the belief that the fetal body parts did not develop simultaneously at conception but were built up by successive accretions. The male sperm was the organizer or creative element which fashioned the menstrual discharge into an identifiable being, as the carpenter fashions a table from wood. Aristotle theorized that the testicles were not necessary for reproduction.

In keeping with the Greek belief in the inherent superiority of the right side, the male was advised to tie a knot around his left testicle to render it inoperative, and to thrust with gusto until ejaculation took place. By this means a male offspring was assured. Alternatively the Hippocratic 'school' advocated intercourse directly after menstruation to achieve a similar result. Male offspring resided in the warmer right part of the uterus having been formed from the rich, thicker sperm, while females were conceived with watery semen and their intrauterine life was spent in the darker left side. In society men retained their superiority, while females were mainly used for their reproductive qualities. Hippocrates maintained that frequent intercourse kept women healthy as it moistened the womb and improved both their general and mental health.

The Greek writers opined that procreation should follow intercourse between females in their late teens and males in their early thirties. However, in practice most women became married soon after their menarche, which occurred in the 13th or 14th year of life. For conception to occur it was thought necessary that the woman should close the cervix immediately after seminal ejaculation in order to retain the male seed. It was a common belief that deformed children came from deformed parents or from those mothers who

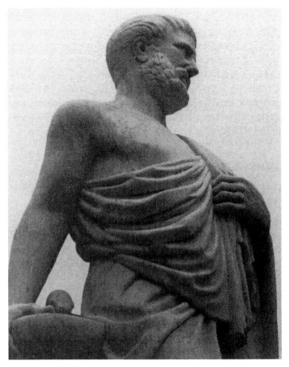

Figure 3 Hippocrates. Sculpture by Kostos Nikolau Georgakas. Reproduced with kind permission from the Lister Hill Library and the University of Alabama, Birmingham, USA

were unfortunate enough to gaze on a monstrous human or animal during their pregnancy. It was further believed that the child's physical appearance could be modified by gazing at beautiful statues or pictures. Twin pregnancy was considered a normal event, as women had two breasts with which to feed the infants. Births of higher multiple order, however, were said to portend disaster.

The theory of superfetation was common. In this situation a second pregnancy was thought to occur in the presence of a previous conception. The second pregnancy could be delivered as a stillborn fetus or lost at miscarriage. Pregnancy was divided into three phases, comparable to the modern concept of zygotal, embryonic and fetal life. The length of gestation could last from 7 to 11 months. Quickening was thought to occur at 3 months in males, or 4 months in females. It was observed that the baby born during the 8th month was liable to be imperfect and would die from the effects of prematurity. Miscarriage was thought to be unlikely after the first 40 days of healthy pregnancy.

Throughout pregnancy, expectant mothers were advised to take exercise, eat well, and avoid alcohol and excessive salt. Intercourse during pregnancy was considered beneficial by some writers. Aristotle advised coitus prior to labour, which he believed shortened the birth process. His observation was brought to fruition in this century with the discovery and use of prostaglandins.

Labour and birth took place in the home. The labouring woman was attended by a midwife, and three or four female friends or members of her family. Physicians were only called when complications occurred. The midwives were generally parous women and were postmenopausal. The midwife supervised the cleaning of the birth chamber and probably visited the pregnant woman prior to labour. Various grades of midwife were recognized and those with a knowledge of dietetics, surgery and pharmacy were highly prized. During labour the midwife supervised drug administration, and led incantations to the goddesses of pregnancy, Eileithyia, Artemis and Hera. Some types of drugs were used to accelerate labour and prior to delivery the birth canal was moistened with warm oil. Both Hippocrates and Aristotle advocated breathing exercises to relieve pain and hasten the birth.

A birthing chair was used during the delivery process although on some occasions the pregnant mother sat on a helper's lap. The midwife delivered the baby with her left hand, placed the baby on a sheet and cut the umbilical cord four finger breadths from the infant's stomach. She then examined the infant carefully to see whether it was worth rearing or not. The infant was bathed, and in some parts of Greece was wrapped in swaddling bands.

The earliest description of a normal birth was presented in the Hippocratic work, *Nature of the Child*. It was theorized that the fetus adopted a cephalic presentation as its weight measured from the navel to the scalp was greater than that from navel to feet. Spontaneous rupture of the membranes was ascribed to the fetus who used hand or foot movement to rupture the amniotic sac. The fetus itself was thought to force a wide passage to the pelvic outlet. In the Hippocratic works it was stated that the pelvic bones separated in labour. In consequence it was thought that obstructed labour was due to the child being too weak to separate the pelvic bones, and the importance of disproportion went unrecognized. When labour was prolonged and the child was undelivered, a physician was called. Transverse lie and stillbirth

were sometimes diagnosed. Delivery was effected by means of various hooks and instruments to which traction was applied, and the child was stillborn or died soon after. Maternal injury with consequent haemorrhage and sepsis would have been potent causes of maternal death. The maternal mortality rates may have been in the region of 10–20% for all births.

The Greeks practised exposure of unwanted newborn children, many of whom were premature, deformed, illegitimate, or the offspring of slaves. Girls were also more likely to be abandoned as boys were thought to offer a more economic return. However, boys were also at risk because in some of the Greek states, a father's wealth was divided equally among the male offspring. The laws militated against a large number of male offspring. Eventually legislation was introduced which regulated the practice of exposure, or banned it altogether.

Family size was regulated in part by perinatal and infant mortality, which was very high. Most deaths occurred in the 1st week of life, and the practice of naming the baby in the 2nd or 3rd postnatal week evolved. The laws of inheritance, and also state population policy, played an important role in determining family size.

Infertility was thought to be a form of divine retribution for offences committed against the gods. Rivers and streams, and the god Dionysol, were thought to promote human fertility. These ideas were replaced about the beginning of the fifth century when scientific explanations were proffered. Hippocrates held the opinion that there was a channel between the vagina and mouth. He proposed that incense be burned to fumigate the vagina. If the smell of incense appeared in the woman's mouth or nostrils, the passage was clear, and the woman was capable of conception. Various fertility treatments or medications were offered, including garlic and fresh beavers' testicles. It was thought that women who were excessively thin tended to miscarry, while those who were overweight had difficulty conceiving due to irregularity of menses or inability to open the mouth of their womb. Men with large penises were thought to be less fertile as the sperm cooled down and lost its generative capacity on its long journey.

The Greeks used a variety of concoctions which they applied to the vagina and cervix as contraceptive methods. These included olive oil, honey and various juices which formed a barrier, or had a spermicidal effect. A form of rhythm method was used as the Greeks believed that a short abstinence from coitus at the end of menstruation increased the likelihood of conception. The use of coitus interruptus was not mentioned until the first century BC.

Abortion was resorted to when other methods failed. Aristotle in *Politics*, XI, Verse 14, said 'there must be a limit fixed to the appropriation of offspring, and if any people have a child . . . in contravention of these regulations, abortion must be practised on it before it has developed sensation'. Although Hippocrates had advised against the use of abortifacient pessaries, Greek law did not forbid induced abortion. By law the husband's consent was necessary. The Pythagoreans opposed abortion as they believed that life began at the time of conception.

The word 'menstruation' was introduced by the Greeks and menstrual blood was said to be a fatal poison which could kill insects, flowers, grass and fruits, and could cause a dog to go mad. Despite that, it was used as a therapeutic agent which was said to be particularly effective in the treatment of gout. As the menstrual woman was dangerous, a custom of wearing a bandage around the head was instituted to warn others in the vicinity. Despite its toxic effect women were apparently immune, although contact with menstrual blood was said to cause miscarriage. The first pad worn by healthy virgins was mixed with wine or vinegar and was highly prized as a medication. The Greeks noted the duration and character of menstruation, and also measured the amount of menstrual blood.

Various forms of prolapse and malpositions of the uterus were noted and fumigation was commonly used in the treatment of genital disorders. Dilators and sounds were used to stretch the cervix or cure displacements. The uterus was considered to be a wandering organ and fragrant odours or semen were offered to attract it back to the pelvis.

The menopause occurred after the 40th year and changed the woman's status. As women were no longer capable of supplying heirs less protection was required, so menopausal women were allowed more freedom and could appear in public unattended. They also adopted the role of midwife and for the first time gained a source of income from their duties.

Hippocrates (c. 460–377 BC)

Hippocrates was born on the island of Cos. He received his initial training from his father (who

was a doctor), and later studied medicine in Athens. He is known to have travelled extensively and soon built a reputation for his great humanity and professional skill. One of his great contributions was his belief in the ethics which governed the practice of medicine. The Oath which is ascribed to him, may have derived from ancient Indian sources. The Hippocratic school of medicine became famous and left for posterity 72 books, which were housed in the Alexandrian Library under the title 'Corpus Hippocraticus' during the third century BC. Most of the texts were written by disciples rather than by the man himself, with the exception of the book *Prognosticon* which is attributed to Hippocrates. The modest knowledge of anatomy is evidenced by the Hippocratic notion that the clear or white liquid in the intestinal lymphatic vessels was mother's milk en route to the breasts. The growing uterus was said to squeeze this milk from the abdomen to the lactating mammae.

Aristotle (c. 384–322 BC)

Aristotle was born in Macedonia and his father was a royal physician. He became a scientist and philosopher and studied in Athens where he later founded his school (Figure 4). Aristotle was accustomed to delivering his lectures while strolling along the shaded arcades (*peripatoi*) of the lyceum

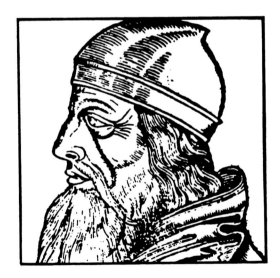

Figure 4 Aristotle – the first known Greek writer to mention contraceptive methods. Reproduced with kind permission from the IPPF

(a gymnasium and grove beside the Temple of Apollo) so his school became known as the 'peripatetic' school. He was the private tutor of Alexander, later Alexander the Great, who founded Alexandria in Egypt. As a scientist he had a keen interest in zoology and was the first to categorize the parts of the body into their component tissues. Aristotle forged a bridge between biology and medicine. He was a prolific author who also gathered a large library of philosophical and scientific works. He conceived many new terms, thus building the terminology of science and philosophy. Aristotle developed many theories relative to menstruation, conception, pregnancy and infertility.

ALEXANDRIA

As the power and influence of classical Greece waned the medical centre moved to North Africa and the city of Alexandria. This city was founded by Alexander the Great c. 332 BC and was sited on the Mediterranean coast of Egypt, at the northwest corner of the Nile delta. Alexandria became the leading capital in the Greek world. A large museum and library were built and many thousands of books were stored there. The city became an ideal centre for medical research. The library of Alexandria was the most famous library of antiquity. The idea of founding it came from Alexander The Great and it was maintained as a royal library by the Ptolemy rulers from the third century BC. It was also a museum, a school and a centre of scholarly research. An enormous collection of Greek books was gathered, edited and classified there. The library eventually contained about 700 000 books. It was burnt in the third century AD by a mob of fanatics, who destroyed it in order to found a 'new order'. In this way the world lost the finest collection that had been assembled in a single library at the time of Jesus. Eight hundred years after its foundation Aetius used texts derived from the library during research for his book *Diseases of Women*. A systematic study of anatomy was begun in the newly formed medical shool. Dissection of human remains was allowed for the first time in the Old World, thus setting the scene for many new discoveries.

The Ptolemites, who were a science-loving people, succeeded Alexander and under their influence the medical school flourished. Herophilus of Chalcedon studied there and was known for his anatomical research. Among his many accurate discourses on human anatomy he described the blood supply to the brain, duodenum and the reproductive tract. Herophilus is said to have been the first to describe accurately the ovaries and was the author of a book on obstetrics c 300 BC. Another famous anatomist was Erasistratus. Both he and Herophilus taught midwifery and were considered to be the founders of the medical school at Alexandria. The Alexandrian school was one of the best known medical schools of antiquity. Many of its graduates became famous. Egypt was conquered by Caesar in 47 BC and through his efforts many of the great medical men moved from Alexandria to Rome. Alexandria however continued to flourish for many more years although Alexander's empire disintegrated in the first century BC.

ROME

Rome came into prominence as the power and influence of Greece and Alexandria slowly declined. The Roman empire dominated much of the Western world and lasted from the first century BC to about AD 500. In the early period of Roman history there were no doctors as such. Each householder had his own treatments, and an array of gods to appeal to for help. Physicians slowly moved in from Greece and Alexandria and despite initial disapproval were gradually accepted. One of the first Greek physicians to practise in Rome was Archagathus, who had trained in Alexandria. He proved so successful that many followed to fill the demand for Greek or Alexandrian medicine. Asclepiades of Bithynia may have founded the first medical school and in his treatments used dietary measures, massage, bathing and bleeding. As the last pagan centuries drew to a close, a number of physician scientists came to prominence. Their work influenced medicine for well over 1000 years.

Aurelius Cornelius Celsus (27 BC–AD 50)

Celsus was a 'scientist' who compiled the works of previous and existing physicians. In AD 30 he published his work *De Re Medicina* in which he described the size of the uterus and noted various medications for menstrual disturbances. The treatment for prolapse was astringent washes, replacement of the uterus, and application of medicated pessaries to prevent further prolapse. Celsus described a cruciate incision for imperforate hymen and also detailed the procedure of podalic version. He described various surgical instruments including the speculum, and was probably the first to document the ligation of blood vessels to effect haemostasis. His *De Re Medicina* covered a wide variety of topics and survived right through to the fifteenth century. It was rediscovered by Pope Nicholas and printed in movable type in 1478. Celsus wrote in Latin rather than the customary Greek used in medicine at that time.

Gaius Plinius Secondus (Pliny the Elder AD 23–79)

Pliny was born in northern Italy and educated in Rome. He also was a compiler and wrote extensively on a wide array of topics including medicine. He compiled a large work entitled *Historia Naturalis* which was an encyclopaedia of the time. Pliny followed the Greek teachings when he referred to menstruation, and reported that menstrual fluid could make dogs 'go mad'. Even ants were frightened by it and discarded their food and fled. He described the symptoms of early pregnancy which he said had their onset 10 days after cohabitation. 'Giddiness of the brain, wambling in the stomach, abhorrence of meat', and other symptoms could be noted. If pregnant with a male offspring the woman perceived quickening earlier. The female fetus was responsible for late quickening and caused a more difficult pregnancy.

Pliny wrote on sterility and also referred to Caesarean section. He advised application of various drugs which would keep breasts firm, and also suggested the smearing of blood from amputated lambs' testicles to reduce armpit odour. He claimed that physicians, and Greeks in particular, experimented with patients for their own gain.

Soranus of Ephesus (AD 98–138)

Soranus studied at Alexandria and practised in Rome during the reigns of Trajan and Hadrian. He wrote almost 20 works on biology and medical science including texts on surgery and gynaecology. He also wrote a biography of Hippocrates. His scientific books included his own experiences and research, combined with the existing knowledge of the day. His book on gynaecology (in four parts) was translated and copied by many famous authors. A short version was translated into Arabic, and Muscio translated it into Latin. It was also published in the main European languages during the post-renaissance period, and Rösslin's *The Byrth of Mankynd* was based on it. His *Gynaecology* was translated into English by Temkin in 1956.

Soranus illustrated the fetal positions *in utero*

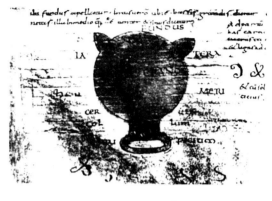

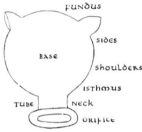

Figure 5 Earliest known representation of the anatomy of the uterus. It embodies Soranus' conception of the organ and appears in a Muscio text of the ninth century. From Weindler (1908). Courtesy of the National Library of Medicine, Bethesda, Maryland, USA

(Figure 5), and advocated internal version, a procedure revived by Paré in the sixteenth century. He distinguished between primary and secondary amenorrhoea and believed that conception was most likely to occur directly after menstruation. Soranus gave the first scientific account of gynaecological anatomy. He treated puerperal sepsis and uterine prolapse, and his writings show that he was familiar with the use of the speculum.

Rufus of Ephesus (c. AD 110–180)

Rufus of Ephesus also trained at Alexandria and was a physician and investigator who made many original observations in anatomy. He described the course of the optic nerves, the various parts of the eye, and also realized that the pulse and heartbeat were synchronous. In his book entitled *The Names of the Parts of the Body* he described both the male and female reproductive organs including the oviducts (in animals) and the various parts of the vulva.

Claudius Galen (AD 131–201)

Galen was born in Pergamus (Pergamum) in Asia Minor. He studied at Alexandria and became the most influential writer of all time on medical subjects. His anatomical knowledge was gained from the Barbary ape and other animals, and he thus perpetrated mistaken ideas which were only corrected in the sixteenth century. Despite that, he made many valid observations and was the first to discover that arteries contained blood and not air. He brought drug therapy to a fine art and developed 'theriac' – an antidote to snake bite and other poisons. Galen's work on therapy, the *Ars Magna*, was central to medical practice for centuries. He wrote over 500 works, of which 83 survived. Galen gave a definitive description of breast cancer and described its surgical treatment. He described the cervical softening of early pregnancy but did not appear particularly interested in practical obstetrics or gynaecology.

Obstetrics and gynaecology in Rome

Menstruation

Menarche was said to occur between the 13th and 14th year with menopause occurring between the 40th and 50th years. Impending menstruation was diagnosed by various physical and psychological complaints. Treatments were offered for dysmenorrhoea, menorrhagia, oligo- and amenorrhoea.

Pregnancy

Soranus advised that first intercourse should not take place before the menarche. Marriage occurred at the early age of 15 or 16 years, and a family size of two to five children was normal. Fruitful intercourse was best planned for the direct postmenstrual days. When pregnancy occurred, 'preservation of the seed' was important and the mother was not subjected to undue physical stress so as to avoid loss of the seed, or miscarriage. Early pregnancy sickness and pica were noted, but Soranus advised against eating for two. Births were planned to take place in the home, where the parturient was attended by a midwife and helpers. Soranus discussed the qualities required of a midwife but did not require that she should have given birth herself. The patient was nursed in bed until delivery was imminent and she was then moved to the birthing chair. The midwife sat opposite the labouring woman and allayed her anxiety, also directing the mother to push without crying out. An assistant would exert mild fundal pressure and a third protected the anus. The midwife dilated the birth passage and received the infant onto scraps of thin papyrus or pieces of cloth.

Dystocia in labour was thought to be due to psychological causes or those which arose from the fetus or birth canal. When dystocia occurred the bladder was catheterized, the rectum evacuated, and greasy substances were applied to the birth canal. Any obvious tumours or membranes were divided. If manual traction failed to deliver the infant, various forms of hooks and other instruments were used. Haemorrhage and sepsis were the main dangers in childbirth and although no maternal mortality figures are available, maternal deaths may have occurred at a rate of 25 per 1000.

Breastfeeding

Maternal breastfeeding was advocated, but Soranus believed that there should be a lapse of 3 weeks to allow the mother to recover from her labour. In the meantime a wet nurse *(nutrix)* was employed. Breastfeeding was continued for up to 2 years and it was known that those infants who were fed with cow's or goat's milk were more likely to succumb to enteritis and die. Contraception was used and abortion was attempted in some cases of unwanted pregnancy. Weak or deformed infants were sometimes exposed and allowed to die – similiar to the Greek practice of infanticide.

The emperor Constantine moved from Rome to Byzantium in AD 300 (this city later became Constantinople and then Istanbul). The centre of medicine had thus returned close to its origins.

CHINA

The development of gynaecology

It is very difficult for a Westerner to find out much about old obstetric history in China. Medicine existed in China, of course, a very long time ago; and according to legend it commenced with Fu Hsi about 3000 BC. Huang Ti, who died about 2598 BC, was known as the 'Yellow Emperor'. He is said to have written a canon of internal medicine called the *Nei Ching*. Much later in about the seventh century AD came the Tantras, texts dealing with practices of different sects – some Hindu, some Buddhist and some Jaina. The most famous medical work of these is the *Four Tantras* compiled under the Tibetan medical master in the late eighth century. The *Four Tantras* was translated into Mongolian, English, French and other languages, but it did not contain much about obstetrics.

From 200 BC onwards Chinese medicine progressed rapidly. In 1972, a woman's body was discovered in a Han Dynasty tomb at Mawangdui in Hunan Province. It was very well preserved and flexible after 2100 years of interment. This shows that Chinese pharmacology had already then effective ways of preventing the decay of interred corpses. On the same site, instructions, including some on acupuncture, surgery, obstetrics and diagnosis, were found.

Gynaecology and obstetrics have had a long history of development since the *Canon of Internal Medicine* appeared, giving names to women's diseases and treatments for conditions in pregnancy. In the thirteenth Century Chen Ziming (AD 1190–1270) compiled *Elections of Effective Prescriptions for Women*. This summarized practice in the field and is still worth reading.

Acupuncture originated in China; and until recently was confined to China and Tibet. At the turn of the millennium there were bronze figures to illustrate the acupuncture points made by Wang Weiyi (about 987–1067).

Infertility was, and for many still is, a curse. The attitude of the Chinese to women was such that if the wife of an only son failed to carry on her husband's ancestral line, she would be likely to suffer unbearable discrimination and maltreatment.

Not only in Western society and in biblical society has infertility been the subject of much literature but also in Chinese society. There is a splendid book by R. H. van Gulik who worked as a diplomat in the Dutch Embassy in Japan in 1949 and collected a great deal of literature which he used to write *Sexual Life in Ancient China – a Preliminary Survey of Chinese Sex and Society from C.A. 1500 BC to AD 1644*. It contains sections about books and documents of instruction written during the time of the Sui Dynasty AD 519–616. van Gulik points out that there had already in previous centuries been popular handbooks of sex. In the Sui Dynasty *Principles of Nurturing Life* by Chang Chan in two books explained various ways of having intercourse and the timing of intercourse to ensure fertility. Remarkable prescriptions are

given for failure of erection (4 g each of deer horns, cedar seeds, *Cuscuta japonica* and *Plantago major* var. *asiatica*, *Polygala japonica*, *Schizandra sinensis* and *Boschniakia labourer*). This is not only helpful for the man who fails to have an erection, but it could prevent shrinking of the member during the act. Furthermore, 'involuntary emissions, excess of urine, and aches in the back and middle will also be cured'. There is a medicine to shrink a woman's vagina; this consists of 2 g sulphur, 2 g incense, 2 g seeds of *Evodia rutaecarpa*, B. Th. and 2 g of *Cridium japonica*. Alternatively, three pinches of sulphur powder and 1 pint and a half of water will do the trick. More interesting however, is the timing of intercourse which should not be during menstruation; and for preference it should be 5 days after the end of menstruation. Boys are conceived on alternate days after the end of menstruation and girls on even days after the end of menstruation!

It is sad in a way that no matter how many books are consulted none except Garrison's first book mentions much about Chinese medicine, and even he who is full of admiration for Egyptian medicine, Sumerian and Oriental medicine and Greco-Roman medicine, finds little to say about Chinese medicine and nothing about Chinese obstetrics and gynaecology.

It is quite clear that acupuncture and herbalism were the big contributions made by Chinese medicine; and William Osler in his *Evolution of Modern Medicine* pointed out that the Chinese had also invented pulse diagnosis which apparently depended on great delicacy of touch.

CHRONOLOGY

Mesopotamia

6000 BC	The area between the Tigris and Euphrates became populated.
4000 BC	The Sumerians came to prominence.
2400 BC	The Semitic influence began.
1900 BC	Babylon was built and Hammurabi ruled supreme.
1100 BC	The Assyrian era began. Diseases were thought to be caused by demons.
606 BC	The Chaldean Empire began. Hebrews were taken captive. Nebuchadnezzar was the outstanding figure.
539 BC	The Persians conquered Babylonia and Egypt.

Egypt

c.4000 BC	Ancient Egyptians farmed the valley of the Nile.
c.3100 BC	The Royal Dynasties began.
c.3000 BC	Memphis became capital.
2680 BC	The Old Kingdom period began and medical thought flourished.
2280 BC	The Middle Kingdom began.
c.2000 BC	Papyral texts were copied from older versions, and were rediscovered 3800 years later.
1980 BC	The New Kingdom flourished until 1085 BC.

Greece

2000 BC	Greeks were present on the Balkan peninsula.
1500 BC	The Thera volcano erupted, and soon after the Greek people dispersed.
800 BC	Greeks established colonies along the Mediterranean coasts.
460 BC	Hippocrates was born on the island of Cos.
5th C. BC	The Hippocratic School of Medicine was established.
384 BC	Aristotle was born.

Alexandria

c.332 BC	Alexander the Great founded Alexandria. It became the new centre of Greek medicine.
c.300 BC	Erasistratus and Herophilus dissected human remains, and began a series of anatomical discoveries. They also taught midwifery.
47 BC	Caesar conquered Egypt and the centre of medicine moved to Rome.

Rome

1st C. BC	Rome became the capital of the medical world.
27 BC–AD 50	Aurelius Cornelius Celsus compiled the available knowledge of medicine.
AD 23–79	Pliny the Elder, another compiler, included items on gynaecology in his texts.
AD 98–138	Soranus of Ephesus studied at Alexandria and became Rome's most famous physician.

AD 110–180	Ruphus of Ephesus also trained at Alexandria, and worked in Rome. He gave an accurate description of the oviduct in animals.
AD 131–201	Claudius Galen wrote texts on general medicine and included some of the available gynaecological knowledge.
AD 300	The Emperor Constantine moved from Rome to Byzantium thus creating a new capital and a new era.

China

3000 BC	Fu Hsi was the 'Father' of medicine.
2598 BC	Huang Ti wrote the first canon of internal medicine.
2100 BC	Preservatives were used to mummify bodies. Some instructions on obstetrics date from this time.
AD 519	Handbooks of sexual etiquette were available.
7th C.	The 'Four Tantras' were written.
13th C.	Chen Ziming summarized the medical practice available for women.

ACKNOWLEDGEMENTS

The authors are very greatly indebted to Dr Barbara Watterson, of Liverpool, for permission to quote from Chapter 5 of her book *Women in Ancient Egypt* published by the British Museum. The chapter in Dr. Watterson's book ends with an extremely helpful and very full bibliography of the sources. We are also very grateful to Mr Edwin L. Holland MA, MB, FRCOG, of Newry, County Down, who clarified the dates of the various papyri mentioned above.

BIBLIOGRAPHY

Brown, W.G. (1799). *Travels in Africa, Egypt and Syria in the Years 1792–98*, p. 347. (London)

Cianfrani, T. (1960). *A Short History of Obstetrics and Gynaecology*. (Springfield, Illinois: Charles C. Thomas)

Clayton, P. (1990). *Great Figures in Mythology*. (Leicester: Magna Books)

Cowen, D.L. and Helfand, W.H. (1990). *Pharmacy: An Illustrated History*. (New York: Harry N. Abrams Inc. Publishers)

Estes, J. (1989). *The Medical Skills of Ancient Egypt.* (USA: Science History Publications)

Garland, R. (1990). *The Greek Way of Life.* (London: Duckworth)

Garrison, F.H. (1929). *An Introduction to the History of Medicine.* (Philadelphia: W.B. Saunders Co.)

Graham, H. (1950). *Eternal Eve.* (London: W. Heinemann)

Haeger, K. (1988). *The Illustrated History of Surgery.* (London: Harold Starke)

Jackson, R. (1988). *Doctors and Diseases in the Roman Empire.* (London: British Museum Publications)

Lyons, A.S. and Petrucelli, R.J. (1978). *Medicine: an Illustrated History.* (New York: Harry N. Abrams Inc. Publishers, Abradale Press)

McGrew, R. (1985). *Encyclopedia of Medical History.* (London: MacMillen Press)

McKay, W.J.S. (1901). *The History of Ancient Gynecology.* (London: Ballière Tindall Cox)

Osler, Sir W. (1921). *The Evolution of Modern Medicine.* (New Haven: Yale University Press)

Peoples and Places of the Past (1983). *The National Geographic Illustrated Cultural Atlas of the Ancient World.* (Washington, D.C.: The National Geographic Society)

Rhodes, P. (1985). *An Outline History of Medicine.* (Cambridge: Butterworth)

Ricci, J.V. (1950). *The Genealogy of Gynaecology,* 2nd edn. pp. 9–24. (Philadelphia: Blakiston)

Temkin, O. (1956). *Soranus Gynaecology.* (Translated with an introduction by O. Temkin). (Baltimore: Johns Hopkins Press)

van Gulik, R. H. (1961). *Sexual Life in Ancient China – a Preliminary Survey of Chinese Sex and Society from C.A. 1500 BC to AD 1644,* pp. 119–69. (Leiden: E. J. Brill)

Venzmer, G. (1972). *5000 Years of Medicine.* (London: MacDonald & Co.)

Ward, A. (1977). *Adventures in Archaeology.* (London: Hamlyn)

Whigham Price, A. (1964). *Ladies of Castlerae, the Life of A.S. Lewis and M.D. Gibson.* (Durham: Presbyterian Historical Society of England)

Anatomy

INTRODUCTION

Our early ancestors gained knowledge of anatomy from the slaughtering of animals; from the birth process; and also from the observation of injuries to the human. The surface anatomy, and various structures of the body, were gradually recognized in the Egyptian, Alexandrian, Grecian and Roman eras. Dissection of the human body was not allowed in antiquity, except for a short time in Alexandria. Medieval anatomists formalized the knowledge of the female reproductive organs transmitted to them from antiquity, but no new detail was added. This situation remained unchanged until the advent of the Renaissance when artists and anatomists produced drawings and paintings of high quality, from anatomical dissections.

The illustrations employed for the study of anatomy were of three kinds. The first was 'schematic', and this form of illustration was used when precise knowledge of the individual organs was lacking. It presented an outline of the main characteristics of one or more parts. A second form, that of 'individually correct presentations', illustrated with exactness a particular subject, and first appeared when dissatisfaction was expressed with schematic drawings. The third form showed an 'ideal human figure' constructed from the constant mean proportions of several types. This ideal and invariable norm, required exact and extensive dissection. It was the form of illustration most suitable for both artistic anatomy and teaching purposes, and was developed in the seventeenth and eighteenth centuries (Choulant, 1920).

Throughout history plagiarism of written and illustrated anatomy was common, so both correct and incorrect ideas were perpetuated. Many of the illustrations from the 'middle ages' were actually copies of the work of ancient scribes. Gross anatomical structures were generally well researched and documented by the end of the nineteenth century. Microscopy allowed even more detailed analysis of body parts and thus the emphasis switched to the structure, function and physiology of the various structures.

PREHISTORY

The earliest representations of the human body, in the form of cave drawings and stone figures, date back to the middle Aurignacian period (40 000–16 000 BC), so called because the archaeological finds were made in Aurignac. An ice-age illustration of a birth, 21 cm high, was recovered in 1911 among the artefacts from the latter part of the ice age, on a cliff at Laussel, Dordogne, France, a part of Europe referred to as the 'cradle of prehistory'. The people who lived there were cave dwellers, and their main source of food was caribou meat. They populated the area for a span of 17 000 years – from c.32 000 to 15 000 BC. (Speert, 1973; Leonardo, 1944).

The earliest known anthropomorphic figure was excavated from a 32 000-year-old level in a cave at Hohlenstein, West Germany. It was the carved body of a man with striations on the upper arm (Putmann, 1988). An 8-cm male head carved of mammoth ivory and dated c.25 000 BC was discovered recently (Marashank, 1988).

The earliest female representations, the so-called 'Venus figures' were discovered in France, Austria and Malta, the oldest of which was a carved female head, the Venus of Brassempouy c. 24 000 BC. Another famous statuette which dates from around the same time was the Venus of Willendorf. The effigy was carved in limestone. The Sumerians who lived in the eastern cradle of civilization, depicted their birth godess Nintu in the shape of a uterus (Gruhn and Kazer, 1989).

ANTIQUITY

Egypt

The earliest anatomic records are contained in the Ebers Papyrus (c.1550 BC). The Egyptians were aware of surface anatomy and they distinguished between the uterus, vagina and external genitalia, but dissection of human remains was forbidden. The ancient Egyptians buried their dead in the sands of the desert. The dry climate and preservative effects of direct contact with the sand led to mummification. Eventually the Egyptian custom of embalming the dead evolved. That custom however, gave very little useful information on anatomy.

Prior to the embalming process, evisceration was carried out through slits in the body, rather than through a substantial opening. The Paraschistes made the preliminary abdominal incision. The Taricheutae passed their hands through the opening and removed the intra-abdominal organs, which were later placed in four stone canopic jars. Preservatives and bandaging were then applied to the body. The art of mummification familiarized its users somewhat with the internal structure of the body, and also with chemical preservatives. The practice, which developed a religious significance, continued for about 3000 years.

The Egyptian knowledge of internal anatomy was incomplete and was based mainly on animal dissection. The uterus was depicted as the bifid uterus of the cow. The ancient Egyptian scribes used hieroglyphics and the SA or ankh, depicted like tresses of hair on the birth goddess Taurt, resembled a uterus (Gruhn and Kazer, 1989).

The Hindus

The ancient Hindus c. 900 BC were aware of the oviducts, and their Ayur-Veda stated 'the menses have two canals. When they are wounded, barrenness is caused'. Dissection was permitted and the uterus, vagina, external genitalia and ovaries were distinguished. Many important Hindu works on medicine were housed in the Alexandrian Library which was founded by Alexander the Great under the influence of his Athenian friend Demetriose.

Greece

The early Greeks based their anatomical knowledge on dissection of animals, as dissection of the human was forbidden. A Greek work on anatomy was written in Crotono, Italy, by the Pythagorean philosopher Alcmaeon, in the sixth century BC. The external genitalia were examined and the perineum, vagina, cervix and labia were described. Hippocrates did not write on gynaecological anatomy but theorized that the uterus went wild when not fed with semen. His followers practised gynaecology and described internal examinations. They believed that the uterus could wander extensively in the body cavity and that when the organ

was displaced the woman developed the symptoms of hysteria. The term hysteria was originally applied to 'affections of the womb' and was believed to be a specifically female condition. Various treatments were used, including the intravaginal application of squashed bed bugs or charred deer's horn, and the insertion of a pipe to blow air from a blacksmith's bellows which thus distended the birth canal and ensured the safe return of the nomadic organ to the pelvis. No doubt males were glad that the prostate was well tethered. The Pythagoreans believed that the uterus was bifid. The left side represented the west, or darkness from which females arose, and the right side represented the east, or light in which male offspring developed.

Aristotle (384–322 BC) described the uterus in various animals and is recognized as the founder of comparative anatomy. In his *de Generatione Animalium* he alluded to the cervix but was not well versed in human anatomy. He imagined that the human uterus was made up of seven cells; three to the left, three to the right, and one between and on top. The same erroneous belief of a seven-cell uterus appeared in the *Anatomia Mundini* which was written 1600 years later, in AD 1311. Aristotle carried out some early work on embryology and investigated dog, fish, and chick embryos (Ramsey, 1989). Arateus the Cappadocian, a Greek physician (second century AD), described the uterus as resembling an animal which wandered throughout the body cavity and was subject to prolapse. The uterus was altogether erratic and delighted in fragrant smells, but was adversely affected by fetid smells and fled from them.

Alexandria

Alexander the Great, who was a pupil of Aristotle, founded the city of Alexandria in 331 BC. The Alexandrian school was founded about 320 BC. A library and museum which were built there became world famous. Dissection of the human body was permitted at the school until the second century AD. Herophilus of Chalcedon (335–280 BC) worked in Alexandria and wrote a book on obstetrics which contained anatomical detail, but his writings were lost. Herophilus was one of the originators of gross dissection and is regarded as the first anatomist to describe the mammalian ovaries, which he called female testicles. His original writings were lost but Claudius Galen copied extracts of them into his own *De Seminae* thus saving them for posterity. Herophilus described the cervix as a definite region of muscular and cartilaginous character 'like the head of a cuttlefish' (Bodemer, 1973), and also reported his observations on the uterine body, oviducts and ovaries.

Rome

Cornelius Celsus (27 BC–AD 50) was a non-medical compiler who summarized the medical and scientific knowledge available at that time. Some of his work survived, including his *De Re Medicina*, and was later rediscovered by Pope Nicholas during the Renaissance. Celsus was the first medical author to have his writings printed (in the year 1478) in movable type after Johannes Gutenberg's invention of the printing press in about 1454/5 (Lyons and Petrucelli, 1978). He gave a short description of the uterus in which he referred to it as 'vulva' and was aware that the organ was small in girls and larger in adult females. He referred to the vagina as the 'canal'.

Soranus of Ephesus (AD 98–138) lived for some time at Alexandria and later practised as a physician in Rome. His treatise *On The Nature of the Uterus and Female Pudendae* was discovered in the library of the College of Physicians in Edinburgh. It was published in Paris in 1554. The work was not illustrated, but his anatomical description of the female organs was accurate, and was the earliest scientific account of gynaecological anatomy.

Soranus described the uterus and pelvic organs in great detail from his observations on the dissection of cadavers. The earliest known illustration of the anatomy of the uterus dates from the ninth century and embodied Soranus' teaching on the appearance of the organ. He reported the relationships of the bladder and rectum to the uterus and found that the os uteri was about 4 inches from the labia. In his description he noted that the uterus contained arteries, veins and flesh. He documented the presence of uterine ligaments and described that when inflamed, they could become shorter.

Soranus described the size and shape of the uterus; named the various parts; and he discovered that the uterus was made up of two coats which differed in their arrangement. The outer was fibrous and smooth, firm and white, and the inner more fleshy and villous, soft and red, intertwined throughout with vessels. He noted that the menstrual discharge came from the latter. Soranus disagreed with those who claimed that the uterus had nipple-like outgrowths for the fetus to practise

suckling, and he also theorized that the uterus was not essential to the continuing life of a woman. In his description of the female pudenda he described the vulva in detail and noted similarities between the vagina and intestine (McKay, 1901).

Soranus indicated that the ovaries were attached to the uterus and were not of firm consistency, but glandular and covered with a membrane. He found that they were similar to testicles, and he called them *didymi* (twins) (Temkin, 1956). He also described the suspensory ligaments of the ovaries, but held the opinion that the 'female seed' did not play a part in the production of life. Soranus did not believe in the existence of the hymen, and also theorized that the cervix elongated during intercourse, in a fashion similar to the penis. He described an enlarged clitoris, the treatment for which was removal of the excess tissue. In labour he theorized that the pelvic bones separated. Soranus' *Gynaecology* later served as the original of Rösslin's *Der Swangern Frawen Und Hebammen Roszgarten* (1513) and Raynold's published translation *The Byrth of Mankynde* (1540).

Rufus of Ephesus was born in AD 110 and trained in Alexandria. He later practised in Rome during the reign of Trajan. He dissected sheep and described varicose vessels which he found on either the side of the uterus, attached to the uterine body and running toward the ovaries. This was an early description of the oviducts.

Claudius Galen (AD 130–200) was born in the city of Pergamon in Asia Minor. He studied in Alexandria and later went to Rome. During his time at Alexandria, dissection was not allowed so his knowledge of anatomy was essentially that of the lower animals. However, his teachings were accepted as fact for a thousand years. Although he wrote many articles, few contained any reference to gynaecology. One of these was *On the Anatomy of the Uterus*, an early work which he dedicated to a midwife (Jackson, 1988). He mentioned displacements of the womb and also noted that the cervix became soft in early pregnancy. Galen described the vagina and labia which he considered to be similar to the prepuce in men, and was aware of the existence of the ovaries and uterine tubes.

Galen's interpretation of the female reproductive anatomy was through analogy with the male. He considered that the uterus corresponded to the scrotum, the cervix to the penis and the vagina to the prepuce. By turning a woman's reproductive organs outwards he considered that the male and female organs were the same in every respect.

He did not believe in the theory that uterine migration caused hysteria, but attributed that condition to seminal retention or suppression of the menses. Galen considered that the uterus had two cavities. The right uterine cavity received warm pure blood from the aorta and vena cava and in consequence the male developed on that side. The left side of the uterus received impure blood from vessels passing to the kidneys and gave rise to the female.

After the death of Galen, Rome was captured by the Barbarians and Constantinople became the cultural centre of the world. The Christian religion forbade anatomical dissection and no progress was possible. Oribasius (AD 325–403) was a leading writer at that time and his book contained a chapter on the anatomy of the uterus and vulva, which had been copied from Soranus.

The Hebrews

Development of anatomical knowledge was not possible among the ancient Jews because of their prohibition against dissection of the dead. Later, when the Babylonian Talmud was written (AD 352–427) the Rabbis showed considerable knowledge of the generative organs.

Anatomical Terms in Antiquity (Tables 1–3)

Egyptian

The uterus was called *met-ret*; the vagina was *sed*; the term *at* was used for the vulva.

Jewish Talmud

The female body was compared to a larder with the uterus the sleeping chamber; the cervix uteri, the porch; the 'seed vessels', the store room; the vagina, the outer house; the hymen, the virginity; the labia majora, the hinges; the labia minora, the hinges or doors; and the clitoris, the key.

Greek

Aristotle may have used the terms 'vagina' and 'placenta' and Hippocrates named the mouth of the womb for its resemblance to the circles of iron on a plough. Hymen or Hymenaios was the god of marriage, but was also used as a term for membrane, from the fourth century BC. The words myrtleberry and acorn were used to describe the clitoris.

Rome

Cornelius Celsus referred to the uterus as *vulva* and the vagina as *canalis*. Soranus gave a detailed description of the uterus which he called 'mother'. The shape of the uterus was likened to a cupping glass or gourd. The first and projecting part was 'the mouth'. Other parts were 'the neck', meaning cervix; and the 'narrow neck', meaning isthmus. The neck and narrow neck formed the stem. Where it broadened out beyond the constriction of the neck the uterus had 'shoulders', 'ribs', 'fundus' and 'base'. Soranus remarked that the outer parts (labia) were called 'wings', and where they met was the clitoris. He also described the opening of the urethra. The word vulva (or volvo) was derived from Latin, and meant wrapping or covering, or womb. Rufus of Ephesus referred to the pubic hair, vulva, and clitoris as 'the comb, the cleft and the myrtleberry'.

Table 1 Terms which signified 'womb', and the authors who used them

Alvus	(Cicero)	Arvum	(Virgil)
Bulga	(Lucilius)	Fovea	(Tertullianus)
Loci/Loca	(Cicero)	Matrix	(Vegetius)
Uter	(Statius)	Uterus	(Plautus)
Venter	(Juvenal)	Cavum	(Soranus)
Vulva	(Celsus)		

Table 2 Terms which signified 'vagina'

Cunnus	Vagina
Canalis	Concha
Sinus	Tubus

Acunulate – prostitutes with gonorrhoea were not allowed to work and were referred to as acunulate (McKay, 1901)

Table 3 Terms which signified 'vulva' and the authors who used them

Crista	(Juvenal)	Sulcusa	(Virgil)
Muliebria	(Tacitus)	Navis/Saltus	(Plautus)
Hortulus	(Cuplidinis)	Porcus	(Varro)
Perineum	(Rufus)	Pubes	(Laertius)
Specus	(Auctor Prioapeiorum)		

General terms for vulva: pudendum – the part about which to be ashamed; groin or pudenda (McKay, 1901)

THE MIDDLE AGES

From the days of Cornelius Celsus to the end of the thirteenth century, the writings of earlier scientists were copied or revised, but virtually no progress was made in surgery, gynaecology, or anatomy. Scholasticism and spiritualism were judged more important and ancient writers were thought to be authorities, so their works were not challenged. Dissection was forbidden for Christians, and the Koran forbade the faithful Mohammedan from interfering with the dead. The Arab writings were transcriptions of the works of ancient authors but were of great importance, as it was through them that the science of ancient times was reintroduced to Europe during the Renaissance.

In the sixth century Aetius was a compiler, copyist and author of medical and surgical treatises. One of his books was devoted to the diseases of women. His work was of great importance as it contained much of the writings of Soranus and other authors whose texts did not survive. Aetius followed the teachings of Galen and was aware of the position of the uterus within the peritoneum between the bladder and rectum. However, he held the erroneous view that the unimpregnated uterus could reach close to the umbilicus. He mentioned the increased size of the uterus during pregnancy and prescribed treatment for dealing with retroversion of the uterus by placing the patient in a knee–elbow position. In the seventh century Paulus of Aegina again compiled the work of ancient authors.

The earliest illustrations of the uterus, and pictures of the fetus *in utero* are to be found in a ninth century Moschion Codex (3701–3714) in the Royal Library at Brussels. The oldest known drawing shows a flask-shaped uterus with the corpus sharply demarcated from the cervix. The Copenhagen Codex, which dates from the twelfth century, contains 15 pictures, one of which shows a twin pregnancy. The fetuses are depicted enclosed by membranes in a flask-shaped uterus, and surrounded by a double circle which represented the peritoneum. Coloured illustrations of the pregnant uterus with fetus, from the twelfth century, are contained in the Thatt Collection in Copenhagen. Further illustrations of the pregnant uterus are contained in the thirteenth century Palatine Codex at Rome, and also in the Latin Munich Codex.

The Arabian medical books were translated into Latin by Constantine, a monk at Monte Cassino (1018–1085). His texts contained anatomical descriptions and were used at the famous medical school at Salerno. The anatomy taught there was based on dissections of the pig, but that was an advance on the attempts to study anatomy from old manuscripts.

The first dissection of a cadaver in modern times was authorized and carried out at the University of Bologna by Mondino Dei Luzzi in 1315. His *Anathomia*, a book on human dissection, became the standard work for the next two centuries (Ramsey, 1989). Mondino (1275–1326) however, perpetuated some of Galen's mistakes and believed that the uterus was divided into seven compartments or cells, with three on the right for males, three on the left for females and a central one retained for hermaphrodites.

The female genital tract as illustrated by Mondino showed vessels which conveyed menstrual blood to the mammary glands, which was later to be converted to milk during pregnancy. He accurately observed however that the uterus was situated in the pelvic cavity, where it was held and surrounded by ligaments, thereby correcting the earlier teaching which claimed that the uterus could wander around the body cavity. Henri De Mondeville (1260–1320) stated that the uterus had as many compartments as the animal had breasts, and assumed that as the human species had two breasts, the uterus had two compartments. The Papacy eventually allowed postmortems with the advent of the black death about 1348.

Probably the oldest illustration of a pregnant woman was that of a miniature, c. AD 1400, contained in the Leipzig M.S. Codex 111–2. It represented a nude female figure without external genitalia in squatting positon. The vagina was demonstrated as a tube-like structure and the uterus as an inverted flask containing a fetus presenting by the feet. A similar common model may have existed in antiquity and come down through the middle ages to the Renaissance. Matteo de Gradi of Milan (died 1418) applied the name ovary to the female testes and theorized that the ovaries were the site of egg formation, similar to those in the bird (Leonardo, 1944). However, Niels Stensen may have first applied the term 'ovary' to the female gonads in 1667 (Medvei, 1982).

RENAISSANCE

There was no definable cut-off point for the end of the long doze of the Middle Ages. By convention, the fall of Constantinople to the Ottoman Turks in 1453 is usually accepted as the beginning of the

Renaissance in Europe. The term 'Renaissance', a French word meaning rebirth, is used to mark the beginning of the Modern Period of history, during which there was a rebirth of learning following the darkness of the Medieval period. In the anatomical sense however, the Renaissance had started with Mondino's dissection of the human body in 1315.

With the upsurge of interest in anatomy many names came to the fore, and Benedetti da Legnano (1460–1525) was the first to use the terms cervix, perineum and procidentia. Luigi Bonacciuoli, who was his contemporary, worked at the university of Ferrara and gave detailed descriptions of the mons veneris, clitoris and hymen.

The development of printing by movable type in 1454/5 had a major impact on learning, through its effect on dissemination of medical and other knowledge. Until that time texts were copied by hand, and were so expensive that only royalty or religious communities could afford them. The first illustrated medical work was that of Johannes von Kircheim, a Swabian physician who used the pen name de Ketham. His text *Fasciculus Medicinae* of 1491 was a collection of popular Latin medical tracts, mainly of the fourteenth century, and its figures were the first didactic medical wood cuts. The illustrations were simple (schematic) and displayed the first representation of the female viscera in a printed book (Speert, 1973).

The Italian artist Leonardo da Vinci (1452–1519) (see Biographies) dissected animals and also some human remains. He made careful anatomical drawings from his own personal observation and produced the first correct drawings of the uterus. He outlined the uterine arteries with their cervico-vaginal branches, and proved that the uterus had a single cavity – prior to this the uterus was thought to consist of several chambers. In 1510 Leonardo was the first to depict the fetus *in utero* in realistic fashion showing fetal membranes and placental site. Despite the accuracy, he had not actually seen the fetus *in utero* and his study was based on the transposition of details from the bovine embryo. The artist is considered the founder of iconographic anatomy. His method of drawing from nature was a landmark and from that time on was never to be abandoned. Many of his anatomical drawings, which number 779, notable for their simplicity and clarity, lay forgotten in Windsor Castle from the time of Charles I, until their rediscovery in 1778. Leonardo was also the architect, inventor and visionary who painted the *Mona Lisa* and *The Last Supper* (Mathe, 1984).

Working at the same time as da Vinci was Eucharius Rösslin (q.v. in Biographies) who in 1513 published his Treatise on midwifery *Der Swangern Frawen und Hebammen Roszgarten* which was based on the work of Soranus of Ephesus of the second century AD. The title was derived from the fabled Rose Gardens at Worms. Rösslin probably got his inspiration for illustrations of the fetus *in utero* from the Heidelberg codex of the Vatican Library in Rome and had them produced as wood cuts by Erhard Schon of Strassburg. The *Roszgarten* was translated into English by Richard Jones and published by Thomas Raynold as *The Byrth of Mankynde* in 1540. It became a standard textbook for over 200 years until the works of Smellie and Hunter became available.

Jacobus Berengarius of Carpi (1470–1530) who was Professor at Bologna and Pavia gave a relatively accurate anatomical description of the uterus in his book *Isagoge Breves* (1522). The uterus was depicted in coronal section and disproved the 'seven-cell compartment' uterine cavity theory. However, Berengarius was of the opinion that the uterus was divided into two parts close to the fundus, with males being 'bound fast' in the right, and females in the left part. His work was considered to make the transition from medieval to modern medicine and he endeavoured to make his anatomical drawings direct from nature. His contemporary, Nicolaus Massa (1499–1569) also disputed the seven-cell theory and described the three layers of the uterus, with its inner lining, muscular layer and peritoneal covering.

Andreas Vesalius (1514–1564) (q.v. in Biographies) was the founder of modern systematic anatomy. He was born in Brussels, educated at Louvain in Paris, and eventually settled in Padua. About 1540 he assisted in editing a Latin edition of Galen, and found discrepancies in the text when compared with his own dissections of the human body. This led him to believe that Galen's anatomy was based on that of animals. His monumental *De Humani Corporis Fabrica* (1543), with a text of 663 pages was illustrated with numerous wood engravings by the artist Jan Kalkar. A shorter version, the *Epitome* (a collection of specimen pages), was produced in the same year. His work had great appeal as it was systematic, relatively complete, and well illustrated. Vesalius dissected nine female corpses and dispensed with the Galenian notion, to which he himself had previously subscribed, of the existence of uterine horns. His book which contained the first good illustrations of the internal female genitalia also showed the left ovarian vein entering the renal vein for the first time.

It was at the this time that the anatomic wood cut achieved its highest perfection, but copper plate engraving was developed soon afterwards and replaced the wood cut in illustration. Ambroise Paré (1510-1590) (q.v. in Biographies) who studied at the Hotel Dieu in Paris, made major contributions to obstetrics as well as surgery, and also translated large tracts of Vesalius into French. By the end of the sixteenth century Vesalian anatomy had become the standard for anatomical studies throughout Europe.

Pope Clement VII finally endorsed the teaching of anatomy by dissection in 1537. In England anatomy was taught by readers chosen from the Barber surgeons, and the first anatomy text written in English was the *The Englishman's Treasure* by Thomas Vicary in 1548 (Leonardo, 1944).

Bartolommeo Eustachio (1520-1574), who is remembered for his description of the tube running from the middle ear to the naso-pharynx, carried out detailed dissection of the female reproductive tract. He injected coloured dyes into the intra-abdominal blood vessels and demonstrated the hypo-gastric and ovarian arteries leading to the uterus, ovaries, bladder and clitoris, and also the numerous anastomoses in the pelvic vasculature. Eustachius' anatomical copper plates of 1552 were hidden, but were discovered 162 years later in 1714, and published.

Another great anatomist of that time was Gabrielle Falloppio (q.v. in Biographies) who in 1561 described the human oviduct in his *Observationes Anatomicae* (Speert, 1958). He was born in 1523 in Modena, Italy, was appointed Professor of Anatomy at the University of Pizza in 1548, and later moved to Padua where he succeeded Vesalius. He gave the first precise description of the clitoris, and the skeletel system of the fetus. Falloppio also introduced the anatomic use of the term vagina and he used the word *luteum* in his description of the ovary. He also used the name placenta (a term which may have previously been used by the ancient Greeks) and described its cotyledons. During his anatomic investigations he corrected numerous errors and discovered many new structures in the body.

Despite all the advances made by da Vinci, Vesalius, Eustachius and Falloppius, texts were produced which perpetuated the old ideas. In 1575 Georg Bartsich produced his *Kuntsbuch*, in which the female anatomy was grossly inaccurate and bore a strong resemblance to the external male genitalia. Jacob Rueff wrote his *de Concepto et Generatione Hominis* in 1580 which included the depiction of a uterus with uterine horns. His work may have been based on Vesalius' early work of 1538, the *Tabulae Anatomicae*, which closely followed the teaching of Galen and was quite inaccurate. In 1595 Scipione Mercurio published *La Commare O'Raccoglitrice* in which illustrations of the uterus and vagina closely resembled the male anatomy. His dissections showed a heart-shaped uterus with a phallic-type vagina (Speert, 1973).

The earliest illustrations of the vulva were by Leonardo Da Vinci, and also Severinus Pineus (1550-1619). However, the external female genitalia were displayed on sculpted figurines which can be traced back to ancient Babylonia and the near east. The Indian Tantric tribes venerated the vulva in the seventh century AD. A more modern form of female with exposed vulva, the so-called Sheela-na-Gig, was carved in stone and adorned the walls of Christian churches in Europe from the twelfth century (Andersen, 1977).

SEVENTEENTH CENTURY

Caspar Bauhin produced an illustrated compendium of anatomy at the beginning of the century. A new departure was introduced in 1619 by Remmelin where pictures were superimposed on each other and could be turned like the pages of a book, thus allowing the various layers of anatomy to be exposed. Three years later the polychrome woodcut–print (chiaroscuro) was introduced by Aselli, in his depiction of the chyliferous vessels. This was a very detailed work on scientific anatomy with numerous illustrations. In 1627 Giulio Casserio produced a set of copper plates which comprised the whole of human anatomy as understood at that time. Casserio, who was a student of Fabricius, portrayed the female form and internal genitalia with beauty and accuracy in his *Placenti Tabulae Anatomicae*.

One of the great investigators of the seventeenth century was William Harvey (q.v. in Biographies) (1578-1657) who was born at Folkestone, graduated from Cambridge and studied at Padua. He later became physician to King Charles I. His major publication *De Mortu Cordis* of 1628 revolutionized medical thought. Due to his discovery of the circulation, he is judged to be 'the founder of physiology'. Because he did not have a microscope he could not see the capilliary anastomosis between arteries and veins. Later, in 1651, his *De Generatione Animalium* was published with a chapter entitled *De Partu.* In this chapter on labour, he recommended patience and gentleness in all things. Harvey carefully observed the development of the chick embryo and also made dissections of the human embryo, using a simple lens for magnification. He described the size of the uterus in relation to age and pregnancy (Cianfrani, 1960).

Although the lymph nodes had been recognized in Greco-Roman times, their structure was first detailed by the Englishman Thomas Wharton (1656) and the Italian Marcello Malpighi (1666). The lymphatic valves were described by Rudbeck in 1653. Thomas Bartholin named the lymphatic system in 1653. The term was derived from the Latin *lympha*, which referred to clear transparent spring water, supposedly similar to the watery fluid found within lymphatic vessels.

The gelatinous material of the umbilical cord was first described by Thomas Wharton (1656) in his book *Adenographia.* He qualified in Oxford and later served as physician to St Thomas's Hospital, London. He is mainly remembered for his interest in anatomy and his description of the various glands in the body. He is eponymously related not only to the Wharton's jelly of the umbilical cord but also to the duct of the submaxillary salivary gland.

The terms 'fourchette' and 'fossa navicularis' were introduced by Francois Mauriceau (q.v. in Biographies) (1637–1709) of Paris, a noted obstetrician of his time. In Mauriceau's *Traite des Maladies des Femmes Grosses, et de Celles Qui Sont Accouchées* (1668) were published anatomical plates of the female pelvic organs. The anatomy of the bony pelvis was also studied and described by Hendrik van Deventer (q.v. in Biographies) (1651–1724). Born in the Hague, he studied medicine at Groningen. He described inlet contraction of the pelvis and also the pelvis which was generally contracted. He was aware of the axis of the birth canal and described its course.

The human placenta, cord and fetal membranes were described and personally illustrated by Nicolaas Hoboken (1632–1678) in his text the *Anatomia Secundinae Humanae* (1669). In it he described his dissection of the umbilical cord. Within the umbilical vessels he demonstrated intraluminal folds or projections which were also called valves or nodes. These 'nodes of Hoboken' did not form functionally competent valves. Valvulae and plicae of the umbilical vessels were described by contemporaries of Hoboken, but his description was the first accurate account.

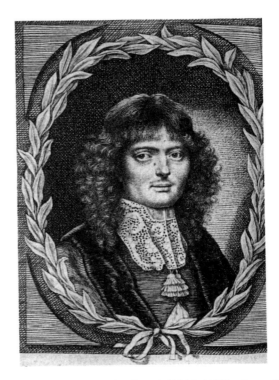

Figure 1 Regnier de Graaf (1641–1673). Portrait (1666) from the first edition (1668) of his *Virorum Organis Generationi* (*see* text)

Regnier de Graaf (Figure 1) (q.v. in Biographies) (1641–1673) was born in Holland and after early studies there and in France, he entered practice in Delft. His *De Mulierum Organis Generationi Inservientibus* (1672) contained a detailed account of the pelvic blood supply, the lymphatic system of the uterus, the crura of the clitoris, and the structure of the ovary. He concluded that the ovarian follicle was the egg. Jan Swammerdam and Van Horn of Leiden had developed a similar theory some 6 years previously but had not published their conclusions. De Graaf gave a detailed description of the corpus luteum which he called the substantia glandulosa and also made the first discovery of tubal impregnated ova.

Caspar Bartholin (1655–1738) was born in Copenhagen and became Professor of Philosophy at the age of 19 years. In his *De Ovariis Mulierum, et Generationis Historia* (1677) he described the vulvovaginal glands and ducts which are still called by his name. Until that time it was believed that the coital fluid in the female was produced by the ovaries and discharged through the urethra. Much of his investigation was carried out in the cow.

The development of microscopy in this century led to many new discoveries. Marcello Malpighi (1628–1694) was Professor of Medicine at Messina and Bologna. He discovered the blood capillaries and described mucus glands in the uterus and the muscle fibres of the uterine wall. He also described a structure in the cow, now known as Gartner's duct (see later), and also carried out studies on descriptive embryology (Cianfrani, 1960). His contemporary, Antony van Leeuwenhoek of Delft (q.v. in Biographies) (1632–1723) carried out detailed microscopic examinations and contributed many observations of note. With his student Haman, he first described spermatozoa in semen (1678).

Cystic irregularities on the cervix were discovered by Guillaume Desnoues who reported his findings in the journal *Zodiacus Medico–Gallicus* in 1681. Desnoues, a French surgeon who became Professor of Anatomy in Genoa, was of the opinion that he had discovered the site of a reservoir for a spermatic substance which was secreted at the time of intercourse and deposited close to the male semen. The glands he discovered were later attributed to Naboth as the Nabothian glands. Aetius of Amida (sixth century AD) may also have referred to the 'Nabothian' follicles, and used astringent pessaries to cure them (McKay, 1901). The broad and round ligaments, vaginal rugae and the plicae palmitae of the cervix were accurately

displayed by Govert Bidloo (1649–1713) of Amsterdam in his published work *Anatomia Humani Corporis* in 1685 (Speert, 1973).

The inguinal canal was investigated by Anton Nuck (1650–1692) of the Netherlands. Cysts of the canal had been noted in females many years previously and Swammerdam in 1692 had shown the round ligament encased in a sheath of peritoneum coursing its way into the canal. Nuck's description of the canal appeared in his *Adenographia* (1691). The narrow inguinal canal in women was found to contain strands of the round ligament which end at the labium majus. (During fetal development the round ligament is surrounded by a sheath of peritoneum, which occasionally persists into adult life. The diverticulum may provide a channel for hernial development or cyst formation and was later termed the canal of Nuck.) He also decribed the lymphatic network of the ovary, and the glandular structure of the female breast.

One of the most interesting ways of teaching obstetric anatomy was by the use of ivory models (Figures 2 and 3). An extremely beautiful one is

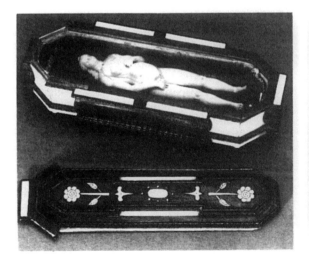

Figure 2 An ivory model of a pregnant woman used for teaching purposes, in its ornate original box. Reproduced with kind permission from the Städtisches Museum Schloß Rheydt, Mönchen-Gladbach

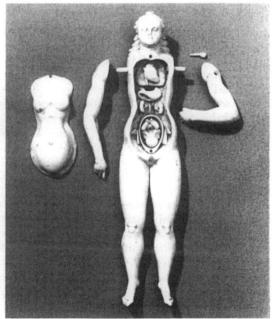

Figure 3 Same ivory model with the abdominal wall put on one side to reveal internal organs that can also be taken out. The arms have also been detached (*see* text). Reproduced with kind permission from the Städtisches Museum Schloß Rheydt, Mönchen-Gladbach

illustrated here with the kind permission of the Städtisches Museum, Schloß Rheydt. This was made by Stefan Zwick at the end of the seventeenth century and is part of the Theodor Meyer Steineg collection of the History of Medicine, collected between 1910 and 1933 and still on exhibition in Mönchen-Gladbach. It is an ivory model kept in a wooden box with inlaid ivory. The ivory model represents a young woman who is about 20 weeks pregnant and the abdominal wall can be taken away to show ivory models of her heart, liver, kidneys and uterus containing a 20-week fetus in the cephalic position which also lifts out from the model.

These ivory models were used for teaching purposes not only in Germany but throughout Europe in the seventeenth and eighteenth centuries. William Hunter's atlas of 1774 was prepared from engravings made from coloured illustrations of post-mortem models of women in many stages of pregnancy with many obstetric abnormalities such as breech presentations and placenta praevia, as well as ectopic pregnancy. The models in wax can be found in the Hunterian Museum in Glasgow.

EIGHTEENTH CENTURY

In the early part of the century, Martin Naboth (1675–1721) investigated the structures of the cervix. He was aware that they were previously described by Desnoues in 1681. While Desnoues considered that the cystic structures were the site of male semen formation, Naboth disagreed and regarded the cysts as sacs which contained eggs. Naboth, who was born in Saxony, became Professor of Chemistry in Leipzig. In his *De Sterilitate Mulierum* (1707) he described in detail his dissection findings of the cervical cysts which were later called after his name.

A notable event in this century was the publication of G.H. Eisenmann's *Tabulae Anatomical Quatour Uteri* (1725) in Strasbourg. His Atlas of the Uterus was an important advance in the history of gynaecological anatomy.

The peritoneal cavity was first described by the Egyptians in the Ebers Papyrus but the modern interpretation of the peritoneal cavity and its lining, depends on the work of James Douglas (1675–1742) who first described its structure in his treatise *A Description of the Peritonaeum* (1730). Douglas, who was born in Scotland, graduated from medical college in Rheims, and later settled in London. He developed a large obstetric practice and carried out anatomic investigations. In his treatise there was only a short reference to the pelvic peritoneal cul-de-sac. The term 'cul-de-sac' was first used by Alexander Munro, Professor of Anatomy at the University of Edinburgh in 1737, but the 'Pouch of Douglas' was soon substituted for it.

Douglas was involved in the exposure of Mary Toft who claimed to have given birth to litters of rabbits. Toft was helped and advised by a woman accomplice who promised to continually supply her with rabbits. King George I ordered an investigation and Nathaniel St Andre, a Swiss anatomist who was attached to the Royal Court, examined the patient. He reported that he delivered her of the entire trunk of a rabbit, stripped of its skin, of about 4 months growth. Unknown to St Andre, Mary kept inserting bits of rabbits which she had hidden in her pockets, into her vagina. Eventually she confessed to the hoax when questioned by James Douglas and another 'man midwife', Sir Richard Manningham (Speert, 1973).

The mesonephros of the early embryo was investigated by Caspar Friedrich Wolff (1734–1794) who reported his finding of the primitive kidneys in his *Theoria Generationis* (1759). The nineteenth century embryologist Rathke later called them the 'Wolffian bodies' in recognition of Wolff's discovery. Wolff, who was born in Berlin, was educated both there and at Halle, and held an appointment as an anatomy teacher in Breslau but later returned to Berlin. His views on generation were met with hostility by his colleagues, so he later moved to St Petersburg, Russia. He disputed the theory of 'emboitment', or 'preformation' in which the embryo supposedly resided completely formed in the ovary.

From his microscopic observations he claimed that the particles which constituted all animal organs in their earliest inception were little globules (cells). He attempted to explain early embryogenesis as a process of 'epigenesis', in which the organism developed with gradual building up of its parts.

The bony pelvic canal was first investigated by Hendrik van Deventer, and subsequently by Smellie, Levret and Baudelocque. Van Deventer discovered that the canal was set obliquely on the spine. In 1761 Levret (q.v. in Biographies) first described the three pelvic obstetric planes and noted that they all intersected a parabolic line through which the fetal head passed in labour. His description was erroneous in many respects and was not popularly accepted.

The small fluid-filled cysts sometimes attached to the fimbriae of the Fallopian tubes are called 'hydatids of morgagni'. They were first described by Giovanni Battista Morgagni (1761) who was born in Forli, Italy, and spent most of his medical career at Padua. The word hydatid was derived from the Greek and meant 'drop of water'. Regnier de Graaf had also recognized cystic structures close to the ovary in the seventeenth century.

The Scotsman William Hunter (1718–1783), (q.v. in Biographies) one of the great names in anatomy, obstetrics, and gynaecology, was born in Lanarkshire. He studied for the Ministry but left after 5 years and then worked for Dr William Cullen who later became Professor of Medicine at Glasgow. Hunter studied anatomy and physiology in Edinburgh and London, and was associated for a time with Smellie and Douglas. He finally settled in London and became Surgeon Man-Midwife to the British Lying-In Hospital and the Middlesex. He was the first to use the term 'retroversion'. During trips to the continent he had learned how to preserve bodies and anatomical specimens, and recognized the value of the procedure. He realized that wax models of dissected specimens could be used to great effect for teaching and demonstrating the art of anatomy. In his dissection of the embryo he demonstrated the various stages of its development. Hunter's *The Anatomy of the Human Gravid Uterus* (1774) was the result of 24 years of research. The engravings in his book were by Van Rymsdyk and Robert Strange. His brother John, a renowned surgeon, helped with his dissections and carried out important work on the process of inflammation. John went on to became a pioneer in comparative and pathological anatomy (Venzmer, 1972).

William Smellie (q.v. in Biographies) (1697–1763) was born in Lanarkshire, Scotland, and studied medicine at Glasgow. He later practised and taught obstetrics in London. Among his many observations, the 'Master of British Midwifery' first recognized the influence of rickets on the pelvis. He described the anatomy of the bony parts in that condition, and was responsible for the introduction of clinical pelvimetry. He also investigated the round and broad ligaments, and the changes which occurred in them during pregnancy. Among his important publications was the *Sett of Anatomical Tables* which was published in 1754. The illustrations in the text were by Rymsdyk, although Smellie himself also drew some. He also wrote *A Treatise on the Theory and Practice of Midwifery* (1752).

A common theory of the time was that the cervix was a form of store house for new material which was necessary for uterine growth in pregnancy. Petit (1766) wrote as follows 'I consider the cervix as a magazine in which nature has placed in reserve the quantity of muscular fibres which she needs, to furnish by their development materials for the expansion of the uterus during the course of gestation . . . '. This view was challenged later when it was demonstrated that the primary changes which occurred in pregnancy were due to hypertrophy within the muscular layer of the corpus uteri itself.

A contemporary of Smellie's was Andre Levret (1703–1780), a Parisian. He was known for his work on the bony pelvis, and described the three pelvic planes – the inlet, mid-pelvis and the outlet. Another French obstetrician of note was Jean Louis Baudelocque (1748–1810) who was born in Heilly, and became head of the obstetric department in the Medical School of Paris. He was aware of the work of Smellie and Levret but improved the available knowledge on pelvic diameters. Baudelocque developed techniques for measuring the pelvic diameters in normal and contracted pelves in living women and correlated pelvic measurement with fetal head size.

Among other measurements Baudelocque described the external conjugate of the pelvis 'by measuring the thickness of the woman from the middle of the pubis to the tip of the spine of the last lumbar vertebra . . . ' and this measurement became identified with his name. He later became one of France's best known obstetricians being appointed accoucheur to Empress Marie-Louise the wife of Napoleon, and also to the Queen of Holland. Baudelocque's teaching on pelvic measurement was detailed in *L'Art des Accouchemens* (1781). The investigation of pelvic adequacy by X-ray techniques would later demonstrate the inadequacy of external pelvic measurement.

The first adequate depiction of the lymphatic topography of the female pelvis was contained in Mascagni's *Vasorum lymphaticorum corporis humani* (1787). He used a technique of heavy metal salt injections which had been introduced and perfected by Anton Nuck (1692). Some of Mascagni's work is preserved at the Anatomical Museum at Siena University. He was the first to discover that red blood corpuscles were readily absorbed from the peritoneal cavity. Further work on the lymphatics was carried out by William Hunter, William Hewson and William Cruickshank in the 1770s.

NINETEENTH CENTURY

The axis of the birth canal was investigated and described in the nineteenth century by Karl Gustav Carus (1789–1869). Born in Leipzig, Germany, he obtained his medical degree at the University of Leipzig and later practised in Dresden. He documented his formulation of the parturient axis in Part 1 of his *Lehrbuch Der Gynakologie* (1820). Carus was aware of previous descriptions by Levret and Roderer but disagreed with their ideas, and adopted the principle of a curved line in defining the pelvic axis.

Carus commented, 'one takes the middle of the pubic symphysis where the conjugate of the pelvic cavity begins, and using a radius of two and a quarter inches, describes a circle around the synchondrosis, whereupon it will be seen that the arc of this circle, falling inside the pelvic cavity, transects the middle of the inlet, as well as the outlet. Coursing in general through the middle of the pelvic cavity, it indicates the true axis of the pelvis in the most precise way'.

The mesonephric, or Wolffian, duct was probably recognized by Marcello Malpighi in 1681, but was described in detail by the Danish anatomist Hermann Gartner in 1822 during his dissection of the internal genitalia of the sow (Gartner, 1824). Gartner (1785–1827) was born in the West Indies where his father worked as a tax official, and returned to Copenhagen where he studied medicine. His initial dissections were carried out in the cow, but Gartner later examined the sow where he traced the bilateral ducts along the course of the vagina, to within an inch or two of the ovaries. In the same year of 1822 possibly the most beautiful of all obstetrical atlases was published on behalf of Jacques-Pierre Maygrier (1771–1835).

Dissection of cadavers became accepted practice in the late eighteenth and early nineteenth centuries. The demand for 'subjects' on which to demonstrate anatomy was high and led to illegal acquisition of bodies (Figure 4). The infamous pair William Burke and William Hare, murdered at least 16 people in 1823, and supplied the corpses to Dr Robert Knox of Edinburgh for dissection. The criminals were later apprehended. Burke was hanged and his own body was subjected to a demonstration on dissection. Hare turned King's evidence and was not prosecuted. Knox was unrepentant and left Edinburgh after a large mob set fire to his house. It became legal for custodians of a body to turn it over to a medical school in 1832.

Johannes Muller (1801–1858), who was born

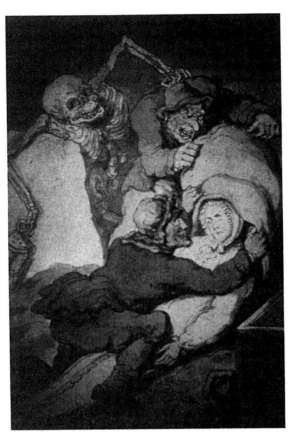

Figure 4 Body Snatchers: an illustration of about 1840 of a model made by Joseph Towne who made coloured wax models by a method that has remained a secret, mostly from dissections carried out by John Hilton (q.v.). Towne was modeller at Guy's Hospital, London for 53 years in the nineteenth century

in Coblenz, became the foremost physiologist of his day. His *Bildungsgeschichte Der Genitalien* (1830) contained his own observations, as well as those of other embryologists, on the development of the mammalian uterus. The female genital tract was known to be a paired structure, and Muller described the union of the ducts to form a single uterus during his dissection of a $3^{1}/_{2}$-inch fetus. During his scientific research Muller was assisted by Theodore Schwann who established the basis of pathologic histology and was later called the founder of the 'cell theory'. Another of his disciples was Rudolph Virchow who became known as 'the father of cellular pathology'.

The lymph nodes of the pelvic wall were found to have constant lymph centres supplied by groups of lymph nodes which occurred at accurately defined locations. Although that concept was introduced by Baum (1926), regional lymph nodes were designated in the nineteenth century by Cruveilhier (1834), Sappey (1879) and Peiser (1898). A previous system of classifying pelvic nodes as groups of plexuses was developed by the anatomist Haase in 1786. Sappey (1885) also demonstrated the lymphatics of the vulva. Bruhns (1898) and Poirier made important contributions to the understanding of lymphatics of the vagina and Bartholin's glands. Sappey and Poirier investigated those from the cervix. Kroemer, who was a contemporary, published work using ether dye mixtures to outline the lymphatic channels in 1904.

The canal for the internal pudendal vessels and nerve in the ischio-rectal fossa was described by Benjamin Alcock in 1836. Born in 1801, he attended Trinity College, Dublin, and later became Professor of Anatomy, Physiology and Pathology at the School of the Apothecaries' Hall, Dublin. In 1849 he became the first Professor of Anatomy at Queens College Cork, but migrated to America in 1855 (Lourie, 1986).

The enlargement of the breasts, and change of colour in the areolae had long been identified with the pregnant state. William Fetherston Montgomery (1797–1859) born and educated in Dublin, qualified as MB in 1825. Through his efforts a Chair of Midwifery was established in the College of Physicians, and he served for 30 years as its first professor. Montgomery wrote his *An Exposition of the Signs and Symptoms of Pregnancy* (1837) which contained a detailed description of the breast changes in pregnancy. He noted that 'a condition of fullness of the breasts may be natural to the individual, or it may take place at the turn of life, when the menses become naturally suppressed, the person grows at the same time fatter, and the breasts under such circumstances become full and are not infrequently painful . . . ' He thus alluded to the lack of specificity of increased breast size in the diagnosis of pregnancy.

Montgomery remarked that it was the alteration in the areolar tissue which was most specifically related to a pregnant state. He disagreed that colour change of the areolae was a good indicator but instead stressed that 'a soft and moist state of the integument (areolae), which appears raised and in a state of turgescence, giving one the idea that, if touched by the point of the finger, it would be found emphysematous . . . and we not infrequently find that the little glandular follicles or tubercules, as they are called by Morgagni, are

bedewed with a secretion sufficient to dampen and colour the woman's inner dress . . . the glandular follicles, which, varying in number from 12 to 20, project from the 16th to the 8th of an inch . . . ' A shorter but similar account was published by Roederer (1753) but it was Montgomery's detailed account which led to the appellation 'Montgomery's follicles'.

Five years after the publication of Carus' book, Franz Karl Naegele (1778–1851) pointed out that the circle, or curve, of Carus did not correctly reflect the track of the fetal head through the pelvis. Naegele (1839) correctly indicated that the bony birth canal was a straight line in its upper half, to the level of the mid-pelvis, and curved in its lower part, to the outlet. Naegele, who was born in Dusseldorf, was Professor and Director of the Lying-In Hospital at Heidelberg where he carried out studies on the obstetric pelvis, and the mechanism of labour. He also described the obliquely contracted pelvis. A 'double Naegele' or 'Robert pelvis' was described soon afterwards by Ferdinand Robert (1842). In this form the sacral alae were lacking bilaterally, thus causing extreme transverse narrowing of the pelvis.

Additional anatomical findings in this century were the discovery of the human ovum by Karl Ernst Von Baer (1827) and Henle's description of the cervix as a distinct histological entity in 1841. Henle concluded that the myometrium was a three-layered structure in his *Recherches sur la Disposition des Fibres Muscularis de L'Uterus Developpé par la Grossesse* which was published in Paris.

Following 12 years of investigation of the uterine body Henle proposed that the external layer contained two longitudinal parts with a transverse sheet arranged between them. He found the middle layer consisted of an interlacing network of fibres curved as figures of eight, which were perforated by blood vessels, and myometrial contraction thus resulted in constriction of blood vessels. Henle documented that the internal layer consisted of two triangular segments, one on the anterior and the other on the posterior wall of the uterus, which were connected at the fundus by an arch.

Despite the previous attempts of other illustrious anatomists, it was eventually Robert Lee (1793–1877) who gave the first good overall description of uterine innervation. Born in Scotland he studied in Paris and later practised obstetrics in London. He was Professor of Midwifery in Glasgow for a short time, but soon moved to St George's Hospital, London, where he spent the rest of his career. Lee's (1842) description of the uterine innervation was supplemented with additional material and further papers were published in the years through to 1856. In his 1842 paper he noted 'the uterus and its appendages are wholly supplied with nerves from the great sympathetic and sacral nerves. At the bifurcation of the aorta, the right and left cords of the great sympathetic nerve unite upon the anterior part of the aorta, and form the aortic plexus'. He then went on to describe the hypogastric nerves and plexus, and also the hypogastric or uterocervical ganglion, later called 'Lee's ganglion'. He concluded that 'it is chiefly by the influence of these nerves, that the uterus performs the varied functions of menstruation, conception, and parturition . . . '

The fact that the placental villi are covered by epithelium was pointed out by Dalrymple (1842). Over the next 30 years the placental architecture and histology were studied by many investigators. It became apparent that there were two types of epithelium in the formative stage of the placenta, the syncytiotrophoblast or syncytium, and the cytotrophoblast. This latter layer was found to contain large cells which were pale staining, with relatively large nuclei and vacuoles which contained glycogen. From this layer, columns arose which secured firm attachment for the developing conception, to the uterine wall. As the placenta matured it was found that the cytotrophoblast slowly disappeared.

The mesonephric remnant, or Wolffian body, was first described in the human by Johann Christian Rosenmüller (1802). Born in Hessburg, Germany, Rosenmüller (1771–1820) became Professor of Anatomy and Surgery at the University of Leipzig. He described the vestigial tubules in a 12-week fetus. He also described canals, which he first thought were lymphatic vessels, merging towards the upper extremity of the ovary. The little canals so described proceeded towards the ovary in a cone-shaped distribution and this structure soon became known as the organ of Rosenmüller. Later anatomists suggested the terms 'epoophoron' and 'parovarian' for the Wolffian body remnant in the female, and the individual tubules were called after George L. Kobelt, who gave a more detailed description of them in 1847.

The prevesical space and its areolar connective tissue was first described by Anders Adolf Retzius (1849). The term *cavum praeperitoneale Retzii* (cave of Retzius) was first used by the Viennese anatomist Hyrtl in 1858. Retzius (1796–1860) first men-

tioned this space in his description of the pubo-prostatic ligament. Born in Lund, Sweden, he had an illustrious academic career and was elected President of the Royal Academy of Sciences of Stockholm 2 years before his death.

During the century many well illustrated books with engravings by artists of note were published. G. Spratt's book, *Midwifery* (1850) contained plates, some of which were in colour. Each plate had superimposed drawings which could be lifted and turned over to reveal the underlying drawing. This method of superimposed plates to represent anatomic relations was previously used in 1627 by Gaspar Aselli in his book *De Lactibus Sine Lacteis Venis*, but the earliest book with superimposed plates was by George Bartsich of Frankfurt in 1584 which contained hand-coloured plates.

In a further investigation of external pelvimetry, Gustav Adolf Michaelis (1798–1848) (Figure 5) compared normal with contracted pelves. Although he doubted the clinical application of those measurements, he defined the 'sacral

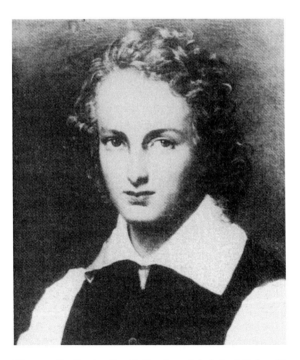

Figure 5 Portrait of Gustav Adolph Michaelis (1798–1848) from an oil painting by Karl Aubel in 1820, Paris. Michaelis was Professor of Obstetrics in Kiel, Germany from 1840–1848. Kiel has had a succession of notable professors of obstetrics. Reproduced with kind permission from Semm, K. (1985). *Universitäts-Frauenklinik Kiel*

quadrangle', an area bounded by the medial borders of the gluteal muscles, the dimples overlying the posterior superior iliac spines, and the depression over the sacrum. He endeavoured to correlate the measurements of the 'sacral quadrangle', later called 'Michaelis' rhomboid' (Figure 6), with the various forms of normal and contracted pelves. His major work *Das Enge Becken* (1851) was published posthumously, and included details on his study of 1000 obstetric pelves. In 72 of those cases, the true conjugate was 8.75 cm or less. He estimated that a third of contracted pelves were due to rickets, while the rest were probably due to heredity. Michaelis concluded that 'only pelvic mensuration can be relied upon as a sure means of recognising pelvic contraction' (Figures 7 and 8). Born in Harbourg, Germany in 1798, he carried out his obstetric practice as Professor in Kiel. He committed suicide by throwing himself under a train in 1848, one year after a beloved cousin of his died of puerperal fever (Semm, 1985).

The development of the ovary was studied in animals by Edward Pfluger (1829–1910). He extended the previous studies by Valentin, who had noted tubular cell masses in the medulla of developing ovaries. Pfluger (1863) demonstrated that the medullary columns originated from the surface layer of cells. He was unable to demonstrate those tubules or cords in the human ovary. However, his study was based on the adult ovary

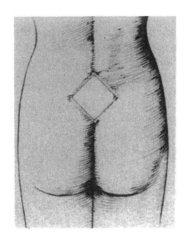

Figure 6 Michaelis' quadrangle (*see* text). Reproduced with kind permission from Semm, K. (1985). *Universitäts-Frauenklinik Kiel*

and a later investigator, Waldeyer (1870) demonstrated that Pfluger's tubules were present in the human ovary during its fetal development.

The innervation of the uterus was studied by Weber (1817); Tiedemann (1822); Kaspar (1840); Kolliker (1844); Beck (1846); and Kilian (1851). In 1874 Goltz and Frusberg demonstrated uterine function and contractility which was independent of its innervation. Further major studies on the uterine innervation were carried out by Ferdinand Frankenhauser (1832–1894). He served as

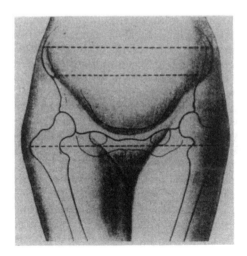

Figure 7 External measurements of the front of the female pelvis. Reproduced with kind permission from Semm, K. (1985). *Universitäts-Frauenklinik Kiel*

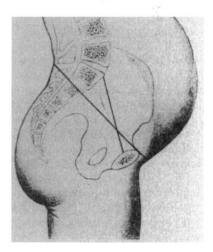

Figure 8 Michaelis' external conjugate and internal true conjugate measurements. Reproduced with kind permission from Semm, K. (1985). *Universitäts-Frauenklinik Kiel*

Professor of Obstetrics and Gynaecology in Zurich. Frankenhauser (1867) redescribed the uterine innervation with its plexuses and ganglia in great detail and the structures are eponymously related to his name.

Wilhelm Waldeyer (1836–1921) the German anatomist, carried out important work on the ovary, pelvis, pelvic viscera, and topographical relations of the pregnant uterus (1870) and Max Brodel in 1897 published his findings on the uterine and ovarian vascular supply. The Viennese anatomist and anthropologist Joseph Hyrtl (1811–1894) also carried out detailed anatomical study of the blood supply to the reproductive tract. Hyrtl was responsible for saving the skull of Mozart for posterity. The famous musician died in 1791 and was buried in a third-class common grave containing about 15 other bodies. Joseph Rothmayer, the sexton of St Marks in Vienna, was a great admirer of the composer. He identified Mozart's corpse with a wire. When the grave was reopened in 1801 Rothmayer removed Mozart's skull and kept it as a sacred relic. The skull found its way into the hands of Joseph Hyrtl, and after his death it was acquired by the Mozarteum in Salzburg (Davies, 1991).

Small cystic spaces which appear similar to ova, are often found among the ovarian granulosa cells. They were first described by Emma Call and Siegmund Exner (1875) and have since been known as Call–Exner bodies. Emma Louise Call (1847–1937) was one of the first women physicians in the United States. She qualified at the University of Michigan and underwent further training in Vienna. Later, she became the first woman to be elected to membership of the Massachussetts Medical Society. Siegmund Exner (1846–1926) was born in Vienna, where he later became Professor. It was while Emma Call was undergoing a period of postgraduate study in his physiology laboratory that the Call–Exner bodies were first demonstrated.

The paraurethral ducts were rediscovered by Alexander Johnstone Chalmers Skene (1838–1900) who was born in Aberdeenshire, Scotland, and migrated to America when he was 19. He practised as a gynaecologist in New York and later became Professor of Gynecology at the Long Island College Hospital. He was also a founding member of the American Gynecological Society in 1880. Skene (1880) detailed his observations on the anatomy and pathology 'of two important glands of the female urethra' in a report to the *American Journal of Obstetrics*.

The first of the two cases documented in his paper involved a 30-year-old woman who was referred to him with subacute vaginitis, perhaps of gonorrhoeal origin, and inflamed papillomata of the urinary meatus. The vaginitis settled with treatment but the inflammation and tenderness of the meatus remained. Skene applied cautery with nitrate of silver, but the treatment was ineffective. Over a period of months he applied caustics and a number of chemicals without success. Eventually Skene probed the elevated points which he had noted close to the urethral meatus, and subsequently milked the urethra from above downwards. Purulent fluid escaped from both ducts. Skene injected each duct with tincture of iodine, and then cauterized them. The inflammation settled. A second case was diagnosed more promptly and also reacted well to treatment.

Stimulated by his initial findings Skene investigated the paraurethral ducts in over 100 patients and observed that gonorrhoeal infection was the cause of mucopurulent discharge from the structures. The paraurethral ducts were previously described by Regnier De Graaf (q.v. in Biographies) (1672) in his book *De Mulierum Organis Generationi Inservientibus*. He also found them to be the foci of gonorrhoeal infection, but Skene was unaware of this previous discovery.

It was Theodor Langhans (1839–1915) who described the cytotrophoblast in detail in his definitive paper on the subject (1882). Born in Usingen, Germany, he began his placental studies while working at Marburg. He also reported the 'Langhans cell' component of the tubercule. His pupil Raissa Nitabuch (1887) described a further placental layer, that of an eosinophilic honeycombed fibrinoid deposition between the invading trophoblast and the maternal decidua.

The triangular ligament, or urogenital diaphragm, was described in detail by Savage (1882). The superficial fascia of the perineum was found to have a superficial fatty layer with a deep membranous layer, termed the 'fascia of Colles'. The deep portion of the superficial fascia was continued anteriorly as the 'fascia of Scarpa' on the lower abdominal wall. Hart and Barbour (1883) were of the opinion that the triangular ligament opened like folding doors, with the anterior wall, urethra, and bladder being lifted up, while the posterior vaginal wall was depressed posteriorly, to allow the fetus to pass. This theory was later shown to be anatomically impossible.

The cardinal ligaments were discovered by Alwin Mackenrodt (1859–1925). In his paper

(1895) Mackenrodt described the transverse cervical ligaments, and stressed their significance in uterine support. This ended years of speculation on the mechanism of uterine support, and the anatomical condition of ante- or retroversion of the uterus. In his description of the dissection of an 8-month-old fetus, he found 'firm band-like fibrous processes . . . which attach directly to the uterine cervix, vagina, rectum and bladder. These bands, arranged systematically, carry complex muscular elements as well as numerous bundles of elastic fibres . . . this whole ligamentous apparatus appears . . . excellent and extensive . . . ' Mackenrodt was born in Germany and after a varied career eventually entered gynaecological practice in Berlin. The Mackenrodt ligaments were also called the 'ligaments of Koch', the 'sustentacula of Bonney' and the 'cervico-pelvic ligaments of Nuylasy'.

The corpus luteum and the ovary were studied extensively in the latter part of the nineteenth century. The monograph *Eierstock und Ei* (1870) was produced by the leading German anatomist, Heinrich W.G. Waldeyer-Hartz (Waldeyer) in which he published the results of his research. Both he and Edward F.W. Pfluger (1863) believed that the corpus luteum formed as a response to emptying of the Graafian follicle at ovulation. Robert H.J. Sobotta introduced serial section studies and examined over 1500 mouse ovaries (1896). He believed that formation of the corpus luteum made ovulation possible again at a later date, by restoring normal blood flow to the ovary. John Beard (1897) and Louis Auguste Prenant (1898) theorized on the endocrine role of the corpus luteum structure. The endometrium was studied by William (1875) and Engelmann (1875). The various types of hymen were described by Testut (1896) as round, crescentic, labial, biperforate, fimbriate and cribriform.

TWENTIETH CENTURY

Fraenkel and Cohn (1901) of Germany reported that the ovary had two functions which were to develop and release ova, and to assist with implantation of impregnated ova in the uterus. During their studies they showed that destruction of corpora lutea caused loss of implanting embryos. In the same year Magnus (1901) reported his work from Norway, where he found that abortion could be caused in pregnant rabbits by removing or destroying their corpora lutea.

Small epithelial cell nests are often found under the serosa of the broad ligaments or in the walls of the Fallopian tubes in infants or young girls. These cell nests were first described by Werth in 1887, but were extensively investigated by Max Walthard (1867–1933). He described them as being arranged compactly with elongated flat dark nuclei pointed at one or both ends, with scarcely any space between nuclei. The cells were flat with scanty cytoplasm. Walthard's description (1903) was based on cell nests found in the ovaries of two girls aged 12 and 14. Pathologists later regarded those tiny bodies as the site from which Brenner tumours of the ovary developed.

Neumann, in 1897, first noted the presence of large isolated cells in the placental villi. The cells were again investigated by Isford Isfred Hofbauer, who was born in Vienna and emigrated to America in 1924. In a detailed description of the placental histology, Hofbauer (1905) described the cells thought to be histiocytes, probably present for their protective function. The cells first appeared towards the end of the 4th week, and were abundant in early pregnancy, but decreased as the placenta matured. The presence of fat in the cells led Hofbauer to speculate that the placental histiocytes possessed a digestive function. His assumption proved correct as they were later shown to have the ability to ingest and destroy bacteria. Hofbauer (1911) pioneered the use of posterior pituitary extract in cases of uterine inertia during labour.

The histology of the endometrium was studied by Leo Loeb (1907; 1908) who stimulated decidual reaction of the endometrium in guinea-pigs, by injecting foreign material into the uterine cavity during the luteal phase of the cycle. Hitschmann and Adler (1908) studied the histologic changes of the endometrium throughout the menstrual cycle and Bouin and Ancel (1909; 1910) published illustrated articles depicting progestational endometrium in the pregnant rabbit. Robert Schroder was the first to use the terms 'proliferative' and 'secretory endometrium' and demonstrated that the endometrium had basal and functional layers. Schroder (1909) produced a number of papers on cyclic endometrial changes between 1909 and 1915 and later described 'endometrial hyperplasia' which he indicated was due to the persistent action of oestrogen. His contemporary, Robert Meyer, assessed the development and eventual disappearance of the corpus luteum (1911).

The pelvic and endopelvic fascia were described by Poirier-Charpy (1923). The pelvic fascia which covers the upper and lower surfaces of the levator ani muscles and that on the mesial surfaces of the two obturator internis muscles were then more accurately described by von Peham and Amreich (1930). Goff (1931) investigated the vesico-vaginal space which separated bladder and vagina and found it to consist of delicate connective tissue which was relatively bloodless and passed between the vaginal and vesical fasciae. Those fasciae were noted to fuse together at what was termed 'the transverse vaginal sulcus' (Shaw, 1947). The vesico-uterine ligament, a thin layer of fascia connecting bladder and uterus, was described by Shaw and Nirula (1951).

Tandler (1926) gave a detailed diagramatic description of the blood supply, venous drainage and innervation of the perineum. It was Cleland (1933) who suggested that the outflow of the sensory nerve supply of the cervix travelled by the parasympathetic and that from the body of the uterus via the sympathetic nervous system.

The process of menstruation focused the attention of investigators on the cyclic changes which occurred in the reproductive tract. Early studies dealt with gross and microscopic change in the vagina, endometrium and ovary. Starting in the 1930s attention switched to the study of the spiral or coiled arteries of the endometrium. George W. Bartelmez (1931;1957) demonstrated that a basic step in endometrial breakdown involved a shut-off of the coiled arteries which supplied it. Similar changes in the endometrial blood supply were demonstrated by John E. Markee (1940) during his study of endometrial transplants in the anterior chamber of the eye of rhesus monkeys.

Further investigations of the vascular patterns of the human adult uterus were carried out by Hasner (1946) who based his observations on anatomical specimens obtained from the necropsy rooms of the University Institute for Forensic Medicine in Copenhagen. The uteri were obtained from women who were killed during street fighting in the Second World War. Schlegel (1946) and Dalgaard (1946) independently found that arteriovenous anastomotic passages existed in the human endometrium. Schlegel used an injection technique under air pressure and thus obtained a high arterial pressure despite collateral leakages, while Dalgaard used a modified benzidine staining technique. Both methods were superior to the injection techniques used by other anatomists who had failed to find the anastomoses.

The first attempt to apply the endometrial cyclical change to dating the menstrual cycle was made by Rock and Bartlett (1937). Their criteria were later modified by Noyes, and eventually Noyes, Hertig and Rock (1950) published their paper *Dating the endometrium*. Their work on the histology of the endometrium became the standard reference and was reinvestigated recently by Li and Cooke (1989). These investigators suggested that 'the traditional methods of dating endometrial biopsy are not precise enough . . . the precision of chronological dating can be improved by the use of the LH (luteinizing hormone) surge as the reference point . . . histological dating can be improved by quantitative histological techniques (morphometry) . . . using these improved methods of dating it is found that a strong correlation ($r = 0.98$) exists between histological dating and chronological dating . . . '.

Thoms (1935) investigated the inclination of the pelvic brim and found that the plane of the pelvic inlet lay at an angle to the spine which could vary from 40–100°, but was more usual at 60°. He detailed the measurements of the pelvic inlet, the plane of greatest pelvic dimensions (mid-pelvis), the plane of least dimensions (from the lower margin of the symphysis to the tip of the sacrum and the ischial spines laterally) and also the outlet.

Caldwell, Moloy and D'Esopo (1940) recognized four 'parent types' of pelvis, although mixed types were common. Thoms had already documented that only one third of women had what could be classified as a normal, or gynaecoid, pelvis. The four parent types were found to be anthropoid, or of a type resembling that of the anthropoid ape; gynaecoid, or the true female type; android, or wedge-shaped, and resembling the male type; or platypelloid, a flat pelvis. Not only could the four parent types present as mixed varieties, but they could also be modified by injury or disease of the pelvic bones or joints, or become altered secondary to abnormalities of the vertebral column or lower limbs. Thoms (1940) in his paper on the use of routine prenatal Roentgen pelvimetry, classified pelvic types as suggested by Turner in 1885: dolichopellic, mesatipellic and platypellic. To these three he added a fourth type, the brachypellic or oval-type pelvis.

Another major study on the pelvis was that of Kenny (1944) of London who described a study of 1000 pelves. The most common subgroup was the gynaecoid variety. The shape of the sacrum in females should be a gradual curve, compared to the shallowness of the sacrum in males. Snow (1949) analysed over 10 000 X-rays and classified the female sacra as curved in 45%, shallow in 30%, and flat to convex in 25%. Snow also described low and high assimilation pelves.

The diagonal conjugate of the pelvis was taken as the distance between the lower border of the symphysis pubis and the sacral promontory. It was measured clinically by pelvic examination with the index and middle finger. The promontory could only be palpated in the unanaesthetized patient if the pelvis was contracted. If the middle finger reached the promontory, the distance between the finger tip and the part of the hand which lay immediately beneath the symphysis pubis was measured. Subtraction of 1.25–1.9 cm, depending on pelvic inclination, gave a measurement for the true conjugate. This measurement was described by William Smellie c.1750, and for many years was taken to be 10.6 cm but radiographic examinations showed that the measurement should be 11.3–12 cm. Biscow (1944) devised a special rubber glove with a scale imprinted on the index finger to measure the true conjugate. DeLee and Greenhill (1950) introduced a classification to determine the position of the fetal head in the pelvis. The level of the tip of the ischial spines was taken as zero station. The position of the head relative to the zero station was measured in centimetres, as being minus for above and plus for below. Alternatively the head was said to be high-, mid-, or low-cavity.

The isthmus of the uterus, that portion which lies between the uterine body and the cervix, was described as a circular borderline area by Aschoff in 1908. It was found to measure 5–10 mm in length and was marked by a slight constriction on the surface of the uterus. It roughly corresponded with the level of the internal os and the reflection of the peritoneum from the body of the uterus to the bladder surface (Smout, Jacoby and Lillie 1969). Frankl (1933) reported that the response of the isthmus to hormonal stimuli was relatively small while Marshall (1939) documented that when supravaginal Caesarean hysterectomy was performed, as much as 4 or 5 cm of lower segment could remain attached to the cervix but menstruation did not recur. Danforth (1947) showed that the non-pregnant cervix was composed almost entirely of fibrous tissue. The uterine wall was composed of smooth muscle and the transition to fibrous was abrupt. The condition of cervical incompetence as a cause of habitual second trimester abortion was recorded by Lash and Lash (1950). They described a remodelling operation of the cervix but this was overtaken by the Shirodkar (q.v. in Biographies) (1955;1963) suture technique.

McDonald (1957) introduced a simplified technique using a purse string suture of braided nylon.

Femoral arteriography and aortography techniques were used by Borell and Fernstrom (1953,1954) to outline the arterial blood supply of the female genital tract. Reich, Nechtow and Bogdan (1964) correlated the radiographic findings with cadaver dissection.

Although radiology greatly enhanced the knowledge of pelvic architecture in the pregnant patient, a cautionary note was sounded in 1956 when a report suggested that antenatal radiology could cause genetic hazard to the gonads of both the *in utero* fetus and its mother (Medical Research Council, 1956). Stewart *et al.* (1956) documented an increased incidence of leukaemia in those children who were subjected to intrauterine radiation from antenatal radiology, and reported that other childhood malignancies were also increased (1958). Radiological examinations were used in a more restricted fashion thereafter.

Our knowledge of anatomy is now embellished by the use of radiology, ultrasound, computerized tomographic scans, and magnetic resonance imaging.

CHRONOLOGY

Antiquity

24000 BC   The Venus figures date from this time.

c.1550 BC   Egyptians gained anatomic knowledge from dissection of animals. The practice of embalming the dead, added little extra.

c.900 BC   The Hindus identified the human uterus, tubes, and ovaries.

6th C. BC   Alcmaeon, a Greek, wrote a text on anatomy.

4th C. BC   Artistotle described the animal uterus.

3rd C. BC   Herophilus of Chalcedon was one of the originators of human dissection at Alexandria.

1st C. BC   Cornelius Celsus, the Roman compiler, described the vulva, vagina, and uterus.

2nd C. AD   Soranus of Ephesus accurately described the female genital organs. His work was reproduced in the 16th C.
Rufus of Ephesus described the oviducts in sheep.
Claudius Galen dissected animals, and transposed the knowledge to the human. His teachings were accepted for over 1000 years.

4th C. AD   The Talmud contained references to the female anatomy.

References: Temkin (1956), McKay (1901), Leonardo(1944)

The Middle Ages

6th C.   Aetius of Amida wrote a text devoted to the diseases of women. He was aware of the uterine position between the bladder and the rectum.

7th C.   Paulus of Aegina copied the work of ancient authors for posterity.

9th C.   The oldest known depiction of the uterus was contained in the Moschion text.

11th C.   The Arabian medical books, copied from the ancient Greek and Roman, were translated back to Latin by Constantine.

1315   Mondino dei Luzzi was first to dissect a cadaver in modern times.

c.1400   Gian Matteo de Gradi of Milan first used the term 'ovary', instead of 'female testes'.

References: Bodemer (1973), Leonardo (1944), Speert (1973), McKay (1901), Ramsey (1989), Graham (1951)

Renaissance

1491   Johannes von Kircheim was responsible for the first illustrated medical work (Speert, 1973).

1510   Leonardo da Vinci accurately depicted the fetus *in utero* and also the uterus with its blood supply (Mathe, 1978).

1513   Eucharius Rösslin produced his *Der Swangern Frawen und Hebammen Roszgarten*, based on the work of Soranus of Ephesus of the 2nd C. AD

1522   Jacobeus Berengaris de Carpi wrote *Isagoge Breves,* and disproved the seven-cell compartment uterine cavity theory.

1543   Andreas Vesalius produced his *De Humani Corporis Fabrica* with illustrations by Jan Kalkar.

1552   Bartolommeo Eustachio described the pelvic blood supply.

1561   Gabrielle Falloppio described the human oviduct in *Observationes Anatomicae.*

Seventeeth century

1651   William Harvey wrote his *De Generatione Animalium* (Aveling, 1873).

1656   Thomas Wharton described the umbilical cord.

1668   Francois Mauriceau introduced the terms 'fourchette' and 'fossa navicularis'. He wrote extensively on female anatomy.

1669   Nicolaas Hoboken dissected the umbilical vessels.

1672   Regnier de Graaf studied the ovarian follicle.

1677   Caspar Bartholin described the vulvovaginal glands.

1677/78   Anton van Leeuwenhoek of Delft, described sperm at microscopy.

1691   Anton Nuck investigated cysts of the inguinal canal.

Eighteenth century

1707   Martin Naboth described cystic structures of the cervix.

1730   James Douglas described the peritoneal cavity and the pelvic cul-de-sac.

1754   William Smellie wrote his *Sett of Anatomical Tables.*

1759   Caspar Friedrich Wolff described the Wolffian bodies.

1761   Levret described the three pelvic obstetric planes.

1766   Petit considered the cervix as a store house which produced fresh muscle fibres for the myometrium in pregnancy.

1774   William Hunter's *The Anatomy of the Human Gravid Uterus* was published.

1781   Jean Louis Baudelocque described pelvic measurement. André Levret, Hendrik van Deventer and Smellie also wrote on pelvic assessment.

1787   Mascagni wrote on the lymphatics of the female pelvis.

Nineteenth century

Dissection of cadavers became accepted practice.

1802   The Wolffian body was described by Johann Christian Rosenmüller.

1820   Gustav Carus described the axis of the birth canal.

1822   Herman Gartner described the mesonephric duct.

1827	Karl Ernst von Baer described his discovery of the human ovum.
1830	Johannes Muller documented his observations on the development of the mammalian uterus.
1834	Cruveilhier described regional lymph nodes. Further work was carried out by Sappey, 1879, and Peiser, 1898. Bruhns and Poirier also contributed.
1836	Benjamin Alcock described the pudendal canal.
1837	William Fetherston Montgomery described signs of pregnancy in the breast.
1839	Franz Karl Naegele added further observations on the axis of the parturient canal.
1842	Dalrymple documented the epithelial covering of the placental villi. Robert Lee described the uterine innervation.
1849	Anders Adolf Retzius described the cavum praeperitoneale Retzii.
1850	G. Spratt wrote his *Midwifery* which contained coloured superimposed drawings.
1851	Gustav Adolf Michaelis described the sacral quadrangle and examined over a thousand obstetric pelves.
1863	Pfluger demonstrated tubular cell masses in the ovarian medulla. He investigated the corpus luteum. Further work in this century was carried out by Waldeyer (1870), Sobotta (1896), Beard (1897), and Prenant (1898).
1864	Henle described the cervix as a distinct histological entity.
1867	Ferdinand Frankenhauser detailed his major studies on uterine innervation.
1870	Wilhelm Waldeyer made important contributions to the description of the female pelvis.
1875	Emma Call and Siegmund Exner documented the small cystic space, similar to ova, in granulosa cells.
1880	Alexander J.C. Skene described the urethral glands.
1882	Theodor Langhans described the cytotrophoblast. Savage described the triangular ligament (urogenital diaphragm).
1895	Alwin Mackenrodt described the transverse cervical ligament.

Twentieth century

1901	Fraenkel and Cohn of Germany and Magnus of Norway reported their work on developing embryos and the relationship to corpora lutea.
1903	Walthard described cell nests, later thought by pathologists to be the area from which Brenner tumours developed.
1907	Leo Loeb studied endometrial histology. Further studies were carried out by Hitschmann and Adler (1908), Bouin and Ancel (1909) and Robert Schroder (1909).
1908	Aschoff described the uterine isthmus in detail.
1923	The pelvic and endopelvic fascia were described by Poirier-Charpey.
1931	George W. Bartelmez studied the arteries of the endometrium.
1935	Thoms investigated the pelvic architecture at radiology.
1937	Rock and Bartlett introduced histological dating of the endometrial cycle.
1940	Caldwell, Moloy and D'Esopo documented the four parent types of pelvis. John E. Markee studied intraocular endometrial transplants.
1944	Kenny of London described a study of 1000 pelves.
1946	Hasner and also Schlegel and Dalgaard studied vascular patterns of the human adult uterus.
1949	Snow analysed over 10 000 X-rays and described pelvic characteristics.
1950	Noyes, Hertig and Rock wrote their paper which became the standard reference for endometrial dating. DeLee and Greenhill introduced their classification to determine fetal head levels in the pelvis.
1956	Reports questioned the safety of radiology in pregnancy.

REFERENCES

Alcock, B. (1836). Quoted by Lourie, J. (1986) *Medical Eponyms: Who was Coude?*, p. 3. (Edinburgh, London, Melbourne, New York: Churchill Livingstone)

Andersen, J. (1977). *The Witch on the Wall. Medieval Erotic Sculpture in the British Isles.* (Copenhagen: Rosenkilde and Bagger)

Aschoff, L. (1908). Quoted by Smout, C.F.V., Jacoby, F. and Lillie, E.W. (1969). *Gynaecological and Obstetrical Anatomy.* (Aylesbury, England: H.K. Lewis & Co. Ltd.)

Aveling, J.H. (1873). Biographical Sketch of Harvey. *Obstet. J. Gr. Br. Irel.*, **1**, 23–31

Baer von, C.E. (1827). *De Ovi Mammalium et Hominis Genesi.* (Lipsiae: L. Vossius)

Bartelmez, G.W. (1931). The human uterine mucous membrane during menstruation. *Am. J. Obstet. Gynecol.*, **21**, 623–43

Bartelmez, G.W. (1957). The phases of the menstrual cycle and their interpretation in terms of the pregnancy cycle. *Am. J. Obstet. Gynecol.*, **74**, 931–55

Bartholin, C. (1677). *De Ovariis Mulierum, et Generationis Historia.* (Rome: Paolo Moneti)

Baudelocque, J.L. (1781). *L'Art des Accouchemens*, Vol. 1 pp. 38–45; 54–8. (Paris: Mequignon)

Baum, H. (1926). Die Benennung der Lymphknoten. *Anat. Anz.*, **61**, 39

Beard, J. (1897). *The Span of Gestation and the Cause of Birth.* (Jena: Fischer)

Beck, T. (1846). On the nerves of the uterus. *Phil. Trans. R. Soc. London*, **136**, 213

Berengario de Carpi, J. (1522). *Isagoge Breves Perlucide ac Uberime in Anatomiam Humani Corporis.* (Bologna: A Communi Medicorum Academia Usitatum)

Biscow, H.B. (1944). Special rubber glove with scale for measuring the true conjugate diameter. *Am. J. Obstet. Gynecol.*, **47**, 430

Bodemer, C.W. (1973). Historical interpretations of the human uterus and cervix uteri. In Blandau, R.J. and Moghissi, K. (eds.) *The Biology of the Cervix*, pp. 1–11. (Chicago: University of Chicago Press)

Borell, U. and Fernstrom, I. (1953). The adnexal branches of the uterine artery. *Acta Radiol. (Stockholm)*, **40**, 562

Borrel, U. and Fernstrom, I. (1954). The ovarian artery. *Acta Radiol. (Stockholm)*, **4**, 253

Bouin, P. and Ancel, P. (1909). Sur la fonction du corps jaune. Action du corps jaune vrai sur l'uterus. *C.R. Soc. Biol.*, **66**, 505–7

Bouin, P. and Ancel, P. (1910). Recherches sur les fonctions du corps jaune gastatif. 1. Sur le determinisme de la preparation de l'uterus a la fixation de l'oeuf. *J. Physiol. Pathol. Gen.*, **12**, 1–16

Bruhns, C. (1898). Uber die Lymphgefasse der Weiblichen Genitalien nebst Bemerkungen uber die Topographie der Leistendrusen. *Arch. Anat. Physiol.*, **57**

Caldwell, W.E., Moloy, H.C. and D'Esopo, D.A. (1940). The more recent conceptions of the pelvic architecture. *Am. J. Obstet. Gynecol.*, **40**, 558

Call, E.L. and Exner, S. (1875). Zur Kenntniss des Graafschen Follikels und des Corpus luteum beim Kaninchen. *Sitzungsb. d.k. Akad. d. Wissensch. Math. naturw. Cl.*, **71**, 321–8

Carus, C.G. (1820). *Lehrbuch der Gynakologie, oder Systematische Darstellung der Lehren von Erkenntniss und Behandlung Eigenthumlicher Gesunder und Krankhafter Zustande, sowohl der nicht Schwangern, Schwangern und Gebarenden Frauen, als der Wochnerinnen und Neugeborenen Kinder*, Part 1, pp. 32–33, Fig.6. (Leipzig: G. Fleischer)

Choulant, L. (1920). *History and Bibliography of Anatomic Illustration: in its Relation to Anatomic Science and the Graphic Arts*, pp. 22 and 83. Translated and edited with notes and a biography by Mortimer Frank. (Chicago: University of Chicago Press)

Cianfrani, T. (1960). *A Short History of Obstetrics and Gynecology.* (Springfield, Illinois: C.C. Thomas)

Cleland, J.G.P. (1933). Paravertebral anaesthesia in obstetrics, experimental and clinical basis. *Surg. Gynecol. Obstet.*, **57**, 51–4

Cruveilhier, J. (1834). *Traite d'Anatomie Descriptive*, Vol. 3. (Paris: Ancienne Maison Bechet Jeune)

Dalgaard, J.B. (1946). The blood vessels of the human endometrium. *Acta Obstet. Gynaecol. Scand.*, **26**, 342

Dalrymple, J. (1842). On the structure and functions of the human placenta. *Med. Chir. Tr.*, **25**, 21–9

Danforth, D.N. (1947). The fibrous nature of the human cervix and its relation to the isthmic segment in gravid and nongravid uteri. *Am. J. Obstet. Gynecol.*, **53**, 541

Davies, P.J. (1991). The death of Mozart. Letter. *J. R. Soc. Med.*, **84**, 246

DeLee, J.B. and Greenhill, J.P. (1950). Diameters of the pelvis. *Br. Med. J.*, **2**, 737

Douglas, J. (1730). *A Description of the Peritonaeum, and of that Part of the Membrana Cellularis Which lies on its Outside*, pp. 37–8. (London: J. Roberts)

Eisenmann, G.H. (1725). *Tabulae Anatomical Quatour Uteri*. (Strasbourg)

Engelmann, G.J. (1875). The mucous membrane of the uterus. *Am. J. Obstet.*, **8**, 30–86

Eustachio, B. (1552). *Tabulae Anatomicae*, quoted by Speert (1973). p. 18

Falloppio, G. (1561). *Observationes Anatomicae* quoted by Graham, H. (1951). pp. 160–1

Fraenkel, L. and Cohn F. (1901). Experimentelle Untersuchungen uber den Einfluss des Corpus Luteum auf die Insertion des Eies. *Anat. Anz.*, **20**, 294–300

Frankenhauser, F. (1867). *Die Nerven der Gebaermutter und ihre Endigung in den Glatten Muskelfasern*. (Jena: Mauke)

Frankl, O. (1933). On the physiology and pathology of the isthmus uteri. *J. Obstet. Gynaecol. Br. Emp.*, **40**, 397

Gartner, H. (1824). *Anatomisk Beskrivelse over et ved Nogle Dyr-Arters Uterus undersogt Glandulost Organ. Det Kongelige Danske Videnskabernes Selskabs Naturvidenskabelige og Mathematiske Afhandlinger*, pp. 277–317. (Copenhagen: Forster Deel) Reprinted from an earlier publication in 1822

Goff, B. (1931). A histological study of the perivaginal fascia in a multipara. *Surg. Gynecol. Obstet.*, **52**, 32

Graaf, R. de (1672). *De Mulierum Organis Generationi Inservientibus*. (Leiden: Hackiana)

Graham, H. (1951). *Eternal Eve: the History of Gynaecology and Obstetrics*. (New York: Doubleday & Co. Inc.)

Gruhn, J.G. and Kazer, R.R. (1989). *Hormonal Regulation of the Menstrual Cycle: the Evolution of Concepts*. (New York, London: Plenum Medical Books Co.)

Hart, B. and Barbour, A.H.F. (1883). *Manual of Gynaecology*, 2nd edn. (Edinburgh: Johnston)

Hasner, E. (1946). *Endometriets Vasculare Cyklus*, with English summary. (Copenhagen: Det Berlingske Bogtrykeri)

Henle, F.G.J. (1864). *Recherches sur la Disposition des Fibres Muscularis de L'Uterus Developpe par la Grossesse*. (Paris)

Hitschmann, F. and Adler, L. (1908) Der Bau der Uterusschleimhaut des geschlechtsreifen Wibes, mit besonderer Berucksichtigung der Menstruation. *Mschr. Geb. Gynäkol.*, **27**, 1–82

Hoboken, N. (1669). *Anatomia Secundinae Humanae, Quindecim Figuris ad Vivum Propria Autoris Manu Delineatis, Illustrata*, pp. 28–34. (Utrecht: Joannes Ribbius)

Hofbauer, J. (1905). *Grundzuge einer Biologie der Menschlichen Plazenta mit besonderer Berucksichtigung der Fragen der Fotalen Ernahrung*, pp. 28–30. (Vienna, Leipzig: Braumuller)

Hofbauer, J. (1911). Hypophysenextrakt als Wehenmittel. *Zentralbl. f. Gynäkol.*, **35**, 137–41

Howkins, J. (1968). *Shaw's Textbook of Operative Gynaecology*, 3rd edn. (Edinburgh, London: E. & S. Livingstone Ltd.)

Hunter, W. (1774). *The Anatomy of the Human Gravid Uterus*. (Birmingham: Baskerville)

Jackson, R. (1988). *Doctors and Diseases in the Roman Empire*, p.87. (London: British Museum Publications)

Kaspar, G. (1840). *De Structura Fibrosa Uteri non Gravidi*. (Bratislava)

Kenny, M. (1944). The clinically suspect pelvis and its radiographical investigation in 1,000 cases. *J. Obstet. Gynaecol. Br. Emp.*, **51**, 277

Kilian, H. (1851). Die Nerven des Uterus. *Z. Rat. Med. Henle Pfeufer*, **10**, 41

Kolliker, A. (1844). *Die Selbstandigkeit und Abhangigkeit des sympathischen Nervensystems, durch anatomische Untersuchungen bewiesen*. (Zurich)

Langhans, T. (1882). Ueber die Zellschicht der menschlichen Chorion. In *Beitrage zur Anatomie und Embryologie als Festgabe Jacob Henle* zum 4, April 1882 dargebracht von seinen Schulern, pp. 69–79. (Bonn: Max Cohen & Sohn)

Lash, A.F. and Lash, S.R. (1950). Habitual abortion: the incompetent internal os of the cervix. *Am. J. Obstet. Gynecol.*, **59**, 68, (quoted by Smout *et al.* (1969) p.229

Lee, R. (1842). *On the Ganglia and the Other Nervous Structures of the Uterus*. (London: Richard & John E. Taylor)

Leeuwenhoek van, A. (1678). De natis e semine genitali animalculis. *Philos. Trans. R. Soc. London*, **XII**, 1040

Leonardo, R.A. (1944). *History of Gynaecology*. (New York: Froben)

Levret, A. (1761). *L'Art des Accouchemens Demontré par des Principes de Physique et de Mèchanique*, 2nd edn. pp. 7–8; 299–303. (Paris: Le Prieur)

Li, T.C. and Cooke, I.D. (1989). Chronological and histological dating of the endometrial biopsy. *Contemp. Rev. Obstet. Gynaecol.*, 1, 266–72

Loeb, L. (1907). Ueber die Experimentelle Erzeugung von Knoten von Deciduagewebe in dem Uterus des Meerschweinchens nach stattgefundener Copulation. *Zentralbl. Allg. Path. Path. Anat.*, 18, 563–5

Loeb, L. (1908). The experimental production of the maternal part of the placenta in the rabbit. *Proc. Soc. Exp. Biol. Med.*, 5, 102–4

Lourie, J.A. (1986). *Medical Eponyms: Who was Coude?* p.3. (Edinburgh, New York: Churchill Livingstone)

Lyons, A.S. and Petrucelli, R.J. (1978). *Medicine: An Illustrated History*, p. 247. (New York: Abradale Press and Harry N Abrams Inc.)

McDonald, I.A. (1957). Suture of the cervix for inevitable miscarriage. *J. Obstet. Gynaecol. Br. Emp.*, 64, 346

McKay, W.J.S. (1901). *The History of Ancient Gynaecology*, pp. 4–14. (London: Balliere Tindall Cox)

Mackenrodt, A. (1895). Ueber die Ursachen der normalen und pathologischen Lagen des Uterus. *Arch. f. Gynäkol.*, 48, 394–421

Magnus, V. (1901). Ovariets betydning for svangerskabet med saerligt hensyn til corpus luteum. *Nor. Mag. Laegevidensk.*, 62, 1138–45

Malpighi, M. (1666). *De viscerum structura exercitatio anatomica.* (J. Montij, Bononiae)

Marashank, A. (1988). An ice age ancestor? *National Geographic*, 174, 478–81

Markee, J.E. (1940). Menstruation in intraocular endometrial transplants in the rhesus monkey. *Contr. Embryol. Carneg. Inst.*, 518, 29, 219

Marshall, C.M. (1939). *Caesarean Section*, quoted by Smout *et al.* (1969) p.218

Mascagni, P. (1787). *Vasorum lymphaticorum corporis humani historia et ichnographia.* (Senis: P. Carli)

Mathe, J. (1978–1984). *Leonardo da Vinci. Anatomical Drawings.* (Geneva, Fribourg: Productions Liber and Editions Minerva)

Mauriceau, F. (1668). *Traite des Maladies des Femmes Grosses, et de Celles Qui Sont Accouchées.* (Paris)

Medical Research Council (1956). *The Hazards to Man of Nuclear and Allied Radiations.* (London: Her Majesty's Stationary Office)

Medvei, V.C. (1982). *A History of Endocrinology.* (Lancaster: MTP Ltd.)

Meyer, R. (1911). Uber Corpus Luteumbildung beim Menschen. *Zentralb. Gynäkol.*, 35, 1206–8

Michaelis, G. A. (1851). In Litzmann, C.C.T. (ed.) *Das Enge Becken nach eigenen Beobachtungen und Untersuchungen.* (Leipzig: Wigand)

Montgomery, W.F. (1837). *An Exposition of the Signs and Symptoms of Pregnancy, the Period of Human Gestation, and the Signs of Delivery.* (London: Sherwood, Gilbert & Piper)

Morgagni, G.B. (1761). *De Sedibus, et Causis Morborum per Anatomen Indagatis, Libri Quinque.* (Venice). English translation from the Latin by B. Alexander, (1769) *The Seats and Causes of Diseases Investiagated by Anatomy, in Five Books*, Vol. 2, book 111, Letter 38, Articles, 35, 36, 37, 38, 42, 44

Muller, J. (1830). *Bildungsgeschichte der Genitalien aus anatomischen Untersuchungen an Embryonen des Menschen und der Thiere, nebst einem Anhang uber die chirurgische Behandlung der Hypospadia.* (Dusseldorf)

Naboth, M. (1707). De Sterilitate Mulierum. (Leipzig). Also published in von Haller, A. (1750). *Disputationum Anatomicarum Selectarum*, Vol.5, pp. 233–59. (Gottingen)

Naegele, F.K. (1839). *Das Schrag Verengte Becken nebst einem Anhange uber die Wichtigsten Fehler des Weiblichen Beckens uberhaupt.* (Mainz: Von Zabern)

Neumann, J. (1897). Beitrag zur Kenntnis der Blasenmolen und des "malignen Deciduoms". *Monatschr. f. Geburtsh. u. Gynäkol.*, 6, 17–36, 157–77

Nitabuch, R. (1887). *Beitrage zur Kenntniss der Menschlichen Placenta. Stampfli'sche Buchdruckerei.* (Bern)

Noyes, R.W., Hertig, A.T. and Rock, J. (1950). Dating the endometrium. *Fertil. Steril.*, 1, 3–25

Nuck, A. (1691). *Adenographia Curiosa et Uteri Foeminei Anatome Nova. Cum Epistola ad Amicum de Inventis Nova*, pp. 130–8. (Leiden: Jordan Luchtmans)

Nuck, A. (1692). *Adenographia curiosa et uteri foeminei anatome nove.* (P. vander Aa, Lugduni Batavorum)

Peham von, A. and Amreich, J. (1930). *Operations-lehre.* (Philadelphia, London: J.B. Lippincott)

Peiser, E. (1898). Anatomische und klinische Untersuchungen uber den Lymphapparat des Uterus mit besonderer Beruchsichtigung der Totalexstirpation bei Carcinoma Uteri. *Z. Geburtsh. Gynäkol.,* **39**, 259

Petit, A. (1766). *Recueil des Pieces Relatives a la Question des Naissances Tardives.* (Paris), quoted by Bodemer (1973)

Pfluger, E.F.W. (1863). *Ueber die Eierstocke der Saugethiere und des Menschen.* (Leipzig: Engelmann)

Poirier-Charpy (1923). *D'Anatomie Humaine,* Vol. 5, quoted by Howkins (1968) p.18

Prenant, A. (1898). La valeur morphologique du corps jaune. Son action physiologique et therapeutique possible. *Rev. Gen. Sci. Pure. Appl.,* **9**, 646–50

Putmann, J.J. (1988). The search for modern humans. *National Geographic,* **174**, 434–77

Ramsey, E.M. (1989). History. In Wynn, R.M. and Jollie, W.P. (eds.) *Biology of the Uterus,* 2nd edn. pp. 1–17. (New York: Plenum Medical Book Co.)

Reich, W.J., Nechtow, M.J. and Bogdan, J. (1964). The iliac arteries. *J. Int. Coll. Surg.,* **41**, 53

Retzius, A. (1849) Om Ligamentum pelvio-prostaticum eller den apparat med Lvilken blasan, prostata och urinroret aro fastade vid nedre backenoppningen. *Hygiea,* **11**, 321–6, translated from the Swedish by Creplin, F. (1849). Ueber das Ligamentum pelvioprostaticum oder den Apparat, durch welcher die Harnblase, die Prostata und die Harnrohre an der untern Beckenoffnung befestigt sind. *Arch. f. Anat. Physiol. u. wissensch. Med.,* 182–90

Robert, F. (1842). *Beschreibung eines im hochsten Grade Querverengten Beckens, bedingt durch Mangelhafte Entwickelung der Flugel des Kreuzbeins und Synostosis Congenialis beider Kreuzdarmbeinfugen.* (Herder, Carlsruhe & Freiburg)

Rock, J. and Bartlett, M.K. (1937). Biopsy studies of human endometrium: criteria of dating and information about amenorrhoea, menorrhagia and time of ovulation. *J. Am. Med. Assoc.,* **108**, 2022–8

Roederer, J.G. (1753). *Elementa Artis Obstetriciae in Usum Praelectionum Academicarum,* p.62. (Gottingen)

Rosenmüller, J.C. (1802). *Quaedam de Ovariis Embryonum et Foetuum Humanorum.* (Leipzig: C. Tauchnitz)

Rösslin, E. (1513). *Der Swangern Frawen und Hebammen Roszgarten.* (Hagenau)

Rösslin, E. (1540). *The Byrth of Mankynde,* translation. (London: Raynold)

Sappey, P.C. (1879). *Traite d'Anatomie Descriptive.* (Paris: A. Delahaye et Cie)

Sappey, P.C. (1885). *Description et Iconographie des Vaisseaux Lymphatiques Consideres Chez l'Homme et les Vertebres.* (Paris: A. Delahaye et E. Lecrosnier)

Savage, H. (1882). *The Surgery, Surgical Pathology and Surgical Anatomy of the Female Pelvic Organs,* 5th edn. (London: Churchill)

Schlegel, J.V. (1946). Arterio-venous anastomoses in the endometrium in man. *Acta Anat., Basel.,* **1**, 1285

Schroder, R. (1909). Die Drusenipithelveranderungen der Uterusschleimhaut in Intervall und Pramenstruum. *Arch. Gynäkol.,* **88**, 1–28

Semm, K. (1985). *Weichert von Hassel.* Universitäts-Frauenklinik Kiel, published privately

Shaw, W. (1947). A study of the surgical anatomy of the vagina with special reference to vaginal operations. *Br. Med. J.,* **1**, 477

Shaw, W. and Nirula, P. (1951). The origin of the lower uterine segment. *J. Obstet. Gynaecol. Br. Emp.,* **58**, 165

Shirodkar, V.N. (1955). A new method of operative treatment for habitual abortions in the second trimester of pregnancy. *Antiseptic,* **52**, 299

Shirodkar, V.N. (1963). *Progress in Gynecology,* p. 260. (New York: Grune and Stratton)

Skene, A.J.C. (1880). The anatomy and pathology of two important glands of the female urethra. *Am. J. Obstet.,* **13**, 265–70

Smellie, W. (1754). *A Sett of Anatomical Tables, with Explanations, and an Abridgment of the Practice of Midwifery.* (London)

Smellie, W. (1752). *A Treatise on the Theory and Practice of Midwifery.* (London)

Smout, C.F.V., Jacoby, F. and Lillie, E.W. (1969). *Gynaecological and Obstetrical Anatomy.* (Aylesbury, England: H.K. Lewis & Co. Ltd.)

Snow, W. (1949). Basic analysis of obstetric pelvis by Roentgen Study. *Am. J. Obstet. Gynecol.*, **58**, 752

Sobotta, R.H.J. (1896). Ueber die Bildung des Corpus Luteum bei der Maus. *Arch. mikr. Anat.*, **47**, 261

Speert, H. (1958). *Essays in Eponymy: Obstetric and Gynecologic Milestones*, p. 4. (New York: The MacMillan Co.)

Speert, H. (1973). *Iconographia Gyniatrica, A Pictorial History of Gynecology and Obstetrics*, p. 1. (Philadelphia: F.A.Davis Co.)

Spratt, G. (1850). *Obstetric Tables in Midwifery*, (with dissected plates), 1st American edn. (from 4th London edn). (Philadelphia: Bill)

Stewart, A., Webb, J., Giles, D. and Hewitt, D. (1956). *Lancet*, **2**, 447, quoted by Smout *et al.* (1969) p.59

Stewart, A., Webb, J. and Hewitt, D. (1958). *Br. Med. J.*, **1**, 1495, quoted by Smout *et al.* (1969) p.59

Tandler, J. (1926). *Lehrbuch der Systematischen Anatomie.* (Leipzig: Vogel)

Temkin, D. (1956). *Soranus' Gynecology*, translation). (Baltimore: Johns Hopkins Press)

Testut, L. (1896). *Traite d'Anatomie Humaine.* (Paris: Doin)

Thoms, H. (1935). Variations of the female pelvis in relation to labour. *Surg. Gynecol. Obstet.*, **60**, 680

Thoms, H. (1940). Roentgen pelvimetry as a routine prenatal procedure. *Am. J. Obstet. Gynecol.*, **40**, 891

Tiedemann, F. (1822). *Tabulae nervorum uteri.* (Heidelberg)

Venzmer, G. (1972). *Five Thousand Years of Medicine*, translated by Marion Koenig. (London: MacDonald & Co. Ltd.)

Vesalius, A. (1543). *De Humani Corporis Fabrica Libri Septem.* (Basel)

Waldeyer, W. (1870). *Eierstock und Ei.* (Leipzig: W. Engelmann)

Walthard, M. (1903). Zur Aetiologie der Ovarialadenome. *Ztschr. f. Geburtsh. u. Gynäkol.*, **49**, 233

Weber, E. (1817). *Anatomia Nervi Sympathici.* (Leipzig)

Wharton, T. (1656). *Adenographia: sive, Glandularum Totius Corporis Descriptio*, pp. 243–4. (London: R. Marriot)

William, J. (1875). The structure of the mucous membrane of the uterus and its periodic changes. *Obstet. J. GB. Ir.*, **23**, 661–767

Wolff, C.F. (1759). *Theoria Generationis*, pp. 96–7. (Hendel: Halle)

FURTHER READING

Andersen, J. (1977). *The Witch on the Wall. Medieval Erotic Sculpture in the British Isles.* (Copenhagen: Rosenkilde and Bagger)

Bodemer, C.W. (1973). Historical interpretations of the human uterus and cervix uteri. In Blandau, R.J. and Moghissi, K. (eds.) *The Biology of the Cervix*, pp. 1–11. (Chicago: University of Chicago Press)

Bowes, K. (ed.) (1950). *Modern Trends in Obstetrics and Gynaecology.* (London: Butterworth & Co. Ltd.)

Choulant, L. (1920). *History and Bibliography of Anatomic Illustration: In its Relation to Anatomic Science and the Graphic Arts*, translated and edited with notes and a biography by Mortimer Frank. (Chicago: University of Chicago Press)

Cianfrani, T. (1960). *A Short History of Obstetrics and Gynecology.* (Springfield, Illinois: C.C. Thomas)

Graham, H. (1951). *Eternal Eve: The History of Gynaecology and Obstetrics.* (New York: Doubleday & Co. Inc.)

Gruhn, J.G. and Kazer, R.R. (1989). *Hormonal Regulation of the Menstrual Cycle. The Evolution of Concepts.* (New York, London: Plenum Medical Book Co.)

Howkins, J. (1968). *Shaw's Textbook of Operative Gynaecology*, 3rd edn. (Edinburgh, London: E.& S. Livingstone Ltd)

Leonardo, R.A. (1944). *History of Gynecology.* (New York: Froben)

McGrew, R.E. (1985). *Encyclopedia of Medical History.* (London: Macmillan Press)

McKay, W.J.S. (1901). *The History of Ancient Gynaecology.* (London: Balliere Tindall Cox)

Mathe, J. (1978/84). *Leonardo Da Vinci Anatomical Drawings*, translated by David Macrae. (Liber)

Plentl, A.A. and Friedman E.A. (1971). *Lymphatic System of the Female Genitalia. The Morphologic Basis of Oncologic Diagnosis and Therapy.* (Philadelphia London Toronto: W.B. Saunders Co.)

Ramsey, E.M. (1989). History. In Wynn, R.M. and Jollie, W.P. (eds.) *Biology of the Uterus,* 2nd edn. pp. 1–17. (New York, London: Plenum Medical Book Co.)

Smout, C.F.V., Jacoby, F. and Lillie, E.W. (1969). *Gynaecological and Obstetrical Anatomy.* (Aylesbury, England: H.K. Lewis & Co. Ltd)

Speert, H. (1958). *Essays in Eponymy. Obstetric and Gynecologic Milestones.* (New York: The Macmillan Co.)

Speert, H. (1973). *Iconographia Gyniatrica. A Pictorial History of Gynecology and Obstetrics.* (Philadelphia: F.A. Davis Co.)

Venzmer, G. (1972). *Five Thousand Years of Medicine,* translated by Marion Koenig. (London: Macdonald & Co. Ltd)

Antenatal care and the early diagnosis of pregnancy

SEVENTEENTH AND EIGHTEENTH CENTURIES

In the seventeenth century the only antenatal treatment was bleeding. A vein was opened with the cut of a scalpel or lancet and a pint or two of blood was allowed to run out. This 'treatment' was not only given to pregnant women, but was widely used to treat a large variety of illnesses in both sexes. In some towns in Austria and Bavaria women would be bled routinely at least once, and sometimes two or three times, during their pregnancies. It is not altogether surprising that bleeding was carried out in pregnancy because it was thought that the body was made up of four humours, blood, phlegm, yellow bile and black bile, and as bleeding was a common treatment for most diseases and as pregnancy with its high mortality and morbidity was like an illness, bleeding had to be considered as correct treatment to put right the balance of the humours that were upset.

Queen Charlotte (Figure 1), after whom the oldest maternity hospital in London is named, was bled in her first pregnancy in 1762, after 'she was taken ill at Chapel with giddiness, palpitation, difficulty of breathing, and with pain round the hypochondria'; for which he (Mr Hawkins, her surgeon) bled her 6 ounces. Later Mr Hawkins thought it would be proper to bleed her (again), but William Hunter, her obstetrician, very skilfully dissuaded Mr Hawkins by writing to him 'I am clear in my opinion that it is judicious practice to take away some blood in the last month of pregnancy when the patient is heated or has symptoms . . . when the patient is cool and has no marks of having too much blood the taking away cannot do good and may do harm' (Hunter, 1762).

TWENTIETH CENTURY

The idea of regular antenatal care was originated by J. W. Ballantyne in about 1913. Already 20 years earlier he had published important volumes on the diseases and deformities of the fetus, and had made an attempt to systematize antenatal pathology (Ballantyne, 1892; 1895). He suggested that there should be a 'pro-maternity' hostel, primarily to enable scientific study of the physiology and quality of pregnancy. Only later, outpatient antenatal care became possible with the setting up of antenatal clinics all over the United Kingdom. The first antenatal outpatient clinic probably opened in Edinburgh in 1915. Although Ballantyne's name is given to it the idea came from a Dr Haig Ferguson (1862–1934).

At the beginning of the twentieth century it was rare for a woman to be examined at all by her

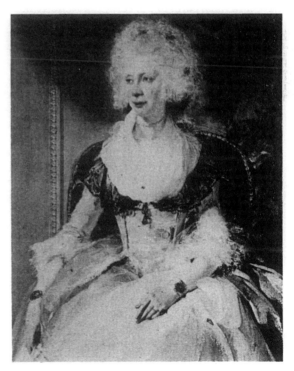

Figure 1 Queen Charlotte

doctor or in the hospital during her pregnancy. In Italy antenatal visits were carried out at the beginning of the century just two or three, or even fewer times during the pregnancy.

Before Ballantyne there was virtually no antenatal care anywhere, although Royalty and the aristocracy did get some as could be seen from Hunter's book of his care of Queen Charlotte (Hunter, 1762). The Municipal Borough of Woolwich in 1915 established a municipal antenatal clinic, and six voluntary experimental clinics were opened in England by the National League for Maternity and Child Welfare soon after. The spread of such care among the general population from the nucleus of Ballantyne's work in Edinburgh at the turn of the century, was mainly due to the energy of Dame Janet Campbell. As a Senior Civil Servant in the Department of Health, she was responsible for starting the National System of Antenatal Clinics and the uniform pattern of visits and routines to be followed. A few private patients had previously received a little antenatal care from their private practitioners.

The patterns suggested by Janet Campbell in the 1920s are still in existence today all over the Western world. Whereas in the early 1990s all women, except those who hide their pregnancies, have antenatal care, in the early 1920s, none had. By the start of the Second World War in 1939 just about 40% of all women in the UK were attending antenatal clinics. One year later the figure had gone up to about 50% and by the end of the war in 1945 nearly 100% (with the exception of those who were hiding their pregnancies, a common occurrence at that time) attended the clinics. Janet Campbell not only set the pattern but did an enormous amount of statistical work. In her book she set out a classical study on obstetric sepsis which had caused 256 deaths all over England in 1921 and 1922 (Campbell, 1924). Some of the septic cases that Janet Campbell assessed had arisen in spite of the fact that no internal examinations had been carried out on the women. Their infection came from sepsis in the wards in which they were delivered or in which they spent the 'lying-in' period.

Before the First World War many women lost babies because of multiparity. Women had the greatest difficulty in controlling their fertility. One of the greatest risks to women was to have to deliver many children. This is still so today in Third World countries, particularly if there is already some underlying disease. This can be true even in socially advantaged families, but the risk

for them is not as great as in socially disadvantaged families. Now there are pre-pregnancy advice centres. These have only recently been adopted, but they may become as important as the antenatal care centres themselves have been. A visit to a cemetery, such as the one in Ullapool in Scotland, to see the graves of the families up to about 1970 is highly instructive. Many gravestones mark the final resting places of mothers of large families. They are buried with several of their newly born or young children in the same grave. It was not only the poor who suffered. In 1879 Lady Edward Cavendish was 'dreadfully low' because she had delivered her fourth dead child (Jallard, 1986).

Janet Campbell was one of the first to advocate that an anaesthetist should be present at most deliveries and that every woman should be offered an anaesthetic if she wished it; and she warned 'the medical attendant may not find it altogether easy to resist the demands of his patient for speedy relief'.

In the 1946 enquiry conducted by the Population Investigation Committee and the Royal College of Obstetricians and Gynaecologists with the help of the National Birthday Trust Fund a reminder was given that Dr J. W. Ballantyne had arranged for expectant mothers booked for delivery at the Edinburgh Royal Infirmary, to be visited at home during the pregnancy. That was in 1913, 2 years before he established the antenatal centre in Edinburgh.

Before the advent of the National Health Service in 1948 antenatal clinics were run mainly by local authorities. They took note of the social, educational and clinical aspects of the pregnant woman. When the National Health Service came, antenatal care was provided in the general practitioner's surgery as well as the hospital clinic, and the local authority municipal clinic attendances fell markedly. In the late 1950s general practitioners were carrying out a lot of antenatal care in their surgeries and conducting many deliveries in patient's own homes. Ann Oakley (1984) has pointed out that antenatal care itself did almost nothing to lower maternal mortality or the stillbirth rate. Gibberd showed that the obstetric interference rate had risen from 1.35% in 1863–1875, to 8.86% in 1928 (Gibberd, 1929). While the maternal mortality had fallen in that time it had not been due to antenatal care nor necessarily because of the obstetric interference by doctors, which had itself given rise to some sepsis. Yet, as Gibberd pointed out, half of all septic deaths had followed normal labours – possibly due to vaginal examinations.

It is not easy to pinpoint which of the scientific and statistical advances has played the major role in improving antenatal care. Certainly the three great nationwide surveys conducted by the National Birthday Trust Fund in 1946, 1958 and 1970 revealed much about the causes of maternal mortality and morbidity and indicated ways of lowering them and perinatal mortality (Douglas, 1948; Butler and Bonham, 1963; Butler and Alberman, 1969; Chamberlain *et al.*, 1975; 1978). Gradually the number of antenatal visits crept up until a routine was established by the 1950s of a visit every 4 weeks for the first 28 weeks, then every 2 weeks until the 36th week and thereafter weekly. The routine tests were of blood for its group and haemoglobin content as well as for the rhesus factor; and the woman was weighed and her urine tested for albumin and sugar at each visit. Her abdomen was also palpated and she had an internal examination at least once and sometimes twice or more during the pregnancy, the first being to detect abnormalities in the pelvis and the shape of the pelvis itself and the second, towards the end of the pregnancy, to assess the descent of the presenting part into the pelvis and to attempt to tell if there was any likelihood of disproportion.

In France it was routine to perform a vaginal examination at every visit to ascertain the state of the cervix as well as the position of the presenting part.

Gradually more tests were added such as susceptibility for rubella, antibody tests for rhesus incompatibility and if antibodies were found, amniocentesis. Later came chromosome testing of the amniotic fluid for congenital abnormalities if these were suspected, and still later, chorionic villus sampling. Radiology was used and abused so that before the dangers were recognized, every woman routinely had an X-ray of her chest to assess the state of her heart and lungs. This rarely showed anything abnormal.

It became clear from the Perinatal Mortality Surveys that social class, smoking, nutrition, avoiding assault in pregnancy by a husband, partner or close relative, adequate rest and the ability to take maternity leave if the woman was in employment were important. So, questioning of the expectant mother about her social conditions became a prominent part of her antenatal care. This was particularly so after epidemiological studies, and especially the 1958 National Birthday Trust Survey, showed what an enormous role the social status played in lowering or raising perinatal mortality and morbidity (Butler and Bonham, 1963; Butler and Alberman, 1969). History taking was also increasingly devoted to seeking out family histories of genetic abnormalities.

Furthermore, instruction in pregnancy became more common, so that following the teachings of Grantly Dick Read (Read, 1942; 1946) women were increasingly told what to expect in labour and their partners were increasingly brought into the picture.

DIAGNOSIS OF EARLY PREGNANCY

In 1923 Allen and Doisy demonstrated that menstrual bleeding followed a fall in the blood oestrogen level (Allen and Doisy, 1923). This was the first time that an oestrogenic hormone had been identified. By 1931 oestrone and oestriol had been separated among the oestrogenic hormones. Dr A. Girard was the first to extract oestrogens from mares' urine. In 1938 Charles Dodds synthesized diethystilboestrol, the hormone that was later given to diabetic pregnant women with disastrous results for their children because of a tendency for their daughters to develop cancer of the vagina and their sons to be sterile. Progesterone, the other hormone of importance, was named in 1935 at a party near the Imperial Hotel in Russell Square on the eve of the Second International Conference on Standardization of Sex Hormones (Oakley, 1984).

Human chorionic gonadotrophin was discovered in 1930 by Collip and his colleagues (1930). Aschheim and Zondek (1928) discovered that pregnant women's urine, being highly oestrogenic, could be used to test for pregnancy. This was done by injecting five female mice 3 and 4 weeks old with the urine twice a day for 3 days. After 100 hours the mice were killed and their ovaries were inspected. If the ovaries were enlarged and congested there was a 98% chance the woman was pregnant. R. W. Johnstone, a Scottish gynaecologist, said that this process raised the rodents to the 'rank of obstetrical consultants'. The accuracy of the test was about 98% and vast numbers (130 000) were carried out in the Animal Breeding and Research Department of the University of Edinburgh. In 1931 rabbits were substituted for mice by Friedman (Cianfrani, 1960). The rabbits were cheaper. The woman who suspected she was pregnant gave her first morning specimen of urine. Some was injected into the rabbits' ear for 2 days and the rabbits' ovaries were then inspected by laporotomy. Later toads were used in the Hogben test. Toads did not need to be killed, they just shed their eggs. The Aschheim–Zondek test was only done when it was very important for a woman to know whether she was pregnant or not (Zondek and Aschheim, 1927). At one time X-rays were used to diagnose early pregnancy, but later it was realized that they could be teratogenic.

Chronology

Very little antenatal care before the twentieth century.

1915	First hostel opened in Edinburgh by J.W Ballantyne.
1920	Antenatal care started.
1924	Janet Campbell was advocating antenatal care in clinics.
1923–1935	Oestrogen and progestogen being discovered.
1928	Aschheim and Zondek described the first test for pregnancy by using pregnant womens' urine causing changes in mice ovaries.
1931	Rabbits' ovaries were used and inspected at laparotomy instead of mice being killed. Later Hogben test.
1946, 1958 and 1970	Enquiries into Maternal Mortality and Perinatal Mortality showed the importance of social factors and the need for improving antenatal care.
1980s	Human assay tests for use in laboratories and still later in patients' own homes.

REFERENCES

Allen, E. and Doisy, E.A. (1923). An ovarian hormone; preliminary report on its location, extraction and partial purification and action on test animals. *J. Am. Med. Assoc.*, **54**, 819–21

Aschheim, S. and Zondek, B. (1928). Schwangerschafts diagnose aus den Harn (Durch Hormonnachweis). *Klin. Wchschr.*, **7**, 8

Ballantyne, J.W. (1892, 1895). *The Diseases and Deformities of the Fetus, An Attempt Towards the System of Antenatal Pathology*, 2 vols. (Edinburgh: Oliver & Boyd)

Butler, N.R. and Bonham, D.G. (1963). *Perinatal Mortality*. (Edinburgh: E. & S. Livingstone Ltd.)

Butler, N.R. and Alberman, E.D. (1969). *Perinatal Problems*. (Edinburgh: E. & S. Livingstone Ltd.)

Campbell, J., (1924). *Maternal Mortality, London,* Reports on Public Health No. 25, pp. 9–10. (London: Ministry of Health)

Chamberlain, R., Chamberlain, G., Howlett, B. and Clareau, A . (1975). *British Births 1970*. (London: Heinemann Medical Books Ltd.)

Chamberlain, G., Philipp, E.E., Howlett, B. and Masters, A. (1978), *British Births 1970*. (London: William Heinemann Medical Books Ltd.)

Cianfrani, T. (1960). *A Short History of Obstetrics and Gynaecology*. (Springfield, Illinois: Charles C. Thomas)

Collip, J.B. (1930). Further observations on an ovary stimulating hormone of the placenta. *Can. Med. Assoc. J.*, **22**, 761

Douglas, J.W.B. (1948). *Maternity in Great Britain*. (London: Oxford University Press)

Gibberd, G.F. (1929). A contribution to the study of the maternal death rate, *Lancet*, 14th September, 535–8

Hunter, W. (1762). *A Journal of Attendance on the Queen*. Manuscript in the Special Collections section of the University Library of Glasgow

Jallard, P. (1986). *Women, Marriage and Politics 1860–1914*, pp. 165–6. (Oxford: Oxford University Press)

Oakley, A. (1984). *The Captured Womb, A History of the Medical Care of Pregnant Women*, p. 96. (Oxford: Basil Blackwell Publishers Ltd.)

Read, G.D. (1942). *Revelation of Childbirth*. (London: William Heinemann Medical Books Ltd.)

Read, G.D. (1946). *Childbirth without Fear*. (London: William Heinemann Medical Books Ltd.)

Zondek, B. and Aschheim, S. (1927). *Berlin Klin. Wchschr.*, **6**, 348–52

Blood transfusions, blood groups, the rhesus factor and haemoglobinopathies

Without the knowledge of how the blood circulates and how different types and groups of blood interact practical obstetrics and gynaecology could not be the subject it is today.

In 1616 William Harvey had discovered how blood circulates. The first edition of his very important book, *Exercitatio Anatomica de Motu Cordis et Sanguinis in Animalibus*, was published in 1628 by Guilielmi Fitzeri of Frankfurt. The English version, *On the Motion of the Heart and Blood in Animals*, appeared only in 1653. It was important to know the way the blood circulates in the body before the idea of transfusion of blood from one animal to another could even be considered.

INTRAVENOUS INJECTIONS

In the 1650s Sir Christopher Wren (1632–1723), whilst a student of science in the University of Oxford, was one of the first to document administering a drug intravenously. He wrote 'I injected wine and ale into the mass of blood in a living dog by a vein, in good quantities till I made him extremely drunk but soon after he passed it out'. Sir Christopher Wren, a polymath if ever there was one, graduated from Oxford in 1651. He was Professor of Astronomy, first in London in 1657 then in Oxford from 1661 to 1673. While occupying the Savilian professorship he designed the Sheldonian Theatre in Oxford (1662–1669) and later designed many other great buildings.

BLOOD TRANSFUSIONS

In 1665 Richard Lower pioneered blood transfusions in dogs. There is a very nice entry in Pepys Diary for the 14 November 1666 (Pepys, 1972) 'Dr Croone told me, that, at the meeting at Gresham College tonight (which it seems they now have every Wednesday again) there was a pretty experiment, of the blood of one dog let out till he died, into the body of another on one side where all his own blood ran out on the other side. The first died upon the place and the other very well and likely to do well. This did give occasion to many pretty wishes, as of the blood of a Quaker to be let into an Archbishop and such like; but, as Dr Croone says "may if it takes be of much use to man's health, for the amending of bad blood by borrowing from a better body". The experiment was conducted on a mastiff and a spaniel and recorded by P. Birch and R. Lower in 1665 or 1666. Samuel Pepys wrote on the 30 November 1667 'I was pleased to see a person who had his blood taken out. He speaks well and did this day give the society a relation thereof in Latin, saying that he finds himself much better since, and as a new man. But he is cracked a little in his head though he speaks very reasonably and very well. He had but 20 S [shillings] for his suffering it, and is to have the same again tried upon him – the first man that ever had it tried on him in England, the one that we hear of in France, which was a porter hired by the virtuosi'. It is recorded in the *Philosophical Transactions and Collections* of the Royal Society that the experiment was performed by Dr Richard Lower on Mr Arthur Coga on 23 November 1667 (Lowthorp, 1712).

Jean-Baptise Denys a few months earlier, in France, experimented on a madman, but the Royal Society experiment on the 30 November 1667 seems to be the first transfusion conducted on a human being in England. According to the minutes of the Royal Society, the official report on it was made on the 28 November 1667. It had been conducted by Drs King and Lower on the 23 November, and was repeated again on the 12 December (Keynes, 1922).

In November 1667 Lower transfused the blood of a lamb into a man and Jean-Baptiste Denys had also been transfusing lamb's blood into human subjects. The result was a fatality and Denys was arrested. The transfusion of blood from other animals into a man was prohibited by an act of the Chamber of Deputies in France in 1668.

James Blundell as part of the vogue, used human blood for transfusion in cases of postpartum haemorrhage, but between 1875 and 1900 physiological saline solution started to be used.

It was in 1875 that a German physiologist Leonard Landois showed that if the red blood cells of an animal belonging to one species were mixed with serum from another species the red blood cells usually clumped. Sometimes the red blood cells burst. He realized that black urine after transfusion of blood from a different species was due to breakdown of the incompatible red blood cells.

Figures 1 and 2 illustrate early nineteenth century blood transfusions.

BLOOD GROUPS AND THE RHESUS FACTOR

In 1609 Loiyse Bourgeois, the midwife of Marie de Medici, described jaundice in twins which Sir Cyril Clarke thinks could possibly have been due to the rhesus factor as they were not the first babies of the mother, and the first child had been born without jaundice. It is just a supposition. In 1900 Karl Landsteiner (1868–1943 born in Vienna and died in USA) an immunologist, discovered the A,B,O blood groups (Landsteiner, 1900). In the years 1939–1940 two teams of physiologists Karl Landsteiner and Alexander S.Wiener, and Philip Levine and R.E. Stetson (all of the USA) conducted a series of animal experiments in which they injected the red blood corpuscles of rhesus monkeys into rabbits or guinea-pigs. The rabbits and the guinea-pigs formed an anti-rhesus antibody (Levine and Stetson, 1939; Landsteiner and Wiener, 1940).

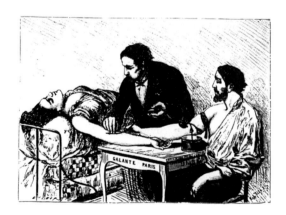

Figure 1 Direct donor-to-patient blood transfusion using Pagot's transfusor

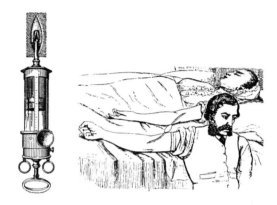

Figure 2 Direct donor-to-patient blood transfusion using Roussei of Geneva's apparatus

In the year 1939 an American woman gave birth to a premature, macerated dead fetus. She needed a blood transfusion and, as was quite customary in those days, her husband was called upon to act as a donor. He was group O and so was she. Unfortunately the result of the transfusion was a severe, utterly unexpected, haemolytic reaction. Levine and Stetson investigated this phenomenon and found that the woman's serum contained an irregular antibody or agglutinin which was quite different from the naturally occurring anti-A and anti-B agglutinins, in that it agglutinated not only the husband's cells but also 83 out of 104 random samples of group O cells from other subjects. They suggested that the fetus had inherited the antigen from the husband, and that the mother had become immunized by the passage of antigen across the placenta from the fetus, and in response to this immunization had produced the corresponding antibody.

The fascinating discovery by Levine and Stetson was that the atypical antigen in the case of the young mother who lost her baby appeared identical to the artificially produced anti-rhesus antibody of Landsteiner and Wiener. When the red cells of 'Europeans' were exposed to this anti-rhesus antibody the cells of about 85% gave a positive reaction by agglutination, while the other 15% gave no reaction. Landsteiner and Wiener therefore called the 85% majority rhesus positive and the rest rhesus negative; and that is how these rather elastic terms originated. In 1940 Wiener and Peters described four cases in which rhesus-negative patients developed haemolytic transfusion reactions after repeated transfusions of rhesus-positive blood which was compatible according to its ABO group and they showed furthermore that all four patients had anti-rhesus antibodies.

Levine and his colleagues meanwhile continued their studies of the occurrence of atypical antibodies in recently delivered mothers and in 1941 announced two very important conclusions. Firstly, they showed that the formation of atypical immune antiglutinins by a woman during pregnancy frequently resulted in the birth of a dead or diseased infant. When born alive it had haemolytic anaemia and jaundice. Secondly, they showed that the atypical agglutinins were anti-rhesus in specificity.

Returning to Landsteiner's discovery of the blood groups in 1900 (Landsteiner, 1900). Landsteiner himself divided blood into three groups. Two years later in 1902 Alfred von de Castello and Adriano Sturli (de Castello and Sturli, 1902) found the fourth group, which was the rarest of the blood groups. Landsteiner labelled blood that he found not to be clumped by serum from other people as blood group O. There were samples of blood clumped by serum from *some* other people and these were labelled A. Red cells from blood, the serum of which clumped A red cells would themselves be clumped by a serum, and were labelled B. So, there is an antigen in the red cells of type A blood that reacts to the serum of people from groups B and AB. It was soon discovered that there are many blood groups other than the A, B and O groups discovered by Landsteiner (1931). They have been named either after the patients in whom they were discovered or after the doctors who discovered them. Research is still continuing to discover new blood groups.

Blood transfusion would not be possible if a substance such as sodium citrate was not used to prevent clotting of the donor's blood during the transfusion. This technique was developed during the First World War, particularly in the casualty clearing stations run by the Americans (Keynes, 1981).

It obviously soon became important to work out the inheritance of blood factors and in particular the rhesus factors and this has now been done.

By about 1946 it had been realized that if 100 European children were taken at random they would include ten rhesus-positive children whose mothers were rhesus negative. The instance of haemolytic disease however was only about 1 in 200 of all pregnancies, whereas if every rhesus-positive child born to a rhesus-negative mother were affected the incidence should be about 20 in every 200. There are two main reasons for this discrepancy, the first being that the disease almost never affects children of a first pregnancy, the second that the capacity of rhesus-negative mothers to produce antibodies varies greatly. Furthermore, before the rhesus factors had been discovered, rhesus-negative women could have been sensitized by transfusions or injections of rhesus-positive blood. Now, precautions are taken to see that rhesus-negative women do not receive blood from rhesus-positive donors.

The Kleihauer test

In 1957 Kleihauer and others discovered a way of detecting whether a fetus's cells had leaked into its mother's blood (Kleihauer *et al.*, 1957). This was by an acid elution technique, in which the fetal red cells could be demonstrated and counted among the population of adult red cells in the mother's blood.

The prevention of rhesus immunization

Rhesus-negative women married to rhesus-positive husbands, and especially those in the same ABO group as themselves, who have positive Kleihauer tests, i.e. who have had blood from their fetuses leak across into their own circulation, are at risk of developing rhesus antibodies. These antibodies behave in the same way as other antibodies from the mother and can cross the placenta to the fetus; and if they are present in any quantity they will do so in a subsequent pregnancy. Antibodies on immunoglobulin G can be useful by crossing the placenta to protect the fetus, in theory at any rate, from certain illnesses from which the mother has suffered. In this way the newborn child is protected from many infectious diseases for the first few months of life.

The first method for the prevention of formation of anti-D γ globulin by a mother is the selection of the right 'mate'. This is easily applicable in countries where the rhesus problem hardly exists. Most Chinese are rhesus-positive. If a rhesus-positive Chinese woman were to marry a rhesus-negative man, nothing bad would happen because only rhesus-negative women make antibodies. In the Chinese population nearly 99% are rhesus positive and less than 1% are negative.

In 1963 a momentous discovery was made by Professor Cyril A. Clarke of Liverpool, working together with Drs D.R. Finn and Vincent Freida.

They took anti-D γ globulin from women who were known to have been sensitized by rhesus-positive pregnancies and who, by testing, had been found to have a very high titre of incomplete anti-D antibody in their blood, and injected it, within 48 hours of delivery, into rhesus-negative women considered to be at risk, i.e. those who had a positive Kleihauer test in the hours following delivery of a rhesus-positive child. This injection protected them against developing rhesus antibodies (Finn *et al.*, 1961; Freida and Gorman, 1962; Clarke *et al.*, 1963; Woodrow *et al.*, 1963).

As the years went by it was realized that not only women who had given birth to full term infants were capable of developing anti-D γ globulin, but also those who had had either intentional or unintentional abortions. As the production of anti-D γ globulin by a rhesus-positive woman is triggered by her reaction to fetal blood cells, it became common practice in the 1980s and later to give doses of anti-D γ globulin to any woman traumatized during pregnancy or who had had an abortion spontaneously or intentionally. Such trauma may occur as the result of a motor car accident or even as the result of an attempt to turn the baby in pregnancy. The protective injection has to be given within 72 hours of the possible leak of blood from the fetus to the mother.

The great discovery by Clarke and his team in Liverpool has not completely wiped out the possibility of the mother carrying a rhesus-affected baby. There is not just one rhesus factor but there are three allelomorphic pairs of genes designated C/c, D/d, and E/e. Usually by the term rhesus-positive one means somebody with the D/d rhesus group.

The anti-D γ globulin which is used to protect women from being sensitized by the blood leaking from their fetuses is obtained from women who have already been sensitized. As the number of sensitized patients who can act as donors of anti-D γ globulin is decreasing, because of the effectiveness of the immunization programme, so volunteers including men have come forward to be sensitized and to make the anti-D γ globulin.

As late as 1938 the cause of severe jaundice in the newborn (erythroblastosis) was completely unknown. Ruth Renter Darrow wrote 'The etiology of Icterus Gravis Neonatorum is still a subject of speculation . . . ' She wrote 33 pages summarizing all the possible hypotheses; but at the very end proposed a hypothesis based on an antigen–antibody reaction between mother and fetus. She put forward the view that fetal haemoglobin may be immunologically different from adult, and that if it gained access to the maternal circulation the mother might become sensitized and the resulting antibody cross the placenta, destroying the fetal erythrocytes. She missed by a hair's breadth the actual mechanism (Darrow, 1938).

Erythroblastosis: a rarer disease than before 1966

The main pathology from rhesus incompatability in the fetus is the haemolysis, or breakdown, of red blood cells which leads to anaemia and to jaundice. This can become very serious when the child is still *in utero*, and may lead to kernicterus, yellow pigentation of basal ganglia and other nerve cells in the spinal cord and brain after birth. Fetuses may develop gross oedema so that they become hydropic. These cases can be diagnosed *in utero* not only by the blood test that is carried out on the mother, but by the appearances on ultrasound; and on the results of amniocentesis, originally very bravely performed for this condition by Douglas Bevis in 1956 (Bevis, 1956). Bevis first suggested in 1950 that examination of the liquor amnii might show iron which had been passed into the liquor from the fetal urine, in cases of pre-eclampsia and postmaturity. The method at that time in 1950 for collecting the liquor was by high rupture of the membranes as a method of inducing labour. The liquor obtained by the rupture was examined for various constituents (Bevis, 1950). In his 1950 paper Bevis had suggested that an attempt should be made to obtain liquor earlier in pregnancy to give some prognosis for the rhesus-affected child. In 1952 he published a paper (Bevis, 1952) showing how he obtained liquor antenatally from the 28th week onwards at fortnightly intervals until delivery, by paracentesis (later known as amniocentesis). He gave details of the technique using a spinal needle (gauge 20) through which he aspirated 3 ml of liquor amnii. The needle was inserted at a point midway between the umbilicus and the symphysis pubis. This was almost certainly one of the first reports of amniocentesis being carried out. He looked in the liquor for urobilinogen and non-haematin iron, and in summary he stated that the results of the analysis of the liquor amnii taken at various times during pregnancy, indicated that the concentration of non-haematin iron and urobilinogen would offer a reliable guide to the outcome for the fetus in cases of haemolytic disease of the newborn (Bevis, 1953).

Bevis elaborated his work in 1956 when he pointed out that he then looked for many other substances including blood pigments that he found in haemolytic disease of the newborn by further examination of the liquor amnii (Bevis, 1956).

A.W. Liley in 1963 was the first to visualize the whole skin surface of a fetus by injecting urograffin into the amnion. He then placed a needle into the fetal peritoneum and transfused blood into the baby that way (Liley, 1963).

Fetoscopy, the direct visualization of the fetus by transabdominal amnioscopy was first described by Charles Rodeck in 1981 (Rodeck, 1981).

It has now become possible, due to this pioneering work, to treat affected babies *in utero*. If it is suspected that a child is affected, amniocentesis is carried out and if it is proven that they are necessary, transfusions are given. This is particularly so if there is a history of a previously affected infant. Furthermore the mother's blood can be checked for the level of rhesus-negative antibodies.

In such cases, amniocentesis should be carried out from about 18 weeks onwards, and can be repeated at intervals of 2–3 weeks. The amniotic fluid is examined for the presence of pigments, in particular bilirubin produced consequent on the haemolysis of the baby's blood. Until effective ways of transfusing babies *in utero* had been perfected, possible damage to the fetus had been minimized by early induction of labour, followed by exchange transfusion, as it still often is. It is very difficult to decide whether the risk of prematurity followed by an exchange transfusion of the baby's affected blood is likely to be greater or less than the risk of leaving the baby inside the uterus.

In 1981 Charles Rodeck also described a technique for transfusing blood directly into the fetus (Rodeck *et al.*, 1981). It requires very great skill to place a catheter into the umbilical blood vessels in the cord and so give the blood transfusion. However, the technique was developed at King's College Hospital in London and the lives of many babies have been saved by the transfusion of fresh O rhesus-negative blood, free from antibodies, and free from contamination by the maternal blood.

A less effective way of transfusing the infant is to inject rhesus-negative blood into the fetus's abdominal cavity in the hope that the cells will be absorbed through the fetal peritoneum. Intra-peritoneal transfusions are not new. The first experimental ones on animals were done in the early 1800s and human beings seem first to have received them in 1857 as described later by Ponfick (1844–1913) (Ponfick, 1875).

The first transuterine intraperitoneal transfusions were described by Liley in 1963. But before these techniques were perfected the rhesus-affected baby was treated by exchange transfusions. The technique for doing this is to wash out the child's blood and to replace it with rhesus-negative blood. A polythene tube is inserted into the umbilical vein and from it blood is withdrawn into a syringe which is then emptied, and a similar quantity of rhesus-negative blood is passed up the polythene tube. Ingenious taps have been designed to make this replacement transfusion less wearisome for the operator.

SICKLE CELL DISEASE

In sickle cell anaemia, which is a genetically determined disease, the red blood cells assume a crescent shape when the oxygen pressure in the environment of the cells is lowered. The illness affects 1 in every 350 American Negroes. Carriers have the trait of both normal and sickle cell haemoglobin. Patients suffering from sickle cell anaemia have crises involving restriction of the blood flow to joints and muscles causing severe pain. Pregnancy and delivery tend to precipitate such crises

. The American chemist Linus Pauling in 1949 discovered the nature of the physical flaw in the haemoglobin in sickle cell anaemia. He found that the blood of a person with sickle cell anaemia had a speed of movement when separated by means of electrophoresis different from that of the blood of a normal individual.

Vernon Ingram the biochemist, later discovered that in sickle cell anaemia valine, an amino acid, is substituted for glutamic acid in the blood.

REFERENCES

Bevis, D.C.A. (1950). Preliminary communication on the composition of liquor amnii in haemolytic disease of the new born. *Lancet*, **2**, 443

Bevis, D.C.A. (1952). The antenatal prediction of haemolytic disease of the new born. *Lancet*, **1**, 395–8

Bevis, D.C.A. (1953). Composition of liquor amnii in haemolytic disease. *J. Obstet. Gynaecol. Br. Emp.*, **60**, 244–51

Bevis, D.C.A. (1956). Blood pigments in haemolytic disease of the new born. *J. Obstet. Gynaecol.*, **63**, 68–75

Birch, P. (1665/6). *123 Philos. Trans.*, ii, 353–8

Clarke, C.A. *et al.* (1963). Further experimental studies on the prevention of Rh haemolytic disease. *Br. Med. J.*, 1, 978–84

Darrow, R. (1938). Icterus gravis (erythroblastosis) neonatorum – a general review. *Arch. Pathol.*, 25, 378–417

de Castello, A. and Sturli, A. (1902). Ueber die Isoagglutinine in Serum Gesunter und Kranker Menschen. *Munch. Med. Wschr.*, 49, 1090–5

Finn, R. *et al.* (1961). Experimental studies on the prevention of Rh haemolytic disease. *Br. Med. J.*, 1, 1468–90

Freida, V.J. and Gorman, J.G. (1962). Current concepts: antepartum management of Rh haemolytic disease. *Bull. Sloane Hosp. Women*, 8, 147–8

Keynes, G. (1922). *History of Blood Transfusion.* (London: Hodder & Stoughton)

Keynes, G.L. (1981). *The Gates of Memory*, p. 144. (Oxford: Clarendon Press)

Kleihauer, E., Braun, H. and Betke, K. (1957). Demonstration von fetalem Haemoglobin in den Erythrocyten eines Blutausstrichs. *Klin. Wchschr.*, 35, 637–8

Landois, L. (1878). *Beitrage zur Transfusion des Blutes.* (Leipzig and Berlin)

Landsteiner, K. (1900). Zur Kenntniss der antifermentationen, Lytischen und agglutinierenden Wirkungen des Blutserums und der Lymphe. *Zbl. Bakt.*, 27, 357–62

Landsteiner, K. (1931). Nobel Lecture. *Science*, 23, 403

Landsteiner, K. and Wiener, A.S. (1940). An agglutinable factor in human blood recognized by immune sera for rhesus blood. *Soc. Exp. Biol. NY.*, 42, 223

Levine, P. and Stetson, R.E. (1939). An unusual case of intragroup agglutination. *J. Am. Med. Assoc.*, 113, 126–7

Liley, A.W. (1963). Intrauterine transfusion of fetus in haemolytic disease. *Br. Med. J.*, 1107–9

Lowthorp, J. (ed.) (1712). *The Philosophical Transactions and Collections of the Royal Society to the end of the year 1700*, Vol. III chapter V pp. 225–35

Pauling, L. *et al.* (1949). Sickle cell anemia, a molecular disease. *Science*, 110, 543–8

Pepys, S. (1972). The Diary of Samuel Pepys, edited by Nathan, R. and Matthews, W., Vol. 7, p. 170; Vol. 8, p. 554. (London: G. Bell & Sons)

Ponfick, E. (1875). Experimentele Beitrage zur Lehre von der Transfusion. *Virchow. Arch. Pathol. Anat.*, 62, 273

Rodeck, C.H. (1981). Fetoscopy at King's College Hospital, London. In Rocker, E.D. and Lawrence, K.M. (eds.) *Fetoscopy*, Chap. 9. (Amsterdam: Elsevier)

Rodeck, C.J., Kemp, J.R., Holman, A. *et al.* (1981). Direct intravascular fetal blood transfusion by fetoscopy in severe rhesus iso-immunisation, *Lancet*, 1, 625–7

Wiener, A.S. and Peters, H.R. (1940). Haemolytic reactions following transfusions of blood of the homologous group with three cases in which the same agglutinogen was responsible. *Ann. Intern. Med.*, 13, 2306–22

Woodrow, J.C. *et al.* (1963). Prevention of Rh haemolytic disease: third report. *Br. Med. J.*, 1, 279–83

FURTHER READING

Clarke, C.A. (1975). *Rhesus Haemolytic Disease, selected papers, extracts and commentaries.* (Lancaster: MTP)

Eclampsia

This dramatic, lethal, frightening illness is well named from the Greek for 'flash' or 'bursting forth'. It is an extremely serious disease which occurs during pregnancy or labour and just occasionally after delivery. It was a very common disease until it became realized that it was preventable. Eclampsia has been known for a long time. It is characterized by fits, similar to epileptic fits, with irregular jerky movements and unconsciousness .

The Kahun (Petrie) Papyrus which dates from about 1850 BC may have contained some kind of description of eclampsia (Menascha, 1927). Menascha cited a paper by F. L. Griffith, quoted from the *British Medical Journal*, 1893. Griffith interpreted the Papyrus in the following way 'to prevent a woman from biting her tongue Auit Pound . . . upon her jaws a day of birth. It is a cure of biting excellent truly millions of times'. Griffith has suggested that an Auit meant a small wooden stick. The translation has been revised to say 'to prevent a woman from biting (her tongue ?) beans pound upon her jaws the day of birth' (Bernhart, 1939).

According to Chesley (1978; 1984) the Greeks recognized pre-eclampsia. He also held that Hippocrates wrote about it in section 5, number 30 of his aphorisms. The translation of this aphorism however by Adams (1952) is 'it proves fatal to a woman in a state of pregnancy if she be seized with any of the acute diseases'. This seems to stretch a little the relationship to eclampsia! Chesley also held that Galen in the second century AD, agreed with Hippocrates and commented that epilepsy, apoplexy, convulsions, and tetanus are especially lethal. He also pointed out that Galen would not have known the difference between eclampsia and epilepsy because it took another 1600 years before the one could be differentiated from the other.

Other writers whom we come across in this book, such as Cornelius (27 BC – AD 50) and Aetius of Amida (AD 500–550) mention women subject to convulsions. Chesley says that there is a possible reference to eclampsia in Rösslin's *Der Swangern Frawen und Hebammen Roszgarten* published in 1513. Mauriceau devoted much attention in later editions of his books to what we now call eclampsia. In his edition of 1694 he set forth several aphorisms dealing with eclampsia, which were that the mortal danger to the mother and the fetus was greater when the mother did not recover consciousness between convulsions; primigravida were at far greater risk of convulsions than multipara. Convulsions during pregnancy were more dangerous than those beginning after delivery, and convulsions were more dangerous if the fetus was dead (Chesley, 1943). Nicolas Puzos stated that if the convulsions were weak and well spaced out there was hope for the woman; if they were worse, in other words lasting longer and occurring more frequently, it was very important to bleed her abundantly, especially if the patient became unconscious. He described the signs of eclampsia very well, as frothing of the mouth, trouble with the throat, and losing consciousness (Puzos, 1759). As well as

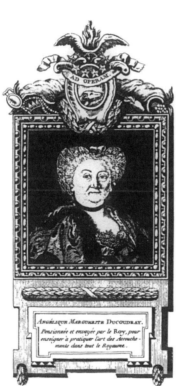

Figure 1 Madame du Coudray

being bled, a patient should be given enemas composed of Lenitif, diaphenic and the leaves of armoise (sage brush) and matricaire.

Madame Le Boursier du Coudray (Figure 1), the Chief Midwife of Paris, in her book of which the second edition appeared in 1769, and the third in 1773, wrote in Chapter 36 about convulsions and lethargy occurring to women in labour and pointed out how dangerous this condition could be. She believed that bleeding was the first treatment that should be used; and she warned against letting any cold water drop on to the woman's face or neck because this would increase the likelihood of convulsions and 'spiritus liquors' would make them still more violent. She wrote that if the cervical os was open and labour pains were coming regularly there was hope for the woman, especially if there was a good presentation. Since it was important to deliver the child early if the head was not down, an internal version should be carried out to bring the legs down to hasten the delivery. She warned however that the manoeuvre should not be carried out with any violence because that would provoke further fits. If the woman were to become unconscious the case was virtually hopeless. The only way the woman could be saved would be to deliver the baby. She said that she, fortunately, had never lost a mother, nor even failed to deliver the babies alive (Le Boursier du Coudray, 1769; 1773). She later published more on convulsions in the 1777 edition of her book.

Alexander Hamilton, Professor in Midwifery at the University of Edinburgh and a member of the Royal College of Surgeons, wrote *A Treatise on Midwifery* of which the first edition appeared in 1781. He wrote 'Convulsions often occur during labour to those who were subject to them while pregnant, and, in some instances they are fore-runners of labour itself. They may arise from fullness when the woman has been over-heated by stimulating food and drink, confined air, or other mismanagements; or they may precede from irritation, by the stretching of the mouth of the womb, or the contraction of the womb itself to expel the child; for sometimes, though rarely, the womb bursts from the violence of the labour throes and the child escapes into the cavity of the belly'.

'When the fits are slight and of short duration, recur at distant periods and the woman is sensible during the interval, there is less danger. But, when they come on steadily, when the face is frightfully distorted with foamings, etc., when the fit continues long, or recurs often, leaving a total stupor behind, the most unhappy event is to be dreaded' (Hamilton, 1781).

In another edition he says 'convulsions – no disease is more dreadful and alarming in appearance than convulsions; tho' they are confined to no particular period of pregnancy, they are most frequent and most dangerous in the latter months'.

'Fits come on very suddenly, generally preceded by pains above the region of the womb, anxiety at the pit of the stomach, and intolerable headache; these are soon succeeded by distortions of the body, foamings, etc. Sometimes the disease terminates fatally in a fit or two. If the woman survives a few fits, and recovers her senses in the intervals there is less danger. The child is often thrown off by the fits, at whatever period of pregnancy they occur'.

'As the disease is always attended with the utmost hazard, and frequently kills the woman like a fit of apoplexy, the most skilful of the medical profession must be immediately consulted . . .'

'These cases are highly dangerous, because they do not often admit of a relief until after delivery. It is also evident, that they may arise from frights, violent passions, and too great evacuations, in the pregnant as well as in any other state, they are then less alarming; and less when they attend profuse floodings.'

Hamilton went on to advocate bleeding, repeated laxative clysters and afterwards keeping the woman cool and quiet and confining her to a spare diet. If there were any symptoms of labour, he said that the membranes should be broken (Hamilton, 1781; 1785). In 1791 Hamilton gave the arguments for and against Caesarean section and quoted several authorities (Hamilton, 1790; 1791).

John Charles Weaver Lever, born in 1811, published in 1843 a paper in the Guy's Hospital Reports on some cases of puerperal convulsions. He was the first to describe swelling of the ankles and puffiness around the eyelids and to find that the urine contained albumin which slowly disappeared following delivery. He only found the albumin in the urine in cases of eclampsia or those that looked as though they were going to develop eclampsia, but none in 50 normal women.

In 1771 an obstetrician by the name of Manning recommended that opium should be administered, and this advice was carried out by Gustav Veit (1825–1903). Veit was more famous for his description of how to deliver the aftercoming head in a breech delivery.

W. Strogonoff wrote a history of the treatment of eclampsia as a preliminary to propounding his own method for the treatment of the condition. He said that a Dr Bland had given large doses of opium in 1794 with good results and that a Dr Bidden in 1892 in the lying-in hospital of Petersburg, gave chloral hydrate, morphia, and used chloroform. By 1908 in view of the urgency of delivery, Caesarean section was being resorted to, but the mortality was 47.97%.

Strogonoff's own methods formed a complete revolution in the subject. He claimed that there had been over 1000 papers written between the years 1909 and 1912, and by 1930 eclampsia was the chief scourge of lying-in women and their unborn children (Strogonoff, 1930).

Professor de Lee in Chicago had said that 5000 women a year died from eclampsia and 6000 from infections (de Lee, 1924). Janet Campbell said in 1922 that 1079 women had died from sepsis and 556 from puerperal albuminuria and convulsions in England in that year (Campbell, 1924). Once Strogonoff had introduced his regimen mortality fell to 2.6% in 300 cases of eclampsia. The secret of his method was to put the patient into a separate and quiet room, to carry out very few examinations and such as were carried out, were performed under light chloroform narcosis. Morphine enemas and injections should be given but always under chloroform narcosis. He discussed the question of how much chloroform to use. As had been noted by previous authors, exposure to cold could bring on fits, so the patient had to be kept warm but only light blankets should be used to cover her.

The regimen was as follows:

(1) In the beginning 0.16 g of morphine was given subcutaneously under light chloroform narcosis;

(2) One hour later chloral hydrate 2 g should be given by mouth in milk if the patient was conscious. If she was unconscious milk and chloral hydrate could be given by enema;

(3) After 3 hours the morphine was repeated and after 7 hours the chloral hydrate was repeated, then after 13 hours and after 21 hours.

Strogonoff said that it was wrong to bleed the patient.

D.F. Corkill in 1961 said that the incidence of eclampsia in 1956 and 1958 as compared with in 1928–33 had declined from 3.2 per 1000 cases delivered in hospital, to 0.80 per 1000 cases. Mortality from eclampsia had declined from 18.9% to 3.5%. The drop in the incidence and mortality was claimed to be due to preventive antenatal care which included the early recognition of the signs of pre-eclampsia and immediate treatment. It was important not to restrict protein and to recognize hypertension before the proteinuria showed itself.

Corkill's paper was delivered at the Seventh Conference of the International Society of Geographical Pathology. Various other authors at the Congress showed that there were great variations in the geographical distribution of eclampsia (Corkill, 1961).

Louis Hellman, a famous obstetrician from Brooklyn, New York, pointed out how difficult it was to diagnose pre-eclampsia (Hellman and Pritchard, 1971).

Following Strogonoff's teachings came the realization that eclampsia was a preventable disease, and antenatal care was therefore directed to searching for patients at risk. This was done by measuring the blood pressure regularly and taking action if it rose. Regular examination of the urine for protein became routine and initially oedema was sought, but it soon became realized that it was relatively unimportant.

The development of new sedatives such as diazepam has made it easier for patients to be sedated.

Hibbard (1988) was able to detail principles for managing pre-eclampsia and eclampsia. It is remarkable how closely these resemble those suggested by the ancient authors, because the essentials were still the use of a quiet room with minimal stimuli given to the patient, and reduction of sensitivity to stimuli by giving a variety of sedative, hypnotic and anticonvulsant drugs.

Hibbard in his book gives a complete summary of a scheme for the management of severe pre-eclampsia/eclampsia. Substances such as magnesium sulphate, that depress the central nervous system and inhibit neuromuscular transmission, have been used widely, particularly in the USA, where magnesium sulphate has been given slowly by the intravenous route (Hibbard, 1988).

Hypotensives are used, as well as hypnotics and anticonvulsants of low toxicity. Phenylthiazines with their ability to depress the arousal mechanism and act as sedatives and antiemetics, have gradually taken the place of 'lytic cocktails', pethidine, chlorpromazine and promethazine, which became popular over the years from 1950 onwards.

Although the condition has not disappeared, when antenatal care is good, its dangers have been dramatically lessened.

CHRONOLOGY

1850 BC   The Kahun Papyrus may have described eclampsia. The Ancient Greeks knew about fits in pregnancy and Hippocrates wrote about it.

6th C. AD Aetius of Amida wrote about fits in pregnancy.

1513   Possibly referred to in Rösslin's famous book.

1694   Mauriceau set forth his Aphorisms dealing with eclampsia.

1759   Nicolas Puzos described eclampsia and its treatment.

1769   Le Boursier du Coudray wrote about eclampsia.

1771   Manning recommended the administration of opium.

1791   Alexander Hamilton wrote about convulsions occurring in pregnancy and in labour.

1930   Strogonoff expounded his regimen and advocated examining women during pregnancy to predict and avoid eclampsia.

1950   Lytic cocktails became fashionable for pre-eclampsia and eclampsia.

All authors for centuries have advocated keeping the patient quiet and in a dark room.

REFERENCES

Adams, F. (1952). Hippocrates Writings translated. In *Encyclopaedia Brittanica*, pp. 137–8. (Chicago: Encyclopaedia Brittanica)

Bernhart, F. (1939). Geschichte, Wesen und Behandlung der Eklampsie. *Wien Klin. Wchschr.*, 52, 1009–13

Campbell, J.M. (1924). *Maternal Mortality Associated with Childbirth. Maternal Mortality Third Report.* Reports on Public Health and Medical Subjects, No. 25 (London: Ministry of Health)

Chesley, L.C. (1943). A short history of eclampsia. *Obstet. Gynecol.*, 74, 599

Chesley, L.C. (1978). *Hypertensive Disorders in Pregnancy*, pp. 17–34. (New York: Appleton-Crofts)

Chesley, L.C. (1984). History and epidemiology of pre-eclampsia-eclampsia. *Clin. Obstet. Gynecol.*, 27, 801–20

Corkill, T.F. (1961). Pathologia and Microbiologia. *7th Conference of the International Society of Geographical Pathology*, Vol. 24, p. 429

de Lee, J.B. (1924). *The Principles and Practice of Obstetrics*, 4th edn. p. 152. (Philadelphia: W.B. Saunders & Co.)

Editorial (1974). *J. Am. Coll. Gynecol.*, 43(4), 599–602

Griffith, F.J. (1893). *Br. Med. J.*, 1, 1172–4

Hamilton, A. (1781). *A Treatise of Midwifery*, pp. 131–3. (London: J. Murray)

Hamilton, A. (1791). *Outlines of the Theory and Practice of Midwifery*, 3rd edn. (London: T. Kay)

Hellman, L.M. and Pritchard, J.A. (1971). *Williams' Obstetrics*, 14th edn. (New York: Appleton-Crofts)

Hibbard, B.M. (1988). *Principles of Obstetrics.* (London: Butterworths)

Le Boursier Du Coudray (1769, 1773). *Abbrégé de l'art des Accouchemens.* (France: Pierre Toussaints Saints)

Le Boursier Du Coudray (1777). *Abbrégé de l'art des Accouchemens.* (Paris: Debusse)

Lever, J.C.W. (1843). Cases of puerperal convulsions, with remarks. *Guy's Hosp. Rep.*, 1(2nd ser.), 495–517

Manning, H. (1771). *A Treatise on Female Diseases, in which are also comprehended those most incident to pregnant and child-bed women.* (London: Baldwin)

Menascha, I. (1927). Geburtshilfe bei den alten Aegypten. *Arch. Gynaekol.*, 131, 425–61

Puzos, N. (1759). *Traites des Accouchemens*, pp. 172–4. corrected and edited by M. Mauriceau. (Paris: Desaint and Saillant)

Rösslin, E. (1513). *Der Schwangeren Frawen und Hebammen Roszgarten.* (Worms)

Strogonoff, W. (1930). *The Improved Prophylactic Method in the Treatment of Eclampsia.* (Edinburgh: E. & S. Livingstone)

Fetal monitoring

INTRODUCTION

Fetal monitoring has mainly evolved in this century. Our increased knowledge of the state of the fetus *in utero* has been coupled with advances in technology to aid our efforts to detect the at-risk fetus and remove it from an apparently hostile maternal environment. Previously, when the fetus at risk was not detected, labour became a testing ground, with the fetus being compromised during uterine contractions, when uterine blood flow is reduced. Some infants were delivered stillborn, while others were in poor condition at birth. Despite efforts at resuscitation, some died, while those who lived developed handicaps, or survived intact.

The initial attempts to preserve and protect the fetus were aimed at a reduction in the incidence of difficult labour and delivery. It was known that the malpresenting fetus was likely to suffer, and that the mother with a malformed or small pelvis would add to its problems. Various methods were used to restore the fetus to cephalic presentation, shorten labour, and expertly assist delivery, thereby reducing the fetal mortality rates in labour.

Intermittent auscultation of the fetal heart rate in labour began in the nineteenth century. Despite early observations of its importance, the full significance of fetal heart changes in labour had to await the clarification which occurred after the commencement of modern electronic fetal monitoring. As changes in the fetal heart rate were found to relate to fetal acidosis, electronic fetal monitoring was introduced (without scientifically controlled trials) on a wide scale in an attempt to reduce the incidence of birth asphyxia.

FETAL MONITORING IN LABOUR

Fetal auscultation and meconium staining

Philippe Le Goust, a physician in the French town of Niort, is credited with first describing the fetal heart as heard by immediate auscultation by his obstetrician colleague Marsac in the late seventeenth century. Nearly 150 years later François Mayor, a forensic physician in Geneva, rediscovered the technique of immediate auscultation while attempting to hear fetal movements *in utero*. His claim to fame was recorded in November 1818 in a Swiss Medical Journal (Pinkerton, 1976).

In the year 1819, René Laennec invented the stethoscope (Laennec, 1819). Prior to that, direct application of the ear to the patient, so called 'immediate' auscultation, was the method used, and was originally described by Hippocrates. Laennec initially used a cyclinder of paper to conduct heart sounds from the patient's chest wall to his ear. This method was called 'mediate' auscultation. Laennec's pupil, Jacques Alexandre Le Jumeau, Vicomte de Kergaradec, held a theory that the intrauterine fetus moving around in the liquor amnii would make a splashing sound. He applied Laennec's stethoscope to a pregnant abdomen and heard the rapid beat of the fetal heart which he called the 'double pulsation'. Kergaradec (1821) reported his findings to the Royal Academy of Medicine in Paris, and Laennec later included those observations in the second edition of his own book on auscultation. While Kergaradec thought that fetal heart sounds would indicate the position of the fetus or placenta, it was later realized that observation of the fetal heart in labour would help the obstetrician to know whether labour was proceeding normally.

William Stokes was still a 21-year-old undergraduate student in Edinburgh when his book *Introduction to the Use of the Stethoscope* (1825) was published. His book was one of the earliest and most widely read on the subject in the English language. Auscultation of the fetal heart was not mentioned in Stokes' book, but the 2nd edition of Laennec's Treatise was translated into English by Dr John Forbes in 1827 and contained Kergaradec's observations on auscultation of the fetal heart (Laennec, 1827).

William Stokes's friend and fellow student, John Creery Ferguson, developed an interest in auscultation. He travelled to Paris where he met both Laennec and Kergaradec, and on his return to Dublin, Ferguson was the first to use mediate auscultation of the fetal heart in the British Isles, on a lady in the Dublin General Dispensary in November 1827. He is known to have retained and developed his interest in the fetal heart. Later he moved to Belfast where he became the first Professor of Medicine in the Queens University in 1849 (Pinkerton, 1980).

On the instigation of Ferguson, fetal auscultation was introduced and developed in the Rotunda Hospital Dublin, during the mastership (1826–1833) of Robert Collins. During that time Nagle (1830), who was one of Collins's assistants, reported to the *Lancet* on the diagnosis of twins by Laennec's stethoscope. O'Brien Adams, also of the Rotunda Hospital, referred to the almost daily employment of the fetal stethoscope in the hospital (Adams, 1833). Soon afterwards Evory Kennedy (Rotunda) published his book *Observations on Obstetric Auscultation* (1833). His text was widely read and subsequently published in New York (Kennedy, 1843).

The Scots became converted to fetal auscultation by Evory Kennedy's reports and also by the investigations of John Moir of the Edinburgh General Lying-In Hospital. Moir wrote on his fetal heart research in an appendix to Professor Hamilton's *Practical Observations on Midwifery* (1836). His observations included the first description of the effect of uterine contractions on the fetal heart.

Mediate auscultation of the fetal heart initially met with some scepticism and even hostility. An elderly obstetrician called Forestier opposed the stethoscope as a 'new fangled and ridiculous plaything' and strongly advised Kergaradec 'to abandon these toys of ignorance truly prejudicial to science and to the well being of an amiable and interesting sex'. In 1828 John Burns, the Regius Professor in Glasgow, wrote that 'it is supposed by some that... the child's heart... can be heard, but not I presume by ordinary ears' (Pinkerton, 1976). Von Hoefft (1836) described the normal range of fetal heart rate.

Eventually fetal auscultation became established throughout Europe and the British Isles during the 1840s and 50s. Kennedy (1833) observed that the most ominous fetal heart sign was delay of its return following a contraction and Bodson (1843) described excessive frequency, great irregularity or marked slowing in the fetal heart rate, as indicative of a fetus in 'articulo-mortis'. By 1849 Kilian had advocated an auditory

indication for forceps delivery (Fogarty and Dornan, 1990). J.Y. Simpson (1855) pointed out that the death of a child was more frequently threatened when the fetal pulse became slower and slower. There were also cases, he added, where the fetal heart became more rapid and at the same time irregular and indistinct.

Meanwhile Schwartz (1858) recognized the value of fetal heart auscultation and advocated its use throughout labour. Fleetwood Churchill (1866) regarded 'weakening' of the fetal heart as an indication for forceps delivery. McClintock (1876) pointed out that the fetal heart beat slowed following labour pains, and that this slowing preceded intrauterine death. Alfred Lewis Galabin (1886) suggested that a good fetal outcome could be expected, if during spontaneous fetal movement its heart rate increased by 20 beats per minute.

In the 1840s two French obstetricians Cazeaux and Tarnier noted fetal heart irregularities which they termed as a 'state of suffering' (Bullock, 1871). Von Winckel (1893) regarded fetal compromise to be present if the fetal heart rate was above 160 or below 100 beats per minute. Eventually the term 'fetal distress' was first used by Hastings Tweedie and his assistant G.T. Wrench in their Rotunda Practical Midwifery book published in 1908 (Pinkerton, 1976). They suggested that the normal fetal heart rate lay between 120 and 160 beats per minute.

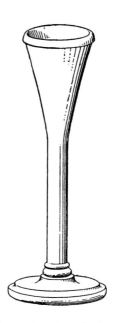

The fetal stethoscope as we know it today, is called after Adolphe Pinard (1844–1934) a French obstetrician – also known for his pioneering work on abdominal palpation (1889) and external cephalic version (Figure 1).

Vaginal stethoscopes were developed by Nauche (1865) and also by Verardini (1878) of Bologna who claimed that the fetal heart was audible in the first trimester. In the USA the obstetric head stethoscope (fetoscope) was popularized by Hillis (1917) and DeLee (1922).

Figure 1 Pinard's fetal stethoscope

Jaggard (1888) proposed that fetal bradycardia which followed Braxton-Hicks contractions indicated fetal asphyxia. The passage of meconium in the liquor was also noted to be an adverse sign, and Schwartz (1858) stated that meconium in the liquor was proof of a reduction in placental activity, and a sign of fetal distress or death. Reed (1918) suggested that passage of meconium was secondary to fetal hypoxia which caused the anal sphincter to relax. Walker (1959) showed that the fetus passed meconium if there was lack of oxygen, and Desmond *et al.* (1957) found meconium staining was more common when the fetus was mature or if anoxia was present. The problems of meconium staining awaited final elucidation until the second half of this century.

Fetal demise

The advent of mediate auscultation was to prove beneficial in determining not only life but also death of the fetus *in utero*. Until mediate auscultation became available the diagnosis of fetal demise was one of the most difficult and unpleasant tasks the obstetrician was called upon to perform. Obstetric texts of the seventeenth to nineteenth centuries were remarkably similar to Rösslins early sixteenth century book, *Der Swangern Frawen und Hebammen Roszgarten* in their listing of the signs and symptoms of fetal death. Thomas Raynold printed Rösslin's book translated from the German to English and published his *The Byrth of Mankynde* (1540). Little progress occurred until the early 1800s.

Although many signs and symptoms of fetal death were noted in Rösslin's book, William Potts Dewees of Pennsylvania in 1830 commented that 'all the commonly enumerated signs have been known to fail, and even when many of the strongest were united'.

Evory Kennedy (1843) wrote that children had been destroyed, or dragged mutilated into the world by the practitioner acting on the supposition that the child was dead; or that the mother was subjected to a difficult delivery in an effort to preserve the child's life when it was already dead; or the practitioner would trust to natural efforts and vainly sit by the bedside for days after fetal death expecting the birth of a living child.

With the advent of mediate auscultation, active interference in prolonged labour became possible. If the fetus was alive a more frequent use of forceps saved the infant and probably also the mother.

The 'fetus at risk'

The concept of the 'fetus at risk' which was based on epidemiological findings, was introduced prior to the introduction of electronic fetal monitoring. Hippocrates of Kos was one of the first in the field with his report in 430 BC when he related fetal outcome to the time of year in his *Airs, Waters, and Places* (Chalmers, 1977). Reliance on epidemiology continued to be important in clinical medicine, but in the seventeenth century concentration on the individual patient increased.

Early in this century Dugald Baird of Aberdeen, reapplied the art of epidemiology to perinatal medicine; and descriptive research on perinatal death and its causation was later carried out in the British Perinatal Surveys of 1946, 1958 and 1970 (Chalmers, 1977).

This form of research became the norm internationally and with the information gained it was possible to place certain women and their unborn babies in 'at-risk' categories. Pregnancies in the 'at-risk' groups were then supervised more carefully, particularly during the stressful time of labour. The various reports highlighted the causes of perinatal mortality and remedial action was undertaken on a broad front. Hypoxia was a major cause of death and its recognition and detection stimulated a vast amount of research directed towards analysis of the fetal heart rate in labour, and the estimation of fetal scalp blood biochemistry. Eventually the advances in cardiotocography during labour were to be applied to fetal health assessment in the antenatal period.

Electronic monitoring begins

Phonocardiography was invented in the early 1880s and the technique was used by Pestalozzo to make a tracing of the fetal heart sound in 1891 (Pinkerton, 1976). Some 12 years later Einthoven first published his work on the adult electrocardiograph (ECG) using the string galvanometer in 1903 (Curran, 1975). Using Einthoven's galvanometer Cremer (1906), while working in Von Winckel's unit, decided to attempt to obtain a fetal ECG. One electrode was placed on the fundus of the maternal uterus and the other in the vagina. Using this technology he obtained the first fetal heart trace and thereby started a revolution in our appreciation of the fetus *in utero*. In 1930 Maekawa and Toyoshima used a radio-valve amplifier and this made the detection of the small fetal signal a practical proposition. The initial traces displayed both maternal and fetal ECG together with background electrical noise. Various techniques were used to eliminate all but the fetal complex.

During the Second World War there was an upsurge in electronics technology. C.N. Smyth (1953) was first to describe the use of an electrode applied directly to the fetus. The signal he obtained had an amplitude of five times that previously obtained from abdominal leads. Sureau (1956a,b) first described a scalp electrode which was manually held on to the fetus. Hunter et al. (1960) used an electrode that could be clipped and retained on the fetal scalp, while a second electrode was placed on the perineum and a third attached to the patient's right leg. Hon (1963a) modified the electrodes and in 1972 the spiral fetal scalp electrode became available. The other popular form of electrode was the Copeland clip which was popularized by Ghosh and Tipton (1976).

While a very satisfactory fetal ECG could be obtained from the fetus during labour by using a fetal scalp electrode and a simple differential amplifier, antenatal monitoring of the fetal ECG was fraught with difficulties. The main problem was that the fetal signal had the much larger maternal ECG superimposed on it. A trace which would be relatively free of maternal elements was desirable. A number of methods were used including 'cancellation', which was a method of removing the maternal element by electronic subtraction, first described by Hon and Hess (1957). Hon and Lee (1963) reported their averaging techniques and noise reduction in fetal electrocardiography. Another commonly used technique to remove maternal signals was one of 'gating' as described by Offner and Moisland (1966). Maternal elements could also be removed by computer (Favret and Caputo, 1963), and soon the use of modern electronics with integrated circuitry simplified the amplifier problems.

Radiotelemetry which was based on single channel fetal ECG complexes was another breakthrough reported by Hess (1962) and Kendall et al. (1962). It allowed for patient ambulation in labour.

Phonocardiography was invented around 1880. Pestalozzo in 1891 was the first to make tracings of the fetal heart. The fetal phonocardiograph (FPCG) was reintroduced by Hofbauer and Weiss (1908), and the first recorded analysis of the FPCG was by Gunn and Wood (1953). The FPCG was adulterated by sounds arising from the maternal abdomen and electronic filters were used to 'clean' the sounds. Saywer in 1959 and Shelley in 1967 carried out research to determine limits at which filters should be set (Curran, 1975).

Hammacher (1966a) decided on a range of 60–120 Hz and it was he who popularized the FPCG more than any other contributor. Hewlett-Packard made his instrument commercially available (Hammacher et al., 1968). Hammacher in 1962 to 1966 developed the phonocardiograph and reported on fetal heart rate characteristics associated with antenatal compromise; and Kubli et al. (1969) noted the association of late decelerations, baseline tachycardia, and loss of variability with fetal compromise. The ultrasonic Doppler effect was used by Bishop (1966a,b) who described the commercial instrument called the Doptone (Smith-Kline Instruments, USA). Fielder (1968) described the first British instrument (Sonicaid) and Brown and Robertson (1968) described the 'ultra-dop'. The Doppler devices were later linked to automated fetal heart monitoring and described by Bishop (1968) and also by Mosler (1969).

While the presentation of fetal heart action via loud speaker or oscilloscope offered advantages over intermittent auscultation, it became apparent that a permanent record of the fetal heart action was desirable. The most popular form of presentation was introduced by Hon (1959) and Caldeyro-Barcia (1961), in which the fetal heart rate was plotted against time on a paper strip recorder, while a second trace on the same paper depicted uterine action from a tocodynamometer or intrauterine catheter.

Hon in 1957 and Larks in 1958 entered the field of cardiotocography. Both were prolific investigators and writers in the field, and Larks (1961) published his book on fetal electrocardiography. Eventually the work of Hon, Caldeyro-Barcia and Hammacher provided the basis for the majority of practical monitoring systems. The nomenclature and significance of transient fetal bradycardias worked out by Hon and Caldeyro-Barcia became generally accepted, although other workers added refinements.

Fetal electrocardiography slowly became the method of choice for accurate monitoring of the fetal heart in labour. The obstetrician who listened and counted the fetal heart for a specified time only ascertained an average rate. By measuring the interval between two fetal R waves however an instantaneous rate could be obtained and the effects of normal and abnormal labour on heart rate patterns could be studied in detail.

Electronic monitoring in labour

In 1963 Hon had described a fetal scalp electrode which could be applied *per vaginam* to record the fetal heart electronically (Hon, 1963b). This technique was later coupled with external uterine pressure readings (tocodynamometry) as first described by Reynolds *et al.* (1948), or with intrauterine pressure catheters as described by Williams and Stallworthy (1952). A composite recording of the fetal heart and intrauterine pressure was thus available for scrutiny and analysis. In 1968 Hon went on to describe three types of fetal heart deceleration which he classified as early, late, or variable decelerations (Hon, 1968). The early decelerations were found to be similar to Caldeyro-Barcia's (1966a) description of type 1 dips, and type 2 dips. Wood *et al.* (1969) compared the classifications of Hon and Caldeyro-Barcia and showed that late decelerations or their equivalent type 2 dips, were associated with low Apgar scores. Tipton (1975) enumerated the many disadvantages of records obtained by intermittent auscultation. He noted that there was a discontinuous record; an average fetal heart rate was obtained; observer error was common; uterine contractions interfered with direct auscultation as did maternal position; pressure of the fetal stethoscope could cause fetal heart irregularities; and finally beat to beat irregularity of the fetal heart could not be detected.

Hammacher (1966b) showed a relationship between reduced variability and chronic hypoxia. He later investigated beat to beat irregularity and noted four basic patterns which he described as saltatory, undulatory, narrowed undulatory, and silent, and correlated them with fetal distress (Figure 2) (Hammacher *et al.*, 1968; Hammacher, 1969).

Beard *et al.* (1971a) found that early decelerations, which were most often due to head compression, were not usually ominous or associated with low Apgar scores. Dip area was investigated by Shelley and Tipton (1971) while sinusoidal patterns which were reported by Manseau *et al.* (1972) were found to be associated with fetal anaemia as a result of rhesus sensitization or cardiac failure. Since then many other parameters have been assessed. Despite these and other innovations, the many irregularities noted on fetal heart tracings approximate poorly with the fetal condition as assessed by scalp pH and Apgar scores (Renou and Wood, 1974).

The conduct of labour

It was Friedman in 1954 who focused attention on the stages of labour and developed his concept of latent and active phases (Friedman, 1954). This later led to changes in the management of labour, including the adoption by Philpott (1972) of the

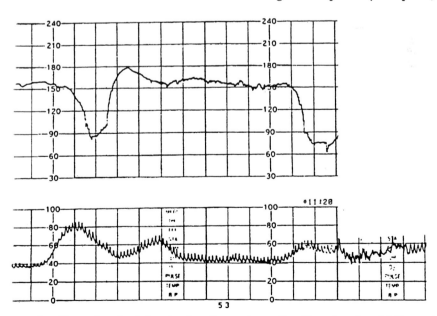

Figure 2 An example of 'overshooting' showing baseline tachycardia with reduced variability and acceleration only following deceleration (associated with birth asphyxia). Paper speed 3cm/min

101

composite partogram and the introduction of a policy of active management in labour (O'Driscoll *et al.*, 1969). These measures helped to increase the quality of care in labour with a resultant decrease in perinatal morbidity and mortality.

Acid–base studies

Fetal scalp blood sampling was introduced in the 1960s. The technique was soon used in an effort to reduce the number of apparently unnecessary Caesarean sections carried out due to changes in fetal heart rate patterns which were interpreted as 'fetal distress'. The work of James *et al.* (1958) first showed a correlation between umbilical cord pH and depression of the human neonate. A logical extension of this finding was to measure fetal scalp blood acid–base parameters. This was made possible when Saling (1961) introduced a technique for obtaining fetal scalp blood samples during labour (Figure 3). Saling (1966) and Saling and Schneider (1967) claimed that acid–base measurements were a reliable and quantitative indicator of the fetal condition, and were of clinical value in predicting the condition of the baby at birth. Despite this apparent advance many obstetric units failed to introduce fetal scalp pH estimation to back up their electronic and or intermittent auscultation fetal monitoring.

Outcome

Virginia Apgar (1953) (Figure 4) devised a scoring system which could be used to assess the condition of the newborn infant. Normal infants with a high

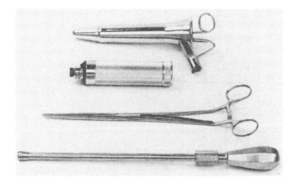

Figure 3 Scalp electrode introducing amnioscope and accessories. Reproduced with kind permission from *Clinics in Obstetrics and Gynaecology* (April 1974), Vol. 1, No. 1, p. 173 (London: W. B. Saunders)

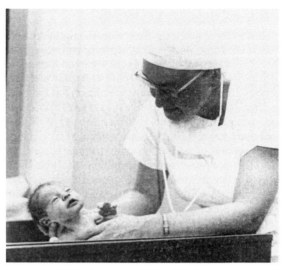

Figure 4 Virginia Apgar (1909–1974)

score were likely to fare well. Those with a low score were more likely to require resuscitation and could suffer perinatal mortality or handicap. The scoring system was universally adopted for appraisal of the newborn infant.

The relationship of the fetal heart rate, meconium in the liquor, scalp pH in labour, and eventual fetal outcome have all been assessed in relation to the Apgar score recorded postdelivery.

Nelson and Ellenberg (1981) found that Apgar scores did not accurately predict the later onset of cerebral palsy. Sykes *et al.* (1982), one of a number of other investigating groups, determined that only 21% of infants with an Apgar score of less than 7 at 1 minute and 19% with an Apgar score of less than 7 at 5 minutes had severe acidosis at birth, while of infants with severe acidosis at birth 73% had had an Apgar score of 7 or more.

Quilligan (1972) observed a slightly lower perinatal mortality amongst 'monitored' high-risk patients than in unmonitored normal patients. It gradually became accepted thought that perinatal mortality was reduced if the fetus was monitored electronically. Later however the enthusiasm was dampened when it was found that none of a series of reported randomized trials demonstrated a reduction in mortality attributable to intensive electronic fetal monitoring in labour (Haverkamp *et al.*, 1976; Renou *et al.*, 1976; Kelso *et al.*, 1978; Haverkamp *et al.*, 1979; Wood *et al.*, 1981; MacDonald *et al.*, 1985).

The use of electronic monitoring led to an increase in intervention, its major effect being an increase in Caesarean section rates for apparent 'fetal distress', as diagnosed from fetal heart dips seen on monitor traces (Haverkamp *et al.*, 1976 ; Banta and Thacker, 1979). The outcome for the individual fetus was not always improved. The machinery involved was complex and removed labour from being a relatively normal process, to one of high technology and hospital care (Figure 5). Attention was often diverted from the mother to the electronic monitors, with loss of the essential person to person contact for the labouring woman. Medico-legally the cardiotocographic trace became a major issue with varying opinion as to possible fetal outcome related to the various changes noted.

It became apparent that fetal monitoring could not always predict the fetus who was at risk, although for a time it was mooted that fetal handicap related in large part to undetected fetal hypoxia in labour. It is now realized however, that less than 10% of handicap in infants is a result of asphyxia

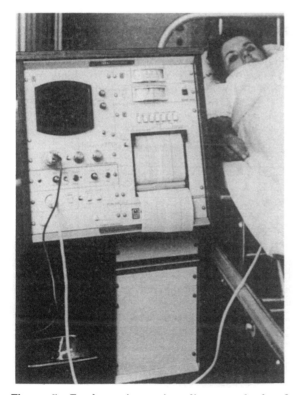

Figure 5 Fetal monitor using direct methods of cardiotocography and with written and recorded display of fetal electrocardiograph configurations (M.G. Electronics). Reproduced with kind permission from *Clinics in Obstetrics and Gynaecology* (April 1974), Vol. 1, No. 1, p. 174. (London: W. B. Saunders)

during labour or at delivery (Nelson and Ellenberg, 1986).

The presence of hypoxic ischaemic encephalopathy in the neonate is a prognostic sign of subsequent development (Amiel-Tieson, 1969). Sarnat and Sarnat (1976) and Fenichel (1983) established a classification and determined outcome according to the grade of severity. Levene *et al.* (1985) determined an incidence of 6 per 1000 births.

Chalmers (1979) predicted from the pooled results of previous trials that electronic fetal monitoring would have a protective effect against the development of early neonatal seizures. This prediction was confirmed by the Dublin trial which demonstrated a doubling for risk for neonatal seizures in low-risk infants when labour was allocated to supervision by intermittent auscultation rather than electronic fetal monitoring (MacDonald *et al.*, 1985). However, on further follow up no differences were found between the two groups when assessed for neurological deficit. Paul *et al.*, (1986) and Mann (1986) pointed out that abnormal fetal heart patterns might be the result of antenatal events, and perhaps not due to the often suspected hypoxia in labour.

Dermot MacDonald (1989) of the National Maternity Hospital, a short distance away from the Rotunda Hospital Dublin where fetal auscultation was pioneered soon after Kergaradec's description, summarized the benefits to date of continuous electronic monitoring of the fetal heart during labour. He pointed out that nine prospective randomized controlled trials involving 53 000 infants demonstrated no advantage from electronic intrapartum fetal surveillance over intermittent auscultation as judged by mortality, neonatal morbidity, or cerebral palsy at the age of 4 years. He quoted the words of Prentice and Lynd (1987) from their *Lancet* article, 'for low-risk mothers there is a good case for a return to the traditional method of intermittent auscultation' and 'even with high-risk pregnancy the benefit of continuous fetal monitoring has not been as clearly demonstrated as the practising obstetrician might suppose'. He also noted that the American College of Obstetricians and Gynaecologists had recommended that when high-risk factors are present in labour or when intensified monitoring is chosen, the fetal heart rate should be monitored by 'one of two equal methods'. So while it would appear that electronic monitoring has not been a major benefit, MacDonald advised further research in intrapartum fetal surveillance, including that of biochemical examination of the fetal blood in labour.

Currently it is appreciated that electronic fetal monitoring is not superior to intermittent auscultation: it increases the Caesarean section rate; leads to an increase in medico-legal claims; and despite all efforts it appears that electronic fetal monitoring has not offered markedly increased protection to the fetus.

ANTENATAL FETAL MONITORING

Fetal movements

It has been appreciated since antiquity that the fetus can move *in utero*. References to fetal movements appear in the Bible (Genesis 25: 22 and Luke 1: 41; 1: 44) and in the early writings of a number of civilizations. Vesalius is said to have observed fetal movement and possibly fetal breathing movement in pigs in 1543, while Ambroise Paré (1634) taught that the presence of fetal movement indicated that the child in the womb was alive. Fetal movement as an early sign of pregnancy was also reported by Wrisberg of Sweden in 1770 (Thacker and Berkelman, 1986). Beclard (1813) reported on fetal breathing activity in the *Bulletin de la Faculté de Medicine de Paris*. Playfair

(1886) advised induction of labour for decreased fetal movements.

Ahlfeld (1905) was one of the first to evaluate scientifically the different types of fetal movement in the human fetus. However, it was not until the 1960s that techniques for studying fetal movement were developed.

Sterman (1967) reported 'passive' methods for fetal movement studies. The most commonly used device to record fetal movements was the tocodynamometer. Boddy and Mantell (1972) introduced their 'active' recording system, in which they used A mode ultrasound, and later Marsal *et al.* (1976) used B mode techniques. Sadovski *et al.* (1977) introduced an instrument using piezoelectric materials, while Birnholz *et al.* (1978) introduced real time sonographic methods of visualizing fetal movements. The types of fetal movements were noted and quantified in an effort to determine a prognostic indicator of fetal health.

Sadovski and Yaffe (1973) suggested that cessation of maternally perceived fetal movements meant impending fetal death, and 3 years later Pearson and Weaver (1976) showed that maternal fetal movement counting was as good a test for fetal assessment as oestriol measurements. Pearson (1977) introduced a 'count-to-10' fetal movement chart which became popular (Figure 6).

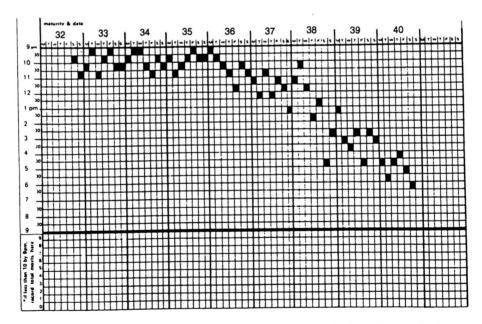

Figure 6 A typical example of a 'Count-to-10' chart showing the gradual diminution in frequency of fetal movements as term approaches. Reproduced with kind permission from Studd, J. (ed.) (1981). *Progress in Obstetrics and Gynaecology*, Vol. 1. (Edinburgh, London: Churchill Livingstone)

Liston *et al.* (1982) prospectively evaluated the fetal movement chart and found that pregnancies in which there were fewer than ten movements in 12 hours were associated with a significant increase in perinatal mortality, fetal distress, and fetal compromise. A false-positive prediction rate of 36% and a false-negative prediction rate of 2%, was recorded.

Fetal breathing

Fetal breathing movements (FBM) were first recorded from the maternal abdomen by Ahlfeld (1888). However, the inaccessibility of the fetus to direct examination delayed development in this area until the 1970s when Dawes *et al.* (1970; 1972) in Oxford, and Merlett *et al.* (1970) in Paris reported on fetal breathing movements in normal fetal lambs. Boddy and Robinson (1971) developed and introduced a gated A mode ultrasound method for recording fetal chest wall movement, while Manning (1976) of Canada developed a B mode ultrasound technique which enabled precise measurement of FBM to be made with ease. Platt *et al.* (1978) showed that if FBM were present in the last test before delivery, the incidence of fetal cardiorespiratory depression at birth was 4%, whereas if FBM were absent then depressed infants were born in 50% of cases. Later, records of fetal breathing movements, fetal movement, fetal tone, the results of a non-stressed cardiotocograph and qualitative amniotic fluid volumes were developed by Manning *et al.* (1980) to achieve a fetal biophysical profile.

Biochemical tests

Arnold Klopper (1989) vividly described how biochemical measurements of fetal metabolism began when Guy Marrian (1930) evaporated great pans of urine from pregnant women on a flat roof at University College London, and isolated a trihydroxyphenol, later called 'oestriol'. Kober (1931) developed a colour reaction for oestrogens in sulphuric acid and James Brown (1955), an ex pupil of Marrian's in Edinburgh, published his assay for oestrone, oestradiol and oestriol in urine.

Beischer *et al.* (1968) showed that oestriol excretion might be low in the absence of abnormal clinical signs and that low levels tended to predict subsequent fetal distress and asphyxial damage in surviving infants. Dickey *et al.* (1972) were able to predict 70% of growth retarded infants using oestriol measurements. Progesterone

the other steroid, was actively investigated but was not found to be as helpful as oestriol.

Ito and Higashi (1961) discovered human placental lactogen – a substance which provoked lactation in laboratory animals, and Josimovich and MacLaren (1962) showed that placental lactogen had features in common with pituitary growth hormone. Human placental lactogen levels were found to rise with advancing gestation. Letchworth and Chard (1972a) found that abnormal levels were associated with poor fetal outcome and Spellacy (1973) defined a fetal danger zone within which few normal values were found to occur.

During the 1970s hormonal tests of placental function were widely adopted. The measurement in maternal blood or urine of specific products of the feto-placental unit were thought to provide a valuable means of assessing the well-being of the child. A number of placental products were tested and used for a time. However, the introduction of fetal biophysical techniques in many units signalled the demise of biochemical testing. Geoffrey Chamberlain (1984) recorded that oestrogen assays for fetal monitoring had been abandoned in his hospital without any consequent rise in perinatal mortality. Human placental lactogen estimations suffered a similar fate.

Modern antenatal cardiotocography

Intrapartum observations on the relationship between the fetal heart rate pattern and uterine activity formed the basis for the contraction stress test (CST). In the non-labouring woman contractions were induced by administration of oxytocin, thus forming the basis of the oxytocin challenge test (OCT). Hammacher (1966a) studied 207 pregnancies and found that late decelerations in the antepartum period were associated with low Apgar scores at delivery. Seventeen of 23 stillbirths in their study manifested late decelerations antenatally. The first American study to evaluate the OCT was published by Ray *et al.* (1972) and was a prospective, blind evaluation, carried out on 66 patients. There were no fetal deaths within a week of a negative test. Of 15 fetuses with a positive test, there were three intrauterine deaths within 72 hours, and 40% of the live births with positive tests had low 5-minute Apgar scores. Slomka and Phelan (1981) noted that repetitive low decelerations were associated with persistence of that pattern in labour in up to 60% of cases.

As the OCT gained popularity, several investigators observed independently that when fetal movements were associated with accelerations the likelihood of fetal death was remote. Subsequently Lee *et al.* (1976) described their new test of fetal well-being which they called fetal activity determination. The test gained popularity and was later called the non-stress test (NST). The NST gained popularity and replaced the OCT as the primary method of cardiotocographic fetal assessment. A normal test was found to be associated with an acceptably low rate of fetal death within 7 days (Freeman, 1982; Phelan and Lewis, 1982). Antepartum cardiotocography became an integral part of the management of high-risk pregnancies.

Fetal biophysical profile

Manning *et al.* (1980) introduced additional surveillance techniques by including ultrasound fetal assessment with cardiotocography, and the resulting test was termed the 'biophysical profile'. Clinical testing of the concept of fetal biophysical profile scoring began with a prospective blind clinical study in 216 high-risk patients. By 1986 the series had expanded to over 19 000 patients and Manning was able to report a corrected perinatal mortality rate of less than 2 per 1000. Based on his fetal biophysical profile, a test score result of 10 out of 10 carried a perinatal mortality risk of less than 1 per 1000, within a week, without intervention.

Blood flow and Doppler studies

The Austrian physicist Johann Christian Doppler (1842) described the phenomenon whereby if a wave source is moving in relation to an observer the perceived wave frequency is different from the emitted frequency. This, the eponymously labelled 'Doppler effect', has been widely used in astronomy, radar and navigation. Satomura (1957) described ultrasonic Doppler methods for the inspection of cardiac function, in the *Journal of the Acoustical Society of America.*

Fitzgerald and Drumm (1977) of Dublin first applied Doppler ultrasound to obstetrics and its employment in the investigation of blood flow velocities made possible the non-invasive study of human fetal circulation dynamics. The Doppler signals obtained are of three types. The 'continuous wave' Doppler was essentially a fetal heart detector with the disadvantage of not being visualized at the time of study. In 1980 Eik-Nes described the first linear array duplex system where an off-set 'pulsed' Doppler was attached to a linear array imaging transducer (Eik-Nes *et al.*, 1980). 'Colour flow' equipment was introduced to fetal cardiology in 1987 by Kurjak *et al.* and appeared to offer major advantages over the other two methods for study of both the utero-placental and fetal circulations.

Various indices were devised to investigate the qualitative features of flow velocity wave forms. The 'resistance index' of Porcelot (1974); the 'pulsatility index' devised by Gosling and King (1974); and the 'A/B ratio' of Stuart *et al.* (1980), were all found to be very highly correlated when studied by Thompson *et al.* (1986). Doppler techniques were applied to both normal and abnormal pregnancies. Abnormal Doppler findings appeared to predate similar findings from standard methods of assessing fetal well-being, with the changes apparent days to weeks before delivery.

Clinical studies have been carried out on the umbilical vessels, the aorta, cerebral blood flow and the utero-placental bed. It was felt that there could be potential clinical uses for patients with multiple pregnancy, diabetes, post-dates pregnancy, rhesus disease and possibly as a general screening procedure. Knowledge of umbilical artery wave forms appeared to improve pregnancy management. The absence of end diastolic frequencies was found to be associated with a marked increase in both perinatal mortality and morbidity. Absent end diastolic frequency in the umbilical artery was associated with an 80% chance of hypoxia, and a 46% chance of acidosis. Results to date are encouraging but the place of umbilical artery flow velocity wave form analysis in obstetric practice is not yet clear.

CHRONOLOGY

History

1634 Ambroise Paré taught that the presence of fetal movements indicated whether the child in the womb was dead or alive.

1819 René Laennec invented the stethoscope (Rhodes, 1985).

1821 Kergaradec discovered that the fetal heart sounds could be auscultated by applying a stethoscope to the maternal abdomen.

1825 Stokes wrote the first Treatise in English on the use of the stethoscope.

1827   In the second edition of his Treatise of mediate auscultation, Laennec acknowledged that it was his friend Kergaradec who thought of applying Laennec's technique of auscultation to the study of pregnancy.

1830   John C. Ferguson was the first to use mediate auscultation of the fetal heart in the British Isles, on a lady in the Dublin General Dispensary, in November of that year.

Nagle reported on the use of the stethoscope to detect twins *in utero*. Collins the then Master of the Rotunda, had been persuaded to use the stethoscope by John C. Ferguson who later became Professor of Medicine in Belfast.

1833   Evory Kennedy of the Rotunda Hospital Dublin, recognized that abnormal fetal heart rate patterns indicated poor fetal well-being, and wrote his book *Observation on Obstetric Auscultation.*

1836   John Moir of Edinburgh, wrote in Hamilton's *Practical Observations on Midwifery,* on the effect of uterine contractions on the fetal heart.

1838   Naegele described fetal heart auscultation in German.

1843   Bodson described fetal heart irregularities.

1855   J.Y. Simpson described slowing of the fetal heart.

1866   Fleetwood Churchill used forceps to expedite delivery when there was 'weakening of the fetal heart'.

1876   McClintock noted poor fetal outcome in association with fetal heart slowing.

1886   Alfred Lewis Galabin suggested a good outcome could be expected if when the fetus moved, its heart rate increased by 20 beats per minute.

1888   Jaggard suggested that fetal bradycardia following Braxton Hicks contractions signified asphyxia and observed that this sign was associated with a 'puny' fetus.

1893   Von Winckel described the association of a slow fetal heart rate with poor neonatal results.

1908   Hastings Tweedie and G.T. Wrench (Rotunda Hospital Dublin) introduced the term 'fetal distress' (Pinkerton, 1976).

Early developments

1903   Einthoven first published his work on the adult electrocardiograph (ECG) using the string galvanometer.

1906   Cremer obtained a fetal ECG (FECG) with one abdominal electrode at the maternal uterine fundus and one in the vagina.

1930   Although a few isolated reports of FECGs were noted in the previous 20 years, it was not until the application of the radio-valve amplifier by Maekawa and Toyoshima that a reasonable degree of amplification became available, and the detection of the small fetal signal a practical proposition.

1934   Easby demonstrated the FECG on a patient who was 18 weeks pregnant.

1938   Strassman and Mussey attempted to assess the clinical significance of FECGs. At the Glasgow Royal Materniity Hospital, Bell was the first to record twin FECG complexes using a valve amplifier and balanced differential input.

1941   Dressler and Mokowitz described clinical information derived from a study of combined maternal and FECG traces. It became clear however, that it was necessary to free the trace of maternal elements. This was eventually achieved by either cancellation or gating.

Later developments

1948   Reynolds *et al.* first described an external tocodynamometer for recording uterine contractions.

1952   Williams and Stallworthy introduced the modern type of intrauterine catheter.

1953   Smyth described a series of cases using an improved valve amplifier.

1957   Hon and Hess described a cancellation system.

1960   Hunter *et al.* described an electrode which could be attached to the fetal scalp.

1961   Sureau and Trocellier described satisfactory results with two-channel cancellation.

107

1962   Hess described radiotelemetry of a single channel fetal ECG.

Kendall *et al.* described their use of telemetry to transmit the fetal heart rate records.

1963   Hon described a fetal scalp electrode (a modified Michelle surgical skin clip) which was applied vaginally and used to record the fetal heart rate electronically (1963b).

1966   Offner and Moisland introduced 'gating' techniques.

Favret and Marchetti described the removal of maternal elements from the trace by using a large digital computer.

1967   Kitahama and Sasaoka introduced the first spiral fetal scalp electrode.

1968   Hon classified fetal heart decelerations as three types, i.e. Early, Late and Variable decelerations.

Hammacher *et al.* classified short-term variability.

Tazawa *et al.* found that the fetal scalp ECG could be recorded by telemetry.

1970   Neuman *et al.* were able to transmit both the fetal heart rate and intrauterine pressure using a two-channel system of telemetry.

1971   de Haan *et al.* noted that fetal sleep, or the administration of sedative drugs to the mother could result in decreased variability.

Beard *et al.* considered that early decelerations were due to head compression and were not usually ominous (1971a).

Cordero and Hon reported an incidence of 0.3% fetal scalp infection from electronic fetal monitoring.

1972   Tatano categorized responses of 50 postpartum women to electronic fetal monitoring; initially 62% were negative, but only 12% of follow-up responses were negative.

Manseau *et al.* reported 'sinusoidal' patterns which were characterized by a regular undulating trace, fluctuating with a range of 5–15 beats per minute, and occurring every 15–30 seconds.

Hon introduced a disposable spiral scalp electrode.

1976   Gabbe and Hon noted that baseline variability had two components.

1976   Flynn and Kelly monitored the fetal heart by radiotelemetry.

Renou *et al.* showed the benefits of electronic fetal monitoring in high-risk patients.

Bernstein *et al.* measured pre-ejection periods of the fetal heart during labour.

1978   Kelso *et al.* failed to show any statistically significant fall in perinatal death in patients who had electronic fetal monitoring.

1979   Banta and Thacker concluded that electronic fetal monitoring resulted in a doubling of the Caesarean section rate.

1981   Johnson *et al.* reported that sinusoidal patterns might be present in fetal anaemia. Ingermarsson *et al.* reported that following the introduction of electronic fetal monitoring the incidence of low Apgar scores decreased significantly.

1987   Raymond and Whitfield reviewed the work carried out on systolic time intervals of the fetal cardiac cycle.

Fetal electrocardiography (FECG)

1906   Cremer recorded the first fetal electrocardiogram by using external electrodes applied to the abdomen of the pregnant woman.

1942   Tarnover and Lattin reported a case of A/V nodal tachycardia diagnosed before birth.

1952   Garvin and Kline diagnosed supraventricula tachycardia from FECG before birth.

1953   Smyth first described the use of an electrode applied directly to the fetus.

1956   Sureau first described a scalp electrode held manually on the fetus.

1957   Southern was the first of several authors to claim that meaningful analysis of the abdominal traces of FECG could be made. Southern found in cases of fetal distress that the P wave was increased, the PR segment lengthened, and the ST segment isoelectric or depressed.

1960 Hunter *et al.* clipped an electrode directly to the fetus, to record the fetal heart.

Hon and Hess reviewed the publications which claimed accuracy in the diagnosis of presentation of the fetus as noted by FECG polarity

Smith *et al.* recognized the persistently slow regular heart rate of congenital heart block.

Larks published the first of his series of papers on the relationship of fetal QRS complexes associated with fetal distress.

Hunter *et al.* described an electrode that could be clipped and retained on the fetal scalp, through the cervix. A similar electrode was placed on the perineum and a third was attached to the patient's right leg.

1961 The earliest recording in pregnancy of the FECG from abdominal leads was at 11 weeks' gestation (Larks).

1962 Larks *et al.* diagnosed triplets by FECG.

Larks and Anderson published proposals on FECG waveforms as predictors of fetal condition.

Larks and Longo and subsequent workers showed that mechanical interference e.g. cord or skull compression, caused slowing of FECG rate.

1963 Cox *et al.* demonstrated that by measuring the interval between two fetal R waves an instantaneous fetal heart rate estimation could be obtained electronically.

Hon placed the second ECG lead in the vagina thereby relieving the discomfort of a perineal clip (1963b).

Hon and Lee recorded the FECG in a 25-week aborting fetus; changes in waveforms occurred very late and even a few minutes prior to death long spells of normal ECG records could be obained.

1964 Friedman and Eckerling diagnosed quadruplets by FECG.

1965 Hellman and Fillisty noted that atropine caused an increase in the fetal heart rate.

1966 Caldeyro-Barcia *et al.* examined the possibility of prognostic information in the FECG waveform (1966b).

1970 Reed *et al.* demonstrated that the Venacaval Obstruction Syndrome caused maternal hypotension and fetal bradycardia.

1972 Hon *et al.* introduced a spiral electrode for application to the fetal scalp.

1976 Ghosh and Tipton described their 4 years' experience with the Copeland clip electrode.

Fetal phonocardiography (FPCG)

1908 Hofbauer and Weis introduced the FPCG.

1953 Gunn and Wood reported the first recorded analysis of FPCG.

1966 Hammacher described his FPCG machine (1966a).

1969 Hammacher helped to design a phonocardiograph which was later commercially developed by Hewlett-Packard and he also extensively reviewed the results of its clinical application.

Huntingford and Pendleton reviewed the phonocardiographic method and confirmed its use in clinical practice.

Ultrasonic fetal cardiotocography

1958 Donald *et al.* began to use pulsed ultrasound in obstetrics.

1959 Hon developed a presentation in which the fetal heart rate was plotted against time on a paper-strip recorder.

1961 Caldeyro-Barcia also developed paper-strip recording of fetal heart traces

1964 The earliest description of an ultrasonic Doppler device was by Callagan *et al.* from the Bethesda National Naval Medical Centre.

1966 Bishop described a commercial instrument called the Doptone (Smith-Kline Instruments, USA).

1968 Bang and Holm described a method for the demonstration of fetal heart movement in early pregnancy.

Brown and Robertson raised the question of safety to the fetus during prolonged use of ultrasound for monitoring the fetal heart.

109

Fielder described the first British instrument (Sonicaid) using the Doppler effect and Brown and Robertson described the Ultradop (Ames Ltd., USA).

The linking of Doppler devices with automated fetal monitoring was described by Bishop.

1971 Shelley showed that the total area of fetal heart rate slowing over an hour of labour was highly predictive of neonatal outcome.

Abdulla *et al.* found no detrimental effect to the fetus from prolonged exposure to ultrasound.

Fetal electroencephalography (FEEG)

1875 Caton first documented the electrical energy of the brain wave from studies on rabbits.

1929 Berger successfully demonstrated the human brain wave.

1937 Jasper *et al.* reported early studies in fetal electroencephalography in their work on the fetal guinea-pig.

1955 Bernstine *et al.* reported the use of both abdominal and vaginal electrodes for recording FEEG.

1965 Rosen and Satran reported recording FEEG during labour, using metal scalp clip electrodes.

1981 Weller *et al.* recorded the FEEG during labour using a newly developed electrode.

Sorokin *et al.* showed that certain patterns on the electroencephalogram are related to the development of neurological disorders after birth.

Modern antepartum cardiotocography (CTG)

1957 Duncan noted that hypoxia as a stress test had been suggested by Meyerscough in the early 1940s.

1961 Hellman *et al.* wrote on the administration of gas mixtures to the mother as another form of stress test.

1962 The history of modern antepartum monitoring of the fetal heart rate to assess fetal condition dates from this time, when Hammacher (1962) published his first and preliminary clinical experience (Kubli *et al.* 1977).

1963 Cox classified fetal heart rates relating anoxia to tachycardia, bradycardia and irregularity.

The concept of fetal distress extending back to the antenatal period was detailed in a classification by Gruenwald.

1966 Caldeyro-Barcia *et al.* (and Hon and Quilligan in 1967) described the type 2 or late decelerations of the fetal heart rate (1966b).

Hammacher was first to demonstrate the fact that inducing uterine contractions stresses the latently compromised fetus (1966b).

1967 Hon (and later Schiffrin and Dame in 1972) found that deviations in the heart rate could predict low Apgar scores with only an accuracy of 30–50%.

1968 Hon and Quilligan observed a relationship between fetal heart rate patterns and the fetal condition.

1969 Kubli, Kaeser and Hinselmann used stress testing. Late decelerations, persistent tachycardia, and a loss of beat to beat fluctuation, were considered abnormal.

Pose *et al.* helped to develop the oxytocin stress test.

1971 Kubli developed a scoring system for antenatal fetal heart rate.

Spurrett found that positive tests correlated highly with stillbirth, growth retardation and fetal depression at birth.

Sanchez-Ramos *et al.* found that in 98 high-risk patients there were no fetal deaths within a week of a negative test.

1972 Ray *et al.* reported the first American study to evaluate the oxytocin challenge test. There were no fetal deaths within a week of a negative test. Of 15 fetuses with a positive test, three had intrauterine deaths within 72 hours of the test. If late decelerations did not occur a low incidence of fetal demise could be expected and 40% of the live births with postive tests had low 5-minute Apgar scores.

Kubli *et al.* found that decelerations which were either late or atypically variable and severe reduction of the amplitude of long-term irregularity, were consistent signs of impending fetal death. However, abnormalities of baseline rate were not consistent.

Goodlin and Schmidt noted the presence of accelerations, and related them to fetal outcome. Lack of accelerations was an ominous sign.

1973 Myers *et al.* showed that hypoxia alone caused late decelerations.

1974 Simmonds took the view that the precise relationship between contractions and decelerations on antenatal CTG were unimportant.

Hammacher *et al.* published an antenatal CTG scoring system.

Baillie evolved a hypoxia stress test but the potential hazard was such that the test was unacceptable for general use.

1975 Paul *et al.* showed that loss of fetal heart rate variability was closely associated with acidosis, especially in the presence of late decelerations.

Lee *et al.* found that when fetal movements were associated with accelerations, the likelihood of fetal death was remote.

1976 Fischer *et al.* (1976), Meyer-Menk *et al.* (1976a, b), and Visser and Huisjes (1977) published scoring systems for antenatal CTGs.

Lee *et al.* introduced a fetal activity determination (FAD) test, later called the non-stress test (NST) and this eventually replaced the contraction stress (oxytocin challenge) test as the primary method of fetal assessment.

1977 Lewis *et al.* showed that the systolic time interval (STI) of the cardiac cycle was of value in predicting cardiovascular malfunction.

1978 Pearson and Weaver evaluated cardiotocography and introduced a scoring system.

1979 The presence of fetal heart rate accelerations associated with fetal movements indicated an intact response of the central nervous system (Paul and Keegan).

Manning and Platt noted that a non-reactive predelivery non-stress test, predicted fetal distress for 31% of patients.

1980 Manning *et al.* added further surveillance techniques and introduced the biophysical profile scoring system.

1981 Slomka and Phelan found that repetitive late decelerations were associated with a persistence of that pattern in labour in up to 60% of cases.

1982 Dawes *et al.* observed that in any 30-minute recording, the fetal heart rate shows at least 10 minutes high variation in over 80% of cases.

Freeman found that a normal antepartum cardiotocograph is associated with acceptably low rate of fetal death within 7 days.

1987 Smith and Paul pointed out that a fetus with reactive non-stress test or negative contraction stress test had a perinatal mortality rate of only 2–5 per 1000.

Fetal health and maturity assessment

1946 McBurney and Western presented the first description of the 'small-for-dates' fetus.

1953 Rumbolz and McGoogan demonstrated the close association between reduced growth of the uterine fundus and intrauterine fetal growth retardation.

1957 Blair Hartley documented the relationship of bony centres of ossification to fetal maturity.

1966 Brosens and Gordon introduced the Nile blue sulphate test in cytological examination of liquor amnii. As fetal skin matures the proportion of desquamated fetal cells in the liquor which contain fat increases. The fat containing cells stain orange, and the percentage of those cells in the sample was taken as an index of fetal maturity.

1967 Pitkin and Zwirek introduced liquor creatinine concentration as a method of testing fetal maturity.

1968 Beischer *et al.* showed that oestriol excretion tended to predict subsequent fetal distress.

Campbell introduced ultrasonic measurements of the biparietal diameter of the fetal head to assess fetal growth.

1970 Beazley and Underhill demonstrated that clinical assessment of the uterine size in relation to abdominal landmarks showed wide variation between women and was not an accurate method of estimating fetal maturity.

Elder *et al.* noted a significant association between the combination of static or falling weight and girth measurements, and the occurrence of a light-for-dates baby.

1971 Winick noted that there is permanent loss of cells, and that the fetal brain is not spared in cases of symmetrical growth-retardation caused by viral infection or chromosomal anomalies.

Gluck *et al.* showed that lecithin concentrations in the liquor increase steeply towards term.

Borer *et al.* introduced a lecithin sphingomyelin area ratio (LSAR).

Where Naegele's rule is applied, Beazley and Underhill demonstrated that in 22% of patients it was not possible to predict the estimated delivery date accurately.

Lind and Billewicz performed biochemical and cytological examination of the amniotic fluid and developed a scoring system to assess fetal maturity.

Gluck *et al.* found that fetal pulmonary maturity could be assessed by quantitative assay of lecithin in liquor amnii, and introduced the lecithin sphingomyelin

(L/S) ratio in amniotic fluid (see also Borer *et al.*).

1972 Dickey *et al.* studied total urinary oestrogen excretion and were able to predict 70% of growth-retarded infants.

Letchworth and Chard found similar results using human placental lactogen and claimed values were predictive of fetal asphyxia (1972a).

Campbell and Kurjak reported that only 30% of growth-retarded babies were diagnosed as such in the antenatal period by clinical means.

Clements *et al.* described the 'bubble test' technique of assessing the concentration of pulmonary surfactant in liquor.

Whitfield *et al.* showed that if the concentration of lecithin in the liquor exceeds 3.5 mg per 100 ml, or the LSAR is greater than 2, respiratory distress is extremely unlikely to occur.

Bennett noted that hormone assays and ultrasonic measurements were widely used to detect fetal compromise but their interpretation depended on knowledge of the gestational age, which was doubtful in up to 40% of patients (Bennett, 1974).

Bennett calculated the uterine volume by clinical means. He found a significant difference between normal weight for gestation and light-for-dates infants from as early as the 32nd week of pregnancy.

1973 Robinson showed that measuring the crown–rump length of the fetus before the 12th week of pregnancy is an accurate method of assessing gestational age.

Rhodes outlined a comprehensive list of 'at risk' pregnancies.

Assali and Brinkman pointed out the brain sparing effect which happens in asym-metrical growth retardation due to placental damage in later pregnancy.

1977 Westin showed that serial measurements of the symphysis–fundus distance, when plotted on an experimentally derived nomogram (gravidogram), were superior to both human placental lactogen and urinary oestriol in detecting growth retardation.

Carrera and Barri indicated that asymmetrical growth-retarded babies have a head to thorax or abdomen ratio of greater than unity.

Myers stated that the use of dextrose infusions in the presence of fetal asphyxia could precipitate fetal cerebral oedema and brain necrosis due to lactate accumulation in the fetal brain.

1979 Varma and colleagues found the head to abdomen area ratio could identify growth retardation in about 80% of cases in late pregnancy. Small-for-dates infants were usually only clearly distinguishable from 33 weeks on.

Spellacy reviewed the world literature and found that human placental lactogen tended to be low in conditions of poor intrauterine growth.

1980   The fetal biophysical score was introduced by Manning *et al.*

1982   Calvert *et al.* devised a chart of symphysis-fundus height based on Cardiff data.

Fetal movements and biophysical profile

1840   Cazeau observed a startle response by the fetus when slapping the uterus.

1905   Ahlfeld evaluated the different types of human fetal movement. Although further work was carried out on animals, fetal movement was treated primarily as a sign of fetal life until the early 1960s. Fetal movements as observed by the mother, electromechanical techniques, and active recording systems were all investigated.

1925   Peiper, a German researcher, demonstrated that the *in utero* fetus responded to sound as early as the 26th week.

1932   Ray recorded fetal movements via a tambour strapped to the maternal abdomen.

1936   Sontag and Wallace noted that the fetus responded to sound.

1965   Rovinsky and Guttmacher suggested that fetal movements were an expression of fetal well-being.

1971   Grimwalde *et al.* showed that 50% of fetuses exhibited fetal heart rate accelerations associated with movement when exposed to an externally applied sound.

1972   Matthews noted that reduced fetal movements were associated with development of intrapartum fetal distress.

1973   Sadovski *et al.* reported good correlation between maternal appreciation of fetal movement and objective assessments. They made the important observation that fetal movements decreased or stopped 12 – 48 hours before the fetal heart ceased to beat.

Sadovski and Yaffe concluded that subjective assessment of fetal movements by the mother provided valuable information regarding the state of the fetus.

1974   Pearson suggested that decreased fetal movements of fewer than ten per 12 hours bear a significant correlation with fetal jeopardy.

The fetus was shown to respond to light by Boddy *et al.*

1975   Polishuk *et al.* noted that the fetus responded to light stimulus.

1976   Pearson and Weaver introduced fetal movement counting to the UK and showed that maternal fetal movement counting was as good a test as oestriol measurements. They published a range of fetal activity as measured by the decreased fetal movement charts (DFMC) and this showed that about 2.5% of DFMCs in women who subsequently gave birth to healthy infants fell below ten movements per 12 hours.

Timor-Tritch *et al.* classified fetal movements as rolling, simple movements, high frequency hiccup-like movements or respiratory movements. A tocodynamometer was used to record fetal movements.

1977   Pearson recommended a 'count to ten' method of assessing fetal activity.

1978   Birnholz *et al.* noted 11 separate spontaneous fetal movement patterns in clinically normal women.

Trudinger *et al.* used a longitudinal ultrasound scan to observe fetal movement.

1979   Sadovski *et al.* found that normal daily fetal movements ranged widely from about 50 to nearly 1000.

Hertogs *et al.* showed that very few major fetal movements involving limbs and trunk were not appreciated by the mother.

Roberts *et al.* introduced the concept of total fetal activity.

1980   Manning and Platt devised a biophysical profile based on five variables i.e. fetal breathing movements, fetal body movements, CTG, fetal tone and amniotic fluid volume.

1981   Marsal reviewed major studies relating to human fetal activity and fetal condition.

1982   Patrick *et al.* showed that fetal activity displayed a diurnal rhythm, with a peak in the hours around midnight.

Liston *et al.*, using the 'Count to Ten' chart, found that pregnancies in which there were fewer than ten movements in 12 hours were associated with a significant increase in perinatal mortality, fetal distress and fetal compromise.

Fetal breathing movements (FBM)

1543   Vesalius observed FBM in pigs.

1787   Winslowius reported rhythmic breathing activity.

1813   Beclard noted rhythmic breathing activity in fetal animals.

1882   Preyer reported on fetal breathing activity.

1888   Ahlfeld made recordings of FBM using a funnel and tambour kymograph.

1938   Bonar *et al.* studied fetal respiratory movements in historical and present day perspective.

1970   Dawes *et al.* reported on their observations of FBM in the fetal lamb.

1971   Boddy and Robinson evolved an ultrasonic method for detection of fetal chest wall movements during the antenatal period.

1972   Boddy and Mantell suggested that FBM *in utero* provided an indication of fetal health.

1974   Boddy *et al.* noted periodicity of FBM. Periodicity was seen to vary with sleep state and the time of the day.

1975   Genser *et al.* found maternal smoking caused a reduction in fetal breathing incidence by 30%.

Boddy *et al.* reported apnoea and gasping in ten of eleven fetuses, 48–72 hours prior to intrauterine death (Griffin, 1984).

1976   Patrick *et al.* noted that fetal breathing was suppressed prior to fetal death.

1977   Wladimiroff *et al.* showed that maternal hyperventilation caused reduction in fetal breathing.

1978   Platt *et al.* showed that if FBM were present in the last test before delivery, the incidence of fetal depression was very low. If FBM were absent, depressed infants were born in 50% of cases.

Lewis *et al.* noted that there was a marked increase in FBM following maternal administration of glucose.

Fetal breathing and its possible clinical significance was extensively reviewed by Wilds.

1979   Richardson *et al.* noted that the incidence of FBM falls during labour, irrespective of sedatives or other factors.

Trudinger *et al.* reported an improvement in the positive predictive value of breathing studies by including an analysis of breathing rate and variability of breath to breath intervals.

1980   Manning and Platt noted that a reactive CTG is as effective as ultrasonic observation of total fetal movement or FBM.

Ritchie and Lakhani noted that maternal hyperoxia had no effect on breathing incidence of normally grown healthy human fetuses (1980a).

Ritchie and Lakhani noted that fetal breathing increased in response to 5% CO_2 (1980b).

1981   Ritchie and Dornan found in the growth-retarded fetus that a reduced incidence of breathing may return to or exceed normal values following administration of 50% oxygen to the mother.

Trudinger confirmed that the breathing rate in normal fetuses becomes slower and more regular with increasing fetal maturity.

Ultrasound

1958   Donald *et al.* first introduced pulsed echo ultrasonic diagnosis to obstetrics.

1961   Donald and Brown demonstrated their use of the contact scanner, so called because the transducer was directly in contact with the skin of the maternal abdomen.

Donald and Brown first described fetal cephalometry by ultrasound.

1963   Holmes and Howry of Denver developed ultrasound techniques in the USA.

1969   Campbell introduced ultrasonic measurement of the biparietal diameter to predict fetal maturity.

1971 Campbell and Newman determined the growth rate of the normal fetal head.

1972 Campbell and Kurjak compared serial ultrasonic cephalometry and urinary oestrogen estimations; and ultrasound was found to be significantly better at diagnosing the small-for-dates fetus.

1973 Robinson introduced sonar measurements of fetal crown–rump length as a means of assessing fetal maturity in the first trimester of pregnancy.

Hansmann and Voigt determined abdominal circumference measurements.

1980 Neilson *et al.* extended ultrasonic examination to 34 or 36 weeks to detect small-for-dates infants.

1981 Manning *et al.* reported on the evaluation of amniotic fluid volume by ultrasound and its relationship to intrauterine growth retardation.

1983 Grannum classified the variable appearance of the placenta throughout pregnancy and noted four grades from immature to mature.

1984 Chamberlain *et al.* further assessed the amniotic fluid volume relationship to perinatal outcome.

In a controlled study, Neilson *et al.* detected 94% of growth retarded fetuses by ultrasonic examination.

1985 Phelan *et al.* reported higher Caesarean section rates for fetal distress, meconium stained fluid and depressed 5-minute Apgar scores in patients with decreased amniotic fluid volume.

Hobbins *et al.* introduced percutaneous umbilical blood sampling under direct ultrasound guidance to obtain fetal blood sampling for rapid karyotyping, and the technique was further used by Daffos *et al.* in France and Nicolaides and colleagues in England in 1986.

1986 The safety of ultrasound was reviewed by a Royal College of Obstetricians and Gynaecologists working party.

1987 The British Institute of Radiology reviewed the safety of ultrasound (Wells, 1987).

Blood flow and Doppler studies

1774 Sabatier described the theory of the preferential distribution of oxygenated blood from the placenta to the left side of the heart.

1842 Doppler first reported that as an observer approaches a stationary source of light the emitted frequency appears to increase. This was later called the Doppler shift.

1843 Buys Ballot described a Doppler shift effect with sound waves.

1934 Barcroft, Flexner and McClurkin described the fetal circulatory pathway by carrying out radiographic studies on the fetal goat.

1951 Greenfield *et al.* first reported attempts to quantify human fetal umbilical blood flow on an exteriorized 15-week fetus.

1954 Lind and Wegelius described the arterial and venous blood trajectory in the human fetus using cardiographic techniques.

1957 Satomura described his investigation of the human circulation with Doppler.

1960 Assali *et al.* carried out flow measurements on 12 fetuses.

1964 Stembera *et al.* carried out haemodilution techniques to determine blood flow directly after birth in term neonates.

1967 Brosens and *et al.* found that in normal pregnancy the trophoblast invades the placental bed and migrates the entire length of the spiral arteries by about the 20th postmenstrual week.

1970 Baker noted that if the pulse repetition frequency is less than half the Doppler shifted frequency an artefact known as 'aliasing' occurs.

1974 McDonald described the distribution of velocities of fluid flowing in a long straight smooth-sided, non-branching tube.

Porcelot introduced the 'resistance index'.

Gosling and King used the 'pulsatility index' to characterize qualitative flow.

1976 Coghlan and Taylor developed the real time spectrum analyser to quantify Doppler frequencies and present them visually in real time.

Brosens *et al.* found failure of invasion by the trophoblast to the myometrial portion of the spiral artery, in placental bed biopsies obtained from patients with pregnancy induced hypertension.

Fitzgerald and Drumm first reported the non-invasive investigation of the fetal circulation by Doppler ultrasound.

1979 Kaufman *et al.* found that the tertiary stem villi are seen in increasing numbers from about the 30th week of gestation.

1980 Stuart *et al.* devised the A/B ratio, the peak systolic frequency to end diastolic frequency.

Eik-Nes *et al.* introduced the linear array duplex system with ultrasound and pulsed Doppler.

1981 Wladimiroff and McGhie calculated fetal left ventricular volumes from a study of two dimensional measurements of real time ultrasonic images of the left ventricle.

Jouppila *et al.* found umbilical vein velocities to be unrecordable in a significant number of growth-retarded fetuses in their study.

Rodeck *et al.* investigated the relationships of fetal blood flow after intravascular fetal transfusion.

Gill *et al.* reported a reduction in umbilical venous flow in six out of ten fetuses with intrauterine growth retardation.

1983 Campbell *et al.* described the 'frequency index profile'.

Griffin *et al.* calculated measurement of angles of insonation.

Campbell *et al.* first reported the use of flow velocity waveforms from the utero-placental circulation in complicated pregnancies.

1984 Joupilla and Kirkinen demonstrated a significant negative correlation between umbilical vein blood flow and the cord haemoglobin level.

Reuwer studied a group of 20 pregnancies with severe intrauterine growth retardation and found that absence of frequencies in end diastole were associated with those fetuses most at risk of intrauterine death or severe fetal asphyxia (1984a).

Schulman *et al.* reported intrauterine death occurring after normal Doppler results in non-compromised fetuses.

1985 Erskine and Ritchie reported intrauterine death following abnormal Doppler results.

Giles *et al.* reported on umbilical artery waveforms in twin pregnancies (1985).

Trudinger *et al.* reported abnormal utero-placental flow velocity waveforms in small-for-dates infants (1985a,b).

Teague *et al.* further developed the duplex scanner system.

1986 Trudinger *et al.* reported that abnormal Doppler results identified fetal compromise more effectively when compared to cardiotocography. They also found that abnormal waveform patterns preceded abnormal fetal heart traces.

1987 Rochelson *et al.* reported that lack of end diastolic flow was a sign of fetal compromise and that there was an increased incidence of abnormal antenatal cardiotocographs when Doppler studies were abnormal (1987a,b).

Raymond and Whitfield, in their review of systolic time intervals of the fetal cardiac cycle, noted that with improvement in technology the pre-ejection period or the ventricular ejection time may prove to be of value in the detection of fetal compromise, particularly in the patient with accurate dates.

Kurjak *et al.* introduced colour flow mapping to fetal cardiology.

1988 Nicolaides *et al.* found a very high incidence of acidosis and hypoxia as determined at cordocentesis, in pregnancies complicated by absent end diastolic flow.

Gudmundsson and Marsal reported an increase in the incidence of operative delivery for fetal distress in Doppler abnormal patients.

Beattie *et al.* in a large prospective double-blind study of 2097 pregnancies suggested that umbilical artery flow velocity waveforms was not a useful screening test in a low-risk population.

Dempster *et. al* reported on increased incidence of fetal distress in labour, in a Doppler abnormal group.

Biochemical methods

1927 Aschheim and Zondek discovered a protein hormone secreted by the placenta which was subsequently named chorionic gonadotrophin.

1930 Guy Marrian isolated oestriol from pregnancy urine.

1931 Kober developed a colour reaction test for oestrogens.

1955 Brown described the method of isolating 24-hour urinary oestrogen.

1961 Ito and Higashi discovered a second placental protein which provoked lactation in laboratory animals. The substance was ultimately named human placental lactogen.

1962 Josimovich and MacLaren showed that the placental lactogen protein had features in common with pituitary growth hormone.

1968 Beischer *et al.* published normal ranges of urinary oestriol levels in pregnancy.

Klopper noted that there were wide normal limits of variation for urinary oestrogen excretion in pregnancy.

1969 Sadovski *et al.* and others used heat stable alkaline phosphatase measurements as a measure of placental function.

Klopper found that the trend of serial estimations of urinary oestrogens was more meaningful than absolute values.

Saxena *et al.* observed that levels of maternal serum human placental lactogen showed close correlation with both fetal and placental weight.

Spellacy reviewed the work carried out on human placental lactogen, in the past decade.

1972 Barnard and Logan emphasized that statistical significance is not the same as clinical significance, as noted for instance with urinary oestriols.

Letchworth and Chard reported on human placental lactogen levels in patients with pre-eclampsia and showed that human placental lactogen estimation had a prognostic ability as regards fetal well-being (1972b).

Beischer and Brown reviewed the then current status of oestrogen assays in obstetrics and gynaecology and commented that 'fetal mortality and morbidity were found to have a significant correlation with low oestriol excretion'.

1973 Mathur *et al.* demonstrated a highly significant correlation with urinary and plasma oestriols.

Low levels of human placental lactogen were reported prior to death by Ward *et al.*

Spellacy designated a fetal danger zone where few normal human placental lactogen levels occurred.

1976 Spellacy found that human placental lactogen was synthesized and stored in the syncytiotrophoblast cells of the placenta.

1980 Goebelsman wrote that daily oestriol assays were mandatory for fetal surveillance in (diabetic) pregnancies.

1984 Geoffrey Chamberlain observed that oestrogen assays for fetal monitoring had been abandoned at his hospital without any consequent rise in perinatal mortality.

Uterine activity and labour

1759 The existence of a uterine labour force was noted by Laurence Sterne in *Tristram Shandy*, Book 11 (Reynolds *et al.*,1954).

1872 Schatz recorded intrauterine pressures in labour with water-filled balloons.

1896 Schaeffer devised an external tocodynamometer.

1927 Bourne and Burn first suggested that the uterine activity required in labour to expel the fetus is best represented by the pressure exerted by contractions and their duration.

1948 Reynolds *et al.* described a multi-channel tocodynamometer.

1950 Caldeyro-Barcia *et al.* reported using a transabdominal open-ended internal catheter and seven-channel recorder to measure the external pressure from various areas over the uterus.

1952 Williams and Stallworthy described their use of intrauterine pressure cathethers.

1954 Friedman described his graphic labour record, consisting of a cervicograph with added clinical comments.

1955 Caldeyro-Barcia *et al.* introduced the 'Montevideo' unit which was a manual method of quantifying uterine activity.

1959 Rosa and Ghilain used simple graphic labour records.

1960 Lish *et al.* showed that β-sympathomimetic agents are effective in reducing uterine activity.

1963 Hon provided the basic terms to describe fetal heart rate patterns in labour (1963a).

1964 Bishop quantified cervical ripeness by assessing the cervical dilatation, effacement, consistency, position of the cervix in the pelvis and station of the presenting part. A score was allocated to each of the five parameters.

1965 Rodesch *et al.* in Brussels changed from using 'fingers' of dilatation to one, two, and five francs, along a linear centimetre scale.

1966 Caldeyro-Barcia *et al.* explored the relationship between uterine activity and fetal heart rate pattern (1966a,b).

1967 Friedman reported his detailed study of over 10 000 labours, and found that labour could be divided into latent and active phases.

1968 Hon and Quilligan detailed their descriptive analysis of fetal heart rate patterns.

Caldeyro-Barcia *et al.* related pH to fetal heart rate patterns.

Hon published an atlas of fetal heart rate patterns.

Caledyro-Barcia *et al.* noted the lag time to recovery with late decelerations was in excess of 18 seconds.

1969 Hammacher classified fetal heart rate recordings.

1971 Shelley and Tipton correlated dip area in the hours prior to delivery with Apgar scores.

Beard *et al.* obtained false patterns when maternal tachycardia was present (1971a,b).

1972 Philpott introduced graphic labour records. Philpott in Salisbury Rhodesia, devised the composite labour record on which details of progress, fetal condition and maternal condition could be annotated on a single page against a time scale.

1973 Hon and Paul developed a concept of uterine acitivy units. This was later replaced by the uterine activity integral.

1975 Tutera and Newman noted hazards due to the use of intrauterine cathethers.

1978 Steer *et al.* introduced the transducer-tipped catheter for estimation of intrauterine pressure.

1984 Steer *et al.* found that the uterine activity integral bears a closer correlation to the rate of cervical dilatation than either the frequency or amplitude of uterine contraction.

Meconium

1858 Schwartz stated that meconium in the liquor was proof of a reduction in placental activity.

1918 Reed suggested that anoxia caused the anal sphincter to relax, and meconium to be passed *in utero.*

1956 Eastman postulated that anoxia weakens the tone of the anal sphincter.

1957 Desmond *et al.* found meconium staining was more common when the fetus was mature or if anoxia was present.

1959 Walker reported that fetuses with meconium passage had lower umbilical vein oxygen saturation than did normal term fetuses.

1968 Saling speculated that fetal hypoxia stimulated vasoconstriction of the gut with hyperperistalsis and subsequent passage of meconium.

1973 The reported perinatal mortality rate with meconium passage alone ranged from 1 to 13.5% (Mandelbaum).

1975   Miller *et al.* reported that Apgar scores were significantly lower in infants with meconium passage compared to a non-meconium group.

1976   Carson *et al.* quoted mortality rates for infants with meconium aspiration as 20 times the expected rate for term size infants. Routine intrapartum pharyngeal suctioning of infants with meconium staining significantly reduces the incidence and severity of meconium aspiration.

1978   Green and Paul reported a meconium incidence of 4.6% at 28 weeks, and 8% at 38 weeks, in patients undergoing amniocentesis.

Meis *et al.* noted that thick meconium, which was present in 25.2% of his cases, was associated with an increased risk of fetal acidosis and perinatal morbidity and mortality.

1979   Knox *et al.* reported that postdate pregnancies have a very high incidence of meconium passage.

1980   Starks reported a significantly higher rate of fetal heart rate abnormalities with meconium staining.

1985   MacDonald *et al.* found the perinatal mortality rate in infants with thick or moderately thick meconium, or where there was oligohydramnios, was 11.4 per 1000 compared to 2.1 per 1000 in those where there was clear amniotic fluid or only light meconium staining of an adequate volume of fluid.

Mitchell *et al.* found that meconium aspiration syndrome was more common if the infant was asphyxiated at any stage.

Acid–base

1912   Hasselbalch and Lundsgaard found that pCO_2 values in the blood of women in late pregnancy were lower than normal.

1915   Hasselbalch and Gammeltoft discovered that the low pCO_2 values were shown to be associated with maternal metabolic acidosis.

1916   Ylppo pioneered the investigation of fetal acid–base balance and recorded that by adult standards the cord blood of the fetus was acidotic.

1928   Blair Bell *et al.* published the first report on umbilical arterial and venous lactate concentrations at birth.

1929   Oard and Peters showed that maternal metabolic acidosis consisted of a reduction of about 5% of total base in the serum of women in late pregnancy.

1931   Eastman and McLane measured blood gas and acid–base components in cord blood. They discovered that asphyxiated babies had significantly higher lactate concentrations at delivery when compared with healthy ones.

1932   Eastman demonstrated a marked fall in cord pH in infants suffering from asphyxia neonatorum.

1956   Clarke devised an electrode to measure pO_2 transcutaneously.

1958   James *et al.* demonstrated that the degree of cord blood acidosis correlated well with the extent of neonatal depression.

James *et al.* first related abnormal pH, pO_2 and buffer base values to low Apgar scores and revealed that these parameters were better indices of neonatal condition than oxygen saturation.

1959   Vedra and later workers developed the concept of maternal infusion of the fetus with products of maternal metabolism, thereby causing fetal acidosis.

1961/64 Saling introduced fetal blood sampling and acid–base determination of the fetus in labour (1964a,b).

Quilligan *et al.* showed that both tachycardia and bradycardia are associated with fetal acidosis.

Huntingford, and later Morris and Beard (1965) further described techniques of fetal scalp blood sampling.

1965   Vector cardiography was studied by Larks showing a shift to the left of electrical axis of fetal heart with fetal acidosis.

1966   Beard *et al.* recorded fetal haemorrhage following scalp blood sampling.

1967   Kubli *et al.* showed that the pH was the easiest parameter to measure as well as being the one with the lowest methodological error, when compared to other biochemical parameters.

Wood *et al.* indicated that abnormal fetal heart rates normally precede pH changes.

Beard *et al.* showed that 92% of babies have an Apgar score greater than 7, when the pH at the time of delivery is in excess of 7.25.

1968 Saling found the average pH of the normal fetus throughout labour averages about 7.3.

Beard showed that evaluation of scalp pH allowed a more accurate diagnosis of fetal distress.

Kirschbaum and DeHaven reviewed the extensive studies which had been carried out to date on acid–base status of the fetus.

1969 Wood *et al.* found that the severity of fetal acidosis and the Apgar score were positively correlated.

1970 Symonds related fetal ECG changes to fetal biochemistry.

1971 Lumley, McKinnon and Wood determined the range of acid–base balance, in a review of the published work of 14 authors.

Beard *et al.* found the fetal scalp pH to be a more reliable indicator of hypoxia than the fetal heart pattern (1971a).

1972 Hull wrote on perinatal coagulopathy complicating fetal blood sampling.

1976 Stamm *et al.* reported on the possibility of recording continuous tissue pH measurement in neonates.

Haverkamp *et al.* in their study at the Denver General Hospital showed an increase in Caesarean sections for fetal distress, when continuous fetal heart monitoring without scalp pH estimation, was carried out.

1977 Huch *et al.* introduced continuous transcutaneous pO_2 measurements of the fetus during labour.

1978 Henner *et al.* applied a pH electrode to the fetus in labour.

1979 Weber and Hahn-Pederson found that the normal values for tissue pH obtained during continuous monitoring, were similar to those taken at intermittent sampling.

1980 Smyth and Soutter reported that pH lactate was the only useful biochemical measure of fetal asphyxia.

1986 Nicolaides *et al.* obtained ultrasound guided sampling of umbilical cord and placental blood to assess fetal acid–base status.

Outcome

1953 Virginia Apgar first proposed her neonatal assessment score.

1965 Honzik *et al.* examined infants with poor Apgar scores at 1 year of age. Apgar scores did not correlate well with the outcome, in individual cases.

1967 Richards and Roberts reviewed the 'at risk' registers, and demonstrated that no sequelae of hypoxia at birth, other than death could be demonstrated.

1970 Windle showed that hypoxia caused central nervous system damage in monkeys. The type of lesions however were not those associated with spasticity.

1976 Sarnat and Sarnat provided a classification of hypoxic ischaemic encephalopathy (HIE) – mild, moderate, and severe, according to clinical behaviour.

1977 Beard reviewed the work of Tutera and Newman in 1975 and of other investigators and concluded that continuous fetal heart rate monitoring appeared to have a favourable effect on perinatal outcome.

1978 Neutra *et al.* used concurrent non-randomized controls in a large study of electronic fetal monitoring versus intermittent auscultation. Electronic fetal monitoring appeared to be of no benefit to the majority of low-risk women but possibly of substantial benefit in the small number of women at high risk.

1979 Chalmers reviewed the work of Havercamp *et al.* (1976); Renou *et al.* (1976); Kelso *et al.* (1978) and Havercamp *et al.* (1979). Based on the above studies he stated that there was no evidence to support suggestions that intermittent auscultation should be replaced by continuous electronic monitoring in cases at lower risk of adverse perinatal outcome. Chalmers found that intensive fetal heart rate monitoring alone resulted in an increase in Caesarean sections.

Lower rates of intrapartum stillbirth, neonatal death and depressed Apgar scores were associated with electronic fetal monitoring as reported by the National Institutes of Health. The studies used historical controls.

The National Institutes of Health Consensus Document (USA) states that periodic auscultation of the fetal heart rate is an acceptable method of assessment of fetal condition for women at low risk of intrapartum fetal distress.

1981   Nelson and Ellenberg found that the Apgar score was a poor predictor of eventual outcome for the fetus.

1982   Dennis and Chalmers found that intractable neonatal seizures following birth asphyxia are the more severe examples of hypoxic ischaemic encephalopathy and are closely associated with long-term neurological handicap. They found that approximately 25% of infants with seizures in the first 48 hours of life die, 25% survive with moderate or severe handicap and 10% survive with mild handicap. The remaining 40% are normal.

1985   Grant and Chalmers reviewed three methods of comparing electronic fetal monitoring to intermittent auscultation – historical controls, concurrent non-randomized controls, and randomized controls.

MacDonald *et al.* reported on the Dublin randomized controlled trial of intrapartum fetal heart rate monitoring of over 12 000 women. This trial showed that the benefit of electronic fetal monitoring was in prevention of seizures in neonates. However at 1 and 4 years the number of cases with severe neurological damage amongst babies who survived seizures was similar in both the study and control groups.

1986   Nelson and Ellenberg reported that hypoxic events in labour contribute perhaps less than 10% to the total population of neurologically damaged infants. They stated that they did not know what caused most cases of cerebral palsy.

1987   MacDonald and Grant noted that six trials showed electronic fetal monitoring was followed by a dramatic increase in the Caesarean section rate unless used in conjunction with fetal scalp blood sampling.

REFERENCES

Abdulla, U., Campbell, S., Dewhurst, C.J., Talbert, D., Lucas, M. and Mullarkey, M. (1971) Effect of diagnostic ultrasound on maternal and fetal chromosomes. *Lancet,* **2,** 829–831

Adams-0'B. (1833). Observations on medical auscultation as a practical guide in difficult labours. *Dublin J. Med. Sci.,* **3,** 65

Ahlfeld, F. (1888). Uber bisher noch nicht beschriebene intrauterine bewegungen des kindes. *Verhandlungen der Deutschen Gesellschaft fur Gynaekologie,* **2,** 203–10

Ahlfeld, F. (1905). Die intrauterine Tatigkeit der Thorax-und Zwerchfellmuskulatur. Intra-uterine Atmung. *Monatsschrift fur Geburtshilfe Gynaekologie,* **21,** 143

Amiel-Tieson, C. (1969). Cerebral damage in full term newborns. Etiological factors, neonatal status and long term follow up. *Biol. Neonate,* **14,** 234–50

Apgar, V. (1953). A proposal for a new method of evaluation of the newborn infant. *Anaesth. Analg. (Cleve.),* **32,** 260–7

Aschheim, S. and Zondek, B. (1927). Hypophysen vorderlappenhormon und ovarialhormon in Harn von Schwangeren. *Klin. Wochenschr.,* **6,** 1322

Assali, N.S. and Brinkman, E.R. (1973). The role of circulatory buffers in fetal tolerance to stress. *Am. J. Obstet. Gynecol.,* **13,** 511

Assali, N.S., Rauramo, L. and Peltonen, T. (1960). Measurement of uterine blood flow and uterine metabolism. VIII. Uterine and fetal blood flow and oxygen consumption in early human pregnancy. *Am. J. Obstet. Gynecol.,* **79,** 86–98

Baillie, P. (1974). Non hormonal methods of antenatal monitoring. In Beard, R.W. (ed.) *Fetal Medicine: Clinical Obstetrics and Gynaecology,* p. 103. (London: W.B. Saunders C. Ltd.)

Baker (1970). Quoted by Pearse, J.M. (1987) Uteroplacental and fetal blood flow. In Whittle, M.J. (ed.) *Fetal Monitoring. Clinical Obstetrics and Gynaecology,* 1.1. p. 160. (London, Philadelphia: Baillière Tindall)

Bang, J. and Holm, H.H. (1968). Ultrasonics in the measurement of fetal heart movements. *Am. J. Obstet. Gynecol.,* **102,** 956–60

Banta, D.H. and Thacker, S.B. (1979). Costs and benefits of electronic fetal monitoring. *Obstet. Gynecol. Surv.,* **34,** 627–42

Barcroft, J., Flexner, L.B. and McClurkin, T. (1934). The output of the fetal heart in the goat. *J. Physiol.*, **82**, 498–508

Barnard, W.P. and Logan, R.W. (1972) The value of urinary oestriol estimation in predicting dysmaturity. *J. Obstet. Gynaecol. Br. Commonw.*, **79**, 1091–4

Beard, R.W. (1968) The effect of fetal blood sampling on caesarean section for fetal distress. *J. Obstet. Gynaecol. Br. Commonw.*, **75**, 1291–5

Beard, R.W. (1977). Is intrapartum monitoring worthwhile? In Beard, R. and Campbell, S. (eds.) *The Current Status of Fetal Heart Rate Monitoring and Ultrasound in Obstetrics*. Proceedings of the Scientific Meeting of the Royal College of Obstetricians and Gynaecologists, p. 2. (London: RCOG)

Beard, R.W., Morris, E.D. and Clayton, S.G. (1966). Haemorrhage following fetal blood sampling. *J. Obstet. Gynaecol. Br. Commonw.*, **73**, 860–1

Beard, R.W., Morris, E.D. and Clayton, S.G. (1967). pH of foetal capillary blood as an indicator of the conditon of the foetus. *J. Obstet. Gynaecol. Br. Commonw.*, **74**, 812–22

Beard, R.W., Filshie, G.M., Knight, C.A. and Roberts, G.M. (1971a). The significance of the changes in the continuous fetal heart rate in the first stage of labour. *J. Obstet. Gynaecol. Br. Commonw.*, **78**, 865–81

Beard, R.W., Brudenell, J.M., Feroze, R.M. and Clayton, S.G. (1971b). Intensive care of the high risk fetus in labour. *J. Obstet. Gynaecol. Br. Commonw.*, **78**, 882–93

Beattie, R.B., Dornan, J.C., Clements, C.W.A. and McGrath, B. (1988). Umbilical artery velocity waveform assessed as an antenatal screening tool for intrauterine growth and poor fetal outcome. *Br. J. Obstet. Gynaecol.*, **95**, 534–5

Beazley, J.M. and Underhill, R.A. (1970). Fallacy of the fundal height. *Br. Med. J.*, **4**, 404–6

Beazley, J.M. and Underhill, R.A. (1971). Confinement date unknown. *Nursing Times*, **67**, 1414–17

Beclard, P.A. (1813), quoted by Griffin, D. (1984). p. 96

Beischer, N.A. and Brown, J.B. (1972). Current status of estrogen assays in obstetrics and gynaecology. *Obstet. Gynecol., Surv.*, **27**, 303–43

Beischer, N.A., Bhargava, V.I., Brown, J.B. and Smith, N.A. (1968). The incidence and significance of low oestriol excretion in an obstetric population. *J. Obstet. Gynaecol. Br. Commonw.*, **75**, 1024–33

Bennett, M.J. (1972). *Antenatal gestational ageing*, M.D. Thesis. University of Capetown, quoted by Bennett (1974)

Bennett, M.J. (1974). Antenatal fetal monitoring. *Br. J. Hosp. Med.*, **12**, 27–32

Berger, H. (1929). Uber das Electroenkephalogramm des Menschen. *Archiv. Psychiatr. Nerven Krankheiten*, **87**, 527–70

Bernstein, A., Organ, L.W., Eisner, L.E., Smith, K.C. and Rowe, I.H. (1976). Measurement of the pre-ejection period during labour with the use of arterial pulse time. *Am. J. Obstet. Gynecol.*, **126**, 238

Bernstine, R.L., Borkowski, W.J. and Price, A.H. (1955). Prenatal fetal electroencephalography. *Am. J. Obstet. Gynecol.*, **70**, 623–30

Birnholtz, J.C., Stephens, J. and Faria, M. (1978). Fetal movement patterns: a possible means of defining neurologic developmental milestones *in utero*. *Am. J. Roentgenology*, **130**, 537–40

Bishop, E.H. (1964). Pelvic scoring for elective induction. *Obstet. Gynecol.*, **24**, 266–8

Bishop, E.H. (1966a). Instrument and method: the Doppler ultrasonic motion sensor. *Obstet. Gynecol.*, **28**, 712

Bishop, E.H. (1966b). Obstetric uses of the ultrasonic motion sensor. *Am. J. Obstet. Gynecol.*, **96**, 863–7

Bishop, E.H. (1968). Quoted by Curran, J.T. (1975) p. 11

Blair Bell, W., Cunningham, L. and Jowett, M. (1928). The metabolism and acidity of the foetal tissues and fluids. *Br. Med. J.*, **1**, 126–31

Blair Hartley, J. (1957). Radiological assessment of foetal maturity. *Br. J. Radiol.*, **30**, 561–76

Boddy, K. and Robinson, J.S. (1971). External method for detection of fetal breathing *in utero*. *Lancet*, **2**, 1231

Boddy, K. and Mantell, C. (1972). Observations of fetal breathing movements transmitted through maternal abdominal wall. *Lancet*, **2**, 1219

Boddy, K., Dawes, G.S. and Robinson, J.S. (1974), quoted by Pearson (1981) p. 105

Boddy, K., Dawes, G.S., Fisher, R., Pinter, S. and Robinson, J.S. (1975). Foetal respiratory movements, electrocortical and cardiovascular responses to hypoxemia and hypercapnia in sheep. *J. Physiol.*, **243**, 599

Bodson, M. (1843). Quoted by Fenton A.N. and Steer, C.M. (1962)

Bonar, B.E., Blumemfeld, C.M. and Fenning, C. (1938). Studies of fetal respiratory movements: historical and present day observations. *Am. J. Dis. Children*, **55**, 1

Borer, R.C., Gluck, L., Freeman, R.K. and Kulovich, M.V. (1971). Pre-natal prediction of respiratory distress syndrome. *Paediatr. Res.*, **5**, 655

Bourne, A. and Burn, J.H. (1927). The dosage and action of pituitary extract of the ergot alkaloids on the uterus in labour with a note on the action of adrenaline. *J. Obstet. Gynaecol. Br. Emp.*, **34**, 249–72

Brosens, I. and Gordon, H. (1966). The estimation of maturity by cytological examination of the liquor amnii. *J. Obstet. Gynaecol. Br. Commonw.*, **73**, 88–90

Brosens, I., Robertson, W.B. and Dixon, H.G. (1967). The physiological response of the vessels of the placental bed to normal pregnancy. *J. Pathol. Bacteriol.*, **93**, 569–79

Brosens, I., Dixon, H.G. and Robertson, W.B. (1977). Fetal growth retardation and the arteries of the placental bed. *Br. J. Obstet. Gynaecol.*, **84**, 656–63

Brown, A.D.G. and Robertson, J.G. (1968). The ultrasonic doppler cardioscope in obstetrics. *J. Obstet. Gynaecol., Br. Commonw.*, **75**, 92–6

Brown, J.B. (1955). A chemical method for the determination of oestriol, oestrone, and oestradiol in urine. *Biochem. J.*, **60**, 185

Bullock, W.R. (ed.) (1871). *Theoretic and Practical Treatise of Midwifery*, 5th edn. (Philadelphia: Lindsay and Blakiston)

Buys Ballot, C.H.D. (1843). Akustische Versuche auf der Niederlandischen Eisenbahn nebst gelegentlichen Bemerkungen zur Theories des Hrn. prof. Doppler. *Poggendorf Annalen B*, **66**, 321–51

Caldeyro-Barcia, R. (1961). Quoted by Curran, J.T. (1975). p. 12

Caldeyro-Barcia, R., Alvarez, H. and Reynolds, S.R.M. (1950). A better understanding of uterine contractility through simultaneous recording with an internal and a seven channel external method. *Surg. Gynecol. Obstet.*, **91**, 641–50

Caldeyro-Barcia, R., Alvarez, H. and Poseiro, J.J. (1955). Normal and abnormal uterine contractility in labor. *Triangle*, **2**, 41–52

Caldeyro-Barcia, R., Pose, S. and Alvarez, H. (1957). *J. Pharmacol. Exp. Ther.*, **121**, 18, quoted by Goodlin (1979) p. 343

Caldeyro-Barcia, R., Mendez-Bauer, C., Poseiro, J., Escarena, L.A., Pose, S.V., Bieniarz, J., Arnt, A., Gulin, L. and Althabe, O. (1966a). Control of the human fetal heart rate during labor. In. Cassels, D.E. (ed.) *The Heart and Circulation in the Newborn and Infant*, pp. 7–36. (New York: Grune and Stratton)

Caldeyro-Barcia, R., Riguero-Longo, J.G., Poseiro, J.J. and Alverez, L.O. (1966b). Fetal electrocardiogram at term labor obtained with subcutaneous fetal electrodes. *Am J. Obstet. Gynecol.*, **96**, 556–64

Caldeyro-Barcia R., Casacuberta, C., Bustos, R. *et al.* (1968). Correlation of intrapartum changes in fetal heart rate with fetal oxygen and acid base balance. In Adamson, K. (ed.) *Diagnosis and Treatment of Fetal Disorders*, pp. 205–25. (New York: Springer Verlag)

Callagan, D.A., Rowland, T.C, and Goodman, D.E. (1964). Ultrasonic doppler observation of the fetal heart. *Obstet. Gynecol.*, **23**, 637

Calvert, J.P., Crean, E.E., Newcombe, R.G. and Pearson, J.F. (1982). Antenatal screening by measurement of symphysis fundus height. *Br. Med. J.* **285**, 846

Campbell, S. (1968). An improved method of fetal cephalometry by ultrasound. *J. Obstet. Gynaecol. Br. Commonw.*, **75**, 568

Campbell, S. (1969). The prediction of fetal maturity by ultrasonic measurement of the biparietal diameter. *Br. J. Obstet. Gynaecol. Br. Commonw.*, **76**, 603–9

Campbell, S. and Newman, G.B. (1971). Growth of the fetal biparietal diameter during normal pregnancy. *J. Obstet. Gynaecol. Br. Commonw.*, **78**, 513–19

Campbell, S. and Kurjak, A. (1972). Comparison between urinary oestrogen assay and serial ultrasonic cephalometry in assessment of fetal growth retardation. *Br. Med. J.*, **4**, 336

Campbell, S., Diaz-Recasens, J., Griffin, D.R., Cohen-Overbeek, T.E., Pearce, J.M., Wilson, K. and Teague, M.J. (1983). New Doppler technique for assessing uteroplacental blood flow. *Lancet*, 1, 675–7

Carrera, J.M. and Barri, P.N. (1977). Diagnosis of intrauterine growth retardation. In Salvadori, B. and Bacchi-Modena, A. (eds.) *Poor Intrauterine Fetal Growth*, p. 277. (Rome: Centro Minerva Medica)

Carson, B.S., Losey, R.W., Bowes, W.H. and Simmons, M.A. (1976). Combined obstetric and paediatric approach to prevent meconium aspiration syndrome. *Am. J. Obstet. Gynecol.*, 126, 712

Caton, R. (1875). The electric currents of the brain. *Br. Med. J.*, 11, 278

Cazeau, P.A. (1840s). Quoted by Bullock, W.R. (1871).

Chalmers, I. (1977) Perinatal epidemiology: strengths, limitations and possible hazards. In Beard, R.W. and Campbell, S. (eds.) *The Current Status of Fetal Heart Rate Monitoring and Ultrasound in Obstetrics*, pp. 12–27. (London: RCOG)

Chalmers, I. (1979) Randomised controlled trials of intrapartum fetal monitoring. In Thalhammer, O., Baumgarten, K. and Pollack, A. (eds.) *Perinatal Medicine, 6th European Congress Vienna*, pp. 260–5. (Stuttgart: Georg Thieme)

Chamberlain, G.V.P. (1984). An end to antenatal oestrogen monitoring. *Lancet*, 1, 1171–2

Chamberlain, P.F., Manning, F.A., Morrison, I. *et al.* (1984). Ultrasound evaluation of amniotic fluid volume.I. The relationship of marginal and decreased amniotic fluid volumes to perinatal outcome. *Am. J. Obstet. Gynecol.*, 150, 245

Churchill, F. (1866). *The Theory and Practice of Midwifery*, 5th edn. (London) quoted by Pinkerton (1976) p. 363

Clarke, L.C. (1956). Monitor and control of blood tissue oxygen tensions. *Trans. Am. Soc. Artificial Internal Organs*, 2, 41–9

Clements, J.A., Platzker, A.C.G., Tierney, D.F., Hobel, C.J., Creasey, R.K., Margolis, A.J., Thibeault, D.W., Tooley, W.H. and Oh, W. (1972). Assessment of the risk of the respiratory distress syndrome by a rapid test for surfactant in amniotic fluid. *N. Engl. J. Med.*, 268, 1077–81

Coghlan, B.A. and Taylor, M.G. (1976). Directional Doppler techniques for detection of blood velocities. *Ultrasound Med. Biol.*, 2, 171–81

Cordero, L. and Hon, E.H. (1971). Scalp abscess: a rare complication of fetal monitoring. *J. Pediatr.*, 78, 533

Cox, L.W. (1963). Foetal anoxia. *Lancet*, 1, 841–3

Cox, L.W., Wall, I.B. and Wood, A.E.R. (1963). (Quoted by Curran, J.T. (1975) p. 26)

Cremer, M. (1906). Uber Die Direkte Ableitung der Aktionstrome des Menschlichen Herzens vom Oesophagus und Uber das Elektrokardiogramm des Fetus. *Munchener Medizinische Wochenschrift*, 53, 811

Curran, J.T. (1975). *Fetal Heart Monitoring*. (London, Boston: Butterworths)

Daffos, F., Capella-Pavlovsky, M. and Forestier, F. (1985). Fetal blood sampling during pregnancy with use of a needle guided by ultrasound: a study of 606 consecutive cases. *Am J. Obstet. Gynecol.*, 153, 655–60

Dawes, G.E., Fox, H.E., Leduc, B.M., Liggins, G.C. and Richards, R.T. (1970). Respiratory movements and paradoxical sleep in foetal lambs. *J. Physiol. (London)*, 210, 47

Dawes, G.S., Fox, H.E., Leduc, B.M., Liggins, G.C. and Richards, R.T. (1972). Respiratory movements and rapid eye movement sleep in the foetal lamb. *J. Physiol.*, 220, 119–43

Dawes, G.S., Houghton, C.R.S., Redman, C.W.G. and Visser, G.H.A. (1982). Pattern of the normal human fetal heart rate. *Br. J. Obstet. Gynaecol.*, 89, 276–84

DeLee, J.B. (1922). Ein Neus Stethoskop fur die Geburtshilfe besonders Geeignet. *Zentralbl. Gynäkol.*, 46, 1688

Dempster, J., Mires, G.J., Taylor, D.J. and Patel, N.B. (1988). Fetal umbilical artery flow velocity waveforms: prediction of small for gestational age infants and late decelerations in labour. *Europ. J. Obstet. Gynaecol. Reprod. Biol.*, 29, 21–5

Dennis, J. and Chalmers, I. (1982). Very early neonatal seizure rate: a possible epidemiological indication of the quality of perinatal care. *Br. J. Obstet. and Gynaecol*, 89, 418–26

Desmond, M., Moore, J., Lindley, J.E., and Brown, C.A. (1957). Meconium staining of the amniotic fluid: the marker of fetal hypoxia. *Obstet. Gynecol.*, 9, 91–103

Dickey, R.P., Grannis, G.F. and Hanson, F.W. (1972). Use of the oestrogen/creatinine ratio and the 'oestrogen index' for screening of normal and 'high-risk' pregnancy. *Am. J. Obstet. Gynecol.*, **113**, 880

Donald, I. and Brown, T.G. (1961). Demonstration of tissue interfaces within the body by ultrasonic echo sounding. *Br. J. Radiol.*, **34**, 539

Donald, I., MacVicar, J. and Brown, T.G. (1958). Investigation of abdominal masses by pulsed ultrasound. *Lancet*, **1**, 1188–95

Doppler, J.C. (1842). Uber das farbige Licht der Doppelsterne und einiger anderer Hestirne des Himmels. *Abhandlungen d. Konigl. Bohmischen Gesellschaft der Wissenschafter. V.* No. 2

Dressler, J. and Mokowitz, L. (1941). Fetal electrocardiography and stethography *Am. J. Obstet. Gynecol.*, **41**, 775–91

Duncan, A.S. (1957). Placental insufficiency. *Medical Press* **238**, 336

Easby, M.H. (1934). Quoted by Curran, J.T. (1975) p. 5

Eastman, N.J. (1932). Fetal blood studies; chemical nature of asphyxia neonatorum and its bearing on certain practical problems. *Johns Hopkins Hospital Bull.*, **50**, 39–50

Eastman, N.J. (1956). *Williams Obstetrics*, 2nd Edn. p.1026. (New York: Appleton-Century Crofts)

Eastman, N.J. and McLane, C.M. (1931). Foetal blood studies 11. The lactic acid content of umbilical blood under various conditions. *Bull. Johns Hopkins Hospital*, **4**, 261–8

Eik-Nes, S.H., Brubakk, A.O. and Ulstein, M. (1980). Measurement of human fetal blood flow. *Br. Med. J.*, **1**, 283–4

Einthoven, W. (1903). Quoted by Curran, J.T. (1975) p. 4

Elder, M.G., Burton, E.R., Gordon, H., Hawkins, D.F. and McClure Browne, J.C. (1970). Maternal weight and girth changes in late pregnancy and the diagnosis of placental insufficiency. *J. Obstet. Gynaecol. Br. Commonw.*, **77**, 481–91

Erskine, R.L.A. and Ritchie, J.W.K. (1985). Umbilical artery blood flow characteristics in normal and growth retarded fetuses. *Br. J. Obstet. Gynaecol*, **92**, 605–10

Favret, A.G. and Caputo, A.F. (1963). Quoted by Curran, J.T. (1975). p. 8

Favret, A.G. and Marchetti, A.A. (1966) Quoted by Curran, J.T. (1975). p. 8

Fenichel, G.M. (1983). Hypoxic-ischemic encephalopathy in the newborn. *Arch. Neurol.*, **40**, 261–6

Fenton, A.N. and Steer, C.M. (1962). Foetal distress. *Am. J. Obstet. Gynecol.*, **83**, 354–62

Ferguson, J.C. (1830). *Dublin Med Transactions*, **1**, 64. Quoted by Pinkerton, J.H.M. (1976) p. 368

Fielder, F.D. (1968). Quoted by Curran, J.T. (1975) p. 11

Filshie, M. (1974). Intrapartum fetal monitoring. *Br. J. Hosp. Med.*, **12**, 33–46

Fischer, W.M., Stude, I. and Brandt, H. (1976). Ein Vorschlag zur Beurteilung des antepartualen Kardiotokogramms. *Zeitschrift Perinatologie*, **180**, 117–23

Fishman, A.P. and Richards, D.W. (eds.) (1964). *Circulation of the Blood: Men and Ideas*, p. 746. (Oxford: Oxford University Press)

Fitzgerald, D.E. and Drumm, J.E. (1977). Non-invasive measurement of the fetal circulation using ultrasound: a new method. *Br. J. Obstet. Gynaecol.*, **2**, 1450–1

Flynn, A.M. and Kelly, J. (1976). Continuous fetal monitoring in the ambulant patient in Labour. *Br. Med. J.*, **2**, 842–3

Fogarty, P. and Dornan, J. (1990). Computerized spectrum analysis of fetal heart rate variability during labour. *Contemp. Rev. Obstet. Gynecol.*, **2**, 69–74

Freeman, R.K. (1982). Contraction stress testing for primary fetal surveillance in patients at risk for uteroplacental insufficiency. *Clin. Perinatol.*, **9**, 265

Freeman, R.K., Garite, T.J. and Nageotte, M.P. (eds.) (1991). *Fetal Heart Monitoring*, 2nd edn. pp.1–6. (Baltimore: Williams and Wilkins)

Friedman, E.A. (1954). The graphic analysis of labor. *Am. J. Obstet. Gynecol.*, **68**, 1568–71

Friedman, E.A. (1967). *Labor. Clinical Evaluation and Management.* (New York: Meredith)

Friedman, S. and Eckerling, B. (1964). Quoted by Curran, J.T. (1975) p. 6 and p. 17

Gabbe, S.G. and Hon, E.H. (1976). New trends in fetal heart rate monitoring. The importance of variability. *5th European Congress of Perinatal Medicine.* (Uppsala: Allinquist and Wicksell Trycheri)

Galabin, A.L. (1886). *A Manual of Midwifery*. (London: J. & A. Churchill)

Garvin, J.A. and Kline, E.M. (1952). Quoted by Curran, J.T. (1975) p. 19

Genser, G., Marsal, K. and Brautmark, B. (1975). Maternal smoking and fetal breathing movements. *Am. J. Obstet. Gynecol.*, **123**, 861–7

Ghosh, A.K. and Tipton, R.H. (1976). Fetal scalp electrodes. *Lancet*, **1**, 1075

Giles, W.B., Trudinger, B.J. and Cooke, C.M. (1985). Fetal umbilical artery flow velocity time waveforms in twin pregnancies. *Br. J. Obstet. Gynaecol.*, **92**, 490–7

Gill, R.W., Trudinger, B.J. and Garrett, W.J. (1981). Fetal umbilical venous blood measured *in utero* by pulsed Doppler and B mode ultrasound. *Am. J. Obstet. Gynecol.*, **139**, 720–5

Gluck, L., Kulovich, M.V., Borer, R.C., Brenner, P.H., Anderson, G.G. and Spellacy, W.N. (1971). Diagnosis of respiratory distress syndrome by amniocentesis. *Am. J. Obstet. Gynecol.*, **109**, 440–5

Goebelsman, U. (1980) Hormonal assessment of fetoplacental function. In Givens, J.R. (ed.) *Endocrinology of Pregnancy*, pp. 364. (Chicago: Year Book Medical)

Goodlin, R. (1979). History of fetal monitoring. *Am. J. Obstet. Gynecol.*, **133**, 323–52

Goodlin, R.C. and Schmidt, W. (1972). Quoted by Kubli *et al.* (1977) p. 29

Gosling, R.G. and King, D.H. (1974). Ultrasonic angiology. In Marous, A. and Adamson, L. (eds.) *Arteries and Veins*, pp. 61–98. (Edinburgh: Churchill Livingstone)

Grannum, P.A. (1983). Ultrasound examination of the placenta. *Clin. Obstet. Gynecol.*, **10**, 459–73

Grant, A. and Chalmers, I. (1985). Some research strategies for investigating aetiology and assessing the effects of clinical practice. In MacDonald, R.R. (ed.) *Scientific Basis of Obstetrics and Gynaecology*, 3rd edn. pp. 49–84. (London: Churchill Livingstone)

Green, J.N. and Paul, R.H. (1978). The value of amniocentesis in prolonged pregnancy. *Obstet. Gynecol.*, **51**, 293

Greenfield, A.D.M., Shepherd, J.T. and Whelan, R.F. (1951). The rate of blood-flow in the umbilical cord. *Lancet*, **2**, 422–4

Griffin, D. (1984) Fetal activity. In Studd, J. (ed.) *Progress in Obstetrics and Gynaecology*, Vol. 4 p. 103. (Edinburgh, London: Churchill Livingstone)

Griffin, D., Cohen-Overbeck, T. and Campbell, S. (1983). Fetal and utero-placental blood flow. *Clin. Obstet. Gynecol.*, **10**, 565–601

Grimwalde, J.C., Walker, D.W., Bartlett, M., Gordon, S. and Wood, C. (1971). Human fetal heart rate change and movement in response to sound and vibration. *Am. J. Obstet. Gynecol.*, **109**, 86

Gruenwald, P. (1963). Chronic fetal distress and placental insufficiency. *Biologica Neonat. v. (Basel)*, **5**, 215

Gudmundsson, S. and Marsal, K. (1988). Umbilical and uteroplacental blood flow velocity waveforms in pregnancies with fetal growth retardation. *Europ. J. Obstet. Gynaecol. Reprod. Biol.*, **27**, 187–96

Gunn, L. and Wood, M.C. (1953). Quoted by Curran, J.T. (1975) p. 8

Hamilton, J. (1836). *Practical Observations on Various Subjects Relating to Midwifery*. (Edinburgh: Hill)

Hammacher, K. (1962). New method for the selective registration of the fetal heart beat. *Geburtshilfe und Frauenheilkunde*, **22**, 1542

Hammacher, K. (1966a). Fruherkennung intrauterineo gefahrenzustande durch electrophonocardiographie und focographie. In Elert, R. and Hates, K. (eds.) *Prophylaxe Frundkindicher Hirnschaden*, p. 120. (Stuttgart: Georg Theime Verlag)

Hammacher, K. (1966b). *Intra-Uterine Dangers to the Fetus*, Monograph. (Amsterdam: Excerpta Medica)

Hammacher, K. (1969). The clinical significance of cardiotocography. In Huntingford, P.J., Huter, K.A. and Saling, E. (eds.) *Perinatal Medicine*, pp. 80–93. (New York: Academic Press)

Hammacher, K., Huter, K.A., Bokelmann, J. and Werners, P.H. (1968). Foetal heart frequency and perinatal condition of the foetus and newborn. *Gynaecologica*, **166**, 349–60

Hammacher, K., Brun del Re, R., Gaudenz, R., de Grandi, P. and Richter, R. (1974). Kardiotokographischer Nachweis einer fetalen Gefahrdung mit einem CTG-Score. *Gynakologische Rundschau*, **14**, (Suppl. 1) 61

Haan, J. de., Van Bemmel, J.H., Stolte, L.A.M., Janssens, J., Ejkes, T.K.A.B., Versteeg, B., Veth, A.F.L. and Braksha, J.T. (1971). Quantitative evaluation of fetal heart rate patterns: (11): The significance of the fixed heart rate during pregnancy and labour. *Europ. J. Obstet. Gynaecol.*, **3**, 103

Hansmann, M. and Voigt, U. (1973). Ultrasonic fetal thoracometry: an additional parameter for determining fetal growth. *J. Perinat. Med.* quoted by Campbell (1974), Fetal growth. In Beard, R.W. (ed.) *Fetal Medicine. Clinics in Obstetrics and Gynaecology*, pp. 41–65. (London: W.B. Saunders Co. Ltd.)

Hasselbalch, K.A. and Lundsgaard, C. (1912). Blutreaktion und Lungenventilation. *Scand. Archiv. Physiol.*, **27**, 13–32

Hasselbalch, K.A. and Gammeltoft, S.A. (1915). Die Ventralitats-regulation des graviden organismus. *Biochemische Zeitschrifte*, **68**, 206–64

Haverkamp, A.D., Thompson, H.E., McFee, J.G. and Cetrulo, C. (1976). The evaluation of continuous fetal heart rate monitoring in high-risk pregnancy. *Am. J. Obstet. Gynecol.*, **125**, 310–20

Haverkamp, A.D., Orleans, M., Langendoerfer, S., McFee, J., Murphy, J. and Thompson, H.E. (1979). A controlled trial of the differential effects of intrapartum fetal monitoring. *Am. J. Obstet. Gynecol.*, **134**, 399–412

Hellman, L.M. and Fillisty, L.P. (1965). Quoted by Curran, J.T. (1975) p. 19

Hellman, L.M., Johnston, H.L., Tolkes, W.E. and Jones, E.H. (1961). Some factors affecting the fetal heart rate. *Am. J. Obstet. Gynecol.*, **82**, 1055

Henner, H., Ruttgers, H., Muliwan, D., Haller, U. and Kubli, F. (1978). A new application tool for the roche pH electrode. *Archiv. Gynecol.*, **226**, 75–7

Hertogs, K., Roberts, A.B., Cooper, D., Griffin, D.R. and Campbell, S. (1979). Maternal perception of fetal motor activity. *Br. Med., J.*, **2**, 1183

Hess, O.W. (1962). Radio-telemetry of fetal heart energy. *Obstet. Gynecol.*, **20**, 516–21

Hillis, D.S. (1917). Attachment for the stethoscope. *J. Am. Med. Assoc.*, **68**, 910

Hobbins, J.C., Grannum, P.A., Romero, R., Reece, E.A. and Mahoney, M.J. (1985). Percutaneous umbilical blood sampling. *Am. J. Obstet. Gynecol.*, **152**, 1–6

Hofbauer, J. and Weis, O. (1908). Quoted by Curran, J.T. (1975) p. 8

Holmes, J.H. and Howry, D.H. (1963). *Am. J. Dig. Dis.*, **8**, 12, quoted by Goodlin (1979) p. 338

Hon, E.H. (1959). Observations on 'pathologic' fetal bradycardia. *Am. J. Obstet. Gynecol.*, **77**, 1084–99

Hon, E.H. (1963a). The classification of fetal heart rate. No 1. A working classification. *Obstet. Gynecol.*, **22**, 137–47

Hon, E.H. (1963b). Electronic evaluation of the fetal heart rate and fetal electrocardiography (11). A vaginal electrode. *Am. J. Obstet. Gynecol.*, **86**, 772

Hon, E.H. (1963c). Quoted by Curran, J.T. (1975). pp. 6, 19 and 30

Hon, E. (1967). Address at the *5th World Congress of Obstetrics and Gynecology*, Sydney, Australia, In Wood, C. and Walters, W.A.W. (eds.) (London: Butterworths)

Hon, E.H. (1968). *An Atlas of Fetal Heart Rate Patterns.* (New Haven: Harty Press)

Hon, E.H. and Hess, O.W. (1957). Quoted by Curran, J.T. (1975) p. 7

Hon, E.H. and Hess, O.W. (1960). The clinical value of fetal electrocardiography. *Am J. Obstet. Gynecol.*, **79**, 1012–23

Hon, E.H. and Lee, H.S. (1963). Quoted by Curran, J.T. (1975) p. 22

Hon, E.H. and Quilligan, E.J. (1967). Classification of the fetal heart rate: II. A revised working classification. *Connecticut Medicine*, **31**, 779–85

Hon, E.H. and Quilligan, E.J. (1968). Electronic evaluation of the fetal heart rate. *Clin. Obstet. Gynecol.*, **11**, 145

Hon, E.H. and Paul, R.H. (1973). Quantitation of uterine activity. *Obstet. Gynecol.*, **42**, 368–70

Hon, H.E., Paul, R.H. and Hon, R.W. (1972). Electronic evaluation of fetal heart rate. XI. Description of spiral electrode. *Obstet. Gynecol.*, **40**, 362

Honzik, M.P., Hutchings, J.J. and Burnip, S.R. (1965). Quoted by Curran J.T. 1975) p. 36

Huch, R., Seler, D., Salster, H., Weinzer, Z. and Lubbers, D.W. (1977). Transcutaneous pCO_2 measurement with a miniaturised electrode. *Lancet*, **1**, 982

Hull, M.G.R. (1972). Perinatal coagulopathies complicating fetal blood sampling. *Br. Med. J.*, **4**, 319–21

Hunter, C.A., Lansford, K.G., Knoebel, S.B. and Braunlin, R.J. (1960). A technique for recording fetal ECG during labour and delivery. *Obstet. Gynecol.*, **16**, 567

Huntingford, P.J. (1964). A direct approach to the study of the fetus. *Lancet*, **1**, 95–6

Huntingford, P.J. and Pendleton, H.J. (1969). The clinical application of cardiotocography. *J. Obstet. Gynaecol. Br. Commonw.*, **76**, 586–95

Ingemarsson, E., Ingemarsson, I. and Svenningsen, N.W. (1981). Impact of routine fetal monitoring during labour on fetal outcome, with long-term follow up. *Am. J. Obstet. Gynecol.*, **141**, 29

Ito, Y. and Higashi, K. (1961). Studies on the prolactin like substance in human placenta. *Endocrinol. Jap.*, **8**, 279–81

Jaggard, W.W. (1888). In Hirst, B.C. (ed.) *A System of Obstetrics*. (Philadelphia: Lea Broth)

James, L.S., Weisbrot, I.M., Prince, C.E., Holaday, D.A. and Apgar, V. (1958). The acid–base status of human infants in relation to birth asphyxia and the onset of respiration. *J. Pediatr.*, **52**, 379–94

Jasper, H.H., Bridgman, C.S. and Carmichael, L. (1937). An ontogenetic study of cerebral electrical potentials in the guinea pig. *J. Exp. Psychol.*, **21**, 63–71

Johnson, F.R.B., Compton, A.A., Rothensch, J., Work, B.A. and Johnson, J.W.E. (1981). The significance of the sinusoidal fetal heart rate pattern. *Am. J. Obstet. Gynecol.* **139**, 446

Josimovich, J. and MacLaren, J. (1962). Presence in the human placenta and term serum of a highly lactogenic substance immunologically related to pituitary growth hormone. *Endocrinology*, **71**, 209–15

Joupilla, P. and Kirkinen, P. (1984). Umbilical vein blood flow in the human fetus in cases of maternal and fetal anaemia and uterine bleeding. *Ultrasound Med. Biol.*, **10**, 365–70

Jouppila, P., Kirkinen, P., Eik-Nes, S. and Koivula, A. (1981). Fetal blood flow in growth retarded pregnancies. In Kurjak, A. and Kratchowil, A. (eds.) *Recent Advances in Ultrasound Diagnosis 3*, pp. 226–30. (Amsterdam: Excerpta Medica)

Kaufman, P., Sen, D.K. and Schweikhart, G. (1979). Classification of human placental villi. I. Histology. *Cell Tissue Res.*, **200**, 409–23

Kelso, I.M., Parsons, R.J., Lawrence, G.F., Arora, S.S., Edmonds, D.K. and Cooke, I.D. (1978). An assessment of continuous fetal heart rate monitoring in labour: a randomised trial. *Am. J. Obstet. Gynecol.*, **131**, 526–32

Kendall, V., Farrell, D.M. and Kane, H.A. (1962). Fetal radio-electrocardiography: a new method of fetal electrocardiography. *Am. J. Obstet. Gynecol.*, **83**, 1629

Kennedy, E. (1833). *Observations of Obstetric Auscultation*. (Dublin: Hodges & Smith)

Kennedy, E. (1843). *Observations on Obstetric Auscultation, with an Analysis of the Evidences of Pregnancy, and an Enquiry into the Proofs of the Life and Death of the Fetus in utero*, pp. 250–1. (New York: J. and H.G. Langley)

Kergaradec De, M.J.A.L. (1821). Memoire sur l'auscultation appliquée a l'etude de la grossesse ou recherches sur deux nouveaux signes propres a faire reconnaitre plusieurs circumstances de l'état de gestation; read at *l'Academie Royale de Medicine* at its General Meeting on 26 December 1821, Paris

Kirschbaum, T.H. and DeHaven, J.C. (1968). Maternal and fetal blood constituents. In Assali, N.S. (ed.) *Biology of Gestation: The Fetus and Neonate*, Vol. 11, p. 143. (New York: Academic Press)

Kitahama, K. and Sasaoka, K. (1967). *Jpn. J. Med. Electron.*, **5**, 27, quoted by Goodlin (1979) p. 329

Klopper, A. (1968). The assessment of feto-placental function by estriol assay. *Obstet. Gynecol. Surv.*, **23**, 813–38

Klopper, A. (1969). Foetus and placenta. In Klopper, A. and Diczfalusy, E. (eds.) *The Assessment of Placental Function in Clinical Practice*, pp. 471–555. (Oxford: Blackwell Scientific)

Klopper, A. (1989). Biochemical methods of fetal assessment. In Turnbull, Sir A. and Chamberlain, G. (eds.) *Obstetrics*, pp. 361–82. (Edinburgh, London, Melbourne, New York: Churchill Livingstone).

Knox, G.E., Huddleston, J.F. and Flowers, C.E. (1979). Management of prolonged pregnancy: results of a prospective randomised trial. *Am. J. Obstet. Gynecol.*, **134**, 376

Kober, S. (1931). Ein Kolorimetrische Bestimmung des Brunshormons. *Biochemische Zeitung,* **239,** 209

Kubli, F. (1971) *Perinatal Medicine,* quoted by Pearson, J.F. (1981). p. 16

Kubli, F.W., Berg, D., Kohnlein, G., Huter, J. and Bretz, D. (1967). Diagnostic management of chronic placental insufficiency. *German Medical Monthly,* **12,** 315

Kubli, F.W., Kaeser, O. and Hinselmann, M. (1969). In Pecile, A. and Finzi, C. (eds.) *The Feto-Placental Unit,* p. 323. (Amsterdam: Excerpta Medica)

Kubli, F., Ruttgers, H., Haller, U., Bogdan, C. and Ramzin, R. (1972) *Z. Gebh. Perinat.,* **176,** 809, quoted by Kubli, F. *et al.* (1977). p. 29

Kubli, F., Boos, R., Ruttgers, H., V.Hagens, C. and Vanselow, H. (1977). Antepartum fetal heart rate monitoring. In Beard, R.W. and Campbell, S. (eds.) *The Current Status of Fetal Heart Rate Monitoring and Ultrasound in Obstetrics,* pp. 28–47. (London: RCOG)

Kurjak, A., Breyer, B., Jurkovic, D., Alfirevic, Z. and Miljan, M. (1987). Colour flow mapping in obstetrics. *J. Perinat. Med.,* **15,** 271–81

Laennec, E.T.H. (1819). Traite de L'auscultation Mediate, quoted by Rhodes, P. (1985) p. 102

Laennec, E.T.H. (1827). *Treatise on Mediate Auscultation and Diseases of the Lungs and Heart,* 2nd edn., translated by J. Forbes, London

Larks, S.D. (1960). Quoted by Curran, J.T. (1975) pp. 29–30

Larks, S.D. (1961). Quoted by Curran, J.T. (1975) p. 14

Larks, S.D. (1965). Estimation of the electrical axis of the fetal heart. *Am. J. Obstet. Gynecol.,* **91,** 46–55

Larks, S.D. and Anderson, G. (1962). The abnormal fetal electrocardiogram. *Am. J. Obstet. Gynecol.,* **84,** 1893

Larks, S.D. and Longo, L.D. (1962). Electrocardiographic studies of the fetal heart during delivery. *Obstet. Gynecol.,* **19,** 740–7

Larks, S.D., Faust, R., Longo, L. and Anderson, G. (1962). Quoted by Curran, J.T. (1975) p. 17

Lee, C.Y., Di Loreto, P.C. and O'Lane, J.M. (1975). A study of fetal heart rate acceleration patterns. *Obstet. Gynecol.,* **45,** 142

Lee, C.Y., Di Loreto, P.C. and Logrand, B. (1976). Fetal activity determination for antepartum evaluation of fetal reserve. *Obstet. Gynecol.,* **48,** 19

Letchworth, A.T. and Chard, T. (1972a). Placental lactogen levels as a screening test for fetal distress and neonatal asphyxia *Lancet,* **1,** 704

Letchworth, A.T. and Chard, T. (1972b). Human placental lactogen levels in pre-eclampsia. *J. Obstet. Gynaecol. Br. Commonw.,* **79,** 680

Levene, M.L., Kornberg, J. and Williams, T.H.C. (1985). The incidence and severity of post-asphyxial encephalopathy in full-term infants. *Early Human Development,* **11,** 21–6

Lewis, P.J., Trudinger, B.J. and Mangez, J. (1978). Effect of maternal glucose ingestion on fetal breathing and body movements in late pregnancy. *Br. J. Obstet. Gynaecol.,* **85,** 86–9

Lewis, R.P., Rittgers, S.E., Forrester, W.F. and Boudoulas, H. (1977). A critical review of systolic time intervals. *Circulation,* **56,** 146

Lind, J. and Wegelius, C. (1954). Human fetal circulation: changes in the cardiovascular system at birth and disturbances in the post-natal closure of the foramen ovale and ductus venosus. *Cold Spring Harbor Symposium on Quantitative Biology,* **19,** 109–25

Lind, T. and Billewicz, W.Z. (1971). A point-scoring system for estimating gestational age from examination of amniotic fluid. *Br. J. Hosp. Med.,* **5,** 681–5

Lish, P.M., Hillyard, I.W. and Dungan, K.W. (1960). Uterine relaxant properties of isoxsuprine. *J. Pharmacol. Exp. Therap.,* **129,** 438–44

Liston, R.M., Cohen, A.W., Mennuti, M.T. and Gabbe, S.G. (1982). Antepartum fetal evaluation by maternal perception of fetal movement. *Obstet. Gynecol.,* **60,** 424

Lumley, J., McKinnon, L. and Wood, C. (1971). Lack of agreement on normal values for fetal scalp blood. *J. Obstet. Gynaecol. Br. Commonw.,* **78,** 13–21

McBurney, R.D. and Western, J. (1947). *J. Surg. Obstet. Gynecol.,* **55,** 363

McClintock, A.H. (1876). In *Smellie's Treatise on the Theory and Practice of Midwifery,* Vol. 1, p. 291. (London: New Sydenham Society)

McDonald, D.A. (1974). *Blood Flow in Arteries.* (London: Edward Arnold)

MacDonald, D. (1989). Supervision of the fetus during labour. *Irish Med. J.*, **82**, 104

MacDonald, D. and Grant, A. (1987). Fetal surveillance in labour – the present position. In Bonnar, J. (ed.) *Recent Advances in Obstetrics and Gynaecology*, No. 15 pp. 83–100. (Edinburgh, London: Churchill Livingstone)

MacDonald, D., Grant, A., Sheridan-Pereira, M., Boylan, P. and Chalmers, I. (1985). The Dublin randomized controlled trial of intrapartum fetal heart rate monitoring. *Am. J. Obstet. Gynecol.*, **152**, 524–39

Maekawa and Toyoshima (1930). Quoted by Curran, J.T. (1975). p. 5

Mandelbaum, B. (1973). Gestational meconium in the high risk pregnancy. *Obstet. Gynecol.*, **42**, 87

Mann, L.I. (1986). Pregnancy events and brain damage. *Am. J. Obstet. Gynecol.*, **155**, 6–9

Manning, F.A. (1976). Fetal breathing as a reflection of fetal status. *Postgrad. Med.*, **61**, 116

Manning, F.A. and Platt, L.D. (1979). Fetal breathing movements: antepartum monitoring of fetal condition. In Quilligan, E.J. (ed.) *Update on Fetal Monitoring. Clinics in Obstetrics and Gynaecology*, Vol. 6, pp. 335–49. (London, Toronto: W.B. Saunders Ltd.)

Manning, F.A. and Platt, L.D. (1980). Human fetal breathing monitoring – clinical considerations. In Patrick, J. (ed.) *Fetal Breathing Movements. Seminars in Perinatology*, Vol. **4**, pp 311–18

Manning, F.A., Platt, L.D. and Sipos, L. (1980). Antepartum fetal evaluation: development of a fetal biophysical profile. *Am. J. Obstet. Gynecol.*, **136**, 787

Manning, F.A., Hill, L.M. and Platt, L.D. (1981). Qualitative amniotic fluid volume determination by ultrasound: antepartum detection of intrauterine growth retardation. *Am. J. Obstet. Gynecol.*, **139**, 254–8

Manseau, P., Vaquies, J., Chavinie, J. and Sureau, C. (1972). Fetal sinusoidal heart rate. Monitoring of fetal distress in pregnancy. *J. Gynaecol. Obstet. Biol. Reprod.*, **1**, 343

Marrian, G.F. (1930). The chemistry of oestrin. *Biochem. J.*, **24**, 1021

Marsal, K. (1981). Fetal movements and fetal breathing movements in the second half of pregnancy. In Kurjack, A. and Kratochwil, A. (eds.) *Recent Advances in Ultrasound Diagnosis*, Vol. 3, pp. 174–80. (Amsterdam: Exerpta Medica)

Marsal, K., Genner, G., Hansson, G., Lindstrom, K. and Mauritzson, L. (1976). New ultrasonic device for monitoring foetal breathing movements. *Biomed. Eng.*, February

Mathur, R.S., Chestnut, S.K., Leaming, A.B. and Williamson, H.O. (1973). Application of plasma estriol estimations in the management of high risk pregnancies. *Am. J. Obstet. Gynecol.*, **117**, 210–19

Matthews, D.D. (1972). Measuring placental function. *Br. Med. J.*, **1**, 439

Meis, P.J., Hall, M., Marshall, J.R. and Hobel, C.J. (1978). Meconium passage: a new classification of risk assessment during labour. *Am. J. Obstet. Gynecol.*, **131**, 509

Merlet, C., Hoeter, J., Devilleneuve, C. and Tchubrutsky, C. (1970). Mise en evidence de movements respiratoires chez le foetus d'agneu 'in utero' au cours du dernier mois de la gestation. *C.R. Acad. Sci.*, **270**, 2462

Meyer-Menk, W., Ruttgers, H., Lorenz, U., Henner, A. and Kubli, F. (1976a). Lecture presented at the *41st Meeting of the Deutsche Gesellschaft Fur Gynakologie und Geburtshilfe.* quoted by Kubli, F. *et al.* (1977) p.34

Meyer-Menk, W., Ruttgers, H., Boos, R., Wurth, G., Adis, B. and Kubli, F. (1976b). A proposal for a new method of CTG evaluation. In Rooth, G. and Bratteby, L.E. (eds.) *Abstracts of the 5th European Congress of Perinatal Medicine*, p.138. (Uppsala: Alinquist and Wicksell Trycheri)

Mitchell, J., Schulman, H., Fleischer, A., Farmakides, G. and Nadeau, D. (1985). Meconium aspiration and fetal acidosis. *Obstet. Gynecol.*, **65**, 352–5

Miller, F.C., Sacks, D.Z., Yeh, S.Y., Paul, R.H., Schifrin, B.S., Martin, C.B. and Hon, E.H. (1975). Significance of meconium during labour. *Am. J. Obstet. Gynecol.*, **122**, 573

Morris, E.D. and Beard, R.W. (1965). The rationale and technique of foetal blood sampling and amnioscopy. *J. Obstet. Gynaecol. Br. Commonw.*, **4**, 489–95

Mosler, K.H. (1969). *Experientia*, **25**, 222, quoted by Curran (1975) p. 11

Myers, R.E. (1977). Experimental models of perinatal brain damage: relevance to human pathology. In Gluck, L. (ed.) *Intrauterine Asphyxia and the Developing Fetal Brain*, chap. 4 p. 37. (Chicago: Year Book Medical Publishers)

Myers, R.E., Mueller-Heubach, E. and Adamsons, K. (1973). Predictability of the state of fetal oxygenation from a quantitative analysis of the components of late deceleration. *Am. J. Obstet. Gynecol.*, 115, 1083–94

Naegele, H.F.J. (1838). *Die geburtshülfliche Auscultation*. (Mainz: V. von Zabern)

Nagle, D.C. (1830). On the use of the stethoscope for the detection of twins *in utero*. *Lancet*, 1, 232–4

National Institutes of Health (1979). Report of a Task Force on Predictors of Fetal Distress. In *Antenatal Diagnosis*. (Washington, D.C.: US Department of Health, Education and Welfare)

Nauche (1865), quoted by Goodlin (1979) p. 323

Neilson, J.P., Whitfield, C.R. and Aitchinson, T.C. (1980). Screening for the small-for-dates fetus: a two-stage ultrasonic examination schedule. *Br. Med. J.*, 1, 1203–6

Neilson, J.P., Munjanja, S.P. and Whitfield, C.R. (1984). Screening for small for dates fetuses: a controlled trial. *Br. Med. J.*, 289, 1179–82

Nelson, K.B. and Ellenberg, J.K. (1981). Apgar scores as predictors of chronic neurological disability. *Pediatrics*, 68, 36–44

Nelson, K.B. and Ellenberg, J. (1986). Antecedants of cerebral palsy: multivariate analysis of risk. *N. Engl. J. Med.*, 315, 81–6

Neuman, M.R., Picconnatto, J. and Roux, J.F. (1970). A wireless radio telemetry system for monitoring fetal heart rate and intrauterine pressure during labour and delivery. *Gynaecol. Invest.*, 1, 92

Neutra, R.R., Fienber, S.E., Greenlands, S. and Friedman, E.A. (1978). Effect of fetal monitoring on neonatal death rates. *N. Engl. J. Med.*, 299, 324–6

Nicolaides, K.H., Soothill, P.W., Rodeck, C.H. and Campbell, S. (1986). Ultrasound-guided sampling of umbilical cord and placental blood to assess fetal well-being. *Lancet*, 1, 1065–7

Nicolaides, K.H., Bilardo, C.M., Soothill, P.W. and Campbell, S. (1988). Absence of end diastolic frequencies in umbilical artery: a sign of fetal hypoxia and acidosis. *Br. Med. J.*, 297, 1026–7

Oard, H.C. and Peters, J.P. (1929). The concentration of acid and base in the serum in normal pregnancy. *J. Biol. Chem.*, 81, 9–27

O'Driscoll, K., Jackson, R.J.H. and Gallagher, J.T. (1969). Prevention of prolonged labour. *Br. Med. J.*, 2, 447–80

Offner, F. and Moisland, B. (1966). A coincidence technique for fetal electrocardiography. *Am. J. Obstet. Gynecol.*, 95, 676–80

Paré, A. (1634). By what signs it may be knowne whether the childe in the wombe bee dead or alive. In Johnson (translator and editor) *The works of the famous Chirugian Ambrose Paré 24th Book "Of the Generation of Man"* p. 913. (London: T. Coltes and R. Young)

Patrick, J., Dalton, K.J. and Dawes, G.S. (1976). Breathing patterns before death in fetal lambs. *Am. J. Obstet. Gynecol.*, 125, 73–8

Patrick, J., Campbell, K., Carmichael, L., Natale, R. and Richardson, B. (1982). Patterns of gross fetal body movements over 24 hour observation intervals during the last 10 weeks of pregnancy. *Am. J. Obstet. Gynecol.*, 142, 363

Paul, R.H. and Keegan, K.A. (1979). Nonstress antepartum fetal monitoring. In Quilligan, E.J. (ed.) *Update on Fetal Monitoring: Clinical Obstetrics and Gynaecology*, Vol. 6, 351–8

Paul, R.H., Suidan, A.K., Yeh-S-Y., Schifrin, B.S. and Hon, E.H. (1975). Clinical fetal monitoring VII. The evaluation and significance of intrapartum baseline FHR variability. *Am. J. Obstet. Gynecol.*, 123, 206–10

Paul, R.H., Yonekura, M.L., Cantrell, C.J., Turkel, S., Pavlova, Z. and Sipos, L. (1986). Fetal injury prior to labor: does it happen? *Am. J. Obstet. Gynecol.*, 154, 1187–93

Pearson, J.F. (1974). Personal communication. In Clayton, S.G. and Beard, R.W. (eds.) *Methods for Monitoring the Fetus in Pregnancy and Labour*. Report of the Study Group of the RCOG. (London: RCOG)).

Pearson, J.F. (1977). Fetal movements – a new approach to antenatal care. *Nursing Mirror*, 144, 49–56

Pearson, J.F. (1981). The value of antenatal fetal monitoring. In Studd, J.W. (ed.) *Progress in Obstetrics and Gynaecology*, Vol. 1, pp. 105–24. (Edinburgh London: Churchill Livingstone)

Pearson, J.F. and Weaver, J.B. (1976). Fetal activity and fetal well-being: an evaluation. *Br. Med. J.*, **1**, 1305–7

Pearson, J.F. and Weaver, J.B. (1978). A six point scoring system for antenatal cardiotocographs. *Br. J. Obstet. Gynaecol.*, **85**, 321

Peiper, A. (1927). *Monatsschr. Kinderheilkd.*, **29**, 236, quoted by Goodlin (1979) p. 340

Phelan, J.P. and Lewis, P.E. (1982). The nonstress test: the false negative test. *Am. J. Obstet. Gynecol.*, **142**, 293–6

Phelan, J.P., Platt, L.D., Yeh, S-Y. *et al.* (1985). The role of ultrasound assessment of amniotic fluid volume in the management of the post dates pregnancy. *Am. J. Obstet. Gynecol.*, **151**, 304

Philpott, R.H. (1972). Graphic records in labour. *Br. Med. J.*, **4**, 163–5

Pinard, A. (1889). *Traite de Palper Abdominal au Point de Vue Obstetrical, et de la Version par Manoeuvres Externes*, 2nd Edn. (Paris: H. Lauwereyns)

Pinkerton, J.H.M. (1976). Fetal auscultation – some aspects of its history and evolution. *Irish Med. J.*, **69**, 363–8

Pinkerton, J.H.M. (1980). John Creery Ferguson. Friend of William Stokes and pioneer of auscultation of the fetal heart in the British Isles. *Br. J. Obstet. Gynaecol.*, **87**, 257–60

Pitkin, R.M. and Zwirek, S.J. (1967). Amniotic fluid creatinine. *Am. J. Obstet. Gynecol.*, **98**, 1135–8

Platt, L.D., Manning, F.A., LeMay, M. and Sipos, L. (1978). Human fetal breathing: relationship to fetal condition. *Am. J. Obstet. Gynecol.*, **132**, 514–18

Playfair, N.S. (1886). *A Treatise on the Science and Practice of Midwifery*, p. 458. (Philadelphia: Lea Brothers)

Polishuk, W.Z., Laufer, N. and Sadovsky, E. (1975). Fetal response to external light stimulus. *Harefuah*, **89**, 395

Porcelot, L. (1974). Applications cliniques de l'examen Doppler transcutané. In Peronneau, P. (ed.) *Velocimetric Ultrasonor Doppler*, Inserm 7–11, pp. 213–40. (Paris: Inserm)

Pose, S.V., Castillo, J.B., Mora-Rojas, E.O. and Sotoyances, A. (1969). *Perinatal factors affecting human development*, **185**, 96. (Washington, DC.: Pan American Health Organization)

Prentice, A. and Lynd, T. (1987). Fetal heart rate monitoring during labour – too frequent intervention, too little benefit. *Lancet*, quoted by MacDonald (1989) p. 104

Preyer, W. (1882). Ueber die erste athembewegungen des neugeborenen. *Z. F. Geburtshilfe*, **7**, 241–53

Quilligan, E.J. (1972). The Obstetrical Intensive Care Unit. *Hospital Practice*, **7**, 61–9

Quilligan, E.J., Katigbak, E., Norwacek, C. and Nezarnecki (1964). Correlation of fetal heart rate patterns and blood gas values. Normal heart rate values *Am J. Obstet. Gynecol.*, **90**, 1343–9

Ray, W.S. (1932). *Child. Dev.*, **3**, 173 quoted by Goodlin (1979) p.323

Ray, M., Freeman, R., Pine, S. and Hesselgesser, R. (1972). Clinical experience with the oxytocin challenge test. *Am. J. Obstet. Gynecol.*, **114**, 1–9

Raymond, S.P.W. and Whitfield, C.R. (1987). Systolic time intervals of the fetal cardiac cycle. In Whittle, M.J. (ed.) *Fetal Monitoring. Clinical Obstetrics and Gynaecology*, Vol. 1, pp. 185–201. (London, Philadelphia: Bailliere Tindall)

RCOG (1986). *Safety of Diagnostic Ultrasound: Report of a Working Party London.* (London: RCOG)

Reed, C.B. (1918). Physiology of meconium passage. *Surg. Gynecol. Obstet.*, **26**, 550

Reed, N.E., Teteris, W.J. and Essig, G.F. (1970). Quoted by Curran, J.T. (1975) p. 25

Renou, P. and Wood, C. (1974). Interpretation of the continuous fetal heart rate record. In Beard, R.W. (ed.) *Fetal Medicine: Clinical Obstetrics and Gynaecology*, Vol. 1, pp. 191–216. (London: W.B. Saunders)

Renou, P., Chang, A., Anderson, I. and Wood, C. (1976). Controlled trial of fetal intensive care. *Am. J. Obstet. Gynecol.*, **126**, 470–6

Reuwer, P.J.H.M., Bruinse, H.W., Stoutenbeek, P. and Haspels, A.A. (1984a). Doppler assessment of the fetoplacental circulation in normal and growth retarded fetuses. *Europ. J. Obstet. Gynaecol. Reprod. Biol.*, **18**, 199–205

Reuwer, P.J.H.M., Nuyen, W.E., Beijer, H.J.M. *et al.* (1984b). Characteristics of flow velocities in the umbilical artery, assessed by Doppler ultrasound. *Europ. J. Obstet. Gynaecol. Reprod. Biol.*, **18**, 397–408

Reynolds, S.R., Heard, O.O., Bruns, P. and Hellman, L.M. (1948). A multi-channel strain-gauge tocodynamometer: an instrument for studying patterns of uterine contractions in pregnant women. *Bull. Johns Hopkins Hospital*, **82**, 446

Reynolds, S.R.M., Harris, J.S. and Kaiser, I.H. (1954). *Clinical Measurement of Uterine Forces in Pregnancy and Labor*, p. 180. (Springfield: Charles C. Thomas)

Rhodes, P. (1973). Obstetric prevention of mental retardation. *Br. Med. J.*, **1**, 399

Rhodes, P. (1985). *An Outline History of Medicine.* (London, Boston: Butterworths)

Richards, I.D.J. and Roberts, C.J. (1967). The 'at risk' infant. *Lancet*, **2**, 711–13

Richardson, B., Natale, R. and Patrick, J. (1979). Human fetal breathing activity during electively induced labour at term. *Am. J. Obstet. Gynecol.*, **133**, 247–55

Ritchie, J.W.K. and Lakhani, K. (1980a). Fetal breathing movements and maternal hyperoxia. *Br. J. Obstet. Gynaecol.*, **87**, 1084–6

Ritchie, J.W.K. and Lakhani, K. (1980b). Fetal breathing movements in response to maternal inhalation of 5% carbon dioxide. *Am. J. Obstet. Gynecol.*, **136**, 386–8

Ritchie, J.W.K. and Dornan, J.C. (1981). Maternal hyperoxia and its effect on fetal breathing movements in the growth retarded human fetus. *8th International Conference on Fetal Breathing and other Measurements.* State University Limburg. Maastricht. October 29,30

Roberts, A.B., Little, D., Cooper, S. and Campbell, S. (1979). Normal patterns of fetal activity in the third trimester. *Br. J. Obstet. Gynaecol.*, **86**, 4–9

Robinson, H.P. (1973). Sonar measurement of fetal crown-rump length as means of assessing maturity in first trimester of pregnancy. *Br. Med. J.*, **4**, 28–31

Rochelson, B.L., Schulman, H., Farmakides, G., Bracero, L., Ducey, J., Fleischer, A., Penny, B. and Winter, D. (1987a). The significance of absent end diastolic velocity in umbilical artery velocity waveforms. *Am. J. Obstet. Gynecol.*, **156**, 1213–18

Rochelson, B.L., Schulman, H., Fleischer, A., Farmakides, G., Barcero, L., Ducey, J., Winter, D. and Penny, B. (1987b). The clinical significance of Doppler umbilical artery velocimetry in the small for gestational age fetus. *Am. J. Obstet. Gynecol.*, **156**, 1223–6

Rodeck, C.H., Kemp, J.R., Holman, C.A., Whitmore, D.N., Karnicki, J. and Austin, M.A. (1981). Direct intravascular fetal blood transfusion by fetoscopy in severe rhesus isoimmunization. *Lancet*, **1**, 625–7

Rodesch, F., Ehman-Ellinger, C., Wilkin, P. and Hubinont, P.O. (1965). Introduction, use and results of a new partogram. *J. Obstet. Gynaecol. Br. Commonw.*, **72**, 930–5

Rosa, P. and Ghilain, A. (1959). The use of a partogram in labour. *Bull. Soc. Belge Gynecol. Obstet.*, **29**, 1–4

Rosen, M.G. and Satran, R. (1965). Fetal electroencephalography during labour. *Obstet. Gynecol.*, **26**, 740–5

Rösslin, E. (1540). *The Byrth of Mankynde, otherwyse named the Woman's Booke. Newly set Furth, Corrected and Augmented. Whose Contentes Ye Maye Rede in the Table of the Booke, and most playnly in the Prologue.* By Thomas Raynold Phisiton. London.

Rovinsky, J.J. and Guttmacher, A.F. (1965). *Medical, Surgical and Gynecological Complications of Pregnancy*, p. 805. (Baltimore: Williams and Wilkins)

Rumbolz, W.L. and McGoogan, L.S. (1953). Placental insufficiency and the small undernourished full-term infant. *Obstet. Gynecol.*, **1**, 294

Sabatier, R.B. (1774). *Memoires Academie Royal des Sciences, Paris* pp. 198

Sadovski, E. and Yaffe, H. (1973). Daily fetal movement recording and fetal prognosis. *Obstet. Gynecol.*, **41**, 845–50

Sadovski, E., Zuckerman, H., Diamant, Y.Z. and Polishuk, W.Z. (1969). Leukocyte alkaline phosphatase and fetal prognosis in placental dysfunction. *Am. J. Obstet. Gynecol.*, **108**, 979

Sadovski, E., Polishuk, W.Z., Mahler, Y. and Malkin, A. (1973). Correlation between electromagnetic and maternal assessment of fetal movement. *Lancet*, **1**, 1141–43

Sadovski, E., Polishuk, W., Yaffe, H., Adler, D., Pachys, F. and Mahler, Y. (1977). Fetal Movements recorder, use and indications. *Int. J. Gynecol. Obstet.*, **15**, 20

Sadovski, E., Evron, S. and Weinstein, D. (1979). Daily fetal movement recording in normal pregnancy. *Rivrista Obstetrica Ginecol Practica Medicina Perinatal.*, **59**, 395

Saling, E. (1964a). Die Blutgasverhaultnisse und der Saure-Basen-Hanshalt des Feten bei ungestortem Geburtsablauf. *Zeitschrifte fur Geburtschilfe und Gynaekologie*, **161**, 262–92

Saling, E. (1964b). Technick der endoskopischen Mikrobluhentnahme am Fetus. *Gerburtshilfe und Frauenheilkunde*, **24**, 464

Saling, E. (1961). *Geburts. Frauenheilkd.*, **21**, 694 quoted by Goodlin (1979) p. 334

Saling, E. (1966). Fetal blood gas and acid-base status. In Edward, S.E. (ed.) *Neonatal Hypoxia*, pp. 29–41. (London: Edward Arnold)

Saling, E. (1968). *Fetal and Neonatal Hypoxia in Relation to Clinical Obstetrical Practice*, pp. 83–4. (London: Edward Arnold)

Saling,E. and Schneider, D. (1967). Biochemical supervision of the foetus during labour. *J. Obstet. Gynaecol. Br. Commonw.*, **74**, 799–811

Sanchez-Ramos, J., Santisimo, J.L. and Peman, F.C. (1971). La prueba del la Oxitocina en el Diagnostico del estado fetal anteparto. *Acta Genecologica (Madrid)*, **22**, 697

Sarnat, H.B. and Sarnat, M.S. (1976). Neonatal encephalopathy following fetal distress: a clinical and electroencephalographic study. *Archiv. Neurol.*, **33**, 696–705

Satomura, S. (1957). Ultrasonic Doppler method for the inspection of cardiac functions. *J. Acoustical Soc. Am.*, **29**, 1181–5

Saxena, B.N., Emerson, K. and Selenkow, A.A. (1969). *N. Engl. J. Med.*, **281**, 225

Schaeffer, O. (1896), quoted by Goodlin (1979) p. 342

Schatz, F. (1872). *Arch. Gynäkol.*, **3**, 58, quoted by Goodlin (1979) p. 342

Schiffrin, B.S. and Dame, L. (1972). Fetal heart rate patterns. Prediction of Apgar score. *J. Am. Med. Assoc.*, **219**, 1322–5

Schulman, H., Fleischer, A., Stern, W., Farmakides, G., Jagani, N. and Blattner, P. (1984). Umbilical velocity wave ratios in human pregnancy. *Am. J. Obstet. Gynecol.*, **148**, 985–90

Schwartz, H. (1858). Die Vorzeitigen Atembewgungen Leipzig, quoted by Fenton, A.N. and Steer, C.M. (1962) pp. 354–62.

Shelley, T. (1971). Quoted by Curran, J.T. (1975) p. 13

Shelley, T. and Tipton, R.H. (1971). Dip area. A quantitative measure of fetal heart rate patterns. *J. Obstet. Gynaecol. Br. Commonw.*, **78**, 694–701

Simmonds, S.C. (1974). Organisation of fetal intensive care. *Clin. Obstet. Gynecol.*, **1**, 217

Simpson, J.Y. (1855). *Edinburgh Monthly Journal in Medicine*

Slomka, C. and Phelan, J.P. (1981). Pregnancy outcome in the patient with a nonreactive nonstress test and a positive contraction stress test. *Am. J. Obstet. Gynecol.*, **139**, 11–15

Smith, C.V. and Paul, R.H. (1987). Antepartum cardiotocography. In Whittle, M.J. (ed.) *Fetal Monitoring. Clinical Obstetrics and Gynaecology*, pp. 17–28. (London, Philadelphia: Baillière Tindall)

Smith, J.J., Schwartz, E.D. and Blatman, S. (1960). Quoted by Curran, J.T. (1975) p. 19

Smith, N.C. and Soutter, W.P. (1980). Intrapartum fetal scalp lactate measurement as an indicator of fetal hypoxia. Abstract. *Scientific Programme of the British Congress of Obstetrics and Gynaecology*, Edinburgh, 1980

Smyth, C.N. (1953). Experimental electrocardiography of the fetus. *Lancet*, **1**, 1124

Smyth, D.H. (1953). Quoted by Curran, J.T. (1975) p. 5

Sontag, L. and Wallace, R. (1936). Changes in the rate of the human fetal heart in response to vibratory stimuli. *Am. J. Dis. Child.*, **51**, 583

Sorokin, Y., Rosen, M.G. and Sokol, R.J. (1981). Fetal electroencephalography. In Barson, A.J. (ed.) *Laboratory Investigation of Fetal Disease*, pp. 97–108. (Bristol: J. Wright)

Southern, E.M. (1957). Fetal anoxia and its possible relation to changes in the prenatal fetal electrocardiogram. *Am. J. Obstet. Gynecol.*, **73**, 233

Spellacy W.N. (1969). Human placental lactogen (hPL): the review of a protein hormone important to obstetrics and gynecology. *Southern Med. J.*, **62**, 1054–7

Spellacy, W.N. (1973). Human placental lactogen in high-risk pregnancy. *Clin. Obstet. Gynecol.*, **16**, 298–312

Spellacy, W.N. (1976). Monitoring of high-risk pregnancies with human placental lactogen. In *Management of the High-Risk Pregnancy*, pp. 107–35. (Baltimore: University Park Press)

Spellacy, W.N. (1979). The use of human placental lactogen in the antepartum monitoring of pregnancy. In Quilligan, E.T. (ed.) *Clinical Obstetrics and Gynaecology*, 6, Part 2, p. 245. (London: W.B. Saunders & Co. Ltd)

Spurrett, B. (1971). Stressed cardiotocography in late pregnancy. *J. Obstet. Gynaecol. Br. Commonw.*, **78**, 894–900

Stamm, O., Latscha, U., Janecek, P. and Campana, A. (1976). Development of a special electrode for continuous subcutaneous pH measurement in the infant scalp. *Am. J. Obstet. Gynecol.*, **124**, 193–5

Starks, G.C. (1980). Correlation of meconium-stained amniotic fluid, early intrapartum fetal pH and Apgar scores as predictors of perinatal outcome. *Obstet. Gynecol.*, **56**, 604

Steer, P.J., Carter, M.C., Gordon, A.J. and Beard, R.W. (1978). The use of catheter-tip pressure transducers for the measurement of intrauterine pressure in labour. *Br. J. Obstet. Gynaecol.*, **85**, 561–6

Steer, P.J., Carter, M.C. and Beard, R.W. (1984). Normal levels of active contraction area in spontaneous labour. *Br. J. Obstet. Gynaecol.*, **91**, 211–19

Stembera, Z.K., Modr, J., Ganz, V. and Fronek, A. (1964). Measurement of umbilical cord blood flow by local thermodilution. *Am. J. Obstet. Gynecol.*, **90**, 531–6

Sterman, M. (1967). Relationship of intrauterine fetal activity to maternal sleep stage. *Exp. Neurol.*, **19**, 98

Stokes, W. (1825). *An Introduction to the use of the Stethoscope.* (Edinburgh and Dublin)

Strassman, N.E.O. and Mussey, R.D. (1938). Technique and results of routine fetal electrocardiography during pregnancy. *Am. J. Obstet. Gynecol.*, **36**, 986–97

Stuart, B., Drumm, J., Fitzgerald, D.E. and Duignan, N.M. (1980). Fetal blood velocity waveforms in normal pregnancy. *Br. J. Obstet. Gynaecol.*, **87**, 780–5

Sureau, C. (1956a). *Obstet. Gynecol.*, **53**, 3 quoted by Filshie, M. (1974) p. 33

Sureau, C. (1956b). Fetal cardiotocogram during gestation and childbirth. *Gynecol. Obstet. (Paris)*, **551**, 21

Sureau, C. and Trocellier, R. (1961). Quoted by Curran, J.T. (1975) p. 7

Sykes, G.S., Molloy, P.M., Johnson, P., Gu, W., Ashworth, F. and Stirrat, G.M. (1982). Do Apgar scores indicate asphyxia?. *Lancet*, **1**, 494–6

Symonds, E.M. (1970). M.D. Thesis submitted to University of Adelaide, quoted by Filshie, M. (1974) p. 34

Tarnover, H. and Lattin, B. (1942). Quoted by Curran, J.T. (1975) p. 19

Tatano, C.L. (1972). *Patients' cognitive and emotional responses to fetal monitoring.* Masters Thesis, Yale School of Nursing

Tazawa, H., Wada, T., Oguni, C. and Yoshimoto, C. (1968). Quoted by Curran, J.T. (1975) p. 8

Teague, M.J., Willson, K., Battye, C.K. *et al.* (1985). A combined ultrasonic linear array scanner and pulsed Doppler velocimeter for the estimation of blood flow in the fetus and adult abdomen – I: technical aspects. *Ultrasound Med. Biol.*, **11**, 27–36

Thacker, S.B. and Berkelman, R.L. (1986). Assessing the diagnostic accuracy and efficacy of selected antepartum fetal surveillance techniques. *Obstet. Gynecol. Surv.*, **41**, 121–41

Thompson, R.S., Trudinger, B.J. and Cook, C.M. (1986). A comparison of Doppler ultrasound waveform indices in the umbilical artery – I. Indices derived from the maximum velocity waveform. *Ultrasound Med. Biol.*, **12**, 835–44

Timor-Tritch, I., Zador, I., Hertz, R.H. and Rosen, M.H.G. (1976). Classification of human fetal movement. *Am. J. Obstet. Gynecol.*, **126**, 70–7

Tipton, R.H. (1975). Fetal heart rate monitoring in labour. In Beazley, J.M. (ed.) *The Active Management of Labour: Clinical Obstetrics and Gynaecology*, pp. 153–72. (London Philadelphia: W.B. Saunders and Co. Ltd)

Trudinger, B.J. (1981). Fetal breathing movements – an index of fetal maturation and health. In Kurjak, A. and Kratochwil, A. (eds.) *Recent Advances in Ultrasound Diagnosis*, Vol. 3, pp. 187–92. (Amsterdam: Exerpta Medica)

Trudinger, B.J., Lewis, P.J., Mangez, J. and O'Connor, E. (1978). Fetal breathing movements in high risk pregnancy. *Br. J. Obstet. Gynaecol.*, **85**, 662–7

Trudinger, B.J., Lewis, P.J. and Pettit, B. (1979). Fetal breathing patterns and intrauterine growth retardation. *Br. J. Obstet. Gynaecol.*, **86**, 432–6

Trudinger, B.J., Giles, W.B. and Cook, C.M. (1985a). Uteroplacental blood flow velocity-time waveforms in normal and complicated pregnancy. *Br. J. Obstet. Gynaecol.*, **92**, 39–45

Trudinger, B.J., Giles, W.B. and Cook, C.M. (1985b). Uteroplacental blood flow velocity-time waveforms in normal and complicated pregnancy. *Br. J. Obstet. Gynaecol.*, **92**, 39–45

Trudinger, B.J., Cook, C.M., Jones, L. and Giles, W.B. (1986). A comparison of fetal heart rate monitoring and umbilical artery waveforms in the recognition of fetal compromise. *Br. J. Obstet. Gynaecol.*, **93**, 171–5

Tutera, G. and Newman, R.L. (1975). Fetal monitoring: its effect on perinatal mortality and caesarean section rates and its complications. *Am. J. Obstet. Gynecol.*, **122**, 750–4

Varma, T.R., Taylor, H. and Bridges, C. (1979). Ultrasound assessment of fetal growth. *Br. J. Obstet. Gynaecol.*, **86**, 623–32

Vedra, B. (1959). Acidosis and anaerobiosis in full term infants. *Acta Paediatrica (Uppsala)*, **48**, 60–9

Verardini (1878), quoted by Goodlin (1979)

Vesalius, A. (1543). De humani corporis fabrica libri septum. *Generations Organorum Basilieae*, p. 660

Visser, G.H.A. and Huisjes, H.J. (1977). Diagnostic value of the unstressed antepartum cardiotocogram. *Br. J. Obstet. Gynaecol.*, **84**, 321–6

Von Hoefft, (1836). Beobachtungen uber Auskultation der Schwengeren. *Zeitschrift fur Geburtskund*, **vi**, 1

Von Winckel, F. (1893). *Lehrbuch der Geburtshilf* Leipzig

Walker, J. (1959). Fetal distress. *Am. J. Obstet. Gynecol.*, **77**, 94

Ward, H., Rochman, H., Varnavides, L.A. and Whyley, G.A. (1973). Hormone and enzyme levels in normal and complicated pregnancies. *Am. J. Obstet. Gynecol.*, **116**, 1105

Weber, T. and Hahn-Pedersen, S. (1979). Normal values for fetal scalp tissue pH during labour. *Br. J. Obstet. Gynaecol.*, **86**, 728–31

Weller, C., Dyson, R.J., McFadyen, I.R., Green, H.L. and Arias, E. (1981). Fetal EEG using a new, flexible electrode. *Br. J. Obstet. Gynaecol.*, **88**, 983–6

Wells, P.N.T. (1987). The safety of diagnostic ultrasound. *Br. J. Radiol.*, Suppl. 20

Westin, B. (1977). Gravidogram and fetal growth, comparison with biochemical supervision. *Acta Obstet. Gynecol. (Scandinavica)*, **56**, 273

Whitfield, C.R., Chan, W.H., Sproule, W.B. and Stewart, A.D. (1972). Amniotic fluid lecithin: sphingomyelin ratio and fetal lung development. *Br. Med. J.*, **11**, 85–6

Wilds, P.L. (1978). Observations of intrauterine fetal breathing movements – a review. *Am. J. Obstet. Gynecol.*, **131**, 315–38

Williams, E.A. and Stallworthy, J.A. (1952). A simple method of internal tocography. *Lancet*, **1**, 330

Windle, W.F. (1970). Quoted by Curran, J.T. (1975) p. 36

Winick, M. (1971). Cellular changes during placental and fetal growth. *Am. J. Obstet. Gynecol.*, **109**, 166

Winslowius (1787). Quoted by Griffin, D. (1984) p. 96

Wladimiroff, J.W. and McGhie, J. (1981). Ultrasonic assessment of cardiovascular geometry and function in the human fetus. *Br. J. Obstet. Gynaecol.*, **88**, 870–5

Wladimiroff, J.W., Van Weering, H.K. and Roodenburg, E. (1977). The effects of changes in maternal blood gases on fetal breathing movements. In Beard, R.W. and Campbell, S. (eds.) *The Current Status of Fetal Heart Rate Monitoring and Ultrasound in Obstetrics*, pp. 221–37. (London: RCOG)

Wood, C., Lumley, J. and Renou, P. (1967). A clinical assessment of foetal diagnostic methods. *J. Obstet. Gynaecol. Br. Commonw.*, **74**, 823–5

Wood, C., Newman, W., Lumley, J. and Hammond, J. (1969). Classification of fetal heart rate in relation to fetal scalp blood measurements and Apgar score. *Am. J. Obstet. Gynecol.*, **105**, 942

Wood, C., Renou, P., Oats, J., Farrell, E., Beischer, N. and Anderson, I. (1981). A controlled trial of fetal heart rate monitoring in a low-risk obstetric population. *Am. J. Obstet. Gynecol.*, **141**, 527–34

Ylppo, (1916). Neugeborenen, hunger und intoxikations-acidosis in ihren Beziehungen Zueinander. *Zeitschrift fur Kinderheilkunde*, **14**, 268

FURTHER READING

Beard, R.W. and Campbell, S. (eds.) (1977). Antepartum fetal heart rate monitoring. *The Current Status of Fetal Heart Rate Monitoring and Ultrasound in Obstetrics,* pp. 28–44. A Scientific Meeting of the Royal College of Obstetricians and Gynaecologists, December, 1977. (London: RCOG)

Bennett, M.J. (1974). Antenatal fetal monitoring. *Br. J. Hosp. Med.,* **12,** 27–32

Curran, J.T. (1975). *Fetal Heart Monitoring.* (London and Boston: Butterworths)

Filshie, M. (1974). Intrapartum fetal monitoring. *Br. J. Hosp. Med.,***12,** 1, 33–46

Flynn, A.M. and Kelly, J. (1982). Fetal monitoring in labour. In Bonnar, J. (ed.) *Recent Advances in Obstetrics and Gynaecology,* Vol. 14 pp. 25–45. (Edinburgh, London: Churchill Livingstone)

Freeman, R.K., Garite, T.J. and Nageotte, M.P. (1991). History of fetal monitoring. In *Fetal Heart Rate Monitoring,* 2nd edn. pp. 1–16. (Baltimore: Williams & Wilkins)

Goodlin, R.C. (1979). History of fetal monitoring. *Am. J. Obstet. Gynecol.,* 133, 323–52

Griffin, D. (1984). Fetal activity. In Studd, J. (ed.) *Progress in Obstetrics and Gynaecology,* Vol. 4, pp. 92–117. (Edinburgh, London: Churchill Livingstone)

Hutchinson, R.S. and Crawford, J.W. (1985). Intrapartum fetal monitoring – present status. In Studd, J. (ed.) *The Management of Labour,* chapter 14, pp. 195–212. (Oxford: Blackwell Scientific Publications)

Kubli, F., Boos, R., Rutgers, H., Hagens, C.V. and Vanselow, H. (1977). Antepartum fetal heart rate monitoring. In Beard, R.W. and Campbell, S. (eds.) *The Current Status of Fetal Heart Rate Monitoring and Ultrasound in Obstetrics,* pp. 28–45. (London: RCOG)

MacDonald, D. and Grant, A. (1987). Fetal surveillance in labour – the present position. In Bonnar, J. (ed.) *Recent Advances in Obstetrics and Gynaecology,* No. 15, pp. 83–100. (Edinburgh, London: Churchill Livingstone)

Pearson, J.F. (1981). The value of antenatal fetal monitoring. In Studd, J. (ed.) *Progress in Obstetrics and Gynaecology,* Vol. 1, pp. 105–24. (Edinburgh, London: Churchill Livingstone)

Pinkerton, J.H.M. (1976). Fetal auscultation – some aspects of its history and evolution. *J. Irish Med. Assoc.,* **69,** 363–8

Pinkerton, J.H.M. (1980). John Creery Ferguson, friend of William Stokes and pioneer of auscultation of the fetal heart in the British Isles. *Br. J. Obstet. Gynaecol.,* **4,** 257–60

Pinkerton, J.H.M. (1984). Evory Kennedy: a master controversial. *Irish Med. J.,* **77,** 77–81

Labour and delivery

Positions of the child inside the uterus, the development of the obstetric forceps, the vacuum extractor, ergot and oxytocics

The vast majority of babies are born with the head emerging first, with the back of the head facing the front of the mother, and with the shoulders, the rest of the body and the afterbirth following. Labour is divided into stages, the first being the opening up of the neck of the womb, the second being the actual emergence of the baby, and the third being the delivery of the placenta, which because it normally comes after the baby, is called the afterbirth.

When the position of the baby's head in the pelvis is unusual (Figure 1), so that the back of the head faces the side of the mother or is towards the mother's back, there may be delay in the first and in the second stages of labour. Until the discovery of oxytocics there was little that could be done to hasten the first stage of labour, although throughout history well-meaning people had tried. When the delay was in the second stage of labour, originally filets, crotchets and other devices to pull the baby's head out were tried, but the greatest advance was the invention of the obstetric forceps, and then later the increasing safety of the Caesarean operation.

When it was realized that the fetus was lying in the uterus in an abnormal position it was known that if labour started with the position persisting, delivery might be impossible. This was particularly so if an arm should come down through the vagina first. Attempts were therefore made to turn the baby into a more favourable position, and from the time of Soranus (AD 98–138; q.v. in Biographies) chapters had been written in books explaining how to turn the baby. Attempts were made to turn it from outside the womb through the abdomen, and from inside the womb. It was realized by Soranus (1955) and after the Dark Ages by Ambroise Paré (1655) that it was easier, if turning the baby from inside the womb to reach for one or both feet and turn it round to deliver with feet first rather than to try to turn the head so that this would emerge first.

At some other places in the book internal podalic version, which is the operation of bring-

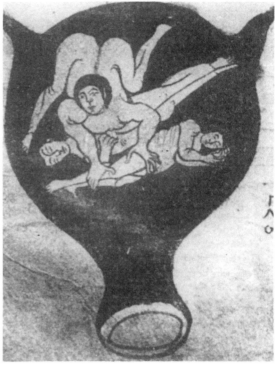

Figure 1 Positions of the fetus after Moschion Muscio circa 500 AD. Drawn after Soranus of Ephesus (98–138 AD). This M.S. is considered to be of about 900 AD

ing the feet down, is discussed; but this chapter will be concentrating on the development of the obstetric forceps, the ventouse and oxytocics.

THE DEVELOPMENT OF THE OBSTETRIC FORCEPS AND OF THE VACUUM EXTRACTOR

The secret of a successful delivery of a baby through the mother's pelvis and vagina lies in the ability of the *forces*, these being the contractions of the mother's uterine muscles and of her abdominal wall muscles when she is pushing in the second stage of labour, to overcome the resistance of the bony pelvis and sometimes of the muscular part of the pelvis. The bony pelvis may be resistant because of its small size. This was especially so in the days of malnutrition with attendant rickets – common in the United Kingdom until the 1940s. The two main ways of overcoming the resistance of the pelvis due to disproportion of the baby's size and the diameters through which it has to pass are the forceps or ventouse applied to the baby's head to pull it through the birth canal, and Caesarean section to deliver it through an incision in the abdomen.

The reasons for choosing forceps to effect delivery may lie in the size of the baby, in the weakness of the forces or misdirection by the mother of her expulsive efforts, or in the position of the baby's head so that the smallest possible diameter is not available to go through the mother's pelvis. Other reasons are rigidity of the soft tissues of the mother's pelvis or tiredness of the mother, or the baby suffering distress. Forceps are instruments curved so as to fit round the baby's head and not compress it too much. Most forceps, after the original ones, had a second curve, the so-called pelvic curve, to enable the baby's head to be pulled through the mother's pelvis, which is itself curved (Figure 2).

The county of Essex plays a very important part in the history of the invention of the forceps, in particular because the Chamberlen family lived there. A Mr Edmund Chapman, of South Halsted in Essex, wrote a book in 1733 describing the

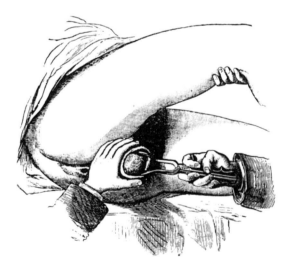

Figure 2 A French illustration (late nineteenth century) of a forceps delivery with the mother in the left lateral position ('the English position')

forceps, but he may have obtained the idea of them from a publication by a Mr William Giffard, a surgeon and man-midwife of London, whose writings were published by a Mr Edward Hody in 1734. Chapman's forceps were made of soft metal and easily became distorted and so were apt to slip off the baby's head.

It seems that Mr Drinkwater, a surgeon and man-midwife of Brentford, had a pair of forceps which after his death passed to a Dr Robert Wallace Johnson, one of Hunter's pupils, who mentioned it in his book on midwifery published in 1769. There is also the work of a local obstetrician Benjamin Pugh, of Chelmsford in Essex, who published a book in 1754 in London entitled *A Treaty of Midwifery Chiefly with Regard to the Operation. With several improvements of that art, to which is added: some cases and descriptions with place of several new instruments both in midwifery and surgery.*

Before forceps were invented, ingenuity was applied to find methods of extraction of the fetus when it was stuck in the pelvis, or above the pelvis. Amand designed a net or filet and this was placed over the head of the fetus (Witkowski, 1906). There were small loops for the fingers of the operator to be inserted and a thread to close the neck of the net around the baby's head when it had been applied. Thereafter traction was exerted on four stud tapes buried into the net. This was an adaptation of Smellie's filet shown in one of his tables, which was merely a string to be tied around the baby's head. The Japanese also invented different kinds of filets. Poullet invented a similar kind of apparatus with a rather more robust construction to be placed around the fetal head with thicker tapes for traction.

Forceps – derivation of the word

The word 'forceps' probably derived from the words *formus* which means 'hot' and *capere* which means 'to seize'; therefore forceps were instruments with which to seize hot things. They are something like fire tongs used to rearrange the coals on an open coal fire. There is an Egyptian carving which illustrates an instrument similar to obstetric forceps; but this was probably designed to hold sacrifices. Virgil described Cyclops handling hot iron with forceps while working at their forges on Mount Etna. Ovid also mentioned the instrument. So the name of the obstetric instrument may well have derived from the instrument used for handling hot iron or coal. The *Ayurveda* (science of life) written in India about

1500 BC clearly described some obstetric instruments, but no definite forceps. The earliest instruments, hooks and knives, were clearly used to deliver only dead children, to be used only when the labour was completely obstructed, the infant had perished and there was no hope of delivering it.

It appears that an instrument called a 'wombpin' was used in Tibet. It was described in the German publication on Tibetan Medicine by Heinreich Laufer in Leipzig in 1900 and by a Russian, A. Pozdeniev, in St Petersburg in 1908. Destructive instruments seem to have been known for a very long time and appear in Sanskrit texts. The *Sushruta Sanhita* is one such old text. Our knowledge of these old instruments is scanty; even Das, who made a profound study of obstetrical instruments (Das, 1929), could not describe them. Hippocrates seemed to possess an instrument to compress a dead child, and Soranus had 7 instruments for breaking up dead children before delivering them with hooks (Soranus, 1955). Aetius (q.v.) employed two hooks to grasp a dead child's head from the opposite sides. Albucasis (q.v.) (AD 936–1013) described a variety of obstetrical instruments, but none of them were true forceps.

Ambroise Paré described crotchets, kinds of forks with long pointed teeth bent back in the middle to grasp the dead child (Paré, 1655). The first mention of forceps that could possibly have been used on a live child was by Jacques Jacob Rueff of Zurich in 1554, but we have no record of the dimensions of his instrument nor what they really looked like, although they do seem to have been some sort of grasping instrument, more like long thin spoons with long handles held together at the hinge by some kind of a screw. Rueff's name is also associated with the speculum but he never claimed he was the inventor of it, although he did publish a drawing, apparently of a speculum, in 1554. It seems according to Das that 'Rueff completely amended Rösslin's chapter on the extraction of the retained fetus but Rösslin did not mention his speculum in his *Roszgarten* which was published in 1515.

Mauriceau (q.v.) invented a perforator and another instrument to extract a dead baby after having made a hole in its head so that the brain could come out and the bones collapse.

In his book on the Chamberlens and the midwifery forceps, subtitled *Memorials of the Family and an Essay on the Invention of the Instrument*, J-H. Aveling in 1882 stated 'it is beyond doubt a fact that Arabian surgeons used forceps to deliver the fetal head in difficult labours. Avicenna mentions them, and Albucasis gives drawings of barbarous instruments which were intended to be used as cranioclasts' (Das, 1929; p. 19). Aveling also mentions Rueff only to dismiss him entirely as the inventor of midwifery forceps and says 'in 1554 he published a book on midwifery, which bears no evidence of his being an obstetrician of exceptional talent'! He also compares it adversely to Rhodion's book and he deplores the fact that it was translated into English under the title of *The Expert Midwife* because it would have been much better if midwives had remained ignorant!

Das, on page 49 of his book, wrote 'a struggle was now about to begin, however, between them (the midwives who read Rueff's book) and the members of our profession as to whether the midwife or the doctor should be paramount in the delivery room, in which the gradually extending power of the printing press gave the men who wrote and read the works on science and art an advantage over the women'. He does mention the work of Louise Bourgeois (q.v.), Marguerite de Tertre, the Chief Midwife of the Hotel Dieu, Justine Sigmundin of Germany, and Mrs Jane Sharp and Mrs Nihell of England.

It was the development of the forceps which gave men an edge over the midwives. Jean Palfyn of the City of Ghent demonstrated a rudimentary pair of forceps in 1720, but the Chamberlens had already been using forceps for four generations by that time. As so often happens, Palfyn's claim to be an inventor of an instrument was disputed by Gilles le Doux who designed two blades with handles which he held together by thread. A full account of Palfyn's demonstrations is given by Das (1929) but no publication by Palfyn is now available.

Thomas More Madden (1875) wrote that he had devoted a great deal of attention to the question (of whether the Chamberlens had invented the forceps) and came to the conclusion that they had not, but that they were already being used 1800 years earlier as, claimed Madden, they had been discovered in the excavations at Pompeii, and he said that Avicenna had written about forceps in the tenth century and Albucasis (q.v.) in the eleventh century.

It appears, according to Rueff, that Avicenna's forceps like those of Jacobus (Jacques) Rueff had a cardinal fault in that the blades were united by a fixed point, and had to be introduced articulated into the vagina which must have been extremely difficult. It was only after they had been

141

introduced that they were opened to try to catch the baby's head (Das, 1929; p.18 Figure 16).

There does seem to have been a time when forceps of a rather primitive type were made and then there was a big hiatus until the Chamberlens came up with the forceps which could be introduced one blade at a time: that was their great invention. Many of the obstetricians mentioned in this history (see Biographies) invented or modified forceps. Mauriceau did, as did Mesnard and Palfyn with his 'mains de fer' and probably Gilles le Doux; although his may have been copied from Palfyn. It is possible that some confusion arises from the invention of cranioclasts which are very much like forceps, but designed to crush the baby's head and not to bring it out undamaged.

A reviewer of Aveling's book claimed that Avicenna, Albucasis and even Jacob Rueff all designed craniotomy forceps that resembled, but were not nearly up to the standard of Chamberlen's forceps (Anon., 1883). Das's book has the great merit of giving almost 200 references to articles and books on the history of the forceps before the Chamberlens.

It would have been strange if the Chamberlen family had been able to keep their secret watertight for 100 years or more. There was some acrimony between Mauriceau and Chamberlen; and Mauriceau without good evidence pointed out that the women of England were the easiest to deliver, easier than the women of France, when they had a narrow pelvis. It was claimed that the Chamberlens' forceps was designed to meet that need. Mauriceau according to Das, wrote that Chamberlen was asked by Mauriceau to deliver a baby through an impossibly deformed contracted pelvis and failed, 'Moy', declares Mauriceau, with all that Frenchman's untranslatable vanity, 'qu'il disoit assuroit être le plus habile homme de ma profession qui fort a Paris', which loosely translated is 'I who is claimed to be the most clever in my profession in Paris' was told by Chamberlen that he was surprised he could not deliver a baby. Not only was his vanity exposed, but the crude chauvinism of his time. There seems no doubt that nationalistic pride played a large role in the discussions and especially in the issues between Mauriceau and the Chamberlens.

The country where the production of forceps flourished most after 1693, when Chamberlen may have divulged the secret to Roger Roonhuysen was Holland. The Roonhuysen family kept the forceps as a monopoly in Amsterdam for 60 years between 1693 and 1753; but there were assistants and associates who knew about the secret and they formed themselves into a sort of company – The Medico-Pharmaceutical College of Amsterdam – and maintained the monopoly by having the sole right to licence physicians to practise in Holland. Those given the licence had to buy the secret. Inevitably the secret leaked out by a mixture of cunning and, to put none to fine a word on it, thievery. Van de Smorren a student of Roonhuysen, saw Roonhuysen, who had been called urgently to see the Burgermaister, put the instrument into a bag. He opened the bag and saw the design of the forceps. Armed with this design, which he copied, he met another obstetrician, Rathlau, who had been unable to obtain a licence to practise because he refused to pay for the secret, and Rathlau must have made some form of forceps from it. Of course those who had paid to be in the know, claimed that Rathlau's forceps were useless. Eventually the whole thing came out in Holland because one of Roonhuysen's pupils Jean de Bruin gave his daughter Gertrude the secret and she communicated it to her husband Thomas de Heide. This couple sold it on. There was obviously money – big money – in the discovery.

Benjamin Pugh was one of the first inventors of the forceps with a pelvic curve in 1754. He wrote a treatise on midwifery illustrated with plates. He really seems to have copied from the Levret or the Smellie forceps. Anyhow, he describes the forceps quite ingeniously by giving the maximum measurements of the curve as the distance away from a string held tight from the beginning of the curve to the other end of it. 'Thus the distance from the middle of the curve ought to be 1 inch and a half from the string.' He also gives measurements of the upper edge of the curve. His forceps were fenestrated. Benjamin Pugh, although he spent most of his professional life in Chelmsford, was born in Bishops Castle in Shropshire where he inherited an estate from his mother, who was the daughter of Walter Woolaston. In Chelmsford in 1738 he married Amy Evans a widow, who was the daughter of Sherman Wall, an apothecary in Chelmsford. When Wall died the Pugh's inherited Wall's house and built a new one on the site. For a time the Essex Independent was published from that house. In 1747 Pugh became apothecary 'to the poor of the Chelmsford district and up to 2 miles distant'. Pugh's house became known as the Mansion House, though there is nothing very striking about it either in shape or size, and it would now be called a 'town house'.

The Chamberlen forceps really were astoundingly cleverly designed, with a beautiful curve (the cephalic curve) to fit round the baby's head. They were however, missing the all important pelvic curve. But before we get to that, it is important to mention another feature of the forceps which could cause trouble, and this was the screw. The screw designed by the Chamberlens was a fixed one. One day Edmund Chapman the man-midwife from South Halstead in Essex lost the screw in the patient's sheets and was constrained to invent some other way of locking the forceps together and so he designed the Chapman's lock which later became known as the English lock. He did not join the parts together; and quite honestly recounted that having lost the screw he had to find some other way to use the instrument which 'did its office much better without the screw or without the two parts being fixed'. With the invention of the English lock the shanks which connected the blades to the handles on each side could be slotted one into the other. This was a great advance.

In France Palfyn had designed two large spoons that were neither screwed together nor locked together, but tied together by strips of napkins, and later by a mobile hook (Figure 3). The locking forceps had the advantage that the shanks crossed over one another and allowed much stronger traction (without the risk of the blades slipping off), than forceps such as Palfyn's that did not cross over.

The development of a pelvic curve in order to allow the forceps which had been applied to the baby's head to follow the axis of the pelvis, followed on the first description of this invention, by Hendrik van Deventer (q.v.), the famous Dutch obstetrician, in 1701. His book was published in Latin by Dyckuisen. There was an English translation published in 1716 (Deventer, 1716).

Levret, the famous French obstetrician, took up Deventer's idea. Levret described his invention to the Academie de Sciences on the 7 January 1747 and again in 1761 he gave a description of the various planes of the pelvis. He got it slightly wrong as did so many other people, thinking that the inlet of the pelvis was virtually horizontal (which it is not in the standing woman) and that there was an angle of about 35 degrees from the top of the pubic symphysis to the middle of the lower edge of the last lumbar vertebra (actually about 55 degrees from the horizontal) and that there is a line parallel with it from the tip of the coccyx and extending to the lower part of the vulva. Levret was the first to show that the fetal head had to go down the pelvis through a curve and he illustrated such a pelvis in his book which showed the curve. There were plenty of mistakes; and in fact the legend that he wrote under his illustration does not correspond with the features demonstrated in the illustration. Levret's confused drawing and descriptions were corrected much later by a German gynaecologist Carl Gustav Carus (1789–1869) (Carus, 1820). Long before Carus's accurate description Levret, and soon after him Smellie, both designed forceps with a pelvic curve, probably at about the same time. It is known that Smellie was in Paris to learn from Gregoire in 1739 having travelled there for a short time. He had arrived in London from Scotland only in 1738. Not only did Smellie design, or co-design, the pelvic curve (Figure 4), but he also almost certainly modified or redesigned the English lock that allowed the shanks of the forceps to fit into one another and to stay articulated without the need for a screw. He also designed a straight forceps, and a double-curved crotchet with scissors. The crotchet was for use only when the fetus had already died; and his double-curved crotchet, like his forceps, had the English lock incorporated in them.

Smellie designed his forceps after he had read a description of Edmund Chapman's forceps. This description was published without illustrations in 1733; and after Giffard had published his illustrated *Midwifery* in 1734. But Chapman had already made forceps for several years before 1733, probably about a dozen years after the secret of the Chamberlen forceps had leaked out.

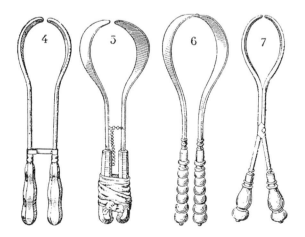

Figure 3   Palfyn's forceps. ('Hands of iron' 1721)

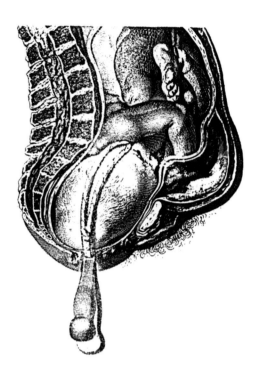

Figure 4 Smellie's forceps (*see* text). Note the blades have strips of durable leather wound round them

It is very difficult now to know exactly the priorities in the various inventions and discoveries (and who copied ideas from whom), but it is certain that the great names from the early days of forceps are Chamberlen, Chapman, Levret and Smellie. It is not necessary at this stage to decide between Levret and Smellie as to who copied from whom. It is just as likely that they both had similar ideas at the same time as so often happens in science today.

Once the curve of the bony pelvis had been understood and forceps with a curve to follow the anatomical bony structure had been designed, techniques had to be worked out to use them to the maximum effect with the minimum of trauma to the mother. Pajot in Paris (details of his life are to be found in Fasbender (1906) and in Witkowski (1887)) who was a wonderful technician, developed a method of pulling on the handles of the Levret forceps, while at the same time depressing the shank with his other hand, so it is today called Pajot's manoeuvre.

It was not always easy, however, manually to make the forceps follow the pelvic curve; and

obstetrics had to wait until Tarnier in Paris invented his axis traction forceps first published in 1877 in a monograph (Figure 5). The way Tarnier described the new forceps was to claim for them, correctly, that traction need not be as strong as with the ordinary forceps and the pull need be no more than to overcome a resistance of 17 kg. He also claimed that with the new forceps all the applied force brought the head into the axis of the pelvis without producing any compression of the maternal tissues as was done with conventional forceps. Furthermore, there was less likelihood of the fetal head slipping out from between the blades. The handles of Tarnier's forceps were horizontal and therefore much easier for the operator to grip.

Etienne Stephane Tarnier (1828–1897) really understood the mechanical principles that had to be applied. He wrote 'all obstetricians know that in a proper application of the forceps, traction ought to be directed as far as possible, in the axis of the pelvis; but all acknowledge that at the superior strait and above the strait it is impossible to pull far enough back, because the instrument is unavoidably maintained in the wrong direction by the resistance of the perineum. I would go further and say that at the level of the imperial strait and at the vulval orifice, traction is always misdirected when one uses ordinary forceps, because of the very shape of the instrument whether its blade be crossed or parallel.' He added that when obstetricians try to overcome the harmful effects of the wrong direction they fail

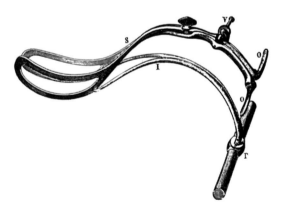

Figure 5 Tarnier's axis-traction forceps. The 1877 model. (I) Parallel traction rods; (S) blades, or as called by Tarnier, prehension branches, which cross over; (O) wings of forceps handles; (r) axis traction handle; (V) screw lock (*See* text)

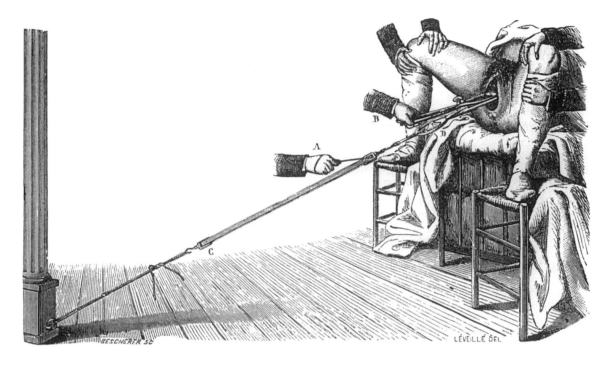

Figure 6 Delore's method of axis traction using pulleys and cords attached to the axis traction rod handle of Tarnier's forceps (after Witkowski)

and damage the mother. Pajot's manoeuvre was helpful, but Tarnier's instrument was designed to satisfy the requisites of the ideal forceps:

(1) 'To enable the operator to pull at all times in the axis of the pelvis, whatever the position of the head in the pelvic canal,

(2) To allow the fetal head enough mobility to follow the curve of the pelvis freely,

(3) To carry a needle indicator showing the obstetrician the direction that he should give his traction in order that it be absolutely correct'.

Tarnier designed his instrument after another obstetrician named Pros had shown him his forceps with a hinge in the pelvic curve which allowed the pelvic curve to become greater or less as the forceps came down the cavity of the pelvis. Pros's forceps were complicated and required a long tractor to be attached to the ends of the handles of the forceps after their application to the baby's head.

Tarnier's forceps had axis traction rods attached to the lower edges of the blades (which he called branches of prehension) parallel to one

another and able to articulate freely (Figure 6). Aubenas in 1877 described Tarnier's forceps as 'it is composed of two handles and of two traction rods. The rods are inserted into a transverse bar at 'p' and 'a' parallel as in the forceps of Thenance. The fenestre are not as long as in the classic forceps; the instrument has a perineal curve, that of Morales modified; the traction rods and the handles are united by a freely movable articulation. To apply these forceps; articulate each traction rod to its corresponding blade and it is easily done. Holding both in the hand the blade is applied to the head in the usual fashion. When both blades have been introduced, the forceps are locked with the traction rods below, compression is applied to the head by means of a screw working from one handle to the other. The traction rods are inserted into the transverse traction bar. During traction on this bar, the handles act as an index of the direction in which traction should be made and the operator has only to follow the oscillations of these handles keeping the traction rods about one half an inch apart from the handles.' There are more technical details about the forceps but the principle is quite simply that traction is made on the rods; and the blades around the baby's head follow the pelvic curve automatically while the rods indicate to the operator exactly how he should pull.

Tarnier's contribution to obstetrics was greater than the invention of his forceps, for he also worked very closely with Paul Dubois to defeat puerperal sepsis in the Maternité Hospital in Paris. He had the satisfaction of succeeding Pajot who had criticized his forceps as unnecessary if Pajot's manoeuvre was followed. Tarnier introduced the idea of heated cots to put premature babies in and also instituted the idea of delaying tying the umbilical cord after delivery of the baby. He wrote a text book on obstetrics. Tarnier's forceps or modifications of them are still in use today in the 1990s.

Another look at the Chamberlen forceps

Thomas Denman (1733–1815) wrote in 1793: 'It behoveth every person who may use the instrument in the practice of midwifery to be well convinced of the necessity before they are used, and to be extremely careful in their use that he does not create new evils or aggravate those that might be existing'.

Historically the most famous and most valuable of all forceps are those invented by the Chamberlen family and now in the Royal College of Obstetricians and Gynaecologists in Regent's Park in London. In 1813 a Mrs Campbell, whose son occupied Woodham Mortimer Hall (Figure 7) near Maldon in Essex, found underneath the floorboards in an upper room on the second floor at the Hall a box containing ladies' gloves, some books, some old trinkets, Mrs Chamberlen's husband's last tooth and a few coins, as well as unusual instruments shaped like tongs and hooks. She showed them to a Mr Henry Cawardane, a retired surgeon, who realized that they were midwifery instruments. Since Peter Chamberlen (q.v.) had occupied Woodham Mortimer Hall after the restoration of the Monarchy when Charles II came back to England, it was very likely that these were the original Chamberlen forceps kept hidden 100 years after Peter's death. Mr Cawardine in 1818 deposited them with the Medico-Chirurgical Society in London. He also gave a dissertation on the history of the forceps to the Society. There are many stories concerning the dealings of the first Peter Chamberlen and his descendants which do not reflect well on their professional behaviour according to the ethics of today, but may have been slightly more acceptable in the seventeenth century. For several generations over at least 100 years they kept their invention of forceps a secret although they did try to sell it to various fellow obstetricians, including Francois Mauriceau (1637–1709) (q.v.) in Paris. Mauriceau would not buy the forceps until he had had a demonstration of their use by Chamberlen. He, unfortunately for Chamberlen, picked a labouring patient with a pelvis that was very contracted and distorted due to rickets. Chamberlen claimed he would be able to deliver the child without trouble to the mother or to the baby within 10 minutes, but he laboured underneath a sheet, which served as a curtain to hide his instrument from Mauriceau, for 3 hours before he had to admit defeat. The woman died the next day, when it became quite obvious at the post-mortem examination that Chamberlen's manipulations had inflicted grievous damage to her uterus. Not surprisingly, therefore, Mauriceau refused to buy the invention; and Peter Chamberlen returned to England with his forceps.

It had been the practice of the Chamberlens when they were called into a difficult case to bring their instruments in a very large wooden box, and insist that everybody else should leave the room while they performed the forceps delivery under a large sheet which hid the instruments even from the labouring mother herself. Hugh Chamberlen, a member of the family, translated Mauriceau's first book D*es Maladies des Femmes Grosses* which was published in France in 1668 into English in 1672, under the title *The Accomplisht Midwife.*

It is not known exactly when the first Chamberlen forceps were made although they were certainly the forerunners of forceps that are used all over the world today (Figure 8).

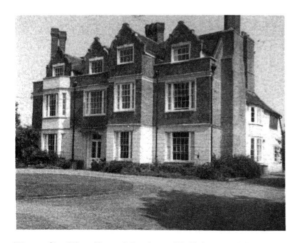

Figure 7 Woodham Mortimer Hall (*see* text)

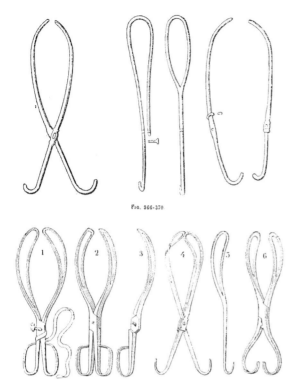

FIG. 366-370

Figure 8 Experimental designs of metal rivets to unite the two portions of the early Chamberlen's forceps (1–4). Various Chamberlen's forceps are illustrated as is Chamberlen's lever (5) and Giffard's forceps (6)

The Chamberlen family are often blamed for the fact that they kept their invention secret, taking large sums of money when called in to deliver mothers whose labours had become obstructed. It is not known which member of the family actually invented the forceps. Dr Walter Radcliffe, an Essex General Practitioner (Radcliffe, W. 1967) has written a splendid account of the invention, in a small book published in 1947, entitled *The Secret Instrument*. There is a family tree on page 72 of this book. There is quite a lot of confusion as to who is who, because William Chamberlen, who died in the seventeenth century, came to England from France as a Huguenot refugee from the religious persecution then present in France, landing in Southampton in 1569. The persecution resulted from the order given by Catherine de Medicis (1519–1589), one of the most influential personalities in the Wars of Religion, to slaughter all Huguenots. The famous massacre on St Bartholomew's Day in August 1572 was the result. It was William Chamberlen's grandson, born in 1630 and died in London 1720,

who exploited the forceps more than anybody in England and in France. In 1670 he offered the secret to the French Government. He had translated the book on midwifery by Francois Mauriceau and there was a reference to the forceps in the preface. Peter Chamberlen the older, was in continuous trouble with the College of Physicians, particularly for missing meetings when he went to the Netherlands. He was the obstetrician to Henrietta Maria, the wife of Charles I, who became the mother of Charles II.

The Medico-Chirurgical Society in London became the Royal Society of Medicine by its amalgamation with various other societies in London. It is situated in a very fine building in the West End of London. The Medico-Chirurgical Society handed the instruments down to the Royal Society of Medicine, where during the 1939–1945 war they were stored in the basement. Later, Dr Walter Radcliffe, of Essex arranged with the late Mr R. Alan Brews that they should be handed on to the Royal College of Obstetricians and Gynaecologists, but not before Mr Brews himself had carried out a low forceps operation at the London Hospital (where he was on the staff) with one pair of them, and found them quite efficient. Thanks to the work of Professor Bryan Hibbard of Cardiff, they are splendidly housed in the Royal College of Obstetricians and Gynaecologists together with many other obstetric instruments of historic interest.

The Royal College of Obstetricians and Gynaecologists has been responsible for restoring Peter Chamberlen's tomb in the churchyard of Woodham Mortimer Parish Church (Figure 9).

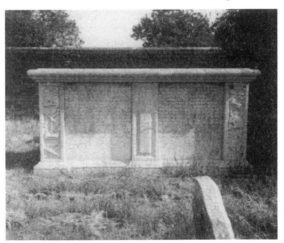

Figure 9 Peter Chamberlen's tomb almost next door to Woodham Mortimer Hall (*see* text)

The Kielland forceps: the resurrection of the straight forceps and the invention of a sliding lock

Christian Caspar Gabriel Kielland (1871–1941) designed a forceps with practically no pelvic curve. It might seem a retrograde step to have done this, since all recognized the benefit that the development of the pelvic curve in forceps, particularly that by Levret, brought. But the purpose of Levret's pelvic curve was to allow the fetal head with the forceps pulling it to come round the lowest strait of the pelvis with the minimum of damage to the soft tissues. Once local anaesthesia and general anaesthesia were effective, the need for preserving the soft tissues on the floor of the pelvis diminished, as episiotomies became almost routinely performed and indeed had to be when Kielland's forceps were used.

Kielland often journeyed to Germany; and in 1915 first demonstrated his forceps at the University Clinic in Munich, Germany, at a meeting of the Munich Gynaecological Society under the auspices of Professor Doederlein (Kielland, 1915). A year later he published a paper in the German Journal of Obstetrics pointing out that the application of his forceps was particularly indicated for the presenting head that needed rotation. The main point, therefore, of Keilland's forceps was in order to deliver an incompletely rotated head from the upper pelvis. In this position it is very difficult to grasp the head with standard forceps which are ideally used when the head is lower in the pelvis and correctly rotated. If the head is not rotated and ordinary forceps are applied with the blades parallel to the sides of the pelvis, one blade will find itself over the brow, the top of the nose, or one of the eyes, and the other over the occiput. This can be highly damaging for the fetus.

Kielland's forceps being straight could be applied either by a wandering method so that each blade came to lie over the side of the baby's head, or by a straight method, particularly suitable for the posterior blade which, after the anterior blade had been applied correctly to the fetal head, is inserted just in front of, or beside the promontory of the sacrum. The blades can be rotated around so that they come to fit well against the fetal head, and because the lock is a sliding lock the blades can find different levels, particularly when there is asynclitism of the fetal skull.

The method of application of the anterior blade can be by inserting it into the anterior part of the pelvis with the fetal curve of the forceps facing anteriorly, i.e. away from the baby's head, and then rotating it 180 degrees and pulling it down gently until it comes to be well applied to the fetal head. The absence of a pelvic curve makes it relatively easy to rotate the fetal head either in the upper part of the pelvis, or allow it to rotate as traction is exerted and it comes down through the pelvis.

The increasing safety of Caesarean operations in the 1980s led to a lessening need for forceps deliveries, particularly from the upper part of the pelvis and gradually Kielland's forceps, which in the hands of careless obstetricians could do great damage, became less popular in obstetric departments (Speert, 1958; Hibbard, 1987).

Lyman G. Barton had, in 1925, made a very interesting forceps, the design of which he published in January 1928 in the *American Journal of Obstetrics and Gynecology*. The difference in his and his colleagues forceps was that the blades joined the shanks at an angle. 'This angle was the normal angle between the axis of the superior strait of the pelvis and the axis of the pelvic outlet... Owing to the peculiar shape of the anterior blade, for the purpose of application it is necessary to incorporate a joint at the junction of the blade and shank. By means of this joint, the blade can be swung through an arc of a circle until it is nearly parallel with the shank. The lock of the forceps is so constructed that a gliding motion of one member on the other is permitted; this ensures the adaptability of the blades to heads of varying sizes without destroying the symmetry of the space between the blades', (Das, 1929). Das's book contains a full description by Barton explaining how he had obtained the idea from dentists using different types of extraction forceps for the molar teeth from those used for the incisor teeth. In one letter quoted by Das, Barton says that he had not heard of the Keilland forceps until several years after his drawings were made. He suggested that his were an improvement on the Kielland forceps.

There is a splendid resume of Doran's *A Chronology of the Founders of Forceps* (1569–1799) from the *Journal of Obstetrics and Gynaecology of the British Empire* (Das, 1929, pp. 765–771). This chronology, in seven closely printed pages, outlines all the important forceps designed between 1669 and the end of the eighteenth century. Besides this there is an interesting breakdown of Laurence Sterne's *Life and Opinions of Tristram Shandy, Gentleman*, which contains numerous paragraphs on midwives and midwifery, and in particular on the discovery and improvements made to the forceps.

Tristram Shandy is written in a sarcastic manner. There are very interesting caricatures in the chronology.

It can be said that abuse of the obstetric forceps was one of the reasons why Grantley Dick Read wrote his extremely popular book *Natural Childbirth* (Dick Read, 1933).

The history and development of the vacuum extractor, or ventouse

Much of the history of this apparatus for delivering babies vaginally is recounted in the monograph by Chalmers (Chalmers, 1971).

The idea of using vacuum to assist vaginal delivery was developed from the discovery by Ambroise Paré (q.v.) that compressed fractures of the skull in infants could be corrected by using a leather sucker (1632). Hildanus made several such suckers in 1632, including one of plaster constructed from a sturgeon's bladder and other exotic substances (Eustace, 1991). Paré had applied the same principle as Hildanus, using a cupping-glass to correct a depressed fracture of the skull in an adult (Paré, 1655). It was James Young (1706) who in November 1705, 'called to deliver a woman four days in labour' wrote that he could neither 'fasten the crotchet nor draw it out by a cupping glass fixed to the scalp with an air pump' (Young, 1706). James Young may have been the first to attempt to deliver a baby by a vacuum extractor. Because he failed he directed his son to open and crush the baby's head which allowed a rapid delivery. A Doctor Saemann apparently had a dream in which he saw an air pump made of brass, with a covering of rubber, with ventilators, wherewith one could seize the head of the infant without injury to mother and child. Saemann thought that this was a dream that might one day come true (Saemann, 1794).

Neil Arnott (1788–1874), was said, to have described in 1829 the principle derived from the application by small boys of wet leather to dried stone to make a vacuum and to lift the stone to make a 'pneumatic tractor', but there is no record that he actually made one. The first really practical suggestion for the use of the vacuum extractor was made by the great James Young Simpson (q.v.) who had the wonderful gift of introducing and adapting into obstetrics many other discoveries such as, above all, anaesthesia, a practical forceps for mid-cavity application in order to accomplish vaginal delivery, acupressure and so on (Simpson, 1849; 1867). Simpson said that in 1836

he had thought of sucking the baby out after he had seen a group of Edinburgh schoolboys playing a game of 'suckers' to see who could lift the largest stone with a piece of wet leather threaded to a string. He may had got the idea from Arnott. A few years later Simpson wrote 'the instrument is now nearly perfect, I showed it last Wednesday to the Medical Chirurgical Society . . . there was a great crowd . . . the experiment went off beautifully. I fixed a small tractor to the palm of my right hand and lifted up with it an iron weight of 28 pounds. One of the physicians of the St Petersburg court is here. He admired the work but doubted that it would work in practice. Well, I took him and others to see a baddish case and fixed the tractor on. The operation was most successful. The Russian cried "C'est superbe; c'est immortalité a vous".' Simpson acknowledged his debt to Arnott.

The first instrument Simpson designed was a round metal speculum which was fitted over a piston. It had a large handle to obtain a good practical grip. The broader, trumpet-shaped end was covered with leather and greased with lard. It was this end that was attached to the head of the fetus. The piston made the vacuum and Simpson 'sucked' the baby out. Apparently he also occasionally used it on breech births (Figure 10).

Simpson developed his ideas and in December 1848 he presented a paper at the Edinburgh Obstetrical Society suggesting the use of a metal

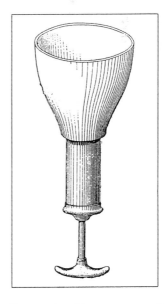

Figure 10 Simpson's rubber ventouse with a vacuum pump handle – this was a gift from Simpson to the French Professor Pajot in 1848

vaginal speculum whose 'cephalic end was covered with leather, was applied to the head of the child, well greased with lard'. This applicator was then evacuated by a syringe. Simpson being the man he was, tried a variety of forms of cup, some of metal, and one of which had a deeper cup of caoutchouc (rubber) inside it (Simpson, 1848).

So often with discoveries of an original nature someone else, in this case a Dr James Mitchell, claimed that he had suggested the use in an answer to an examination question which Simpson is said to have corrected.

A Dr John Haddy James of Exeter became interested in the same principle, and in 1857 Soubhy Saleh from Paris, designed an instrument which could not only assist delivery, but also, following perforation of the head, could evacuate brain matter from the skull. In 1875 Stillman seemed to be the first to suggest the use of a vacuum extractor before full dilatation of the cervix, and in 1890 McCahey of Philadelphia again described a vacuum extractor. Until McCahey's day the apparatus that made the vacuum and the cup on the baby's head were all in one instrument, but McCahey was able to separate the two by means of a pipe.

In 1912 a Dr Kuntch of Potsdam near Berlin, designed a vacuum helmet with a separate pump and with a manometer fitted. Torpin of Georgia who was a most inventive obstetrician, in 1937 designed a suction cup which he made from a toy rubber ball cut in half and evacuated by a pump attached to a rubber tube, sealed onto the half ball. He filed a patent in that year for a system of gradually reducing the pressure so as to make a Chignon on the baby's head.

Torpin was also, to digress, the inventor of a tank for the examination of the placenta. His tank was filled with water; and the membranes of the amniotic sac were attached to a circular ring by small clothes hooks so the maternal side of the membranes together with the placenta could be inspected easily through the walls of the tank which had electric lights in it. Torpin's suction instrument was not dissimilar to one later made by Oedenberg and Herbert Thoren in 1953 from a design by Malmström. This instrument has proved to be such an important invention that in many countries, and in particular Belgium, where a Professor Snoek was a great advocate, vacuum extraction has replaced the obstetric forceps as a method of delivering babies, even when the end of the first stage of labour is delayed. This also true of China today. Malmström's extractor consists of two metal cups inside one another, with a rubber cover outside the external metal cup. The inside cup prevents the baby's head being sucked too deeply into the outside cup and the rubber allows a very good application and minimizes the risks of leakage.

One of the great advantages of the extractor over forceps is that it does not take up room between the fetal and maternal tissues, and another advantage is that it can be applied before full dilatation of the cervix. Malmström's recent vacuum extractors have cups with in-curved margins to apply to the fetal head and to make it possible to form an artificial caput succedaneum within the cup following Torpin's methods.

Various modifications have been made over the years but the principle is still the same. The cup is attached to the fetal head. There is a chain that either goes through or beside the tubing through which the vacuum is obtained using a pump. A bottle intervenes between the pump and the tubing attached to the cup to catch liquor and any blood which may be sucked out. Pumps may be made like ordinary bicycle pumps or much more elaborate electrical pumps.

Bird in 1969 (Bird, 1969) modified the Malmström vacuum extractor by attaching the tubing, through which the vacuum is made, laterally on the cup, while the chain through which traction is applied was placed centrally on the cup. Some of Bird's cups are more shallow than those of Malmström of Göteborg, Sweden (Malmström, 1954; 1957).

There have been many further developments in the ventouse notably by Hawkin in 1964 and Lovsett who in 1965 altered the shape of the cup. The cups of Geoffrey Bird of Australia have the suction tube at an eccentric angle, at the edge or side of the cup. In Romania a doctor designed a foot-operated pump, and another doctor later in 1989 used the vacuum system attached to many labour wards in hospitals to evacuate air from the cup but this required manometers to be put into the system (Carter, 1990).

In the 1970s and the 1980s manufacturers developed pliable silastic vacuum extractors which were thought to be less traumatic for the fetal scalp and caused less chignon formation (Carter, 1990).

There has been a splendid historical lecture on the origins and the development of the ventouse given by Mr D.L.S. Eustace of St Thomas' Hospital, London, to the Royal College of Obstetricians and Gynaecologists in December 1991.

ERGOMETRINE AND OXYTOCICS

Ergot has a long history. The effects of ergot on the contractions of the uterus have been known for a very long time. Its effects on the extremities, especially the fingers and toes, characterized by intense burning in these digits and later sometimes by gangrene, were known as St Anthony's Fire; because St Anthony and his followers centuries back, provided help for the victims of poisoning caused by the eating of bread made from diseased corn which was contaminated with black spurs of the Ergot fungus, *Claviceps purpurea.*

There is a story that in 1822 a Dr Hosack wrote that the introduction of ergot had caused the number of stillborn children to increase so much in New York that the Medical Society there had instituted an inquiry. He said 'the Ergot has been called . . . *Pulvis ad partum;* as regards the child it may with almost equal truth be denominated *Pulvis ad mortem'.*

J. Chassar Moir has written the story and his book (Chassar Moir, 1970) contains all other relevant references. In the Middle Ages there was an epidemic disease that ravaged Europe. It was particularly likely to occur in corn-producing districts of South Germany and France where instead of wheat the farmers grew rye. In wet seasons fungus appeared on the rye-grass, causing it to blacken and produce slightly curved spurs three or four times the length of the natural grain. By the sixteenth century it was known that eating bread made from rye affected by the fungus could lead to a disease called 'cold fire'. One of the main features of the disease was tingling of the skin a burning sensation in the fingers which sometimes, together with the toes and occasionally even the whole limbs, turned black and were sloughed off. Sometimes convulsions occurred as well as mental frenzy and hallucinations. It also caused pregnant sows to litter before their time. As early as the year 945 a plague of 'the fire' occurred in and around Paris. Brotherhoods of monks who were dedicated to St Anthony established hostels in the stricken areas and possibly because of this association the disease came to be called 'St Anthony's fire'. By the end of the sixteenth century ergot was used medicinally. It could 'awaken the pains of labour'.

Dr John Stearns, a general practitioner working in Saratoga County in New York State, was asked by the midwife with whom he was working to make a powder from the black corns found in a rye granary. In 1808 he wrote a letter which said among other things 'previous to its exhibition it is of the utmost consequence to ascertain the presentation as the violent and almost incessant action which it induces in the uterus precludes the possibility of turning . . . you would be surprised at the suddenness of its operation; it is therefore necessary to be completely ready before you give the medicine'.

It was indeed remarkable how very violently and how very fast the uterus reacted to the giving of ergot powder by mouth so that Dr Hosack was driven to write his well-known phrase about ergot being a killer. Ergot used to speed up labour could kill both the baby and the mother whose uterus might rupture. Once the baby was out, ergot was invaluable, and still is at speeding up the delivery of the placenta and making the uterine muscle contract to stop haemorrhage.

J. Chassar Moir, the Nuffield Professor of Obstetrics and Gynaecology in the University of Oxford, together with the head of the Therapeutics Trials Committee of the Medical Research Council, Sir Henry Dale and a chemist Dr H.W. Dudley, first investigated the active substance derived from the fungus which affected rye grass used to make bread. Sir Henry Dale (q.v.) had been working on ergot in relation to the activities of ergotoxine, an alkaloid that he had extracted from ergot. He had found that it abolished the motor effects of sympathetic stimulation and of adrenaline. Sir Henry went on investigating the activity of particular extracts that he had isolated, which effects were contrary to those he had been expecting. Already in 1906 a Doctor Barger and a co-worker Kerr (Barger, 1931) found another alkaloid ergotoxine which stimulated the muscle action of the isolated uterus and which had the same sort of effect in producing gangrene as ergot had.

Professor F.J. Browne of University College Hospital was approached by the Medical Research Council Therapeutic Trials Committee to investigate the action of two of the alkaloids of ergot; ergotoxine and ergotamine. They did make the uterus contract, but slowly, much more slowly than would be expected from reading Dr Stearn's letter which talked about the surprising suddenness of the action. Chassar Moir, who worked with F. J. Browne, was disappointed with the action of ergotoxine and ergotamine and went back to the aqueous extract of ergot which then appeared as a preparation in the British Pharmacopoeia. It was known not to contain ergotamine or ergotoxine. He found that when he gave liquid extract of ergot by mouth to a woman who had delivered her baby the action of her uterus, as measured by an apparatus introduced into her uterus to record the intrauterine pressure, was very fast. Professor Moir wrote 'then felt I like some watcher of the skies, when a new planet swims into its ken'. Professor Moir realized that there must be a third alkaloid in the watery extract of ergot that he had been using. His recording apparatus was a small bag placed in the uterus and connected by a pipe to a recording system in the side room adjacent to the labour ward. He had actually put the bag into a woman 7 days after delivery because he thought the risk of sepsis would be least then. He made tracings of the action of ergot on the uterus recording contractions by a needle moving up and down on a rotating drum. Because there was not room in the labour ward for his apparatus he had to put it into the lying-in ward next to the labour ward. He first tried to conduct the tubing which was connected to a balloon in the patient's uterus through an iron pipe outside the window of the labour ward and running in through the window in the lying-in ward but when this was not very successful he bored a hole through the very thick wall separating the two rooms and ran the gas piping with his rubber tubing inside it through to the recording machine.

J. Chassar Moir first described his early work on ergometrine in 1932. At that time he was first assistant to F. J. Browne in the Obstetric Unit at University College Hospital London where together they carried out a classical experiment with analytical chemists to isolate the active alkaloid of ergot and to test it on patients in the hospital. There is a nice story of Chassar Moir going round chemist shops to buy ergot and being asked, because he looked very young at that time, in one 'Young man what do *you* want ergot for?' Chassar Moir did not discover the effects of ergot on the uterus because it had been known for a long time, but he did make the first scientific measurements of the active alkaloid. Chassar Moir's other very great contribution to gynaecology, incidentally, was improving the techniques for the repair of vesico-vaginal and other fistulae.

Dr Dudley, a chemist, after some disappointments isolated the third alkaloid which they named ergometrine. They first announced their discovery in the *British Medical Journal* of the 16 March 1935. Refining the substance had been difficult and Dudley had worked for 3 years before he produced a pure substance obtained from infected rye harvested in Spain.

Not only does ergometrine contract the uterus but hormone extracts of the posterior pituitary do so as well. Sir Henry Dale had been examining the effects of some pituitary extracts on blood pressure in cats. He found that a certain pituitary extract had the property of causing an instant and intense contraction of the uterus that was totally unexpected. Blair Bell (q.v.) was the first man to publish a report on the clinical use of the extract which Sir Henry had sent him 3 years previously.

When unstandardized preparations of pituitary were used to hasten labour the effects were similar to using undiluted extracts of ergot, namely fetal asphyxia and rupture of the uterus as well as the awful side-effect of pituitary shock which was sudden pallor, collapse and sometimes even death when an overdose of pituitary extract was given. This side-effect was overcome by separating the pituitary extract into fractions, the one causing contraction of the uterus and the other causing a rise in blood pressure. Pitocin was the name given to the former and pitressin to the latter.

The next step was the synthesis of Syntocinon a synthetic substance related to the posterior pituitary extract but free from any vasopressor effect (Chassar Moir, 1964). Moir showed that the uterine response to vasopresssin and oxytocin is not constant but varies with the biological state of the uterus.

CHRONOLOGY

16th C.	Midwives were making infusions from 'Black Spurs' found on diseased grains in local granaries 'to expedite lingering labour'.
1808	Dr John Stearns of New York State published an account of how ergot could be used to hurry labour. In the enthusiasm that followed many obstetric tragedies resulted.
1932	J. Chassar Moir and colleagues isolated the active alkaloids of ergot.
1935	Ergometrine was isolated.
1930–1940	Sir Henry Dale and others carried out research work on ergot alkaloids.

Obstetric forceps

An ancient Egyptian frieze shows an instrument shaped like a pair of forceps, probably used to handle pieces of sacrificial animals.

1500 BC	The Ayurveda (India) mentioned obstetric instruments.
AD 98–138	Soranus and AD 500–550 Aetius mentioned destructive instruments, as did Albucasis an Arabian doctor (936–1013).
16th C.	Ambroise Paré described bent forceps to grab a dead child in the womb (according to Paré, 1655).
17th C.	The Chamberlen family had designed forceps which they used, and managed to keep the design a secret for probably three generations.
1693–1753	The Roonhuysen family had a monopoly in the use of the forceps in Holland.
1721	Palfyn a Belgian barber-surgeon made crude 'hands of iron' to grasp the baby's head on both sides but there was no lock.
1733	Chapman designed the English lock after losing the screw from a Chamberlen's forceps in a patient's bed clothes.
1753 and 1761	Levret, a French obstetrician, first described the various planes of the pelvis.
1754	Benjamin Pugh invented a forceps with a pelvic curve.
1877	Tarnier a Parisian obstetrician published his description of axis-traction forceps.
1915	C.C.G. Kielland (1871–1941) introduced a new forceps with no pelvic curve to rotate the head in the upper pelvis.

Vacuum extractors

16th C.	Ambroise Paré (1510–1590) discovered that depressed fractures of the skull in infants could be corrected by using a leather sucker.
1705	James Young may have been the first to try to deliver a baby using a cupping glass fixed to the skull with an air pump.
1836	Simpson (q.v.) thought of sucking the baby out and in 1848 he demonstrated his invention.
1953	Malmström designed the first modern vacuum extractor.
1969	Baird of Australia modified it.

REFERENCES

Anonymous (1883). Review of The Chamberlen's and the Midwifery Forceps by J.H. Aveling. *Am. J. Med. Sci.*, 483–94

Aveling, J.H. (1882). The Chamberlens and the Midwifery Forceps. (London: J. & A. Churchill)

Barger, G. (1931). *Ergot and Ergotism.* (London: Gurney & Jackson)

Barton, L.G., Caldwell, W.E. and Studdiford, W.E. (1928). A new obstetric forceps. *Am. J. Obstet. Gynecol.*, **15**, 16–26

Bird, G.C. (1969). Modification of Malström's vacuum extractor. *Br. Med. J.*, **3**, 526

Carter, J. (1990). The vacuum extractor. In Studd, J. (ed.) *Progress in Obstetrics and Gynaecology*, Vol. 8, pp. 107–26. (Edinburgh: Churchill Livingstone)

Carus, C.G. (1820). *Lehrbuch der Gynakologie, oder Systematisch Darstellung der Lehren von Erkenntniss und Behandlund Eigenthunlicher Gesunder und Krankhafter Zustande, Sowohl der Nicht Schwangern, Schwangern und Gebarenden Frauen, als der Wochnerinnen und Neugeborenen Kinder*, Part I, pp. 32–3, and Figure 6. (Leipzig: G. Fleischer)

Chalmers, J.A. (1971). *The Ventouse – The Obstetric Vacuum Extractor.* (London: Lloyd-Luke Medical Books Ltd)

Chamberlen, H. (1672). *The Diseases of Women with Child and in Childbed*, translation of Mauriceau, F. (1668) (London: Bell)

Chapman, E. (1773). *A Treatise on the Improvement of Midwifery, chiefly with regard to the operation.* (London: Brindley)

Chassar Moir, J. (1955). The history and present day use of ergot. *Canad. Med. Assoc. J.*, **72**, 727–34

Chassar Moir, J. (1964). The obstetrician bids, and the uterus contracts. *Br. Med. J.*, **2**, 1025–9

Chassar Moir, J. (1970). In Philipp, E.E., Barnes, J. and Newton, N. (eds.) *Scientific Foundations of Obstetrics and Gynaecology*, 1st edn., pp. 649–52. (London: William Heinemann Medical Books Ltd.)

Das, K. (1929). *Obstetric Forceps – History and Evolution.* (Calcutta: The Art Press); Facsimile reprint (1933) (Leeds: Medical Museum Publishing)

Denman, T. (1793). *Aphorisms on the applications and use of the forceps and vectis; on preternatural labours, on labours attended with haemorrhage, and with convulsions*, 4th edn. (London: Johnson)

Deventer, H. (1716). *The Art of Midwifery Improv'd, 'fully and plainly laying down whatever instructions are requisite to make a complete midwife. And the many errors in all the books hitherto written on this subject clearly refuted. Illustrated with 30 cuts curiously engraven on copper plates, representing in their due proportion the several positions of a fetus . . .'* (London: E. Curll, J. Pemberton and W. Taylor)

Dick-Read, G. (1933). *Natural Childbirth*, (subsequent editions entitled *Childbirth Without Fear*). (London: Heineman)

Eustace, D.L.S. (1991). Lecture at the Royal College of Obstetricians and Gynaecologists, December 1991, unpublished

Fasbender, H. (1906). *Geschichte der Geburtshilfe.* (Jena: Gustav Fischer)

Giffard, W. (1734). *Cases in Midwifery.* (London: Edward Hody-Motte)

Hibbard, B.N. (1987). *The Obstetric Forceps. A short history and descriptive catalogue of the forceps in the Museum of the Royal College of Obstetricians and Gynaecologists*, pp. 58–9. (London: RCOG)

Hildanus, G.F. (1632). *Guildhelmi Fabricii, Hiladani Opera*, p. 84

Johnson, R.W. (1769). *A new system of midwifery; founded on practical observations.* (London: for the author, Wilson & Nichol)

Keilland, C. (1915). Eine Neuen Form und Einfuhrungsweise der Geburtszange, Stets Biparietal an den Lindlichlen Schadel gelegt. *Munchen. med. Wchnschr.*, **62**, 923

Laufer, H. (1900). *Beitrage zur Kenntnis der Tibetischen Medicin*, 41 pp. (Berlin: Gebr. Unger)

Levret, A. (1753). *Guides des Accouchements.* (Paris: De laguette)

Levret, A. (1761). *L'Art des Accouchements et de Mechanique.* (Paris: Didot)

McCahey, P. (1890). *Med. Surg. Rep. Philadelph.*, **43**, 6319

Madden, T.M. (1875). Puerperal convulsions. *Obstetrical Journal of Great Britain and Ireland. Abstracts of Societies' Proceedings*, 236

Malström, T. (1954). *Acta Obstet. Gynaecol. Scand.*, **36**, Suppl. 3

Malström, T. (1957). *The Vacuum Extractor, An Obstetrical Instrument.* (Gothenberg: Elanders Boktryckeri AB)

Mauriceau, F. (1668). *Des Maladies des Femmes Grosses et Accouchées.* (Paris: Henault)

Paré, A. (1655). *The Works of that Famous Chirurgion Ambroise Parey*, p. 243, translated by Thomas Johnson. (London)

Pugh, B. (1754). *A Treaty of Midwifery, chiefly with regard to the operation. With several improvements of that art, to which is added: some cases and descriptions with place of several new instruments both in midwifery and surgery.* (London: Buckland)

Radcliffe, W. (1947). *The Secret Instrument (The Birth of the Midwifery Forceps)* (London: William Heinemann Medical Books Ltd.)

Radcliffe, W. (1967). *Milestones in Midwifery.* (Bristol: John Wright Ltd.)

Rösslin, E. (1513). *Der Swangern Frawen und Hebammen Roszgarten* (Hagenau)

Rueff, J. (1554). *De Conceptu et Generatione Hominis*, Libriisex Tiguri Zurich Froschoverus

Saemann, J.F. (1794). *Stark's Arch Jena*

Simpson, J.Y. (1848). *Proc. Edin. Obstet. Soc.*, December, 124

Simpson, J.Y. (1849). *Edin. London Monthly J. Med. Sci.*, **9**, 193

Simpson, J.Y. (1867). *Notes on the Progress of Acupressure.* (Edinburgh: Adam & Charles Black) (Extracted from the *Lancet*, 23 February 1867 with additional annotations)

Smellie, W. (1754). *A Sett of Anatomical Tables with Explanations and an Abridgement of the Practice of Midwifery with a view to illustrate a Treatise on the subject and collection of cases*, Table 38. (London)

Soranus (1955). *Gynecology*, translated by Owsei Temkin, pp. 189–92. (Baltimore, MD: Johns Hopkins Press)

Speert, H. (1958). *Obstetric and Gynecologic Milestones*, pp. 150–160, 457–468, 492–500. (New York: Macmillan Company)

Stillman, H.L. (1875). U.S. Patent Office, no. 160037

Tarnier, E.S. (1877). *Description de deux nouveaux Forceps.* (Paris: Martinet)

Witkowski, G.J. (1887). *Histoire des Accouchements.* (Paris: G. Steinheil)

Witkowski, G.-J. (1906). *Appendix to Histoire des Accouchements chez tous les peuples (L'arsenal obstetrical)*, pp. 55–6

Young, J. (1706). *Philosophical Transactions of the Royal Society*

Caesarean section

The idea of delivering a baby through the abdominal wall of the mother goes back into deep mythology. Zeus is supposed to have torn the premature Dionysus out of the abdomen of his dead mistress Semele and implanted him into his own thigh. Apollo is supposed to have killed his mistress Coronis when he discovered that she had been unfaithful to him and while she was lying on the pyre that was meant to consume her, he removed his unborn child Aesculapius from her abdomen and asked the wise Centuar Chiron to bring up the child. This is mentioned in Rousset's book (Rousset, 1581). The handsome Adonis was born from the trunk of the Myrrha into which his mother was turned after she had conceived incestuously from her father Kin Cinyra who was either King of Cyprus or King of Assyria.

Brahma was said to have been delivered from the umbilicus of his mother, and in 563 BC Buddha from his mother Maya's right flank . . . . Buddha's mother, who was a virgin, had become pregnant when she dreamed that a great white elephant pierced her side with its tusk.

There is an undated illuminated manuscript in the National Library in Paris, France, depicting the birth of Gaius Julius Caesar. There is also a miniature from *Les Anciennes Hystoires Romaines, Traduit de Latin en Francois Selonc Lucan et Suestoines et Saluste*, dated 1364, with the same theme. Rustam the legendary Persian hero was said to have been delivered abdominally, and

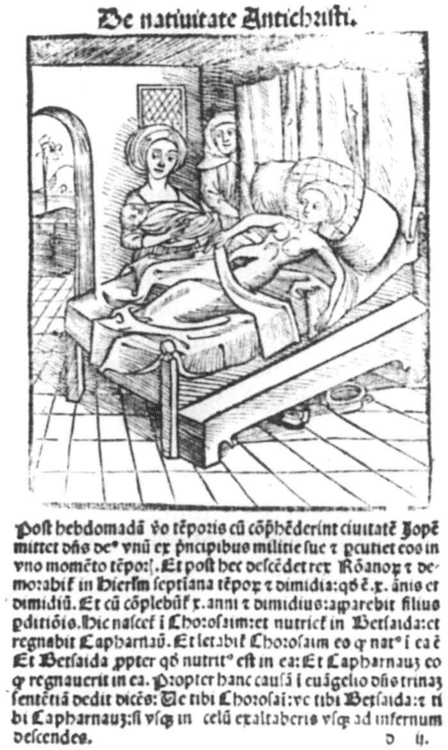

Figure 1 Saint Methodius: birth of Anti-Christ from a live mother by Caesarean section (from an illustration printed in Basle in 1516)

there is an illuminated manuscript in the National Library in Naples depicting this delivery. The manuscript is dated AD 1010.

The Mishnah, the first large commentary on the Hebrew bible compiled in the second century (135–175) mentions the operation several times.

Maimonides (1135–1204) (q.v.) who wrote a commentary on the tractate Nidda when he was classifying the Talmud, said that if the baby was to be delivered from the mother's abdomen the cut should be made in the woman's side (Figure 1).

Jacob Nufer in AD 1500 cut open his wife as recounted later and delivered the baby with his wife's survival. An account of the operation was given 82 years after its performance by Caspar Bauhin (1550–1624) in an appendix to his Latin translation of Francis Rousset's book (Rousset, 1581, 1591) and recounted again in 1751 by John Burton (Burton, 1751). Rousset advocated the operation when the baby was dead and might decompose and cause an infection in the uterus, or when the baby had escaped from the uterus into the abdominal cavity giving rise to an abscess which could be opened without danger to the mother. Rousset managed to prove that a pregnancy could follow the operation. Apparently the operation had been performed on Anne Goddard six times by a Dr Guillet. However, she unfortunately died when she became pregnant for a seventh time because there was no other surgeon willing to undertake the operation. Rousset in his book described at least six different Caesarean operations by different surgeons, but about 2 years before his book was published Ambroise Paré (1510–1590) (q.v.) had criticized the Caesarean operation in his book on surgery published in 1579. In the translation into English in 1678 it was said that it was insolent to claim that the operation could be done and he did not know of any that could be done without the death of the mother. Apparently, according to Jacques Guillemeau, Paré had seen the operation done twice, but both patients had died. Caspard Bauhin described other Caesarean operations that had been performed successfully. One woman, Elizabeth Turgois, who had a successful Caesarean operation, was subsequently delivered vaginally of four children. Jacques Guillemeau (1550–1630) (q.v. in Biographies) surgeon to Henry IV, wrote to Rousset to oppose the operation, but it does not seem that Rousset himself had ever done the operation and nearly all his reports were anecdotal. In Guillemeau's book, translated into English by Thomas Hatfield in 1612 there is a chapter devoted to the Caesarean operation. He said that he had seen the operation carried out by various surgeons on five different women, all of whom had died.

There is no mention of the operation in Rösslin's *Byrth of Mankynde* (1540), but in 1604 Scipio Mercurio (1540–1616) (q.v. in Biographies) a surgeon of Padua, in an Italian work, did write about successful cases of Caesarean section and there are two chapters on Caesarean section in his book. He suggested that the operation should be performed for a large baby trying to issue from a woman with a small pelvis. In the seventeenth century Hendrik van Roonhuyze was an advocate of the operation and said that a physician of Bruges called Sonnius performed the operation seven times on his own wife. Roonhuyze was a pioneer gynaecological surgeon. It was to his son, Roger van Roonhuyze, that Hugh Chamberlen the elder, sold the secret of the obstetric forceps in about 1663. There are many other authors who wrote about the subject and claimed successes including Theophilus Raynaud who wrote about it in 1637.

The first definitely authenticated report of the operation intentionally performed on a woman was carried out on the 21 April 1610 by Trautmann of Wittenberg; and it was recorded by Professor Sennert of Wittenberg who was present at the operation. The baby was healthy but the woman died on the 25th day following the operation because her wound became septic. Mauriceau was such a determined opponent of the Caesarean section that he said 'that which Rousset reports of the Caesarean section, is nothing but the ravings, capriciousness and menposture . . . ' Mauriceau did not hesitate to attack Paré and Guillemeau, although he did agree to the operation being carried out if the mother had died. It was possibly Mauriceau who held back the development of the operation. He was later roundly condemned by Burton in his book – 'to neglect to save a person when it is in your Power is to be accessary to his Death – in this case to be accessary to the Death of two persons is unpardonable'.

Giulio Cesari Aranzio (1530–1589) carried out one of the first Caesarean operations in 1578, delivering a live child from a woman who had been killed in the last month of her pregnancy. Guillemeau (q.v.) in the sixteenth century seems to have discussed with Ambroise Paré the possibility of carrying out the operation in the living – knowing that it had been performed on the dead mother – but he eventually came out in opposition to the idea .

It would seem that the birth of an heir presumptive was already in the third edition of Mauriceau's book (1681) considered to be an indication for the delivery of a child abdominally if he was going to be the king because 'public interest was more important than that of an individual'; so he did relent a little.

John Harley Young of Edinburgh has written a short history of the operation (Young, 1944). Young's history was submitted to the Faculty of Medicine of the University of Edinburgh in 1942 as a thesis for the degree of M.D. He says that the origin of the name 'Caesarean' is unclear. It almost certainly is not derived from the myth that Julius Caesar was delivered this way, because his mother Aurelia was alive when he undertook the invasion of Britain, and in early times no woman delivered in this way was at all likely to survive the operation. Some histories suggest that Scipio Africanus may have been delivered from his mother by this operation in 237 BC, but this also seems unlikely, and it is unlikely also that Scipio Africanus was the first to be called Caesar. It has also been suggested that Caesar was the name given to the Julia family because one of them may have killed or kept an elephant, and Caesar in Punic is an elephant. Caesar seems to have had a profile of an elephant crushing a serpent beneath his feet on the reverse of some of his coins. Others have suggested that the term is derived from the Latin verb *caedare* which means to cut, and this is quite possible. When women died the children were sometimes delivered from them by an abdominal cut, and they were known as *caesones*.

In 715 BC the King of Rome made a law stating that no pregnant woman who died could be buried until the child had been removed from her abdomen. Only a few of these children could have survived. The operation was a 'grand' operation and therefore it may have been called after Caesar; just as in Germany where until the end of the First World War, the operation was called Kaiserschnitt, after the Kaisers who were important. Caesarean birth, as a term, was first used by Rousset in 1581, and published in his book in 1591 (Rousset, 1581, 1591). Jacques Guillemau, who wrote a book on midwifery which was first published in 1598 and translated into English in 1612 (Guillemeau, 1612), apparently was the first to use the term 'section'. However, Caesarean operation was the term used until the beginning of the twentieth century.

It seems almost certain that the operation was performed on dead women if there was any movement whatsoever of the fetus after the woman died. The great Aescalapius was delivered, according to some mythology by this operation from his mother; and the operation was performed by Apollo himself. Bacchus, the God of Wine was also said to have been delivered by the same operation as Aesculapius.

In Shakespeare's play *Macbeth*, Macbeth's enemy MacDuff was said to have been born by the operation. The famous phrases being:

MACBETH   I beare a charméd life which must not yield to one of woman borne,

MACDUFF   Dispaire thy charm
And let the angell whom thou still has't served
Tell thee, MacDuff was from his mother's womb
Untimely ript.

'Untimely' may have meant post-mortem.

It is possible that Edward VI, the son of Henry VIII and Jane Seymour was born by Caesarean operation on 12 October 1537 and that Jane Seymour died 4 days after the delivery. However, there is little evidence that this rumour was based on truth, and it is possible that she died of puerperal sepsis. According to other versions she died 12 days after the delivery, but it is highly unlikely that she would have survived a Caesarean operation for 12 days; and 12 days seems to agree with all the records.

There is mention of Caesarean section in the Talmud in the Tractate Nidda, which deals with 'uncleanliness' consequent upon vaginal bleeding or menstruation; and according to Young there is a passage that says 'it is not necessary for women to observe the date of purification, after removal of a child through the wall (parieties) of the abdomen'. The operation is certainly mentioned many times in Rabbinical writings, so it probably was performed in the Middle Ages but most probably only on dead women.

It does seem that the operation was performed in Uganda as early as 1879, and it was witnessed by Felkin in (Felkin, 1884). There are instances of women conducting Caesarean operations on themselves. The one that has received the most publicity was that of a peasant woman of Viterbo who, aged 23, was so provoked by the angry members of her family that she was determined to rid herself of her pregnancy. In the middle of the night, with a not very sharp kitchen knife, she cut into her abdomen. She decapitated the fetus when cutting into the uterus. Later, she bound a bandage tightly round her body to bring the edges of the wound together. The next morning the intestines prolapsed out of the wound, but doctors were called, replaced them, turned the patient on her side to allow blood and serum to escape, and closed the wound with twisted sutures. The patient was well enough to be able to walk quite well on the 48th day after the procedure. Carbolic acid, 4%, was injected through the drainage tube which had been inserted after the repair to the abdominal wall. This was removed after 10 days because it seemed to irritate. The stitches were removed on the 14th day.

There are other cases recorded of women carrying out Caesarean sections on themselves. Women have been ripped open by the horns of bulls, cows and other mammals. In 1647 the wife of a farmer at Zaandam in Holland was gored by a bull; a child issued from the wound. The mother died very soon after (Felkin, 1884).

John Burton (1751) tells the story of how in 1500 the wife of the sow gelder, Jacob Nufer, went into labour and was unable to deliver herself of a child. 'One Elizabeth Alice Pachin, wife to James Nufer in the village of Sigershaufen could not be delivered in the natural Way, after several Days spent in Labour-Pains, though she had with her thirteen Midwives and some Surgeons who used to cut for the stone; her Husband (a Gelder) an illiterate Fellow, and without the least Experience in Surgery, having previously obtained Leave of the Magistrate, the President of Fravenfelden, and implored the Almighty's Assistance, performed this Operation upon his own Wife in the Presence of those Surgeons and two of the Midwives (the others he turned out, because they opposed the Operation) and by this Means saved both the Mother and Child. This child lived to be 77 years old; the mother was afterwards delivered of twins in the natural way, and of four other children successively, and lived to be upwards of 60 years old: one of the twins was Judge of Sigershaufen and was alive in 1583'. Recently there has been some question as to whether Jacob Nufer's wife did not have a full-term extrauterine intra-abdominal pregnancy.

In the late eighteenth and early nineteenth centuries, obstetricians such as Charles White and John Hull of Manchester both advocated Caesarean section over other methods such as craniotomy which could only result in a dead baby. The first Caesarean section performed in the Rotunda Hospital, Dublin, was in 1854 and Dr Henry Briggs performed the first operation in Liverpool in 1894. It was not until after the turn of the century in 1902 that more than ten Caesareans were done in 1 year, and nearly all of these were emergency operations.

In J.H. Young's book there are many references to Caesarean operations carried out with the patient held down by assistants (Young, 1944). The abdomen was opened by incisions in the side, lateral to the rectus muscle. The assistants tried to hold the intestines back with their hands, and the wound in the uterus was not stitched but was left gaping open although the edges of the abdominal wall were put together with a few stitches. The names of the surgeons reported by Young to have performed the operation, or else to have described it, included Olaus Rudbeck, (second half of the seventeenth century), Saviard (1692), Chaubert (1692), Vater (1695), Churchill (1741), Ruleau (1704), de la Motte (1656–1737, writing in 1721; English translation by Thomas Tomkyns 1746).

The first Caesarean section performed in Great Britain was on 29 June 1737 by Mr Smith, a surgeon of Edinburgh, on a woman who had been in labour for 6 days and who had a very distorted pelvis. The patient was delivered of a stillborn child and she herself died 18 hours after the operation. The first successful case in Ireland was performed by a midwife in January 1738. The patient's name was Alice O'Neale who was 33 years of age and she was the wife of a farmer of Charlemont in Ireland. She had already had several children. She had been in labour for 12 days and the operation was performed by Mary Donally, 'an illiterate woman eminent among the common people for extracting births'. She cut the abdominal wall and then the uterus with a razor with an incision 6 inches long on the right side of the umbilicus, then she stitched the wound with silk and a tailor's needle. She dressed the wound with the white of an egg. The woman made a good recovery and was able to walk a mile on the 27th postoperative day. Like very many others who had this operation she later developed a ventral hernia. Many of the authorities whose names appear in this book, including William Harvey, Percival Willoughby and Ould wrote about the operation, mainly to condemn it (Figure 2).

There was, of course, the ethical and theological aspect, and this raged on the question of the priority of life of the mother or the child. The operation was carried out several times in France in the 1750s when vaginal delivery was impossible, but mainly to deliver dead babies and to save the life of the mother, but many of these women are reported to have had vaginal deliveries following the operation.

The great Smellie is said to have written in his *Treatise* (second edition, 1752), of which there were nine English editions and French, German and Dutch translations, 'of the Caesarian operation . . . When a woman cannot be delivered by any of the methods hitherto described and recommended in laborious and praeternatural labours, on account of the narrowness or distortion of the Pelvis, into which it is sometimes impossible to introduce the hand; or from large excrescences and glandular swellings that fill up the Vagina and cannot be removed; or from large cicatrices and adhesions in that part . . . if the woman is strong and in good habit of body, the Caesarean operation is certainly advisable and ought to be performed; because the mother and child have no other chance to be saved, and it is better to have recourse to an operation which hath sometimes succeeded than leave them both to inevitable death'. He says it would be rash to try the operation on a woman who was weak and exhausted and in fruitless labour.

Smellie's advocacy of the operation in such conditions coincided more or less in time with that of John Burton who was an antiquary and man-midwife born in Colchester in 1710. After

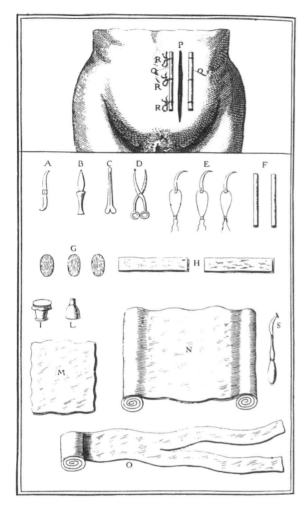

Figure 2 Upper illustration – incision to carry out Caesarean section and the method used to close it. Lower illustration – instruments, the bandages, the compresses, pots containing ointments and balsam and the instrument to dilate the cervix from above to allow the lochia to be passed. All French eighteenth century after Mesnard

describing the case of Nufer, as mentioned earlier, he went into minute details concerning the operation, particularly whether the fetus was alive or dead and advocated it for what we would now call disproportion where other instruments were of no value. He thought the risks of the operation were exaggerated, especially that of haemorrhage, but they were well worth undertaking when the alternative was 'to neglect to save a person' as he had written when condemning Mauriceau and his attitude. He felt that skilful surgeons should not be deterred from performing the operation

when absolutely necessary and he described how the incision should be made and how the baby should be extracted. He quoted Rousset's publication of 1581 and Caspard Bauhin. Benjamin Pugh a surgeon of Chelmsford, Essex, published his *Treatise on Midwifery* in 1754 and considered that the Caesarean operation should not be carried out because of its dangers 'sporting with lives'.

Lebas (1719–1797) the French surgeon, was the first surgeon to stitch the wound in the uterus in 1769, and in spite of the patient recovering he was highly criticized!

If the operation of symphysiotomy had been discovered earlier than 1768, when Sigault described it (inevitably, like all new procedures, it was criticized), some Caesarean operations in the eighteenth century might have been avoided. Jean René Sigault carried out symphysiotomy on the 1 October 1777 on a lady whose first baby had died after a craniotomy. Support all round included a medal to Sigault together with a pension, a medal to his assistant Monsieur Alphonse le Roi, and a pension to the patient! Inevitably there were heated disputes about the propriety of doing the operation, which had an enormous mortality. Cutting into the bony structure of the pelvis to divide it and symphysiotomy where the cartilage is divided, were alternatives that were practised, but were almost as barbaric, if not more so, than the Caesarean operation in the eighteenth century.

Pupils of William Hunter, namely William Osborn (1736–1808) and Thomas Denman (1733–1815) together founded a successful school of midwifery where they were heartily opposed to the Caesarean operation, except in the case of women with the most extreme forms of contracted pelvis.

The first successful Caesarean section in England, after that by Mary Donally in Ireland, was performed in 1793 but not published until 1798. The patient was a Jane Foster,who was about 40 years of age and had had several children. She had a fractured pelvis after falling from a loaded cart the wheel of which passed over her pelvis, causing the bony structures great damage. However, she managed to become pregnant and went into labour on the 22 November 1793. When she had been in labour for 3 days a surgeon, James Barlow of Blackburn in Lancashire, was called in by Mr Hawarden of Wigan who examined the lady and found that the pelvis was very much distorted. Mr Hawarden when the decision was made to carry out a Caesarean section, walked out on the patient. Mr Barlow called on Mr Hawarden's brother, a practitioner in a local village (Blackrod) and delivered a dead child through a 5 inch incision to the left of the midline. He then delivered the placenta and membranes and secured the wound by seven stitches, but did not include the peritoneum. The stitches were removed on the 6th postoperative day and this may have been the first operation from which the mother made a full recovery.

The next successful operation was apparently 40 years later in April 1834, and was performed by a surgeon by the name of Greaves. Only very few more were carried out in the nineteenth century. John Howell (1799) of Manchester, and Mr Wood (1799) also of Manchester, and Mr John Bell (1819) performed the operation; the child was saved in Mr Bell's case. The operation was very slowly becoming slightly more popular, or perhaps slightly less unpopular, and indications of when the operation should be done were being laid down. They were always for disproportion. France was the country where more operations were carried out than in most other countries; it was performed in Germany or Holland more readily than in England. Accounts of the operation, and the pros and cons for it, were published by such authors as William Hunter (1778) and Ambroise Paré (1678), A. Hamilton (1791), J. Bell (1826) and van Deventer (1734). Gradually the operation spread from France to other countries and the first Caesarean section in Denmark was performed by Schlegal, an Army surgeon, on 26 October 1813, at the behest of the parents who refused to allow a forceps delivery; The child survived but the mother died 2 days later from peritoneal infection and intestinal paralysis (Trolle, 1982).

A most important date in the development of Caesarean section was 1876 because on 21 May 1876 Porro introduced an operation to avoid the development of haemorrhage and sepsis. Eduardo Porro (1842–1902) was Professor of Obstetrics in Pavia and in Milan, Italy. The operation Porro performed had already been advocated by Cavallini in 1768 and by Michaelis in 1809. In 1828 Blundell recommended the operation after he had removed an inverted uterus some months after a woman had delivered. In Porro's operation he carried out Caesarean section as had previously been done, then tied a strong iron wire round the cervix. He amputated the body of the uterus and both ovaries and Fallopian tubes, and then brought the stump of the cervix to the lower end of the wound in the abdomen. Both mother and child

survived. The mother was the first woman in Pavia to survive a Caesarean operation. The Church was initially against the operation, judging it immoral, but the Bishop of Padua issued a decree that acquitted Porro of having offended morality because the Church said it was permissible to make a woman barren in order to save her life and to sacrifice a part to save the whole. Porro had only considered doing the operation on a woman after he had removed the uterus from three pregnant rabbits all of whom recovered.

Joseph Cavallini had published a paper in Florence in 1768 entitled *Medico-Chirurgical experiments in the successful excision of the uterus in certain animals, etc.* He concluded after he had experimented on dogs and sheep, including a dog from whom he had removed the uterus with nine pups in it, that the uterus was not necessary for life. Dr G.P. Michaelis of Harburg, Germany in 1809 suggested amputation of the uterus after removing the fetus and pointed out that opium was needed for treatment when the uterus was cut away, and a Dr James Blundell, who lectured on obstetrics in Guy's Hospital, speculated in 1828 whether the dangers of the Caesarean operation 'might not be considerably diminished by the removal of the uterus'. He published his lectures in 1832.

Dr Horatio Storer in 1869 in Boston, USA, had removed the uterus from a woman because she was haemorrhaging so badly during a Caesarean operation. The fetus was already dead and the woman died 68 hours after the operation.

Porro's patient of May 1876 was a 25-year-old dwarf, named by coincidence Cavallini. She had not delivered a baby before and she had a small pelvis, deformed by rickets. After the patient had been anaesthetized with chloroform, Porro and his assistants washed their hands in a diluted solution of carbolic acid. The child was removed alive through an incision in the uterus and after the placenta had been removed a constrictor was passed over the neck of the uterus to include both ovaries and Fallopian tubes. This was really a large snare that was successfully applied, before the uterus was cut away. The abdominal cavity was cleaned out with carbolized sponges, and drainage tubes were passed through the abdominal wall and the Pouch of Douglas to come out through the vagina. The abdominal wall, through which the stump of the uterus had been brought out, was closed with silver wire sutures. The snare was left outside the abdominal wound under the dressing for 4 days. The sutures in the abdomen were removed after a week and the strangulated portion of the cervix sloughed off at the end of another 7 days. The patient was well in 40 days. Porro (1876) published details of his operation in the same year. Others tried to copy him but they lost their patients, and others followed until a Professor Spath of Vienna successfully performed the operation. By 1884 a table was produced of 134 operations carried out in Italy, Austria, Germany, France, Great Britain, USA, Belgium, Switzerland, Spain, Holland and Russia. Italy led the way with 53 operations out of the 134 with Austria and Germany second and third in the table. The maternal mortality, however, was 55.97%. In 1881 Professor A.R. Simpson of Edinburgh (not to be confused with James Young Simpson) performed the Porro operation for the first time in the United Kingdom with a senior team of assistants on a woman with a very small pelvis. The patient died 3 days after the operation from peritonitis. Professor Tarnier, the famous French obstetrician who gave his name to a maternity hospital in Paris, as well as to axis-traction forceps, carried out his first successful Porro operation on 20 May 1879. Gradually the results of the Porro operation improved.

In 1890 Lawson Tait of Birmingham, modified the Porro operation. He carried a loop of drainage tube over the uterus and down into the pelvis and tightened it to strangle the circulation. He then opened the uterus with a small cut sufficient to admit a finger, and this was enlarged by moving the finger up and down. The child was delivered feet first. The placenta was then removed and the contracted uterus pulled out of the wound and the ligature tightened. He flattened the elastic tube through which needles were passed through the uterus and out the other side and the uterus was cut off close to the needles and the strangulating rubber tube. Tait as always was enthusiastic and claimed that figures of a very low mortality would soon be obvious, but they were not.

Inevitably some objected on religious grounds to removal of the uterus and with that the capacity to procreate.

The next development was the Sanger operation (Sanger, 1882; 1886). In 1882 he changed the technique of the operation completely. Max Sanger (1853–1903) was a German surgeon whose modification was to preserve the uterus and to suture the incision in it very carefully so as to minimize the bleeding and the chance of liquor coming from it into the peritoneal cavity. Furthermore, he put a large number of Lembert's intestinal sutures into the peritoneum of the uterus to seal it off. Sanger's operation was the first truly conservative Caesarean section. It not only saved the life of the mother, and of the child, but also the genital organs. Sanger insisted that the operation should be performed early in labour before the patient was ill or septic and that the precautions taken at the operation should be fully aseptic. During his operation, Sanger used every precaution to prevent liquor from the uterus going into the peritoneal cavity, including putting a sheet of waterproof material moistened with a 5% solution of carbolic acid around the cervix. He pulled the body of the uterus out of the abdominal wound before opening it. After the uterus had been well contracted he put a drainage tube down through the cervix so that the contents of the uterus could drain out into the vagina. He used a very careful suturing technique placing eight or ten stitches superficially and up to 20 stitches in the peritoneum, which he had dissected from the anterior wall of the uterus.

Kehrer of Heidelburg in 1882, independently from Sanger, used Listerian principals. As often in history we find disputes as to who published his paper first, or who, in spite of priority of publication, first performed the operation. It does not matter, but it seems likely that Kehrer did his first operation on 25 September 1881 and Sanger insisted on Leopold doing his operation for the first time on 25 May 1882. Sanger however, published slightly earlier than Kehrer. Although there was still quite a high mortality (somewhere around 28%) the improvement on Porro's operation was great, as even in the best hands the Porro operation had a maternal mortality of 44%.

In 1890 Halsted in the USA introduced the wearing of rubber gloves. Also at that time it was realized that the earlier a Caesarean operation was performed the less likelihood there would be of infection in the uterus, so Sanger's operation slowly took over from the Porro operation.

John Martin Munro Kerr, 1868–1960, Professor of Obstetrics of Gynaecology and Obstetrics in the University of Glasgow in Scotland, together with Eardley Holland (1879–1967) introduced the lower segment Caesarean operation to the United Kingdom in 1921. Holland was the first to carry out nine cases and Munro Kerr followed with 22 cases. They favoured the lower segment operation for its lower risk of rupture in a subsequent pregnancy, its lower risk of causing peritonitis because the incision is extra-peritonealized by covering with peritoneum from the utero-vesical fold, and because haemorrhage is less than with a classical incision. Furthermore, it is possible for a 'trial of scar' to be carried out in subsequent labours because of the lesser risk of rupture. It was also reported that intestinal distension after the operation was less with the lower segment incision than with the classical upper segment scar (Holland, 1921; Kerr, 1921).

A more recent innovation has been the substitution of epidural anaesthesia for the operation instead of general anaesthesia. This has the advantages of allowing the mother to take part in the delivery and 'be present' at the time. She can hear her baby give its first cry and her husband can be present and share the joy of their new parenthood. Furthermore the child will not be anaesthetized and will therefore breathe more easily; and if the mother wishes, it can be placed to her breast even before the closure of the abdominal wound is completed.

CHRONOLOGY

In mythology Greek gods and some demi-gods claimed to have been born through cuts made in their mothers' sides.

563 BC	The Buddah was said to have been born from his mother's right flank. Rustam a hero in Persian mythology was born to Rudaba, the wife of King Sal after his mother's body was cut open, she having been given Hyoscyamus by Simurg and fallen asleep.
AD 1500	Jacob Nuffer is said to have delivered his wife, using his sow-gelding instruments, of a large child and both wife and child are said to have survived. This was reported in 1582 by Caspar Bauhin.
1578	Guilio Cesari Arantius performed a Caesarean operation delivering a live child from a woman who had been killed in the last month of her pregnancy.
1579	Ambroise Paré criticized the operation.
1610	Trautman of Wittenburg did the first intentional Caesarean section.
1612	Thomas Hatfield's translation of a book by Jacques Guillemeau (q.v.) had a chapter devoted to the operation.
1637	Theophilus Raynaud wrote about it.
1681	'To be a future king' would be sufficient reason for operating on a mother to get a live child even at the risk of her life.
1769	Lebas was the first to stitch the wound in the uterus.
1876	Porro developed his operation.
1881–1882	Sanger and Kehrer adopted Lister's principles for the operation.
1890	Lawson Tait (q.v.) modified Porro's operation.
1921	Munro Kerr introduced the lower segment operation.

REFERENCES

Bell, J. (1826). *The Principles of Surgery*, 4 Vol., new edition with commentaries and a critical enquiry into the practice of surgery. (London: Charles Bell)

Blundell, J. (1832). *Lectures on Midwifery, and the diseases of women and children as delivered at Guy's Hospital.* (London: Field and Bull)

Burton, J. (1751). *An Essay Towards a Complete New System of Midwifry*, pp. 260–70. (London: James Hodges)

Cavallini, J. (1768). *Tentamina Medico-Chirurgica de felici in quibusdam Animantibus Uteri Extractione.* (Florence: Josephum Allegrini & Socios.)

Felkin, R.W. (1884). *Edin. Med. J.*, **29**, 928

Guillemeau, J. (1612). *Childbirth or a Happy Deliverie of Women*, English translation. (London: K. Hatfield)

Hamilton, A. (1791). *Outlines of the Theory and Practice of Midwifery*, 3rd edn. pp. 314–19. (London: Kay; Edinburgh: Greach)

Holland, E. (1921). (a) Methods of performing Caesarean section. (b) Results in Great Britain and Ireland 1911–1920. *J. Obstet. Gynecol. Br. Emp.*, **28**, 349–446

Hunter, W. (1778). Reflections occasioned by a decree of the Faculty of Medicine at Paris: relative to the operation of cutting the symphysis of the ossa pubis. In Vaughan, J. Cases and Observations on the hydrophobia

Kehrer, F.A. (1882). *Arch Gynäkol.*, **19**, 196

Kerr, J.N.M. (1921). The lower uterine segment incision in conservative Caesarean section. *J. Obstet. Gynecol. Br. Emp.*, **28**, 475–87

Leopold, G. (1882). *Arch Gynäkol.*, **19**, 400

Mauriceau, F. (1681). *Traites des Maladies des Femmes Grosses*, 3rd edn. (Paris: chez l'auteur)

Mercurio, S. (1601). *La Commare Oriccoglitrice Divisa in tre libri, Ristampata, Correta et Acclescuita.* (Venice: Ciotti)

Paré, A. (1545). *La Methode de traiter de les playes faites par les arquebuses et autres bastions a feu.* (Paris)

Porro, E. (1876). Della amputazione utero-ovarica come complemento di taglio Cesario. *Ann. Univ. Med. Chirurg.*, 273, 289–350

Pugh, B. (1754). *A Treatise on Midwifery, chiefly with regard to the operation. With several improvements in that art.* (London: Buckland)

Raynaud, R.P.T. (1637). *De Ortu Infantium contra Naturam per Sectionem Caesaream.* (Lugduni: Gariel Boissat)

Rösslin, E. (1540). *The Byrth of Mankynde, otherwise named the woman's book.* Newly set forth by Thomas Raynold. (London: Raynold)

Rousset, F. (1581). *Traite Nouveau de l'hysterotomokie ou l'enfantement Caesarienne, qui est extraction de l'enfant par incision laterale de ventre et matrice de la Famme Grosse. Pouvant Autrement Accoucher, et ce sans Prejudicer a la vie de l'un et de l'autre ni l'empecher la Fecondite Maternelle par apres.* (Paris: Demeys Duval)

Rousset, F. (1591). *Foetus vivi ex matre viva sine alterutrius vitae periculo caesura a Franciso Rousset . . . conscripta Caspara Bauhino latio reddita . . .* (Basle: Waldkirch)

Sänger, M. (1882). *Arch. f. Gynäkol.*, **19**, 370 (*Intern. Encyclop. Surg.*, 1886, **3**, 768)

Sänger, M. (1886). *Am. J. Obstet.*, **19**, 883

Smellie, W. (1752). *Treatise on the Theory and Practice of Midwifery*, 2nd edn. pp. 380–4. (London: D. Wilson and T. Durham)

Trolle, D. (1982). *The History of Caesarean Section*, p. 39. (Copenhagen: C.A. Rietzel Booksellers)

van Deventer, H. (1734). *Observations importantes sur le manuel des accouchemens.* Premiere partie, translated from the Latin by Ablaincourt, J.J. (Paris: Cavelier)

Young, J.H. (1944). *Caesarean Section, The History and Development of the Operation From Earliest Times.* (London: H.K. Lewis)

FURTHER READING

Craigin, E.B. (1916). Conservation in Obstetrics. *N.Y. Med. J.*, **I**, 104

Encyclopaedia Britannica (1981). Caesarean Section. Vol. II, p. 698.

Ferguson, I.L.C., Taylor, R.W. and Watson, J.M. (1982). *Records and Curiosities in Obstetrics and Gynaecology*, p. 107. (London: Bailliere Tindall Ltd.)

Hall, M.H. (1987). The Patient Demanding a Caesarean. *Br. Med. J.*, **294**, 201

Kiwanuka, A.I. and Moore, W.M.O. (1987). The changing incidence of Caesarean section in the health district of Central Manchester. *Br. J. Obstet. Gynecol.*, **94**, 440–4

Lao, T.T., Leung, B.F.H. and Young, S.S. (1987). Trial of scar of Caesarean operation. *Br. J. Clin. Practice*, **41**, 594–600

Moir, J.C. and Myerscough, P.R. (1971). *Monro Kerr's Operative Obstetrics*, 8th edn. pp. 527–8. (London; Bailliere, Tindall & Cassell)

Ploss, H.H., Bartels, M. and Bartels, P. (1935). *Woman III*, pp. 81–94. (London: Heinemann Medical Books)

Rosenbaum, J. (1836). *Analecta quaedam ad Sectionis Caesareae Antiquitates.* (Halle)

Shiono, P.H., Fielden, J.G., McNellis, D., Rhoades, G.G. and Pearse, W.D. (1987). Recent trends in Caesarean birth and trial of labour rates in the United States. *J. Am. Med. Assoc.*, **257**, 4

Spencer, H.R. (1927). *The History of British Midwifery from 1650–1800.* (John Bail Sons and Danielson Ltd.)

Midwives in history

According to Towler and Bramall (1986) it is possible that men helped deliver their wives as early as 40 000 BC but by 6000 BC women were delivering the babies. Gradually, some women became more experienced than others in the art of delivering babies. They were the ancestors of the present day midwives.

In Genesis 38:28 onwards it is recounted how Tamar, who had become pregnant after seducing her dead husband's father, had twins in approximately 1700 BC. 'When the time for her delivery came, there were twins in her womb and when she was in labour, one put out a hand; the midwife took and bound on his hand a scarlet thread saying "this came out first". But as he drew back his hand and behold his brother came out; and she said "what a breach you have made for yourself". Therefore he was called Perez, and the one with a thread on his hand was called Zera.' So it was clear that a midwife was present who was competent to deal with such a difficult delivery and what is known as a compound presentation.

Unfortunately, today many traditional birth attendants confronted with a hand would pull on it and the end result would be great trauma with probable death of both the infants and the mother. This is regularly seen today in Pakistan and other countries.

The Bible in Exodus tells us that birthing stools were used by Shiphrah and Puah the midwives who delivered Jewish babies in Egypt: and it also mentions that women gave birth in the sitting or squatting positions, as they did in Egypt, often crouching upon a pair of bricks or upon a birth stool.

It is quite clear that in Greece (800–500 BC approximately) midwives enjoyed a very high social status, but this declined within a few hundred years so that Agnodike, the midwife of Athens had to disguise herself as a man to study midwifery under Herophilus. It is presumed that the influence of Greece spread in time to Rome where in the second century Soranus produced his textbook in which he says 'so she (the midwife) must also be literate in order to comprehend the art through theory also'. A Chinese translation of Soranus was probably made. This appeared in Japan in 1661 entitled *Tat Shang Pin* (Midwifery Made Easy).

TRADITIONAL BIRTH ATTENDANTS

Women have delivered babies since time immemorial; men have not. In most countries of the world (now excluding parts of the USA) the great majority of all babies are delivered by women, and in particular by midwives. An account is given here of the present status of the traditional birth attendant because it is very likely that the training, behaviour, habits, status and role of midwives in societies where traditional birth attendants work has not changed much in the last 1000 or more years.

In 1975 a book was published by the World Health Organization in Geneva (Verderese, 1975). This book is based on analysis of information on traditional birth attendants from investigations carried out by a number of people in different countries. It is clear that rural areas in many so-called developing countries are poorly covered by personnel with any scientific training in antenatal care and in delivering women.

It is not known how far back the concept of traditional birth attendants goes, but probably it reaches the depths of pre-history. Verderese states that the traditional birth attendant is usually 'an older woman, almost always past menopause, and who must have borne one or two children herself. She lives in the community in which she practises. She operates in a relatively restricted zone, limited to her own village, but sometimes immediately adjacent. Many of her beliefs and practices related to the reproductive cycle are dependent on religious or mystic sanctions and are re-enforced by rituals which are performed with traditional ceremonies which are intended to maintain the balance between the absence of ill health and a state of ill health'.

The traditional birth attendant adheres rigidly to the dietary rules of her community and assumes an important role in the transmission of ideas concerning the nature and effects of food. Traditional birth attendants are often accomplished herbalists, whose knowledge and use of herbs, roots and barks may be quite extensive. Infusions of herbs are frequently prescribed to relieve discomfort during pregnancy, to speed up delivery, as abortifacients, and for treating dysmenorrhoea and certain types of illness. The following description of the traditional birth attendant is given because of its roots in history. Typically she is illiterate and has had no formal training. She learns her craft from other traditional birth attendants; and inherits as clients the daughters of the women attended by her traditional birth attendant–sponsor. In most countries she is practising outside the law; but at a local level there appears to be no restriction or interference with her practice. 'She is a reassuring, familiar figure, who is unhurried and patient in the assistance given to her clients. She speaks in a language and concepts they can understand and accept, and learns by experience the proper approach to the village people. She is usually not rewarded financially in any way'. She usually carries out the deliveries in the homes of her clients and she stays with the client until after the birth has taken place. In countries such as Senegal the delivery takes place outside the house in the backyard, as it is considered essential for the infant to be in contact with the earth which is considered to be the source of nourishment and the burial ground after death.

The traditional birth attendant may herself wear talismans and charms and say prayers or get her clients to do so. She may apply heat to the abdomen of the woman, make her run up and down steps, or maintain certain positions and push externally on the uterus. She may also forcibly extract the baby if it is lying wrongly or if the placenta is not coming out quickly. In some societies the woman is placed in a kneeling position at the time of childbirth; in others she squats, sits or lies down, depending on tradition. It is considered that the position adopted is more in keeping with the woman's sense of modesty than a modern obstetrical position. Even exposure of the lower part of the body in some traditional cultures is considered to be immodest.

Traditional birth attendants often cut the cord with the bark of a bamboo, a hard and sharp stalk of a plant, or a razor blade, or two sharp stones between which the cord is crushed. Hygienic precautionary measures are not always observed. Such interesting objects as cow dung and ashes from the heart of a stove may be applied to the stump of the umbilical cord. It is important that the traditional birth attendant should herself have experienced childbirth and its attendant 'pain', so that she can assist others in a judicious and sympathetic way. Unless she has had a painful childbirth she is not accepted in the community of mothers. Her legal status and her role differ very much from country to country, as does her name. This varies from 'accoucheuse traditionelle' (in Senegal) to 'bush midwife', 'bundo Mamy', 'dai' (in Afghanistan, Bangladesh, India, Mauritius and Pakistan), and 'daya dukun buja' in Indonesia, where there are many different kinds of dukuns. She is called 'matrone' in French-speaking countries, and 'Wata Sitong' in Timor.

It is not only in Third World countries that midwives attend maternity cases; but even in Europeanized countries like Croatia and Tunisia, a large proportion of the babies are born in unsupervised hospitals or unsupervised domiciliary settings attended by traditional birth attendants as they have been for centuries. In many countries traditional birth attendants are unable to read or write and in some countries they are quite young; as for instance in Togo; there they must have some standard of literacy.

'Then the King of Egypt spoke to the Hebrew midwives, whose names were Shiphrah and Puah "when you are attending the Hebrew women in childbirth" he told them "watch that the child is delivered and if it is a boy, kill him; if it is a girl, let her live" but they were God fearing women' (Exodus 1:15). There seems to be no question in the Bible of men delivering babies. For instance in Genesis 35:17 speaking about Rachel 'while her pains were upon her, the midwife said "do not be afraid, this is another son for you".'

Almost all ancient historical records show that babies were delivered only by women. Initially they were instructed by other women in their societies in the arts of delivery. Men entered the scene only when the idea developed that labour had a 'mechanism'. It does seem that the control of midwifery was almost entirely in the hands of women who called in male doctors to deal with complicated cases only when they had become very difficult. In consequence, the role of midwives as against that of doctors has always been somewhat competitive and in many civilizations midwives have always been recruited from classes socially inferior to doctors. Even when midwives fought hard for recognition and brilliant midwives such as Loyse Bourgeois (1563–1636), who published a notable book (Bourgeois, 1609), were highly respected as midwives to the Queens of France, their position was, if not antagonistic, somewhat subservient to men (Witkowski, 1890).

Some of the reasoning behind the fact that midwives were more popular was that it would be immodest for a woman patient's genitalia to be seen by a man. There are illustrations which have been reproduced many times, of men delivering women, particularly where forceps have been used, hidden under large sheets draped over the patients' nether parts and legs. There is a famous wood cut from an eighteenth century Dutch work on midwifery showing the bed sheet pinned around the obstetrician's neck so that he could not see the woman's genitalia (Donnison, 1988) (Figure 1).

A summary of the position of midwives and their battle, which does not yet seem to have been won, to have equal status with doctors, is recounted brilliantly in Donnison's book, which has as its subtitle *History of the Struggle for the Control of Childbirth.* Indeed it does seem that particularly in countries like the United States, there has been a continuous struggle to determine who should deliver the baby. Towards the end of the twentieth century, the majority of babies in the USA are certainly delivered by men, while on the other hand in the UK about 80% are still delivered by female midwives and a midwife is present at every delivery.

From Donnison's book it is clear that up to the sixteenth century midwives indulged in what she calls 'the female mysteries'. It was only in the middle of the fifteenth century that municipalities took over the regulation of midwives. This

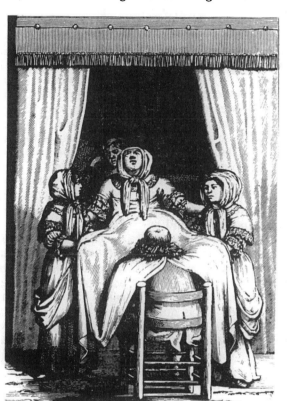

Figure 1 Man-midwife delivering a baby (*see* text)

started in the city of Ravensburg in Germany, where doctors were also appointed to control medical practice. These are the first records of a municipality controlling midwifery and exhorting the midwives to call for the assistance of a doctor or surgeon when the births were being difficult.

CONTROLLING THE WORK OF MIDWIVES

The first arrangements for the control of midwives in England were made under the Henry VIII Act of 1512 for the Regulation of Physicians and Surgeons, which was initiated by Thomas Linacre who was responsible with others, for founding the College of Physicians of London in 1518.

In all British Hospitals that concerned themselves entirely with midwifery, such as lying-in wards at the Middlesex Hospital (see William Hunter, 1747) and the British and City of London Lying-in Hospitals (1749–1750) as well as the General Lying-in Hospital (Queen Charlotte's, 1752), the day to day delivery of women was conducted by midwives who called in doctors for difficult cases. The doctors, together with the board of governors, supervised the running of the hospitals. The list of doctors attached to these hospitals founded by humanitarian philanthropists was published on the noticeboard at the entrance to the hospital, and included most of the very fashionable obstetricians and accoucheurs of the time. The pupils at the City of London Lying-in Hospital (for married women) were always female until the twentieth century when a few male students were attached from London teaching hospitals. The preponderance of the teaching however, was always by the midwives and these were until 1974, always women. A few men have been admitted as pupil midwives for some years.

There always seems to have been a rise and fall in the fortunes of female midwives who, in spite of conducting the majority of deliveries never achieved a status, except in France, equal to that of doctors of medicine. It is probable that the invention by the Chamberlens of forceps marked the start of the ascendancy of men in midwifery. Yet, Peter Chamberlen had, in the first half of the seventeenth century when he was physician to the Queen, suggested a scheme for instructing midwives. These schemes to instruct midwives were alternately supported by the midwives themselves and opposed by them. One of the troubles was that male doctors seldom, unless attending Royalty, saw normal deliveries and were only called in when things were going wrong.

Furthermore, the church had the task of issuing licences to midwives. In the sixteenth century licences to practise midwifery were granted by Bishops; for instance in 1567 the Archbishop of Canterbury granted a licence to Eleoner Pead to be a midwife. Midwives were enjoined not to lay 'supposititious children in place of the true natural ones', nor could they use sorcery and enchantments. They also had to christen children because taking a frail and perhaps dying child by road to a priest might have been too dangerous for the child's life.

In 1686 the midwife's licence was granted by the Bishop of London, to Helen Perkins, in which it was stated that she had been examined by 'diverse, honest and discreet women'. It is quite clear that the Bishop had power to grant licences to midwives and to supervise their work which, of course, had to be in accordance with the teachings of the Church.

In Elisabeth Bennion's illustrated book *Antique Medical Instruments* (Bennion, 1979), we see illustrations of what appear to be catheters, but which were in fact tubes to be introduced into the uterus by the midwife if she thought the infant was going to die so that it could be baptised before birth if necessary, to save its soul.

SOME FAMOUS MIDWIVES IN HISTORY

In the Bible we have the midwives mentioned in Genesis and Exodus, including the two who defied Pharoah.

In Greece there was a woman called Elephantis who has gone down in history as much for being a pornographer as for being a midwife, but evidence of her pornographic writings are hard to come by. Another famous midwife of antiquity was Olympias Anastasia who may also have had as a surname 'the Navel!' She was said to be the mistress of Sirus the younger. It is recounted that when she grew a tumour on her chin, neither she nor her father Hermotine, had the money to pay for its removal so, acting on a vision she had in a dream, she applied a bouquet of roses prepared to be offered to Venus, to the tumour, and it disappeared (Witkowski, 1887).

In the Middle Ages midwives were often accused of witchcraft and were either burnt at the stake or put in the pillory. A famous French midwife who suffered this was Perette who lived at the beginning of the fifteenth century. She was condemned to death for sorcery, but because of her great reputation as an accoucheuse had the sentence commuted to being exposed on the pillory in Rouen. Perette died in 1411.

Elizabeth Woodeville, the wife of Edward IV and mother of the two Princes who disappeared in the Tower, of whom the elder was Edward V, was delivered of these Princes by her midwife Marquerite Cobbe. Edward V was born in 1470 in Westminster, possibly in the Abbey (Aveling, 1872); the second Prince was Richard, Duke of York.

There was no doubt that being a Royal midwife carried enormous professional as well as financial advantages. One of the most famous of all was Loyse (or Louise) Bourgeois who was also called Boursier (her married name) in the seventeenth century. She delivered Marie de Medicis (Figure 2) six times. After her first delivery Marie was allowed out of bed on the second day, and her husband Henri IV of France wrote to Sully 'It is impossible to believe how well my wife is. Seeing the suffering she underwent, she does her own hair and already speaks about getting up'. Sully (1560–1641) incidentally was a covert Protestant, fortunate to escape the massacre of the Protestants on St Bartholomew's Day 1572 (as had been the Chamberlens, see chapter 9). He had helped to arrange the marriage between Henry and Marie de Medicis.

Loyse Bourgeois was an extremely handsome woman as is testified by the engraving of her portrait when she was 45 years of age. She wrote an account of the delivery of the royal children with the title *The True Story of the Birth of The Infants of France, with Particulars* . . . This was published in 1652 and she signed herself as Loyse Bourgeois dit Boursier, 'mother' of the king. Her book

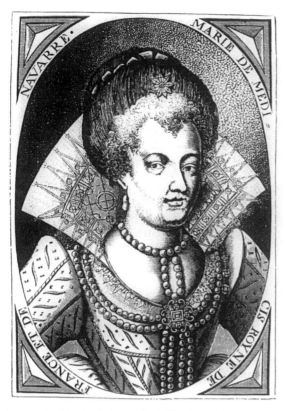

Figure 2 Marie de Medicis (1573–1642) Queen consort of Henry IV of France (ruled 1589 to 1610, when assassinated) then Regent for her son King Louis XIII (ruled 1610–1643). She was a Florentine Princess who had her six children (*see* text) in eight years starting in 1601

recounts how she became the Queen's midwife after being recommended by Madame de Thou, wife of the president of Thou, a district of France. Although there were five doctors looking after the Queen it was Loyse who delivered the children. There is a long account of her relationship with the Queen in her book that is quoted in Witkowski (Witkowski, 1887). Her reign as royal midwife ended with the unfortunate death of Madame de Gaston d'Orleans in June 1627, possibly of puerperal fever.

Another reason why Loyse Bourgeois is so famous is that she wrote a text book, 'in a style that is not without merit' under the title *Instruction to my Daughter* (1609). This book of instruction was on methods of delivery and went into several editions. She even delivered babies in malpositions or with malpresentations.

Fasbender (1906) states that Loyse Bourgeois was the first to describe prolapse of the umbilical

cord, after rupture of the membranes, and to emphasize how important it was to return the cord into the uterus. She also seems to have been the first to describe quite clearly face presentations, and she says that there should be no interference when the face comes down onto the perineum.

In England in the first half of the sixteenth century Alice Massey delivered Elizabeth of York, the wife of Henry VII, in 1603, and charged handsomely for it. More famous was Jane Sharp who in 1671 published her *Treatise of Obstetrics* which went into several editions. It does seem that she stole many of the secrets from Loyse Bourgeois.

At the same time, the midwife Elizabeth Cellier really went outside her field by meddling in politics: and on 30 April 1680 she was accused of having 'diabolically and traitorously conspired against King Charles II, having tried to introduce the Catholic religion into the Kingdom'. She was tried before Chief Justice Scroggs. She defended herself and was acquitted (Cellier, 1680). The jury 'as was customary, applied for a guinea a piece' from Mrs Cellier. She declined to pay it and offered her services if any of their wives were to become pregnant!

Of her was written the following quatrain

'you taught the judges to interpret laws;
showed Sergeant Maynard how to plead a cause;
you turned and wound and roguedem at your will;
'twas trial, not of life or death, but skill'.

She then published a libellous work for which she was put in the pillory

'poor Cellier, you had better brought to bed anything, than have a plot and triumph led, and thus to be received into the world's arms by dirt and stones, and other warlike arms'.

For her malicious libel, sentence on 13 September 1680 was passed by the Recorder of London. She was fined £1000.00, to be kept in prison until the £1000.00 was paid, and to be put on the pillory. She tried all sorts of tricks to avoid the last, including pretending she was pregnant and in labour.

'So . . . an able physician and several discrete women were sent for. They searched her so narrowly that they discovered the whole cheat, and found that the good lady was no more with bairn than the town-bull, but only having overnight privately gotten a bladder of blood, had used her skill in creating the necessary symptoms, and, preparing certain clots of it, had put them in her body . . .'

She had been married for 20 years but then 'she received into her house an Italian and his negro servant, and fell in love with both, and was delivered soon after of a tawny-faced boy, to the great amazement of all beholders' (Aveling, 1872, p. 73). She married again and had several children. Her second husband escaped from her and went to live in Barbados where he died. Mr Cellier was her third husband. Aveling concludes his description of Mrs Cellier with the following sentence 'had it only been properly directed she might have done for midwifery in England what Justine Siegemundine did in Germany, and Madame Boivin in France'.

The lovely little book, by J.H. Aveling, Physician to the Chelsea Hospital for Women and published by J.N.A. Churchill, 1872, entitled *Some English Midwives* details the history of English midwifery from the sixteenth century onwards and gives short and very pertinent biographies of some midwives. Among the women of whose lives there is a short note, is the Mrs Draper who delivered Queen Charlotte on 12 August 1762, of the future King George IV. Dr William Hunter was 'in waiting in case of his help being wanted'. In 1706, Peter Chamberlen it is clear, was working with a midwife whose name was Mrs Bizzol.

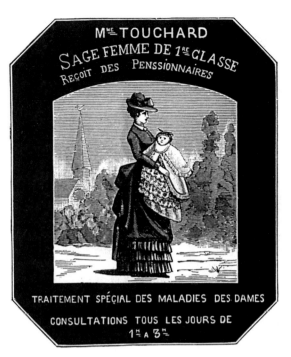

Figure 4 A later advertisement by a French 'first class' midwife

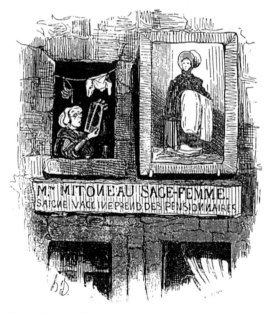

Figure 3 An illustration satirizing the methods used by French midwives to advertise that they took in women for delivery. From H. Daumier's *Nemesis Medicale*

From Aveling's book we know of some othe English midwives. For instance Margaret Cobbe who had a salary of £10 a year granted to her by the Crown on 15 April 1469. She attended the Queen of Edward IV (Elizabeth Woodville) when she was delivered of Edward V in 'the gloomy sanctuary of Westminster'. This was on 1 November 1470. She was given letter patents to continue practising in 1473. A selection of advertisements used by various French midwives is shown in Figures 3–5.

Aveling describes in some detail the midwives oath and the midwives licence to practise.

Another midwife whose name has gone down in history, and whose works are still being republished was Madame Boursier Du Coudray. Her book of which there was a facsimile made in 1989 is entitled *Abrégé de l'art des Accouchements*. It was published first in Chalons-Sur-Marne by Bouchard in 1773. It has as its frontispiece a portrait of a matronly buxom lady. The text contains not only the qualities required by a midwife, but considerable descriptive anatomy of the bony structures and illustrations of such procedures as delivery of the aftercoming head in breech deliveries, shoulders in normal deliveries, dealing with a prolapsed arm, for which the treatment was to find a foot and bring the leg down, and manual removal of the placenta. She writes about a double uterus, a rigid hymen, compound deliveries, twin deliveries and the use of a leather pessary in the case of prolapse! Madame De Coudray who was born Angelique-Marie Le Boursier (not to be confused with the famous Loyse Bourgeois) was, as were so many midwives who received their licences from the Royalty or the Church, concerned with baptism of the newborn baby, especially the baby at risk of dying, and she wrote about that too.

There were two outstanding teachers of midwifery in France in the nineteenth century. One Mrs Lachapelle, who was the midwife in charge of the Maisons D'Accouchements de Paris, wrote a splendid *Practice of Obstetrics* published in Paris in 1825. This also appeared in England in the same year as the French edition. The book was published with the help of her nephew Dr Duges, Professor of Medicine in Montpellier and in Paris. It is somewhat confusing to recount that there were several well-known midwives in France with the name Lachapelle but it was the superintendent midwife of the maternity Hospital of Paris who wrote the book. Her nephew also seemed to have helped another superintendent midwife, Madame Veuve (widow) Marie-Anne-Victoire Boivin (1773–

1841) who wrote a practical thesis on diseases of the uterus, published in English in 1834 in two volumes with many illustrations.

French midwives often had special chairs in their homes, one of which is illustrated in Figure 6.

It would appear that there was bitter jealousy between Madame Lachapelle and Madame Boivin in spite of their having sought the assistance from the same Professor of Medicine to help them publish their books. Madame Lachapelle's book goes to three volumes and Madame Boivin's book has one large volume of text and an accompanying volume of very fine illustrations. The text deals more with gynaecology than with obstetrics.

Mrs Elizabeth Nihell was a formidable opponent of men-midwives and their instruments. Mrs Nihell said the success of he-practisers was due to fashion – 'this silly vanity'. One of Mrs Nihell's opponents was Smellie the 'head of the men-midwives'. She wrote a book against him and his works, published in London in 1760. Not surprisingly Dr William Hunter was also one with whom she quarrelled, when he was called in to assist her in a difficult case and found that the umbilical cord had been separated from the placenta.

A very notable midwife at the end of the nineteenth century was Caroline Tarpley, who was born in 1828 and died in 1925. She was the village midwife of Cropthorne, Worcester.

MEN-MIDWIVES

Certainly medical intervention seems originally to have been as a whole damaging rather than beneficial. Before 1720 almost all babies were delivered by female midwives because there were very few male midwives before then (Aveling, 1872; Wilson, 1984). Some men-midwives did not interfere, as can be seen by the accounts of William Hunter (q.v.), who of course was active after 1720, but others were more likely to intervene. The term man-midwife was first used in England in the early seventeenth century, and man-midwifery became part of surgical practice in that century. Up until then, it was only when a female midwife could not deliver a baby that she would call in a surgeon to use instruments if he could. In the 1720s however, medical practitioners started to attend normal labours by arrangement. Before then it is unlikely that men had any great experience of normal labour. It was in 1720, that the secret of the forceps was wrested from the Chamberlens and they started being used in the

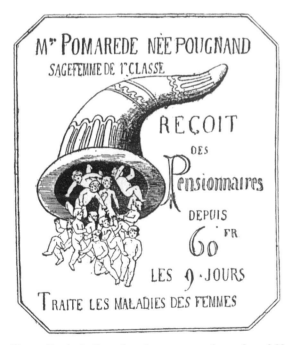

Figure 5 A similar advertisement quoting a fee of 60 Francs for nine days lying-in after delivery. This midwife also treated female disorders

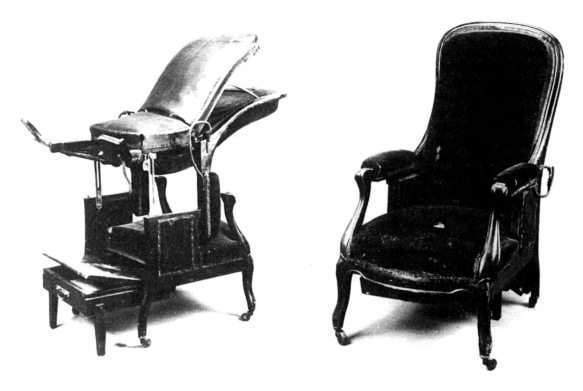

Figure 6 A mid-nineteenth century French midwives' delivery chair. This particular chair was used by a midwife in the village of Tours in the Loire valley, and possibly occasionally by a local surgeon. It is of green velvet and converts to a delivery table which itself is covered in black fibre (left). It folds to become a very presentable dining room arm chair (right) (q.v. Voltaire chair, p.20). Reproduced with kind permission from Christie's, South Kensington, London, UK (C. Keith Wilbur (1987) *Antique Medical Instruments*, Pennsylvania, p.73.)

home counties, but not as far away as Somerset where they had not been used at all even as late as 1800.

Smellie and William Hunter were teaching midwifery to men in the middle of the eighteenth century and Smellie was taking his pupils to attend labours where he was officiating (Brocklebank and Kenworth, 1968). It was after 1750 that medical practitioners attended all complicated labours and some normal ones. It was considered proper obstetric training for medical students to use forceps, but not for midwives. Midwife Sarah Stone, who practised in Bridgewater in Taunton between 1702 and 1730 where there were no men-midwives, found to her intense disgust after moving to Bristol that 'every young man who had serviced his apprenticeship to a barber-surgeon, immediately sets up as a man-midwife; although he is ignorant and indeed much ignorantor than the meanest Woman of the profession' (Stone, 1737).

It seems absolutely clear that the advent of men-midwives into obstetrics, especially in the patients' own homes, meant much more interference with normal labour than was desirable and this in part was due to the very scanty and poor training that men-midwives obtained.

In his book Aveling compared maternal mortality at the hands of men-midwives as against the mortality rate at the hands of lady-(women)-midwives. The men seem to have won on the statistical argument.

OFFICIAL RECOGNITION OF MIDWIVES

The struggle for official recognition of midwives depended on many things. For instance, in France and in England, when the Queen was attended by a midwife rather than an accoucheur, the status of the midwife was clearly raised. When William Hunter had been forced to stand by, either outside the Palace or in an adjoining room while the

Queen was delivering, Mrs Draper her personal midwife clearly 'ruled the roost'. But Hunter had had enough of this by the time the third child had been born and ousted Mrs Draper using the diplomatic excuse that she was too old to continue in her post. Hunter delivered the Queen's remaining 12 children, except the last because he died in the fourth month of that pregnancy.

Other royal midwives from previous centuries were Margaret Cobb, midwife to the Queen of Edward IV who in 1469 was granted a pension of £10.00 a year for life, as was Alice Massey for attending Elizabeth of York in 1503. The midwife of Queen Henrietta Maria, the wife of Charles I, received a remuneration of £300 for her work and £100 for her diet and entertainment. Some midwives, although very few, became very rich (Donnison, 1988).

Peter Chamberlen did not like the fact that the clergy had control over the licensing of midwives and in the time of Cromwell seized an opportunity to increase his criticism of the Bishops' role. He wanted a civil authority to control midwives.

Mrs Jane Sharp's textbook was the first to be written by any English midwife. It could not compare however, with the work of Loyse Bourgeois, of France. At the time of Jane Sharp midwives did hold sway; but when William Smellie, William Hunter, Richard Manningham and Fielding Ould became prominent and the secret of the Chamberlen forceps was revealed, midwives started to lose ground. The noble families were torn between employing a midwife for their deliveries or employing a doctor who was now beginning to be called a 'man-midwife'.

Even before two wards had been set aside at the Middlesex Hospital in 1748 under the control of William Hunter, the Rotunda Hospital was opened in 1745 in Dublin as 'The Lying-in Hospital'. In these hospitals midwives were being trained by older midwives and by man-midwife–accoucheurs. At no stage were midwives encouraged to use instruments, although a very few did have a licence, which allowed them to use them.

Instruction of midwives on the continent of Europe was more thorough and detailed than in England and Madame Du Coudray (Maitresse Sage-Femme) wrote her book in 1760 on commission by the King of France.

As has been said, the release of information about the forceps in 1720 or thereabouts strengthened the hand of the important accoucheurs such as Hunter against the midwives whose status was considered to be lowly; as indeed was the status of accoucheurs as against the elite physicians and the somewhat less elite surgeons. Surgeons, until the Royal College of Surgeons of England was established in 1800, occupied a lower position in the social hierarchy than physicians did.

Part of the decline of female midwives resulted from the fact that forceps were 'machines'. With the advent of machines it was more difficult for women to find honourable employment, and what is more they were being excluded from such typically female occupations as sewing, as machines were introduced for making clothes and suits. This changed fairly soon, but initially women were not considered able to handle machines; not even those which had no moving parts such as the obstetric forceps.

A very fashionable midwife, Mrs T. Beale, was instrumental in founding in 1830 the British Ladies Lying-in Institution. Patrons and patronesses included no less than four Duchesses and two Countesses 'and other ladies of distinction too numerous for insertion'. Mrs Beale apparently had attended all these ladies professionally: and she was the leader of 15 midwives who taught and practised midwifery in the Westminster area. The midwives were all married women or widows. The British Institution took it upon themselves to attend ladies who 'may prefer the attendance of respectable females'. Attendance was assured 'at an hour's notice in town', by addressing a line to the consultant midwife at 10 Chapel Street, Mayfair. Arrangements could be made for a midwife to reside with a family in the country if needed.

What was clear and still is, is that for midwives, childbirth is a 'natural' process, whereas for medical men it is a condition that requires special medical attention.

The discovery of the beneficial use of chloroform also further weakened the status of midwives because it had to be administered by doctors, nearly all of whom were men. What had held the position of men-midwives back a little was the attitude of the Royal Colleges, who thought that as accouchement was a natural process it was unworthy to be considered among the learned disciplines.

When Florence Nightingale established her School of Nursing in St Thomas's Hospital, she hoped also to improve the status of midwives, particularly to supply trained midwives to work among the rural poor.

The status of midwives *vis-à-vis* doctors in some way is linked to the status of women doctors; and a great step forward was the qualifying in medicine of Elizabeth Garrett, later Garrett-Anderson with the licence of the Society of Apothecaries in 1865.

SUPERVISION OF MIDWIVES IN THE TWENTIETH CENTURY

The passage of the Midwives Act in 1902 gave status to and control of midwives. Discussion had taken place as to the status of midwives both inside and outside Parliament, and opinions were voiced not only in the general press but also in the medical press such as the *British Medical Journal* and the *Lancet*. The General Medical Council, who control doctors and their work, was also involved in these discussions. By the turn of the century at least six Midwives Bills had been introduced into the House of Commons concerning whether local registers or state registers for midwives should be kept, and the way in which midwives should be licensed, taught and controlled. Very active lobbying for and against most opinions carried on for 40 years or more. Finally in 1902 the first effective Midwives' Act was passed in Parliament. This involved the setting up of a Central Midwives' Board to supervise the institutes where midwives were trained, the selection of examiners, (by the 1950s equal numbers of midwives and doctors) the setting of the standards for examinations, and the granting of licences throughout the country. One of the most important clauses in the act was that the Central Midwives' Board should be separate from the General Medical Council. In due course, when the Bill was debated in Parliament before it became an Act, discussions were linked to the formation of a nurses' regulatory body, together with a midwives' regulatory body, but this did not come to be at that stage. It was a triumph for those who had agitated to have the Central Midwives' Board set up that it stayed in existence until 1979 when it was abolished.

The position of State-Certified Midwife was established by the 1902 Act, and within 3 years a Midwives Roll of over 22 000 names was available. Not all of these had passed any examination; and in fact quite a proportion of them were illiterate, but had initially to be registered with the Central Midwives' Board as they had been in practice for a long time. Gradually as these retired, the status of the midwife improved and the standard of the examination was raised, but also gradually with the increasing amount of interference in labour because of the increased use of anaesthetics, forceps and Caesarean operation, the midwife became more dependent on her obstetric colleagues than hitherto. Nevertheless, it is obvious to anybody who has gone through training as an obstetrician in British hospitals, that young doctors have to, and do, learn from experienced midwives. The fact that perinatal mortality as well as maternal mortality has dropped so much is greatly due to the increased education and sophistication of the women practising midwifery, now almost entirely in hospital, or following up patients who have been discharged from hospital early in the puerperium to be looked after at home. 'Practice midwives' care for mothers and babies for about 10 or 11 days after the delivery when health visitors, who have not had as intensive a training in midwifery, very often take over; depending on the district (Van Larcome, 1913).

When the Central Midwives' Board was founded it succeeded the London Obstetrical Society which held examinations and issued certificates until 1905. The first examinations of the Central Midwives' Board were held in 1905, and it became the only examining and licensing body in existence. Midwives came from all over the world to obtain its certificate. The Central Midwives' Board had been formed as a direct result of Section III of the 1902 Act; and it consisted of four registered medical practitioners and three other people. Its aims were:

(1) To set the standards to which training schools and instructors must conform in order that their graduates may be eligible for examination;

(2) To give oral and written examinations;

(3) To admonish midwives or revoke their licences; and

(4) To draft rules and regulations controlling midwives and their practice.

After a time those who passed the examinations could put the initials SCM (State-Certified Midwife) after their names. Their status was greatly enhanced by the 1936 Midwives' Act.

THE ROYAL COLLEGE OF MIDWIVES

The Royal College of Midwives was founded in 1881 as a result of agitation by a Miss Zepherina Veitch, who later married a distinguished surgeon

Professor Henry Smith, and a Miss Louisa Hubbard, proprietor and editor of a woman's journal called *Work and Leisure*. It was first called the Midwives' Institute and only later the Royal College of Midwives (Cowell and Wainwright, 1981). Among the functions it carried out was organizing an international midwives' union to look after the affairs of midwives not only in the UK but in other countries as well.

Fortuitously it had its first offices in the same building as the National Birthday Trust Fund and the Queen's Institute for District Nursing. The building, 57 Lower Belgrave Street, had been given to the National Birthday Trust by its chairman Sir Julien Cahn who was very active in its affairs which as we have seen elsewhere played a great role in helping to reduce maternal mortality and perinatal mortality by its great surveys.

The Midwives' Act passed in 1936 to 'secure the organization throughout the country of a domiciliary service and salaried midwives under the control of local supervising authorities,' was an important step in the improvement of the maternity services and in the campaign for reducing maternal mortality. The state of the midwifery profession would be raised 'by providing adequate salaries and secure prospects for those midwives who entered the new service'.

The 1936 Midwives' Act did indeed greatly improve the status of midwives working in hospital-based maternity units as well as in the community under local authorities; and later attached to general practices.

Sir Francis Henry Champneys (1848–1930) a fine obstetrician who worked in St. Bartholomew's Hospital after training in Oxford, Vienna, Leipzig and Dresden as well as various hospitals in London, had been chairman from 1890 of a board set up by the Obstetrical Society of London for the examination of midwives. When the Central Midwives' Board was established in 1902 he became its chairman, and was re-elected year after year for 28 years until he was 80 years of age. His administrative work in this role involved difficult and delicate negotiations and he fought for the midwives fearlessly. Fifty years work for midwives was crowned six years after his death by the passage of the 1936 Act. He had worked very hard indeed towards its achievement and he also had worked hard towards the establishment of the British (later Royal) College of Obstetricians and Gynaecologists. He was a man of broad interests, was deeply religious and extremely conscientious. He was a fine organist, and a member of the council of the Royal College of Music for many years (Peel, 1976).

The Central Midwives' Board's authority which it had exercised from 1902 to 1983 was taken over in that year by the United Kingdom Central Council for Nursing, Midwifery and Health Visiting. This new statutory body became responsible for the rules regulating midwifery practice, framed in accordance with the recommendations of its midwifery committee following the 1979 Act.

In 1979 an Act of Parliament was passed to govern the practice of midwifery, entitled *The Nurses, Midwives, and Health Visitors Act* and this required that:

(1) Midwifery committees are instituted at the United Kingdom Central Council (UKCC) and four national boards which shall consider all matters relating to midwifery;

(2) Midwifery rules should be made under statutory instrument;

(3) Close supervision of midwifery practice should be instituted; and

(4) The only people that should attend a woman in childbirth should be doctors and midwives, or those in training for those professions.

The midwives rules lay down the standards and parameters for midwifery training and the midwife has to be competent to meet the requirements of a European Council Directive.

Under the practice rules the midwife does not have to involve a medical practitioner in the care of clients so long as there is no deviation from normal in the mother or baby. She does however, have to call a doctor if there is an emergency.

BOOKS WRITTEN TO INSTRUCT MIDWIVES

De Partu Hominis was written by Eucharius Rösslin, who was first a physician at Worms, Germany, and later at Frankfurt-am-Main (Graham, 1950). He wrote one of the most, if not the most, influential books on midwifery in 1513. It was published then under the title *Roszgarten* or in full *Der Swangern Frauwen und Hebammen Roszgarten*. It was printed in Worms and then translated into Latin by his son of the same name in 1532. The word Roszgarten was translated into Latin as *De Partu Hominis*, and in Latin the name Rösslin was transliterated into Rhodion. The book was called in English, when it was translated, probably by Thomas Raynold, *The Byrth of Mankynde* but

Raynold also named it in his prologue; *The Womens Booke.* There is considerable confusion as to who actually did the translation because the name of Richard Jonas appears in one of the editions. J.W. Ballantyne (q.v.), the famous twentieth century instigator of antenatal care, has held that Raynold was the publisher and expander of the book. Harvey Graham writes very interestingly about the confusion (Graham, 1950). In any case, Rhodion or Rösslin's work was translated into nearly every European language, and it was practically the only book from which midwives could gain any knowledge of their art. It is difficult to know how many editions of the book appeared and in how many languages, but probably 100 editions appeared altogether. It goes into considerable detail and has illustrations of the different fetal presentations and also of the 'woman's stool'. This is designed so that she can 'sit downe, leaning backward, in manner upright;' then Rhodion goes on to describe stools used in some regions of France and Germany! 'the midwives have stools for the nonce, which being but low are not high from the ground, be so compasse and cave or hollow in the middest, so that may be received from underneath if looked for, and the back of the stoole leaning backward, receiveth the backe of the woman'. He gives figures of the stool and he says that 'the midwife herself shall sit before the labouring woman, and shall diligently observe and waite, how much, and after what meanes the child stirreth itself; and also shall with hands, first anoynted with the oyle of almonds, or the oyle of those white lillies, rule and direct everything as shall seeme best'. He encourages the midwife to instruct and comfort 'the party' not only by giving her 'good meate and drinke', but also with sweet words 'giving her hope of a good speedie deliverance, encouraging and enstomacking her to patience and tolerance, bidding her to hold in her breath as much as she may, also stroking gently with her hands her belly above the Navell, for that helpeth to depress the birth downeward'. He tells the midwife not to let the woman labour before the birth come forward and show itself, (in otherwords not to let her push until the head is at the vulva), because if she does she will labour in vain, her strength will be spent and 'that is a perillous case'.

It is of interest that Professor Hellman, a very cultured professor of obstetrics in New York, acquired a large collection of Rösslin's book, in several editions and several languages. These were bought when Hellman died by the late Alistair Gunn who was the Honorary Librarian at the Royal College of Obstetricians and Gynaecologists. Some were bought for the College, and others mainly as a present for his wife who was very interested in the subject. The College library possesses at least 18 copies ranging from a 1513 edition to the Augsberg-Steiner edition of 1532, and the English *Birth of Mankynde*, newly set forth by Thomas Raynold and published by Raynold in 1545. There are later editions in the College library as well as the Latin *De Partu Hominis* translated in Paris by Foucher in 1532, and also a Frankfurt 1532 edition. There is a 1536 Venice edition and a 1537 Venice edition by the same publisher Perderzoni. There is a 1552 Raynald edition and a 1560 Jugge as well as a 1565 Jugge edition. One can see that the book achieved an enviable circulation very fast indeed.

One of the best known of all midwives was Mrs Sarah Stone whose maiden name was Holmes and whose mother was a midwife, and whose assistant she was for 6 years. She recommended that midwifery had to be taught as an apprenticeship for 3–7 years. She moved to Bristol from Bridgewater because her health would no longer stand driving long distances when she would then sit for long hours in damp clothing. She described how she carried out internal podalic version in a case where the arm was presenting in the vagina. This saved the baby's life and she was able to deliver it quickly. She delivered at least 300 children a year in Taunton before going to Bristol. After being in Bristol for some years she went to London. There in 1737 she published *The Complete Practice of Midwifery*. She dedicated this to the Queen's Most Excellent Majesty. She, like Elizabeth Cellier, campaigned against men-midwives and their instruments. She deplored the fashion for calling in young men-midwives, and said 'I am certain that where 20 women are delivered with instruments (which has now become a common practice) that 19 of them might be delivered without, if not the twentieth, as would appear in my observations'.

It was Peter Chamberlen who in 1616 petitioned King James I 'that some order may be settled by the State for the instruction and civil government of midwives'. Unfortunately the State did not take any notice of what Peter Chamberlen asked. In the first year of the seventeenth century, his son who obtained as big a reputation as his father had and became a Fellow of the College of Physicians in 1628, was taught by his father how to deliver women in difficult cases. He said 'the burthen of all the midwives in and about London lay only on my shoulders'. In 1633 he again attempted, as his father had done before him, to have midwives better educated. His wish was to obtain authority from the Crown to organize female practitioners in midwifery and to form a company with himself as the head as President and Examiner. This angered the College of Physicians.

Aveling says that English midwives 'should always remember that the two Peter Chamberlens were their first champions'. Aveling praises highly, the 'immortal Harvey' and points out that the obstetrical writings of William Harvey were translated into English by Sir George Ent in 1653. A contemporary of Harvey's was Percival Willughby a very distinguished man-midwife. Willughby acknowledged that he owed much to Dr Harvey and wrote . . . 'I wish all midwives to observe and follow (Dr Harvey's directions and method) and often read over and over again'. William Harvey denounced the midwives, and wrote 'the younger and more giddy midwives, who mightily bestow themselves and provoke the expulsive faculty, and who, persuading poor women to their three-legged stool before their time, do weary them out and bring them in danger of their lives'. Both Dr Willughby and Dr Harvey thought midwives could be too officious and not sufficiently trusting to the workings of nature.

Willughby reported that midwives cruelly tortured some patients, but he wished them to be trained and to leave natural labour to the safe conduct of the 'invisible midwife Dame nature'. Not only was Percival Willughby a fine man-midwife himself but he did teach one of his two daughters the art of midwifery. He took her to a case of obstructed labour and although they travelled all night and got soaked through, the mother was dead before they arrived.

Another seventeenth century man-midwife, a Dr William Sermon (1671) also wrote a book *The Labours Companion or The English Midwife*, published in London. He deplored some of the work of midwives who 'desired to excel men, or at least would seem to go beyond them'. It was apparent that midwives ruptured the membranes by tearing at them with their nails and sometimes damaged the child doing this. In his book Dr Aveling (1872) gives a short summary of the background of Peter Chamberlen, William Harvey, Percival Willughby and William Sermon.

In the seventeenth century Jane Sharp dedicated her book on midwifery to Lady Eleanor Talbott. It was published by Simon Miller, of the Star, at the West End of St Paul's in 1671. It was entitled *Midwives Book, or the Whole Art of Midwifery Discovered, Directing Childbearing Women How To Behave Themselves*. Mrs Sharp said that she had been practising midwifery for 30 years before she wrote the book. She recommended midwives to learn anatomy and Aveling quotes at length from Jane Sharp's book which went into four editions, the fourth one being printed soon after her death.

CHANGES IN MIDWIFERY IN THE 1960s AND 1970s

The advances in midwifery in these years was enormous and the term 'Childbirth Revolution' was no exaggeration. Apart from being independent, most midwives considered themselves to be assistants to the doctors who had an ever increasing role in running the maternity units, especially in hospitals. The advent of technological changes was to be far reaching. A very high proportion of labours were induced either by rupturing the membranes or by giving oxytocic transfusions. The drug Pitocin, was replaced by a much safer drug Syntocinon and this made induction of labour both easier and safer. Intravenous automatic counter machines became used routinely with syntocinon because they delivered electronically a pre-set dose of Syntocinon intravenously. Also at that time partograms became more widely used by obstetricans. They replaced, to a certain extent, the verbal descriptions of the progress of each labour and made it possible to see very rapidly what was happening in the way of frequency of contractions, strength of contractions, descent of the presenting part in the pelvis and dilatation of the cervix as well as the heart rates of the mother and fetus. Cardiotocograph machines recorded the fetal heart rate either by the use of a transducer attached by a belt to the mother's abdomen or by an electrode attached to the presenting part of the baby. The use of such machinery meant that the woman had to be confined to bed, usually lying on her back.

The pattern of labour changed chiefly because of the use of Syntocinon and became much more painful. When there were variations in the fetal heart rate as recorded on the machines it was possible to test the effect on the blood gases in the fetus by using the 'Astrup test'. This involved making a prick on the scalp of the fetus and removing a drop or so of capillary blood for testing.

Epidural analgesia also involved setting up an intravenous transfusion. The epidural anaesthetic

179

meant the patient losing the use of her legs while the epidural was working and in any case she was unable to move about as she had an intravenous transfusion going. Furthermore the need for forceps to accomplish the delivery became much more common, because women, especially with their first babies do not have the sensation of needing to push to expel the baby nor do they know how to do it instinctively, as women often do when they have no epidural anaesthesia. Obviously the higher forceps rate, the greater interference rate and the higher Caesarean rate diminished the role of the midwife. It became very worrying by 1974 when the Central Midwives Board in a statement of policy stressed that pupil midwives should receive instruction in the management of natural birth in addition to the new techniques of 'active labour' (Central Midwives Board, 1974). It is quite clear that the role of the midwives *vis à vis* the gynaecologists and obstetricians will change. But then history shows that the relationship has always changed from century to century, if not from decade to decade.

CHRONOLOGY

40 000 BC	Men helped wives to deliver.
6000 BC	Women had taken over all deliveries.
1700 BC	Tamar is delivered (in the Bible) of twins by a midwife.
800–500 BC	Greek midwives enjoyed a very high social status. Traditional birth attendants have worked in the same way for the last 2000 or more years.
15–17 C.	French midwives held in great respect.
1512	An Act passed in Henry VIII's reign helped in the supervision of midwives.
1513	Rösslin's famous book was published.
1518	Foundation of the College of Physicians.
16–17 C.	The Church grants licences to midwives.
15–18 C.	Midwives deliver Royalty.
1720	The secret of Chamberlen's forceps was divulged allowing men to come more often to deliveries.
18 C.	Foundation of British Maternity (Lying-in) Hospitals.

1902	The Midwives Act was passed and Central Midwives' Board established.
1936	The Midwives' Act established a country-wide, comprehensive service of well-trained, qualified, salaried midwives.

REFERENCES

Aveling, J.H. (1872). *English Midwives*. (London: J.N.A. Churchill)

Bennion, E. (1979). *Antique Medical Instruments, Sotheby Parke Bernet*. (California: University of California Press)

Boivin Mme, Veuve and Dugés, A. *A Practical Treatise on the Diseases of the Uterus and its Appendage*, English Edition 1834. (London: Sherwood Gilbert and Paper)

Bourgeois, L. (1609). *Observations diverses sur la sterilitée perte de fruict, foecondite, accouchemens et maladies des femmes et enfants nouveaux naiz*. (Paris: Saugrain)

Brocklebank, W. and Kenworth, F. (ed.) (1968). *The Diary of Richard Kay (1716–1751) of Baldingstone near Bury*. (Manchester: The Chetham Society)

Cellier, E. (1680). *Malice defeated: or a brief relation of the accusation and deliverance of Elizabeth Cellier... together with an abstract of her arraignment and tryal, written by herself for the satisfaction of all lovers of undisguised truth*. (London: for Elizabeth Cellier)

Central Midwives' Board (1974). *Active Management of Labour*. Statement to training schools 1974

Cowell, B. and Wainwright, D. (1981). *Behind the Blue Door, History of the Royal College of Midwives 1881–1981*. (London: Bailliere and Tindall)

Donnison, J. (1988). *Midwives and Medical Men*, pp. 56 and 101; Plate 5. (Historical Publications)

Fasbender, H. (1906). *Geschichte der geburtshilfe*. (Jena: Gustav Fischer)

Graham, H. (1950). *Eternal Eve*. (London: William Heinemann Medical Books Ltd.)

Lachapelle (1825). *Pratique des Accouchemens publiés par Ant Duges, sou neveu*. (Paros: J-B. Bailliere)

Le Boursier de Coudray (1760). *Abrege de l'art des Accouchements*. (Chalons-sur-Marne: Bouchard)

Nihell, E. (1760). *A Treatise on the Art of Midwifery*. (London: Morley)

Peel, J. (1976). *The Lives of the Fellows of the Royal College of Obstetricians and Gynaecologists 1929–1969.* (London: William Heinemann Medical Books Ltd.)

Sharp, J. (1671). *The Midwives Book on the Whole Art of Midwifery Discovered: Directing Child-Bearing Women how to Behave Themselves in Their Conception, Breeding and Nursing of Children.* (London: Simon Muller of the Star at the west end of St Paul's)

Stone, S. (1737). *A Complete Practice of Midwifery.* (London: Cooper)

Towler, J. and Bramall, J. (1986). *Midwives in History and Society.* (Beckenham, Kent: Croom Helm

Van Larcome, C.C. (1913). *Midwife in England,* published in New York City by The Prevention of Blindness (because ophthalmia neonatorum (babies' sore eyes) is the biggest cause of blindness)

Verderese, M. de C. (1975). *The Traditional Birth Attendant and Child Health and Family Planning: a Guide when Training and Utilization,* offset publication no. 18. (Geneva: World Health Organisation)

Wilson, A. (1984). *Childbirth in 17th and 18th century England,* University of Sussex, D. Phil. Thesis

Witkowski, G.J. (1887). *Accoucheurs et Sages Femme Célèbres,* p. 1. (Paris: Steinheil Publishers)

Witkowski, G.J. (1890). *Les Accouchments a la Cour,* pp. 127–70. (Paris: Steinheil Publishers)

Statistics – maternal mortality and perinatal mortality

'A million deaths is a statistic, a single death is a tragedy'.

Although women have been delivering babies since time immemorial and have been dying in the process, as have their babies, it seems that no attempt was made to work out any of the statistics of either maternal or infant mortality until the second half of the eighteenth century.

In 1781 Robert Bland, who was Physician-Accoucheur to the Westminster General Dispensary published the first statistical account of deliveries among the urban poor. He concluded that private patients were more likely to die from childbed fever than the poor who lived in the worst London slums (Bland, 1781). This may well have been because the more prosperous patients were more likely to have been delivered by doctors or man-midwives who might well have come either from the post-mortem room, or from other infected patients. They were also more likely to have been submitted to internal examinations and manipulations, or operative procedures.

Aveling, in his book on midwives of the eighteenth century (Aveling, 1872), pointed out that they had been properly instructed, had taken the oath and had paid fees. Aveling recommended that stillbirths should be investigated as mentioned in the Midwives' Oath, but it was a long time before this recommendation was acted on; 1958 was probably the crucial year for statistical attention to be paid to stillbirths as a result of the National Birthday Trust Perinatal Mortality Survey of that year .

In 1851 J. Roberton of Manchester confirmed the findings of Robert Bland that more women were dying in childbirth in more prosperous areas than in the less prosperous areas in the Manchester district, and in 1898 C.J. Cullingworth showed that the incidence of puerperal fever was much lower in the East End of London than in the more 'salubrious' districts of Hampstead and Islington, St James', Kensington and Chelsea (Loudon, 1986a). The phenomenon of higher mortality and more sepsis in richer areas than in poor ones has been given the name by Loudon of 'the reversed social class relationship'.

Statistics are an extremely important way of ascertaining the health of a nation. Without statistically reviewing the state of health and the work of various places where babies are delivered or cared for there is no way that doctors as a whole can tell whether what they are doing for patients is advantageous to the patients and also to the population as a whole. One of the most important sets of statistics is that concerning childbirth, not only for the country as a whole but from district to district. In these statistics must be included the number of live births, stillbirths, and first week deaths (perinatal mortality) as well as the number of babies dying before 1 year of age.

A change in total population cannot be derived from simply adding up the number of babies born and subtracting from it the number of babies and adults who die, because immigration and emigration have an important effect on populations.

Births were first registered on a national scale in England and Wales in 1837. Before this, records were kept in Parish registers; and these are a fertile source of information. It is only since 1979 that the annual general household survey has divided up to date information about childbearing as inside and outside marriage. The official registration of births followed the passing of the Births and Deaths Registration Act, 1836, which established the General Register Office and provided for the appointment of a Registrar General who in turn appoints local superintendent registrars and registrars. The Act made it a legal requirement for the registrar of births to inform himself within 42 days of any birth occurring within his district. This was done by obliging the parents or occupier of any building in which a birth took place to furnish the local registrar with such particulars about the birth as were required under the Act. These included the child's date and place of birth, and in the case of an illegitimate child the name of the mother; and the rank or profession of the father and the name and residence of the person giving the information.

There was originally no penalty for failure by the parent to register the birth, but this omission was rectified by the Births and Deaths Act of 1974. It was likely therefore that there was under-registration between 1837 and 1974.

In 1938 the Population (Statistics) Act was passed. Under this, informers were required to furnish additional particulars which were used for statistical purposes only. These included: the age of the mother at the time of birth; the date of her marriage; the number of previous children by the present husband; the number of children presently living; and the number of children by any previous husband as well as the number of children at present living.

In 1960 the Act was updated and amended so that in all cases the age of the mother had to be given as well as the age of the person who was entered in the register of births as the father of the child. If the child was not illegitimate information also had to be given about the date of the parents' marriage, whether the mother had been married before she married the father of the child, and the number of children of the mother by her present husband and by any former husband and how many of these were born alive or stillborn.

New regulations were applied in 1969. These took into account not only the mother's date of birth but the father's date of birth, if his name was entered on the register, and, for legitimate births only, the date of the parents' marriage and whether the mother had been married more than once as well as the number of previous children including live and stillbirths born by the mother to the present husband or any other husband.

By law all births, both live and still, must be notified to the District Medical Officer in England and Wales, and the Chief Administrative Medical Officer in Scotland and Northern Ireland within 36 hours of their occurrence to enable a health visitor to visit the mother and baby. This notification is done by the attendant at the birth, usually the midwife, but sometimes an obstetrician or general practitioner or, rarely, the father. Notification is not the same as registration but it is very useful, because an increasing number of health authorities in England and Wales use the information from the notifications to initiate the baby's record on a child health computer system. This is used, for instance, for organizing vaccination and immunization programmes.

In 1948 a book appeared entitled *Maternity in Great Britain* which was written by Dr D.V. Glass. This was a survey of social and economic aspects of pregnancy and childbirth, undertaken by a joint committee of the Royal College of Obstetricians and Gynaecologists and the Population Investigation Committee (Glass, 1948). This survey not only collected a great deal of information, particularly on maternal mortality, but also attempted to find out something about the quality and quantity of antenatal care that was given. It was the first of three great surveys, the other two being the National Birthday Trust surveys of 1958 and 1970 concentrating mainly on perinatal mortality.

W.C.W. Nixon was responsible that the 1958 perinatal mortality survey was carried out by the National Birthday Trust Fund. It was Sir Dougal Baird who led the way by showing that social circumstances had an enormous effect on maternal and fetal mortality. The word 'perinatal' means around the time of birth. Dougal Baird invented that name for mortality occurring as stillbirth and death within the first week (168 hours) of life.

DEFINITIONS AND RESULTS

Maternal mortality is defined as the number of women who die between early pregnancy and delivery, and in the first 42 days after the pregnancy or delivery. 'Late deaths' are those occurring more than 42 days after delivery until 1 year after delivery.

Maternal deaths in England and Wales have been examined very carefully for causation following the initiation of Reports on Confidential Enquiries into Maternal Deaths in England and Wales starting in 1952–1954. There have been tri-annual reports on maternal mortality dating from 1952. The last tri-annual report appeared in 1991 and dealt with the years 1985–1987. It reveals not only a steady drop in maternal mortality in each 3-year interval, but also that the general fertility rate (births per 1000 women aged 15–44 years) has been dropping. The biggest drop was between the years 1965 and 1977; in 1965 it was 90 births per 1000 women aged 15–44 but by 1977 it had gone down to 60 births per 1000 women. Since then it has oscillated a little. The legal abortion rate has steadily risen from 1970 when the first effects of the Abortion Act of 1967 started to be shown, until 1987 when it had risen from 8 per 1000 for the former year in women aged 15–44, to 14 per 1000 women aged 15–44 in 1987.

Stillbirth is defined in Section 41 of the Births and Deaths Registration Act 1953, as 'a child which issued forth from its mother after the 28th week of pregnancy and which has not at any time after being completely expelled from its mother, breathed or shown any other signs of life'.

Perinatal death includes all stillbirths and all babies born alive who die within the first week after birth. The word stillbirth causes some confusion because of the limitation of 28 weeks. It is known that in some cases of twin pregnancies one baby may die very early in the pregnancy and the other survive. The dead baby has to be registered as a stillbirth even though one knows that its demise occurred after only perhaps 16 or less weeks of pregnancy. This causes great anxiety to parents who have to register and bury the stillborn and often macerated fetus.

From the statistics that are collected it is possible to work out a total fertility rate, a gross reproduction rate, a net reproduction rate, and some other interesting statistical information such as the age of parents, the seasonally adjusted numbers of live births as well as figures for legitimacy and illegitimacy. Interesting information about the duration of the marriage before the delivery of the infant has also been compiled. This last figure however, is not very accurate.

Interestingly enough, multiple births arising from a single pregnancy are counted as one maternity/paternity though each child born is reckoned separately in tables relating to births; so that in tables which show the number of previous live born children multiple births are counted as if they had occurred separately as one first and one second birth. Figures have been compiled about whole areas or districts of the United Kingdom. These, of course, vary if there is an institution such as one of the large London teaching hospitals that receives large numbers of patients from all over the country and from abroad. Information is also given of the various types of the places of confinement such as National Health Service hospitals with an obstetric section, or hospitals such as Queen Charlotte's Hospital, London that practise entirely consultant obstetrics.

Information is also obtained about the birthplace of the parents which is not necessarily the same as the ethnic origin or race of the parents.

For instance there are many children born to families resident because of Army service or colonial service, in different countries of the world, e.g. Pakistan or India, but they are not Indian or Pakistani in ethnic origin. Similarly many people who are of Pakistani or Indian ethnic origin or from other new Commonwealth countries are born in the United Kingdom.

More interesting in many ways is the social class of the father and this is found by coding the father's occupation and employment status and giving him an appropriate social class from that. Between 1975 and 1983, one in ten of all paternities were coded for social class. Broadly speaking the classes are as follows:

Class 1 – Professional occupations.

Class 2 – 'White collar' occupations of a managerial or senior administrative status.

Class 3 – N. skilled occupations – non-manual.

Class 4 – M. skilled occupations – manual.

Class 5 – Partly skilled occupations.

Class 6 – Unskilled occupations.

More important, however, is a different category, that of unsupported mothers, the fathers of whose children have abandoned them. They do have a very much higher perinatal mortality than the other groups. This was shown in the Perinatal Mortality Surveys carried out by the National Birthday Trust Fund in 1958 and 1970 (see Further Reading).

In 1838, the 1st year for which there are worthwhile figures, there were 463 797 births of which 236 941 were male and 226 846 were female. The first year for which there are statistics about legitimacy and so on, namely 1842, there were 517 739 total births of which 265 204 were male and 252 535 female and of these total births 482 943 were legitimate and 34 796 were illegitimate, showing an illegitimacy rate of 67.2 per 1000 total of all live births. There is as expected a slight preponderance of male to female births, i.e. 1050 to 1000 .

The highest figure for total births seems to have been in 1920 when there were 957 782 children born and an illegitimacy rate of only 46.9 per 1000. This of course was the first full post-World War One year. Another year with a very high number of births was 1947 with 881 026 births and that was the first full year after the end of World War Two. The figures dropped quite rapidly after the end of World War One reaching their lowest figure of non-war years in 1935 when the total births was 598 756. However, there was a still lower figure in the first full year of World War Two when they dropped to 579 091. The illegitimacy rate in 1918 was 62.6 per 1000 and it dropped considerably until 1945 when it rose to reach 93.3 per 1000. It then dropped again until 1960 when it was 54.4 per 1000 rising rapidly from 1960 so that by the last full year for which figures have recently been published, namely 1983, it had reached 157.7 per 1000 births. It is still rising so that it is estimated that in 1990 270 out of every 1000 births took place outside marriage. These statistics therefore show social trends.

Stillbirth rates given in Table 1:2 in the quoted publication of birth statistics showed a drop from 1931 to 1935, when it averaged 25 826 per year, to 1983 when it dropped very rapidly to 3631. The stillbirth rate dropping from 41 per 1000 in 1931 to 5.7 per 1000 in 1983.

Abortions are pregnancies that are 'legally' terminated under the 1967 Abortion Act. Before then, so-called 'therapeutic abortions' where the mothers health or life was in great danger had been carried out in National Health Service Hospitals only in relatively small numbers so that in 1959 there were only about 10 800 such 'therapeutic abortions' performed in the United Kingdom, compared with well over 100 000 such abortions performed yearly by the late 1980s.

Abortions have been carried out since the earliest recorded times. In 1803 inducing an abortion first became a statutory offence in England and Wales. It remained thus until the 1967 Act came into force, when abortions were allowed up to the 28th week of pregnancy until 1990 when the rules were changed to limit the circumstances in which abortions could be carried out after the 24th week of pregnancy.

Each termination of pregnancy under the 1967 Abortion Act must be notified to the respective Chief Medical Officer. From the notifications an annual volume *Abortion Statistics* is published as well as a report in OPCS monitors, series AB.

About one in five of all pregnancies terminate spontaneously in abortion, apart from those that are induced.

In 1906 the Mayor of Huddersfield offered one pound (£1.00) to mothers who notified a birth at the Town Hall if they could produce their babies alive on their first birthday. He was much surprised that he had to pay out £107 because of the 112 notified births only five babies had died.

Huddersfield immediately applied for a private Act of Parliament to make birth notifications compulsory in that town. One year later an Act of Parliament allowed all other local authorities to enforce notification of births and in 1915 it was made compulsory all over the country.

MATERNAL MORTALITY

The great expert on the history of maternal mortality in England and Wales is Dr Irvine Loudon of the Wellcome Unit of the History of Medicine in Oxford. He has written important papers on the subject, but the most authoritative is his *Deaths in Childbed from the 18th Century to 1935* (Loudon, 1986b). In the introduction to this paper on medical history Loudon states 'maternal morbidity [sic. which he certainly means as mortality] is expressed as the number of deaths per thousand births'. 'Births' meant live births until stillbirth registration was introduced in 1927; thereafter, it meant total births, i.e. live plus stillbirths. In one paper Loudon quotes William Farr in the 39th report of the Registrar General on Maternal Mortality for 1876–1878, (p. 242) 'a deep, dark and continuous stream of mortality'. It is clear that the risk of a mother dying in childbirth, particularly in the north of Britain rather than the south, remained virtually the same from 1850, and probably from 50 years earlier than that until 1935. This was demonstrated by tables in his paper showing that total maternal deaths per thousand births in 1847–1950 was 5.8 per 1000 births, of which about one-third were due to puerperal sepsis (Table 1). The figure did not decline very remarkably until in 1936–1940 it dropped to 3.24 per 1000 of which again one-third were due to puerperal sepsis; then suddenly in 1946–1950 it lowered to 1.09 per 1000 births, with only 15% due to puerperal sepsis. This dramatic drop continued in the following years so that in 1976–1980 it had gone down to 12 per 100 000 births, which is 0.12 per 1000 births. By 1987 the figure had dropped to 7.6 per 100 000 births which, incidentally, for women aged between 24 and 25 is lower than their mortality would be if they were not pregnant and delivering during that year! This is because of the special attention given to women in antenatal care and the extra care they take of themselves when pregnant with the avoidance of risk activities such as mountain climbing or motor cycling.

The Midwives Act of 1936 charged every county-borough-council to provide an adequately salaried domiciliary midwifery service, directly or

Table 1 Maternal mortality 1847–1980 (deaths/1000 births) in England and Wales

Five-year period	Annual mortality averages		
	Puerperal sepsis	Accidents of childbirth*	Total
(1847–50)	1.9	3.9	5.8
1851–55	1.5	3.4	4.9
1856–60	1.5	3.0	4.5
1861–65	1.6	3.2	4.8
1866–70	1.5	3.1	4.6
1871–75	2.4	3.0	5.4
1876–80	1.7	2.2	3.9
1881–85	2.8	2.1	4.9
1886–90	2.4	2.1	4.5
1891–95	2.5	2.9	5.4
1896–1900	2.0	2.6	4.6
1901–05	1.9	2.3	4.2
1906–10	1.6	2.2	3.8
1911–15	1.5	2.3	3.8
1916–20	1.6	2.3	3.9
1921–25	1.5	2.2	3.7
1926–30	1.8	2.2	4.0
1931–35	1.6	2.7	4.3
1936–40	0.77	2.47	3.24
1941–45	0.36	1.90	2.26
1946–50	0.14	0.95	1.09
1951–55	0.098	0.60	0.70
1956–60	0.06	0.37	0.43
1961–65	0.04	0.28	0.32
1966–70			0.27
1971–75			0.13
1976–80			0.12

*The term 'accidents of childbirth' was used to cover all causes of maternal mortality apart from puerperal sepsis.
Sources: *Report of the Registrar General* and *On the State of the Public Health*; reports of the Chief Medical Officer of the Ministry of Health and Department of Health Copyright the Trustees of the Wellcome Trust and reproduced with their permission from Loudon, 1986a

through voluntary organizations (Towler and Bramall, 1986).

The Second World War between 1939 and 1945 saw an increase in the number of babies born in hospital, the proportion rising from 33% in 1937 to 45% in 1944. The birth rate peaked in 1946, the year after the end of the war. At that time there were antenatal and postnatal beds and at least two delivery rooms and a nursery and a delivery/maternity ward in each hospital. Patients were staying in hospital for 8–10 days after the delivery – the so-called 'lying-in' period (Towler and Bramall, 1986 p. 232).

By 1943 maternal mortality had fallen to half the 1935 rate and went down to 2.30 per 1000 registered births. This was considered to be due in part to antibiotic therapy, to the establishment of the flying-squad and to blood transfusion services. Perinatal mortality also went down.

It is difficult to explain why the maternal mortality was so high in the second half of the nineteenth century and first 40 years of the twentieth century in spite of the improvement in living conditions, nutrition and medical knowledge. There were no reliable estimates on maternal mortality before the late eighteenth century.

One doctor who seems to have had a great effect on reducing maternal mortality was Dr Andrew Topping, the medical officer of health for Rochdale between 1930 and 1932. In those 3 years he reduced the average maternal mortality rate in Rochdale from 9 per 1000 to 3 per 1000 possibly by insisting on better use of asepsis and antisepsis.

It is certainly true that there were very large variations in maternal mortality from district to district. With Halifax, Blackpool and Rochdale having very high figures and Westham and Eastham as well as Worcester having very low figures. There is an excellent survey of the deaths and maternal welfare in England and Wales between the wars by Enid Fox (Fox, 1991). She gives a large number of references quoting extensively from Loudon's writings as well as from earlier surveys, and includes the experimental work carried out by Lady Juliet Rhys-Williams on nutrition in the Rhondda Valley.

It was William Farr in his appendices to the Annual Reports of the Registrar General in the 1870s who stated repeatedly that the level of maternal mortality in England and Wales was far too high and that many puerperal deaths were avoidable. It was not however, until 1924 when Dr Janet Campbell, the medical officer in charge of maternal and child welfare, started serious enquiries into maternal mortality that things started to improve. A maternal mortality committee under the chairmanship of Sir George Newman, the Minister of Health and the Chief Medical Officer in 1929 called for a national maternity service in which a midwife or maternity nurse was to be present at every delivery; and it asked, as well, for a full medical follow-up service.

Sir George Newman was committed to strengthening the health services centred upon local authorities (Fox, 1991). The Maternal Mortality Committee examined 5805 maternal deaths occurring between November 1928 and July 1932 and came to the conclusion that many deaths were avoidable so that the maternal mortality rate could be halved.

In 1929 the British Medical Association seemed to want to centre maternity services on general practitioners rather than on local health authority departments and a *British Medical Journal* supplement of 1935, recommended this. Maternal mortality was dropping at this time due to the advent of sulphonamides and later antibiotics. Dr Zarrina Kurtz, (Kurtz, 1991) has traced the history of ill health in infancy and childhood from the sixteenth century onwards . . . By the middle of the nineteenth century one-third of the children still died before the end of childhood, so survival was the key concern. During the twentieth century death rates have fallen considerably, probably due to better social and environmental conditions and the reduction in the incidence and sequelae of infectious diseases. There is still a marked difference in the statistics for the disadvantaged social classes 4 and 5. Higher social class women are having babies later, and they are having fewer, and therefore proportionately more are surviving. There were no reliable estimates on maternal mortality before 1847. Sudden infant death syndrome is a very important cause of mortality.

Dr A.H. Rinsler has kindly made available the figures for the causes of maternal mortality for England, Wales and Scotland in the year 1877. These are as shown in Table 2.

Dr Irvine Loudon, who very kindly extracted figures from the Parliamentary Papers in the basement of the Radcliffe Camera in Oxford, has estimated the population of Great Britain in 1870 to be: 21 869 607 in England and Wales (1869), 3 222 837 in Scotland (1870) (giving a total for Great Britain of 25 092 444), and 5 416 170 in Ireland (1870) giving a total for the United Kingdom of 30 508 614.

The figures that have been given in this chapter are those for the United Kingdom, but similar figures apply throughout the Western World and in most developed countries, although even in Europe there are differences. The perinatal mortality rate in Portugal at about 15 per 1000 total births is double that in Germany which has about the lowest rate in Europe. In the developing world however the figures are vastly different; and in the 1990s reflect what the situation may have been like in Europe 500 years ago. In Pakistan in 1980 it was known, in spite of poor keeping of records, that only about half of all babies born in that country were alive by the age of 1 year – some being stillborn and many others dying within the first week or months after delivery.

The statistics given by Dr Sheldon Segal for maternal mortality throughout the world in 1985 in a lecture which won him the Axel–Munthe Prize, demonstrated that in Northern Europe one mother died in every 9500 deliveries and in North America one in every 6344. In the Caribbean one in 740 deliveries resulted in maternal death, in Latin America one in 75 deliveries, in Asia one in 54 deliveries and in Africa one in 21 deliveries. In the developed world there is a one in 4000 to one in 10 000 chance in a lifetime of a woman dying of a pregnancy-related cause, whereas in the undeveloped world the relative risks are one in 15 to

Table 2 Causes of death in relation to childbirth, 1877; these figures are derived from the Registrar General's Annual Report

Childbirth	475
Miscarriage	85
Abortion	41
Puerperal mania	92
Convulsions*	359
Extrauterine fetation	21
Caesarean operation	1
Placenta praevia	237
Retention of placenta	52
Flooding**	469
Rupture of uterus	28
Phlegmasia dolens***	105
Breast abscess	11
Deformed pelvis	23
Total	1999
Puerperal fever	1444

Total births in 1877 = 888 200 (451 896 male; 436 304 female)
Maternal mortality rate per 1000 live births = 2.25 excluding puerperal fever
Maternal mortality rate per 1000 live births = 1.60 for puerperal fever
Total maternal mortality rate per 1000 live births = 3.8
* Toxaemia
** Postpartum haemorrhage
*** Deep femoral vein thrombosis (Phlegmasia alba dolens = white leg)

one in 50 (Royston and Armstrong, 1989). The causes, according to Dr Sheldon, in these countries with such a high maternal mortality and enormous perinatal mortality were poor socioeconomic development, excessive fertility, high-risk pregnancy and inadequate care. A woman having her eighth or subsequent baby had in 1987 more than four times the chance of dying, than during, or soon after delivering her first or second baby. Medical care together with adequate nutrition, warmth and spacing of children within the family, all contributed throughout the centuries in the West, to lowering maternal and perinatal mortality.

Dr Irvine Loudon has analysed the effects of obstetric care and social class on maternal mortality, and in another important paper in December 1992 described how maternal mortality dropped between 1920 and 1960. He has produced very interesting figures for maternal mortality in different countries of the Western world. In 1920 it was highest in the United States at 689 per 100 000 live births and lowest in Denmark with 235 deaths per 100 000 births. By 1980 the figures for all Western countries had dropped to fewer than nine deaths per 100 000 births.

CHRONOLOGY

1836	Births and Deaths Registration Act making it a legal requirement to register all births and deaths with the Registrar General.
1919	Illegitimacy rate was 62.6 per 1000 total births.
1924	Dr Janet Campbell initiated great improvements.
1938	The Population (Statistics) Act was passed giving more details about women and their fertility.
1946–1950	Sudden lowering of maternal mortality from a fairly constant figure of 5.8 per 1000 births to 1.09 per 1000 births. Again further lowering in the years 1976–1980 to 0.12 per 1000 births.
1946, 1958 and 1970	Nationwide surveys were carried out to try to pinpoint the causes of maternal and perinatal death.
1953	In a new Births and Deaths Registration Act definitions were given.
1974	The Births and Deaths Act was passed to close loopholes in previous legislation.

1990	Illegitimacy rate was 270 per 1000 total births.

REFERENCES

Aveling, J.H. (1872). *English Midwives*. (London)

Bland, R. (1781). Midwifery Report at the Westminster General Dispensary. *Philos. Trans.*, **71**, 355–71

Fox, E. (1991). Powers of life and death: aspects of maternal welfare in England and Wales between the wars. *Medical History*, **35**, 328–52

Glass, D.V. (1948). *Maternity in Great Britain*. (London: Oxford University Press)

Kurtz, Z. (1991). Do we value our children? *J. R. Soc. Med.*, **84**, 509

Loudon, I. (1986a). Obstetrics care, social class, and maternal mortality. *Br. Med. J.*, **293**, 606

Loudon, I. (1986b). Deaths in childbed from the 18th century to 1935. *Medical History*, **30**, 1–41

Loudon, I. (1992). The transformation of maternal mortality. *Br. Med. J.*, **305**, 1557–60

Roberton, J. (1851). *Essays and Notes on the Physiology and Diseases of Women and on Practical Midwifery*. (London: John Churchill)

Royston, E. and Armstrong, S. (1989). *Preventing Maternal Death* (Geneva: WHO)

Towler, J. and Bramall, J. (1986). *Midwives in History and Society*. (Beckenham, Kent: Croom Helm)

Stillbirth references

Births and Deaths Registration Act Section 41 (1953) (London: HMSO)

Extracts from the Proceedings of the General Assembly of the International federation of Gynaecology and Obstetrics Mexico City, 1976.

(1976). *Int. J. Gynaecology Obstet.*, **14**, 570–6

Birth statistics

(1987). Historical Series Statistics from the Registrations of Births in England and Wales 1837–1983. (London: HMSO or the Office of Population Censuses & Surveys)

FURTHER READING

Barnes, R. (1886). *Lectures on Obstetric Operations.* (London: J. & A. Churchill)

Bickerton, T.H. (1936). *A Medical History of Liverpool from the Earliest days to the year 1920.* (London)

Butler, N.R. and Bonham, D.G. (1963). *Perinatal Mortality.* (Edinburgh: E. & S. Livingston Ltd.)

Butler, N.R. and Alberman, E.D. (1969). *Perinatal Problems.* (Edinburgh: E. & S. Livingston Ltd.)

Campbell, Dame J., Cameron, I.D. and Jones, D.M. (1932). *High maternal mortality in certain areas, Reports on public health and medical subjects,* No. 68, Ministry of Health

Chamberlain, G. (1992). *ABC of Antenatal Care.* (London: BMJ)

Chamberlain, G., Philipp, E.E., Howlett, E. and Masters, K. (1978). *British Births 1970.* (London: Heinemann)

Chamberlain, R., Chamberlain, G., Howlett, E. and Claireau, A. (1975). *British Births 1970,* Vol. 1. (London: Heinemann)

Cullingworth, C.J. (1898). On the undiminished mortality from puerperal fever in England and Wales. *Trans. Obstet. Soc. London,* **40,** 91–114

Douglas, C.E. (1924). Some observations on seventy years of country midwifery practice. *J. Obstet. Gynaecol. Br. Emp.,* **31,** 622–46

Dudfield, R. (1924). A survey of the mortality due to childbearing in London from the seventeenth century. *Proc. R. Soc. Med. (section of epidemiology and state medicine),* **17,** 59–72

Fairbairn, J.S. (1931). The medical and psychological aspects of gynaecology. *Lancet,* **2,** 999–1004

Joint Committee of the Royal College of Obstetricians and Gynaecologists and the Population Investigation Committee (1948). *Maternity in Great Britain.* (London: Oxford University Press)

Kerr, J.M. (1933). *Maternal Mortality and Morbidity.* (Edinburgh: E. & S. Livingston)

Kinloch, J., Smith, J.P. and Stephen, J.A. (1928). *Maternal Mortality in Aberdeen 1918–1927 with special reference to puerperal sepsis.* (Edinburgh: Scottish Board of Health, HMSO)

Miller, A. (1899). Twenty years' obstetric practice. *Glasgow Med. J.,* **51,** 216–27

Ministry of Health (1932). *Report on the Departmental Committee on Maternal Mortality and Maternal Morbidity.* (London: HMSO)

Oxley, W.H.F., Phillips, M.H. and Young, J. (1935). Maternal mortality in Rochdale, an experiment in a black area. *Br. Med. J.,* **1,** 304–7

Roberton, J. (1851). *Essays and Notes on the Physiology and Diseases of Women,* pp. 434–7. (London)

Topping, A. (1936). Maternal mortality and public opinion. *Public Health,* **49,** 342–9

Williams, W., (1904). *Deaths in Childbed,* being the Milroy Lectures delivered at the Royal College of Physicians of London. (London: H.K. Lewis)

The breast

In most of the countries of the continent of Europe gynaecologists treat breast conditions including those that require surgery; whereas in the United Kingdom surgery of the breast has been the province of general surgeons. That is why only a very short survey of the history of the breast and its diseases is given in this book.

Human breasts are situated much higher in the body than those of other mammals, whose breasts tend to lie in front of their abdomens rather than their chests. The reason for this is said to be so that breastfeeding women can better kiss, hug, talk to and caress their babies.

The female breasts have been illustrated in rock drawings and in paintings from the earliest possible times. They have been proudly displayed in drawings and paintings and statues for more than the past 2000 years. The prophet Mohammed said 'a wife's breast will nourish the infant and rejoice the father'.

In 1787 a certain Mr Emmanuel wrote 'a gallant madrigal to his wife who was breastfeeding her child'.

Very loosely translated his little doggerel verse said:

> 'Reveal dear wife and mother
> this breast that we must share
> Nature has there placed two buds
> one for the father and one for the heir.'

It is recounted that Louis XIII used a small pincers to draw from her cleavage notes written to him by his mistress Mlle de Hautfort, and Louis XVIII, who was less gallant, used his mistress' cleavage as a snuff box!

There have been different phases in history when the popularity of breastfeeding waxed and waned. As recently as the nineteenth century, upper class ladies thought it was beneath their dignity to breastfeed and employed, 'wet-nurses' who nourished their babies for them. Later came 'formulas' which added and subtracted various substances from cow's milk to make it more digestible for newborn infants.

Jean-Jaques Rousseau (1712–1778) described a Countess who had nipples not long enough to allow her infant to suckle, and so had artificial nipples made to cover her own natural ones. He also described a woman whose breasts were of markedly unequal size. The purpose of the artificial nipple was not only to make breastfeeding easier, but to protect the wet nurse from any risk of catching syphilis from the child that she was feeding. The first ones were made like wooden cups with teats made of cork for which rubber was later substituted (Figure 1).

Deneux who was obstetrician to the Duchess of Berry, had teats made of silver, beautifully engraved with such subjects as the wolf feeding

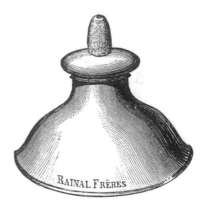

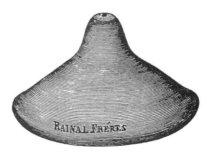

Figure 1 Artificial nipples (*see* text). The top nipple was made of wood with a cork teat, the lower, a nipple made of rubber

Remus and Romulus, and another of a baby suckling from a nanny-goat, and a third showing a pelican, the symbol of maternal love (Witkowski, 1898).

Supernumerary nipples and breasts were described as early as 1675 by Georges Hannaeus; and Witkowski in his book *Histoire des Accouchements Chez Tous les Peuples*, illustrated a woman breastfeeding two of her children, one from her breast in the normal position, and the other from a breast on the lateral aspect of her left thigh four thumb-breadths below the great trochanter (Figure 2).

THE BREAST IN PREGNANCY

Credit goes to W.F. Montgomery, Professor of Midwifery in the King and Queens College of Physicians in Ireland, for beautiful illustrations of the changes in the breasts during pregnancy. His book entitled *An exposition of the signs and symptoms of pregnancy, the period of human gestation, and the signs of delivery* (Montgomery, 1837) is beautifully illustrated and contains eight plates illustrating

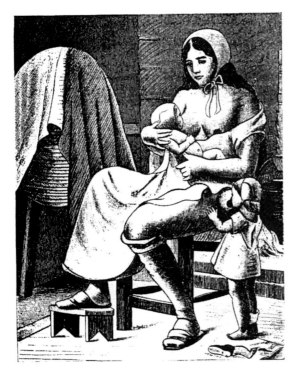

Figure 2 Woman breast-feeding two infants (Witkowski). Note: the supernumery breast is more likely to be on the inside of the thigh (*see* text)

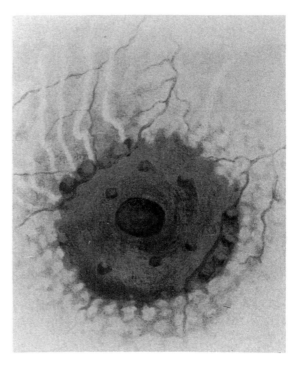

Figure 3 One of Montgomery's illustrations of the changes occurring in the breast during pregnancy

the changes in the areola of the breast month by month from the 3rd month onwards in pregnancy (Figure 3). He speaks about 'mammary sympathies' and he pointed out that there were differences of opinion between Denman (q.v. in Biographies) who did not believe that the changes in the areola occurred only in pregnancy, and Smellie (q.v. in Biographies) and William Hunter (q.v. in Biographies) who did, as did Montgomery himself.

The name of Montgomery has gone down in history because the tubercles that develop in the areola are named Montgomery's tubercles.

CANCER OF THE BREAST

The Edwin Smith Papyrus (q.v.), translated by J.H. Breasted, pointed out that it was useless to try to treat a woman with bulging tumours spreading over her breast, and Hippocrates in 400 BC wrote 'It is better to give no treatment in cases of hidden cancer. Treatment causes speedy death'.

Celsus in the first century tried to describe, classify and stage carcinoma of the breast, and he thought some treatment could be useful in early malignancy.

Galen, who followed Hippocrates' humoral theories of disease, thought cancer was related to the accumulation of black bile that coagulated in the breast. In the Renaissance Ambroise Paré (1510–1590) advised women against gossip in order to avoid suffering from cancer of the breast. He apparently operated on cancer of the breast and advised ligatures to staunch surgical bleeding (Baum, 1986).

Gabrielle Falloppio (1523–1562), who was the Professor of Anatomy at Padua, thought abscesses of the breast were a blend of blood and melancholic humours. He was the first to describe pectoral fixation in advanced cancer of the breast.

Thomas Bartholin (1616–1680) first described the lymphatic system in 1652. It was in his century and the next that the humoral theory of the disease started to wane.

Rembrandt, famous for 'The Anatomy Lesson' showing Dr Tulp dissecting a body, also painted a portrait of his mistress Hendrickje Stoffles as 'Bathsheba at her toilet'. There is a dimple in the upper quadrant of her left breast which may presage the cancer from which she died some years after the painting was made.

John Hunter (1728–1793) favoured the coagulated lymph theory as a preliminary to cancer. It was probably William Cheselden (1688–1752) of St George's Hospital in London, who first advocated lumpectomy rather than removal of the whole breast (de Moulin, 1983).

Radical surgery of the breast has been practised for a very long time and for a variety of reasons. The Amazons in Greek mythology were known as women warriors. The Amazon river is named after warrior women because in the sixteenth century, the Spanish explorer Francisco de Orellana said he had battled with fighting women in South America on the Maranon River, which he renamed after the fighting women 'The Amazon'.

Even if they were only mythical beings, it is reported that the original Amazons were the first to remove a breast surgically; and Hippocrates said some tribes burned their daughters' right breasts with hot irons, so that 'all vigour would flow into the right arm and shoulder'.

The early Romans performed extensive surgery for carcinoma of the breast, including removal of the pectoral muscles; but Celsus (25 BC – AD 50) advised against medicines, caustics, cautery and excision. It may be that Galen was the first to liken the appearance of a cancer to that of a crab, and it is said that he excised breast tumours widely, cutting through healthy tissue surrounding them.

Albucasis (936–1013) an Arabic surgeon, produced the first illustrated treatise on cautery; but he knew of no case of cancer of the breast that had been cured by cautery (Donegan, 1988).

Astley Paston Cooper (1768–1841) in about 1829, wrote a wonderful book *The Anatomy and Diseases of the Breast* which was published after his death in 1845. He described for the first time the suspensory ligaments that extend from the deeper breast tissue to the inner side of the skin. He dissected the breast to show the various ducts and lobules as well as illustrating the human nipple (Cooper, 1845).

James Syme (1799–1870) was a very eminent Scottish surgeon, who later practised at University College Hospital London for a short time, where he managed to quarrel with several of his colleagues. He is said to have performed a mastectomy in 1830 without any form of anaesthesia. Syme was the first to associate involved axillary nodes with a poor prognosis, because in 1842 he wrote that when the glands were involved, even if they were removed, the results tended to be poor.

It is interesting for gynaecological historians that Syme managed to quarrel with his opposite number in gynaecology, James Y. Simpson. Yet when Simpson himself developed an axillary abscess which could have proved fatal, Mrs Simpson insisted that it should be Syme to operate on it, and this he did successfully.

Radical mastectomy

The idea of carrying out radical removal of the breast may have derived from the teachings of Jean Louis Petit (1674–1750) who was director of the French Academy of Surgery and a Foreign Fellow of the Royal Society, a very great surgeon. He wrote 'the roots of a cancer were the enlarged lymph nodes . . . the glands should be looked for and removed, and the pectoral fascia and even some fibres and muscle should also be removed'. The name of W.S. Halsted of Johns Hopkins University in Baltimore (1895), is irrevocably associated with the radical operation; but he had been preceded in performing this operation by Pancoast, and by Samuel W. Gross, both of Philadelphia (Halsted, 1895). It has to be said that American surgery was inspired by German surgery. In the seventeenth century Bidloo performed the operation of mastectomy 20 times in the year 1679 and Henri le Dran (1656–1720) carried out a great number of mastectomies, of which many

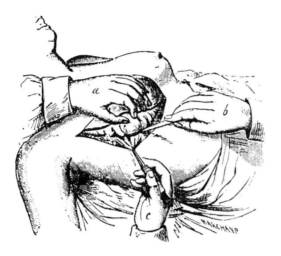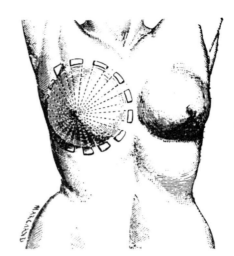

Figure 4 Illustrations of the removal of a breast using a scalpel (left), by cauterizing it with applications of zinc chloride mixed with wheat (right) (A. Guerin), eighteenth century

operations were met with success (Figure 4). C.H. Moore of the Middlesex Hospital (1867) was doing radical operations, and the two Handleys, father and son, carried on the tradition of radical surgery at that hospital for another 80 years. Of the son R.S. Handley (Dick Handley) it is said that he used to recount that visitors said that it was surprising that Mr Handley the surgeon, should have been writing on the same subject for 80 years!

Removal of a breast using a scalpel is illustrated in Figure 4.

THE PRESENT DAY

In the 1970s and 1980s there have been two marked changes. Whereas in earlier years it was women of the lower social classes who out of necessity breastfed their children, and women of the higher social classes who could afford and did have wet nurses for their children, and later formula feeds, in the 1970s there was a switch so that it was the less advantaged women who did not breastfeed or stopped very early, in some cases because of the need to go out to work, whereas women of better means were able to breastfeed. The other great change was the move away from radical surgery of the Halsted type, to much less destructive surgery named 'lumpectomy'. This was nearly always accompanied by exploration and clearance of the axillary nodes, both from the point of view of making a prognosis and possibly effecting a cure.

The other great advance was in reconstructive

surgery to replace the removed breast tissue. Perel wrote a history of the reconstruction of the breast after its removal for cancer in which he gave credit to Professor Louis Ombredanne (1871–1956) for using the pectoralis minor muscle to reconstruct a semblance of a breast in 1905 at the Hôpital Saint Louis in Paris. Ombredanne is supposed to have carried out the procedure at the conclusion of the operation for the removal of a breast and axilliary clearance for cancer.

REFERENCES

Baum, M. (1986). The history of breast cancer In Forbes, J.F. (ed.) *Breast Disease*, pp. 95–105. (Edinburgh: Churchill Livingston)

Cooper, A.P. (1845). *Anatomy and Diseases of the Breast*. (London: Longmans)

de Moulin, D. (1983). *A Short History of Cancer*. (Boston, The Hague, Lancaster: Martinus Neijhoff Publications)

Donegan, W.L. (1988). *Cancer of the Breast*. (Philadelphia, London, Toronto: W.B. Saunders Co.)

Halsted, W.S. (1895). The results of operations for the cure of cancer of the breast performed at the Johns Hospital from June 1889 to January 1894. *Johns Hopkins Rep.*, **4**, 297 (54 pp. with 6 plates)

Montgomery, W.F. (1837). *An Exposition of the Signs and Symptoms of Pregnancy*. (London: Sherwood, Gilbert & Piper)

Witkowski, G-J. (1898). *Tetoniana*, pp. 10–11. (Paris: A. Maloine)

Paediatrics

INTRODUCTION

Paediatrics is a modern specialty which has evolved from medicine, obstetrics and midwifery, starting in the mid-nineteenth century.

In the ancient world the Egyptian Papyri were a valuable source of medical information and the 'Lesser Berlin Papyrus' contained the ritual incantations which were used for sick children. Common children's ailments were noted by the Greek Hippocratic writers. Soranus of Ephesus of the second century AD, who made such an enormous contribution to obstetrics, also wrote on childrens' diseases and child care. In the twelfth century an anonymous Latin manuscript *The Childrens Practice* was an important medieval text. The first printed book on children's disease was written by Paulus Bagellardus and was published in 1472. The first book in English to deal exclusively with paediatric illness was the *Boke of Children* and was a translation by Thomas Phare in 1545 of an earlier French work. In the seventeenth century Thomas Sydenham identified measles and his contemporaries Donald Whistler and Frances Goisson identified the clinical characteristics of rickets.

William Harvey (1578–1657) (q.v. in Biographies), a physician, obstetrician, and fetal physiologist, first described the circulation of the blood in his *On the Motion of the Heart and Blood in Animals* in 1628. He wrote *On the Generation of Animals* in 1651 and also an essay on *Parturition*, the first original work on midwifery. He introduced the experimental and observational approach and wrote about the fetal circulation and placenta, the independent life of the fetus, the nature of respiration, and fetal suckling (Dunn, 1990a). In the eighteenth and nineteenth centuries, perinatal and infant mortality were very high. This led William Cadogan to write *an Essay upon Nursing and the Management of Children from their Birth Through Three Years of Age* in 1750. In this treatise, Cadogan supported breastfeeding and gave advice on cleanliness, diet and clothing. The London Foundling Hospital was opened in 1745 and the first infant poor dispensary opened there 24 years later. The next children's dispensary was opened by John Bunnell Davison in 1816 and in the following year he published his *Cursory Enquiry into Some of the Principle Causes of Mortality among Children.* He trained volunteers to assist and counsel new mothers.

In Europe, Nicholas Andry, Jan C. des Essartez and Jan J. Rousseau published texts on childhood disease and development. In 1784 Michael Underwood, a London physician who specialized in obstetrics, gynaecology, and children's diseases, wrote his Treatise on the diseases of children and described malignant familial jaundice of the newborn and congenital heart disease. In 1828 Charles-Michel Billard correlated autopsy findings with clinical descriptions of children's diseases.

During the nineteenth century the gentle art of breastfeeding came under attack. Infants were fed animal milk, and various formulated milks. Enteritis frequently occurred and mortality rates escalated sharply. In Europe and the New World 'sanitary visitors' were recruited to instruct mothers in cleanliness and in the newer methods of feeding. Milk stations were set up to provide clean, disease-free milk for baby feeding. Formal organizations which promoted child hygiene and welfare were instituted in the early twentieth century.

In France Adolph Pinard began a 'Maternal Dispensary' in 1890 and this idea was soon copied in the UK and America. The United States Childrens Bureau published a pamphlet on prenatal care in 1913, and by 1935 one-third of all babies born in the USA were delivered in hospital. By 1956, 95% of women were delivered in hospital, with physicians attending in 97% of cases. In the UK during the early 1940s, 75% of British mothers had received antenatal care (Cone, 1979; McGrew, 1985).

EVOLUTION OF NEONATOLOGY

The French physician Charles-Michel Billard (1800–1832) was one of the pioneers of neonatal medicine. During 1826 he worked at the Hospice des Enfants in Paris, and 2 years later wrote a book on his experiences, which was the first systematic clinical pathological text on newborn infants (Dunn, 1990b). Billard advocated the use of postmortem examinations and among other subjects wrote on polyhydramnios, jaundice and kernicterus, and the establishment of respiration.

In 1872 Alexandre Gueniot was the first to diagnose prematurity as 'not over 2300 g and may be below 1500 g'. Nikolay F. Miller (1847–1897) of Moscow increased the upper weight limit to 2500 g in the 1880s and that figure was eventually adopted by the World Health Organization in 1950 (Dunham 1957).

The further development of neonatal paediatrics was due in part to the research of the nineteenth century French physicians Etienne Tarnier and Budin, and Germany's Finkelstein and Leo Langstein (Dunham, 1957). Tarnier (1885) first employed incubators for the nursing care of premature and sick newborn infants at the Paris Maternity Hospital in 1880 (Figure 1). August Ritter von Reuss became the first 'neonatal paediatrician' when he was appointed to the directorship of the newborn department at the University Women's Clinic in Vienna in 1911 (Dunn, 1990c). His book *Diseases of the Newborn* was published in Germany in 1914 and was translated into English 7 years later.

Budin outlined the special care needs of premature infants when he wrote that 'with weaklings we shall have to consider three points: (a) their temperature and their chilling, (b) their feeding,

(c) the diseases to which they are susceptible'. In America the Rotch incubator was introduced in 1903 and Hess designed his water-jacketed incubator in 1914. Julius H. Hess (1922) of Chicago (1876–1955) wrote his *Premature and Congenitally Diseased Infants* – the first book which dealt solely with those problems. Stewart H. Clifford (1936) showed that although the infant mortality rate had declined, the infant death rate within the first 2 weeks of life had remained at 30 per 1000 during the period 1910–1934. It became obvious that the major cause of death in the 1st year of life was prematurity, which was responsible for over 40% of early deaths in 1946.

In the UK the first full time neonatologist was appointed in 1959. Modern neonatology began in the 1960s, at a time when umbilical catheterization was first introduced, and when safe management of oxygen therapy was instituted.

RESUSCITATION OF THE NEWBORN

Mouth to mouth insufflation (Figure 2) was used by the prophet Elisha in the Old Testament. More interesting methods were employed by William Smellie in the eighteenth century when he rubbed the 'slow to respond' infant's nose with onions and 'smacked it well', in an effort to make it cry. Inflating the intestine with tobacco smoke via an enema tube was also advocated at that time. In the nineteenth century Schultze described swinging the baby above his head and causing it to jack-knife so as to compress its chest. Other methods

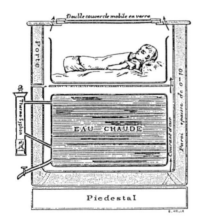 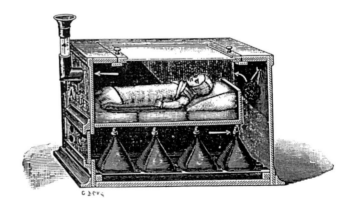

Figure 1 Tarnier's incubator. The left illustration shows that the cover was made of two layers of glass; the walls were made of layers of wood with sawdust between as an insulating material, and heat was provided by hot water circulating underneath the cot. The right illustration is cut vertically to show the construction of the incubator and how warm air circulated through it

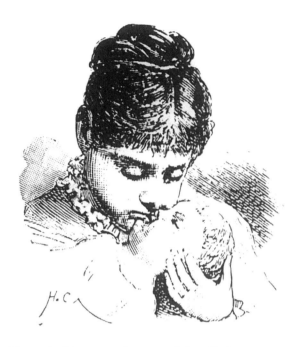

Figure 2 Direct mouth-to-mouth insufflation

included subcutaneous injection of Irish whiskey mixed with tincture of belladona or, failing that, the application of brandy to the baby's gums.

Donald (1974) quoted the words of Buist from 1885, 'standing in a space cleared in the midst of a small room, whose other denizens were withdrawn into the corners, my feet planted well apart and arms extended I taught the neonatus to perform a series of grand circles, while the meconium distributed itself in trajectories for which the room and its inmates, including the physicians, formed a comprehensive recording surface'. Contrast that with the words of James Blundell (1834) 'never hastily despair of the means of resuscitation. Many a fetus is laid aside as dead which, by diligent use of resuscitants, might have been saved . . . In performing artificial respiration on newborn children, I have frequently observed, that while the respiration was continued, the cord pulsated, ceasing to beat in a few seconds, when the operation was suspended . . . when the fetus is stillborn, the artificial respiration should be diligently tried . . . by means of a small instrument, the tracheal pipe, which I think every accoucheur should carry along with him to a labour'. Blundell went on to describe a tracheal catheter which was a small silver tube. He slid his finger over the baby's tongue and directed the tube along his finger. In this way he directed the instrument into the baby's trachea

and then inflated the infant's lungs with his own breath (Figure 3).

Blundell's treatment was echoed by Gibberd and Blaikley (1935). They described in detail the method of introduction of a laryngoscope, suction to clear the airways, and application of oxygen via an endotracheal tube with manometric pressure limited to 35 cms of water. Various drugs including lobeline, nikethamide, vanillic acid, diethylamide, adrenaline, naloxone, nalorphine, and tromethamine or sodium bicarbonate were used.

THE APGAR SCORE

Virginia Apgar (1953) introduced a new method for evaluation of the newborn infant. She evolved a scoring system of two points each for respiratory effort, reflex irritability, muscle tone, heart rate, and colour. A baby with 10 points was in the best possible condition. This quantitative assessment of the newborn provided a simple method to evaluate the infant at birth. The score was recorded at 1- and 5-minute intervals, and 15 minutes after a Caesarean operation. The first score indicated the need for active resuscitation while the second was shown to have some correlation with subsequent brain damage.

POSTMORTEM

Infants who died from hypoxia were subject to postmortem and found to have capillary haemorrhages which were likely to occur throughout the body. The petechiae seen on the liver, lungs, suprarenals and heart muscle were termed

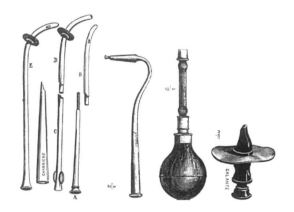

Figure 3 A variety of French insufflators used in resuscitation of the newborn

197

'Tardieu's spots'. A French physician who was born and died in Paris, A.A. Tardieu (1818–1879) investigated postmortem changes relevant to various occupations, and also showed interest in medico-legal affairs.

CONTINUOUS POSITIVE AIRWAYS PRESSURE

Ventilation of the lung fields with expansion during expiration was described by Hoerder (1909). The insufflating pressure was regulated by a water valve.Engelmann's (1911) method of insufflation differed in that an endotracheal catheter was not used. A mask was applied to the infant's face and insufflating pressure was modulated by a ball valve and water chamber. August Ritter von Reuss of Vienna (1921) in his *Diseases of the Newborn* wrote about continuous positive airways pressure (CPAP). With this technique positive pressure not exceeding 8 cm H_2O was applied continuously to the airways. This distending pressure held the alveoli open, thus preventing their collapse during expiration. Four different methods of delivering CPAP evolved – nasal, endotracheal, face mask, or by headbox (Gregory *et al.*, 1971). Various methods of ventilation for the management of respiratory failure also evolved. Herman and Reynolds (1973) suggested peak inflating pressures (PIP), while the other methods of end expiratory pressure (PEEP), and mean airway pressure (MAP) were also found useful.

RESPIRATORY DISTRESS SYNDROME

This condition was first described as a specific pathologic entity in 1953, and was referred to as Hyaline Membrane Disease. Prior to that it was diagnosed as 'congenital atelectasis' or thought to be due to aspiration of amniotic fluid. During the early 1950s the clinical and radiographic features became known and it was realized that the major predisposing factors were prematurity, birth asphyxia, and Caesarean section. Mary Ellen Avery and Jere Mead (1959) discovered that infants who died of the condition were deficient in surfactant. Inadequate surfactant levels led to decreased lung compliance, atelectasis, alveolar instability, and transudation of fluid into the alveoli. The lecithin sphingomyelin area ratio (LSAR) was determined by Louis Gluck *et al.* (1974) to be the best method of assessing fetal lung maturity and the 'shake', 'bubble' or 'foam stability test' was developed by Clements *et al.* (1972). Liggins and Howie (1972)

first suggested that antenatal glucocorticoid administration might reduce the incidence of respiratory distress syndrome. Surfactant replacement therapy began with the proposal of Alarie and Robillard (1963) who suggested treatment with inhalation of α-lecithin aerosol. Further work in the 1960s was carried out by Robillard *et al.* (1964) and Rufer (1968). Enhorning and Robertson (1972) pioneered the use of natural surfactant replacement therapy.

TRANSIENT TACHYPNOEA OF THE NEWBORN

This condition was described by Avery *et al.* (1966). The affected neonates were usually mature and often delivered by Caesarean section. The condition was characterized by a very rapid respiratory rate and chest radiographs showed fluid in the horizontal fissure with shadows radiating out from the hilum. Avery (1977) suggested that transient tachypnoea of the newborn was due to delayed clearance of pulmonary fluid.

HYPOXIC ISCHAEMIC ENCEPHALOPATHY

Serious neurological disease was indicated by a number of signs including irritability, floppiness, hyperexcitability and convulsions. With improved neonatal facilities more infants survived, despite being in poor condition at birth. Neonatal seizures were found to be the most frequent of the major manifestations of neonatal neurologic disease, and Volpe (1981) indicated that hypoxic ischaemic encephalopathy secondary to perinatal asphyxia, was the most common cause. With better methods of management the prognosis improved dramatically. Mortality rates before and after 1969 were reported as 40 and 15% respectively. Long-term neurologic sequelae were found in approximately 30% of hypoxic ischaemic encephalopathy infants.

INTRAVENTRICULAR HAEMORRHAGE

This condition occurred in approximately 40% of infants whose birth weight was below 1500 g. Ultrasound scanning was an important aid in the diagnosis of intraventricular haemorrhage and the subsequent ventricular dilatation which was likely to occur. Periventricular leukomalacia, described at pathology examination by Banker and Larroche (1962), was also detectable by ultrasound.

RETROLENTAL FIBROPLASIA

In the early 1940s aggressive oxygen therapy for infants with respiratory difficulties was begun. Soon afterwards Theodore L. Terry (1942) described the first case of retrolental fibroplasia in a 6-month-old infant who had bilateral blindness. The child was born 8 weeks prematurely and was exposed to high levels of oxygen. Terry believed that the condition was a congenital abnormality but in 1951 Dame Kate Campbell reported that excess oxygen exposure was the main cause of blindness in preterm infants (Reese, 1955). It was estimated that 12% of all premature infants with a birth weight of less than 1360 g suffered the effects of retrolental fibroplasia, which became the single largest cause of child blindness in the USA. After 1955 the inspired oxygen concentration for newborn infants was kept below 40% and the epidemic of retrolental fibroplasia was arrested.

However, Avery and Oppenheimer (1960) and Cross (1973) asserted that oxygen restriction for all premature infants was illogical and was probably responsible for many neonatal deaths and neurologic damage among survivors. Oxygen therapy was eventually rationalized with the advent of umbilical catheterization and titration of inspired oxygen against arterial oxygen tension.

HYPOTHERMIA

The induction of hypothermia for preterm infants with respiratory failure was common medical practice in the early part of this century. Day (1943) pointed out the hazard of a cold environment to the newborn, noting that infants had a large surface area in proportion to body weight, and Hill (1959) demonstrated that cooling actually increased oxygen requirements. Silverman *et al.* (1958) demonstrated (in controlled trials) that there was a higher mortality rate for premature infants nursed in cool incubators.

RADIANT HEAT

Radiant heat sources placed over open incubators were introduced by Levison *et al.* (1966). They demonstrated that radiant heat was as effective as closed heated incubators in maintaining infants' temperatures. Radiant heaters were introduced in a general way in the early 1970s. Wu and Hodgman (1974) warned against the risk of dehydration in heated, exposed infants.

FEEDING

Until 1950 human milk was the food of choice for sick infants and was administered with medicine droppers on a 1–2 hourly basis. In 1950 indwelling nasogastric polyethylene tubes were introduced and feeding via that route was a major advance in sustaining preterm infants.

ARTERIAL CATHETERIZATION

Arterial catheterization allowed access to the aorta for blood sampling of oxygen tension and other vital measurements but Goetzman *et al.* (1975) pointed out that thrombi developed quickly and frequently around the catheter tips.

NECROTIZING ENTEROCOLITIS

Necrotizing enterocolitis became a major problem in the 1970s, with a 15% incidence in infants weighing less than 1500 g. Theories on its causation at that time included the occurrence of virus infections, hypotension, apnoea, the involvement of plasticizers in catheters, and exchange blood transfusions (Harding *et al.*, 1975; Editorial, *Lancet*, 1977).

ERYTHROBLASTOSIS FETALIS

The problem of neonatal jaundice was addressed by John Burns (1817). He described obstructive jaundice and also a non-obstructive form which caused death within a few days. Despite other reports the condition was not fully understood until Diamond *et al.* (1932) first recognized that hydrops fetalis, icterus gravis, and congenital anaemia of the newborn were all due to a single condition which they termed 'erythroblastosis fetalis'.

The serologic basis for materno-fetal blood grouping compatibility was demonstrated by Philip Levine and Rufus Stetson (1939) and the rhesus system was identified by Landsteiner and Alex S. Wiener (1940). Further work by Levine *et al.* (1941) detailed the mechanism of materno-fetal blood grouping incompatibility.

The first successful exchange transfusion for 'familial icterus gravis' was carried out by Alfred P. Hart (1925). He removed blood from the anterior fontanelle while at the same time transfusing 335 ml of blood into the internal saphenous vein of the left ankle. Further work was carried out by Wiener and Wexler (1946) and Wallerstein (1946).

Diamond et al. (1951) introduced umbilical vein catheterization for exchange transfusion.

DRUGS AND KERNICTERUS

Vitamin K was introduced as a treatment modality to prevent haemorrhagic disease of the newborn in 1935. It was soon discovered that the administration of water-soluble vitamin K led to haemolytic anaemia and kernicterus. Further iatrogenic disease was caused by the sulphonamides which were introduced in the mid-1930s. Sulphonamides displaced bilirubin from plasma albumin binding sites and were responsible for an epidemic of kernicterus. (Other drugs were responsible for serious side-effects. When chloramphenicol was introduced it was found that high doses caused the 'gray' syndrome, with collapse and death of low-birth-weight infants, which had also been caused by use of a mixture of powdered ipecacuanha, opium and lactose, used to calm babies with catarrh (Dover's powder).)

PHOTOTHERAPY

Cremer *et al.* (1958) reported that improved lighting in a nursery was associated with a low incidence of jaundice. It was subsequently discovered that bilirubin was photodecomposed as it circulated through skin capillaries – this led to the introduction of phototherapy for jaundice in the newborn. Exposure of premature infants to sunlight or blue fluorescent light was effective in lesser degrees of jaundice and was apparently safe. Dacon-Vontetakis and Anagnostakis (1976) however, indicated that infants who were exposed to prolonged phototherapy showed disorders in hormonal rhythms.

FLUID REPLACEMENT

Parenteral fluid replacement was pioneered towards the end of the nineteenth century and was initially used for infants with diarrhoea. The fluid, usually a saline solution, was injected into the cellular tissue of the abdomen, buttocks, thighs or back. Non-diarrhoeal, sick infants were treated with intraperitoneal or rectal fluids. Intravenous therapy began at the end of the nineteenth century but the procedure was difficult due to the lack of cannulas at the time. By the 1920s blood transfusions had become more common. The blood was administered intraperitoneally and it was shown that red blood cells reached the thoracic lymph stream within 10 minutes of transfusion. James Sidbury (1923) first described umbilical vein cathetherization and blood transfusion in a case of haemorrhagic disease of the newborn, and this method was to become the safest route for exchange transfusion.

The peripheral veins were fragile, but those on the scalp became a common site for cannulation and the superior saggital sinus was sometimes used. The limb veins were more commonly used after the 1970s.

GRIEF

In the Old Testament, the prophet Isaiah admonished his followers to 'bind up the broken hearted' thus equating grief with a physical illness. Over the centuries people looked to their religious leaders, families and friends, to help them cope with the loss of a loved one. With the drift away from religion, and the isolation of families in built up areas away from their ancestral homes, the grief reaction became more difficult to contend with. Couples sought help and support from their family doctor, social worker or mental health worker, or tried to come to terms with their grief in isolation.

The normal grieving reaction was outlined by Eric Lindemann (1944) in a study of families who had experienced sudden death, and his findings were applicable to both perinatal death and miscarriage. At one time parents were pressurized to conceive in an effort to replace a lost child but Cain and Cain (1964) and also Rowe *et al.* (1978) found that parents who conceived too soon after their loss were at risk of morbid grief reactions.

Feelings of guilt or responsibility for the bad outcome were very common. Helmrath and Steinitz (1978) found the reaction was more intense and prolonged in women. The grief reaction following miscarriage could be as intense as that following perinatal death (Leppert and Pahlka, 1984), but little professional support was offered until recent times.

Davidson (1977) interviewed women who had experienced perinatal death. He found that mothers were vulnerable to psychological upset due to difficulty in obtaining emotional support. Other trauma occurred when those women compared their feelings with others in whom empathy was lacking. For some, the infant death retained a dream-like quality, which inhibited their emotional healing.

Various Stillbirth and Neonatal Death Societies began in the late 1970s. In many instances the organizations were founded by parents who themselves had suffered a perinatal death. As awareness of the psychological problems engendered by normal and abnormal grief reactions grew, the scientific study of perinatal death and miscarriage grief reactions became more common. In a recent editorial, Bourne and Lewis (1991a) remarked that 'attitudes to perinatal bereavement have changed profoundly in the past 25 years' and in another paper (Bourne and Lewis, 1991b) an annotated bibliography on the psychological aspects of perinatal death was published which included almost 400 recent papers.

CHRONOLOGY

c. 1500 BC	Ritual incantations for the sick child were contained in the Lesser Berlin papyrus.
c. 400 BC	The Greek Hippocratic writers described common children's diseases.
AD 200	Soranus of Ephesus wrote on child care.
12th C.	A medieval text, *The Childrens Practice*, was used.
1472	The first book on children's disease was printed.
1545	The *Boke of Children* became available in English.
1651	William Harvey wrote on the nature of fetal respiration and suckling.
1745	The London Foundling Hospital was opened.
1816	John Davison investigated the causes of mortality in children.
1828	Charles Billard correlated children's diseases with autopsy findings. Breastfeeding waned. 'Milk stations' were set up in the latter part of the century.
1890	Adolf Pinard started a Maternal Dispensary and Antenatal care began.

References for above: Cone (1979); McGrew (1985)

Neonatology

1828	Charles Billard wrote a clinico-pathological text on the newborn.
1872	Alexander Gueniot defined prematurity by weight.
1880s	Nikolay Miller introduced the 2500 g upper weight limit for prematures.
1880	Tarnier introduced incubators to neonatal care.
1911	August Ritter von Reuss became the first Neonatal Paediatrician.

References for above: Dunham (1957); Dunn (1990 a,b)

Some important events

1909	Hoerder pioneered ventilation therapy.
1923	James Sidbury described umbilical vein cathetherization.
1925	Alfred Hart carried out the first successful exchange transfusion.
1932	Diamond *et al.* introduced the term 'erythroblastosis fetalis'.
1935	Vitamin K therapy was instituted.
1942	Theodore Terry described blindness due to 'retrolental fibroplasia'.
1943	Day disputed hypothermic treatment for the preterm infant.
1953	Virginia Apgar pioneered the newborn evaluation score. Hyaline membrane disease was first described.
1958	Cremer *et al.* discovered the benefits of phototherapy.
1959	Avery and Meade discovered that hyaline membrane disease was due to deficient surfactant levels.
1966	Avery *et al.* described transient tachypnoea of the newborn. Levison *et al.* introduced radiant heat sources.
1970s	Necrotizing enterocolitis became a major problem. Intensive neonatal care began in earnest.
1972	Clements *et al.* introduced the bubble stability test.
1974	Gluck *et al.* introduced the lecithin/ sphingomyelin ratio. Liggins and Howie suggested antenatal glucocorticoid therapy.
1979	Perinatal death and grief reactions were studied. National 'Stillbirth and Neonatal Death' organizations were formed.
1980s	Neonatal care facilities increased. Smaller obstetric units closed.

1980s	Medical and nursing work became more complex.
	Surfactant therapy continued.
	Ultrasound diagnosis of intraventricular haemorrhage.
	About 5% of brain damage in infants were due to hypoxia in labour or difficult delivery.

REFERENCES

Alarie, Y. and Robillard, E. (1963). Modifications of pressure volume curves in rat lungs after inflation of surface active extracts and agents. *Physiologist*, **6**, 128

Apgar, V. (1953). A proposal for a new method of evaluation of the newborn infant. *Anesth. Analg. (Cleve.)*, **32**, 260

Avery, M.E. (1977). In Schaffer, A.J. and Avery, M.E. (eds.) *Diseases of the Newborn*, 5th edn. p. 171. (Philadelphia: W.B. Saunders)

Avery, M.E. and Mead, J. (1959). Surface properties in relation to atelectasis and hyaline membrane disease. *Am. J. Dis. Child.*, **97**, 517

Avery, M.E. and Oppenheimer, E.H. (1960). Recent increase in mortality from hyaline membrane disease. *J. Pediatr.*, **57**, 552–9

Avery, M.E., Gatewood, O.B. and Brumley, G. (1966). Transient tachypnoea of the newborn. *Am J. Dis. Child.*, **111**, 380

Banker, B.Q. and Larroche, J-C. (1962). Periventricular leukomalacia in infancy. *Arch. Neurol.*, **7**, 386–410

Blundell, J. (1834). In Castle, T. (ed.) *Principles and Practice of Obstetrics*, pp. 246–50. (London: E.Cox)

Bourne, S. and Lewis, E. (1991a). Perinatal bereavement. A milestone and some new dangers. *Br. Med. J.*, **302**, 1167–8

Bourne, S. and Lewis, E. (1991b). *Annotated Bibliography on the Psychological Aspects of Perinatal Death.* (London: Tavistock Clinic)

Burns, J. (1817). *The Principles of Midwifery: Including the Diseases of Women and Children*, p. 602. (London: Longman)

Cain, A.C. and Cain, B.S. (1964). On replacing a child. *J. Am. Acad. Child Adolesc. Psychiatr.*, **3**, 443–55

Clements, J.A., Platzker, A.C.G., Tierney, D.F., Hobel, C.J., Creasey, R.K. and Margolis, A.J. *et al.* (1972). Assessment of the risk of respiratory distress syndrome by a rapid test for surfactant in amniotic fluid. *N. Engl. J. Med.*, **286**, 1077–81

Clifford, S.W. (1936). A study of neonatal mortality. *J. Pediatr.*, **8**, 367

Cone, T.E. (1979). *History of American Pediatrics*, pp. 151–228. (Boston: Little, Brown & Co)

Cremer, R.J., Perryman, P.W. and Richards, D.H. (1958). Influence of light on the hyperbilirubinemia of infants. *Lancet*, **1**, 1094–7

Cross, K.W. (1973). Cost of preventing retrolental fibroplasia? *Lancet*, **2**, 954–6

Dacon-Vontetakis, C. and Anagnostakis, D. (1976). Phototherapy and serum L-H levels in newborns. *Abstract of paper presented at the European Society for Paediatric Research Meeting, June 1976*, (Abstract no. 21)

Davidson, G. (1977). Death of the wished-for child: a case study. *Death Education*, **1**, 265–75

Day, R. (1943). Respiratory metabolism in infancy and in childhood XXVII Regulation of body temperature of premature infants. *Am. J. Dis. Child.*, **63**, 376

Diamond, L.K., Allen, F.H. and Thomas, W.O Jr. (1951). Erythroblastosis fetalis, VII: Treatment with exchange transfusion. *N. Engl. J. Med.*, **244**, 39

Diamond, L.K., Blackfan, K.D. and Baty, J.M. (1932). Erythroblastosis fetalis and its association with universal edema of the fetus, icterus gravis neonatorum and anemia of the newborn. *J. Pediatr.*, **1**, 269

Donald, I. (1974). *Practical Obstetric Problems*, p. 627. (London: Lloyd-Luke Medical Books Ltd.)

Dunham, E.C. (1957). Evolution of premature infant care. *Ann. Paediatr. Fenniae*, **3**, 170

Dunn, P.M. (1990a). Dr. William Harvey (1578–1657). physician, obstetrician, and fetal physiologist. *Arch. Dis. Child.*, **65**, 1098–100

Dunn, P.M. (1990b). Charles-Michel Billard 1800–1832: pioneer of neonatal medicine. Perinatal lessons from the past. *Arch. Dis. Child.*, **65**, 711–12

Dunn, P.M. (1990c). Dr. von Reuss on continuous positive airway pressure in 1914. Perinatal lessons from the past *Arch. Dis. Child.*, **49**, 68

Editorial (1977). The Lords on the Court Report. *Lancet*, 1, 495

Engelmann, F. (1911). Die Sanerstoffdruckatmung sur Bekampfung des Scheintodes Neugeborener *Zentralbl. Gynäkol.*, 35, 1–13

Enhorning, G. and Robertson, B. (1972). Lung expansion in the premature rabbit fetus after tracheal deposition of surfactant. *Pediatrics*, 50, 58–64

Gibberd, G.F. and Blaikley, J.B. (1935). *Lancet*, 1, 138, quoted by Donald, I. (1974) p. 648

Gluck, L., Kulovich, M.V., Borer, R.C. and Keidal, W.N. (1974). The interpretation and significance of the L/S ratio in amniotic fluid. *Am. J. Obstet. Gynecol.*, 120, 142–55

Goetzman, B.W., Stadalnik, R.C., Bogren, H.G., Blankenship, W.J., Ikeda, R.M. and Thayer, J. (1975). Thrombotic complications of umbilical artery catheterization: a clinical and radiographic study. *Pediatrics*, 56, 374–6

Gregory, G.A., Kitterman, J.A., Phibbs, R.H., Tooley, W.H. and Hamilton, W.K. (1971). Treatment of idiopathic respiratory distress syndrome with continuous positive pressure. *N. Engl. J. Med.*, 284, 1333–40

Harding, R., Johnson, P., Johnston, B.E., McCleland, M.F. and Wilkinson, A.R. (1975). Cardiovascular changes in newborn lambs during apnoea induced by stimulation of laryngeal receptor with water. *Proc. Physiol. Soc.*, 256, 35–6

Hart, A.P. (1925). Familial icterus gravis of the newborn and its treatment. *Can. Med. Assoc. J.*, 15, 1008

Helmrath, T.A. and Steinitz, E.M. (1978). Death of an infant: parental grieving and the failure of social support. *J. Fam. Pract.*, 6, 785–90

Herman, S. and Reynolds, E.O.R. (1973). Methods for improving oxygenation in infants mechanically ventilated for severe HMD. *Arch. Dis. Child.*, 48, 612–17

Hess, J.H. (1922). *Premature and Congenitally Diseased Infants*. (Philadelphia: Lea & Febiger)

Hill, J.R. (1959). The oxygen consumption of newborn and adult mammals; its dependence on the oxygen tension in the inspired air and on the environmental temperature. *J. Physiol.*, 149, 346–73

Hoerder, C. (1909). Wesen und Bekampfungsmethoden der Asphyxia neonatorum. *Med. Klin.*, 44, 1657–61

Landsteiner, K. and Wiener, A.S. (1940). An agglutinable factor in human blood recognizable by immune sera for rhesus blood. *Proc. Soc. Exp. Biol.*, 43, 223

Leppert, P.C. and Pahlka, B.S. (1984). Grieving characteristics after spontaneous abortion: a management approach. *Obstet. Gynecol.*, 64, 119–22

Levine, P. and Stetson, R. (1939). An unusual case of infra-group agglutination. *J. Am. Med. Assoc.*, 113, 126

Levine, P., Burnham, L., Katzin, E.M. and Vogel, P. (1941). The role of isoimmunization in the pathogenesis of erythroblastosis fetalis. *Am. J. Obstet. Gynecol.*, 42, 925

Levison, H., Linsao, L. and Swyer, P.R. (1966). A comparison of infra-red and convective heating for newborn infants. *Lancet*, 2, 1346–8

Liggins, G.C. and Howie, R.N. (1972). A controlled trial of antepartum glucocorticoid treatment for prevention of the respiratory distress syndrome in premature infants. *Paediatrics*, 50, 515–25

Lindemann, E. (1944). Symptomatology and management of acute grief. *Am. J. Psychiatr.*, 101, 141–8

McGrew, R.E. (1985). *Encyclopedia of Medical History*, pp. 241–5. (London: MacMillan Press)

Reese, A.B. (1955). Editorial: an epitaph for retrolental fibroplasia. *Am. J. Ophthalmol.*, 40, 267

Robillard, E., Alarie, Y., Dagenaise-Peruse, Baril E, and Guilbeault, A. (1964). Micro-aerosol administration of synthetic dipalmitoyl lecithin in the respiratory distress syndrome: a preliminary report. *Can. Med. Assoc. J.*, 90, 55–7

Rowe, J., Clyman, R., Green, C. *et al.* (1978). Follow-up of families who experience a perinatal death. *Paediatrics*, 62, 166–70

Rufer, R. (1968). The influence of surface active substances on alveolar mechanics in the respiratory distress syndrome. *Respiration*, 25, 441–57

Sidbury, J.B. (1923). Transfusion through the umbilical vein in haemorrhage of the newborn. *Am. J. Dis. Child.*, 25, 290

Silverman, W.A., Fertig, J.W. and Berger, A.P. (1958). The influence of the thermal environment on the survival of newly born premature infants. *Paediatrics*, **22**, 876–86

Tarnier, E.S. (1885). Des soins a donner aux enfants nes avant terme. *Bull. Acad. Med. Paris* (2nd ser.), **14**, 944

Terry, T.L. (1942). Retrolental fibroplasia. *Am. J. Ophthalmol.*, **25**, 203

Volpe, J.J. (1981). *Neurology of the Newborn.* (Philadelphia, London, Toronto, Sidney: W.B. Saunders)

Von Reuss, A.R. (1921). *The Diseases of the Newborn,* p. 286. (London: John Bale, Sons and Danielsson)

Wallerstein, H. (1946). Treatment of severe erythroblastosis by simultaneous removal and replacement of the blood of the newborn infant. *Science*, **103**, 583

Wiener, A.S. and Wexler, J.B. (1946). The use of heparin when performing exchange blood transfusions in newborn infants. *J. Lab. Clin. Med.*, **31**, 1016

Wu, P.Y.K. and Hodgman, J.E. (1974). Insensible water loss in preterm infants: changes with postnatal development and non-ionizing radiant energy. *Paediatrics*, **54**, 704–12

FURTHER READING

Chard, T. and Richards, M. (1977). *Benefits and Hazards of the New Obstetrics. Clinics in Developmental Medicine*, No. 64. (London, Philadelphia: Lippincott & Co., William Heinemann Medical Books)

Cone, T.E. (1979). *History of American Pediatrics.* (Boston: Little Brown & Co.)

McGrew, R.E. (1985). *Encyclopedia of Medical History.* (London: MacMillan Press)

Roberton, N.R.C. (1986). *Textbook of Neonatology.* (Edinburgh London Melbourne New York: Churchill Livingstone)

Studd, J. (1985). *The Management of Labour.* (Oxford, London, Edinburgh, Boston, Palo Alto, Melbourne: Blackwell Scientific Publications)

Worden, J.W. (1982). *Grief Counselling and Grief Therapy.* (London, New York: Tavistock Publications)

Zuspan, F.P. (1990). (ed.-in-chief) *Obstetrics/Gynecology Report*, Vol. 2 No. 4. (St. Louis, Missouri: Mosby-Year Book Inc.)

Genetics and congenital malformations

INTRODUCTION

Gregor Johann Mendel (1822–1884) was an Austrian botanist and monk who formulated the basic laws of heredity. At the age of 21 Mendel entered the monastery of St Thomas in Brunn, Austria (now Brno, Czechoslovakia) and took his vows in 1847. Four years later he enrolled at the University of Vienna where he studied science and mathematics. On his return to Brunn he taught biology and physics for the next 14 years. During that time he studied the inheritance of seven pairs of traits in garden pea plants and their seeds in the monastery garden. Pea plants reproduce sexually and their offspring are a product of male and female gametes. Mendel concluded from his studies, that plant traits were handed down through hereditary elements in the gametes. These traits were later called 'genes'. He introduced the concept of dominant and recessive hereditary elements and concluded that the elements (genes) separated in random fashion during gamete formation. Mendel also reasoned that plants inherited each of their traits, independently of other traits. These conclusions became known as Mendel's 'Law of Segregation' and his 'Law of Independent Assortment'. Mendel's (1866) published findings remained unnoticed for 34 years. Details of mitosis were described in 1882 and chromosomes were named by 1888 (Dunn, 1965).

Johannsen (1909), a Danish botanist, coined the term 'gene' and in 1910 Thomas Hunt Morgan, an American biologist, determined that genes were located on structures called 'chromosomes'. The occurrence of 'mutations' was documented around the same time by Hugo de Vries, a Dutch botanist (1900). In 1927 the American genetecist Hermann J. Muller discovered that artificial mutations were produced when organisms were irradiated with X-rays. In the early 1940s two American geneticists George W. Beadle and Edward L. Tatum studied genes and the chemical activity of cells. They concluded that genes exerted their control through the production of the enzymes which directed chemical reactions in the cell. In 1944 the American bacteriologist O.T. Avery of New York demonstrated that the transmission of hereditary characteristics from one bacterium to another takes place due to the intermediary deoxyribonucleic acid (DNA) molecules. This led to the realization that genes were made up of DNA. James Watson of America and Francis Crick of England described the exact structure of the DNA molecule in the British Magazine, *Nature* (Watson and Crick, 1953). Genetic finger printing was developed by Alec J. Jeffreys of the University of Leicester in 1985 based on the principle that DNA varies from person to person.

CONGENITAL MALFORMATIONS

The term 'congenital malformation' has replaced the word 'teratology', which was the original name used for the science dealing with monstrosities. However the word teratogen is still applied to environmental causes of congenital malformation. Warkany (1971) wrote a history of teratology in his *'Congenital Malformations. Notes and Comments'*, which provides an excellent background to the subject.

The oldest congenital abnormality depicted in sculpture was discovered in Southern Turkey and dates from c. 6500 BC. The marble statuette is of a double-headed twin goddess. Other artefacts showing double-headed human figures and conjoined twins date from about the same time and were discovered in Australasia and Central America. The earliest form of writing developed in ancient Bablyonia. Records from that time which were imprinted on clay tablets were discovered during excavations at the Royal library of Nineveh. Sixty-two malformations were detailed and described in five groups dealing with the ears, head, upper limbs, intestines and reproductive tract, and lower limbs.

The birth of a malformed infant was believed to be an omen. Soothsayers predicted future happenings based on individual types of abnormalities. This led to the development of 'divination' which was to play an enormous role in Roman history. The birth of twins for instance prompted those who dealt in augury to expound that food shortage would follow. The birth of a hermaphrodite was a sinister omen, and in Roman times an infant of dubious gender identity was slain.

In ancient times the theory that maternal impressions had a formative effect on the fetus was common. Pregnant mothers in Greece, were advised to gaze on beautiful statues or pictures so that their children in turn would be strong and beautiful. There was also a belief that members of different species could produce monstrous offspring. The theories may have originated in India and Egypt and were common in Greek mythology. Pliny the elder, of the first century AD, recorded many congenital malformations in his *Natural History*. Ambroise Paré wrote a section on the classification and explanation of monsters in his *Chyrurgerie* which was published in 1579.

William Harvey's *De Generatione Animalium* was published in 1651. He described the 'hare-lip' deformity and theorized that arrested development was the cause. This theory was echoed by von Haller and C.F. Wolff in the following century. Many scientific contributions were made to teratology in the nineteenth century and investigators of note were J.F. Meckel, Etienne G. Saint-Hilaire, Otto, Forster, Ahlfeld and C. Taruffi. The *Manual of Antenatal Pathology and Hygiene* (Ballantyne, 1904) was based on the observations of the afore-mentioned workers (Warkany, 1971).

The first demonstration of Mendelian dominant inheritance in man was by Farabee (1905) in his description of digital malformations. Tjio and Levan (1956) determined the correct chromosome number for humans which is 46, comprised of 23 pairs. Ford *et al.* (1959), also Jacobs and Keay (1959) and Lejeune *et al.* (1959a), discovered that some patients with congenital malformations had abnormal chromosome numbers. Carr (1967) documented chromosomal abnormalities in miscarriage tissue.

Goldschmidt (1938) introduced the term 'phenocopy'. Experimental teratology began in the 1930s, and the original studies were based on diets which were deficient in vitamins. Sows who were fed a vitamin A-free diet, delivered piglets who were born without eyeballs. The first positive teratogens, nitrogen mustard and trypan blue, were discovered by Haskin (1948). The Barr body, which later became important in the investigation of intersexuality, was described by Barr and Bertram (1949).

During this century an enormous amount of information has been amassed and the classification of congenital malformations runs to several pages of detailed script. Investigative tools which have proved of great importance are amniocentesis, fetoscopy, chorion villus biopsy, ultrasound, X-ray, amniography, chromosome analysis and determination of α-fetoprotein levels and other components in serum.

Brock (1982) estimated that 8% of pregnancies are sufficiently at risk to require some form of prenatal diagnostic technique. MacLachlan *et al.* (1989) documented 75 disorders that could be diagnosed prenatally, and predicted that rapid developments of new techniques such as the polymerase chain reaction, pulsed field electrophoresis, ribonuclease cleavage and oligonucleotide probes for specific mutant sites would add more genetic conditions which would fall within current diagnostic capabilities.

DIAGNOSTIC METHODS

Amniocentesis

Transabdominal amniocentesis was reported by Prochownick in 1877. Its use in modern times was first reported by Menees *et al.* (1930). The amniotic fluid was tapped by transabdominal needling. Menees injected radio opaque contrast to outline the fetus and placenta by amniography. Bevis (1953) obtained samples of liquor amni by abdominal paracentesis, at fortnightly intervals, in the management of rhesus isoimmunization and found that if the blood pigments bilirubin and oxyhaemoglobin were present in high concentration, kernicterus in the newborn was likely.

Liley (1961) in Auckland, New Zealand discovered a correlation between the deviation on the spectral absorption curve of liquor amnii due to bilirubin, and the severity of rhesus disease in the isoimmunized infant. Following that report, amniocentesis became commonplace and the technique was used in antenatal genetic diagnosis, management of rhesus isoimmunization, determination of fetal maturity, in fetoscopy, and at intrauterine fetal transfusion.

The first use of amniotic fluid examination in the prevention of genetic disease and congenital abnormalities, was by Fuchs and Riis (1956). They determined fetal sex from chromosome material of cells suspended in amniotic fluid, and thus were able to identify some fetuses who were at risk. Steele and Breg (1966) demonstrated that cultured amniotic fluid cells were suitable for karyotyping. Brock and Sutcliffe (1972) discovered that excessive amounts of α-fetoprotein (AFP) were present in the amniotic fluid surrounding an infant with neural tube defects. Raised amniotic AFP levels during the mid-trimester proved an effective method of detecting neural tube defects. Qualitative electrophrosesis of acetylcholinesterase was introduced by Smith *et al.* (1979) and Buamah *et al.* (1980), and in combination with AFP levels provided further valuable information. Indications for genetic amniocentesis included the detection of chromosomal abnormalities, X-linked conditons, inborn errors of metabolism, and the neural tube defects.

The estimation of fetal maturity by analysis of amniotic fluid attracted the attention and expertise of many investigators. Brosens and Gordon (1966) introduced the 'nile blue sulphate test' where fetal squames were stained with the substance. A combined amniotic fluid cytology with a creatinine and urea content scoring system was developed by Lind and Billewicz (1971). Fetal lung maturity was found to be related to the surface active phospholipid lecithin (Gluck *et al.*, 1971). When compared with another phospholipid, sphingo-myelin (Gluck and Kulovich, 1973), the lecithin: sphingomyelin area ratio (LSAR) evolved. The LSAR reading was found to be predictive of severe idiopathic respiratory distress syndrome when a value of less than 1.5 was reported, but was uncommon over a value of 2 (Whitfield and Sproule, 1974). The 'foam stability', 'shake' or 'bubble' test, was devised by Clements *et al.* (1972) and was almost as reliable as LSAR in the prediction of fetal lung maturity.

α-Fetoprotein

Abelov *et al.* (1963) first demonstrated the glycoprotein AFP in the serum of mice. Obstetric interest in AFP began when Brock and Sutcliffe (1972) reported elevated AFP levels in amniotic fluid samples from pregnancies with open neural tube defects – both spina bifida and anencephaly. Ruoslahti and Seppala (1971) demonstrated AFP levels less than 5 ng/ml in non-pregnant females. AFP concentrations were found to rise from the 12th to the 30th week of gestation with a steep rise in the second trimester. The accuracy of gestational dating was therefore critical in the interpretation of amniotic fluid AFP levels.

The report of a UK collaborative study in 1977 indicated that at a gestational age of 16–18 weeks, 88% of cases of anencephaly and 79% of spina bifida could be detected by elevated levels of AFP in maternal serum. Following this, serum AFP levels were introduced as a screening device to detect women who should have intensive genetic screening. Seppala and Ruoslahti (1973) first reported that maternal serum AFP levels could be elevated in rhesus isoimmunization, intrauterine fetal demise and fetal distress. It was later found that high levels were also produced in a number of other congenital abnormalities and in multiple gestations.

Fetoscopy

The first attempts at fetoscopy were carried out by Westin (1954; 1957) using a 10 mm diameter hysteroscope introduced through the cervix. A transabdominal approach was used by Mandelbaum *et al.* (1967) during attempts at intrauterine fetal transfusion for haemolytic disease. Fetal blood and skin samples were obtained during fetoscopy, prior to termination of pregnancy by Valenti (1972; 1973). The term fetoscopy, derived from the Latin word *fetus* and the Greek word *episkopion*, to inspect, was introduced by Scrimgeour (1973). He exposed the uterus at laparotomy and introduced a 2.2 mm telescope to view the amniotic cavity and fetus. The procedure was performed in six women whose offspring were at high risk of recurring fetal neural tube defect. Three healthy infants were delivered but a fourth had spina bifida. This form of fetoscopy was a major procedure, and was outdated by the advent of ultrasound examination and serum AFP estimation. Kan *et al.* (1972) suggested the possibility of prenatal diagnosis of haemoglob-inopathy. This group (Kan *et al.*, 1974) were the first to describe placentacentesis (blind needling of the placenta).

The technique of placental aspiration at fetoscopy via a transabdominal approach under local anaesthesia was pioneered by Hobbins and Mahoney (1974). Fetal vessels on the surface of the chorionic plate were punctured and samples obtained. Rodeck and Campbell (1978; 1979) introduced puncture of the fetal end of the umbilical cord as an alternative, and this proved to be the superior technique. As confidence with the procedure grew, fetoscopy was used for visual assessment of the fetus and for sampling of fetal blood, skin and liver. The risks to the mother were low, but fetal loss occurred in both normal and abnormal pregnancies.

Ultrasound-guided fetal blood sampling by puncture of the umbilical cord (cordocentesis) was pioneered by Daffos *et al.* (1983) and Nicolaides *et al.* (1986). The technique was performed as an outpatient procedure and was used in prenatal treatment of fetal anaemia, and in the detection of intrauterine fetal hypoxia.

Ultrasound

Professor Ian Donald *et al.* (1958) (q.v.in Biography) of Glasgow and his colleagues first experimented with ultrasound in gynaecological diagnosis. The original techniques of assessing fetal maturity in the first trimester were described by Donald and Abdulla (1967). Early studies in the diagnosis of fetal abnormality were carried out for cranial defects (Donald and Abdulla, 1968; Campbell *et al.*, 1972); spinal defects (Campbell, 1974; Campbell *et al.*, 1975); renal agenesis (Campbell *et al.*, 1973); and polycystic kidneys (Garrett *et al.*, 1970). It was discovered that a large range of abnormalities could be detected. The malformations were classified into the general groups cranio-spinal, gastrointestinal, renal, limb deformities, fetal tumours, cardiac anomalies and a miscellaneous group.

Chorionic villus biopsy

Chorionic villus biopsy allowed antenatal diagnosis of genetic disorders in the first trimester. An early application of the procedure was detection of haemoglobinopathy. The technique was based on an ability to carry out chromosome analysis on material obtained from the placental plate. An important publication was that of Evans *et al.* (1972) who reported their work on the isolation of chromosomes from mouse embryos. Further advances were documented by Kullander and Sandahl (1973) and also Hahnemann (1974) who recorded fetal chromosome analysis from transcervical placental biopsy prior to termination of early pregnancy. The first successful prenatal diagnosis attributed to the technique was reported from the Department of Obstetrics and Gynaecology, Tietung Hospital, China (1975) when fetal sex was diagnosed.

Niazi *et al.* (1981) at St Mary's Hospital, London reported successful methods for culture of fibroblasts from trophoblast villi. Kazy *et al.* (1982) of the, then, USSR reported fetal sexing and also enzyme assay on chorion biopsies taken at 6–12 weeks' gestation. The earliest application of the technique was for diagnosis of haemoglobinopathy.

Simoni *et al.* (1983) described a technique for direct chromosome and biochemical analysis on first trimester chorionic villi, without preliminary culture. Chorionic villi were obtained by aspiration or direct biopsy from the chorion frondosum, at the edge of the placental disc, with the procedure being performed under ultrasound control. The procedure caused moderate bleeding in under 10% and perforation of the amniotic sac in 1–2%. Pregnancy loss rates due to subsequent miscarriage were about 10%.

Gene probe analysis

Gene analysis was carried out by E.M. Southern (1975) and he invented the methodology which is central to the procedure. The technique allowed first trimester antenatal diagnosis in a large range of genetic disorders including sickle cell anaemia, the thalassaemias, haemophilia, polycystic kidney disease, myotonic and Duchenne muscular dystrophy, cystic fibrosis, phenylketonuria and other disorders.

SOME COMMON DISORDERS

There are a large variety of central nervous system malformations. Obstetric interest in central nervous system defects increased when it was discovered that many of them could be diagnosed by antenatal ultrasound examination.

Hydrocephalus and spina bifida

Hydrocephalus was known to the ancients and Hippocrates is said to have tapped the hydrocephalic ventricle. The mechanism of production of the condition was elucidated by Dandy *et al.* at the John Hopkins Hospital in 1914. A congenital form caused by the Arnold-Chiari malformation, in which the acqueduct of Sylvius is occluded in part or whole, was noted to be rare. In this condition there was displacement of parts of the cerebellar brain stem through the foramen magnum into the upper part of the vertebral canal (Dandy, 1919; Dandy and Blackfan, 1914).

The acquired form of hydrocephalus was found to be obstructive or non-obstructive. The former was the commoner type and was communicating or non-communicating. In the non-communicating variety obstruction was usually in the form of adhesions blocking the foramina of Magendie and Luschka.

The condition of *holoprosencephaly*, also termed arhinencephaly or holotelencephaly, was first described by Hans Kundrat (1882). He described absence of the olfactory bulbs, failure of cleavage of the developing brain into two hemispheres, and a variety of facial malformations. De Myer (1964) suggested the term 'holoprosencephaly' and divided the entity into three separate types – alobar, semilobar or lobar holoprosencephaly.

Heschl (1859) introduced the term porencephaly for a condition of cerebral defects involving cortical tissue and the ventricular system. He considered it a congenital anomaly, but it was later discovered that labour and postnatal events could cause the condition.

Thomas Willis, described microcephaly in the seventeenth century. The occurrence of iniencephaly was documented around the same time. Hydranencephaly was described by Cruveilhier (1835) while the actual term was introduced by Spielmeyer (1905). Anencephaly, also described some centuries ago, was found to occur more frequently in the autumn months and was particularly common in Northern Ireland. Peak incidences were noted in the early 1940s and early 1960s.

An early reference to spina bifida was that of Morgagni (1769) who explained that spina bifida was a watery tumour of the vertebrae. Von Recklinghausen (1886) carried out detailed examination of the condition and evolved a theory on the pathogenesis of myelomeningocoele. Spina bifida, was due to failure of the neural arches to close and was accompanied by protrusion of the contents of the spinal canal. The lower part of the canal was most often involved with about six or five vertebrae affected. Three forms of spina bifida sac were identified, meningocoele, meningomyelocoele and syringomyelocoele. Spina bifida occulta, a bony defect not accompanied by protrusion of spinal canal contents was also described.

The Arnold–Chiari malformation was described by Julius Arnold and Hans von Chiari (1894). Arnold was professor of pathological anatomy at Heidelberg and Chiari held the chair of pathological anatomy at Strasburg. The malformation describes a hind brain anomaly in which the roof of the fourth ventricle lies below the level of the foramen magnum and causes outflow obstruction to cerebrospinal fluid with consequent hydrocephalus. Their observations were complemented by Russel (1935) and that of Donald (1935) who reported ten cases of spina bifida with myelomeningocoele, all of whom showed the malformation, and in eight of whom hydrocephalus was present.

The surgical treatment of myelomeningocoele was introduced in 1959. Prior to that 70–100% of infants with the malformation died within 6 months of birth (Rickham and Mawdsley, 1966; Laurence and Tew, 1967). Lorber (1971) reported operative treatment of myelomeningocoele by operation with a 2–year survival rate of 64%. The infants did not fare well at follow up, but Lorber indicated those features which could be used to predict survival with acceptable degrees of handicap.

Congenital dislocation of the hip

This deformity was recorded by Hippocrates who recognized the abnormal gait of the condition. The hereditary tendency was noted by Ambroise Paré (1510–1590). The first attempts at replacing the femoral head were made in 1701 by Verduc. Congenital dislocation of the hip was first adequately described by Guillaume Dupuytren (1777–1835), who wrote on its clinical presentation, 'the infirmities that spring therefrom do not attract the attention of the parents until the child first attempts to walk' (Figure 1). Dupuytren described the anatomy and pathology of the condition and attempted the use of traction to treat the condition. He was aware that the disorder was frequently bilateral and occurred most commonly in females (Dunn, 1989). Lorenz (1896) introduced the method of treatment which became standard, of reduction, with retention of the femoral head in its normal location.

The most reliable method for diagnosing congenital dislocation of the hip was described by Ortolani (1937; 1948). The test was one of hip reduction. The femoral head was made to return to the acetabulum with the Ortolani manoeuvre. Barlow (1966) introduced an examination in 1962 where the femoral head was located within the acetabulum. The dislocatable hip was demonstrated by gentle hip flexion and thigh adduction. Von Rosen (1962) pioneered the method of X-ray examination where the procedure was carried out with the femoral head dislocated. In the newborn with marked instability a secure restraint such as the Pavlik harness or von Rosen's splint maintained reduction until joint structure had returned to normal. The Craig splint was popularly used.

Heart disease

Cyanotic heart disease with pulmonary stenosis, ventricular septal defect, right ventricular hypertrophy, and over-riding of the aorta was described by Fallot (1888). Previous descriptions by the Danish scientist Niels Stensen in 1671, Sandiforte of Leiden in 1777, William Hunter of Glasgow and London in 1774 and Peacock in 1866 failed to achieve eponymic distinction (Warkany, 1971).

Cleft lip and palate

Cleft lip and palate was recognized from earliest times. William Harvey (q.v. in Biography) offered the first explanation for the defect in the seventeenth century, and Trew (1757) described familial facial clefts. Fogh-Andersen (1942) established risk figures for recurrence. He also documented three forms of lesion–harelip, harelip with cleft palate, and isolated cleft palate.

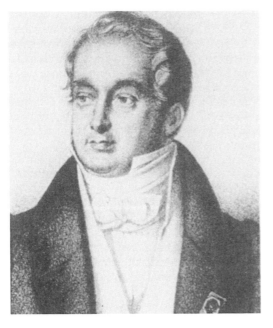

Figure 1 Baron Guillaume Dupuytren of Paris, 1777–1835 (*see* text). Reproduced with kind permission from Dunn, P.M. (1989). *Arch. Dis. Child.*, **64**, 969

Down syndrome (trisomy 21)

Down syndrome was first described by Seguin (1846), who considered the disorder to be a form of hypothyroidism. The characteristics of the syndrome were further described by John Langdon Haydon Down (1866), a physician who practised in London. He was impressed by their similarity to the Mongol race and referred to their 'mongolian racial' characteristics. Shuttleworth (1909) first recorded the association of advanced maternal age at conception with the birth of Down syndrome infants. The pinpoint spots on the outer margin of the iris in Down syndrome were described by Brushfield (1924). Eventually the chromosomal abnormalities of the condition trisomy 21, were discovered by Lejeune *et al.* (1959a,b).

Potter's syndrome

The condition of bilateral renal agenesis was described by Potter (1946) in a report to the *Journal of Paediatrics*. In a further paper (Potter, 1965) he recorded the condition in 50 cases. Potter described the condition in detail, and noted the facial characteristic of 'premature senility'. The infants were found to be small for dates and rarely survived longer than the first 24 hours. The appelation 'Potter's syndrome' was used by Welch (1958). Later reports documented the method of ultrasound diagnosis in pregnancy with small for dates fetus and gross oligohydramnios.

Edwards syndrome (trisomy 18)

Edwards *et al.* (1960) described trisomy 18, a condition of retarded mental development, rockerbottom feet, loose skin, short thorax and an abnormally shaped head. The condition was previously described by Emed (1956) as the Pterygium syndrome. Abnormalities of the cardiovascular system, gastrointestinal and urogenital tracts were also reported in this condition.

Pierre-Robin syndrome

The condition of micrognathia with glossoptosis may cause extreme breathing difficulties in newborn children. Attempts at surgical correction were carried out in the early twentieth century. The condition became eponomously related with Pierre Robin (1923), although he was not the first to describe the abnormality.

Kartagener syndrome

Kartagener or the immotile cilia syndrome, is of importance in infertility practice. Congenital bronchiectasis was first recognised by Laennec in 1819 and the condition was reported by a number of observers during the nineteenth century. Kartagener (1935) described 142 cases. An association with situs inversus and sinus disease was termed the Kartagener syndrome.

Rhesus isoimmunization

The conditions of hydrops fetalis, icterus gravis neonatorum and anaemia of the newborn were well documented but it was a paper by Diamond, *et al.* (1932) which first suggested that the three conditions were manifestations of the same disease. An atypical agglutinin was discovered by Levine and Stetson (1939) and the rhesus antigen on red cells was discovered by Landsteiner and Wiener (1940). The amniotic fluid of affected pregnancies was investigated by Bevis (1953) who demonstrated that analysis of the increased blood pigment in the liquor, provided a method of predicting severity of the disease.

Von Willebrand's disease

A rare cause of menorrhagia is that of Von Willebrand's disease. The disorder was first described by Eric von Willebrand, a Finnish physician in 1926 (Schulman and Simpson, 1981). He documented a family in which five of seven daughters bled to death at an early age. This hereditary haemorrhagic disorder can affect males or females and is related to classical haemophilia.

Phenylketonuria

The condition of phenylketonuria (PKU) was discovered by Folling (1934). The disease is caused by a metabolic disorder in which the conversion of phenylalanine to tyrosine is impaired due to the reduced activity of the enzyme phenylalanine hydroxylase. The disease causes mental retardation and other stigmata of brain damage. Dent (1957) reported the case of a woman with PKU whose children had severe mental retardation. Newborn screening for PKU began in the 1960s, and blood was obtained by 'heelprick' for the Guthrie test. Low-phenylalanine diet which controlled the biochemical abnormalities, and prevented mental retardation and most of the other neurologic manifestations, was found to treat the condition effectively if begun in early infancy.

The adreno-genital syndrome

The manifestations of the congenital adreno-genital syndrome, (a cause of female pseudohermaphroditism) were known since antiquity and were described by Pliny The Elder (translation, 1939) in his *Natural History*. The condition was also documented by Regnier de Graaf in the seventeenth century. Precocious puberty was found to be associated with adrenocortical hyperplasia by Marchant in 1801, while adrenal tumours were found causative by Tilesius in 1803 (Krabbe, 1921). The condition was noted with alarming frequency in the late 1950s. It was subsequently discovered that mothers who had been prescribed synthetic steroids for the treatment of recurrent or threatened miscarriage were involved. The drugs were found to contain testosterone.

Non-genetic congenital diseases

Congenital rubella

Rubella was recognized as a distinct entity in the early nineteenth century. Maton (1815) noted that its symptoms were slight. The infection was known as Rotheln. Veale (1866) suggested that the German name be replaced in the English literature by the term rubella. The separate identity of rubella was finally recognized at an International Medical Congress in London in 1881 (Waterson and Wilkinson, 1978). The disease received scant attention however, due to its mild clinical manifestations until Gregg (1942) noted the association between intrauterine rubella infection and congenital cataract. His suggestion was greeted with caution and an editorial in the Lancet commented that 'the possibility remains but he cannot yet be said to have proved his case' (1944). The congenital rubella syndrome was studied in great detail by Dr Lou Cooper from St Luke's Roosevelt Hospital Central New York, who conducted a long-term follow up of 20 000 children born with the congenital rubella syndrome in the USA during the rubella epidemic of 1964–1965. One-third of the patients were found to be profoundly handicapped and required institutional care. Selective rubella immunization was introduced to the UK in 1970 (*Lancet*, 1991).

Thalidomide abnormality

McBride (1961) first brought attention to the association of thalidomide and congenital abnormalities, documenting the fact that almost 20% of infants delivered to women who had taken the drug were affected.

CHRONOLOGY

General

1866	Mendel published his findings on inheritance in plants.
1882	Mitosis was described. Chromosomes were named.
1909	Johannsen used the term 'gene'.
1930s	Experimental teratology began.
1938	Goldschmidt introduced the term 'phenocopy'.
1944	Hereditary transmission via DNA molecules was determined.
1949	Barr and Bertram described the 'Barr body'.
1953	Watson and Crick described the structure of DNA.
1956	Tjio and Levan determined the correct chromosome number for humans.

Congenital malformations

c. 6500 BC	A double-headed twin goddess discovered in Turkey dates from this time.
3000 BC	Babylonian records documented 62 malformations.
400 BC	Greek mothers believed that maternal impressions helped form the fetus.
1st C. AD	Pliny the Elder recorded congenital malformations. The birth of congenital malformed infants was thought to be a portent.
1579	Paré classified abnormalities.
1751	Harvey described 'hare-lip'.
19th C.	Meckel and others contributed their observations.

Reference: Warkany (1971)

Diagnostic methods

Amniocentesis

1877	Prochownick first reported transabdominal amniocentesis.
1930	Menees *et al.* re-investigated the technique.
1953	Bevis popularized the procedure in the management of rhesus disease.
1956	Fuchs and Riis determined fetal sex from amniocentesis.
1961	Liley studied the spectral absorption curve of liquor.
1966	Brosens and Gordon pioneered the Nile blue sulphate test.
1971	Lind and Billewicz introduced their scoring system. Gluck *et al.* studied lecithin.
1972	Brock and Sutcliffe discovered excess α-fetoprotein in the presence of neural tube defects. Clements introduced the 'shake test'.
1973	Gluck and Kulovich compared lecithin with sphingomyelin.
1979	Smith *et al.* introduced acetylcholinesterase measurements.

Other tests

1954	Westin pioneered fetoscopy.
1958	Donald *et al.* introduced ultrasound imaging.
1975	Prenatal diagnosis at chorionic villus biopsy was first documented. Southern devised a procedure to carry out gene analysis.

Some common disorders

Ancient Rome	Pliny the Elder described signs of congenital adreno-genital hyperplasia.
1671	Stensen (Warkany, 1971) described what was later termed the tetralogy of Fallot (1888).
1701	Verduc attempted replacement of congenital dislocation of the hip (Warkany, 1971).
1846	Seguin first described Down syndrome.
1866	Down described the syndrome of Mongolism.
19thC.	Dupuytren described congenital dislocation of the hip, a condition previously noted by the ancient Greeks (Dunn, 1989).
1894	Arnold, and also Chiari in 1895, described hydrocephalus and spina bifida.

1914	Dandy and Blackfan elucidated the causation of hydrocephalus.
1923	Pierre Robin redescribed a previously known syndrome.
1926	Von Willebrand described the haemorrhagic syndrome (Schulman and Simpson, 1981).
1932	Diamond *et al.* associated hydrops, icterus and anaemia of the newborn.
1934	Folling discovered phenylketonuria.
1935	Kartagener described congenital bronchiectasis – first recognized by Laennec (1819).
1937	Ortolani described a reliable method of diagnosing congenital dislocation of the hip.
1939	Levine and Stetson discovered atypical agglutinins in blood.
1940	Landsteiner and Weiner described the red cell rhesus antigen.
1942	Gregg documented the association of congenital cataract and intrauterine infection with rubella.
1946	Potter described bilateral renal agenesis.
1956	Emed described pterygium syndrome, later called Edwards syndrome (1960).
1961	McBride related congenital abnormalities to maternal thalidomide ingestion.

REFERENCES

Abelov, G.I., Perova, S.D., Khramkova, N.I., Postnikova, Z.A. and Irlin, I.S. (1963). Production of embryonal alpha-globulins by mice with transplanted hepatome. *Transplantation*, 1, 174–80

Arnold, J. (1894). Quoted by Boyd, W. (1955), p.468

Ballantyne, J. W. (1904). *Manual of Antenatal Pathology and Hygiene: The Embryo.* (Edinburgh: W. Green & Son)

Barlow, T.G. (1966). Congenital dislocation of the hip in the newborn. *Proc. R. Soc. Med.*, 59, 1103–8

Barr, M.L. and Bertram, E.G. (1949). A morphological distinction between neurones of the male and female and the behavior of the nucleolar satellite during accelerated nucleoprotein synthesis. *Nature (London)*, 163, 676

Bevis, D.C.A. (1953). The composition of liquor amnii in haemolytic disease of the newborn. *J. Obstet. Gynaecol. Br. Emp.*, 60, 244–51

Boyd, W. (1955). *Pathology for the Surgeon*, 7th edn. pp. 467. (Philadelphia, London: W.B. Saunders Co.)

Brock, D.J.H. (1982). Early Diagnosis of Fetal Defects. *Current Reviews in Obstetrics and Gynaecology*, Vol. 2. (London: Churchill Livingstone)

Brock, D.J.H. and Sutcliffe, R.G. (1972). Alpha-fetoprotein in the antenatal diagnosis of anencephaly and spina bifida. *Lancet*, 2, 197–9

Brosens, I. and Gordon, H. (1966). The estimation of maturity by cytological examination of the liquor amnii. *J. Obstet. Gynaecol. Br. Commonw.*, 73, 88–90

Brushfield, T. (1924). Mongolism *Br. J. Child. Dis.*, 21, 241

Buamah, P.K., Evans, L. and Wilford Ward, A. (1980). Amniotic fluid acetylcholinesterase isoenzyme pattern in the diagnosis of neural tube defects. *Clin. Chim. Acta*, 103, 147–51

Campbell, S. (1974). The antenatal detection of fetal abnormality by ultrasonic diagnosis. In Motulsky, A.G. and Lentz, W. (eds.) *Birth Defects*, pp. 240–7. (Amsterdam: Excerpta Medica)

Campbell, S., Johnstone, F.D., Holt, E.M. and May, P. (1972). Anencephaly: early ultrasonic diagnosis and active management. *Lancet*, 2, 1226–7

Campbell, S., Wladimiroff, J.W. and Dewhurst, C.J. (1973). The antenatal measurement of fetal urine production. *J. Obstet. Gynaecol. Br. Commonw.*, 80, 680–6

Campbell, S., Pryse-Davies, J., Coltart, T.M., Seller, M.J. and Singer, J.D. (1975). Ultrasound in the diagnosis of spina bifida. *Lancet*, 1, 1065–8

Carr, D.H. (1967). Chromosome anomalies as a cause of spontaneous abortion. *Am. J. Obstet. Gynecol.*, 97, 283

Clements, J.A., Platzker, A.C., Tierney, D.F., Hobel, C.J., Creasy, R.K., Margolis, A.J. *et al.* (1972). Assessment of the risk of the respiratory distress syndrome by a rapid test for surfactant in amniotic fluid. *N. Engl. J. Med.*, 286, 1077–81

Cruveilhier, J. (1835). *Anatomie Pathologique du Corps Humain.* (Paris: J.B. Bailliere)

Daffos, F., Cappella-Pavlovsky, M. and Forestier, F. (1983). Fetal blood sampling via the umbilical cord using a needle guided by ultrasound. Report of 66 cases. *Prenat. Diagn.*, 3, 271–7

Dandy, W. (1919). *Ann. Surg.*, **70**, 129, quoted by Boyd, W. (1955), p.500

Dandy, W. and Blackfan, K. (1914). *Am. J. Dis. Child.*, **8**, 406, quoted by Boyd, W. (1955), p.500

DeMyer, W. (1964). The face predicts the brain. *Paediatrics*, **34**, 256

Dent, C.E. (1957). Discussion of M.D. Armstrong. Relation of biochemical abnormality to development of mental defect in phenylketonuria. In *Etiologic Factors in Mental Retardation*, pp. 32–3. (Columbus, Ohio: Ross Laboratories)

Department of Obstetrics and Gynaecology, Tietung Hospital, Anshan (1975). Fetal sex prediction by sex chromatin of chorionic villi cells during early pregnancy. *Chinese Med. J.*, **1**, 117–26

Diamond, L.K., Blackfan, K.D. and Baty, J.M. (1932). Erythroblastosis fetalis and its association with universal edema of the fetus, icterus gravis neonatorum and anaemia of the newborn. *J. Paediatr.* **1**, 269

Donald (1935). Quoted by Boyd, W. (1955). p. 468

Donald, I. and Abdulla, U. (1967). Ultrasonics in obstetrics and gynaecology. *Br. J. Radiol.*, **40**, 604–11

Donald, I. and Abdulla, U. (1968). Placentography by sonar. *J. Obstet. Gynaecol. Br. Commonw.*, **75**, 993–1006

Donald, I., MacVicar, J. and Brown, T.G. (1958). Investigation of abdominal masses by pulsed ultrasound. *Lancet*, **1**, 1188–95

Down, J.L.H. (1866). Observations on an ethnic classification of idiots. *Clin. Lect. Rep. Lond. Hosp.*, **3**, 259

Dunn, L.C. (1965). *A Short History of Genetics.* (New York: Tubor Publishing Co.)

Dunn, P.M. (1989). Baron Dupuytren (1777–1835) Congenital dislocation of the hip. Perinatal lessons from the past. *Arch. Dis. Child.*, **64**, 969–70

Editorial (1944). Rubella and congenital malformations. *Lancet*, **1**, 316

Edwards, J.H., Harnden, D.G., Cameron, A.H., Crosse, V.M. and Wolff, O. (1960). A new trisomic syndrome. *Lancet*, **1**, 787

Emed, A. (1956). Pterygium syndrome *J. Pediatr.*, **48**, 73

Evans, E.P., Burtenshaw, M.D. and Ford, C.E. (1972). Chromosomes of mouse embryos and newborn young: preparations from membranes and tail tips. *Stain Technol.*, **47**, 229–34

Fallot, E.A. (1888). Contribution a l'anatomie pathologique de la maladie bleu (cyanose cardiaque). *Marseille-med.*, **25**, 77, 138, 207, 270, 341 and 403

Farabee, W.C. (1905). Inheritance of digital malformations in man. *Papers, Peabody Museum, Harvard University*, **3**, 69

Fogh-Andersen, P. (1942). *Inheritance of Harelip and Cleft Palate.* (Copenhagen: Arnold Busck)

Folling, A. (1934). Phenylpyruvic acid as a metabolic anomaly in connection with imbecility. *Hoppe-Seyler's Z. Physiol. Chem.*, **227**, 169–76

Ford, C.E., Jones, K.W., Miller, O.J., Mittwoch, U., Penrose, L.S., Ridler, M. and Shapiro, A. (1959). The chromosomes in a patient showing both mongolism and the Klinefelter syndrome. *Lancet*, **1**, 709

Fuchs, F. and Riis, P. (1956). Antenatal sex determination. *Nature (London)*, **177**, 330

Garrett, W.J., Robinson, D.E. and Gruenwald, G. (1970). Prenatal diagnosis of fetal polycystic kidney by ultrasound. *Austr. N. Z. J. Obstet. Gynaecol.*, **10**, 7–9

Gluck, L. and Kulovich, M.V. (1973). Lecithin/sphingomyelin ratios in amniotic fluid in normal and abnormal pregnancy. *Am. J. Obstet. Gynecol.*, **115**, 539–46

Gluck, L., Kulovich, M.V., Borer, R.C., Brenner, P.H., Anderson, G.G. and Spellacy, W.N. (1971). Diagnosis of respiratory distress syndrome by amniocentesis. *Am. J. Obstet. Gynecol.*, **109**, 440–5

Goldschmidt, R. (1938). *Physiological Genetics.* (New York: McGraw-Hill Book Co. Inc.)

Gregg, N.M. (1942). Congenital cataract following German measles in mother. *Trans. Ophthalm. Soc. Austr.*, **3**, 35

Hahnemann, N. (1974). Early prenatal diagnosis: a study of biopsy techniques and cell culturing from extra-embryonic membrane. *Clin. Genet.*, **6**, 294–306

Haskin, D. (1948). Some effects of nitrogen mustard on the development of external body form in the fetal rat. *Anat. Rec.*, **102**, 493

Heschl (1859). Quoted by Warkany, J. (1971), p. 246

Hobbins, J.C. and Mahoney, M.J. (1974). *In utero* diagnosis of haemoglobinopathies. Technique for obtaining fetal blood. *N. Engl. J. Med.*, **290**, 1065

Jacobs, P. and Keay, A.J. (1959). Somatic chromosomes in a child with Bonnevie-Ullrich syndrome. *Lancet*, **2**, 732

Johannsen, W.L. (1909). *Elemente der Exakten Erblichkeitslehre*. (Jena: Gustav Fischer)

Kan, Y.W., Dozy, A.M., Alter, B.P., Frigoletto, F.D. and Nathan, D.G. (1972). Detection of the sickle cell gene in the human fetus. Potential for intrauterine diagnosis of sickle cell anaemia. *N. Engl. J. Med.*, **287**, 1

Kan, Y.W., Vanenti, C., Guidotti, R., Carnazza, V. and Rieder, R.F. (1974). Fetal blood-sampling *in utero*. *Lancet*, **1**, 79

Kartagener, M. (1935). Das Problem der Kongenitalitat und Hereditat der Bronchiektasien. *Ergebn. inn. Med. u. Kinderh.*, **49**, 378

Kazy, Z., Rozousky, I.S. and Bakharev, V.A. (1982). Chorion biopsy in early pregnancy: a method of early prenatal diagnosis for inherited disorders. *Prenat. Diagn.*, **2**, 39–45

Krabbe, K.H. (1921). The relation between the adrenal cortex and sexual development. *N. Y. J. Med.*, **114**, 4

Kullander, S. and Sandahl, B. (1973). Fetal chromosome analysis after transcervical placental biopsies during early pregnancy. *Acta Obstet. Gynaecol. Scand.*, **52**, 355–9

Kundrat, H. (1882). *Arhinencephaly als Typische Art von Missbildung*. (Graz: von Leuscner & Lubensky)

Lancet (1991). Notice board: congenital rubella – 50 years on. **337**, 668

Landsteiner, K. and Wiener, A.S. (1940). An agglutinable factor in human blood recognizable by immune sera for rhesus blood. *Proc. Soc. Exp. Biol.*, **43**, 223

Laurence, K.M. and Tew, B.J. (1967). Follow-up of 65 survivors from 425 cases of spina bifida born in South Wales between 1956 and 1962. *Develop. Med. Child Neurol.*, **Suppl. 13**, 1–3

Lejeune, J., Gautier, M. and Turpin, R. (1959a). Etude des chromosomes somatiques de neuf enfants mongoliens. *Compt. Rend. Acad. Sci. (Paris)*, **248**, 1721

Lejeune, J., Gautier, M. and Turpin, R. (1959b). Les chromosomes humains en culture de tissus. *Compt. Rend. Acad. Sci. (Paris)*, **248**, 602

Levine, P. and Stetson, R. (1939). An unusual case of infra-group agglutination. *J. Am. Med. Assoc.*, **113**, 126

Liley, A.W. (1961). Liquor amnii analysis in management of pregnancy complicated by rhesus sensitization. *Am. J. Obstet. Gynecol.*, **82**, 1359–70

Lind, T. and Billewicz, W.Z. (1971). A point scoring system for estimating gestational age from examination of amniotic fluid. *Br. J. Hosp. Med.*, **5**, 681–5

Lorber, J. (1971). Results of treatment of myelomeningocele. *Develop. Med. Child Neurol.*, **13**, 279–303

Lorenz, A. (1896). Uber die unblutige Behandlung der angeborenen Huftverrenkung. *Zentralbl. Chir.*, **23**, 1014

McBride, W.G. (1961). Thalidomide and congenital abnormalities. *Lancet*, **2**, 1358

MacLachlan, N.A., Rooney, D.E., Coleman, D. and Rodeck, C.H. (1989). Prenatal diagnosis: early amniocentesis or chorionic villus sampling. In Chamberlain, G. and Drife, G. (eds.) *Contemporary Reviews in Obstetrics and Gynaecology*, Vol. 1, pp. 173–80. (London: Butterworths)

McNay, M.B. and Whitfield, C.R. (1984). Amniocentesis. *Br. J. Hosp. Med.*, **31**, 406–16

Mandelbaum, B., Pontarelli, D. and Brushenko, A. (1967). Amnioscopy for prenatal transfusion. *Am. J. Obstet. Gynecol.*, **98**, 1140

Maton, W.G. (1815). Some account of a rash, liable to be mistaken for scarlatina. *Med. Trans. R. Coll. Phys.*, **5**, 149–65 (**65**, 148)

Mendel, G. (1866). Versuche an Pflanzen-Hybriden. *Verh. Naturf. Ver. Brunn*, **4**, 3

Menees, T.O., Millar, J.D. and Holly, L.E. (1930). Amniography. Preliminary report. *Am. J. Roentgenol.*, **24**, 353–66

Morgagni, J.B. (1769). *The Seats and Causes of Diseases Investigated by Anatomy*, translated by Benjamin Alexander, Vol. 3. (London: A. Miller and T. Cadell)

Niazi, M., Coleman, D.V. and Loeffler, F.E. (1981). Trophoblast sampling in early pregnancy. Culture of rapidly dividing cells from immature placental villi. *Br. J. Obstet. Gynaecol.*, **88**, 1081–5

Nicolaides, K.H., Soothill, P.W., Rodeck, C.H. and Campbell, S. (1986). Ultrasound-guided sampling of umbilical cord and placental blood to assess fetal wellbeing. *Lancet*, **1**, 1065–7

Ortolani, M. (1937). Um segno poco noto e sua importanza per la diagnosi precore di prelussazione congenita dell'onca. *Pediatria (Napoli)*, **45**, 129–36

Ortolani, M. (1948). *Lussazione Congenita Dell'Anca.* (Bologna: L. Capelli)

Pliny (The Elder) (1939). *Natural History*, translated by Rackham, H., Vol. 11. (Cambridge Mass.: Harvard University Press)

Potter, E.I. (1946). Bilateral renal agenesis. *J. Paediatr.*, **29**, 68

Potter, E.L. (1965). Bilateral absence of ureters and kidneys. A report of 50 cases. *Obstet. Gynecol.*, **25**, 3

Recklinghausen, von F. (1886). Untersuchungen uber die Spina Bifida. *Virchows Arch. Path. Anat.*, **105**, 243

Rickham, P.P. and Mawdsley, T. (1966). The effect of early operation on the survival of spina bifida cystica. *Develop. Med. Child Neurol.*, (Suppl.) **11**, 20–6

Robin, P. (1923). La chute de la base de la langue considerée comme une nouvelle cause de gene dans la respiration naso-pharyngienne. *Bull. Acad. Med (Paris)*, **89**, 37

Rodeck, C.H. and Campbell, S. (1978). Sampling pure fetal blood by fetoscopy in second trimester of pregnancy. *Br. Med.* J., **2**, 728

Rodeck, C.H. and Campbell, S. (1979). Umbilical cord insertion as source of pure fetal blood for prenatal diagnosis. *Lancet*, **1**, 1244

Rosen, S. Von (1962). Diagnosis and treatment of congenital dislocation of the hip joint in the newborn. *J. Bone Joint Surg.*, **44–B**, 284

Ruoslahti, E. and Seppala, M. (1971). Studies of carcino-fetal proteins III. Development of a radioimmunoassay for α-fetoprotein. Demonstration of alpha-fetoprotein in serum of healthy adult humans. *Int. J. Cancer*, **8**, 374–83

Russell (1935). Quoted by Boyd, W. (1955), p.468

Schulman, J.D. and Simpson, J.L. (eds.) (1981). *Genetic Diseases in Pregnancy: Maternal Effects and Fetal Outcome*, p.138. (New York, London, Toronto, Sydney, San Francisco: Academic Press)

Scrimgeour, J.B. (1973). Other techniques for antenatal diagnosis. In Emery, A.E.H. (ed.) *Antenatal Diagnosis of Genetic Disease*, p.49. (Edinburgh: Churchill Livingstone)

Seguin, E. (1846). *Traitement Moral Hygiene et Education des Idiots.* (Paris & London)

Seppala, M. and Ruoslahti, E. (1973). Alphafetoprotein in maternal serum: a new marker for detection of fetal distress and intrauterine death. *Am. J. Obstet. Gynecol.*, **115**, 48–52

Shuttleworth, G.E. (1909). Mongolian imbecility. *Br. Med. J.*, **2**, 661

Simoni, G., Brambati, B., Danesino, C., Rossella, F., Terzoli, G.L., Ferrari, M. and Fraccaro, M. (1983). Efficient direct chromosome analysis and enzyme determinations from chorionic villi samples in the first trimester of pregnancy. *Hum. Genet.*, **63**, 349–57

Smith, A.D., Wald, N.J., Cuckle, M.S., Stirrat, G.M., Bobrow, M. and Lagercrantz, H. (1979). Amniotic fluid acetylcholinesterase as a possible diagnostic test for neural tube defects in early pregnancy. *Lancet*, **1**, 686–8

Southern, E.M. (1975). Detection of specific sequences among DNA fragments separated by gel electrophoresis. *J. Mol. Biol.*, **98**, 503–17

Spielmeyer, W. (1905). Ein hydranencephales Zwillingspaar. *Arch. Psychiatr. Nervenkr.*, **39**, 807

Steele and Breg (1966). Quoted by McNay, M.B. and Whitfield, C.R. (1984)

Tjio, J.H. and Levan, A. (1956). The chromosome number of man. *Hereditas*, **42**, 1

Trew, C.J. (1757). Sistens plura exempla palate deficientis. *Nova Acta Physico-Medica Academiae Caesareae Leopoldino-Carolinae* (Norimbergae), quoted by Warkany, J. (1971)

Valenti, C. (1972). Endoamnioscopy and fetal biopsy: a new technique. *Am. J. Obstet. Gynecol.*, **114**, 561

Valenti, C. (1973). Antenatal detection of haemoglobinopathies. *Am. J. Obstet. Gynecol.*, **115**, 851

Veale, H. (1866). History of an epidemic of Rotheln, with observations on its pathology. *Edinb. Med. J.*, **12**, 404–14 (**65**,148)

Vries De (1900). Quoted by Dunn, L.C. (1965). p. 28

Warkany, J. (1971). *Congenital Malformations: Notes and Comments*, pp. 646, 494 and 992. (Chicago: Year Book Medical Publishers Inc.)

Waterson, A.P. and Wilkinson, L. (1978). *An Introduction to the History of Virology*. (London, New York, Melbourne: Cambridge University Press)

Watson, J.D. and Crick, F.H.C. (1953). The structure of DNA. *Cold Spring Harbor Symp. Quant. Biol.*, **28**, 123

Welch, R.G. (1958). The Potter Syndrome of renal agenesis. *Br. Med. J.*, **1**, 1102

Westin, B. (1954). Hysteroscopy in early pregnancy. *Lancet*, **11**, 872

Westin, B. (1957). Technique and estimation of oxygenation of the human fetus *in utero* by means of hystero-photography. *Acta Paediatr.*, **46**, 117

Whitfield, C.R. and Sproule, W.B. (1974). Fetal lung maturation. *Br. J. Hosp. Med.*, **12**, 678–90

FURTHER READING

Brock, D.J.H. (1989). Gene probe analysis. In Studd, J. (ed.) *Progress in Obstetrics and Gynaecology*, Vol. 7, pp. 39–52. (Edinburgh, London, Melbourne, New York: Churchill Livingstone)

Crawford, M.d'A. (1989). Diagnosis of chromosomal abnormalities. In Turnbull, Sir A. and Chamberlain, G. (eds.) *Obstetrics*, pp. 309–26. (Edinburgh, London, Melbourne, New York: Churchill Livingstone)

Dornan, J.C. and Sim, D. (1990). Early amniocentesis. In Studd, J. (ed.) *Progress in Obstetrics and Gynaecology*, Vol. 8, pp. 141–8. (Edinburgh London, Melbourne, New York: Churchill Livingstone)

Gerbie, A.B. (ed.) (1980). Antenatal diagnosis of genetic defects. In *Clinics in Obstetrics and Gynaecology*, Vol. 7 No. 1. (London, Philadelphia, Toronto: W.B. Saunders Co. Ltd)

Haldane, J.B.S. (1942). *New Paths in Genetics*. (New York: Harper & Row Publishers)

Loeffler, F.E. (1985). Chorionic villus biopsy. In Studd, J. (ed.) *Progress in Obstetrics and Gynaecology*, Vol. 5. pp. 22–35. (Edinburgh, London, Melbourne, New York: ChurchillLivingstone)

Nicolaides, K.H. and Soothill, P.W. (1989). Cordocentesis. In Studd, J. (ed.) *Progress in Obstetrics and Gynaecology*, Vol. 7. pp. 123–44. (Edinburgh, London, Melbourne, New York: Churchill Livingstone)

Ritchie, J.W.K. and Thompson, B. (1982). A critical review of amniocentesis in clinical practice. In Bonnar, J. (ed.) *Recent Advances in Obstetrics and Gynaecology*, no. 14, pp. 47–70. (Edinburgh, London, Melbourne, New York: Churchill Livingstone)

Robinson, H.P. (1977). The current status of sonar in obstetrics and gynaecology. In Stallworthy, J. and Bourne, G. (eds.) *Recent Advances in Obstetrics and Gynaecology*, no. 12 pp. 239–90. (Edinburgh, London, Melbourne, New York: Churchill Livingstone)

Rodeck, C.H. (1981). Fetoscopy. In Studd, J. (ed.) *Progress in Obstetrics and Gynaecology*, Vol. 1. pp. 79–91. (Edinburgh, London, Melbourne and New York: Churchill Livingstone)

Schulman, J.D. and Simpson, J.L. (1981). *Genetic Diseases in Pregnancy: Maternal Effects and Fetal Outcome*. (New York, London, Toronto, Sydney, San Francisco: Academic Press)

Warkany, J. (1971). *Congenital Malformations: Notes and Comments*. (Chicago: Year Book Medical Publishers)

Willius, F.A. (1948). Cardiac clinics: comments on historical aspects of certain congenital anomalies of heart and great vessels. *Proc. Staff Meet. Mayo Clinic*, **23**, 99

Microbiology

INTRODUCTION

The possibility that a micro-organism could cause disease, was speculated on by Varrow, a Roman author in the first century BC. Girolamo Fracastoro in 1546 theorized that 'disease seeds which could cause infection' were present in the atmosphere, but could not prove his assertion. A theory of 'spontaneous generation', which held that infection occurred in the absence of an infecting agent, was common.

With the discovery of the microscope came proof that organisms did exist. Antony van Leeuwenhoek was one of the first to report the existence of micro-organisms and parasites. Abbé Lazaro Spallanzani (1729–1799) of Pavia disproved the 'spontaneous generation' theory in 1767 when he showed that broth heated above boiling point and sealed directly afterwards would keep indefinitely without generating life (Spallanzani, 1767; 1776).

Theodor Schwann reported in 1877 that yeast cells were responsible for fermentation, and 7 years later Louis Pasteur of France proved that fermentation could only occur when air could reach a previously sterile substance. His work on the heating of wine to 55 °C, thereby eliminating the souring of wine which occurred secondary to infection with *Mycoderma aceti*, was later applied to beer and milk, and the process of 'Pasteurization' was born. Pasteur (q.v. in Biography) developed the germ theory of infection and reported that micro-organisms were responsible for disease, infection, fermentation and putrefaction. The term 'microbe' was first used by Sedillot in 1878 and Pasteur in 1882 suggested that the science of microbial life should be known as 'microbie' or 'microbiology' (Leadbetter and Poindexter, 1985).

Robert Koch firmly established the bacterial concept of disease, and published *The Etiology of Traumatic Infective Diseases* in 1879. He introduced the use of solid culture media for growing bacteria and was renowned for his laboratory techniques and methodology. His laboratory methods were quickly adopted and many micro-organisms, including streptococci, staphylococci and those responsible for gonorrhoea and syphilis, were soon identified. The first system of 'typing' streptococci was developed in 1897 and the modern system was established by J.H. Browne in 1919. About the same time Rebecca Lancefield developed a 'grouping system' which was combined with Griffith's system' in 1934. Griffith had previously carried out research on pneumococcal typing between 1920 and 1928 (McGrew, 1985).

MICROSCOPY

It was Witelo, a Polish scholar, who introduced the Greek and Arab achievements in the science of optics to Western Europe in the thirteenth century. John Peckham, an English theologian, mathematician and physicist, became interested in the science, and wrote a textbook on optics which remained standard for the next 300 years (McGrew, 1985).

By the end of the sixteenth century, lenses were available, and simple magnifying glasses had been in use for a long time. Hans Jansen and his son Zacharias, who were spectacle makers in the town of Middleberg in the Netherlands, introduced the compound microscope somewhere between 1590 and 1610. This first microscope was an adaptation of Galileo's telescope, and used a biconcave lens for the ocular with a biconvex lens for the objective, thereby producing a 60-fold magnification. The lenses were chromatic and without spherical correction. Hans Lippersky claimed priority in the introduction of the microscope, but does not get the credit. He was responsible however, for a binocular telescope (McGrew, 1985; Rhodes, 1988; Grunze and Spriggs, 1983).

Athanasius Kircher (1602–1680), a monk and professor of mathematics at Wurzburg, published a book on the properties of light in 1646. In the second edition of his book, published in 1671, he described a cylindrical instrument with a light aperture, mirror, and a lens mounted in a tube, which he used to magnify objects. This early form of microscope he called his *microspium parastaticum*. Robert Hooke, an English scientist of the Stuart Restoration and curator of the Royal Society, was an early microscopist, and in 1665 designed an instrument which could be adjusted to focus with a screw mechanism (Hooke, 1665).

The next major development was introduced by Antony van Leeuwenhoek (q.v. in Biographies) of Delft in Holland, who began his series of *Reports on Microscopy* to the Royal Society, London, in 1674. He developed the art of lens polishing and built a series of very effective instruments with lenses of short focal length. The simple lens microscope used by van Leeuwenhoek allowed magnification of around 275 times and made possible the first extensive research beyond the limits of the visible world (Figure 1). Another technical advance was introduced in 1712, when Hertel invented the illuminatory mirror for the microscope thus increasing and concentrating the available light, with consequent improvement in microscopic technique (Grunze and Spriggs, 1983).

The first achromatic lenses were made by Francis Beeldsnyder around 1791, but their resolving power was poor. Objects could appear 'fibrillar' or 'globular' under high magnification, due to diffraction haloes. The lens distortion was responsible for many inaccurate observations and much controversy in the eighteenth century. Joseph Jackson Lister, Lord Lister's father, designed a new microscope system which was almost free from spherical and chromatic abberations during the years 1826–1830 (Lister, 1829; Grunze and Spriggs, 1983). His design was a major development and was based on a formula which determined the optimum distance between the lenses in order to eliminate both abberations. Prior to that, the positioning of the lens was by a process of trial and error. Lister's discovery brought an end to the era of early microscopy and opened the way to modern applications of the instrument. His paper on microscopy was probably the most important ever published on the subject (McGrew, 1985).

The next improvements were the polarization microscope, which was designed by Talbot in 1834, and the construction of the oil immersion lens. Carl Zeiss established a mechanical workshop in Jena to serve university scientists in 1846, and Matthias Jacob Schleiden, a botanist, persuaded him to concentrate on assembling microscopes. Ernst Abbe later joined Zeiss and due to his expertise in lenses and optics their microscopes became world famous. They constructed the oil immersion lens in the early 1870s. Abbé, Zeiss and Schott, introduced the 'Abbe system of illumination' with iris shutter and focusable condenser, and produced the apochromatic lens in 1882 (Grunze and Spriggs, 1983).

The first significant change from light microscopy came in the twentieth century. The theoretical foundations for the electron microscope were laid down by Hans Busch of

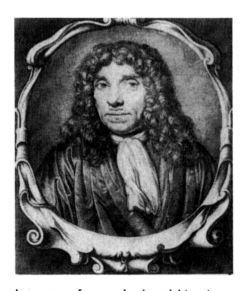

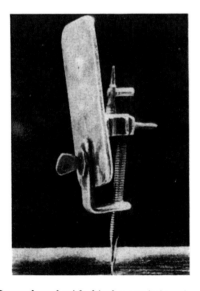

Figure 1 Antony van Leeuwenhoek and his microscope. Reproduced with kind permission from Museum Boerhaave, Leiden, The Netherlands

Germany in 1926, and 2 years later Max Knoll and Ernst Ruska of Berlin carried out experiments based on his research which led to the development of the first operational electron microscope, in 1933. A three-dimensional electron microscope, by which living cells could be viewed, was developed at the Massachusetts Institute of Technology under the direction of Alan Nelson in 1985. A tunnel effect microscope with magnification of a hundred million times, was perfected and introduced by Gerd Binning of West Germany and Heinrich Rohrer of Switzerland between 1980 and 1986. The instrument has produced images of DNA and viruses (Giscard d'Estaing, 1990).

EARLY MICROSCOPISTS AND CELL THEORY

Pierre Borel (1656) reported microscopic studies of many objects, during which he probably visualized the human red cell. Marcello Malpighi (1661), Professor at Bologna and Pisa, discovered blood capillaries thus providing the 'missing link' between arteries and veins, and may have referred to cells when he spoke of 'utricles, globules and saccules'. He is widely considered to be the founder of scientific microscopy and his method of examining the finer structures of organs ushered in a new era in medical history.

Robert Hooke (1665) published a summary of his observations and techniques in his *Micrographia*. He was the first microscopist to use the term 'cell'. The cells he saw were the distinct smallest units in elder pith and in cork (Figure 2). This observation of the basic unit of plant structure was not fully understood until much later when it was appreciated that the cell was the basic 'building block' of both plant and animal tissue. He was probably also the first to use thin sections of objects to reveal their microscopic structure.

Athanasius Kircher (1671) described his microscope and was able to see 'little worms' in the blood of plague victims; this report aroused an early interest in the 'germ cell' theory of disease. In the following year Nehemiah Grew (1672) published an illustrated volume on the microscopic anatomy of plants, and described minute 'utricles' or 'vesicles' which he had found in their substance.

Antony van Leeuwenhoek (1674) reported his discovery of protozoa by microscopy in a letter to the Royal Society of London. In other letters he detailed his discovery of bacteria and other microscopic organisms. With his pupil, Johann Ham (Hamen), he investigated semen and discovered spermatozoa in 1678 (Lammers, 1974). Three years later he was elected a foreign member of the Royal Society. Jan Swammerdam (1637–1680) examined insects and made detailed drawings of them in his *Biblia Naturae*. He was one

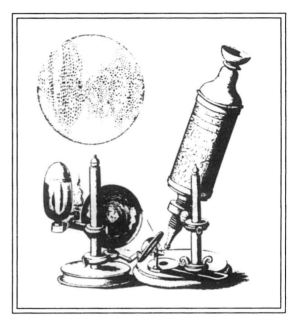

Figure 2 Robert Hooke's drawing of the microscopic structure of cork, and the microscope with which he observed it.

"I took a good clear piece of Cork, and with a Pen-knife sharpen'd as keen as a razor, I cut a piece of it off, and thereby left the surface of it exceeding smooth, then examining it very diligently with a Microscope, me thought I could perceive it to appear a little porous; but I could not so plainly distinguish them as to be sure that they were pores . . . I with the same sharp pen-knife cut off from the former smooth surface an exceeding thin piece of it, and placing it on a black Object plate . . . and casting the light on it with a deep plano-convex Glass, I could exceedingly plainly perceive it to be all perforated and porous, much like a Honey–comb, but that the pores of it were not regular . . . these pores, or *cells*, were not very deep, but consisted of a great many little Boxes, separated out of one continued long pore by certain Diaphrams . . . Nor is this kind of texture peculiar to Cork only; for upon examination with my Microscope, I have found that the pith of an Elder, or almost any other Tree, the inner pulp or pith of the Cany hollow stalks of several other Vegetables: as of Fennel, Carrets, Daucus, Bur-docks, Teasels, Fearn . . . & c. have much such a kind of Schematisme, as I have lately shewn that of Cork." Reproduced with kind permission from Macleod, A. G. (1973 and 1975). *Cytology. A Scope Publication*, p.13. (The Upjohn Company) of the first to visualize red blood corpuscles by microscopy. Swammerdam was acquainted with van Leeuwenhoek, and like him also reported his findings to the Royal Society (Grunze and Spriggs, 1983).

Caspar Friedrich Wolff was born in Berlin in 1734. He studied natural science and medicine there, and at Halle. At the age of 26 he produced his doctoral thesis *Theoria Generationis: 1. De Generatione Plantarum, 11. De Generatione Animalium,* (1759) and noted that all animal organs in their earliest inception were 'little globules' or cells, which may be distinguished under the microscope. He proved that the embryo was a 'simple' structure without organs, which later developed to become the complex fetal organism. Prior to that it was assumed that the embryo was a miniature edition of the fetus, with all its organs 'preformed' and present on a tiny scale.

Felix Fontana (1767) published his work on microscopy and this was translated into French in 1781. His drawings showed that cells contained 'a little body within', but he did not call it a nucleus.

Francois Xavier Bichat of Paris described (without microscopy) the different tissues from which organs were composed. He also used the microscope to define the histological changes produced in tissues by disease, and his findings were detailed in his book *Traité des Membranes* (1802/3). He later abandoned microscopy because he was aware that lens distortion introduced visual inaccuracies.

Charles Francois Brisseau de Mirbel observed in his *Traité d'Anatomie et de Physiologie Vegetales* (1802), that 'plants appear to be entirely composed of cells and of tubes all parts of which are continuous' and 3 years later, Lorenz Oken, hypothesized in *Die Zengung* that 'animals and plants are throughout nothing else than manifoldly divided or repeated vesicles'.

Karl E. von Baer (1827) during his research on the embryology of mammals, was the first to describe the human ovum. He concluded that 'every animal which springs from the coition of male and female is developed from an ovum . . . the male semen acts through the membrane of the ovum . . . '.

F.J.F. Meyen (1830) wrote in his work *Phytotomie,* that 'plant cells appear either singly . . . or they are united together . . . to constitute a more highly organized plant'. Two years later B.C. Dumortier reported his observations on cell division in algae in *Recherches Sur la Structure Comparée Developpement des Animaux et des Vegetaux* (1832).

Robert Brown (1833) in his report to the Linnean Society interpreted Felix Fontana's observation of 1767 correctly, and properly described for the first time the cell nucleus, 'this areola or nucleus of the cell as it perhaps might be termed . . . '. He found that the fine structures of plants and animals were remarkably similar.

The cell theory, which held that cells are the ultimate units of plant and animal life, was developed by Schleiden and Schwann. Mathias Jacob Schleiden (1838) published his *Beitrage Zur Phytogenese* explaining the derivation of plant tissues from cells. Theodor Schwann applied Schleiden's cell theory to animal tissues (1839) and emphasized that 'cells are organisms and entire animals, and plants are aggregates of these organisms arranged according to definite laws'. Karl Nageli (1842) saw and described chromosomes, but he did not appreciate their significance.

Friedrich Miescher (1869) took the initial steps in the biochemistry of the nucleus by separating 'nuclein' from cells in pus and salmon sperm. He found that nuclein was a combination of nucleic acid and protein. Eduard Strasburger (1875) described in great detail the process of cell division in plant cells. He termed the process 'mitosis' or 'karyokinesis' and named the various stages of the process. Walther Flemming (1876–1879) accurately described mitosis in animal cells and applied the term 'chromatin' to the deep-staining material in the nucleus. Paul Ehrlich (1882) developed staining methods for dry preparations.

PUERPERAL FEVER

The condition of puerperal fever was described by Hippocrates in his *Epidemics*, but there is little reference to it again until the mid-seventeenth century. The fever, which was due to sepsis, was often fatal. Epidemics of the disease appeared with the shift towards hospital birth, and the increasing involvement of doctors and medical students in the process. Although traditional midwives were probably no cleaner, mothers who delivered at home were not exposed to the infective environment of hospital wards, and therefore escaped sepsis and death (McGrew, 1985).

William Harvey (1578–1657), who was famed for his work on the circulation of the blood and his studies on embryology, also reported cases of high fever and offensive lochial discharge in women after normal delivery. In the same century other reports came from Thomas Willis (1662) who coined the phrase *Puerperarum Febris*, and also Richard Morton who used the phrase *Febris Puerpera* in 1691. The term 'puerperal fever' was finally introduced in 1716 by Edward Strother and replaced the previously used descriptive terms 'Childbed Fever' and 'Lying-In Fever'. Clinical and post-mortem studies of the disease were described by Paul Jacques Maloruin of the Hotel Dieu in 1746, and 8 years later Thomas Kirkland wrote his *Treatise on Childbed Fevers*. Thomas Denman (1733–1815) graduated from Aberdeen and his *Essay on Puerperal Fever* was published in London in 1768. He is credited with first suggesting that puerperal fever was contagious in nature, and was probably caused by attending physicians. This observation did not increase his popularity (Cianfrani, 1960).

Charles White (1728–1813) of Manchester, physician surgeon and male-midwife, believed that puerperal fever resulted from the absorption of 'infective matter' into the damaged uterine tissue, after delivery. He advocated the use of an adjustable tilting bed, and also a special chair, to enhance the flow of lochia. He also argued for the isolation of infected patients, good ventilation, and the necessity for cleanliness. In 1772 his book *A Treatise on the Management of Lying In Women, and The Means of Curing, but More Especially of Preventing the Principal Disorders to Which They are Liable* was published. The book later appeared in French and German editions, and also became popular in America (Graham, 1950).

Alexander Gordon (1752–1799) of Aberdeen wrote his *Treatise on the Epidemic, Puerperal Fever of Aberdeen* (1795). During his investigations he was influenced by the work of a Dr John Clarke who had related erysipelas to puerperal fever in lying-in women. Gordon realized that the disease occurred only after delivery and that an infecting agent entered through 'the wounds of childbirth'. He was aware that infection could be carried from one case to another, and advocated fumigation of rooms, bedding, and clothes worn by nursing and medical staff.

Robert Collins (1801–1896) who was Master of the Dublin Lying-In Hospital from 1826 to 1833, was faced with an epidemic outbreak of puerperal fever in 1829. He introduced a purification and intensive cleansing plan. Rooms were filled with chlorine gas and left for 48 hours. Chloride of lime in water was painted onto floors and woodwork, and each room was then washed out with fresh lime. Blankets and linen were cooked in a stove at 130 °F. All rooms were kept thoroughly ventilated and infected patients were isolated. His measures proved effective in combating the epidemic (O'Donel Browne, 1947).

Hugh Lenox Hodge (1796–1873) graduated from the University of Pennsylvania, and wrote several papers on puerperal fever including the *Observations Regarding Puerperal Fever* paper of 1833. He did not believe that puerperal fever was contagious (Hodge, 1852).

In America, Oliver Wendell Holmes (1809–1894) prepared a discussion paper for the Boston Society for Medical Improvement (1843), on the topic of the contagiousness of puerperal fever. He concluded that the disease was contagious and could be carried from patient to patient by physician and nurse alike. He advised doctors not to treat other patients if they had assisted at post-mortem examinations or treated a case of puerperal fever. Charles D. Meigs of Jefferson Medical School and Hugh L. Hodge disputed the conclusion and declared that doctors did not communicate the disease.

In Europe, Ignaz Philipp Semmelweiss (q.v. in Biography) (1818–1865) investigated the condition, and is the person most commonly associated with the exposition of its specific character (Sinclair, 1909). Semmelweiss was a Hungarian physician and surgeon who worked as an assistant obstetrician in Vienna's general hospital. A close friend, Jacob Kolletschka died from 'cadaver fever' soon after an infection accidentally contracted while dissecting a corpse. Semmelweis noted the similarity of symptoms in Kolletschka's case to those of puerperal fever victims.

Semmelweiss observed during his first year at the hospital that a maternity ward run by midwives had a lower maternal mortality rate compared to a separate ward which was served by medical students. He concluded that infection was carried by the medical students and doctors from the dissecting room where they had recently conducted dissections and post-mortem examinations. In 1847 he introduced a handwashing routine using liquid chlorate, for which he later substituted chlorinated lime. Those who had recently worked with cadavers were instructed thoroughly to wash their hands with soap and water, and then rewash using 'chlorina liquida', before examining postnatal patients. A rapid drop in mortality occurred.

Although Semmelweiss successfully reduced the maternal mortality due to puerperal sepsis, his theories were not universally popular, and he was attacked by leading members of the profession.

Undaunted, Semmelweiss published his major work on the disease in 1861. Soon afterwards he developed depression with periods of excitement and in 1865 he was admitted to a Viennese mental hospital. It is said that prior to admission he sustained a cut to his right hand during gynaecological surgery, and became a victim himself of the same infection which he had identified with puerperal fever, and died soon afterwards (Venzmer, 1972).

Louis Pasteur (1822–1895) was a major contributor to the knowledge of puerperal pyrexia. He believed that specific microbes caused specific diseases and that infection did not occur spontaneously. He discovered the streptococcus (1860;1879) and demonstrated that (haemolytic) streptococcus was the cause of puerperal infection (Cianfrani, 1960). The treatment of puerperal fever was primarily by prevention, and no effective treatment was available until the introduction of antibiotics. The maternal mortality and incidence of the disease fell significantly during the 1930s, and remained at a low rate thereafter (Lyons and Petrucelli, 1978, McGrew, 1985).

ANTISEPTICS

The term antiseptic was first used by a Mr Place who wrote on *Problems of the Plague* in 1721. However, resins, balsams, gums and spices, with antiseptic properties were used to arrest decomposition in ancient Egypt and Greece. Turpentine, frankincense and myrrh were used in the middle ages. Styrax and benzoin were popularly used in wound dressings, as were wine and vinegar. Auguste Nelaton introduced alcohol soaks to disinfect wounds in the mid-nineteenth century. Iodine was discovered by Bernard Courtois in 1811, and the chemical became popular for treatment of wounds and as a finger dip for surgeons. Ignaz Semmelweiss used carbolic acid to good effect in 1847 (McGrew, 1985).

The name of Joseph Lister (q.v. in Biography) (1827–1912) is associated with a major breakthrough in antiseptic therapy. Although he did not invent antisepsis he developed a successful method of achieving it. Joseph Lister graduated from the University of London and became Professor of Surgery at the University of Glasgow. He observed that almost half of all surgical cases treated by amputation, died from infection. He also found that simple fractures healed but compound fractures were nearly always fatal. Lister theorized that organisms in the air caused putrefaction in the wound which led to severe illness with death. He evolved his treatment methods with that theory in mind. (Lyons and Petrucelli, 1978: Rhodes, 1985). Lister covered all wounds of compound fractures with a dressing soaked in carbolic acid. As a result the wounds did not become infected. In 1867 Lister devised an 'antiseptic curtain' of carbolic acid spray which he used when operating. This proved to be a major success, although he abandoned it himself in 1880. Operating room techniques were improved from then on and linens were regularly cleaned. The area to be operated on, or the diseased tissue, was sprayed with carbolic acid. Rubber gloves were first introduced by William Halsted in the early twentieth century to protect the hands of his operating room nurse, whom he later married (Lyons and Petrucelli, 1978). Masks were introduced at a later date. Robert Koch (1843–1910) found that chemical sterilization of instruments was less effective than heat, and this observation led to the introduction of heat sterilizing units. Chemotherapy began with the work of Paul Ehrlich (1854–1915), who in 1907 discovered that the dye known as 'trypan red' when injected into the blood of animals infected with trypanosomes destroyed the organisms. He then prepared an arsenical salvarsan or '606' which was the first effective treatment for syphilis (Cowen and Helfand, 1990). Later, neo-salvarsan or 914 was an improvement.

TUBERCULOSIS

This disease was known as 'consumption' until 1839 when J.L. Schoenlein, Professor of Medicine at Zurich, introduced the term tuberculosis. The condition had been described in the ancient world and the word 'phthisis' was coined by the Greeks. During the middle ages, a tuberculous infection of lymph nodes of the neck called 'scrofula' was common and 'the King's touch' was a popular ritual remedy to relieve it. The Parisian physician Jean Fernel carried out post-mortem studies on 'consumption' victims in the sixteenth century and identified the disease in the chest cavity.

It was estimated that 20% of all deaths from disease at that time were due to tuberculosis. By the mid-1750s the incidence of the disease was rising and in the early 1800s the Charité Hospital in Paris reported that tuberculosis was the cause of over a third of their deaths. *Mycobacterium tuberculosis*, the bacterial agent responsible, was isolated by Robert Koch in 1882.

No treatment was available, but a 'sanitarium movement' advocating rest, sunshine and good nutrition began in the 1850s and was popular until the Second World War. Surgical treatment, by inducing lung collapse, became popular in the 1920s and was extensively used for 30 years. Calmette and Guerin produced a strain of *M. tuberculosis* named Bacillus Calmette–Guerin (BCG) in 1921. A vaccine was introduced, which by 1928 had become widely available. Chemotherapy in the form of streptomycin was introduced by Selman A. Waksman (1944) of Rutgers University. Para-amino salicylic acid (PAS) was developed by Jorgen Lehmann of Sweden between 1946 and 1948, and isoniazid was isolated in 1950 and 1951 in Germany and the USA (McGrew, 1985).

Tuberculosis affected the genital tract, but until the mid-1950s the only form of treatments available were vitamin D, radiotherapy, heliotherapy and surgery. The reproductive tract could be affected by miliary, ulcerative, papillary or interstitial forms of the disease. Tuberculosis of the vagina was the rarest form while that of the Fallopian tubes accounted for 90% of all tuberculous lesions of the genital tract. The endometrium was infected on a cyclical basis by spread from the oviducts. Evidence of the disease was found in 1–6% of endometrial biopsies obtained from women complaining of sterility. Tuberculosis was a rare form of infection or cause of sterility in the developed countries in the late 1980s but was still common in Third World countries. Tuberculous peritonitis occurred from blood or lymph spread from a distant or nearby focus, and also by direct spread from an intestinal or tubal lesion. It presented in miliary, ascitic, or fibroplastic forms. The cure rate was low (Browne, 1950).

Pulmonary tuberculosis was the most frequent cause of death among women of childbearing age in the 1940s. Some improvement in the condition occurred during pregnancy and it was often quoted that Hippocrates believed that pregnancy was the best cure for 'phthisis' (Bamforth, 1950; Cohen, 1950).

VENEREAL AND SEXUALLY TRANSMITTED DISEASES

The word venereal is derived from the Latin, *venerus* - Venus, Veneris, the Goddess of love; connected with the Latin *venerari*, to worship. Venereal or sexually transmitted diseases, were

recorded for thousands of years. The most common forms were gonorrhoea and syphilis.

The ancient Egyptians were aware of genital infection and the Kahun Papyrus c.1850 BC mentioned itching of the vulva, medication for putrefaction of the womb, and the 'roast meat' smell of vulval inflammation (Ricci, 1943). A word that can be translated as 'inflammation' was used several times in the Smith Papyrus, a scroll written about 1550–1700 BC but possibly derived from an original that was perhaps a thousand years older. The word reads *schememet* and conveys the idea of 'hot thing'. The Hearst Papyrus consisted of 204 sections which referred to genito-urinary diseases in women.

Prostitution existed in those days and to judge by the recorded symptomatology Bartholinitis, vulvitis, vaginitis and salpingitis were recorded. Therapy was by local application of drugs, by rubbing, insertion of medicated tampons, or fumigations of medicinal herbs. Vaginal injection with medicated fluids was also common practice. Some cities such as Naucratis owed their wealth and fame to the beauty of their courtesans (Sanger, 1895).

The Ebers Papyrus c.1550 BC had several sections devoted to diseases of the female genitalia. Remedies were presribed for pustular eruptions of the vulva and vagina and to disperse inflammation of those parts. Watery discharges were noted, and pessaries of impregnated linen were used in treatment. Garlic and the powdered horn of a cow in solution were used to protect against vaginal diseases. If inflammation developed, the irrigating fluid was altered to bile of a cow, cassia and oil. Prescriptions for leucorrhoea in virgins were noted (McKay, 1901), and dried liver of swallow was a specific remedy.

The earliest direct references to a disease that may have been gonorrhoea probably occur in the Bible. Leviticus 15 contains the following passage 'when any man hath a running issue out of his flesh, because of his issue he is unclean'. Moses may have recognized that the disease was transmitted by sexual contact, as he advised washing the genitals after sexual intercourse. Numbers 31 describes how a victorious Israelite army was quarantined for 7 days on their return from a war with the Midianites, and every Midianite woman prisoner who was a possible source of genital infection was killed. There is also reference in Deuteronomy 24:1 'when a man hath taken a wife and married her, and it comes to pass that she finds no favour in his eyes because he hath found some uncleanness in her, then let him write her a bill of divorcement'. In Psalm 38, King David lamented that his loins were filled with 'a loathsome disease' and in Numbers the children of Israel, 'were to put out of the camp every leper, and every one that hath an issue'.

Ancient Chinese and Japanese sources mentioned venereal disease, and in Hindu mythology the God Shiva was described as suffering a disease of the genitals, which may have been gonorrhoea. There were also references in the Talmud to a sexual discharge which may have been gonorrhoea. In some instances the issue or discharge, may have referred to spermatorrhoea. The Hippocratic writers of the fifth century BC referred to 'strangury', or urethral blockage. Hippocrates himself was aware of pelvic abscess and pyometra (McKay, 1901). In Greek medicine inflammation was called *phlegmone* which meant 'the burning thing'.

Cornelius Celsus, the Roman writer (27 BC–AD 50), gave an account of balanitis and phymosis, and mentioned a purulent urethral discharge. He described inflammation of the testicle and genital warts. Celsus also described rabies and may have been the first to use the term 'virus', which at that time was used to mean venom or poison (Waterson and Wilkinson, 1978). He also provided a clinical definition of inflammation *Rubor et Tumour cum Calore et Dolore*- redness and swelling with heat and pain which were later called the 'cardinal signs' of inflammation.

Women who could not have intercourse, either on account of menstruation or due to disease of the genitals, were termed *ancunulentae*. They prayed to Juno Gluonia, and used the 'Aster Atticus', which was a remedy for diseases of the groin. The Romans called this venereal disease *Bubonium*, and from that came the origin of our term 'bubo'.

Gonorrhoea

Soranus of Ephesus (q.v. in Biographies) (AD 99–138) described rectal examination to discriminate between uterine and rectal inflammation, and treatment for inflammation of the vagina and uterus (Graham, 1950). Galen (AD 131–201) was the first to use the term 'gonorrhoea' and is said to have used 'theriac' for inflammation. In the sixth century AD Aetius described *thymus* of the genital organs and detailed the treatment of pelvic abscess (McKay, 1901). He also recounted his discovery of the cystic irregularities of the cervix which were later called the Nabothian follicles.

In the ninth and tenth centuries gonorrhoea, cystitis and inflammation of the testicle were described by Rhazes (AD 852), Mesue (AD 904) and the Persian Ali Abbas (AD 980) (McKay, 1901).

In England gonorrhoea was officially recognized by a 'London Act of 1161' which forbade brothel keepers to house 'women suffering from the perilous infirmity of burning' and in 1162 the Bishop of Winchester directed that 'no stew holder keep no woman within his house that hath any sickness of brenning (burning)'. The English disease of burning, was known in France as 'la chaude pisse' (hot piss) and the word 'clap' was first coupled with the 'burning disease' in a manuscript by John of Arderne in 1378. He and Henri de Mondeville provided the first detailed diagnostic picture of the disease. Gonorrhoea and 'soft chancre' were the dominant venereal diseases in Europe until 1493 when the syphilis epidemic began (McGrew, 1985).

Lazarus Riverius (1589–1655) described 'the woman's flux' or *flour albus* and went on to describe that that of gonorrhoea was of thicker consistency and whiter colour. However, if the discharge was 'virulent', it was the cause of 'sharpness' of urine, and ulcers of the 'privi parts'. It was commonly believed at the time that neglected leucorrhoea led to the condition of gonorrhoea, which when it became chronic led to a syphilitic infection (Cianfrani, 1960). Regnier de Graaf (1641–1673) distinguished between gonorrhoea and leucorrhoea by the presence of purulent discharges from the paraurethral ducts. In 1713 William Cockburn wrote *The Symptoms, Nature, Cause and Cure of a Gonorrhea* and believed that gonorrhoea and syphilis, (also called lues), were two separate entities. Jean Astruc (q.v. in Biographies) (1684–1766) wrote on venereal infection and inflammatory diseases of the adnexae. He also described the chancre, secondary lesions and contagiousness of syphilis.

In 1793 Dr Benjamin Bell argued that gonorrhoea and syphilis were separate infections, clearly distinct in their incubation periods and clinical appearance. Philippe Ricord, working at L'Hôpital du Midi, in Paris, experimented with both diseases in 1838 and also concluded that they were separate. In 1864 the British Government passed a Contagious Diseases Act which attempted to protect military personnel from 'venereal disease, including gonorrhoea'. Women suspected of spreading venereal diseases could be compelled to wear yellow clothes for identification. Five years later a Mrs Josephine Butler formed the Ladies

National Association, and they campaigned against the Diseases Act. It was eventually repealed in 1886.

During the years 1841–1872 T. Gaillard Thomas (1831–1903) published his works on pelvic infection (Cianfrani, 1960) and a contemporary, Emile Noeggerath (1827–1895) who emigrated from Bonn to New York, published observations on gonorrhoea (1872) and documented its relationship to sterility. He advocated treatment of both partners. Noeggerath was a co-founder of the American Gynecological Society, and the *American Journal of Obstetrics.*

The relationship between gonorrhoea and pelvic sepsis was first demonstrated by Bernutz and Goupil (1857). The gonococcus was discovered by the Breslau bacteriologist Albert Neisser (1879), and the causal agent of syphilis was found 26 years later. Ernst Hallier (1869) had described intra- and extracellular cocci in gonorrhoeal pus prior to Neisser, but his observation failed to attract the attention of the medical world. Lawson Tait (1845–1899) introduced a surgical procedure to remove 'pus tubes'. Incision with drainage by colpotomy was used for pelvic abscess. Leo Leistikow (1882) successfully isolated *Neisseria gonorrhoeae* and 3 years later Bumm (1885) successfully cultivated the *Neisseria* organism. No effective cure for gonorrhoea was found until 1937 when sulphonamides became available. Sulpha resistance soon occurred but penicillin, to which the organism was sensitive, became available around the same time.

Syphilis

The history of syphilis dates from about 1493. In that year Colombus and his men returned from their voyage of discovery to the Americas. One theory held that they carried the disease which they had contracted there back to Europe. A second theory argued that syphilis was a form of disease called Yaws which was common in the tropics and which adapted to the colder climate of Europe by invading warm moist areas of the body. Yaws itself slowly died out in the early seventeenth century. Alternatively syphilis could have existed in a mild form for centuries and suddenly developed a new virulence.

The first major appearance of syphilis was during the siege of Naples in 1495. The invading army of Charles VIII of France included many European mercenaries. On the opposing side were the Holy League and Spanish forces. Both sides were so infected by 'The Indian Disease' (syphilis) that the campaign was abandoned, and Charles' troops dispersed across Europe, carrying infection with them. Syphilis reached Paris by 1496, London by 1497, and within the next few years had spread to India and China. A Spanish physician Rodrigo Ruiz de Isla wrote about the disease in his *Treatise on the Serpentine Malady* in the early 1500s and claimed that he had treated victims of the syphilis epidemic in Barcelona during 1493 (McGrew, 1985).

A Spanish physician Francesco Lopez de Villalobos wrote a poem in Latin at Salamanca in 1498 concerning syphilis which he called *Las buvas*, but which was called the 'French Pockes' by his editor. He described a sore (chancre) of the genitals and the pestilence which he believed was punishment for a dissolute life.

The French called syphilis 'the Italian Disease', the English and Germans called it 'the French Pockes'. In Japan it was described as 'the Portuguese sickness'. Syphilis was also known as 'the Great Pockes', and later, 'the Pox'. Between 1494 and 1516 syphilis was reported to begin its spread with a small genital ulcer, followed by a body rash, and then the many other signs which affected all parts of the body and led to early death. The new disease was at its most virulent during the first hundred years, when it was of epidemic proportions. Tens of thousands died, but by the early seventeenth century it had become a more chronic illness, with lower mortality rates.

The name syphilis arose from a poem written in 1530 by an Italian physician Girolamo Fracastoro (1484–1553) who was born in Verona and graduated from Padua. His poem *Syphilis Sive de Morbo Gallico* was published in Venice about 1530. Syphilus was the hero of the legend, and was a Greek shepherd. He offended the god Apollo and was struck down by a terrible disease. The symptoms were those of the syphilis epidemic which was then rampant throughout Europe. Fracastoro borrowed the name Syphilus from Ovid. The birth place of Niobe, the daughter of Tantalus and wife of the Theban King, Amphion, was a hill called Sipylus near Magnesia. Niobe's second son Sipylus, was named after the hill. Fracastoro altered the name and called the shepherd of his poem Syphilus. The disease, from which he was the first to suffer, was called syphilis. Fracastoro later wrote a work in three volumes entitled *De Syphilide Sive de Morbo Gallico* (About Syphilis or the French Sickness) (Venzmer, 1972).

In 1495, Emperor Maximilian I of the Holy Roman Empire wrote 'An Edict Against Blasphemers', and warned against the *Posen Plattern* or 'Evil Pocks', which he said was heaven's punishment on blasphemers. Medical inspection of prostitutes began in 1496, with expulsion of those who were infected. The only forms of treatment available were prayer or isolation. Saint Denis, the patron saint of Paris, was the favoured saint of syphilitics. In 1496 Georgio Sommariva, a Veronese physician, used mercury to treat syphilis and it was later stated that 'a night with Venus meant a lifetime with mercury'. Mercury could be rubbed in, taken by mouth, or administered by fumigation. It was effective but poisonous, and caused symptoms as bad as the disease. Its effects were known as 'salivation', or the 'salivary cure', and the heavy flow of saliva induced by the mercury was thought to wash out the syphilitic poison. A substance called guaiacum, which was grown in the West Indies, was a popular form of treatment for a time, and it is said that a banking house, the Augsburg Fuggers, made a fortune from shipping the substance to Europe.

In 1579 the London surgeon William Clowes reported that seldom fewer than 15 out of every 20 patients admitted to St Bartholomew's Hospital, suffered from syphilis (Newman, 1988). Fallopius in his *de Morbo Gallico*, published posthumously in 1563, wrote the first description of the condom which he claimed was a prophylactic device against the disease; and the chapter introducing it was entitled 'On Preservation from French Caries (Syphilis)' (Graham, 1950).

In 1786 John Hunter wrote on venereal disease and is known to have experimented with gonorrhoeal pus to determine whether gonorrhoea and syphilis were separate entities (Lyons and Petrucelli, 1978). In 1833 Ehrenberg described a large flexible motile organism in water which he called 'spirochaetae', and Edwin Klebs was the first to see spirochaetal bodies in syphilitic material in the year 1875 (Klebs, 1878).

In 1889 Felix Bazzer used bismuth which he found could kill spirochaetes, and about the same time an Irish physician William Wallace introduced potassium iodide as a treatment for some forms of late syphilis (Waugh, 1990).

In 1904 Paul Ehrlich (q.v. in Biographies) of Frankfurt developed the arsenic-based compound 606 (salvarsan) to treat syphilis, and arsenic compounds soon replaced mercury. In the following year two Germans, Dr Fritz Schaudin and Dr Erich Hoffmann (1905), discovered *Treponema pallidum*, the causative organism of the disease. August von Wassermann and associates developed a basic blood test for syphilis in 1906 (Thomas, 1983). Three years later Dr Paul Ehrlich of Germany discovered arsphenamine. The arsenical preparations were highly effective although a course of treatment could last for up to 2 years.

Penicillin was isolated by Alexander Fleming (later Sir) of St Mary's Hospital, London in 1928 (Fleming, 1929), and clinical testing began in 1941. John F. Mahony of New York used the antibiotic, which soon became the standard treatment for syphilis. Barrier methods of contraception were found to be effective in controlling spread of the disease.

The introduction of penicillin had a dramatic effect and it appeared that both syphilis and gonorrhoea would be eradicated. However, by the early 1950s, the world-wide drop of infection rates had ceased. In 1954 the World Health Organization reported that there were 20 million syphilitics in the world and by 1967 the estimate was about 50 million. In the early 1960s it was estimated that gonorrhoea effected at least 60 million people world-wide, and by the early 1970s the number had doubled. The growing number of venereal disease victims was caused by escalating populations world-wide, increased opportunity of travel, and changes in attitudes to sexual activity. In 1961 the US Public Health Department established a task force whose aim was to eradicate syphilis from the United States.

In a recent paper Clarke (1989) reported that sexually transmitted diseases were the commonest group of infectious diseases in the UK. The numbers had tripled compared with 15 years previously. Syphilis was no longer a major problem, but gonorrhoea and non-specific chlamydial infections were the commonest conditions seen. The condition of non-specific urethritis tripled in incidence between 1950 and 1970. The proportion of young people (age 15–19 years) who had had intercourse, increased from 16% in 1964, to 51% in the same age group in 1974 (Schofield, 1965; Farrell, 1978). Women between 15 and 39 years had a 1% incidence of pelvic inflammatory disease (Westrom, 1980). By 1990 27% of all babies born in the UK were born out of wedlock – a reflection on the changing attitudes of the era.

Viral diseases

The term virology has only recently come into common use. The first text book and journal on the subject were published in 1953 and 1955 respectively (Waterson and Wilkinson, 1978). However, the term virus, and various illnesses attributed to this pathogenic agent, had been recognized for centuries. The term itself is derived from the Latin for venom, but an alternative meaning was 'slimy liquid', a reference to saliva which transmitted rabies from infected dogs. Rabies was described by Aristotle, who noted that it was fatal to the animal but not necessarily to humans. Cornelius Celsus wrote a chapter on rabies in which he stated that 'if the dog was rabid, the virus must be drawn out with a cupping glass'. Over the following years the term virus was used to mean poison or venom. Its association with infection was gradually recognized during the eighteenth and nineteenth centuries (Waterson and Wilkinson, 1978).

The acquired immune deficiency syndrome

The aetiologic agent associated with the acquired immune deficiency syndrome (AIDS) was first discovered in 1983, and has been known by a variety of names since then (Gallo *et al.*, 1983; Barré-Sinoussi *et al.*, 1983). In 1986 The International Committee for the Taxonomy of Viruses suggested the name human immunodeficiency virus (HIV). AIDS was first recognized in Los Angeles and New York in 1981 with an outbreak of pneumocystis carinii and Kaposi's sarcoma in previously fit young homosexual men (Center for Disease Control, 1981). Prior to that, pneumocystis carinii was confined to immuno-compromised patients and Kaposi's sarcoma was usually found in those of Jewish or Mediterranean origin. The cases occurred in special risk groups, suggesting that infection occurred from a blood or serum borne infection (Farthing *et al.*, 1986). The syndrome was later found to be part of a spectrum of disease caused by HIV. The origin of the retrovirus HIV is uncertain, but from analysis of stored sera, HIV is known to have first appeared in the USA and Western Europe in 1978, and in Central Africa about 1972.

At least 5–20% of people infected with HIV progress to AIDS; about 25% develop persistent generalized lymphadenopathy; the remainder are either asymptomatic, or have minor lymphadenopathy; or develop minor opportunistic infections such as oral candidiasis and/or cytopaenias, such as thrombocytopaenia. Persistent lymphadenopathy was first described by Mildvan *et al.* (1982). A prodromal syndrome or AIDS-related complex (ARC) was described which

progressed to AIDS in 77% of cases, at a mean interval of 4 months (Mathur-Wagh and Mildvan, 1984). Oral candidiasis was found to be a good clinical indication of immunosuppression.

AIDS was associated with a greatly increased incidence of malignant tumours particularly Kaposi's sarcoma. That tumour was first described in 1872 by Moritz Kaposi, a Hungarian dermatologist. Its occurrence in epidemic fashion among homosexual and bisexual males, was recognized from 1981. In the early 1980s a dramatic rise in the incidence of non-Hodgkin's lymphoma was also found in young homosexual men (Baughan and Phillips, 1987). AIDS was still uncommon in the UK in 1986 with only 328 cases being notified by March of that year.

An important investigation was carried out in the USA where a cohort of 6705 men was recruited from the Municipal Sexually Transmitted Disease Clinic of San Francisco. They were included in a study of the incidence and prevalence of sexually transmitted hepatitis B from 1978 to 1980 but the study continued on. Testing for HIV-1 antibodies was added to the investigations of the members of the study from 1984. By December 1989, 75% of the cohort members were infected with HIV-1, and 22% of the total group developed AIDS (Rutherford *et al.*, 1990). The Centers for Disease Control (1987) revised the case definition for AIDS.

The risk of progression from HIV-1 infection to AIDS was prospectively studied in cohorts of the following high-risk groups: homosexual and bisexual men; parenteral drug users; transfusion recipients; haemophiliacs; and 'vertically infected' (transplacental or at delivery) infants.

Although women were not regarded initally as a high-risk group, an increasing number were infected by heterosexual contact or drug taking. Cervical abnormalities were found to be common in women infected with HIV (Bradbeer, 1987; Byrne *et al.*, 1988).

At first it seemed as though AIDS occurred after a lengthy incubation of the virus, affecting mainly homosexuals; and this was particularly so in homosexual communities in California and later in New York. However, by the late 1980s it was quite clear that world-wide the most common cause of infection was unprotected vaginal intercourse and that increasingly large numbers of women were being infected and were infecting their casual or permanent partners with this deadly virus. Pneumocystis carinii pneumonia outbreaks still occur in HIV infections and it is the greatest killer of people infected with AIDS, who of course have insufficient immunological protection, not only for the virus causing the disease, but for other opportunistic infections. Many of these infections are acquired before the appearance of HIV disease and several, such as salmonellosis, herpes simplex and cytomegalovirus colitis were recognized in the 1970s and 1980s, not only in homosexuals but in their partners appearing in gynaecological clinics.

A major cause for concern is the plight of the pregnant AIDS victim. Perinatal transmission of HIV occurs in 15–33% of their pregnancies (Webster and Johnson, 1990), but there is no evidence that babies born in 'the West' are at increased risk of prematurity or growth retardation (John et al, 1988).

The European Collaborative Study (ECS) (1988; 1991) reported their findings of 600 children born to HIV-infected mothers. The children were examined at birth, then every 3 months up to 18 months of age, and every 6 months thereafter. When last reviewed, 64 children were judged to be HIV-infected, while 343 had lost antibody and were presumed uninfected. An estimated 83% of the infected children showed laboratory or clinical features of disease by 6 months of age; by 12 months 26% had AIDS; and 17% had died of an HIV-related disease. The vertical transmission rate was 12.9%. The mode of vertical transmission remained unknown, but early onset of clinical and immunological features pointed to intrauterine transmission, rather than transmission at delivery. There was also evidence that infection was transmitted in the breast milk of mothers who sero-converted after the birth (Oxtoby, 1989).

The commonly used laboratory tests to diagnose AIDS infection were summarized by Schochetman (1990) and included; the enzyme-linked immunosorbent assay; the Western blot assay; detection of HIV antigen; and detection of viral DNA and RNA from cells of infected persons.

Hepatitis B

The development of jaundice in the wives of two men who themselves had just recovered from the illness was discovered by Bradley (1946). The first observations that hepatitis B was common in male homosexuals were reported in 1970 and Hersh et al. (1971) reported six cases of heterosexual transmission. Heathcote and Sherlock (1973) estimated that a quarter of hepatitis B patients acquired the disease at heterosexual coitus. Mazzur

(1973) demonstrated viral antigen in menstrual blood and Darani and Gerker (1974) demonstrated its presence in vaginal secretions. The hepatitis B virus was also discovered in seminal fluid (Heathcote et al., 1974). The hepatitis B hepatotrophic DNA virus is spread by blood contamination and is common among drug addicts. It has also been described in patients following kidney dialysis and blood transfusion. A number of gynaecologists themselves have become infected after acquiring small injuries while operating or administering injections.

Wart virus

Genital warts were a recognized entity in the ancient world. They were a known form of hetero- and homosexual venereal disease. The term condyloma acuminatum, derives from the Greek, kondulos, a knuckle and the Latin, acuminare, to make pointed. Alternative terms were ficus and thymus (Butler and Stanbridge, 1984). While it was known that warts were infectious, Jadassohn (1896) first produced them in the human by experimental inoculation. In this century, Wile and Kingery (1919) produced warts by intracutaneous inoculation of human beings with a Berkefeld filtrate of a suspension of ground-up wart material. Findlay (1930) noted that venereal warts or condyloma acuminata were infective, apparently caused by a virus, and occasionally became cancerous. Further evidence for viral aetiology was noted by Strauss et al. (1949), who documented crystalline virus-like particles which they obtained from aqueous extracts of skin wart tissue. Particles resembling human papillomavirus (HPV) were discovered in genital wart material by Von Melczer (1965).

Oriel and Almeida (1970) demonstrated virus particles in human genital warts. Their similarity to common skin warts was noted but no antigenic cross-reactivity was found to occur between the two types. The wart virus was assigned to the papovavirus family. Four types of HPV – types 6, 11, 16 and 18, were found to account for almost all HPV of anogenital lesions (Gismann et al., 1983; Ferenczy et al., 1985). The possible malignant potential of vulval condyloma acuminata was found by Charlewood and Shippel (1953).

Ayre (1949) first noted the cytological cellular changes caused by HPV and suggested a link with neoplasia. The term 'koilocytotic atypia' was introduced by Koss and Durfee (1956) who pointed out that these cell patterns were associated with precancer. Meisels and Fortin (1976) described dyskaryotic changes in cytological samples from the cervix and vagina, in association with condyloma acuminatum. They observed 'balloon cells' with a perinuclear halo. Meisels *et al.* (1981) noted the similarity between HPV-induced epithelial abnormality and that of intraepithelial neoplasia. The Center for Disease Control USA (1983) reported a 500% increase in the incidence of genital warts in the previous 15 years.

Herpes genitalis

Herpes genitalis was described by Astruc and Morbis (1736) but isolation of herpes virus from herpetic vulvo-vaginitis had to await until this century and the work of Slavin and Gavett (1946). Nahmias and colleagues discovered the two types of herpes simplex virus (HSV), types 1 and 2, and found that the latter was more responsible for genital infection (Nahmias *et al.*, 1967; Nahmias and Dowdle, 1968). Rawls *et al.* (1971) and Duenas *et al.* (1971) demonstrated that the infection was sexually transmitted. Nahmias *et al.* (1967; 1971) investigated the effect of herpes neonatorum following delivery through an infected birth canal and discovered that of those infants who were infected, 50% died and the remainder had residual neurological deficit. Naib *et al.* (1972) first proposed an association between HSV type 2 and carcinoma of the cervix.

Cytomegalovirus

This DNA virus was found to be a cause of widespread infection, causing 0.3–2.4% of intrauterine infections. The majority of infants were asymptomatic. Diosi *et al.* (1969) found that 5–10% of those shedding virus at birth were symptomatically infected. The illness was fatal in 20%. Fifteen per cent of the survivors developed major sequelae (Griffiths, 1991). Maternal immunity did not appear to prevent the infection nor protect against its harmful sequelae. Although there was no obvious genital lesion, Wilmott (1975) isolated cytomegalovirus from the cervices of almost 7% of women in a venereal disease clinic.

Molluscum contagiosum

Bateman (1814) first described molluscum contagiosum and Juliusberg (1905) determined that the disease was caused by a virus. A circulating antibody to the virus was demonstrated by Epstein *et al.* (1963).

Rubella

W.G. Maton (1815) described rubella infection and noted that its symptoms were slight.

Chlamydia trachomatis

Chlamydia trachomatis was first described by Halberstaedter and Prowazek (1907). The organism was found to be implicated in a large number of sexually tramsmitted disease processes and caused lymphogranuloma venereum, a disease which was described in the eighteenth century by John Hunter. Lindner (1911) documented the association of chlamydial cervical infection and non-gonococcal urethritis. Thygeson and Mengert (1936) noted its relationship to ophthalmia neonatorum.

Bacterial vaginosis (Gardnerella vaginalis) and Mobiluncus

This entity was defined by Gardner and Dukes (1954; 1955), who reported their discovery of non-specific vaginitis due to a single facultative organism which they termed haemophilus vaginalis in 1955. The term corynebacterium was proposed for the same organism by La Page (1961). However, Greenwood and Pickett (1980) officially named the organism *Gardnerella vaginalis* in honour of its principal discoverer. Gardner and Dukes described 'clue cells' on wet smear examination from patients with bacterial vaginosis. Pus cells were few and lactobacilli were lacking. Chen *et al.* (1979) identified amines in the discharge which they felt contributed to the characteristic 'fishy' odour. An associated organism, in the form of small motile anaerobic rods, was discovered by Curtis (1913). His observation went unheeded, but Durieux and Dublanchet (1980) rediscovered the organisms which were called 'mobiluncus', a term introduced by Spiegel and Roberts (1984). Mardh *et al.* (1984) showed that bacterial vaginosis occurred only when both organisms were present.

Trichomonas vaginalis

Trichomoniasis was first described by Donné (1836) (Figure 3) when he reported 'animalcules' in infected discharges from the genital tracts of both men and women. Ehrenberg *et al.* (1838) suggested the term *Trichomonas vaginalis*. Hoehne (1916) described the characteristic vaginal disease, with the presence of trichomonads. Karnaky (1937)

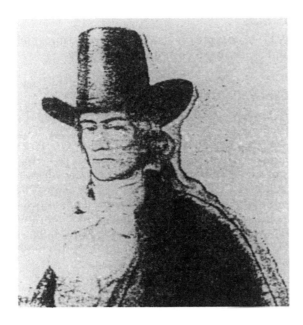

Figure 3 Alfred Donné (1801–1878) originally thought that the *Trichomonas* he found and described in Paris in 1836 was 'the pernicious agent' in gonorrhoea. He was the first to describe living organisms in pathological conditions. Reproduced with kind permission from Thornburn, A. L. (1974). J. Vener. Dis., **50**, 377

documented the clinical and pathologic findings in 4000 cases. Stuart (1944) introduced a transport medium for carriage of swabs taken from possible *T. vaginalis* discharges. Trussell and Plass (1940) isolated *T. vaginalis* in pure culture.

Bacterial infection

The story of gonorrhoea and syphilis is already told, but a new disease called granuloma inguinale was documented by McLeod (1882). Charles Donovan (1905) described the causative organism, *Calymmatobacterium granulomatis* which until recently was referred to as *Donovania granulomatis*. This infection was found to be the most prevalent sexually transmitted disease in developing countries.

Chancroid was first described by Ducrey (1889). The disease was found to be highly contagious and was caused by *Haemophilus ducreyi*. It presented as a genital ulcer with soft edges (the so-called 'soft sore') and was usually accompanied by a characteristic 'bubo'. Chancroid was also found to more common in developing countries.

The β-haemolytic streptococcus rarely caused vulvovaginitis, but did cause cystitis. Of particular importance was the risk of neonatal infection following delivery through a birth canal colonized by the β-haemolytic streptococcus. Infection could show itself in one of two ways. Early-onset disease caused a form of respiratory distress and bacteraemia (Baker and Barrett, 1973). The late onset manifestations occurred between the 2nd and 14th days of life, its most common presentation being meningitis.

Mycoplasma

Borrel (1910) described this organism, which was first isolated from the human by Dienes and Edsall (1937) in pure culture from a Bartholin's abscess. Originally mycoplasmas were called pleuro-pneumonia-like organisms (PPLO). *Mycoplasma hominis* was found mainly in the genitourinary tract and to a lesser extent in the oropharynx. Twelve different species had been isolated from the human by the late 1980s. Shepard (1954) first described the T-strain mycoplasmas. The prefix T (T for tiny) was introduced to describe the small colonies which were produced by those organisms on agar medium. Shepard *et al.* (1974) found that the organisms had the ability to hydrolyse urea and the T mycoplasma was then placed in the genus and species *Ureaplasma urealyticum.*

Pediculosis pubis

A lesser form of sexually transmitted disease, the *Pediculosis pubis*, is described as an infestation of the hairy part of the vulva by 'phthirus pubis', an insect of about 1.5 mm in length. The lice deposit eggs (nits) at the bases of pubic hairs and live on blood which they obtain from the vulval skin.

Actinomyces

This organism was described in animals by Carter van Dyke (1874). Colonies of *Actinomyces* were identified in cervical smears by Gupta *et al.* (1976) and were found to be commonly associated with the use of intrauterine contraceptive devices, particularly those of the plastic variety (Duguid *et al.*, 1980).

Candida and **Lactobacilli**

Robert Hooke (1665) first described a fungus by microscopy. There is a brief mention of possible thrush infection in one of Samuel Peyps' diaries of 1660–1669. The term candida was officially adopted in 1939 at the Third International Microbiological Congress, but diseases due to fungi have been known for many centuries. Wilkinson (1849) was the first to describe their isolation from the vagina. In this century Plass *et al.* (1931) and Hesseltine *et al.* (1934) investigated moniliasis and also the relationship between yeast vaginitis and oral thrush in the newborn. Hausmann (1875) and Hesseltine (1937) inoculated normal patients with cultured organisms and produced vaginal candidiasis.

Lactobacilli were first described in vaginal secretions by Döderlein (1892) and were later found to be aerobes and facultatively anaerobic. Cruickshank and Sharman (1934) determined that they were the dominant flora of the vagina under acid conditions. Lactobacilli form part of the normal flora of the vagina.

Toxic shock syndrome

Case reports of a syndrome similar to that which was later called 'toxic shock syndrome' (TSS) were published intermittently from 1927. A variety of staphylococcal toxins were studied in many laboratories since Billroth (1874), and Ogston (1880) discovered the organism in pus. Neisser and Wechsberg (1901) reported on the toxins of staphylococci and Reme (1930) reported cutaneous reactivity of staphylococcal filtrates.

Stevens (1927) reported the occurrence of *Staphylococcus aureus* infection with a scarlatiniform rash in children, and this is believed to be the first report of TSS. Aranow and Wood (1942) recorded the case of a 15-year-old girl who presented with the symptoms and signs of TSS. The patient was a known sufferer from osteomyelitis of the trochanter. Coagulase-positive staphylococci were isolated from blood cultures, and also from the infected bone.

Todd *et al.* (1978) were the first to use the term 'toxic shock syndrome' in a report which detailed the case histories of seven children aged 8 – 17 years, in whom TSS occurred between June 1975 and November 1977. The syndrome was characterized by high fever, headache, confusion, conjunctival hyperaemia, scarlatiniform rash, subcutaneous oedema, vomiting, watery diarrhoea, oliguria, acute renal failure, hepatic abnormalities, disseminated intravascular coagulation, severe prolonged shock, and desquamation with peeling of the palms and soles which occurred later.

Schrock (1980) reported three cases of menstrual TSS each complicated by herpes virus infections. The Centers for Disease Control (1980a) in the USA documented that by 1 October, 1979, 52 cases of women with TSS had been reported, of whom 95% had menstruation associated TSS. *S. aureus* was isolated from the throat, cervix, vagina or rectum in 73% of the cases. A further report from the Centers for Disease Control (1980b) implicated the use of 'Rely' tampons, and on 22 September of that year, Proctor and Gamble, who had manufactured the product, withdrew the tampons from the market.

Toxic shock syndrome was reported intermittently throughout the 1980s. The Centers for Disease Control (1988) found that only half of the TSS cases were associated with menstruation. However, the pattern of clinical illness was the same wherever the toxin was produced (Reingold *et al.*, 1982). The definition criteria of TSS required: a fever of a least 38 °C; a macular erythema (like sunburn) either generalized, patchy or localized; hypotension, with a systolic blood pressure of 90 mmHg or less (or below the fifth centile by age for children); or a postural drop of diastolic pressure of at least 15 mmHg, causing postural syncope, or dizziness.

Evidence of toxic action on at least three systems had to be shown by either diarrhoea or vomiting; myalgia or raised creatine kinase activity; reddened conjunctivas, oropharynx or vagina; raised creatinine or urea concentrations to at least twice normal; thrombocytopenia or confusional drowsiness without focal neurological signs when the fever and hypotension have been corrected. Hypotension appeared to be a very good diagnostic sign (Williams, 1990).

Treatment for menstrual TSS required removal of vaginal tampons; the administration of parenteral antibiotics; and fluid replacement with crystalloid solutions which countered the effects of toxin. Inotropic support with dopamine or dobutamine was helpful, as were steroids (Todd *et al.*, 1984). The mortality rate of menstrual TSS was about 3%.

CHRONOLOGY

Microscopy

13th C.   Witelo introduced the science of optics to western Europe*.

1590–1610 Hans Jansen and his son Zacharias introduced the first microscope which was a modification of Galileo's telescope*.

1636	Athanasius Kircher wrote on the properties of light and developed an early microscope*.
1674	Anthony van Leeuwenhoek began his reports to the Royal Society, London.
1712	Hertel invented the illuminatory mirror.
1791	Beeldsnyder introduced the first achromatic lens.
1826–1830	Joseph Jackson Lister designed a microscope system almost free of spherical and chromatic abberations.
1870	Abbe, Zeiss and Schott introduced the oil immersion lens and the Abbe system of illumination*.
1926	Hans Busch laid theoretical foundations for development of the electron microscope†.
1933	The first operational electron microscope was used†.
1985	A three-dimensional electron microscope was developed†.
1980–1986	A tunnel effect microscope with extreme magnification was perfected†.

*References: McGrew (1985); Grunze and Spriggs (1983)
†Reference: Giscard d'Estaing (1990)
All others in reference section under named author

Early microscopists and cell theory

1656	Pierre Borel may have visualized the human cell.
1661	Marcello Malpighi described utricles, globules and saccules.
1665	Robert Hooke first used the term 'cell'.
1671	Athanasius Kircher described 'little worms' in the blood of plague victims.
1674	Anthony van Leeuwenhoek reported his discovery of protozoa.
1675	Swammerdam described the microscopic appearance of red blood cells.
1759	Caspar F. Wolff noted that all animal organs were made up of cells.
1767	Felix Fontana noted the cell nucleus, and called it 'a little body within'.
1802/3	Francois X. Bichat defined histological changes produced by disease.
1802	Charles F.B. de Mirbel stated that plants were entirely composed of cells.
1827	Karl E. von Baer described the human ovum.

1830	F.J.F. Meyen noted that plant cells were united together to constitute a highly organized plant.
1833	Robert Brown first used the term nucleus.
1838	Mathias J. Schleiden explained the derivation of plant tissues from cells.
1839	Theodor Schwann applied cell theory to animal tissues.
1842	Karl Nageli described chromosomes.
1869	Friedrich Miescher isolated nuclein.
1875	Eduard Strasburger described cell division and termed the process mitosis.
1876–79	Walther Flemming used the term chromatin.
1882	Paul Ehrlich developed staining methods for dry preparations.

Puerperal fever

Hippocrates described puerperal fever in his *Epidemics*.

17th C.	Francois Mauriceau (1637–1709) described an epidemic of puerperal fever*.
1662	Thomas Willis described 'puerperarum febris'.
1691	Richard Morton described the condition*.
1716	Edward Strother introduced the term 'puerperal fever'*.
1746	Jacques Maloruin of the Hotel Dieu described the clinical and post-mortem findings*.
Mid-1700s	Smellie blamed anomalies of the lochia for puerperal fever*.
1773	Charles White penned a treatise on the topic and suggested methods for prevention and treatment*.
1774	Thomas Kirkland, London, composed his *Treatise on Childbed Fevers*.
1795	Alexander Gordon of Aberdeen wrote a *Treatise on the Epidemic Puerperal Fever of Aberdeen*.
1828–1987	Etienne Stephene Tarnier worked in the Maternité Hospital, Paris where puerperal fever was rampant*.
1833	Hugh Lenox Hodge wrote his *Observations Regarding Puerperal Fever*. Robert Collins, Master of the Dublin Lying-In Hospital, began a system of chlorine disinfection*.

1842–1843 Oliver Wendell Holmes presented his paper on *The Contagiousness of Puerperal Fever.*

1860 Semmelweiss wrote his *Die Aetiologie, Der Begriffe, und Die Prophylaxis des Kindbettfiebers**.
Louis Pasteur discovered the streptococcus.
Ogston of Aberdeen identified streptococci in surgical pyemia.

1863–1865 Mayerhofer isolated organisms from the air of the wards, which were similar to those in the lochia of puerperal women.

1868 Hausmann discovered organisms in vaginal secretions of women who were not ill.

1871 Waldeyer of Breslau investigated the bacteriology of puerperal fever*.

1879 Pasteur blamed haemolytic streptococcus as the cause of puerperal infection.

1880 Doleris of France wrote a thesis on *Antiseptic Midwifery**.

*References: Venzmer (1972); Lyons and Petrucelli (1978); McGrew (1985); Cianfrani (1960); Graham (1950)

Antiseptics

Various antiseptics were used in ancient Egypt, Greece and Rome.

19th C. Auguste Nelaton introduced alcohol soaks.

1811 Bernard Courtois discovered iodine.

1847 Ignaz Semmelweiss popularized the use of chlorate of lime.

1867 Joseph Lister devised his antiseptic curtain of carbolic acid spray.
Lister published a paper *On the Antiseptic Principle in Surgery.*

20th C. William Halsted introduced operating gloves. Sterilization units were developed following the observation by Robert Koch that heat was more effective than chemical methods of sterilization.

References for above: Lyons and Petrucelli (1978); McGrew (1985); Cianfrani (1960)

Tuberculosis

Ancient Greece Tuberculosis was called 'phthisis'.

Middle Ages Scrofula was described.
Early 1800s Tuberculosis caused one-third of hospital deaths.

1850 The sanitarium movement began.

1882 Robert Koch isolated *Mycobacterium tuberculosis.*

1920 Surgical lung collapse was popular as a treatment.

1921 The bacillus Calmette–Guerin (BCG) vaccine was introduced.

1944 Streptomycin was introduced by Selman A. Waksman.

1946–48 Para-amino salicylic developed by Jorgen Lehmann (McGrew, 1985).

1950–51 Isoniazid was isolated.

Toxic shock syndrome

1927 Stevens first reported the occurrence of *Staphylococcus aureus* infection with scarlatiniform rash in children.

1978 Todd *et al.* were the first to use the term toxic shock syndrome.

1980 The Centers for Disease Control in America documented 52 cases of women with toxic shock syndrome. 'Rely' tampons were implicated and withdrawn from the market following which the disease was less commonly reported.

Venereal and sexually transmitted diseases

Gonorrhoea

There were references from ancient Egypt, Greece, Rome and Alexandria to this condition which was also mentioned in the Bible.

2nd C. AD Galen first used the term gonorrhoea*.

6th C. Aetius and his followers described symptoms of a disease which was probably gonorrhoea*.

1161 The disease was officially recognized in England.

1378 John of Arderne introduced the term 'clap'*.

1640s Regnier de Graaf distinguished between leucorrhoea and gonorrhoea*.

1713 William Cockburn theorized that gonorrhoea and syphilis were two separate entities*.

1841 T. Gaillard Thomas investigated pelvic inflammatory disease*.

1857	Bernutz and Goupil noted a relationship between pelvic sepsis and gonorrhoea.
1872	Emile Noeggerath related gonorrhoea to sterility.
1879	Albert Neisser discovered the causal agent.
1882	L. Leistikow isolated *Neisseria gonorrhoea*.
1885	Bumm cultivated the organism.

*References: Ricci (1943); Speert (1958); McGrew (1985)

Syphilis

1493	The first outbreak dates back to this year when Columbus and his men returned from the Americas.
1495	The first major appearance of syphilis was during the Siege of Naples.
1496	Georgio Sommariva introduced mercury treatment*.
1498	Francesco L. de Villalobos wrote a poem on the 'French pockes'*.
1530	Girolamo Fracastoro named the disease after a shepherd in his poem *Syphilis Sive de Morbo Gallico*.
1564	Gabriele Falloppio introduced the condom as a prophylactic device against the disease*.
1786	Hunter investigated the disease*.
1833	Ehrenberg first described a flexible motile organism in water which he called spirochaete. He also developed classifications of genera and species and introduced the genus 'bacterium'.
1875	Edwin Klebs noted spirochaetal bodies in syphilitic material.
1888	Felix Bazzer introduced bismuth treatment and William Wallace used potassium iodide*.
1904	Paul Ehrlich developed salvarsan*.
1905	Fritz Schaudin and Erich Hoffman discovered *Treponema pallidum*.
1906	August von Wassermann developed his blood test.
1929	Alexander Fleming isolated penicillin.

*References: Speert (1958); Graham (1950); Cianfrani (1960); Wilson and Miles (1955); McGrew (1985); Venzmer (1972); Waugh (1990)

The acquired immune deficiency syndrome (AIDS)

1972	The human immunodeficiency virus (HIV) virus may have first appeared in Central Africa.
1981	An outbreak of *Pneumocystis carinii* and Kaposi's sarcoma heralded the worldwide recognition of the disease (Centers for Disease Control, 1981).
1982	Mildvan *et al.* described persistent lymphadenopathy.
1983	Gallo *et al.* and Barré-Sinoussi *et al.* discovered the aetiological agent associated with AIDS.
1984	Mathur-Wagh and Mildvan described AIDS-related complex (ARC).
1987	Cervical abnormalities were found in infected women.
1988	The European Collaborative Study reported on 600 children born to HIV-infected mothers.
1989	Oxtoby indicated that infection could be transmitted through breast milk.

Hepatitis B

1946	Bradley documented the occurrence of jaundice in wives of two men with the disease.
1970	The occurrence of hepatitis B in male homosexuals was reported.
1971	Hersh *et al.* documented heterosexual transmission.
1982	Francis *et al.* reported on prevention by vaccine.

Wart virus

1896	Jadassohn recorded evidence that common warts were infectious.
1911	Rous discovered tumour-inducing viruses.
1930	Findlay documented that venereal warts, (condylomata acuminata) are infective and are apparently caused by a virus. Occasionally warts became cancerous.
1935	Stanley crystallized virus.
1949	Strauss *et al.* demonstrated wart virus in aqueous extracts of skin wart tissue.
1954	Barrett *et al.* reported venereal transmission of genital warts in servicemen returning from the Far East.
1960	Ito discovered that the possible tumour-producing factor of papillomavirus resided in its nucleic acid, and was probably DNA.

1963	Dulbecco found that cells became transformed by virus.
1965	Von Melczer discovered intranucleur and intracytoplasmic clumps of particles resembling human papillomavirus in genital wart material.
1967	Baeferstedt associated genital warts with homosexual practices.
1969	Teokharov found skin warts uncommon in patients with genital warts.
1971	Oriel found a high incidence of sexual contact in patients with genital warts.

Herpes

1714	Daniel Turner described herpes simplex.
1736	Jean Astruc and D.E. Morbis first documented herpes genitalis as a clinical entity.
1832	Dupercque further described herpes genitalis.
1853	Legendre described further cases of herpes genitalis.
1869	Rollet was the first to implicate herpetic ulceration of the cervix as a cause of vaginal discharge.
1883	Unna recorded that 1% of prostitutes attending the Hamburg General Hospital had herpes genitalis.
1906	Tyzzer found nucleur inclusions in skin lesions of varicella which later were proven typical of the herpes virus group.
1920/24	Gruter successfully isolated herpes virus on rabbit corneal tissue.
1921	Lipschutz described the aetiology of genital herpes.
1940	Sharlit documented a case of penile herpes infection in which the female consort developed vulvovaginitis within 5 days of venereal contact.
1946	Slavin and Gavett isolated herpes virus from three cases of herpetic vulval vaginitis.

Cytomegalovirus

1969	Diosi *et al.* implicated the infection with fetal and neonatal compromise.

Gardnerella vaginalis

1954	Gardner and Dukes first described *Haemophilus vaginalis.*
1980	Greenwood and Pickett renamed *Haemophilus vaginalis* as *Gardnerella vaginalis* in honour of Gardner and Dukes.

Trichomonas vaginalis

1836	Alfred Donné described *Trichomonas,* so called because of its similarity to the other protozoa, trichodes and monas.
1838	Ehrenberg confirmed the studies by Donne on *Trichomonas,* and reported that the vagina was the organism's normal habitat. The organism was first reported in the male urethra by three separate workers, Mariehand, Mivera, and Dock (Hare, 1988).
1944	Stuart introduced his transport medium for swabs of exudates with possible *Trichomonas vaginalis.*

Chlamydia

1907	Conjunctivitis was attributed to infection later discovered to be caused by *Chlamydia trachomatis* (Hare, 1988).
1911	Lindner noted chlamydial infection of the cervix, while non-gonococcal urethritis was described in 1910.
1935	Busacca described *Chlamydia trachomatis.*
1936	Thygseon and Mengert related cervical chlamydial infection and non-gonococcal urethritis to non-gonococcal forms of ophthalmia neonatorum.
1945	Jones, Rake and Stearns named chlamydia from chlamys, or cloak (Krieg and Holt, 1984).

Actinomyces

1874	Carter van Dyke described actinomyces and implicated it as a cause of infection in animals.
1976	Gupta *et al.* identified actinomyces in cervical smears.
1980	Duguid *et al.* noted an association with intrauterine contraceptive devices.

Corynebacterium

1883	Klebs described corynebacterium

which may be a secondary invader of skin and vaginal wounds.

Mycoplasma

1910   Borrel *et al.* described mycoplasma.

1937   Dienes and Edsall reported the isolation of mycoplasma from a Bartholin's abscess. Mycoplasma were found to be the smallest free-living micro-organisms.

1974   Shepard *et al.* first described *T.* strain *Mycoplasma.*

Fungi/yeast

1665   Robert Hooke described a fungus at microscopy 'there are a multitude of other shapes of which these microscopical mushrooms are figured'.

1834–1837   Theodore Schwann reported that yeast cells were responsible for fermentation.

1849   Wilkinson recorded the first description of vulvo-vaginal candidiasis and its treatment with a hypochlorite solution.

1875   Hausmann inoculated infected material and produced vaginal candidiasis in a healthy pregnant woman.

Staphylococci

1878   Staphylococcal organisms were noted in pus.

1880   Pasteur cultivated micrococci (staphylococci) in a liquid medium.

1881   Ogston discovered micrococci (staphylococci) present in acute and chronic abscesses.

1884   Rosenbach adopted the term staphylococcus (previously suggested by Ogston).

Streptococcus

1883   Fehleisen described a chain-forming coccus as the causative organism of erysipelas (streptococcus).

1884   Rosenbach first used the term streptococcus (previously suggested by Ogston).

1973   Baker and Barrett implicated vaginal colonization with β-haemolytic streptococcus as a cause of neonatal complications.

Proteus vulgaris

1885   Hauser described proteus vulgaris.

Escherichia coli

1895   Migula discovered this organism.

1919   Castellani and Chalmers named *Escherichia coli* after Theodor Escherich who first isolated the type species of the genus.

Bacteroides

1898   An organism first described by Veillon and Zuber, was later renamed *Bacteroides fragilas.*

Bacteriophage

1915   D'Herelle and Twort independantly showed the existence of bacteriophage.

Rubella

1815   W.G. Maton described rubella.

Lactobacillus

1881   Kern described the lactobacillus organism in milk.

1892   Doderlein observed a similar organism in vaginal fluid.

General

1730–1784   Muller described and classified organisms now known to be bacteria and protozoa.

1877   Robert Koch detailed methods for microscopic examination of bacteria in dried fixed films stained with analine dyes.

Pasteur and Joubert described the *Clostridium* species.

Sedillot first used the term microbe.

Four years later Pasteur suggested that the science of microbial life be known as 'microbie' or 'microbiology'.

1929   Kuester discovered that vaginal secretions had a moderate bactericidial effect.

Antibiotics

1929   Alexander Fleming discovered penicillin.

1935   Domagh discovered sulphonamides and introduced prontosil rubrum which was the first of the sulphonamides.

1939   Ernst Boris Chain first discovered the chemical properties of penicillin and, together with Lord Florey, established principles for its commercial manufacture (Chain *et al.*, 1940).

1944   Sellman A. Waksman discovered streptomycin (Schatz *et al.*, 1944).

REFERENCES

Aranow, H. Jr. and Wood, W.B. Jr. (1942). Staphylococcic infection simulating scarlet fever. *J. Am. Med. Assoc.*, **119**, 1491–5

Aristotle. *Historia Animalium*, Vol. IV, Book VIII, 604a (2)

Astruc, J. (1736). 'De morbis venereis libri sex', quoted by Hutfield, D.C. (1966)

Astruc, J. and Morbis, D.E. (1736). *Veneris* Paris, quoted by Kaufman *et al.* (1989) p.122

Ayre, J.E. (1949). The vaginal smear: "Precancer" cell studies using a modified technique. *Am. J. Obstet. Gynecol.*, **58**, 1205–19

Baeferstedt, B.O. (1967). Condylomata acuminata past and present. *Acta Dermato Venereologica*, **47**, 376–81

Baer von, K. (1827). *De ovi mammalium et hominis genesi epistolam ad Academiam Imperialem Scientiarum Petropolitanam.* (Leipzig: Leopold Voss) *: Deutsche Ubersetzung durch B. Ottow, Uber die Bildung des Eies der Saugetiere und des Menschen. Mit einer Einfuhrung. Faksimiledrucj.* (Leipzig: Leopold Voss 1927)

Baker, C.J. and Barrett, F.F. (1973). Transmission of group B streptococci among parturient women and neonates. *J. Pediatr.*, **83**, 919

Bamforth, J. (1950). Latent tuberculosis of the endometrium. In Bowes, K. (ed.) *Modern Trends in Obstetrics and Gynaecology*, pp. 506–11. (London: Butterworth & Co.)

Barré-Sinoussi, F., Cherman, J.C., Rey, F. *et al.* (1983). Isolation of T. lymphotropic retrovirus from a patient at risk of acquired immune deficiency syndrome (AIDS). *Science*, **220**, 868–70

Barrett, T.J., Silbar, J.D. and McGinley, J.P. (1954). Genital warts – a venereal disease. *J. Am. Med. Assoc.*, **154**, 333–4

Bateman, T. (1814). *Practical Synopsis of Cutaneous Disease*, 3rd edn. (London)

Baughan, C.A. and Phillips, R.H. (1987). The clinical presentation of AIDS: Kaposi's sarcoma and other tumours. In Farthing, C. (ed.) *AIDS in Clinical Medicine*, pp. 11–17. (Middlesex: Barker Publications Ltd)

Beeldsnyder, F. (c.1791). quoted by Harting (1866). Vol.3, p.132

Bernutz, G. and Goupil, E. (1857). Recherches cliniques sur les phlegmons periuterins. *Arch. Gen. de Med.*, **9**, 285–308, 419–32

Beswick, T.S.L. (1962). The origin and the use of the word herpes. *Med. Hist.*, **6**, 214–32

Bichat, M.F.X. (1802/1803). *Traie de l'anatomie Descriptive.* (Paris: Brosson, Gabon & Cie)

Billroth, T. (1874). Untersuchungen uber die Vegetationsformen von Coccobacteria septica, und den Antheil, welchen sie an der Entstehung und Verbreitung der accidentellen Wundkrankheiten haben. *Versuch einer wissenschaftlichen Kritik der verschiedenen methoden antiseptischer Wundbehandlung.* (Berlin: G. Reimer)

Borel, P. (1656). quoted by MacLeod (1973) p.10

Borrel, J. (1910). Le microbe de la peripneumonial. *Ann.. Inst. Pasteur (Paris)*, **24**, 168–79

Bradbeer, C. (1987). Is infection with HIV a risk factor for cervical intraepithelial neoplasia? *Lancet*, **21**, 1277–8

Bradley, W.H. (1946). Homologous serum jaundice. *Proc. R. Soc. Med.*, **39**, 649–54

Brisseau de Mirbel, C.F. (1802). quoted by MacLeod (1983) p.10

Brown, R. (1833). On the Modes of Fecundation in Orchidaceae and Asclepiadaceae. *Transactions of the Linnean Society*, **16**, 685

Browne, F.J. (1950). *Postgraduate Obstetrics and Gynaecology*, pp. 125–140. (London: Butterworth & Co)

Bumm, E. von (1885). Der Mikro-organismus der Gonorrhoischen Schleim hauterkrankungen Gonococcus Neisser. *Dtsch. Med. Wchschr.*, 11, 508

Busacca, A. (1935). Un germe caracterisé de rickettsies (Rickettsies Trachome) dans tissus trachomateux. *Arch. Ophthalmol*, 52, 567–72

Butler, E.B. and Stanbridge, C.M. (1984). Condylomatous lesions of the lower female genital tract. In Fox, H. (ed.) *Clinics in Obstetrics and Gynaecology*, Vol. 11, No. 1, pp. 171–87. (London, Philadelphia, Toronto: W.B. Saunders Co.)

Byrne, M., Taylor-Robinson, D. and Harris, J.R.W. (1988). Cervical dysplasia and HIV infection. *Lancet*, 1, 239

Carter van Dyke (1874). quoted by Wilson and Miles (1955) p.1467

Castellani, A. and Chalmers, A.J. (1919). *Manual of Tropical Medicine*, 3rd edn. (New York: Williams Wood & Co.)

Celsus. *De Medicina* English translation by W.G. Spencer, (1938). (London: William Heinemann)

Center for Disease Control (1980a). Toxic-shock syndrome – United States. *Morbid. Mortal. Weekly Rep.*, May 23 29, 220–30

Center for Disease Control (1980b). Follow-up on toxic-shock syndrome. *Morbid. Mortal. Weekly Rep.*, Oct. 3 29, 470

Center for Disease Control (1981). Pneumocystis pneumonia – Los Angeles. *Morbid. Mortal. Weekly Rep.*, 30, 250–2

Center for Disease Control (1983). Condyloma acuminatum – United States 1966–1981. *Morbid. Mortal. Weekly Rep.*, 32, 306–8

Center for Disease Control (1987). Revision of the case definition for acquired immunodeficiency syndrome *Morbid. Mortal. Weekly Rep.*, 36, 1–15

Center for Disease Control (1988). Summary of notifiable diseases. United States 1988. *Morbid. Mortal. Weekly Rep.*, 37, 40

Chain, E.B., Florey, H.W., Gardner, A.D., Heatley, N.G., Jennings, M.A., Orr-Ewing, J. and Sanders, A.G. (1940). Penicillin as a chemotherapeutic agent. *Lancet*, 2, 226–8

Charlewood, G.P. and Shippel, S. (1953). Vulvar condyloma acuminatum as a premalignant lesion in the Bantu. *South Afr. Med. J.*, 27, 149

Chen, K.C.S., Forsyth, P.S., Buchanan, T.M. *et al.* (1979). Amine content of vaginal fluid from untreated and treated patients with nonspecific vaginitis. *J. Clin. Invest.*, 63, 828–35

Cianfrani, T. (1960). *A Short History of Obstetrics and Gynaecology*, pp.174; 300; and 316. (Springfield Illinois: Charles C. Thomas)

Clarke, M. (1989). Unsafe sex: the case for a primary health care initiative. In Chamberlain, G. and Drife, J. (eds.) *Contemporary Reviews in Obstetrics and Gynaecology*, Vol. 1, No. 4, pp. 261–5. (London: Butterworths & Co. Ltd.)

Cohen, R.C. (1950). Tuberculosis and pregnancy. In Bowes, K. (ed.) *Modern Trends in Obstetrics and Gynaecology*, pp. 392–402. (London: Butterworth & Co. Ltd.)

Colebrook, L. (1954). Puerperal infection. In Munro Kerr, J., Johnstone, R.W. and Phillips, M.H. (eds.) *Historical Review of British Obstetrics and Gynaecology*, pp. 202–22. (London: Livingstone)

Cowen, D.L. and Helfand, W.H. (1990). *Pharmacy. An Illustrated History*, p. 199. (New York: Harry N. Abrams)

Cruickshank, R. and Sharman, A. (1934). The biology of the vagina in the human subject. *J. Obstet. Gynaecol. Br. Commonw.*, 41, 190–226

Curtis, A.H. (1913). A motile curved anaerobic bacillus in uterine discharges. *J. Infect. Dis.*, 12, 165

Darani, M. and Gerker, M. (1974). Hepatitis B antigen in vaginal secretions. *Lancet*, 2, 1008

D'Herelle and Twort (1915). quoted by Wilson and Miles (1955) p.386

Dienes, L. and Edsall, G. (1937). Observations on the L-organism of Klieneberger. *Proc. Soc. Exp. Biol. Med.*, 36, 740–4

Diosi, P., Moldovan, E. and Tomesu, N. (1969). Latent cytomegalovirus infection in blood donors. *Br. Med. J.*, 4, 660

Döderlein, A. (1892). *Das Scheidensekret und Seine Bedeutung für das Puerperalfieber*. (Besold: Leipzig)

Domagh, G. (1935). quoted by Wilson and Miles (1955) p.171

Donne, A. (1836). Animalcules observes dans les matieres purulentes et le produit des secretions des organes genitaux de l'homme et de la femme. *Comptes rendus hebdomadaires des seances de 'Academie des Sciences, Paris*, **3**, 385

Donne, A. (1844). Cours de Microscopie complementaire des Etudes Medicales. *Anatomie microscopique et Physiologie des Fluides de l'Economie.* (Paris: Baillière)

Donovan, C. (1905). Medical cases from the Madras General Hospital. *Indian Med. Gaz.*, **40**, 411

Ducrey, A. (1889). quoted by Wilson, G.S. and Miles, A.A. (1955)

Duenas, A., Adam, I. and Melnick, J. (1971) Herpes virus type 2 in a prostitute population. *Am. J. Epidemiol.*, **95**, 483

Duguid, H.L.D., Parrott, D. and Traynor, R. (1980). Actinomycetes-like organisms in cervical smears from women using intrauterine contraceptive devices. *Br. Med. J.*, **281**, 534–41

Duguid, J.P., Marmion, B.P. and Swain, R.H.A. (1978). *Mackie & McCartney's Medical Microbiology*, 13th edn. (London: Churchill Livingstone)

Dulbecco, R. (1963). Transformation of cells *in vitro* by viruses. *Science*, **142**, 932–6

Dumortier, (1832). quoted by MacLeod (1973) p.11

Dupercque, R. (1832). quoted by Unna (1883)

Durieux, R. and Dublanchet, A. (1980). Les vibrions anaerobies des leucorrées. 1. Technique disolement et sensibilite aux antibiotiques. *Med. Mal. Infect.*, **10**, 109

Ehrenberg (1833). quoted by Wilson, G.S. and Miles, A.A. (1950) p. 1031

Ehrenberg, (1838). Die infusiontheirchen als vollkommene organismen: *Ein Blick in Das Tiefere organische Leben der Natur.* (Leipzig: L Voss)

Ehrlich, P. (1882). quoted in Schnell (1973) p.8

Epstein, W.L. *et al* (1963). Viral antigens in human epidermal tumors. *J. Invest. Dermatol.*, **40**, 51

European Collaborative Study (1988). Mother-to-child transmission of HIV infection. *Lancet*, **2**, 1039–43

European Collaborative Study (1991). Children born to women with HIV-1 infection: natural history and risk of transmission. *Lancet*, **1**, 253–60

Faro, S. (1989). In Kaufman, R.H., Friedrich, E.G. and Gardner, H.L. (eds.) *Benign Diseases of the Vulva*

and Vagina, 3rd edn., pp. 73–105. (Chicago, London, Boca Raton: Year Book Medical Publishers Inc.)

Farrell, C. (1978). *My Mother Said.* (London: Routledge and Kegan Paul)

Farthing, C.F., Brown, S.E., Staughton, R.C.D., Cream, J.J. and Muhlemann, M. (1986). *A Colour Atlas of Acquired Immunodeficiency Syndrome (AIDS)*, p.6. (London: Wolf Medical Publishers Ltd; Year Book Medical Publishers, Inc.)

Fehleisen (1883). *Aetiologie des Erysipels.* (Berlin)

Ferenczy, A., Mitao, M., Nagi, N. *et al.* (1985). Latent papillomavirus and recurring genital warts. *N. Engl. J. Med.*, **313**, 784–8

Findlay, G.M. (1930). *A System of Bacteriology in Relation to Medicine*, p. 252 (London: HMSO, MRC)

Fleming, A. (1929). The antibacterial action of cultures of a penicillium with special reference to their use in the isolation of B Influenzae. *Br. J. Exp. Pathol.*, **10**, 226–36

Flemming, W. (1876). quoted by MacLeod (1973) p.12

Fontana, Fe. (1767). *Ricerche fisiche sopra il veleno della vipera. Lucca-Firenze:I. Giusti.* Translation: *Traite sur le venin de la vipere*, Florence 1781. (Paris: Nyon l'Aine: London: Emsley)

Forster, S.M. (1987). Clinical syndromes associated with the human immunodeficiency virus. In Farthing, C. (ed.) *AIDS in Clinical Medicine*, pp. 24–27. (Middlesex: Barker Publications Ltd)

Francis, D.P., Hadler, S.C., Thompson, S.E. *et al.* (1982). The prevention of hepatitis B with vaccine: report of the Center for Disease Control multi-centre efficacy trial among homosexual men. *Ann. Intern. Med.*, **97**, 362–6

Gallo, R.C., Savin, P.S., Gelman, E.P. *et al.* (1983). Isolation of human T-cell leukaemia virus in acquired immune deficiency syndrome (AIDS). *Science*, **220**, 865–7

Gardner, H.L. and Dukes, C.D. (1954). New etiologic agent in nonspecific bacterial vaginitis. *Science*, **120**, 853

Gardner, H.L. and Dukes, C.D. (1955). *Haemophilus vaginalis* vaginitis: a newly defined specific infection previously classified "nonspecific" vaginitis. *Am. J. Obstet. Gynecol.*, **69**, 962–76

Giscard d'Estaing, V.A. (1990). *The Book of Inventions and Discoveries*, p. 90. (London: Queen Anne Press, MacDonald & Co. Ltd)

Gissmann, L., Wolnik, L., Ikenberg, H. *et al.* (1983). Human papillomavirus types 6 and 11 DNA sequences in genital and laryngeal papillomas and in some cervical cancers. *Proc. Nat. Acad. Sci. USA*, **80**, 560–3

Gordon, A. (1795). quoted by Colebrook (1954). pp. 202–25

Graham, H. (1950). *Eternal Eve*, pp. 71; 131; 378–85; 617 and 659. (London: Heinemann)

Greenwood, J.R. and Picket, M.J. (1980). Transfer of haemophilus vaginalis of Gardner and Dukes to a new genus, Gardnerella: *G. Vaginalis* (Gardner and Dukes) *Comb. Nov. Int. J. Syst. Bacteriol.*, **30**, 170–8

Grew, N. (1672). *The Anatomy of Vegetables.* (London: Hickmann)

Griffiths, P.D. (1991). In Philipp, E. and Setchell, M. (eds.) *Scientific Foundations of Obstetrics and Gynaecology*, pp. 609–11. (Oxford: Butterworth/ Heinemann)

Grunze, H. and Spriggs, A.I. (1983). *History of Clinical Cytology: A Selection of Documents*, 2nd edn., G-I-T p.9. (D-6100 Darmstadt West Germany: Verlag Ernst Ghebelar)

Gruter, W. (1920) quoted by Skinner, G. (1976)

Gruter, W. (1924). Das Herpes Virus, Seine Aetiologische und Klinische Bedeutung. *Munch. Med. Wchschr.*, **71**, 1058

Gupta, P.K., Hollander, D.H. and Frost, J.K. (1976). Actinomyces in cervico-vaginal smears; an association with IUCD usage. *Acta Cytol.*, **20**, 295–7

Halberstaedter and Prowazek (1907). quoted by Faro, S. (1989)

Hallier, E. (1869). Die Parasiten der Infectionskrankheiten. *Z. f. Parasitenk.*, **1**, 117–84

Hare, M.J. (1988). Diagnosis of lower genital tract infection. In Hare, M.J. (ed.) *Genital Tract Infection in Women*, pp. 112–33. (London: Churchill Livingstone)

Harting, P. (1866). *Das Mikroskop*, Vol.3. (Braunschweig: Vieweg & Sohn)

Hauser, G. (1885). Uber faulnisbakterien und beren beziehungen zur septicamie. *Ein Beitrag zur Morphologie der Spaltpilze.* (Leipzig: Vagel)

Hauser, G. (1885). Ueber Faulnisbakterien. *J. Pathol. Bact.*, **31**, 185

Hausmann, D. (1868). quoted by Cianfrani (1960) p.311

Hausmann, D. (1875). *Parasites des organes sexuels femelles de l'homme et de quelques animaux avec une notice sur development de l'Oidium albicans.* (Paris: Baillere)

Heathcote, J. and Sherlock, S. (1973). Spread of acute hepatitis B in London. *Lancet*, **1**, 1468–70

Heathcote, J., Cameron, C.H. and Dare, D.S. (1974). Hepatitis B antigen in saliva and serum. *Lancet*, **1**, 71–3

Hersh, T., Melnick, J.L., Goyal, R.K. and Hollinger, F.B. (1971). Non-parenteral transmission of viral hepatitis type B. *N. Engl. J. Med.*, **285**, 1363–4

Hertel, (Halle) (1712). Quoted by Grunze and Spriggs (1983). p.16

Hesseltine, H.C. (1937). Biologic and clinical import of vulvovaginal mycoses. *Am. J. Obstet. Gynecol.*, **34**, 855–67

Hesseltine, H.C., Borts, I.C. and Plass, E.D. (1934). Pathogenicity of the Monilia (Castellani), vaginitis and oral thrush. *Am. J. Obstet. Gynecol.*, **27**, 112–16

Hodge, H.L. (1852). *On the non-contagious character of puerperal fever: an introductory lecture.* (Philadelphia: T.K. and P.G. Collins)

Hoehne, O. (1916). Trichomonas Vaginalis also Haufiger Erreger Einer Typischen Colpitis Purulenta. *Zentralbl. Gynaekol.*, **40**, 4

Holmes, O.W. (1843). The contagiousness of puerperal fever. *Boston Q. J. Med. Surg.*, **1**, 503–30

Hooke, R. (1665). *Micrographia.* (London: J. Martyn & J. Allestry)

Ito, Y. (1960). A tumor producing factor extracted by phenol from papillomatous tissue (shape) of cotton tail rabbits. *Virology*, **12**, 596–601

Jadassohn (1896). quoted by Wilson and Miles (1955) p.2243

John, F.D., MacCullum, L., Brettle, M., Inglis, J.M. and Peutherer, J.M. (1988). Does infection with HIV affect the outcome of pregnancy? *Br. Med. J.*, **296**, 467

Juliusberg, M. (1905). Zurkenntnis des Virus der Molluscum contagiosum des Menschen. *Dtch. Med. Wchschr.*, **31**, 1598

Karnaky, K.J. (1937). Trichomonas vaginalis vaginitis pathognomonic lesions and pathologic findings in 4000 cases. *Tex. Med.*, **32**, 803

Kaufman, R.H., Friedrich, E.G. and Gardner, H.L. (1989). *Benign Diseases of the Vulva and Vagina.* (Chicago, London: Year Book Medical Publishers Inc.)

Kern (1881). quoted by Wilson and Miles (1955) p.857

Kircher, A. (1671). quoted by McGrew (1985) p.200

Klebs, E. (1875). quoted by Wilson and Miles (1955) p.2027

Klebs, E. (1878). Ueber Syphilis-impfung bei Thieren und uber die Natur des syphilischen Contagiums. *Prager Med. Wchschr.*, **3**, 409

Klebs, E. (1883). quoted by Wilson and Miles (1955) p.536

Koch, R. (1877). quoted by McGrew (1985) p.28

Koch, R. (1878). quoted by Wilson and Miles (1955) p.699

Koch, R. (1882). quoted by Wilson and Miles (1955) p. 489

Koss, L.G. and Durfee G.R. (1956). Unusual pattern of squamous epithelium of uterine cervix: cytologic and pathologic study of koilocytotic atypia. *Ann. N.Y. Acad. Sci.*, **63**, 1235–61

Krieg, N.R. and Holt, J.G. (1984). *Bergeys Manual of Systematic Bacteriology*, Vol. 1. (Baltimore: Williams and Wilkins)

Kuester (1929). *Hdb Path. Mikroorg. Kolle and Wasserman 3TE Anfl.*, **6**, 372

La Page, S.P. (1961). Hemophilus vaginalis and its role in vaginitis. *Acta Pathol. Microbiol. Scand.*, **52**, 34

Lammers, J.W.J. (1974). Johan, Ham, de ontdekker van de zaaddiertjes. *Nederl. Tijdsch. Geneesk.*, **118**, 784

Leadbetter, E.R. and Poindexter, J.S. (eds.) (1985). *Bacteria in Nature: Bacterial Activities in Perspective*, Vol.1, pp.4 and 16. (New York, London: Plenum Press)

Leeuwenhoek, A. van (1678). De natis e semine genitali animalculis. *Philos. Trans. R. Soc. London*, **XII**, 1040

Leeuwenhoek, A. van (1674, 1679, 1702). Letters to the Royal Society. *Philos. Trans. R. Soc. London*, **9**, 121: **12**, 1040: **22**, 552

Legendre, F.L. (1853). *Archiv. Gen. Med.* **5**, 171

Leistikow, L. (1880). Ueber Bacterien bei den venerischen Krankheiten. *Charité Ann.*, **7**, 750

Lindner, K. (1911). Gonoblennorrhoe, Einschlussblennorrhoe, und Trachoma. *Albrecht von Graef's Archives of Ophthalmology*, **78**, 380

Lipschutz, B. (1921). Untersuchungen uber die aetiologie der krankheiten der herpes gruppe (Herpes Zoster, herpes genitalis, herpes febritis). *Arch. Dermatol. Syph.*, **136**, 428–82 (152)

Lister, J.J. (1829). On some properties in achromatic object glasses applicable to the improvement of the microscope. *Philos. Trans.*, **130**, 187

Loeffler, L. (1882). quoted by Wilson and Miles (1955) p. 1649

Lyons, A.S. and Petrucelli, R.J. (1978). *Medicine. An Illustrated History*, p. 482. (New York: H.N. Abrams, Inc.)

McGrew, R.E. (1985). *Encyclopedia of Medical History*, pp. 116; 200–2; 291–94; 329. (London: MacMillan Press)

McKay, W.J.S. (1901). *The History of Ancient Gynaecology.* (London: Bailliere Tindall Cox)

MacLeod, A.G. (1973). In Baird, T.A. (ed.) *Cytology*, pp. 10–13. (Michigan Kalamazoo: The Upjohn Co.)

McLeod, K. (1882). Precis of operations performed in the wards of the first surgeon medical college hospital during the year 1881. *Indian Med. Gaz.*, **17**, 113

Malpighi M. (1661). quoted by MacLeod (1973) p.10

Mardh, P-A., Holst, E. and Moller, B.R. (1984). The Grivet monkey as a model for study of vaginitis. In Mardh, P-A. and Taylor-Robinson, D. (eds.) *Bacterial Vaginosis*, p. 201. (Stockholm: Almquist and Wiksell International)

Mathur-Wagh, U. and Mildvan, D. (1984). Prodromal syndromes in AIDS. *Ann. N.Y. Acad. Sci.*, **437**, 184–91

Maton, W.G. (1815). Some account of a rash, liable to be mistaken for scarlatina. *Med. Trans. R. Coll. Phys.*, **5**, 149–65

Mayerhofer (1863). quoted by Cianfrani (1960) p.311

Mazzur, S. (1973). Menstrual blood as a vehicle of Australian antigen transmission. *Lancet*, 1, 749

Meisels, A. and Fortin, R. (1976). Condylomatus lesions of the cervix and vagina. 1. Cytologic appearance. *Acta Cytol. (Baltimore)*, 20, 205

Meisels, A., Roy, M., Fortier, M. *et al.* (1981). Human papillomavirus infection of the cervix – the atypical condyloma. *Acta Cytol. (Baltimore)*, 25, 16

Melczer von, N. (1965). Uber die aetiologische identitat der gewohnlichem Warzen and Spitzen kondlyome. *Der Hautarzt*, 16, 150–3

Meyen, F.J.F. (1830). quoted by MacLeod (1973) p.11

Miescher, F. (1869). quoted by MacLeod (1973) p.12

Migula, W. (1895). Bacteriaceal (Stabchenbacterien). In Engler and Prantl (eds.) *Pflanzen Familien*, Teil 1, Abt. 1A, pp.20–30. (Leipzig: W. Englemann)

Mildvan, D. *et al.* (1982). quoted by Forster, S.M. (1987)

Mirbel de, C.F.B. (1802). quoted by MacLeod (1973) p.10

Muller (1730 –1784). quoted by Leadbetter and Poindexter (1985) p.4

Nageli, K. (1842). quoted by MacLeod (1983) p.12

Nahmias, A.J. and Dowdle, W.R. (1968). Antigenic and biologic differences in herpes virus hominis. *Prog. Med. Virol.*, 10, 110

Nahmias, A.J., Josey, W.E. and Naib, Z.M. (1967). Neonatal herpes simplex infection *J. Am. Med. Assoc.*, 199, 132

Nahmias, A.J., Josey, W.E., Naib, Z.M. *et al.* (1971). Perinatal risk associated with maternal genital herpes simplex infection. *Am. J. Obstet. Gynecol.*, 110, 825–37

Naib, Z.M., Nahmias, A.J. and Josey, W.E. (1972). Cytology and histopathology of cervical herpes simplex infection. *J. Cancer Res.*, 29, 1026–31

Neisser, A. (1879). Ueber eine der Gonorrhoe eigentumliche Micrococcusform. *Centralbl. f. d. med. Wissensch.*, 17, 497–500

Neisser, M. and Wechsberg, F. (1901). Ueber das Staphyltoxin. *Z. Hygiene und Infektionskrankheit*, 36, 299

Newman, A. (1988). *The Illustrated Treasury of Medical Curiosa*, p.141. (New York London: McGrew Hill Book Co.)

Noeggerath, E. (1872). *Die latente Gonorrhoe im Weiblichen Geschlecht.* (Bonn: Max Cohen & Sohn)

Odds, F.C. (1988). *Candida and candidosis*, 2nd edn. p.1 (London, Philadelphia, Toronto: Balliere Tindall)

O'Donel, T.G. Browne (1947). *The Rotunda Hospital. 1745–1945*, pp. 109–12. (Edinburgh: Livingstone)

Ogston (1860). quoted by Cianfrani (1960) p.311

Ogston (1881). quoted by Wilson and Miles (1955) p.699

Ogston, A. (1880). Uber Abscesse. *Archiv Klin. Chirurg.*, 25, 588

Oriel, J.D. (1971). Natural history of genital warts. *Br. J. Vener. Dis.*, 47, 1–13

Oriel, J.D. and Almeida, J.D. (1970). Demonstration of virus particles in human genital warts. *Br. J. Vener. Dis.*, 46, 37

Oxtoby, M.J. (1989). HIV and other viruses in milk. Placing the issues in broader perspective. For 'CDS: Current Issues in Pediatrics'. In Orenstein, W.A. (ed.) *Paediatric Infectious Diseases Journal*, quoted by Royal College of Obstetricians and Gynaecologists (1990) p. 4

Pasteur, L. (1860). quoted by Cianfrani (1960) p.311

Pasteur, L. (1879). quoted by Cianfrani (1960) p.311

Pasteur, L. (1880). quoted by Wilson and Miles (1955) p.699

Pasteur, L. and Joubert, J. (1877). Etude sur la maladie charbonneuse. *C.R. Acad. Sci, Paris*, 84, 900–6

Peyps, S. (1665). Diary, quoted by Odds, F.C. (1988) p. 1

Plass, E.D., Hesseltine, H.C. and Borts, I.H. (1931). Monilia vulvovaginitis. *Am. J. Obstet. Gynecol.*, 21, 320–34

Rawls, W.E. Gardner, H.L., Flanders, R.W. *et al.* (1971). Genital herpes in two social groups. *Am. J. Obstet. Gynecol.*, 110, 682

Reingold, A.L., Hargrett, N.T., Dan, B.B., Shands, K.N., Strickland, B.Y. and Broome, C.V. (1982).

Nonmenstrual toxic shock syndrome. *Ann. Intern. Med.*, **96**, 871–4

Reme, G. (1930). Hautreaktionen mit Staphylokokkenkulturfiltraten. *Z. Immunitatsforschung und experimentelle Therapie*, **69**, 25

Rhodes, P. (1985) reprinted (1988). *An Outline History of Medicine*, p. 8. (London, Boston: Butterworths)

Ricci, J.V. (1943). *The Genealogy of Gynecology*, pp.9; 321. (Philadelphia: Blakiston Co.)

Ricci, J.V. (1945). *One Hundred Years of Gynaecology 1800–1900.* (Philadelphia: Blakiston)

Rollet, J. (1869). quoted by Hutfield, D.C. (1966) p. 203

Rosenbach, F.J. (1884). *Mikroorganismen bei den wundinfektionskrankheiten des menchen.* Wiesbaden.

Ross, F.C. (1983). *Introductory Microbiology.* (Columbus: Merrill Publishing Co.)

Rous, Peyton, F. (1911). Transmission of a malignant new growth by means of a cell free filtrate. *J. Am. Med. Assoc.*, **56**, 198 (46;159)

Royal College of Obstetricians and Gynaecologists (1990). *HIV Infection in Maternity Care and Gynaecology.* (London: Chameleon Press)

Rutherford, G.W., Lifson, A.R., Hessol, N.A., Darrow, W.W., O'Malley, P.M., Buchbinder, S.P., Barnhart, J.L., Bodecker, T.W., Cannon, L., Doll, L.S., Holmberg, S.D., Harrison, J.S., Rogers, M.F., Werdegar, D. and Jaffe, H.W. (1990). Course of HIV-1 infection in a cohort of homosexual and bisexual men: an 11 year follow up study. *Br. Med. J.*, **301**, 1183–8

Sanger, W.W. (1895). *The History of Prostitution*, pp. 40–41. (New York: The Medical Publishing Co.)

Schaudin, F. and Hoffman, E. (1905). Vorlaufiger Bericht uber das Vorkommen von Spirochaeten in Syphilitischen Krankheitsprodukten und bei Papillomen. *Arbeiten aus dem Kaiserlichen, Gesundheitsamte*, **22**, 527–53

Schatz, A., Bugie, E. and Wacksman, S.A. (1944). quoted by Wilson and Miles (1955) p. 196

Schleiden, M.J. (1838). Beitrage zur Phytogenesis. *Mullers Arch. Anat. Physiol. u. Wiss.*, p. 137. (Medizin: Berlin)

Schnell, J.D. (1973). *Cytology and Microbiology of the Vagina. A Brief Atlas for Doctors and Medical Students.* (Basle: Karger)

Schochetman, G. (1990). Laboratory diagnosis of infection with the AIDS virus. *Hospimedica*, June, 58–68

Schofield, M. (1965). *The Sexual Behaviour of Young People.* (London: Longmans)

Schrock, C.G. (1980). Disease alert [letter]. *J. Am. Med. Assoc.*, **243**, 1231

Schwann, T. (1833). quoted by McGrew (1985) p.52

Schwann, T. (1839). quoted by MacLeod (1973) p.10

Sedillot, C. (1878). De l'influence des decouvertes de M. Pasteur sur le progres de la chirurgie. *C.R. Acad. Sci.*, **86**, 634–40

Sharlit, H. (1940). Herpes progenitalis as a venereal contagion. *Arch. Dermatol. Syphil.*, **42**, 933–6

Shepard, M.C. (1954). The recovery of pleuropneumonia-like organisms from Negro men with and without nongonococcal urethritis. *Am. J. Syphilis*, **38**, 113–24

Shepard, M.C., Lunceford, C.D., Ford, D.K. *et al.* (1974). *Ureaplasma urealyticum* gen. nov., sp. nov.: proposed nomenclature for the human T (T-strain) mycoplasmas. *Int. J. System. Bacteriol.*, **24**, 160–71

Sinclair, Sir. W.J. (1909). *Semmelweiss, his Life and his Doctrine*, p. 234. (Manchester: Manchester University Press)

Skinner, G. (1976). Viral infection in the cervix. In Jordan, J.A. and Singer, A. (eds.) *The Cervix*, p.269. (London: W.B. Saunders)

Slavin, H.B. and Gavett, E. (1946). Primary herpetic vulvovaginitis. *Proc. Soc. Exp. Biol. Med.*, **63**, 343–6

Spallanzani, L. (1767). *Saggio di osservazioni microscopische relative al sistema della generazione.* (Modena: Soc. Tipografica)

Spallanzani, L. (1776). *Opusculi di fisica animale e vegetabile*, 2 vols. (Modena: Soc. Tipografica)

Speert, H. (1958). *Essays in Eponymy*, pp.358; 363. (New York: The MacMillan Co.)

Spiegel, C.A. and Roberts, M. (1984). *Mobiluncus* gen. nov., *Mobiluncus curtisii* subsp., *curtisii* sp. nov., *Mobiluncus curtisii* subsp., *holmesii* subsp. nov., and *Mobiluncus mulieris* sp. nov., curved rods from the human vagina. *Int. J. Syst. Bacteriol.*, **34**, 177–84

Stanley (1935). quoted by Ross (1983) p.17

Stevens, F.A. (1927). The occurrence of *Staphylococcus aureus* infection with a scarlatiniform rash. *J. Am. Med. Assoc.*, **88**, 1957–8

Strasburger, E. (1875). *Zellbildung und Zellteilung.* (Jena: Dabis)

Strauss, M.J., Shaw, E.W., Bunting, H. and Melnick, J.L. (1949). 'Crystaline' virus-like particles from skin papillomas characterised by intranuclear inclusion bodies. *Proc. Soc. Exp. Biol. Med.*, **72**, 46–50

Stuart, R.D. (1944). Transport medium for specimens in public health bacteriology. *Public Health Reports*, **74**, 431

Swammerdam, J. (1675). quoted by Grunze and Spriggs (1983) p.9

Swammerdam, J. (1737). *Biblia naturae sive historia insectorum in classes redacta.* (Leiden: J.Severinus and B. and P van der Aa)

Talbot Fox, H. (1834). quoted by Grunze and Spriggs (1983) p.16

Teokharov, B.A. (1969). Non–gonococcal infections of the female genitalia. *Br. J. Vener. Dis.*, **45**, 334–9

Thomas, C.G.A. (1983). *Medical Microbiology*, 5th edn. (London: Balliere Tindall)

Thygeson, P. and Mengert, W.F. (1936). The virus of inclusion conjunctivitis: further observations. *Arch. Ophthalmol.*, **15**, 377–410

Todd, J., Fishaut, M., Kapral, F. and Welch, T. (1978). Toxic-shock syndrome associated with phage-group-1 staphylococci. *Lancet*, **2**, 1116–18

Todd, J.K., Ressman, M., Castle, S.A., Todd, B.H. and Wiesenthal, A.M. (1984). Corticosteroid therapy for patients with toxic shock syndrome. *J. Am. Med. Assoc.*, **252**, 3399–402

Trussell, R.E. and Plass, E.D. (1940). The pathogenicity and physiology of a pure culture of *Trichomonas vaginalis*. *Am. J. Obstet. Gynecol.*, **40**, 883

Turner (1714) quoted by Beswick, T.S.L. (1962) p. 214

Tyzzer, E.E. (1906). The histology of the skin lesions in varicella. *Philip. J. Sci.*, **1**, 349–72

Unna, P.G. (1883). On herpes progenitalis, especially in women. *J. Cutaneous and Venereal Dis.*, **1**, 321–7

Veillon, A. and Zuber, A. (1898). Recherches sur quelques microbes strictement anaerobies et leur role en pathologie. *Arch. Med. Exp.*, **10**, 517–45

Venzmer, G. (1972). *Five Thousand Years of Medicine,* Translated by M.Koenig pp.135; 150 (London: MacDonald)

Waksman, S.A. (1944). quoted by McGrew (1985) p.344

Wassermann von, A. (1906). quoted by Wilson and Miles (1955) p.2033

Waterson, A.P. and Wilkinson, L. (1978). *An Introduction to the History of Virology*, p. 1. (London, New York, Melbourne: Cambridge University Press)

Waugh, M.A. (1990). History of clinical development of sexually transmitted diseases. In Holmes, K.K. *et al.* (eds.) *Sexually Transmitted Diseases*, 2nd edn. pp. 3–16. (New York: McGraw-Hill)

Webster, A. and Johnson, M. (1990). Human immunodeficiency virus infection. In Studd, J. (ed.) *Progress in Obstetrics and Gynaecology*, Vol. 8, pp. 175–90. (London: Churchill Livingstone)

Westrom, L. (1980). Incidence, prevalence and trends of pelvic inflammatory disease and its consequences in industrialised countries. *Am. J. Obstet.*, **138**, 880

Wile, U.J. and Kingery, L.B. (1919). The aetiology of common warts. Preliminary report of an experimental study. *J. Am. Med. Assoc.*, **73**, 970–3

Wilkinson, J.S. (1849). Some remarks upon the development of griphytes with the description of new vegetable formation found in connection with the human uterus. *Lancet*, **2**, 448

Williams, G.R. (1990). The toxic shock syndrome: many cases are not associated with menstruation. *Br. Med. J.*, **300**, 960

Willis, T.G. (1662). quoted by Cianfrani (1960) p.305

Wilmott, F.E. (1975). Cytomegalovirus in female patients attending venereal disease clinics. *Br. J. Vener. Dis.*, **51**, 278

Wilson, G.S. and Miles, A.A. (1955). *Topley and Wilson's Principles of Bacteriology and Immunity*, 4th edn., Vol. 11, p.1040. (London: Edward Arnold Ltd.)

Wolff, C.F. (1759). *Theoria Generationis.* Inaug. Diss. Med. Fac. Halle/Saale. Hallae ad Salam. Litteris Hendelianis.

FURTHER READING

Bettmann, O.L. (1956). *A Pictorial History of Medicine.* (Springfield: Thomas)

Cianfrani, T. (1960). *A Short History of Obstetrics and Gynecology.* (Springfield, Illinois: Charles C. Thomas)

Hare, M.J. (ed.) (1988). *Genital Tract Infection in Women.* (Edinburgh, London, Melbourne, New York: Churchill Livingstone)

European Collaborative Study (1991). Children born to women with HIV-1 infection: natural history and risk of transmission. *Lancet*, **1**, 253–60

Farthing, C. (1987) AIDS in Clinical Medicine. (Middlesex: Barker Publications Ltd)

Grunze, H. and Spriggs, A.I. (1983). *History of Clinical Cytology: A Selection of Documents*, 2nd edn. G-I-T. (D-6100 Darmstadt, West Germany: Verlag Ernst Ghebelar)

Kaufman, R.H., Friedrich, E.G. Jr. and Gardner, H.L. (1989). *Benign Diseases of the Vulva and Vagina.* (Chicago, London, Boca Raton: Year Book Medical Publishers Inc.)

McGrew, R.E. (1985). *Encyclopedia of Medical History.* (London: MacMillan Press)

MacLeod, A.G. (1973). In Thomas, B.A. (ed.) *Cytology*, pp. 10–13. (Kalamazoo Michigan: Upjohn Co.)

Norman, S., Studd, J. and Johnson, M. (1990). HIV infection in women. *Br. Med. J.*, **301**, 1231–2

Reviews of Infectious Diseases (1986). Vol. 8, Suppl. 1. (Chicago, Illinois, London: University of Chicago Press)

Rutherford, G.W., Lifson, A.R., Hessol, N.A., Darrow, W., O'Malley, P.M., Buchbinder, S.P., Barnhart, J.L., Bodecker, T.W., Cannon, L., Doll, S.L., Holmberg, S.D., Harrison, J.S., Rogers, M.F., Werdegar, D. and Jaffe, H.W. (1990). Course of HIV-1 infection in a cohort of homosexual and bisexual men: an 11 year follow up study. *Br. Med. J.*, **301**, 1183–8

Schochetman, G. (1990). Laboratory diagnosis of infection with the AIDS virus. *Hospimedica*, June 1990 58–68

Speert, H. (1958). *Essays in Eponymy.* (New York: The MacMillan Co.)

Waterson, A.P. and Wilkinson, L. (1978). *An Introduction to the History of Virology.* (London, New York, Melbourne: Cambridge University Press)

Williams, G.R. (1990). The toxic shock syndrome. *Br. Med. J.*, **300**, 960

Wilson, G.S. and Miles, A.A. (1955). *Topley and Wilson's Principles of Bacteriology and Immunity*, 4th edn., Vols. I and II. (London: Edward Arnold Ltd.)

Antibiotics

DEFINITION

The word antibiosis was coined at the end of the nineteenth century. It means a relationship between two organisms, or among the members of a group of organisms, which results in harm to one of them, owing to the production of an antibiotic by the other. Selman Waksman was the first person in the twentieth century to recall the word 'antibiotic' for daily use; it probably was first used in 1876 by John Tyndall (1820–1893). One of the definitions of an antibiotic is: any of the specific substances produced *in vitro* by certain bacteria and fungi which are capable of killing or inhibiting the growth of certain other bacteria and viruses *in vitro* and *in vivo*.

John Tyndall who did the original research work on *Penicillium* showed that certain members of the group could inhibit some bacteria (Mann, 1984). Already in 1877 Pasteur and Jules Joubert had shown that one organism, *Bacillus anthracis*, was antagonistic to other bacteria. In 1899 Rudolph Emmerich (1852–1914) and Oscar Low had prepared an enzyme from cultures of *Pseudomonas aeruginosa* that could destroy bacteria.

THE SULPHONAMIDES

In 1935 an enormously important discovery was made by Gerhard Domagk (1895–1964). This was based partly on the brilliant research work that had been carried out by Paul Ehrlich (1854–1915) who had discovered Salvarsan (Compound no. 606), which was first used in 1911 to treat human syphilis. It revolutionized the handling of this killer illness. The compound was so called because it was the 606th arsenical compound Ehrlich had tested. Ehrlich's assistant Sahachiro Hata (1873–1938) retested 606 on rabbits infected with *Treponema pallidum* and found it was effective against the organism. 606, and later 914 (Neo-Salvarsan, also developed by Ehrlich), was highly effective but was later replaced by penicillin which had fewer side-effects and acted much more rapidly.

Domagk studied biologically effective dyes and showed that his new substance named Prontosil Red protected mice experimentally infected with streptococci. For their research Ehrlich received the Nobel Prize in 1908 and Domagk in 1939. It was the discovery of Prontosil Red and its introduction in 1932, but only published in 1935, that enabled Colebrook to check whether mice infected with streptococci from cases of puerperal fever could be protected. He found that they could not, because they had human- and not mouse-virulent strains.

In January 1936 a woman with very severe puerperal fever was admitted to Queen Charlotte's Hospital isolation block, and given Prontosil Red. Colebrook was working with the clinician Dr Maeve Kenny, a resident medical officer to the isolation block. They treated 38 cases with a mortality of 8%, whereas of the preceding 38 with puerperal fever, 23.7% had died. It was found by Colebrook's team when following up work that had been done in the Pasteur Institute in Paris that Prontosil Red was broken down to para-aminobenzine-sulphonamide. Colebrook and Kenny (1936) gave this substance to 121 patients and the mortality dropped to 6.5%. Not only were maternity patients treated; but two of Leonard Colebrook's assistants, the first with an infected thumb and the second with very severe tonsillitis, were also treated. Both men turned bright red, but both men were cured.

Although the early sulphonamides were fairly effective, they could be and were improved on, so that when M&B 693 had been perfected it was used to treat Winston Churchill, who had developed pneumonia in North Africa during the war (Colebrook, 1954). Special care could be given in an isolation unit, or better still in units where good asepsis was practised, and this was reflected in the figures. In a new unit of Queen Charlotte's Hospital in the west of London, the maternal mortality in booked cases was less than one per

1000 deliveries, although in unbooked cases it was as high as four per 1000; but women who were admitted as emergencies and who had had no effective antenatal care, could have the terribly high mortality rate of 82 per thousand. Some of these had had forceps deliveries attempted in their own homes causing trauma to the genital passages, which then became infected.

PENICILLIN

Sir Alexander Fleming (1881–1955) of St Mary's Hospital London discovered that there was a substance that could kill bacteria in the mucus from the nose of a person suffering from an acute cold. He called this substance 'Lysozyme' and he described some of its properties in 1932. Fleming (1929) discovered penicillin and in his first paper on it noted 'that around a large colony of contaminating mould the *Staphylococcus* colonies became transparent and were obviously undergoing lysis'. He summarized his paper with a description of 10 qualities of *Penicillium* and he suggested that 'it may be an efficient antiseptic for application to, or injection into, areas infected with penicillin-sensitive microbes'.

There were other scientists working on other antibiotics, especially that produced by *Penicillium griseofulvum*. It required a biochemist, which Fleming was not, to work on the chemical structure of the active substance in the mould that had come into the window of Fleming's laboratory at St Mary's Hospital, Paddington. Fleming admitted that he had become discouraged about the problem of isolating chemical substances in penicillin. Perhaps as Sir Henry Dale wrote 'time . . . nor . . . the scientific atmosphere of the laboratory in which Fleming worked, was propitious to such further enterprise as its development would have needed'. In fact Chain wrote that Sir Almroth Wright, Fleming's 'boss' was very antagonistic to any thoughts of the use of penicillin for treating infections (Clark, 1985).

It was fortunate that Fleming had left his culture dish in a warm enough temperature (18–20°C) to allow the *Penicillium* but not the staphylococci and its neighbours in the Petri dish, to grow reasonably fast. Luck played a large role too. Chain had unbelievable luck because he had many fruitful discussions with Florey, the head of his laboratory in Oxford, about how to investigate the chemical nature of microbes that were antagonistic towards each other. As a result he studied many papers and fortuitously came across

Fleming's 1929 report on penicillin. There was another piece of luck that Chain had because he saw a young lady, a Miss Campbell-Renton, walking down the corridor in their laboratory building carrying a mould which happened to be *Penicillium notatum*. It was the mould that Fleming had given to Florey's predecessor in Oxford, who had not done anything serious with it. Chain, seeing the mould in the dish, felt that he must investigate its biochemistry. He thought that the active principle of the *Penicillium notatum* was an enzyme similar to the Lysozyme that Fleming had described.

Chain and Florey determined to undertake a thorough study of the antibacterial substances that could be found in moulds and bacteria, starting with Miss Campbell-Renton's *Penicillium* mould of which they obtained a sample, and they published their paper from the Sir William Dunn School of Pathology in Oxford (Chain *et al.*, 1940). Chain and his co-workers very quickly recognized penicillinase, a substance found in some bacteria that made those bacteria resistant to the penicillin and they reported that finding in December 1940 (Abraham and Chain, 1940). The team had to go to America for volume production of penicillin to be undertaken by pharmaceutical houses there. All this fresh penicillin was produced from subcultures of Fleming's original mould.

Penicillin in obstetrics and gynaecology

The first use of penicillin in obstetrics seems to have been, not for the treatment of staphylococcal or streptococcal infections, but for syphilis. It had already been used to treat syphilis in members of the armed forces who it seems, because of the war effort, had priority in the use of big batches of penicillin to treat the venereal diseases which made them *hors de combat*. Goodwin and Moore (1946) treated 57 pregnant syphilitic women with penicillin; their babies were born without any of the stigmata of syphilis. This was in spite of warnings by Levitt (1945) that penicillin might have an abortifacient action and that it could cause uterine cramps. This belief was contradicted by Speiser and Thomas (1946) and by Olansky and Dick (1947). To achieve rapid treatment of antenatal syphilis they treated some cases with intravenous arsenic and others with penicillin, and the penicillin was shown to be superior, with more rapid onset of action.

Cole *et al.* (1946) treated the first large series of 730 syphilitics with penicillin. Forty-seven of these women were pregnant and only one delivered a stillborn child. One other infant was born with the stigmata of congenital syphilis. By the end of 1946 arsenicals (marpharside) and quinine were being used together with the penicillin. Penicillin and penicillin-like substances were supplementing or even taking over from the sulphonamides as treatment for maternal and postoperative bacterial infections; as well as for syphilis. The syphilis spirochaete was to prove to be almost the only organism that never became resistant to penicillin, which was almost invariably effective in cases of syphilis. So, obstetricians acquired a very powerful weapon against some of the worst infections their patients suffered.

OTHER ANTIBIOTICS

An often fatal infection that remained was tuberculosis, mainly affecting the lungs, but also causing peritonitis and salpingitis. Sellman Abraham Waksman (1888–1973) (Figure 1), a Russian migrant to the USA had discovered a new species of actinomycete from which he and H.W. Woodruff isolated actinomycin. Although actinomycin was strongly antimicrobial it was also highly toxic. Waksman searched further and in 1944 he discovered a new species of fungus which he called *Streptomyces griseus*, and he later isolated streptomycin from it. He and his colleagues' first paper on streptomycin was published in 1944 (Schatz *et al.*, 1944).

There is a very interesting review paper by Philip D'Arcy Hart and D'Arch Montagu (1946) on the chemotherapy of tuberculosis. Philip D'Arcy Hart was in charge of the English clinical trials for streptomycin. Since it was proving to be a lifesaver he had to contend with some very strong ethical problems in deciding to whom the drugs should be given. The selection was made randomly. The first injection of streptomycin to be given in Europe was by one of the authors of this book, on the 21 July 1946 (Philipp, 1947). The patient's treatment was later supervised by William Hugh Feldman who set up clinical trials in the UK in 1946. After a time, streptomycin – unlike penicillin with syphilis – was found not always to be effective against tuberculosis; the effect might and could wear off after a few weeks, so research was instituted for new moulds and different substances to treat tuberculosis and other organisms that had become resistant.

One remarkable preparation is metronidazole (Flagyl). This was the first important drug for relieving one of the most annoying and widespread of gynaecological infections, *Trichomonas vaginalis. Trichomonas* causes a persistent vaginal discharge, sometimes white, but more often yellow or light green in colour, accompanied by itching, and an unpleasant smell. Although the infection is never severe it certainly is an irritation for patients, destroying their self-respect and self-confidence, as well as their interest in a sex life, because the vagina becomes for them something of which to be ashamed. *Trichomonas vaginalis* has been known to be a single-celled organism since 1836. Although men can harbour the organism and certainly infect their sexual partners, they rarely themselves suffer any symptoms or signs.

In 1954 the pharmaceutical house of Rhone-Poulenc in Paris began a research programme to find a drug which was active against this infection. Yet one more fungus of the *Streptomyces* group was found to contain an active substance. This fungus had been isolated from a soil sample collected on the French Isle of Reunion in the Indian Ocean. A substance very much like the active substance in this fungus was synthesized in July 1957 and the formula published in 1959. It is quite a complex compound; its first successful use was reported by Durel *et al.* (1959). Unlike previous treatments for vaginal infections, it was administered by mouth and not vaginally, although in resistant cases vaginal application could be helpful.

Elizabeth Keighley (1962) tried it on 102 prisoners suffering with *Trichomonas* infection in Holloway prison. (She, incidentally, was the first

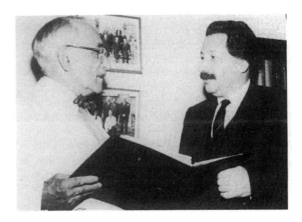

Figure 1 Ernst Chain (right) who elucidated the biochemistry of penicillin together with Sellman Abraham Waksman (left) who discovered streptomycin. Reproduced with kind permission from Clark, R.W. (1985). *The Life of Ernst Chain, Penicillin and Beyond.* (London: Weidenfeld and Nicolson)

person to conduct a prospective trial of Papanicolaou smears in 1000 patients in the same prison.) She found that the cure rate for *Trichomonas* infection in Holloway was 100%, although ten out of the 102 prisoners required a second course of treatment. When there were failures in the outside world these were nearly all due to reinfection by consorts (Keighley, 1962).

Serendipitously a dental registrar at King's College Dental Hospital in London, David Shinn, noticed that the mouth of one of his patients who had acute ulcerative gingivitis improved rapidly as did her *Trichomonas vaginalis* infection when she was given Flagyl for the latter. He wondered whether Flagyl had affected the gingivitis as well; it had. Shinn published his paper in the *Lancet* in 1962 (Shinn, 1962). When the research workers at Rhone-Poulenc's subsidiary factory, May and Baker, heard of the activity of Flagyl against *Trichomonas* and the bacteria of gingivitis they investigated whether the bowel-infecting protozoan *Giardia intestinalis* (formerly *G. lamblia*), which in common with the *Trichomonas* and the gingivitis-causing organisms is anaerobic, was susceptible.

When later Flagyl was given prophylactically by surgeons who were operating on the bowel and who often found their cases to be complicated by anaerobic infection, it worked; markedly lowering the postoperative sepsis rate; so in time, metronidazole was given prophylactically pre- and intraoperatively to many patients undergoing bowel surgery and to large numbers of women who were undergoing hysterectomy. It also worked in amoebic dysentery. By 1991, *Trichomonas* was far less commonly found than earlier. Many vaginal discharges are caused by other anaerobic bacteria which nearly all respond to metronidazole.

Metronidazole has even been tried in combination with irradiation for tumours. Apparently it does have a chemotherapeutic effect if given 36 hours before irradiation, causing a reduction in the dose necessary to destroy some tumours in mice. So, a drug developed originally to cure a gynaecological condition has proved its worth in general surgery and in other infectious conditions (McFadzean, 1986).

As has been seen, even in the 1980s there were patients dying of sepsis and of septic shock. Efforts to reduce this mortality included cardiorespiratory resuscitation developed over the second half of the twentieth century. But the 1990s brought further hopeful progress in the shape of monoclonal antibodies used against the toxic products of infecting organisms. Thus the last decade of the twentieth century has brought hope of further improvements in the fight against sepsis (Heinz, 1992).

CHRONOLOGY

1876	John Tyndall coined the term antibiotic.
1877	Pasteur and Jules Joubert discovered antagonism between bacteria.
1899	Emmerich and Low prepared bactericidal enzymes.
1910	Paul Ehrlich discovered Salvarsan, and the drug was used to treat syphilis in the following years. He developed a more refined drug called Neosalvarsan in 1914 and it became known as the 'magic bullet' (Duin and Sutcliffe, 1992).
	Carell and Burrows using Rous sarcoma were the first to grow a malignant tissue *in vitro* for experimental purposes.
1929	Alexander Fleming discovered penicillin.
1935	Domagk published his discovery of Prontosil red, introduced 3 years previously.
1940	Chain *et al.* used penicillin as a chemotherapeutic agent.
1943	Mahoney used penicillin in the treatment of early syphilis.
1944	Sellman A. Waksman and H.W. Woodruff isolated actinomycin (Schatz *et al.*, 1944).
1946	Goodwin and Moore used penicillin to treat pregnant syphilitic women.
1959	Durel *et al.* reported the successful use of Flagyl.

REFERENCES

Abraham, Sir E.P. and Chain, Sir E.B. (1940). An enzyme from bacteria able to destroy penicillin. *Nature (London)*, **146**, 837

Carell, A. and Burrows, M.T. (1910). Cultures de Sarcoma en dehors de l'organisme. *C.R. Soc. Biol. (Paris)*, **69**, 332–4

Chain, E.B., Florey, H.W., Gardner, A.D., Heatley, N.G., Jennings, M.A., Orr-Ewing, J. and Sanders, A.G. (1940). Penicillin as a chemotherapeutic agent. *Lancet*, **2**, 226–8

Clark, R.W. (1985). *The Life of Ernst Chain... Penicillin and Beyond*, p. 30. (London: Weidenfeld & Nicholson)

Cole, H.N., Ayres, S., Barr, J.H., Genatios, T., Held, B., Murphy, W.W., Printz, D.R. and Strauch, J. (1946). Use of penicillin in the treatment of syphilis in pregnancy. *Archiv. Derm. Syphilol.*, **54**, 225–64

Colebrook, L. (1954). Puerperal infection. In Munro-Kerr, J., Johnstone, R.W. and Philips, M. (eds.) *Historical Review of British Obstetrics and Gynaecology 1800–1950*, pp. 202–26. (Edinburgh: Livingstone)

Colebrook, L. and Kenny, M. (1936). Treatment of human puerperal infections and of experimental infections in mice with prontosil. *Lancet*, **1**, 1279–86

Domagk, G. (1935). Ein Beitrag Zur Chemotherapie der Bakterielle Infektionen. *Dtsch. Med. Wchschr.*, **61**, 250

Duin, N. and Sutcliffe, J. (1992). *A History of Medicine from Pre-History to the Year 2020*, pp. 100–1. (London: Simon and Schuster Ltd.)

Durel, M.P., Roiron, V., Siboulet, A. and Borel, L.J. (1959). *C.R. Soc. Fr. Gynecol.*, 29–36

Ehrlich, P. *et al.* (1910). *Die Experimentelle Chemotherapie der Spirillosen.* (Berlin: J. Springer) quoted by Waugh (1990)

Fleming, A. (1929). The antibacterial action of cultures of a *Penicillium* with special reference to their use in the isolation of B influenzae *Br. J. Exp. Pathol.*, **10**, 226–36

Goodwin, M.S. and Moore, J.E. (1946). Penicillin in prevention of prenatal syphilis *J. Am. Med. Assoc.*, **130**, 688–94

Hart, P.D.A. and Montagu, D'Arch, (1946). Chemotherapy of tuberculosis – researchers during the past 100 years. *Br. Med. J.*, **2**, 805–10; 849–55

Heinz, C.J. (1992). Monoclonal antibodies in a sepsis and septic shock. *Br. Med. J.*, **304**, 132–3

Keighley, E.E. (1962). Trichomoniasis in closed community: 100% follow-up *Br. Med. J.*, **2**, 93–5

Levitt, H. (1945). Penicillin in gonorrhea *Ven. Dis. Inform.*, **2**, 93

McFadzean, J.D. (1986). *Flagyl – The Story of a Pharmaceutical Discovery.* (Carnforth: Parthenon Publishing)

Mahoney, J.F. *et al.* (1943). Penicillin treatment of early syphilis. A preliminary report. *Vener. dis. Inf.*, **24**, 355

Mann, R.D. (1984). *Modern Drug Use*, pp. 558–64. (Lancaster: MTP Press)

Olansky, S. and Beck, R. (1947). Rapid treatment of prenatal syphilis. *Am. J. Syph. Gonorrhea VD*, **31**, 51–7

Philipp, E.E. (1947). MRCOG Commentary

Schatz, A. *et al.* (1944). Streptomycin, a substance exhibiting antibiotic activity against Gram-positive and Gram-negative bacteria. *Proc. Soc. Exp. Biol. (N.Y.)*, **55**, 66–9

Shinn, D.L.S. (1962). Metronidazole in acute ulcerative gingivitis. *Lancet*, **1**, 1191

Speiser, M.P. and Thomas, E.W. (1946). Regarding unusual effect of penicillin therapy upon uterus. *J. Ven. Dis. Inform.*, **27**, 20–1

Waugh, M.A. (1990). History of sexually transmitted disease. In Holmes, K.K., Mardh, P.A., Sparling, P.F. and Wiesner, P.J. (eds.) *Sexually Transmitted Diseases*, 2nd edn., pp. 3–16. (New York: McGraw-Hill)

Hormones and the menstrual cycle

HORMONES AND REPRODUCTIVE ENDOCRINOLOGY

The term endocrine derived from the Greek (*Endon*, within; *Krinein*, to separate) and means inwardly secreting, while hormone also derived from the Greek, *hormao*, means to excite, arouse, or put into quick motion. The term *hormone* was suggested by Sir William B. Hardy of Cambridge, UK, and his colleague W.T. Vesey, and was first used by Professor Ernst Henry Starling in 1905 during his Croonian Lecture on the *Chemical Correlation of the Functions of the Body* (Gruhn and Kazer, 1989).

Although the subject of endocrinology belongs almost entirely to the present century, the endocrine glands were described many years ago. Physicians were aware of the thyroid and reproductive glands from ancient times and Bartolommeo Eustachio described the adrenal glands in 1543. Ruysch, c. 1690, was one of the first to speculate that organs such as the thyroid gland produced substances which were released into the blood stream and in 1830, Johannes Müller opined that the endocrine glands secreted their fluids directly into the blood stream rather than through a duct to the exterior.

Due to the growth of scientific medicine many important discoveries were made in the nineteenth century, and the area of endocrinology attracted the attention of some famous investigators. One of the early researchers in the field was Arnold Adolph Berthold (1849) a physiologist from Gottingen, who carried out his experiments with testicular transplantation and found that removal, but subsequent regrafting of the testicles to another part of the body prevented atrophy of the castrated Cock's (Capon) comb. In the same year Thomas Addison of Guys Hospital London, described the symptoms of the disease which bears his name and implicated the adrenal glands as the source of the disorder (Harkness, 1962). Claude Bernard, a Frenchman, and experimental physiologist, was the first to introduce the new concept of 'internal secretion' in 1855 (Harkness, 1962). A fellow countryman, Charles Eduoard Brown-Sequard (1890) experimented with the effects of self-injection of animal testicular extract and reported 'a radical change back to his former character of many years before'. He suggested that an ovarian extract could be used for rejuvenation of women.

Aqueous extracts of adrenal glands were produced by Oliver and Schafer (1895) and Abel and Crawford isolated epinephrine in 1897 – the first chemically pure endocrine substance to be obtained. Secretin, the first hormone to be recognized by name, was discovered by the English physiologists Bayliss and Starling in 1897. Meanwhile in 1891 Murray had introduced the oral administration of thyroid substance; and the active principle, thyroxin, was isolated by an American research scientist called Kendall (1915). Takamine (1901) of Japan produced 4g of a crystalline active substance of the adrenal glands from 8000 bovine adrenal glands and named it adrenaline, while in 1922 Banting and Best of Canada isolated insulin from the pancreas (Harkness, 1962). The parathyroid glands were discovered by Sandstrom (1880) and an American research scientist called Collip (1925) extracted a hormone from the parathyroids (parathyroid hormone) which raised blood calcium levels.

The endocrine function of the ovaries and testicles was the subject of much investigation, and the effects of gonadal removal and subsequent transplantation, or that of administration of aqueous or lipid extracts of the gland in castrate animals was documented by many workers in the early twentieth century. Edgar Allen and Edward Doisy (1923) are credited with the isolation of an 'ovarian hormone' from the liquor folliculi, and Doisy *et al.* (1929) prepared a crystalline extract of it in 1929, which was later called 'oestrogen'.

Progesterone was isolated and its hormonal action discovered by George Corner and Willard Allen (1929) and the male hormone androsterone was isolated from urine by the German chemist and Nobel prize winner, Adolf Butenandt (1931).

The concept of the pituitary as conductor of an endocrine orchestra was to come later.

THE OVARY AND OVULATION

The ovaries were discovered in ancient times, possibly by Herophilus in the fourth century BC, and were called the female testicles or didymi (twins). In the second century AD. Soranus of Ephesus, who practised in Rome, gave a detailed description of the organs noting their size, shape, and position. However, very little advance in anatomic knowledge was made between the second and sixteenth centuries as the conditions for anatomical dissection and demonstration were rigidly proscribed by the civil authorities, and it was difficult to obtain cadavers for dissection. During those years all anatomical knowledge was based on the writings of Galen (from the second century AD), who had gained most of his knowledge from dissection of animals. Leonardo da Vinci (1452–1519), turned his artistic talent to anatomical drawings and was the first to represent the uterus as having a single uterine cavity; prior to that it had been thought to consist of several distinct chambers. His drawings of the ovaries were not detailed but do show a knowledge of their structure. During Leonardo's lifetime another Italian, Gian Matteo De Gradi of Milan also known as Ferrari D'Agrate, theorized that the mammalian female testicles, like the ovaries of birds, were the site of egg formation.

The first anatomist to display the ovaries and the contained follicles adequately, was Andreas Vesalius, the 'Father of Modern Anatomy'. In the 1555 edition of his book, *De Humani Corporis Fabrica*, he described the ovary as containing 'sinuses' with thin watery fluid, and also what may have been a corpus luteum (Corner, 1933). The first edition of his book was published in 1543, and the anatomical illustrations therein were prepared by Jan Kalkar, a pupil of the famous Venetian and Italian Renaissance painter Titian (1477–1576).

Gabrielle Falloppio is said to have been the most brilliant of Vesalius's pupils; and went on to become professor of anatomy at Padua (Speert, 1958). He dissected the female 'testes' and searched for the semen which he thought was stored in them. In 1621, Falloppio's successor, Fabricius deAquapendente described the hen's ovary, and recognizing it as the organ of egg formation, gave it the name *ovarium*. He did not use the same term for the human ovary, and apparently was unaware of its egg-making function. The prevalent teaching was that of Aristotle, which claimed that the human egg was formed in the uterus.

In 1666 Jan Swammerdam and Johann van Horne, who were working together in Leiden, developed the theory that the mammalian female testes, like the ovaries in birds, were the site of egg formation. A Danish anatomist Niels Stensen, in 1667, developed the same idea. Regnier de Graaf (1672) published his *De Mulierum Organis Generationi Inservientibus* in which he described the ovaries and follicles which have since been eponymously associated with his name, but he assumed that the entire follicle was the ovum. In 1674, Anton van Leeuwenhoek, a Dutch draper and lens grinder, published his discovery of spermatozoa in semen using a hand held microscope for magnification. The term corpus luteum was introduced around 1681 by Marcello Malpighi the pioneer microscopist (Gruhn, 1987; Gruhn and Kazer, 1989; Speert, 1958).

Hermann Boerhaave (1668–1738) was a professor at Leiden for many years, and was not a great researcher but he greatly influenced students who subsequently accomplished greatness. He did speculate that the egg on leaving the ovary left a corpus luteum behind and that sperm fertilized the egg before its entry to the uterus (Short, 1977). One of his own pupils Albrecht von Haller, a Swiss, rejected that idea in 1744, but at a later date was responsible for introducing the term 'Graafian follicle'. William Hunter (1718–1783) (q.v. in Biography) carried out dissection on a large number of human gravid uteri. He described the corpus luteum, and in the case of twins note that two corpora were present. Percival Pott (1714–1788) and later John B. Davidge (1769–1829) linked removal of the ovaries to the cessation of menstruation and shrinking of the breasts (Pott, 1775) while Haighton (1797), in his experiments on rabbits, found that coitus induced ovulation. Prevost and Dumas (1824) who were working with dogs, detailed their observations of ovulation and formation of the corpus luteum.

The search for the mammalian ovum concluded about 1 May, 1827. Karl Ernst von Baer of Germany (Figure 1) while working on the reproductive tract of the dog, noted that the tubal ova were smaller than the Graafian follicles as William Cumberland Cruikshank (1745–1800) of Edinburgh, who had worked with William Hunter, had noted in 1778; and he turned his attention to the ovary (Speert, 1973). He noticed a yellowish white point in each ovarian follicle and led by curiosity he opened one of the follicles to take up the minute object on the

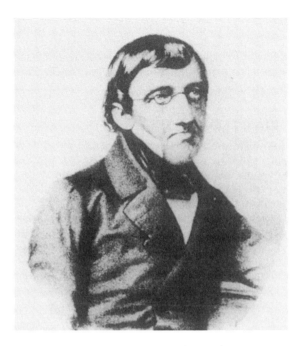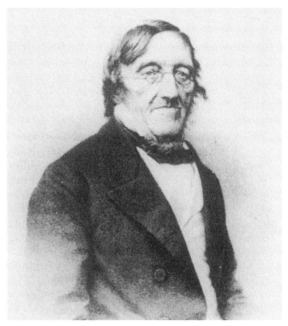

Figure 1 Karl Ernst von Baer (1792–1876) was the first to describe the mammalian ovum in 1827. Left, after a photograph by Dauthendy of St. Petersburg, probably 1829–1830, when he was 38 or 39 years old. Right, painting showing von Baer as an older man. Reproduced with kind permission from Meyer, A. W. (1956). *Human Generation.* (Stanford, California: Stanford University Press)

point of his knife (Von Baer, 1827). He later wrote 'when I placed it under the microscope I was utterly astonished, I saw an ovule . . . and so clearly that a blind man could hardly deny it. It is truly wonderful and surprising to be able to demonstrate to the eye, by so simple a procedure, a thing that has been sought so persistently and discussed *ad nauseam* in every text book of physiology as insoluble'.

In 1840 Negrier and in 1893 Rivelli demonstrated that a follicle ruptures each month, and that ovulation does not occur before the onset of menarche or after the menopause. In 1877 Herman Fol, a Swiss zoologist was the first to observe fertilization, as it occurred in a starfish egg (Gruhn and Kazer, 1989).

Lataste (1886; 1887) in France correlated the cyclic changes in the ovary with cytological changes in the vaginal epithelium. The corpus luteum was investigated by many workers and Louis-Auguste Prenant (1898a,b) suggested that it was a gland of internal secretion. Ludwig Fraenkel and F. Cohn (1901) in Germany and Vilhelm Magnus (1901) in Norway showed that destruction of the corpora lutea in pregnant rabbits led to abortion or resorption of embryos and this underlined the

importance of the corpus luteum in the maintenance of early pregnancy. Hitschmann and Adler (1907; 1908) described the histological changes of the endometrium throughout the menstrual cycle and Meyer (1911) and Ruge (1913) outlined the stages of development of the corpus luteum. The development in America of the vaginal cytological technique by Stockard and Papanicolaou (1917) provided a simple method of studying the menstrual cycle and this proved to be a very helpful bioassay for investigators studying the reproductive hormones.

For a time the 'continuous oogenesis theory' was prevalent and claims were made that new ova and follicles arose from the germinal epithelium of the ovary in a manner similar to that described for the embryo, so that the ova reaching maturity were of recent origin and possibly only a few weeks old (Robinson, 1918; Allen, 1923; Papanicolaou, 1923–24). The alternative or 'storage' theory held that the oocytes were laid down during the embryonic period and from that time on underwent a process of maturation and degeneration.

Simkins (1932), who was investigating the development of the human ovary from birth to

257

sexual maturity, noted that during childhood the stroma of the ovary dominated and only a few follicles were visible on individual sections of the gland. Block (1952) carried out counts and calculations on the ovaries of 43 human females ranging in age from 6 to 44 years. The total number of primordial follicles in both ovaries showed a mean of 439 thousand in girls up to 15 years of age and steadily decreased thereafter, until in a 10-year group, from age 36 onwards, only 34 000 follicles were noted. Meanwhile Ohler (1951) had criticized and refuted the continuous oogenesis theory and Mandl and Zuckerman (1951) in the same year, investigated the effects of destruction of the germinal epithelium on the number of oocytes in rats and found no significant difference between treated and control ovaries.

The general process of ovulation was detailed by Robinson (1918) and Allen et al. (1930). The Graafian follicle was found to grow to a size of about 15 mm diameter and gradually reach the surface of the ovary. The growth of the follicle accelerated prior to rupture but Hartman (1939) noted that the actual rupture of the follicle, which was aided by a rise in intrafollicular pressure, was not an explosive process but a gradual opening. The ovum with its zona pellucida and attached follicular epithelial cells was then discharged (ovulation) into the peritoneal cavity to be caught by the fimbriae of the uterine tube. Hartman (1929) noted that the human ovum varied from 0.133 mm to 0.140 mm in diameter. Allen et al. (1930) observed that the fully grown living human ovum is very transparent when viewed at microscopy, and has a finely granular and almost colourless cytoplasm.

From the histologic study of sexually mature ovaries it became clear that a number of follicles start to grow, but usually just one succeeds and the others become atretic. Westman (1934) showed that the non-ovulatory follicles perform an important function in aiding, by their oestrogenic activity, one of their number to mature and ovulate.

Portes et al. (1938) noted that there was little difference between the corpus luteum of pregnancy and that of menstruation except for its size and life span. The presence of globules of colloid in and around the luteal cells indicated a corpus luteum of pregnancy. Brewer (1942) observed that the first signs of regression and degeneration of the corpus luteum, in a non-pregnancy menstrual cycle, occurred about the 10th day of its existence. During the follicular phase of the menstrual cycle the waking temperature remained low. Barton and Wiesner (1945) showed that postovulatory progesterone secretion was responsible for the raised temperature level, characteristic of the luteal phase of the cycle.

MODERN CONCEPTS

Radioimmunoassay was introduced by Berson et al. (1956), and the technique greatly simplified the quantification of the various hormones which exert their influence on the process of ovulation and the menstrual cycle.

Richards and Midgley (1976) showed that oestrogen played a key role in maintaining the growth and division of granulosa cells, while also increasing their sensitivity to circulating levels of follicle stimulating hormone (FSH). Gougeon (1982), calculated that the time taken from entry of the primordial follicle through the active growing phase, to ovulation was about 85 days. In the same year McNatty (1982) reported that by day 7 of the menstrual cycle, the follicle which would ovulate could be identified by its full complement of healthy granulosa cells and the high concentration of oestradiol in the follicular fluid. In another report of that year Skarin et al. (1982) showed that continuous support is required from gonadotropins throughout the follicular phase.

Baird and Fraser (1975) found that the dominant follicle was the source of over 90% of the oestradiol produced in the body, and the same workers later showed that both granulosa and theca cells synthesized oestrogens. Espey (1974) theorized that follicle rupture occurred because of destruction of the collagen matrix in the ground substance of the follicle wall, due to the action of collagenases.

Although measurements of oestrogens were found to reflect follicular development, their value in the prediction of ovulation was limited by several factors which included the low amount produced; the pulsatile nature of secretion; production of oestrogen from extraovarian sources; and variability in the relationship of ovulation to the oestradiol peak (WHO, 1980). Despite those limitations, oestrogen measurement became the standard method of monitoring follicular development during induction of ovulation.

Hackeloer (1977) used ultrasound imaging to monitor follicular development during the menstrual cycle and 2 years later correlated ultrasonic and endocrine assessment of human follicular development (Hackeloer et al., 1979).

The use of high-resolution ultrasound was a major advance in the ability to monitor ovarian activity. Brown pointed out in 1978 that development of more than one follicle was usual in drug-stimulated cycles, and without knowledge of the number of follicles it was difficult to interpret the given level of oestradiol. Kerin *et al.* (1981) found that the mean follicular diameter just prior to ovulation was 23 mm and that there was good agreement between ultrasound results and direct measurement of follicles at operation.

Edwards (1981) measured luteinizing hormone (LH) levels and found that the time interval between the onset of the plasma LH surge and ovulation was between 32 and 40 hours. Within 6 hours of the start of the LH surge granulosa cells luteinize and commence secreting progesterone. Fleming and Coutts (1982) documented their prediction of ovulation in women using a rapid progesterone radioimmunoassay.

THE PREDICTION OF OVULATION

Calendar method

Practical methods for determining the time of ovulation were introduced in the 1930s when Ogino in Japan (1930) and Knaus in Austria (1933) independently observed that irrespective of cycle length, the time of the occurrence of ovulation was relatively constant in days prior to the succeeding menstruation and not related constantly to the previous one. Their work gave rise to the calculation or 'calendar' method for determining the fertile period. Linzenmeier (1947) analysed a large number of rape cases and found that forced coitus between the 19th and 29th day of the cycle did not result in pregnancy, thus adding support to the concept of the so-called 'safe period' of Knaus.

Temperature method

Squire (1868) had observed that the basal body temperature (BBT) showed a biphasic pattern during the menstrual cycle and the Dutch gynaecologist Van de Velde (1905) suggested a possible relationship between ovulation and change of BBT. Tompkins (1944) noted that there was a rise in body temperature directly after ovulation and in the following year Barton and Wiesner (1945) conclusively showed that the temperature rise and its maintenance were due to progesterone activity. Moghissi *et al.* (1972) found

that the BBT rose soon after the LH surge. The rise in BBT was mirrored by a rise in plasma progesterone. Vollman (1977) was a major contributor to our knowledge of BBT and the menstrual cycle.

Mittelschmerz (mid-cycle pain)

In a report to the *British Medical Journal* Krohn (1949) drew attention to the close correlation between 'Mittelschmerz' and the change in waking oral temperature which he observed through many cycles, in a well-recorded case. O'Herlihy *et al.* (1980) showed that 'Mittelschmerz' pain occurred from 24 to 48 hours before the ultrasonically determined time of ovulation and that the mean diameter of the follicle at that time was 19.3 ± 2.2 mm.

Cervical mucus

Seguy and Simonet (1933) and Seguy and Vimeux (1933), determined that cervical mucus becomes more fluid in consistency and also more easily penetrable by spermatozoa prior to and at the time of ovulation. Further contributions to this work were made by Lamar *et al.* (1940), and Aberbanel (1946). Insler *et al.* (1972) evolved their cervical score and found it to be a reliable method for detecting ovulatory cyles.

John and Evelyn Billings of Melbourne developed their ovulation detection method based on cervical mucus change and reported that cervical mucus symptoms and signs appeared at a mean of 6.2 days before ovulation (Billings *et al.*, 1972). Moghissi *et al.* (1972) agreed that the cervical mucus changes provided an excellent guide to hormonal events in the menstrual cycle.

Gonadotropins

Farris (1946) found an increased concentration of pituitary gonadotropin in human urine about the mid-cycle, prior to and including the day of ovulation, and this demonstrated that urine (and later blood) gonadotropin levels could accurately predict events in the menstrual cycle.

OVUM TRANSPORT AND FERTILIZATION

After its extrusion from the ovary, the ovum with its zona pellucida and cumulus cells normally enters the tube on its own side. Morphological

259

alterations within the tube have been noted, with the epithelium being at its highest in mid-cycle. Butomo (1927) found that intracellular fat was more abundant in the tubal epithelium during mid-cycle. Snyder (1924) and also Novak and Everett (1928) found that the tubal epithelium was highest during the ovulatory part of the cycle. Joel (1939) noted that tubal secretion was more pronounced and that glycogen content was increased during the premenstruum. The rhymythic muscular contractions observed in the tube were found to be most vigorous at the time of ovulation (Seckinger and Snyder, 1923–24; Geist et al., 1938). Westman (1937) investigated human ovulation and showed that the infundibulum of the tube moved in the direction of the ovary, and that the ovary itself rotated on its long axis in preparation for the event.

Brown (1944), while working with freshly excised and perfused human uteri and tubes in 1944 found that the average migration rate of spermatozoa was 2.7 mm per min. Austin (1950) and Chang and Pincus (1951) found that the number of spermatozoa at the site of fertilization was in the order of a thousand or so, although less in some species of mammal.

The early stages of human development were shown by the Miller ovum, discovered by Miller in 1913 (Novak, 1947), and demonstrated histologically by Streeter (1926). It was thought to represent a stage corresponding to the 10th or 11th postfertilization day. Hertig and Rock in 1942 discovered a 7–7.5-day-old fertilized egg implanting as a blastocyst in the endometrium. Over a number of years Hertig and Rock (1944;1945) in collaboration with Heuser (Heuser et al., 1945) provided information on the development of the human fertilized ovum, and found that implantation occurred about 6 days after fertilization. Hertig and Rock (1949) gave an account of potentially abortive ova which they recovered through operation from fertile impregnated women prior to the first missed period. It appeared to them that only a small percentage of fertilized ova developed normally and many early abortions occurred unnoticed.

Once successfully fertilized the ovum undergoes cleavage on its journey down the tube to the uterus. Hertig et al. (1956) found that by the time the fertilized ovum arrived in the uterine cavity, it was in the late morula or early blastocyst stage, and varied in cell number from 16 to 58 or more cells. Noyes and Dickmann (1961) showed that accurate synchronization of fertilized ova and endometrial age was a prerequisite for normal subsequent development, and from this it was deduced that any factor which rushed fertilized eggs prematurely through the tubes, into the uterine cavity, exerted a contraceptive effect.

Adams and Chang (1962) showed that the acquisition of the capacity of spermatozoa to penetrate ova took place gradually in the tube and uterus. Greenwald (1963) investigated tubal transport in the rabbit and found that oestrogen levels appeared to dictate the length of time the ova spent in the tube. Chang (1964) showed that the tubal transport of ova could be modified by certain anti-fertility agents. Chang (1959a,b) reported the fertilization of rabbit ova in vitro, and 10 years later Edwards et al. (1969) reported the early stages of fertilization in vitro of human oocytes which had been matured in vitro.

MENSTRUATION

The ancient Greeks assumed that menstruation was a cleansing process, and the Bible refers to the woman as being 'unclean' at that time. The process was thought to be tidal in nature, being governed by the lunar phases, and Pouchet (1847), Professor of Zoology at Rouen, considered that the menstrual flow appeared at the fertile time of the cycle. However, he correctly deduced that the higher mammals ovulated spontaneously, unlike the rabbit where ovulation was induced by coitus.

Percival Pott (1714–1788), was a famous English surgeon who is eponymously related to several surgical conditions. He first described the relationship of scrotal cancer in chimney sweeps to their constant exposure to soot. Pott (1775) carried out bilateral oophorectomy for correction of 'ovarian herniae', and noted afterwards that the patient's breasts shrank, and menstruation ceased. John B. Davidge (1794;1814) while working in Edinburgh, evolved his theory that menstruation was due to a condition of the ovaries which 'excited' the uterus to bleed. Augustine Nicholas Gendrin (1839) was among the first to suggest that ovulation could control menstruation. Edward F. W. Pfluger (1863) of Germany, outlined his own ideas (later called the German Theory) of menstruation. He believed that during the cycle increasing pressure was set up in the growing Graafian follicle. This caused a reflex irritation which sent nerve impulses via the ovarian nerves to the spinal cord, and this in turn caused pelvic congestion which led to menstruation.

The early work on the menstrual cycle in the human was carried out on endometrial samples obtained at autopsy. Kundrat and Engelmann (1873), Williams (1876) and Leopold (1885) investigated the tissue changes during the menstrual cycle.

The modern curette became available in the mid-1850s and was introduced by the Parisian, Recamier (Zondek, 1966). The first to obtain endometrial samples from living women using a curette was Moricke (1882) and his interpretation of the cycle became well known and generally accepted. Hitschmann and Adler (1908) published a paper with detailed illustrations in which they outlined the various stages of the cycle as determined by histopathological analysis of endometrial samples, and they accurately described the histology of the menstrual cycle for the first time.

The changes in the endometrial cycle were correlated with those in the corpus luteum by the Germans Robert Meyer (1911), and Carl Ruge Jr. (1913). Robert Schroder also of Germany (1909;1913;1915) was active in the same field at that time and it was he who first used the terms 'proliferative' and 'secretory' endometrium. The former was found to correspond to the ovarian follicular phase and the latter to the luteal phase.

Charles R. Stockard and George Papanicolaou (1917) demonstrated the cyclical cytological changes which occurred in the reproductive tract during the oestrus cycle. Lataste (1886;1887) of Bordeaux had carried out similar but less well-known studies. As a result of their work, a simple inexpensive method (bioassay) became available for the investigation of the hormonal status at various stages in the cycle. George Corner (1923; 1935; 1938) carried out experimental studies on the endometrial cycle of the rhesus monkey which was known to closely resemble that of the human. Corner (1939; 1943) discovered that progesterone could inhibit menstruation if given continuously and in sufficient quantities, but that oestrin would prevent bleeding only as long as the endometrium was in the proliferative phase. George W. Bartelmez (1931) defined changes in the spiral arteries of the endometrium which lead to menstruation.

Starting in 1932, John E. Markee began a study of intraocular transplants of endometrium in the rhesus monkey (Markee, 1940; Markee *et al*, 1948). He observed the vascular changes leading up to menstruation and found that the coiling of the endometrial arterioles increased markedly. This was followed by a period of slowed circulation, then vasoconstriction, 4–24 hours before bleeding. Jones (1949) described patients in whom the endometrium was not properly prepared for nidation; and those patients with 'luteal phase defects' who might have regular or irregular cycles, were found to be infertile. When Noyes *et al.* (1950) documented their observations of the histological changes in the endometrium during the menstrual cycle, this became the standard reference work for dating the endometrium.

Arey (1939) determined that the cycle length was 28.4 days, and this observation was substantiated by Haman's (1942) investigations. The blood loss at menstruation was quantified by Barker and Fowler (1936), and the estimated loss of 25–60 ml. noted in a series of reports during the subsequent 30 years was taken to be the normal range of menstrual flow.

OESTROGENS

The French physiologist Charles Edouard Brown-Sequard (1817–1894), who was born in Mauritius, was the son of an American sea captain and a French mother, and is considered to be one of the founders of endocrinology. He claimed, before proof was available, that the adrenals, thyroid, pancreas, liver, spleen and kidneys had secretions (later to be called hormones) which entered the blood stream to exert their actions at a distant site, and asserted that those secretions had the potential to be used in treatment. He believed that injections of extracts of testis would produce rejuvenation and maintained that aqueous extracts of ovaries would prove helpful to women (Brown-Sequard, 1890). Although Brown-Sequard and some of his older medical colleagues benefited from the administration of a testicular extract prepared by himself, the ovarian extracts were not effective in women. Brown-Sequard was greatly honoured as the discoveror of the 'internal secretions' and was made FRCP and a Fellow of the Royal Society.

Emil Knauer (1896), a Viennese gynaecologist, removed ovaries from rabbits, grafted pieces back and demonstrated that the grafts prevented castrate atrophy of the uterus, and 4 years later (Knauer, 1900) he referred to ovarian 'secretions'. In the same year Josef Halban (1900) concluded that the ovaries produced a substance which was essential for the development and maintenance of the genital organs and mammary glands. Marshall and Jolly (1906) stated that the ovary was an organ of 'internal secretion' which induced menstruation and heat in animals. By 1910 there was no doubt about the existence of gonadal hormones, but as yet no active principle had been obtained.

During the years 1911 to 1918 ovarian hormones were extracted by various workers in Europe and America who used a lipid solvent technique. It was Henry Iscovesco (1912a,b) of France who first published on the discovery of an ovarian extract which contained oestrogen. Iscovesco practised as a gynaecologist in Paris and used his ovarian extract, which he called 'gynocrinol', for the treatment of dysmenorrhoea and amenorrhoea.

Charles R. Stockard and George Papanicolaou (1917) demonstrated that the hormonal changes of the oestrus cycle could be detected by cytological examination of vaginal smears. It was soon obvious that the cytologic method provided a simple, rapid, accurate, reproducible, and reliable method for studying the menstrual cycle in animals or humans. Edgar Allen and Edward Doisy (1923) reported their preliminary findings on the localization, extraction, partial purification, and action in test animals, of an 'ovarian hormone'. They indicated that the substance was produced in the Graafian follicles; was probably produced in all ovaries as the ova matured; and was probably common to all female animals. Doisy suggested the term 'theelin' (*thelys*, Greek, female) but other terms including 'feminin', 'folliculin', 'menformin', and 'progynon', were used by other investigators. Parkes and Bellerby (1926) proposed the name 'oestrin'.

The extraction of oestrogen from ovarian tissue proved difficult. However, Loewe and Lange (1926) discovered an oestrogenic substance in human urine and Sellman Aschheim (1927) extracted large amounts of the hormone from pregnant women's urine. Pure crystalline oestrogenic hormone was eventually isolated by four groups of investigators during 1929 and 1930. Doisy *et al.* (1929;1930) and Allen in America (Gruhn and Kazer, 1989), and Butenandt (1929a,b) in Europe proposed the chemical formula for the substance which was later designated as 'oestrone'. Browne (1930) isolated a less potent oestrogenic steroid from the placenta. This was later termed 'oestriol'; and MacCorquodale *et al.* (1936) while working in Doisy's laboratory, crystallized the active ovarian hormone known as 'oestradiol'. In 1936 the Council on Pharmacy and Chemistry of the American Medical Association adopted the term 'estrogen' for all substances which produced the typical changes of oestrus. The first synthetic oestrogen, 'stilboestrol' was synthesized by Dodds *et al.* (1938a–d) in England.

Karl R. Moore and Dorothy Price (1932) introduced the concept of 'negative feedback'. Two years later Walter Hohlweg (1934) provided the first evidence that a positive feedback system existed, and George Corner (1939) proposed his theory that a pituitary–gonad–endometrium axis existed.

It was shown that there was an increased production of oestrin with follicular growth and that the liquor folliculi was rich in this hormone. Oestrin injection in oophorectomized female primates, including the human, produced a proliferative uterine mucosa, but not a secretory one; thus oestrin was shown to control the proliferative phase of the cycle. If oestrin injections were followed by administration of corpus luteum extract (progesterone) or preferably progesterone combined with oestrin, secretory (progestational) endometrium was produced. Frank (1940) proposed that moderate doses of oestrogen would stimulate, and in large doses inhibit, the gonadatropic activity of the anterior pituitary. Smith and Ryan (1962) summarized the available knowledge which showed that cholesterol was the precursor of progesterone, androgens and oestrogens.

PROGESTERONES

Edward Pfluger (1863), a leading German physiologist, published his (erroneous) theory on the mechanism of menstruation. He correctly deduced, however, that the corpus luteum developed due to the loss of the Graafian follicle. The structure and function of the corpus luteum attracted the attention of many investigators from that time on; and Louis-Auguste Prenant (1898a,b) of Nancy in France suggested that the corpus luteum was a 'gland' which produced internal secretions.

Ludwig Fraenkel in Germany (Fraenkel and Cohn, 1901), and Vilhelm Magnus (1901) in Norway, working independently showed that the corpus luteum supported early pregnancy and that destruction of the corpora lutea in pregnant rabbits caused abortion or resorption of embryos. Magnus noted that removal of corpora lutea alone did not cause uterine atrophy, and theorized that the ovary produced more than one hormone. In 1908 Hitschmann and Adler (1908) of Vienna, demonstrated the histological changes of the endometrial cycle and suggested that the ovary went through a corresponding cyclic change.

Robert Meyer (1911), Carl Ruge (1913) and Robert Schroder (1913;1915) related structural changes in the endometrium to gross and histologic changes in the corpus luteum. Eventually in 1928 George Corner, Willard Allen and Walter Bloor obtained crude oily extracts of corpora lutea. Corner is credited with the discovery of the hormonal effect of the extract (progesterone), which he called 'progestin' (Corner and Allen, 1929). Butenandt and Westphal (1934), who had isolated androsterone from male urine (1931), were among groups of investigators who isolated crystalline progesterone from corpora lutea in 1934 and they suggested the term 'luteosterone' for the active principle. In 1935 a compromise term 'progesterone' was introduced during the second International Conference on the Standardization of Sex Hormones, in London (Parkes, 1966). Marrian in 1930 (Gruhn, 1987) and Butenandt (1930) identified a progestational sterol excreted in large amounts in the urine of pregnant women. This substance was later termed 'pregnanediol'. Venning and Browne (1936) established that the substance was a metabolite of progesterone, which when quantified provided a reasonably accurate measure of that hormone's secretion.

THE PITUITARY

The term 'pituitary' (Latin: *pituita*, slyme) perpetuates an ancient theory that this gland was the receptacle of phlegm discharged into it from the brain. Early workers discovered that the pituitary body, like the adrenal, consisted of two parts of different origin and function, which were fused together. The adenohypophysis (Greek: *aden*, acorn; *hupo*, under; *phuein*, to grow) was found to arise from the ectoderm of the roof of the buccal cavity from which a blind pocket (Rathke's pouch) extended upwards. The leading edge becomes invaginated by, and wrapped around, the tip of the neurohypophysis which arises as a down growth (infundibulum, funnel, Latin: *infundere*, pour) from the floor of the third ventricle of the brain. The neurohypophysis was found to begin as a protuberance on the lower surface of the hypothalamus, the median eminence of the tuber cinereum (Latin: *tuber*, swelling: *cinarus*, ashen), while the posterior lobe was thought to contain neuroglia (Greek: *glia*, glue) or connective tissue cells. John G. Gruhn of Chicago (1987) summarized the early studies of the pituitary and noted that Vesalius in 1543 had described *glandula*

pituitam cerebri excipiens and in 1742 Liutaud had described the 'pituitary portal vascular system'. In 1760 DeHaen documented the occurrence of amenorrhoea in a patient with a pituitary tumour and in 1898 Compte found that the pituitary gland increased in size during pregnancy.

The posterior pituitary was investigated by Oliver and Schafer (1895) who prepared active extracts of the gland. Two types of material were obtained, which on investigation were found to have either pressor or oxytocic effects. These materials initially proved difficult to separate from each other. Oxytocin was found to act specifically on uterine muscle, the smooth muscle of the ducts of mammary glands, and on the myoepithelium which surrounds the milk alveoli. Vasopressin and oxytocin were isolated, analysed, and then synthesized by Du Vigneaud and *et al.* (1954). It was later found that the nonapeptide oxytocin was synthesized in the paraventricular and supraoptic nuclei of the hypothalamus, bound to its neurophysin and transported in neurosecretory granules into the posterior pituitary gland where these granules were stored until released by appropriate stimuli. An analogue was synthesized by Otto Schild in London and tried out in the labour wards of University College Hospital by W.C.W. Nixon. The great advantage of synthetic oxytocin over the naturally occurring substance was that it contained no vasopressin substance that raised blood pressure. It was Sir Henry Hallett Dale (q.v. in Biographies) (1875–1968) who had discovered that the initial effect of vasopressin was to raise blood pressure, but if a second dose was given then blood pressure dropped. Oxytocin is now used to induce or accelerate labour.

Frohlich reported the case of a 14-year-old boy with infantilism which was associated with a destructive pituitary lesion and underdevelopment of the reproductive organs in 1901 (Jones and Jones, 1981). This, and other reports, noted that destructive lesions of the anterior pituitary were associated with genital atrophy.

Crowe *et al.* (1910) performed the first experimental hypophysectomy on dogs, and so the laboratory investigation of the control of the reproductive function by the pituitary was begun. Herbert Evans and Joseph Long (1921) experimented with the intraperitoneal placement of anterior pituitary extract and its effect on the oestrus cycle in rats. Philip Smith and Earl Engle (1927) described their work with pituitary extracts, and postulated that two gonadotropic hormones were necessary, one for follicular growth and the other for luteinization. In the same year Zondek and Aschheim demonstrated that extracts of anterior pituitary produced precocious puberty in immature mice.

Aschheim and Zondek (1927) went on to show that the urine of pregnant women contained a substance with gonadotropic effect similar to that of pituitary gonadotropin, and this later formed the basis of a urinary pregnancy test. Four years later Fevold *et al.* (1931) presented evidence that two different pituitary hormones influenced the ovarian cycle, and soon afterwards the separation of follicle stimulating hormone (FSH) and LH was documented.

The term 'Prolan' was used for chorionic gonadotropin. The follicle stimulating principle obtained from the anterior lobe of the pituitary gland by acid extraction was named prolan A, and the luteinizing principle, prolan B. The pituitary gonadotrophic principles were later renamed FSH and LH respectively. Smith (1930) showed that removal of the pituitary gland before maturity caused a cessation of sexual development in animals, and in the mature animal the reproductive system was found to atrophy, after pituitary ablation.

Highly active preparations with follicle stimulating activity were prepared from the pituitary glands of sheep by Li *et al.* (1949) and Li (1958) went on to report the purification of FSH from human pituitaries. In the same year Gemzell *et al.* (1958) also reported the isolation of gonadotropin from human pituitaries. The preparation was administered to women with amenorrhoea and was found to be a highly potent hormone substance. Midgely and Jaffe (1971) discovered that LH, and FSH to a lesser extent, were secreted from the pituitary in episodic bursts on an approximate hourly cycle.

Three groups of investigators determined the amino acid sequence for human LH – Sairam *et al.* (1972) detailed the structure of the α subunit in 1972; Shome and Parlow defined the β and α subunits (1973; 1974), while Closset, Hennon and Lequin (1973) and Saxena and Rathnam (1976) also documented the amino acid sequence of the β subunit. The amino acid sequence of human chorionic gonadotropin was also detailed by Morgan *et al.* (1973).

PROLACTIN

The initiation and continuation of lactation, or galactopoiesis (Greek: *galaktos*, gen. of Gala; milk; *poiesis*, formation) are influenced by many factors,

but prolactin plays a central role. It was discovered that hypophysectomy during breastfeeding led almost immediately to cessation of lactation. Stricker and Grueter (1928) of France described how administration of a pituitary extract caused secretion of milk. George Corner (1930) demonstrated that injections of anterior pituitary lobe extract caused hypertrophy of mammary tissue and secretion of milk, in oophorectomized virgin rabbits, and also documented the lactogenic properties of ovine pituitary extracts. Riddle and Braucher (1931) introduced a pigeon crop bioassay for the milk hormone and 2 years later Riddle *et al.* (1933) reported on their preparation, identification, and assay, of a hormone from the anterior pituitary which was named 'prolactin'. Prolactin was isolated from the pituitary of sheep and cattle in 1940. Emmart *et al.* (1963) used a flourescent antibody technique and confirmed the earlier work of Pearse and Severinghous (Jones and Jones, 1981) which indicated that prolactin was synthesized in the acidophilic (α) cells. Those cells were found to be peripherally located in the pituitary, thus making a surgical approach to prolactinomas relatively feasible.

The fact that ovarian activity is depressed during breastfeeding was scientifically confirmed by Topkins (1943), who showed that endometrial biopsies obtained during lactation were lacking in oestrogen effect. Lyon (1946) showed that in the non-breastfeeding mother there is early resumption of ovarian activity and menstruation could return as early as 6 weeks after delivery.

THE HYPOTHALAMUS

Early observations of the effects of environmental stimuli on ovulation led to the hypothesis that central nervous system reflexes could influence the pituitary secretion of gonadotropic hormones. A portal system joining the hypothalamus and pituitary was first described by Popa and Fielding (1930; 1933). In 1936 a Harvard anatomist named Harry Friedgood proposed the hypothesis that hypothalamic releasing 'factors' controlled anterior pituitary function, and that these 'factors' reached their target cells via the portal blood vessels (Gruhn and Kazer, 1989).

Later Harris showed that stimulation of the tuber cinereum and pre-optic area evoked ovulation (Harris and Naftolin, 1970), and he found that transecting the portal vessels in rats resulted in cessation of reproductive function. Harris (1955) showed that if the pituitary cells from an immature animal were placed in the fossa of an adult animal, the transplanted cells were capable of producing gonadotropic hormones. This suggested that the initiation of puberty was caused by maturation of the nervous system and not the pituitary. McCann and his colleagues were responsible for much of the early physiological work which demonstrated that hypothalamic extracts contained substances which stimulated pituitary function (McCann *et al*., 1960; McCann, 1962). The naming of the 'hypothalamic releasing factors' was by Murray Saffran and Andrew Schally in 1955.

Matsuo *et al.* (1971) elucidated the structure of the porcine LH and FSH releasing hormone (LHRH) and Burgus *et al.* (1971) reported on the ovine hypothalamic luteinizing hormone releasing factor. The structure of LHRH was determined to be a decapeptide. Many of the important discoveries relating to hypothalamic factors came from the laboratories of Andrew Schally and Roger Guillemin and in 1977 they were awarded the Nobel Prize in Medicine, in recognition of their work. Andrew Victor Schally was born in 1926 in Wilno, Poland. He graduated from being a professional footballer, to obtaining a Ph.D. in science and later worked in New Orleans, USA where he isolated LHRH. Roger Guillemin was born in 1924 in Dijon, France and later came to head the laboratories for neuroendocrinology in the Salk Institute, La Jolla, California. The rivalry and the race to elucidate the hypothalamic hormones between Schally and his team and Guillemin and his associates is beautifully described in Medvei's book (1982) on the *History of Endocrinology*.

THE PLACENTA

Halban (1904; 1905) first suggested a secretory function of the placenta. Aschheim and Zondek (1927; 1928) isolated a gonadotropin, and an ovarian hormone (oestrogen) from pregnancy urine. Collip (1930) in a preliminary communication to the *Canadian Medical Journal* indicated that the placenta may produce an ovarian stimulating hormone. The placenta was proven to be an endocrine organ when Gey *et al.* (1938) demonstrated production of chorionic gonadotropin (hCG) by trophoblastic cells growing in culture, and Claesson *et al.* (1948) reported the crystallization of hCG. Wislocki and Bennett, (1943) using histochemical techniques, indicated

that the syncytium was the source of placental steroids. Thiede and Choate (1963) and also Pierce and Midgley (1963) localized chorionic gonadotropin production to the syncytium. Wynn and Davies (1965) used electron microscopy techniques and confirmed that the cytotrophoblast was structurally simple. They regarded the syncytium as a differentiated form of trophoblast capable of synthesis of complex molecules and responsible for the production of all placental hormones.

Ito and Higashi (1961) first described the presence of human chorionic somatomammotropin, later called human placental lactogen (HPL) or chorionic growth hormone. Josimovich and MacLaren (1962) characterized the hormone as a polypeptide, and isolated it from extracts of human placenta and retroplacental blood. Li *et al.* (1968) indicated that the hormone consisted of a single polypeptide chain with a molecular weight of 20 kDa. Eventually Morgan *et al.* (1973) proposed the amino acid sequence of human chorionic gonadotropin. (There are further details about placental hormones in the chapter on Fetal Monitoring.)

RELAXIN

Hisaw in 1926, experimented with mice and guinea-pigs, and discovered that the administration of ovarian extract or blood plasma from pregnant animals, if injected into female guinea-pigs at oestrus, could induce the well-known softening and relaxation which affects the pelvic ligaments in pregnancy. The active principle which caused the ligamentous change was termed 'relaxin' (Hisaw and Zarrow, 1950)

POLYCYSTIC OVARY SYNDROME

In 1830 J. Lisfranc described an entity for which Chereau introduced the term 'sclerotic disease of the ovary' or sclerocystic disease in 1844 (Katz, 1981). The technique of laparotomy became popular in the late 1800s and reports of ovarian microcystic degeneration in sclerotic ovaries with associated abnormal bleeeding patterns appeared in the early 1900s. Irving Stein and Michael Leventhal (1935) of Chicago, described women with amenorrhoea who also had cystic ovaries, and found that menstruation resumed after bilateral ovarian wedge resection. Ten years later, Stein (1945) defined the syndrome of oligoamenorr-

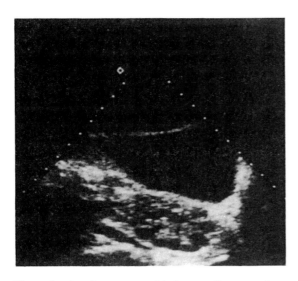

Figure 2 An ultrasonographic image of an ovary in a patient with polycystic ovary syndrome. Note the dense echogenic core produced by stromal hyperplasia and the rim of small cysts. Reproduced with kind permission from *Clinics in Obstetrics and Gynaecology* (Sept. 1985), Vol. 12, No. 2, p.657

hoea, hirsutism, infertility and polycystic ovaries. The appelation 'Stein–Leventhal Syndrome' was first used in 1949 by Dr Jo.V. Meigs. Investigating the eponymous Stein–Leventhal syndrome Keetel *et al.* (1957) noted increased concentrations of androgens and LH in women with polycystic ovaries. The investigation of the polycystic ovary syndrome in recent times has benefited from ultrasound technology. Swanson *et al.* (1981) first defined the ultrasound appearance of polycystic ovaries (Figure 2) and Adams *et al.* (1985) added further detail, thus allowing for ready diagnosis without the benefit of laparoscopy or laparotomy.

HYPERPROLACTINAEMIA

The condition of persistent lactation with atrophy of the uterus was described by Chiari *et al.* (1855) in their report from the gynaecology department of the Municipal Clinic in Vienna. Frommel (1882) concluded that about 1% of women developed persistent lactation with uterine atrophy after the puerperium. David Krestin (1932) reported his observation of patients, not previously pregnant, with amenorrhoea, persistent lactation and enlargement of the pituitary. Ahumada and del Castillo (1932) of Buenos Aires described similar findings and Argonz and del Castillo (1953)

indicated that the disorder was due to anterior pituitary hyperfunction. In the following year Forbes and co-workers at Harvard described similar findings in a number of patients, who were found to have radiological evidence of a pituitary tumour (Forbes *et al.*, 1954). Meites *et al.* (1972) found that the secretion of prolactin was governed by inhibitory control exerted from the hypothalamus. It was later discovered that dopamine was the prolactin inhibitory factor (PIF) and Besser *et al.* (1972) reported that the ergot derivitive, bromocriptine, by virtue of its dopaminergic activity, was effective in lowering prolactin levels.

The pituitary tumours which caused hyperprolactinaemia were found to be either micro- or macroadenomas, the latter referring to tumours which were greater than 1 cm in diameter. Hyperprolactinaemia was also found in patients who were being treated with drugs such as anti-depressants and tranquillizers which had anti-dopaminergic activity.

INDUCTION OF OVULATION

Davis and Koff (1938) were the first to succeed in inducing ovulation in women by the intravenous injection of an extract of pregnant mares' serum. Hamblen et al. (1941) experimented with equine and chorionic gonadotropins in cases of 'ovarian' sterility. Parkes (1942) produced superovulation in rabbits. The ovaries were first primed by injection of horse pituitary extract, and this was followed a few days later by an intravenous injection of chorionic gonadotropin. Hamblen and Davis (1945) combined equine and chorionic gonadotropin in a cyclic fashion. Figueroa Chases (1958) reported ovarian hyperstimulation.

IN VITRO FERTILIZATION

Menkin and Rock (1948) obtained eggs from human ovarian follicles and exposed them *in vitro* to spermatazoa suspensions. They treated 138 eggs in this way and subsequently the development to a three-cell stage occurred in four of them. Chang and Pincus (1951) reported successful experiments with *in vitro* fertilization of mammalian eggs.

STILBOESTROL

The first nearly pure oestrogenic compound was prepared by Doisy *et al.* (1929). During the 1930s oestrogenic preparations became commercially available but the efforts to purify and standardize those products led to many errors. Cook *et al.* (1933) synthesized the first artificial oestrogen. At that time E.C. Dodds was the Courtauld Professor of Biochemistry in the Middlesex Hospital, London, and following the initial publication there were many papers from the unit, which related to synthetic oestrogens. In 1938, Dodds and Robinson of Oxford, prepared various combinations of substituted stilbenes and found that the diethyl derivative was the most effective. Unlike the other compounds, diethylstilboestrol (DES) was found to be effective when administered orally. The potency of the compound was five times that of oestradiol; it was easy to prepare in pure form, and was cheap to produce. Dienestrol and Hexestrol were two other compounds which showed only minor structural and therapeutic difference from DES, and they also became available through the work of Dodds *et al.* (1938a–d). The many therapeutic applications of DES included that of lactation suppression (Winterton and MacGregor 1939; Connally *et al.*, 1940); control of menopausal symptoms (Huberman and Colmer, 1940); control of breast carcinoma (Ellis *et al.*, 1944); control of prostatic cancer (Herbst 1941); hormonal support in threatened miscarriage (Burdick and Vedder, 1941); and morning-after contraception (Board and Bhatnagar, 1972). During the years 1945–1955, DES was frequently prescribed for threatened abortion (Davis and Fugo, 1950) and it has been estimated that up to two million women received the drug during pregnancy.

Soon after the introduction of DES, Castrodale *et al.* (1941) reported toxic effects of the compound in laboratory animals. Then Clinch and Tindall (1969), who studied postpartum women receiving DES to suppress lactation, noted a significant transitory change in liver function. Hepatotoxicity, which was possibly due to hypersensitivity had been documented by Elias and Schwimmer (1945).

Two very important studies were published in the early 1970s, which unfortunately associated maternal DES treatment in pregnancy with neoplasia in their female children. Herbst *et al.* (1971) presented a case–control study which linked maternal DES treatment with the development of vaginal clear cell adenocarcinoma in daughters. This was the first human example of possible transplacental carcinogenesis (Folkman, 1971; Miller, 1971). One year later Nolle *et al.* (1972) found an association between stilboestrol and cervical adenocarcinoma. These and other reports led to a rapid decline in the use of DES after 1955.

Lanier *et al.* (1973) published a report on their follow-up of 1719 girls born between 1943 and 1959 who had been exposed to synthetic oestrogens *in utero*, and estimated that about 4 per 1000 women exposed to the drug *in utero* were likely to develop cancer. Abnormalities of the vagina and cervix were frequently found to be diagnostic of *in utero* DES exposure. Vaginal adenosis was the most common abnormal finding. A cervical hood or 'cock's comb' appearance was described along with other abnormalities of the cervix and vagina, all of which varied in their frequency and severity. Abnormalities of the uterine cavity (in particular a T-shaped irregularity of the cavity) or of the Fallopian tubes, were reported in up to two-thirds of DES-exposed women by Kaufman *et al.* (1984). Conflicting reports were published concerning the fertility of DES-exposed women (Siegler *et al.*, 1979: Berger and Goldstein, 1980: Schmidt *et al.*, 1980: Herbst *et al.*, 1980) but there was general agreement that late pregnancy complications, preterm delivery and perinatal death, were increased in those women who clearly exhibited the changes due to *in utero* exposure to DES.

PROSTAGLANDINS

The prostaglandins are a group of cyclic fatty acids with potent biological effects which involve almost every organ in the body. Early investigation showed that extracts of seminal vesicles or human semen caused contraction of uterine muscle and vasodilatation with lowering of blood pressure. Kurzrok and Lieb (1930) were the first to report this discovery. Von Euler (1934) used the term 'prostaglandin' (PG) to characterize the group of chemicals. Further research was carried out by Goldblatt (1933) who reported the presence of a depressor substance in seminal fluid. Pickles (1957) was the first to demonstrate prostaglandin activity in human menstrual fluid. Bergstrom and Sjovall (1960a,b) documented their isolation of prostaglandin E and F from seminal sheep vesicles. A third class of prostaglandin, PGA, was discovered in rabbit kidney medulla by Lee *et al.* (1963). PGE_2 and $PGF_{2\alpha}$ and six other PGs were isolated from rabbit kidney medulla subsequently. The PGs were found to have stimulatory or inhibitory effects on a large range of biological processes. The role of PGs has been extensively researched in reproductive medicine. Treatment with prostaglandin agents has been most useful for induction of labour. The compounds have also been used for the induction of therapeutic abortion. Inhibitors of prostaglandin synthesis have proved most useful in dysmenorrhoea and menorrhagia.

Karim *et al.* (1968) first reported the use of PGs in the induction of labour, and found that they were potent oxytocics whether administered orally, intravaginally or parenterally. Later work was to prove their efficiency as a preinduction agent when used as intravaginal pessaries, tablets or gel. The intravenous route was abandoned due to side-effects.

Karim and Filshie (1970) and also Roth-Brandel *et al.* (1970) first observed the high success rates for induction of therapeutic abortion by intravenous injection. Later research work showed that a single injection of $PGF_{2\alpha}$ into the amniotic cavity was more successful and had fewer side-effects. The extra-amniotic route was also used.

Karim and Hillier (1979) reviewed the role of PGs in the control of animal and human reproduction, and documented that Schwartz *et al.* (1974) found that PG synthesis inhibitors (indomethacin and fenamic acids) produced symptomatic relief in primary dysmenorrhoea.

The following details of procedures in the induction of labour are extracted from an article by Ian Donald (1972) (q.v. in Biographies) Professor of Midwifery, Glasgow

In 1595 a Reverend Maister Alexis of Piemont advocated medications such as juniper berries, cinnamon, castor oil, white amber in wine and other products which were said to stimulate the uterus. Dr Henry Bracken wrote his *Midwives Companion – Wherein the Whole Art is Explained* in 1735 and recommended that 'oil of sweet almonds be applied warm with a bunch of feathers to the privities and vagina'. Nicholas Culpepper in 1684 stated that 'the child is no better able long to subsist in the womb after these skins are broken than a naked man in an heap of snow ' and was obviousely aware that rupture of membranes could cause labour.

A mid-nineteenth century translation of Aristotle's work advised that the woman with ruptured membranes take 'a swallows nest and dissolve it in water, strain it and drink it warm' to induce labour. In the eighteenth century, William Smellie wrote about artificial rupture of the membranes thus 'the common method of breaking the membranes is by thrusting the fingure against them when they are protruded with the waters during the pain, or by pinching them with the fingure and thumb'. In the same century Denman, of the Middlesex Hospital,

advocated induction of labour to avoid disproportion and secure an easier delivery with a smaller baby. Krause's bougies were introduced in 1855 and were inserted transcervically. Stomach tubes, hydrostatic bags, and pigs' bladders were pushed into the lower uterine segment, and de Lee recommended packing the cervix with gauze. Otherwise Willett's forceps were applied to the presenting part, in the hope of stimulating labour.

Oxytocin was discovered in the early part of the twentieth century and introduced a reliable safe method of stimulating uterine action.

Many of the above procedures probably worked by releasing PGs from the uterine and cervical tissues, as did the time-honoured methods of sweeping the membranes and stretching the cervix.

THE PINEAL

Gutzeit (1896) described the association of precocious puberty with the occurrence of a pinealoma in a boy. Lerner *et al.* (1959) reported isolation of melatonin from the pineal gland and Vaitukaitis *et al.* (1972) showed that pinealomas could contain hCG.

CHRONOLOGY

Ovulation and the ovary

1672 Regnier de Graaf described the mature follicle and erroneously considered it to be the ovum.

1824 Prevost and Dumas described ovulation in the dog.

1827 Karl Ernst von Baer, usually credited with the first description of the ovum, described its development and that of the Graafian follicle.

1858–61 Karl Ludwig found that removal of the ovaries in humans caused amenorrhoea.

1878 Alfred Hegar removed sows' ovaries and caused castration atrophy.

1890 Charles Edouard Brown-Sequard claimed that an aqueous extract of ovarian tissue could have a rejuvenating effect on women.

1895 Robert Tuttle Morris first transplanted human ovarian tissue.

1896 Knauer demonstrated that ovarian grafts prevented the devolopment of castrate atrophy.

1900   Josef Halban concluded that the ovary produced a substance which had a specific influence on the genital organs.

1906   Marshall and Jolly noted the positive effects of ovarian extracts on ovariectomized animals, and predicted the endocrine functions of the ovary.

1917   Stockard and Papanicolaou introduced their vaginal cytology technique for following the stages of the oestrous cycle.

1923   Allen and Doisy found that a hormone (oestrogen) was present in liquor folliculi, which was capable of inducing oestrus in ovariectomized animals.

1929   Hartman noted that the average size of the human ovum varies from 0.133 mm to 0.140 mm in diameter.

Doisy *et al.* produced the first crystalline preparation of oestrogen from the liquor folliculi.

1935   Hill *et al.* described the process of ovulation as observed in the rabbit.

1936   Hartmann detailed ovulation as it occurred in primates.

1963   Baker determined that the pool of primordial follicles was in the region of 200 000–400 000.

Menstrual cycle

It states in the Bible (Leviticus) that the menstruating woman was considered unclean. Hippocrates, Aristotle, Galen, and Pliny, assumed that menstruation was a cleansing process.

1775   Percival Pott claimed to have removed both ovaries from a young woman for correction of 'ovarian herniae'. Menstruation ceased and her breasts shrank.

1794   John B. Davidge, theorized that the ovaries excited the vessels of the womb to menstruate.

1824   Prevost and Dumas described ovulation and corpus luteum formation in the dog.

1847   Pouchet, Professor of Zoology at Rouen, believed that women were fertile during menstruation.

1850s   Recamier developed the modern curette, and obtained samples of endometrium for analysis (Zondek, 1966).

1863   Edward F. W. Pfluger evolved his theory of menstruation. He believed that the enlarged Graafian follicle sent nerve impulses to the spinal cord. In response there was dilatation of uterine and ovarian blood vessels leading to thickening of the endometrium and later menstruation.

1872   Robert Battey performed oophorectomy for various gynaecological problems. When applied to animals, castration uterine atrophy was noted. Later workers used the model of 'castrate uterine atrophy', when experimenting with ovarian and pituitary hormones.

1873   Kundrat and Engelmann studied the endometrium and uterus in cadavers.

1882   Moricke obtained endometrium from live patients and studied the menstrual cycle.

1898   Gebhard described endometrial appearances.

1900   Walter Heape of Cambridge investigated the menstrual cycle in animals and introduced the term 'oestrus'.

1907–08   Leo Loeb reported that injury to, or implanting a foreign substance in, the non-pregnant endometrium, led to a decidual reaction, if the corpus luteum was present.

1908   Hitschmann and Adler were the first to describe in detail the histologic changes which occur in the endometrium throughout the menstrual cycle, and first noted that the endometrium varies in appearance depending on the time it is sampled.

1909–10   Bouin and Ancel documented (progestational) proliferation of the rabbit endometrium.

1909–15   Robert Schroder correlated the endometrial appearance with cyclic changes and introduced the terms 'proliferative' and 'secretory' phase and also described the basal and functional layers of the endometrium.

1911   Loeb reported that removal of corpora lutea hastened the onset of the oestrus cycle in guinea-pigs.

1911–13   Robert Meyer (1911) and Carl Ruge Junior (1913) correlated endometrial change with that happening in the corpus luteum.

1923   Corner studied the menstrual cycle in rhesus monkeys who were known to have a 28-day cycle.

1926–28 Edgar Allen proposed that oestrogen deprivation caused menstruation.

1927 Pratt reported on the corpus luteum and its relation to menstruation and pregnancy.

1930 Schroder wrote a monograph on the endometrial cycle, and also determined that there was a condition of endometrial hyperplasia.

1931 George W. Bartelmez defined changes in the spiral arteries of the endometrium and their link with menstruation.

1932 John E. Markee began his studies on menstruation as it occurred in intraocular endometrial transplants in the rhesus monkey (Markee, 1940).

Smith and Engle demonstrated that crude progestin injections could prevent oestrogen withdrawal bleeding.

1936 Menstrual blood loss was found to range from about 25 to 60 ml (Barker and Fowler, 1936; Millis, 1951; Baldwin et al., 1961; Hytten et al., 1964 Hallberg et al., 1966; 1968;).

1937 Gunn et al. analysed menstrual cycles in 479 British women and found a difference between the shortest and longest cycles of 8 or 9 days.

1938 Hisaw and Greep investigated the inhibition of uterine bleeding with oestradiol and progesterone.

1939 Corner found that both oestrogen and progesterone deprivation were necessary for menstruation to occur.

Arey, in an analysis of 5322 cycles in 485 women, found an average cycle length of 28.4 days.

1942 Haman surveyed 2460 cycles in 150 women and found an average length of cycle of 28–29 days.

1948 Papanicolaou et al. described and illustrated in their monograph, the changes which occur in the cervix and vagina during the menstrual cycle.

1950 Noyes et al. wrote their paper on Dating the Endometrium, which became the standard reference work on the subject.

1957 Chesley and Hellman found an average weight gain of a quarter pound (113 g) throughout the menstrual cycle.

1967 Wynn and Harris gave a detailed account of the ultrastructural cyclical changes in the human endometrium.

Cytology and cyclic changes

1886–87 Lataste studied cytology smears taken from the vagina.

1917 Charles R. Stockard and George Papanicolaou studied the cyclic cytologic changes during the oestrus cycle in the guinea pig, and the technique was later used in humans.

Oestrogens

1896 Knauer demonstrated that ovarian transplants prevented atrophy of the uterus in ovariectomized rabbits.

1912 Although Adler was the first to extract a biologically active substance from ovarian tissue, which caused oestrus in the guinea-pig, Henry Iscovesco was the first investigator to publish the discovery of an ovarian extract (oestrogen).

1922 Frank demonstrated that the active substance of the ovary (oestrogen) was a component of the follicular fluid rather than the whole ovary.

1923 Edgar Allen and Edward Doisy isolated a potent oestrogen from follicular fluid in the sow's ovary and described a method of biologic assay for oestrus producing hormone.

1926 Parks and Bellerby introduced the term 'oestrin' thus displacing the term 'theelin' which was used prior to that (Parkes, 1966).

Loewe and Lange discovered an oestrogenic substance in human urine.

1927 Aschheim found large amounts of oestrogen in urine from pregnant women.

1929 Butenandt, and Doisy et al. announced the crystallization from urine of an oestrogenic substance later called 'oestrone'.

1930 Browne, while working in Collip's laboratory, isolated a less potent oestrogenic steroid called 'oestriol' from placental tissue.

1932 The terminology oestrone, oestradiol and oestriol was officially adopted at the first International Conference on standardization of sex hormones.

1932–35 Two meetings devoted to oestrogen, progesterone, and standardization of hormonal nomenclature, were held in London.

1935   Frank and Salmon showed that the elevated urinary follicle stimulating hormone titre found in menopausal or ovariectomized women could be lowered by the administration of oestrogens.

1936   MacCorquodale *et al.*, working in Doisy's laboratory, crystallized oestradiol, the most potent of the three oestrogenic substances.

The Council on Pharmacy and Chemistry of the Americal Medical Association adopted oestrogen as the collective term for all substances capable of producing the typical changes of oestrus.

1938   Dodds *et al.* reported their discovery of the synthetic oestrogen, 'stilboestrol'.

1943   Dempsey and Bassett using histochemical investigations, indicated that the ovarian thecal cells elaborate estradiol, (also shown by McKay and Robinson, 1947)

1954   Bradbury and White discovered oestrogenic compounds in plants.

Progesterones

1898   Prenant first suggested that the corpus luteum was an organ of internal secretion.

1901   The role of the corpus luteum in maintaining pregnancy was first documented by Fraenkel and Cohn of Germany and Magnus of Norway.

1910   Fraenkel further demonstrated that the activity of the corpus luteum was essential to maintenance of pregnancy.

Bouin and Ancel described the histological characteristics of the endometrium, which occurred due to progesterone activity.

1929   Butenandt found that progestin was a steroid, and suggested that the suffix 'sterone' be added to progestin.

George Corner and Willard Allen, with the assistance of Walter Bloor, obtained crude oily extracts of corpora lutea (progesterone) from sows' ovaries, which they called progestin. They showed that removal of the ovaries or destruction of corpora lutea led to abortion.

1930   Butenandt discovered a urinary steroid secreted in large amounts during pregnancy and named it pregnanediol.

1931   Fels and Slotta obtained almost pure crystalline material from corpora lutea, which was of high progestational activity.

1932   Fevold and Hisaw reported their purification of 'corporin' (progesterone).

Allen documented his preparation of purified progestin.

1934   Crystalline progesterone was isolated, and its structure determined, by four groups: Allen and Wintersteiner, Butenandt and Westphal, Hartmann and Wettstein and Slotta *et al.*

1935   The name progesterone evolved from the terms 'progestin' (proposed by Corner) and 'luteosterone' (Butenandt).

Reynolds and Allen demonstrated the effect of progesterone on uterine muscle.

1936   Venning and Browne isolated pregnanediol, a progesterone derivative, from human pregnancy urine.

1937   Pincus and Werthessen demonstrated that progesterone maintains pregnancy through its protective action on the endometrium.

1938   Venning demonstrated that progesterone appeared in human urine as pregnanediol glucuronide. It was the first of the ovarian hormones or their metabolites for which an assay method was devised.

1939   Joel observed that the glycogen and ascorbic acid content in the human tubal mucosa reached its height during the luteal phase of the cycle.

1948   Hoffman found the first measurable progesterone levels on the 14th day of the menstrual cycle.

1950   Noyes *et al.* described the progestational changes in the endometrium.

Greep and Jones found that progesterone would not suppress the pituitary production of follicle stimulating hormone.

1954   Csapo demonstrated that progesterone has an inhibitory effect upon myometrial function.

The pituitary

1886   The association of the pituitary and acromegaly was first shown by Marie.

1892   Marinescu carried out hypophysectomy on a cat.

1895	Active extracts of the posterior pituitary were first prepared by Oliver and Schafer. Two types of material were found, a pressor and an oxytocic principle.
1898	Howell confirmed the presence of a pressor principle, and found it to be confined to the posterior lobe.
1910	Crowe *et al.* described the effect of hypophysectomy in dogs, and the experimental evidence for a pituitary gonadal axis.
1921	Evans and Long noted that administration of anterior pituitary extract affected growth and the oestrus cycle in rats.
1926	Knaus investigated the action of pituitary extract on the pregnant uterus.
1927	Smith and Engle induced precocious puberty in immature rats by injection of anterior pituitary extract. Phillip Smith, while working with hypophysectomized animals, showed the importance of the pituitary gland in the sexual cycle.
1928	Kamm *et al.* separated the pressor and oxytocic principles of the posterior lobe.
1929	Fluhmann discovered large amounts of pituitary hormone in blood samples from menopausal women.
1931	Fevold *et al.* discovered that the pituitary gonadotropic fraction contained two active components, follicle stimulating hormone and luteinizing hormone – the latter was referred to as interstitial cell-stimulating hormone.
1936	Evans *et al.* described degeneration of the gonads in both sexes following hypophysectomy.
1938	Geneva – Standardization of nomenclature for gonadotropins.
1939	The chemical separation and identification of follicle stimulating and luteinizing hormones were reported by the Evans Laboratory in Berkeley California, and the Squibb Research Laboratory which was directed by Van Dyke (Hellman *et al.*, 1971). Luteinizing hormone was obtained in pure preparation from pituitary glands of sheep and pigs. It was found to be a water soluble glycoprotein.
1949	Although follicle stimulating hormone was one of the first gonadotropic hormones to be identified it was the last to be isolated in pure preparation and was found to be a water soluble glycoprotein.

1954	Vasopressin and oxytocin were isolated and analysed by Du Vigneaud and found to be peptides.
1970	Yussman and Taymor noted a rise in plasma luteinizing hormone levels 12–24 hours prior to ovulation. Van de Wiele *et al.* concluded that luteinizing hormone is essential to maintain the normal life span of the corpus luteum.
1972	Yen and Tsai observed the pulsatility of plasma gonadotropin concentrations.
1972–73	The amino acid sequence for human luteinizing hormone was defined (Sairam *et al.*, 1972; Shome *et al.*, 1973; Clossett *et al.*, 1973).
1974	Shome and Parlow described the amino acid sequence of follicle stimulating hormone.
1976	Saxena and Rathnam carried out further work on the amino acid sequence of follicle stimulating hormone. (Chorionic gonadotropin was referred to as Prolan, the pituitary gonadotropin which caused follicular development was called Prolan A while that which caused luteinization was referred to as Prolan B).
1980	Knobil used pulsatile administration (90-min cycles) of gonadotropin to achieve ovulatory cycles in monkeys with experimentally produced hypothalamic lesions.

Prolactin/hyperprolactinaemia

1855	Chiari *et al.* described persistent lactation with atrophy of the uterus.
1882	Frommel reported that the syndrome described by Chiari occurred in about 1% of 3000 women during and after the purperium.
1928	Stricker and Grueter, using bovine pituitary extracts, induced lactation in oophorectomized rabbits.
1930	George Corner demonstrated the lactogenic properties of bovine pituitary extracts.
1931	Riddle and Braucher introduced a pigeon crop assay for lactogenic hormone.
1932	David Krestin first described persistent galactorrhoea, amenorrhoea and pituitary hyperfunction.

Ahumada and del Castillo described galactorrhoea, amenorrhoea, hypo-oestrogenism and absence of urinary gonadotropins.

1953 Argonz and del Castillo published on the galactorrhoea–amenorrhoea syndrome and its relationship to the anterior pituitary.

1954 Forbes *et al.* described the galactorrhoea amenorrhoea syndrome in patients with evidence of pituitary tumour.

1969 Li *et al.* determined the amino acid sequence for sheep prolactin.

1971 Hwang *et al.* quantified prolactin levels by radioimmunoassay.

1972 Joseph Meites *et al.* and others, noted that prolactin production was under tonic inhibition from the hypothalamus, which produced a prolactin inhibiting factor.
Bromocriptine was introduced by Sandoz Pharmaceuticals. This ergot derivative had potent dopaminergic activity and was very effective in lowering elevated prolactin levels. The prolactin inhibiting factor was thought to be dopamine.

1977 Shome and Parlow elucidated the amino acid sequence for human prolactin.

The hypothalamus

1930 Popa and Fielding described a hypo-thalamic–pituitary portal system.

1938 Wislocki showed that blood flowed from the hypothalamus to the anterior pituitary gland.

1948 Markee *et al.* demonstrated that the release of luteinizing hormone was dependent upon the secretion of certain adrenergic or cholinergic chemicals by cells of the hypothalamic centre.

1952 Harris demonstrated that releasing factors were liberated from nerve endings in the hypothalamic tracts into the capillaries of portal vessels in the median eminence and were then carried through the hypophyseal–portal circulation to the anterior pituitary.
The releasing factors all appeared to be peptides.

1960 McCann *et al.* discovered that hypo-thalamic extracts triggered release of gonadotropins.

1971 The chemical structure of gonadotropin releasing hormone was described by Schally *et al.* and also Burgus *et al.* It was found to release both follicle stimulating hormone and luteinizing hormone.
Matsuo *et al.* showed luteinizing releasing hormone to be a decapeptide.

1980 Leyendecker *et al.* first showed the effectiveness of pulsatile treatment with gonadotropin releasing hormone in stimulating ovulation in women.

The placenta

1927/28 Aschheim and Zondek demonstrated a substance in pregnant womens' urine which was capable of stimulating gonadal function.

1928 Aschheim and Zondek first reported the diagnosis of pregnancy by means of urine testing.

1930 Collip established that the placenta produced an ovarian stimulating hormone.
Cole and Harte described a gonado-trophin in the serum of pregnant mares' (PMSG).

1943 Jones *et al.* showed that chorionic gonadotropin was produced by fragments of placenta grown in tissue culture.

1962 Harkness detailed some commonly used tests for chorionic gonadotropin (pregnancy tests).

Aschheim–Zondek Test:
Urine was injected into female mice and activity was shown by development of haemorrhagic follicles and corpora lutea. This was the first test to be developed but was expensive and slow (5 days).

Friedman Test:
Rabbits were used and ovulation looked for. This was a quicker test (1–2 days).

Kupperman Test:
Urine was injected intraperitoneally into rats and ovarian hyperaemia looked for. This was a rapid test (2–3 h).

Xenopus (Zwarenstein) Test:
Extracts of urine were injected under the skin of the female South African Clawed Toad, (*Xenopus laevis*), and a

positive result was given by the production of ova. This response took place within 24 h of injection.

Galli–Mainini Test:
Urine was injected into the male amphibia and caused expulsion of spermatozoa. This test was quick (2 h).

1973   Morgan *et al.* determined the amino acid sequence of human chorionic gonadotropin.

Pregnancy and lactation

1926   Hisaw first observed that the relaxation changes which occur in the pelvic ligaments in pregnancy could be induced in the non-pregnant by administration of blood plasma from pregnant animals. The active substance was later called 'relaxin' (Hisaw and Zarrow, 1950).

1928   Stricker and Grueter found that extracts of the adenohypophysis would cause secretion of milk.

1933   Riddle *et al.* found that extracts of the adenohypophysis which caused secretion of milk also caused growth and secretion of the crop gland of the pigeon, thus providing a method of biological assay.

1934   Lintzel demonstrated the fact that mammary glands remove neutral fats from the blood and their concentration in blood from a mammary vein is less than in arterial blood.

1935   Grant reported that lactating mammary glands produce lactose from glucose.

1937   Graham established that the concentration of amino acids in venous blood from the mammary gland is lower than in arterial blood.

1940   Li *et al.* obtained pure prolactin from the pituitary of sheep.

Prostaglandins

1930   Kurzrok and Lieb, two New York gynaecologists from Columbia, reported on the effects of fresh human seminal fluid on strips of human uterus.

1933   Goldblatt in England discovered that extracts of seminal vesicles stimulated smooth muscle preparations and also had vasodepressor activity.

1934   Von Euler reported that the active principle was an acidic lipid which he named prostaglandin.

1957   Pickles demonstrated prostaglandin activity in human menstrual fluid.

1960   Prostaglandins were characterized and synthesized by Bergstrom and Sjovall.

1968   Sultan Karim *et al.* were the first to use prostaglandins for the successful induction of abortion, and later for the induction of labour.

1970   It was discovered that a coral off the coast of Florida (*Plexaura homomala*) contained a large amount of prostaglandin materials.

Diethylstilboestrol

1933   Cooke *et al.* synthesized the first artificial oestrogen.

1938   Dodds *et al.* discovered that diethyl derivatives of substituted stilbenes had high oestrogenic activity. It was found that diethylstilboestrol was effective and could be prepared in pure form at very low cost.

1941–50 Burdick and Vedder, and Davies and Fugo and many other workers noted that diethylstilboestrol was frequently prescribed for threatened abortion and up to two million women may have received the drug during gestation.

1941   Morrell noted that in the 2.5 years since its synthesis 257 papers had been written about diethylstilboestrol.

Castrodale *et al.* studied the toxic effect of diethylstilboestrol in laboratory animals.

1971   Herbst *et al.* first linked maternal diethylstilboestrol treatment with the development of vaginal clear cell adenocarcinoma in female offspring. This was the first human example of possible transplacental carcinogenesis.

1972   Noller *et al.* implicated cervical adenocarcinoma with maternal treatment using synthetic oestrogens.

1973   Lanier *et al.* noted that diethylstilboestrol had been administered to 7% of all pregnant patients in the Mayo Clinic, during the years 1943–1959. The use of diethylstilboestrol declined however after 1955, and the US Food and Drug Agency later banned its use in pregnancy.

The thyroid

(Extracted from Harkness, R.D., 1962)

Astley Cooper was the first to remove the thyroid in animals.

1856   Schiff showed that removal of the thyroid, (and the as yet undiscovered parathyroids) was fatal in most species.

1878   The relation of the thyroid to myxoedema was suggested by Ord.

1882   Reverdin showed that the condition of 'cachexia strumipriva' followed thyroidectomy in man.

1883   Kocher confirmed that thyroidectomy induced the cachexia condition.

1884   Horsley removed the thyroid from monkeys.
        Schiff showed that a graft of thyroid relieved the symptoms produced by thyroidectomy.

1889   Iodine was discovered to be an essential constituent of the thyroid by Gley.

1891   Murray introduced oral administration of thyroid extract in man.

1895   Baumann and Roos found that iodine was in organic combination in the thyroid.

1914   Kendall isolated the active principle, thyroxine.

1926   Harington determined the structure of thyroxine.

1927   Thyroxine was prepared synthetically by Harington and Barger.

The parathyroids

(Extracted from Harkness, R.D., 1962).

1880   The parathyroid glands were discovered by Sandstrom.

1897   Gley found that that many of the effects of thyroidectomy were in fact due to removal of the parathyroid glands.

1918   Howland and Marriott investigated the function of the glands, and found that parathyroid tetany was accompanied by a fall in blood calcium levels.

1925   Collip extracted a hormone from the glands which raised blood calcium.

The adrenal glands

(Extracted from Harkness, R.D., 1962).

1543   Eustachius discovered the suprarenal (adrenal) glands.

1849   Addison was the first to point out the function of the adrenal glands and described the symptoms of the disease which bears his name.

1856   Brown-Sequard demonstrated that removal of the glands had fatal consequences.

1894   Oliver and Schafer demonstrated the powerful physiological properties of extracts of the adrenals.

1897   Abel and Crawford isolated a substance which they called epinephrine.

1900   Takamine produced a crystalline active substance of the gland which he called adrenaline.

1901   The actions of adrenaline, and their affinity to effects of stimulating the sympathetic system, were demonstrated by Langley.

1929   Swingle and Pfiffner prepared an adrenal cortical extract, which was capable of suspending the effects of adrenalectomy. Following this Kendall *et al.* showed that a series of steroids were the responsible active ingredients.

REFERENCES

Aberbanel, A.R. (1946). Spermatozoa and cervical mucus. In *The Problem of Fertility*. (Princeton, New Jersey: Princeton University Press)

Adams, C.E. and Chang, M.C. (1962). Capacitation of rabbit spermatozoa in the fallopian tube and in the uterus. *J. Exp. Zool.*, **151**, 159

Adams, J., Polson, D.W., Abdulwahid, N., Morris, D.V., Franks, S., Mason, H.D., Tucker, M. and Price, J. (1985). Multifollicular ovaries: clinical and endocrine features and response to pulsatile gonadotrophin releasing hormone. *Lancet*, **2**, 1375–8

Adler, L. (1912). Zur Physiologie und Pathologie der Ovarialfunktion. *Arch. Gynaekol.*, **95**, 349–434

Ahumada, J.C. and del Castillo, E.B. (1932). Sobre un caso de galactorrea y amenorrea. *Biol. Soc. Ginecol. Obstet.*, **11**, 64–78

Allen, E. (1923). Ovogenesis during sexual maturity. *Am. J. Anat.*, **31**, 439

Allen, E. (1926). The menstrual cycle of the monkey; effect of double ovariectomy and injury to large follicles. *Proc. Soc. Exp. Biol. Med.*, **23**, 434

Allen, E. (1927). The menstrual cycle of the monkey, *Macacus rhesus*; observations on normal animals, the effects of removal of the ovaries and the effects of injections of ovarian and placental extracts into the spayed animals. *Contrib. Embryol. Carneg. Inst.*, **19**, 1

Allen, E. (1928). Effects of ovariectomy upon menstruation in monkeys. *Am. J. Physiol.*, **85**, 471–5

Allen, E. and Doisy, E.A. (1923). An ovarian hormone: preliminary report on its localization, extraction and partial purification, and action in test animals. *J. Am. Med. Assoc.*, **81**, 819–21

Allen, E., Pratt, J.P., Newell, Q.U. and Bland, L.J. (1930). Human tubal ova; related corpora lutea and uterine tubes. *Contrib. Embryol.*, **22**, 45

Allen, W.M. (1932). The preparation of purified progestin. *J. Biol. Chem.*, **98**, 591–605

Allen, W.M. and Wintersteiner, O. (1934). Crystalline progestin. *Science*, **80**, 190–1

Arey, L.B. (1939). The degree of normal menstrual irregularity. An analysis of 20,000 calendar records from 1,500 individuals. *Am. J. Obstet. Gynecol.*, **37**, 12

Argonz, J. and del Castillo, E.B. (1953). A syndrome characterized by estrogenic insufficiency, galactorrhea and decreased urinary gonadotropin. *J. Clin. Endocrinol. Metab.*, **13**, 79–87

Aschheim, S. (1927). Weiterer Untersuchungen uber Hormone und Schwangerschaft. Das Vorkommen der Hormone im Harn der Schwangeren. *Arch. Gynaekol.*, **132**, 179–83

Aschheim, S. and Zondek, B. (1927). Anterior pituitary hormone and ovarian hormone in the urine of pregnant women. *Klin. Wchschr.*, **6**, 248

Aschheim, S. and Zondek, B. (1928). Schwangerschaftsdiagnose aus dem Harn (durch Hormonnachweis) *Klin. Wchschr.*, **7**, 8–9; 1404–11; 1453–7

Austin, C.R. (1950). The fecundity of the immature rat following induced superovulation. *J. Endocrinol.*, **6**, 293

Baird, D.T. and Fraser, I.S. (1975). Concentration of oestrone and oestradiol 17β in follicular fluid and ovarian venous blood of women. *Clin. Endocrinol.*, **4**, 259–66

Baker, T.G. (1963). Quantitative and cytological study of germ cells in human ovaries. *Proc. R. Soc. London, Ser. b.*, **158**, 417–33

Baldwin, R.M., Whalley, P.J. and Pritchard, J.A. (1961). Measurements of menstrual blood loss. *Am. J. Obstet. Gynecol.*, **81**, 739

Barker, A. P. and Fowler, W.M. (1936). The blood loss during normal menstruation. *Am. J. Obstet. Gynecol.*, **31**, 97

Bartelmez, G.W. (1931). The human uterine mucous membrane during menstruation. *Am. J. Obstet. Gynecol.*, **21**, 623–43

Barton, M. and Wiesner, B.P. (1945). Thermogenic effect of progesterone. *Lancet*, **2**, 671

Battey, R. (1872). quoted by Gruhn, J.G. and Kazer, R.R. (1989) p. 32

Berger, M.J. and Goldstein, P. (1980). Impaired reproductive performance in DES-exposed women. *Obstet. Gynecol.*, **55**, 25

Bergstrom, S. and Sjovall, J. (1960a). The isolation of prostaglandin F from sheep prostate glands. *Acta Chem. Scand.*, **14**, 1693

Bergstrom, S. and Sjovall, J. (1960b). The isolation of prostaglandin E from sheep prostate glands. *Acta Chem. Scand.*, **14**, 1701

Berson, S.A., Yalow, R.S., Bauman, A., Rothchild, M.A. and Newerly, K. (1956). Insulin I_{131} metabolism in human subjects; demonstration of insulin binding globulin in the circulation of insulin treated subjects. *J. Clin. Invest.*, **35**, 170–90

Berthold, A.A. (1849). Transplantation der hoden. *Arch. Anat. Phys. Wissen. Med.*, 42–6

Besser, G.M., Parke, L. and Edwards, C.R.W. *et al.* (1972). Galactorrhea: successful treatment with reduction of plasma prolactin levels by bromoergocriptine. *Br. Med. J.*, **3**, 669–72

Billings, E.L., Billings, J.J., Brown, J.B. and Burger, H.G. (1972). Symptoms and hormonal changes accompanying ovulation. *Lancet*, **1**, 282–4

Block, E. (1952). Quantitative morphological investigations of the follicular system in women. *Acta Anat.*, **14**, 108

Board, J.A. and Bhatnagar, A.S. (1972). Postcoital antifertility agents. *South. Med. J.*, **65**, 1390–2

Bonnar, J. (1983). Biological approaches to ovulation detection. In Jeffcoate, S.L. (ed.) *Ovulation: Methods for its Prediction and Detection*, pp. 33–47. (Chichester: John Wiley & Sons, Ltd.)

Bouin, P. and Ancel, P. (1909). Sur la fonction du corps jaune. Action du corps jaune vrai sur l'uterus. *C.R. Soc. Biol.*, **66**, 505–7

Bouin, P. and Ancel, P. (1910). Research on the function of the corpus luteum. *J. Physiol. Pathol. Gen.*, **12**, 1–16

Bradbury, R.B. and White, D. E. (1954). Estrogens and related substances in plants. *Vitam. Horm.*, **12**, 207–33

Brewer, J.I. (1942). Studies of the human corpus luteum. Evidence for the early onset of regression of the corpus luteum of menstruation. *Am. J. Obstet. Gynecol.*, **44**, 1048

Brown, R.L. (1944). Rate of transport of spermia in human uterus and tubes. *Am. J. Obstet. Gynecol.*, **47**, 407

Brown-Sequard, C.E. (1890). Remarques sur les effets produits sur la femme par des injections sous-cutanées d'un liquide retiré d'ovaires d'animaux. *Arch. Physiol. Norm. Pathol.*, **2**, 456–7

Browne, J.S.L. (1930). quoted by Collip, J.B. (1930b)

Burdick, H.O. and Vedder, H. (1941). The effect of stilbestrol in early pregnancy. *Endocrinology*, **28**, 629–32

Burgus, R., Butcher, M. Ling, N. *et al.* (1971). Structure moleculair du facteur hypothalamique (LRF) d'origine ovine controlant la secretion de l'hormone gonadotrope hypophysaire luteinisation (LH) *C. R. Acad. Sci.*, **273**, 1611–13

Butenandt, A.F.J. (1929a). Untersuchungen uber das weibliche Sexualhormon. Darstellung und Eigenschaften des kristallisierten 'Progynons'. *Dtsch. Med. Wchschr.*, **55**, 2171–3

Butenandt, A. (1929b). On 'Progynon' a crystallized female sexual hormone. *Naturwissenschaften*, **17**, 879

Butenandt, A. (1930). On pregnanediol, a new steroid derivative from pregnant urine. *Ber. chem. Ges.*, **63**, 659

Butenandt, A. (1931). Uber die chemische Untersuchung der Sexualhormone. *Z. Angew. Chem.*, **44**, 905–8

Butenandt, A.F.J. and Westphal, U. (1934). Zur Isolierung und Characterisierung des Corpus-Luteum-Hormons. *Ber. Dtsch. Chem. Ges.*, **67**, 1440–2

Butomo, W. (1927). Zur frage von der zyklischen veranderung in den tuben (uber tubenlipoide) *Arch. Gynaekol.*, **131**, 306

Castrodale, D., Bierbaum, O. Helwig, E.B. *et al.* (1941). Comparative studies of the effects of estradiol and stilbestrol upon the blood, liver, and bone marrow. *Endocrinology*, **29**, 363–72

Chang, M.C. (1959a). Fertilization of rabbit ova in vitro. *Nature (London)*, **184**, 466

Chang, M.C. (1959b). Fertilizing capacity of spermatozoa. In Lloyd, C.W. (ed.) *Recent Progress in the Endocrinology of Reproduction*, pp. 131–65. (New York: Academic Press)

Chang, M.C. (1964). Effects of certain antifertility agents on the development of rabbit ova. *Fertil. Steril.*, **15**, 97

Chang, M.C. and Pincus, G. (1951). Physiology of fertilization in mammals. *Physiol. Rev.*, **31**, 1

Chesley, L.C. and Hellman, L.M. (1957). Variations in body weight and salivary sodium in the menstrual cycle. *Am. J. Obstet. Gynecol.*, **74**, 582

Chiari, J., Braun, C. and Spaeth, J. (1855). Report of diseases of women observed during the years 1848 to 1855 inclusive in the Department of Gynecology (Municipal Clinic) in Vienna. *Klin. Geburtsh. Gynaekol.*, 371–2

Cianfrani, T. (1960). *A Short History of Obstetrics and Gynaecology*, p. 392. (Springfield, Illinois: Charles C. Thomas)

Claesson, L., Hoberg, B., Rosenberg, T. and Westman, A. (1948). Crystalline human chorionic gonadotropin and its biological action. *Acta Endocrinol.*, **1**, 1

Clinch, J. and Tindall, V.R. (1969). Effect of oestrogens and progestogens on liver function in the puerperium. *Br. Med. J.*, **1**, 602–5

Closset, J., Hennen, G. and Lequin, R.M. (1973). Human luteinizing hormone: the amino acid sequence of the beta subunit. *FEBS Lett.*, **29**, 97

Cole, H.H. and Hart, G.H. (1930). The potency of blood serum of mares in progressive stages of pregnancy in effecting the sexual maturity of the immature rat. *Am. J. Physiol.*, **93**, 57–68

Collip, J.B. (1925). The extraction of a parathyroid hormone which will prevent or control parathyroid tetany and which regulates the level of blood calcium. *J. Biol. Chem.*, **63**, 395–438

Collip, J.B. (1930). The ovarian-stimulating hormone of the placenta. Preliminary paper. *Can. Med. Assoc. J.*, **22**, 219–20

Connally, H.F.J.R., Dann, D.I., Reese, J.M. *et al.* (1940). A clinical study of the effects of diethylstilbestrol on puerperal women. *Am. J. Obstet. Gynecol.*, **40**, 445–8

Cook, J.W., Dodds, E.C. and Hewett, C.L. (1933). A synthetic oestrus-exciting compound (letter to the editor) *Nature (London)*, **131**, 56–7

Corner, G.W. (1923). Ovulation and menstruation in *Macacus rhesus*. *Contributions to Embryology*, Vol. 15, pp. 75–101, Carnegie Institute of Washington, Publication No. 332. (Washington, D.C.: Carnegie Institute)

Corner, G.W. (1930). The hormonal control of lactation. 1. Non effect of the corpus luteum. 11. Positive action of extracts of the hypophysis. *Am. J. Physiol.*, **95**, 43–55

Corner, G.W. (1933). The discovery of the mammalian ovum. In *Lectures on the History of Medicine: a Series of Lectures at the Mayo Foundation.* (Philadelphia: W.B. Saunders)

Corner, G.W. (1935). Influence of the ovarian hormones oestrin and progestin, upon the menstrual cycle of the monkey. *Am. J. Physiol.*, **113**, 238

Corner, G.W. (1938). The sites of formation of oestrogenic substances in the animal body. *Physiol. Rev.*, **18**, 154

Corner, G.W. (1939). The ovarian hormones and experimental menstruation. *Am. J. Obstet. Gynecol.*, **38**, 862–71

Corner, G.W. (1943). *The Hormones in Human Reproduction.* (Princeton, N.J.: Princeton University Press)

Corner, G.W. and Allen, W.M. (1929). Physiology of the corpus luteum. 11. Production of a special uterine reaction (progestational proliferation) by extracts of the corpus luteum. *Am. J. Physiol.*, **88**, 326

Crowe, J., Cushing, H.W. and Homans, I.J. (1910). Experimental hypophysectomy. *Bull. Johns Hopkins Hosp.*, **21**, 127–69

Csapo, A.I. (1954). The molecular basis of myometrial function and its disorders. In *La Prophylaxie en Gynecologie et Obstetrique, Congres International de Gynecologie et Obstetrique*, p.693. (Geneva: Georg et Cie)

Davidge, J.B. (1794). *Dissertatio physiologica de causis catamenium.* (Birmingham: Pearson)

Davidge, J.B. (1814). Menstruous action. In *Physical Sketches and or Outlines of Correctives, Applied to Certain Modern Errors in Physic*, pp. 31–56. (Baltimore: Warner and Robinson)

Davis, M.E. and Fugo, N.W. (1950). Steroids in the treatment of early pregnancy complications. *J. Am. Med. Assoc.*, **142**, 778–83

Davis, M.E. and Koff, A.K. (1938). The experimental production of ovulation in the human subject. *Am. J. Obst. Gynecol.*, **36**, 183

de Graaf, R. (1672). *De Mulierum Organis Generationi Inservientibus*, p.161. (Leiden. Lugduni Batavorum)

Dempsey, E.W. and Bassett, D.L. (1943). Observations on the fluorescence, birefringence and histochemistry of the rat ovary during the reproductive cycle. *Endocrinology*, **33**, 384

Dodds, E.C., Goldberg, L. and Lawson, W. *et al.* (1938a). Oestrogenic activity of certain synthetic compounds. (Letter to the editor) *Nature (London)*, **141**, 247–8

Dodds, E.C., Golberg, L., Lawson, W. *et al.* (1938b) Oestrogenic activity of alkylated stilboestrols. (Letter to the editor) *Nature (London)*, **142**, 34

Dodds, E.C., Golberg, L., Lawson, W. *et. al.* (1938c). Oestrogenic activity of esters of diethyl stilboestrol. (Letter to the editor) *Nature (London)*, **142**, 211–12

Dodds, E.C., Lawson, W. and Noble, R.L. (1938d). Biological effects of the synthetic oestrogenic substance 4: 4'-dihydroxy-alpha: Beta-diethyl-stilbene. *Lancet*, **1**, 1389–91

Doisy, E.A., Veler, C.D. and Thayer, S. (1930). The preparation of the crystalline ovarian hormone from the urine of pregnant women. *J. Biol. Chem.*, **86**, 499–509

Doisy, E.A., Veler, C.D. and Thayer, S. (1929). Folliculin from urine of pregnant women. (Abstract) *Am. J. Physiol.*, **90**, 329–30

Donald, I. (1972). Review of procedures in induction of labour. In Jacomb, R.G. (ed.) *The Use of Prostaglandins E2 and F2 alpha in Obstetrics and*

Gynaecology, Proceedings of a Symposium held at the RCOG, London, (Upjohn), pp. 5–9. (Miami: Symposia Specialists)

Du Vigneaud, V. (1954). Hormones of the posterior pituitary gland: oxytocin and vasopressin. *Harvey Lect.*, **50**, 1–26

Edwards, R.G. (1981). Test tube babies. *Nature (London)*, **293**, 253–6

Edwards, R.G., Bavister, B.D. and Steptoe, P.C. (1969). Early stages of fertilisation *in vitro* of human oocytes matured *in vitro*. *Nature (London)*, **221**, 632

Elias, H. and Schwimmer, D. (1945). The hepatotoxic action of diethylstilbestrol with report of a case. *Am. J. Med. Sci.*, **209**, 602–7

Ellis, F., Adams, S.B., Blomfield, G.W. *et al.* (1944). Discussion on advanced cases of carcinoma of the breast treated by stilboestrol. *Proc. R. Soc. Med.*, **37**, 731–6

Emmart, E.W., Spencer, S.S. and Bates, R.W. (1963). Localization of prolactin within the pituitary by a specific fluorescent antiprolactin globulin. *J. Histochem. Cytochem.*, **11**, 365

Espey, L.L. (1974). quoted by Henderson, K.M. (1979) p. 134

Evans, H.M. and Long, J.A. (1921). The effect of the anterior lobe administered intraperitoneally upon the growth, maturity and the oestrous cycle of the rat. *Anat. Rec.*, **21**, 62–3

Evans, H.M., Korpi, K., Pencharz, R.I. and Wonder, D.H. (1936). On the separation of the interstitial cell-stimulating, luteinizing and follicle-stimulating fractions in the anterior pituitary gonadotropic complex. *Univ. California Publ. (Anat).*, **1**, 255–73

Fabricius de Aquapendente (1621). De Formatione Ovi et Pulli, quoted by Gruhn and Kazer (1989) p. 15

Farris, E.J. (1946). A test for determining the time of ovulation and conception in women. *Am. J. Obstet. Gynecol.*, **52**, 14

Fels, W. and Slotta, K.H. (1931). Das rein dargestellte Hormon des Corpus Luteum und seine biologischen Wirkungen. *Klin. Wchschr.*, **10**, 1639

Fevold, H.L. and Hisaw, F.L. (1932). Purification of corporin. *Proc. Soc. Exp. Biol. Med.*, **29**, 620–1

Fevold, H.L., Hisaw, F.L. and Leonard, S.L. (1931). The gonad-stimulating and the luteinizing hormones of the anterior lobe of the hypophysis. *Am. J. Physiol.*, **97**, 291–301

Figueroa Chases, P. (1958). Reaccion ovarica monstruosa a las gonadotrofinas: a proposito de un caso fatal. *Anal. Cirug.*, **23**, 116

Fleming, R. and Coutts, J.R.T. (1982). Prediction of ovulation in women using a rapid progesterone radioimmunoassay. *Clin. Endocrinol.*, **16**, 171–6

Fluhmann, C.F. (1929). Anterior pituitary hormone in blood of women with ovarian deficiency. *J. Am. Med. Assoc.*, **93**, 672

Folkman, J. (1971). Transplacental carcinogenesis by stilbestrol. (Editorial) *N. Engl. J. Med.*, **285**, 404–5

Forbes, A.P., Henneman, P.H., Griswold, G.C. *et al.* (1954). Syndrome characterized by galactorrhea, amenorrhea and low urinary FSH: Comparison with acromegaly and normal lactation. *J. Clin. Endocrinol. Metab.*, **14**, 265–71

Fraenkel, L. (1910). New experiments on the function of the corpus luteum. *Arch. Gynaekol.*, **91**, 705

Fraenkel, L. and Cohn, F. (1901). Experimentelle Untersuchungen uber den Einfluss des Corpus Luteum auf die Insertion des Eies. *Anat. Anz.*, **20**, 294–300

Frank, R.T. (1922). The ovary and the endocrinologist. *J. Am. Med. Assoc.*, **78**, 181–5

Frank, R.T. (1940). The sex hormones. *J. Am. Med. Assoc.*, **114**, 1504

Frank, R.T. and Salmon, U.J. (1935). Effect of administration of estrogenic factor upon hypophysial hyperactivity in the menopause. *Proc. Soc. Exp. Biol. Med.*, **33**, 311

Frommel, R. (1882). Ueber puerperale Atrophie des Uterus. *Z. Geburtsh. Gynaekol.*, **7**, 305–13

Gebhard, C. (1898). Die Menstruation. *Veits. Handb. Gynaekol.*, **3**, 1

Geist, S.H., Salmon, U.J. and Mintz, M. (1938). The effect of oestrogenic hormone upon the contractility of the Fallopian tubes. *Am. J. Obstet. Gynecol.*, **36**, 67

Gemzell, C.A., Diczfalusy, E. and Tillinger, K.G. (1958). Clinical effect of human pituitary follicle stimulating hormone. *J. Clin. Endocrinol.*, **29**, 1333

Gendrin, A.N. (1839). quoted by Cianfrani, T. (1960) p. 392

Gey, G.O., Jones, G.E.S. and Hellman, L.M. (1938). The production of a gonadotrophic substance (prolan) by placental cells in tissue culture. *Science*, **88**, 306

Goldblatt, M.W. (1933). Depressor substance in seminal fluid. *J. Soc. Chem. Ind.*, **52**, 1056

Gougeon, A. (1982). Rate of follicular growth in the human ovary. In Rolland, R., Van Hall, E.V., Hillier, S.G., McNaulty, K.P. and Schoemaker, J. (eds.) *Follicular Maturation and Ovulation*, pp. 155–63. (Amsterdam, Oxford, Princeton: Excerpta Medica)

Graham, W.R. (1937). The utilization of lactic acid by the lactating mammary gland. *J. Biol. Chem.*, **122**, 1–9

Grant, G.A. (1935). The metabolism of galactose. 11. The synthesis of lactose by slices of active mammary gland *in vitro. Biochem. J.*, **29**, 1905–9

Greenwald, G.S. (1963). *In vivo* recording of intraluminal pressure changes in the rabbit oviduct. *Fertil. Steril.*, **14**, 666

Greep, R.O. and Jones, I.C. (1950). *Recent Progress in Hormone Research*, Vol. 5. (New York: Academic Press)

Gruhn, J. G. (1987). Historical introduction to gonadal regulation of the uterus and the menses. In Gold, J.J. and Josimovich, J.B. (eds.) *Gynecologic Endocrinology*, 4th edn., pp. 3–10. (New York: Plenum Medical Book Co.)

Gruhn, J.G. and Kazer, R.R. (1989). *Hormonal Regulation of the Menstrual Cycle: The Evolution of Concepts*. (New York: Plenum Publishing Corporation)

Gunn, D.L., Jenkin, P.M. and Gunn, A.L. (1937). Menstrual periodicity: statistical observations on a large sample of normal cases. *J. Obstet. Gynaecol. Br. Emp.*, **44**, 839

Gutzeit, J.P. (1896) quoted by Jones and Jones (1981) p. 23

Hackeloer, B.J. (1977). The ultrasonic demonstration of follicular development during the menstrual cycle and after hormone stimulation. In Kurjak, A. (ed.) *Recent Advances in Ultrasound Diagnosis*, Excerpta Medica International Congress Series no. 436, pp. 122–8. (Amsterdam, Oxford: Excerpta Medica)

Hackeloer, B.J., Fleming, R., Robinson, H.P., Adam, A.H. and Coutts, J.R.T. (1979). Correlation of ultrasonic and endocrinologic assessment of human follicular development. *Am. J. Obstet. Gynecol.*, **135**, 122–8

Haighton, J. (1797). An experimental enquiry concerning animal impregnation. *Phil. Trans. R. Soc. Lond.*, **87**, 159–96

Halban, J. (1900). Uber den Einfluss der Ovarien auf die Entwicklung des Genitales. (Transplantation von Uterus, Tube, Ovarium). *Mschr. Geburtsh. Gynaekol.*, **12**, 496–505

Halban, (1904, 1905), quoted by McKay Hart, D. Jr. (1971)

Hallberg, L., Hogdahl, A.M., Nilsson, L. and Rybo, G. (1966). Menstrual blood loss, a population study: variation at different ages and attempts to define normality. *Acta Obstet. Gynecol. Scand.*, **45**, 320

Hallberg, L., Hallgren, J., Hollender, A., Hogdahl, A.M. and Tibblin, G. (1968). Occurrence of iron deficiency anaemia in Sweden. *Symposia of Swedish Nutrition Foundation*, **6**, 19

Haman, J. O. (1942). The length of the menstrual cycle. A study of 150 normal women. *Am. J. Obstet. Gynecol.*, **43**, 870

Hamblen, E.C. and Davis, C.D. (1945). Treatment of hypo-ovarianism by the sequential and cyclic administration of equine and chorionic gonadotrophins – so-called one-two cyclic gonadotrophic therapy. *Am. J. Obstet. Gynecol.*, **50**, 137

Hamblen, E.C., Cuyler, W.K., Wilson, J.A. *et al.* (1941). Endocrine therapy of functional menometrorrhagia and ovarian sterility IV. One-two cyclic therapy with equine and chorionic gonadotropins. *J. Clin. Endocrinol. Metab.*, **1**, 974

Harkness, R.D. (1962). The provision of special chemical stimulants, and of measures for continuance of the species. In Davson, H. and Grace Eggleton, M. (eds.) With historical notes by Sir C. Lovatt-Evans. *Starling and Lovatt Evans Principles of Human Physiology*, 13th edn. pp. 1387–447;1502. (London: J. & A. Churchill Ltd)

Harris, G.W. (1952). Hypothalamic control of the anterior pituitary gland. *Ciba Foundation Colloquia on Endocrinology*, **4**, 106

Harris, G.W. (1955). *The Neural Control of the Pituitary Gland*. (London: Edward Arnold)

Harris, G.W. and Naftolin, F. (1970). Hypothalamus and control of ovulation. *Br. Med. Bull.*, **6**, No.1, 3–9

Hartman, C.G. (1929). How large is the mammalian egg? *Q. Rev. Biol.*, **4**, 373

Hartman, C.G. (1936). *Time of Ovulation in Women.* (London: Balliere, Tindall & Cox)

Hartman, C.G. (1939). Ovulation, fertilization and the transport and viability of eggs and spermatozoa. In Allen, E. (ed.) *Sex and Internal Secretion*, 2nd edn., chap. IX. (London: Bailliere, Tindall & Cox)

Hartmann, M. and Wettstein, A. (1934). Ein krystallisiertes Hormon aus Corpus Luteum. *Helv. Chim. Acta*, **17**, 878–82

Heape, W. (1900). The "Sexual Season" of mammals and the relation of the "pro oestrum" to menstruation *Q. J. Micr. Sci.*, **44**, 1–10

Hegar, A. (1878). Die Castration der Frauen. *Sammlung. klin. Vortr. Volkmann. Gynekol.*, **42**, 925–1068

Hellman, L.M., Pritchard, J.A. and Wynn, R.M. (1971). *Williams Obstetrics*, 14th edn., pp. 83; 122. (London: Butterworths)

Henderson, K.M. (1979). Gonadotrophic regulation of ovarian activity. *Br. Med. Bull.*, **35**, 164

Herbst, A.L., Ulfelder, H. and Poskanzer, D.C. (1971). Adenocarcinoma of the vagina: association of maternal stilbestrol therapy with tumor appearance in young women. *N. Engl. J. Med.*, **284**, 878–81

Herbst, A.L., Hubby, M.M., Blough, R.R. and Azizi, F. (1980). A comparison of pregnancy experience in DES-exposed and DES-unexposed daughters. *J. Reprod. Med.*, **24**, 62

Herbst, W.P. (1941). The effects of estradiol dipropionate and diethylstilbestrol on malignant prostatic tissue. *Trans. Am. Assoc. Genitourin. Surg.*, **34**, 195–202

Hertig, A.T. and Rock, J. (1944). On the development of the early human ovum with special reference to the trophoblast of the previllous stage: a description of 7 normal and 5 pathologic human ova. *Am. J. Obstet. Gynecol.*, **47**, 149

Hertig, A.T. and Rock, J. (1945). Two human ova in the previllous stage, having a developmental age of about 7 and 9 days respectively. *Contrib. Embryol.*, **35**, 65

Hertig, A.T. and Rock, J. (1949). A series of potentially abortive ova recovered from fertile women prior to the first missed menstrual period. *Am. J. Obstet. Gynecol.*, **58**, 968

Hertig, A.T., Rock, J. and Adams, E.C. (1956). A description of 34 human ova within the first 17 days of development. *Am. J. Anat.*, **98**, 435–93

Heuser, C., Hertig, A.T. and Rock, J. (1945). Two human embryos showing early stages of the definitive yolk sac. *Contrib. Embryol.*, **31**, 85

Hill, R.T., Allen, E. and Kramer, T.C. (1935). Cinemicrographic studies of rabbit ovulation. *Anat. Rec.*, **63**, 239–46

Hisaw, F.L. and Greep, R.O. (1938). Inhibition of uterine bleeding with estradiol and progesterone and associated endometrial modifications. *Endocrinology*, **23**, 1–14

Hisaw, F.L. and Zarrow, M.X. (1950). The physiology of relaxin. *Vitam. Horm.*, **8**, 151–78

Hitschmann, F. and Adler, L. (1907). Die Lehre von der Endometritis. *Z. Geburtsh. Gynaekol.*, **60**, 63–86

Hitschmann, F. and Adler, L. (1908). The structure of the endometrium of sexually mature women with special reference to menstruation. *Mschr. Geburtsh. Gynaekol.*, **27**, 1–82

Hoffman, F. (1948). On the content of progesterone in the ovary and blood during the cycle. *Geburtsh. Frauenh.*, **8**, 723

Hohlweg, W. (1934). Veranderungen des Hypophysenvorderlappens und des Ovariums nach Behandlung mit grossen Dosen von Follikelhormon. *Klin. Wochenschr.*, **13**, 92–5

Howell, (1898). quoted by Harkness, R.D. (1962) p. 1388

Huberman, J. and Colmer, M.J. (1940). The effects of diethyl stilbene (stilbestrol) on menopausal symptoms. *Am. J. Obstet. Gynecol.*, **39**, 783–91

Hwang, P., Guyda, H. and Friesen, H.G. (1971). A radioimmunoassay for human prolactin. *Proc. Natl. Acad. Sci. USA*, **68**, 1902–6

Hytten, F.E., Cheyne, G.A. and Klopper, A.I. (1964). Iron loss at menstruation. *J. Obstet. Gynaecol. Br. Commonw.*, **71**, 255

Insler, V., Melmed, H., Eichenbrenner, I., Serr, D.M. and Lunenfeld, B. (1972). The cervical score: a simple semiquantitative method for monitoring of the menstrual cycle. *Int. J. Gynecol. Obstet.*, **10**, 223–8

Iscovesco, H. (1912a). Les lipoides de l'ovaire. *C.R. Soc. Biol. Paris*, **63**, 16–18

Iscovesco, H. (1912b). Le lipoide uterostimulant de l'ovaire. Proprietes physiologiques. *C.R. Soc. Biol. Paris*, **63**, 104–6

Ito, Y. and Higashi, K. (1961). Studies on prolactin-like substance in human placenta. 11. *Endocrinol. Jap.*, **8**, 279

Joel, K. (1939). The glycogen content of the fallopian tubes during the menstrual cycle and during pregnancy. *J. Obstet. Gynaecol. Br. Emp.*, **46**, 721

Jones, H.W. and Jones, G.S. (1981). *Novak's Textbook of Gynecology*, 10th edn. (Baltimore and London: Williams & Wilkins)

Jones, S.G.E. (1949). Some newer aspects of the management of infertility. *J. Am. Med. Assoc.*, **141**, 1123–8

Jones, S.G.E., Gey, G.O. and Gey, M.K. (1943). Hormone production by placental cells maintained in continuous culture. *Johns Hopkins Hosp. Bull.*, **72**, 26–38

Josimovich, J.B. and MacLaren, J.A. (1962). Presence in human placenta and term serum of a highly lactogenic substance immunologically related to pituitary growth hormone. *Endocrinology*, **71**, 209

Kamm, *et al.* (1928). quoted by Harkness, R.D. (1962). p. 1388

Karim, S.M.M. and Filshie, G.M. (1970). Therapeutic abortion using prostaglandin F2 alpha. *Lancet*, **1**, 157

Karim, S.M.M. and Hillier, K. (1979). Prostaglandins in the control of animal and human reproduction. In Short, R.V. (ed.) *Br. Med. Bull.*, **35**, 173–80

Karim, S.M.M., Trussell, R.R., Hillier, K. and Patel, R.C. (1968). Induction of labor with prostaglandin F2 alpha. *Br. Med. J.*, **4**, 621

Katz, M. (1981). Polycystic ovaries. In Hull, M.G.R. (ed.) *Clinics in Obstetrics and Gynaecology*, Vol. 8, No. 3, pp. 715–31. (London, Philadelphia, Toronto: W.B. Saunders Co. Ltd.)

Kaufman, R.H., Noller, K., Adam, E., Irwin, J., Gray, M., Jefferies J.A. and Hilton, J. (1984). Upper genital tract abnormalities and pregnancy outcome in diethylstilbestrol-exposed progeny. *Am. J. Obstet. Gynecol.*, **148**, 973

Keetel, W.C., Bradbury, J.T. and Stoddard, F.J. (1957). Observations on the polycystic ovary syndrome. *Am. J. Obstet. Gynecol.*, **73**, 954–62

Kendall, E.C. (1915). The isolation in crystalline form of the compound containing iodine which occurs in the thyroid. *J. Am. Med. Assoc.*, **64**, 2042–3

Kerin, J.F., Edmonds, D.K., Warnes, G.M., Cox, L.W., Seamark, R.F., Matthews, C.D., Young, G.B. and Baird, D.T. (1981). Morphological and functional relations of Graafian follicle growth to ovulation in women using ultrasonic, laparoscopic and biochemical measurements. *Br. J. Obstet. Gynaecol.*, **88**, 81–90

Knauer, E. (1896). Einige Versuche uber Ovarientransplantation bei Kaninchen. *Zentralbl. Gynaekol.*, **20**, 524–8

Knauer, E. (1900). Ovarian transplantation *Arch. Gynaekol.*, **60**, 322–76

Knaus, H. (1926). The action of pituitary extract upon the pregnant uterus of the rabbit. *J. Physiol.*, **61**, 383

Knaus, H. (1933). Die periodische Frucht-und Unfruchtbarkeit des Eribes. *Zentralbl. Gynaekol.*, **57**, 24–33

Knobil, E. (1980). The neuroendocrine control of the menstrual cycle. *Rec. Prog. Horm. Res.*, **36**, 53–88

Krestin, D. (1932). Spontaneous lactation associated with enlargement of the pituitary. *Lancet*, **2**, 928–30

Krohn, P.L. (1949). Intermenstrual pain (the "Mittelschmerz") and the time of ovulation. *Br. Med J.*, **1**, 803

Kundrat, H. and Engelmann, G.J. (1873). Untersuchungen uber die Uterusschleimhaut. *Vienna, Med. Jahrbuch*, 43

Kurzrok, R. and Lieb, C.C. (1930). Biochemical studies of human semen. II. *Proc. Soc. Exp. Biol. Med.*, **26**, 268

Lanier, A.P., Noller, K.L., Decker, D.G. *et al.* (1973). Cancer and stilbestrol: a follow-up of 1,719 persons born 1943–1959 and exposed to estrogens *in utero. Mayo Clin. Proc.*, **48**, 793–9

Lamar, J.K., Shettles, L.B. and Delfs, E. (1940). Cyclic penetrability of human cervical mucus to spermatozoa *in vitro*. *Am. J. Physiol.*, **129**, 234

Lataste, F. (1886). Notes prises au jour le jour sur differentes especes de l'ordre des rongeurs observées en captivite. *Actes. Soc. Linn. Bordeaux,* **40**, 293–466

Lataste, F. (1887). Notes prises au jour le jour sur differentes especes de l'ordre des rongeurs observees en captivite. *Actes. Soc. Linn. Bordeaux,* **41**, 201–536

Lee, J.B. *et al.* (1963). Sustained depressor effects of renal medullary extract in the normotensive rat. *Circ. Res.*, **13**, 369

Leopold, (1885). quoted by Cianfrani, T. (1960) p. 394

Lerner, A.B., Case, J.D., Biemann, K., Heinzelman, R.V., Szmuszkovicz, J., Anthony, W.C. and Kriuis, A. (1959). Isolation of 5-methoxyindole-3-acetic acid from bovine pineal glands. *J. Am. Chem. Soc.*, **81**, 5264

Leyendecker, G., Wildt, L. and Hansmann, M. (1980). Pregnancies following chronic intermittent (pulsatile) administration of GnRH by means of a portable pump ("Zyklomat") – a new approach to the treatment of infertility in hypothalamic amenorrhoea. *J. Clin. Endocrinol. Metab.*, **51**, 1214–16

Li, C.H. (1958). *Proc. Soc. Exp. Biol.*, **98**, 839

Li, C.H., Lyons, W.R. and Evans, H.M. (1940). A comparison of the electrophoretic behaviour of the lactogenic hormone as prepared from beef and from sheep pituitaries. *J. Am. Chem. Soc.*, **62**, 2925–7

Li, C.H., Simpson, M.E. and Evans, H.M. (1949). quoted by Sommerville, I.F. (1964)

Li, C.H., Grumbach, M.M., Kaplan, S.L., Josimovich, J.B., Friesen, H. and Cati, K.J. (1968) Human chorionic somatomammotropin (HCS) proposed terminology for designation of a placental hormone. *Experimenta*, **24**, 1288

Li, C.H., Dixon, J.S., Lo, T.B. *et al.* (1969). Amino-acid sequence of ovine lactogenic hormone. *Nature (London)*, **224**, 695–6

Lintzel, W. (1934). Untersuchungen uber den Chemismus der Milchfettbildung in Abhangigkeit von der Futterung. *Z. Sucht, B.*, **29**, 219–42

Linzenmeier, G. (1947). Zur Frage der Empfangniszeit der Frau: Hat Knaus oder Stieve Recht? *Zentrabl. Gynaekol.*, **69**, 110

Loeb, L. (1907). Ueber die Experimentelle Erzeugung von Knoten von Deciduagewebe in dem Uterus des Meerschweinchens nach stattgefundenen Copulation. *Zentralbl. Allg. Path. Anat.*, **18**, 563–5

Loeb, L. (1908). The experimental production of the maternal part of the placenta in the rabbit. *Proc. Soc. Exp. Biol Med.*, **5**, 102–4

Loeb, L. (1911). Ueber die Bedeutung des Corpus Luteum fur die Periodizität des sexuellen Zyklus beim weiblichen Saugetierorganismus. *Dtsch. Med. Wchschr.*, **37**, 17–21

Loewe, S. and Lange, F. (1926). Der Gehalt des Frauenharnes an brunsterzeugenden Stoffen in Abhängigkeit vom ovariellen Zyklus. *Klin. Wchschr.*, **5**, 1038–9

Ludwig, K. (1858–1861). *Lehrbuch der Physiologie des Menschen.* (Leipzig: C.F. Winter)

Lyon, R.A. (1946). Ovulation in non-lactating puerpera. *Proc. Soc. Exp. Biol.*, **63**, 105

McCann, S.M., Taleisnik, S. and Friedman, H.M. (1960). LH-releasing activity in hypothalamic extracts. *Proc. Soc. Exper. Biol. Med.*, **104**, 432–4

McCann, S.M. (1962). A hypothalamic luteinizing hormone-releasing factor. *Am. J. Physiol.*, **202**, 395–400

MacCorquodale, D.W., Thayer, S.A. and Doisy, E.A. (1936). The isolation of the principal estrogenic substance of liquor folliculi. *J. Biol. Chem.*, **115**, 535

McKay, D.G. and Robinson, D. (1947). Observation on fluorescence, birefringence and histochemistry of human ovary during menstrual cycle. *Endocrinology*, **41**, 378

McKay Hart, D. Jr. (1971). Placental function. In MacDonald, R.R. (ed.) *Scientific Basis of Obstetrics and Gynaecology,* pp. 115–143. (London, Edinburgh: Churchill Livingstone)

McNatty, K.P. (1982). Ovarian follicular development from the onset of luteal regression in human and sheep. In Rolland. R., van Hall, E.V., Hillier, S.G., McNatty, K.P. and Schoemaker, J. (eds.) *Follicular Maturation and Ovulation*, pp. 1–18. (Amsterdam, Oxford, Princeton: Excerpta Medica)

Magnus, V. (1901). Ovariets betydning for svangerskabet med saerligt hensyn til corpus luteum. *Nor. Mag. Laegevidensk*, **62**, 1138–45

Mandl, A.M. and Zuckerman, S. (1951). The effect of destruction of the germinal epithelium on the number of oocytes. *J. Endocrinol.*, **7**, 103

Marie, (1886). quoted by Harkness, R.D. (1962) p. 1388

Marinescu, (1892). quoted by Harkness, R.D. (1962) p. 1388

Markee, J.E. (1940). Menstruation in intraocular endometrial transplants in the rhesus monkey. *Contrib Embryol. Carneg. Inst. Wash.*, **28**, 219–308

Markee, J.E., Sawyer, C.H. and Hollinshead, W.H. (1948). Andrenergic control of release of luteinizing hormone from hypophysis of rabbit. *Rec. Progr. Horm. Res.*, **2**, 117

Marshall, F.H.A. and Jolly, W.A. (1906). Contribution to the physiology of mammalian reproduction. *Phil. Trans. R. Soc. Lond.*, **198**, 99–141

Matsuo, H., Baba, Y., Nair, R.M.G., Arimura, A. and Schally, A.V. (1971). Structure of porcine LH and FSH releasing hormone. 1. The proposed amino acid sequence. *Biochem. Biophys. Res. Comm.*, **43**, 1334–9

Medvei, V.C. (1982). *A History of Endocrinology*, pp. 619–22. (Lancaster: MTP Press Ltd.) 2nd edn. (1993). *The History of Clinical Endocrinology*. (Carnforth: Parthenon Publishing)

Meites, J., Lu, K-H, Wuttke, W. *et al.* (1972). Recent studies on functions and control of prolactin secretion in rats. *Rec. Prog. Horm. Res.*, **28**, 471–516

Menkin, M.F. and Rock, J. (1948). *In vitro* fertilization and cleavage of human ovarian eggs. *Am. J. Obstet. Gynecol.*, **55**, 440

Meyer, R. (1911). Uber Corpus Luteumbildung beim Menschen. *Zentralbl. Gynaekol.*, **35**, 1206–8

Midgley, A.R. Jr. and Jaffe, R.B. (1971). Regulation of human gonadotropins. X. Episodic fluctuation of LH during the menstrual cycle. *J. Clin. Endocrinol. Metab.*, **33**, 962–9

Millis, J. (1951). The iron losses of healthy women during consecutive menstrual cycles. *Med. J. Aust.*, **2**, 874

Moghissi, K.S., Syner, F.N. and Evans, T. (1972). A composite picture of the menstrual cycle. *Am. J. Obstet. Gynecol.*, **114**, 405–18

Moore, C.R. and Price, D. (1932). Gonad hormone function and the reciprocal influence between gonads and hypophysis. *Am. J. Anat.*, **50**, 13–67

Morgan, F.J., Birken, S. and Canfield, R.E. (1973). Human chorionic gonadotropin: a proposal for amino acid sequence. *Mol. Cell. Biochem.*, **2**, 97–8

Moricke, R. (1882). Die Uterusschleimhaut in verschiedenen Altersperioden und zur Zeit der Menstruation. *Z. Geb. Gynaekol.*, **7**, 84–137

Morrell, J.A. (1941). Summary of some clinical reports on stilbestrol. *J. Clin. Endocrinol. Metab.*, **1**, 419–23

Morris, R.T. (1895). *Lectures on appendicitis and notes on other subjects.* (New York: G.R. Putnam)

Noller, K.L. and Fish, C.R. (1974). Diethylstilbestrol usage; its past present and future. In Fish, C.R. and Decker, D.G. (eds.) *Medical Gynaecology. The Medical Clinics of North America*, p. 801. (Philadelphia, London, Toronto: W.B. Saunders Co.)

Noller, K.L., Decker, D.G., Lanier, A.P. *et al.* (1972). Clear-cell adenocarcinoma of the cervix after maternal treatment with synthetic estrogens. *Mayo Clin. Proc.*, **47**, 629–30

Novak, E. (1947). *Gynaecological and Obstetrical Pathology, with Clinical and Endocrine Relations*, 2nd edn. p. 479. (Philadelphia: W.B. Saunders Co.)

Novak, E. and Everett, H.S. (1928). Cyclical and other variations in the tubal epithelium. *Am. J. Obstet. Gynecol.*, **16**, 499

Noyes, R. W. and Dickmann, Z. (1961). Survival of ova transferred into the oviduct of the rat. *Fertil. Steril.*, **12**, 67

Noyes, R.W., Hertig, A.T. and Rock, J. (1950). Dating the endometrial biopsy. *Fertil. Steril.*, **1**, 3–25

O'Herlihy, C., Robinson, H.P., De Crespigny, L.J., Ch. (1980). Mittelschmerz is a preovulatory symptom. *Br. Med. J.*, **280**, 986

Ogino, K. (1930). Ovulationstermin und Konzeptionstermin. *Zentralbl. Gynaekol.*, **54**, 464–79

Ohler, I. (1951). Beitrag zur Kenntnis des Ovarialepithels und seiner Beziehungen zur Oogenese. *Acta Anat.*, **12**, 1

Oliver, G. and Schafer, E.A. (1895). The physiological effects of extracts of the suprarenal capsules. *J. Physiol.*, **18**, 230–79

Papanicolaou, G.N., Traut, H.F. and Marchetti. A.A. (1948). *The Epithelia of Woman's Reproductive Organs.* (New York: Commonwealth Fund)

Papanicolaou, G.N. (1923–24). Ovogenesis during sexual maturity, as elucidated by experimental methods. *Proc. Soc. Exp. Biol. Med.*, **21**, 393

Parkes, A.S. (1942). Induction of superovulation and superfecundation in rabbits. *J. Endocrinol.*, **3**, 268

Parkes, A.S. (1966). The rise of reproductive endocrinology 1926–1940. *J. Endocrinol.*, **34**, xix–xxxii

Parkes, A.S. and Bellerby, C.W. (1926). Studies on the internal secretion of the ovary. 1. The distribution in the ovary of the oestrus-producing hormone. J. *Physiol (London)*, **61**, 562–75

Pfluger, E.F.W. (1863). *Uber die Eierstocke der Saugethiere und des Menschen.* (Leipzig: Englemann)

Pickles, V.R. (1957). A plain muscle stimulant in the menstruum. *Nature (London)*, **180**, 1198–9

Pierce, G.B.Jr. and Midgley, A.R.Jr. (1963). The origin and function of human syncytiotrophoblastic giant cells. *Am. J. Pathol*, **43**, 153

Pincus, G. and Werthessen, N.T. (1937). Quantitative method for bioassay of progestin. *Am. J. Physiol.*, **120**, 100

Popa, G.T. and Fielding, U. (1933). quoted by Harris, G.W. and Naftolin, F. (1970)

Portes, Aschheim and Robey (1938). Sur la differenciation des corps jaunes gestatifs et menstruels. *Gynecol. Obstet.*, **37**, 100

Pott, P. (1775). An ovarian hernia. *The Chirurgical Works*, pp. 791–2. (London: James Wilson)

Pouchet, F.A. (1847). *Theorie Positive de l'Ovulation Spontanée et de la Fecondation des Mammiferes et de l'Espece Humaine.* (Paris: Bailliere)

Pratt, J.P. (1927). Corpus luteum in its relation to menstruation and pregnancy. *Endocrinology*, **11**, 195

Prenant, A. (1898a). La valeur morphologique du corps jaune. Son action physiologique et therapeutique possible. *Rev. Gen. Sci. Pure. Appl.*, **9**, 646–50

Prenant, A. (1898b). On the morphologic importance of the corpus luteum, and its physiologic and possible therapeutic action. *Rev. Medicale de Liest.*, **30**, 385

Prevost, J.L. and Dumas, J.A.B. (1824). De la generation dans les mammiferes et des premiers indices du developpement de l'embryon. *Ann. Sci. Nat.*, **3**, 113–8

Reynolds, S.R.M. and Allen, W.M. (1935). Physiology of the corpus luteum. The comparative action of crystalline progestin and crude progestin on uterine motility in unanesthetized rabbits. *Am. J. Obstet. Gynecol.*, **30**, 309–18

Richards, J.S. and Midgley, A.R.Jr. (1976). Protein hormone action: a key to understanding ovarian follicular and luteal cell development. *Biol. Reprod.*, **14**, 89–94

Riddle, O. and Braucher, P.F. (1931). Studies on the physiology of reproduction in birds. XXX. Control of the special secretion of the crop-gland in pigeons by an anterior pituitary hormone. *Am. J. Physiol.*, **97**, 617–25

Riddle, O., Bates, R.W. and Dykshorn, S.W. (1933). The preparation, identification and assay of prolactin – a hormone of the anterior pituitary. *Am. J. Physiol.*, **105**, 191–206

Robinson, A. (1918). The formation, rupture and closure of ovarian follicles in ferrets and ferret-polecat hybrids, and some associated phenomena. *Trans. R. Soc. Edin.*, **52**, 303

Roth-Brandel, U. *et al* (1970). Prostaglandins for induction of therapeutic abortion. *Lancet*, **1**, 191

Ruge, C. (1913). Uber Ovulation, Corpus Luteum und Menstruation. *Arch. Gynaekol.*, **100**, 20–48

Sairam, M.R., Papkoff, H. and Li, C.H. (1972). Human pituitary interstitial cell stimulating hormone: Primary structure of the alpha subunit. *Biochem. Biophys. Res. Commun.*, **48**, 530–7

Sandstrom, I.V. (1880). On a new gland in man and several mammals. *Bull. Inst. Hist. Med.*, **6**, 192–222

Saxena, B.B. and Rathnam, P. (1976). Amino acid sequence of the beta subunit of follicle-stimulating hormone from human pituitary glands *J. Biol. Chem.*, **251**, 993–1005

Schally, A.V., Arimura, A., Kastin, A.J. *et al* (1971). Gonadotropin-releasing hormone: one polypeptide regulates secretion of luteinizing and follicle stimulating hormones. *Science*, **173**, 1036–7

Schmidt, G., Fowler, W.C.Jr., Talbert, L.M. and Edelman, D.A. (1980). Reproductive history of women exposed to diethylstilbestrol *in utero. Fertil. Steril.*, **33**, 21

Schroder, R. (1909). Die Drusenepithelveranderungen der Uterusschleimhaut in Intervall und Premenstruum. *Arch. Gynaekol.*, **88**, 1–28

Schroder, R. (1913). Uber die zeitlichen Beziehungen der Ovulation und Menstruation *Archiv. Gynaekol.*, **101**, 1

Schroder, R. (1915). Anatomische Studien zur normalen und pathologischen Physiologie des Menstruationszyklus. *Archiv. Gynaekol.*, **104**, 27–102

Schroder, R. (1930). Weibliche Genitalorgane. *Handb. Mikros. Anat.*, **7**, 329–556

Schwartz, A., Zor, U., Lindner, H.R. and Naor, S. (1974). quoted by Kairim, S.M.M. and Hillier, K. (1979). p. 178

Seckinger, D.L. and Snyder, F.F. (1923–24). Cyclic variations in the spontaneous contractions of the human Fallopian tube. *Proc. Soc. Exp. Biol. Med.*, **21**, 519

Seguy, J. and Simonet, H. (1933). Recherches des signes directs d'ovulation chez la femme. *Gynecol. Obstet.*, **28**, 657

Seguy, J. and Vimeux, J. (1933). Contribution a l'etude des sterilites inexpliquées: etude de l'ascension des spermatozoides dans les voies genitales basses de la femme. *Gynecol. Obstet.*, **27**, 346

Shome, B. and Parlow, A.F. (1973). The primary structure of the hormone-specific, beta subunit of human pituitary luteinizing hormone (hLH) *J. Clin. Endocrinol. Metab.*, **36**, 618–21

Shome, B. and Parlow, A.F. (1974). Human follicle stimulating hormone (hFSH): first proposal for the amino acid sequence of the alpha subunit (hFSHalpha) and first demonstration of its identity with the alpha-subunit of human luteinizing hormone (hLHalpha) *J. Clin. Endocrinol. Metab.*, **39**, 199–202

Shome, B. and Parlow, A.F. (1977). Human pituitary prolactin (hPRL) The entire linear amino acid sequence. *J. Clin. Endocrinol. Metab.*, **45**, 1112–15

Short, R.V. (1977). The discovery of the ovaries. In Zuckerman, L. and Weir, B.J. (eds.) *The Ovary*, 2nd edn., pp. 1–39. (New York: Academic Press)

Siegler, A.M., Wang, C.F. and Friberg, J. (1979). Fertility of the diethylstilbestrol-exposed offspring. *Fertil. Steril.*, **31**, 601

Simkins, C.S. (1932). Development of the human ovary from birth to sexual maturity. *Am. J. Anat.*, **51**, 465

Skarin, G., Nillius, S.J. and Wide, L. (1982). Pulsatile low dose luteinizing hormone-releasing hormone treatment for induction of follicular maturation and ovulation in women with amenorrhoea. *Acta Endocrinol.*, **101**, 78–86

Slotta, K.H., Rushig, H. and Fels, W. (1934). Reindarstellung der Hormone aus dem Corpus Luteum (Vorlauf Mitteil). *Ber. Dtsch. Chem. Ges.*, **67**, 1270–3

Smith, O.W. and Ryan, K.J. (1962). Estrogen in the human ovary. *Am. J. Obstet. Gynecol.*, **84**, 141–53

Smith, P.E. (1927). The disabilities caused by hypophysectomy and their repair. *J. Am. Med. Assoc.*, **88**, 158

Smith, P.E. (1930) quoted by West, E.S., Todd, W.R., Mason, H.S. and van Bruggen, J.T. (1970)

Smith, P.E. and Engle, E. (1927). Experimental evidence regarding the role of the anterior pituitary in the development and regulation of the genital system. *Am. J. Anat.*, **40**, 159–217

Smith, P.E. and Engle, E.T. (1932). Prevention of experimental uterine bleeding in macacus monkey by corpus luteum extract (progestin) *Proc. Soc. Exp. Biol. Med.*, **29**, 1225–7

Snyder, F.F. (1924). Changes in the human oviduct during the menstrual cycle and pregnancy. *Bull. Johns Hopkins Hosp.*, **35**, 141

Sommerville, I.F. (1964). Methods of hormone assay. In Thompson, R.H.S. and King, E.J. (eds.) *Biochemical Disorders in Human Disease*, 2nd edn., pp. 980–9. (London: J.&A. Churchill Ltd)

Speert, H. (1958). *Essays in Eponymy. Obstetric and Gynecologic Milestones.* p.9, 15. (New York: Macmillan)

Squire, W. (1868) Puerperal temperatures. *Trans. Obstet. Soc. (London)*, **9**, 129

Stein, I.F. (1945). Bilateral polycystic ovaries. *Am. J. Obstet. Gynecol.*, **50**, 385–96

Stein, I.F. and Leventhal, M.L. (1935). Amenorrhea associated with bilateral polycystic ovaries. *Am. J. Obstet. Gynecol.*, **29**, 181–91

Stockard, C.R. and Papanicolaou, G.N. (1917). The existence of a typical oestrus cycle in the guinea pig, with a study of its histological and physiological changes. *Am. J. Anat.*, **22**, 225–84

Streeter, G.L. (1926). The 'Miller' ovum – the youngest normal human embryo thus far known. *Carnegie Contrib. Embryol.*, **18**, 31

Stricker, P. and Grueter, F. (1928). Action du lobe anterieur de l'hypophyse sur la montée laiteuse. *C. R. Soc. Biol. Paris*, **99**, 1978–80

Swanson, M., Salebrei, R.E.E. and Cooperberg, P.L. (1981). Medical implications of ultrasonically detected polycystic ovaries. *J. Clin. Ultrasound.*, **9**, 219–22

Takamine, J. (1901). The isolation of the active principle of the suprarenal gland. *J. Physiol.*, **27**, 29–30

Thiede, H.A. and Choate, J.W. (1963). Chorionic gonadotropin localization in the human placenta by immunofluorescent staining 11. Demonstration of HCG in the trophoblast and amnion epithelium of immature and mature placentas. *Obstet. Gynecol.*, **22**, 433

Tomkins, P. (1944). Use of basal temperature graphs in determining date of ovulation. *J. Am. Med. Assoc.*, **124**, 698

Topkins, P. (1943). The histologic appearance of the endometrium during lactation amenorrhoea and its relationship to ovarian function. *Am. J. Obstet. Gynecol.*, **45**, 48

Vaitukaitis, J.L., Graunstein, G.D. and Ross, G.T. (1972). A radioimmunoassay which specifically measures human chorionic gonadotropin in the presence of human luteinizing hormone. *Am. J. Obstet. Gynecol.*, **113**, 751

Van de Velde, T.H. (1905). *Uber den zusammenhang zwischen Ovarialfunction, Wellenbewegung und Menstrualblütung und Uber die Enstenhung des sogenannten Mittelschmerzes* (On the relationship between ovarian function, periodicity and menstrual flow, and on the origins of the so-called Mittelschmerz), p. 39. (Haarlem: F.Bohn)

Van de Wiele, R.L., Bogumil, J., Dyrenfurth, I., Ferin, M., Jewelewicsz, R., Warren, M., Rizkallah, T. and Mikhail, G. (1970). Mechanisms regulating the menstrual cycle in women *Rec. Prog. Horm. Res.*, **126**, 63

Venning, E.H. (1938). Further studies on the estimation of small amounts of sodium pregnanediol glucuronidate in urine. *J. Biol. Chem.*, **126**, 595–602

Venning, E.M. and Browne, J.S.L. (1936). Isolation of water-soluble pregnanediol complex from human pregnancy urine. *Proc. Soc. Exp. Biol. Med.*, **34**, 792–3

Vollman, R.F. (1977). *The Menstrual Cycle, Major Problems in Obstetrics and Gynecology*, Vol. 7. (Philadelphia: W.B. Saunders)

von Baer, C.E. (1827). *De Ovi Mammalium et Hominis Genesi.* (Lipsiae, L. Vossius)

von Euler, U.S. (1934). Zur Kenntnis der pharmakologischem Wirkungen von nativesekreten und extrakten mannlicher accessorischer Geschlectsdrusen. *Arch. Exp. Pathol. Pharmakol.*, **175**, 78

West, E.S., Todd, W.R., Mason, N.S. and van Bruggen, J.T. (1970). *Textbook of Biochemistry*, p. 1471. (London: Collier-McMillan Ltd)

Westman, A. (1934). Untersuchungen uber die Abhangigkeit der Funktion des corpus luteum von den Ovarialfollikeln und uber die Bildungsstatte der Hormone im Ovarium. *Archiv. Gynaekol.*, **158**, 476

Westman, A.A. (1937). Investigations into the transit of ova in man. *J. Obstet. Gynaecol. Br. Emp.*, **44**, 821

WHO Task Force on Methods for the Determination of the Fertile Period (1980). Temporal relationships between ovulation and defined changes in the concentration of plasma estradiol-17β, luteinizing hormone, follicle stimulating hormone and progesterone. I. Probit analysis. *Am. J. Obstet. Gynecol.*, **138**, 383–90

Williams, (1876). Quoted in Cianfrani, T. (1960) p. 394

Winterton and MacGregor (1939). quoted by Noller, K.L. and Fish, C.R. (1974)

Wislocki, G.B. (1938). The vascular supply of the hypophysis cerebri of the rhesus monkey and man. *Proc. A. Res. Nerv. Ment. Dis.*, **17**, 48

Wislocki, G.B. and Bennett, H.S. (1943). The histology and cytology of the human and monkey placenta with special reference to the trophoblast. *Am. J. Anat.*, **73**, 335

Wynn, R.M. and Davies, J. (1965). Comparative electron microscopy of the hemochorial villous placenta. *Am. J. Obstet. Gynecol.*, **91**, 533

Wynn, R.M. and Harris, J.A. (1967). Ultrastructural cyclic changes in the human endometrium. I Normal preovulatory phase. *Fertil. Steril.*, **18**, 632

Yen, S.S.C. and Tsai, C.C. (1972). Pulsatile patterns of gonadotropin release in subjects with and without ovarian function. *J. Clin. Endocrinol. Metabol.*, **34**, 671–5

Yussman, M.A. and Taymor, M.L. (1970). Serum levels of follicle stimulating hormone and luteinizing hormone and of plasma progesterone related to ovulation by corpus luteum biopsy *J. Clin. Endocrinol.*, **30**, 396

Zondek, B. (1966). Foreword. In Greenblatt, R.B. (ed.) *Ovulation*, p. vii. (Philadelphia: J.B. Lippincott)

FURTHER READING

Armar, N.A., Adams, J. and Jacobs, H.S. (1987). Induction of ovulation with gonadotrophin releasing hormone. In Bonnar, J. (ed.) *Recent Advances in Obstetrics and Gynaecology*, Vol. 15, pp. 259–7. (Edinburgh, London: Churchill Livingstone)

Baird, D.T. (1983). Prediction of ovulation: biophysical, physiological and biochemical coordinates. In Jeffcoate, S.L. (ed.) *Ovulation: Methods for its Prediction and Detection.* (Chichester: John Wiley & Sons, Ltd.)

Brown, J.B. (1986). Gonadotropins. In Insler, V. and Lunenfeld, B. (eds.) *Infertility: Male and Female*, pp. 359–96. (New York: Churchill Livingstone)

Cousins, L., Karp, W., Lacey, C. and Lucas, W.E. (1980). Reproductive outcome of women exposed to diethylstilbestrol *in utero. Obstet. Gynecol.*, **56**, 70

Emmart, E. W., Spincer, S.S. and Bates, R.W. (1963). Localization of prolactin within the pituitary by specific fluorescent antiprolactin globulin. *J. Histochem. Cytochem.*, **11**, 365

Fevold, H.L. (1944). *The Chemistry and Physiology of Hormones*, p. 152. (Washington, D.C.: American Association for the Advancement of Science)

Fish, C.R. and Decker, D.G. (eds.) (1974). *The Medical Clinics of North America. Symposium on Medical Gynaecology*, Vol. 58, No. 4. (Philadelphia, London, Toronto: W.B. Saunders Co.)

Gruhn, J.G. and Kazer, R.K. (1989). *Hormonal Regulation of the Menstrual Cycle. The Evolution of Concepts.* (New York: Plenum Medical Book Company)

Harkness, R.D. (1962). The provision of special chemical stimulants and of measures for continuance of the species. In Davson, H. and Grace Eggleton, M. (eds.) *Starling and Lovatt Evans Principles of Human Physiology*, 13th edn., pp. 1387–516. (London: J. & A. Churchill Ltd)

Hellman. L.M. and Pritchard, J.A. (1971). *Williams Obstetrics*, 14th edn. (London: Butterworths)

Hull, M.G.R. (1989). Polycystic ovarian disease: clinical aspects and prevalence. In Cooke, I.D. and Lunenfeld, B. (eds.) *Research and Clinical Forums. Current Understanding of Polycystic Ovarian Disease*, Vol. 11, No. 4. (England: Royal Wells Medical Press)

Lee, J.B. (1981). The prostaglandins. In Williams, R.H. (ed.) *Textbook of Endocrinology*, 6th edn., pp. 1047–63. (Philadelphia, London, Toronto: W.B. Saunders Co.)

Lyons, A.S. and Petrucelli, R.J. (1978). *Medicine An Illustrated History*. (New York: Abradale Press H.N. Abrams, Inc., Publishers)

Medvei, V.C. (1982). *A History of Endocrinology.* (Lancaster: M.T.P. Press Ltd.)

Niswander, G.D. and Nett, T.M. (1988). The corpus luteum and its control. In Knobil, E. and Neil, J. *et al.* (eds.) *The Physiology of Reproduction*, pp. 489–525. (New York: Raven Press)

Nordenskiold, E. (1936). *The History of Biology.* (New York: Tudor)

Novak's Textbook of Gynecology (1981). Jones, H.W. Jr. and Jones, G.S. (eds.) 10th edn.; Novak, E.R., Jones, G.S. and Jones, H.W. Jr. (eds.) 9th edn. (Baltimore: Williams & Wilkins Co.)

Parkes, A.S. (1966). The rise of reproductive endocrinology, 1926–1940. *J. Endocrinol.*, **34**, xix–xxxii

Shaw, R.W. (1984). Hypothalamic reproductive failure. In Studd, J. (ed.) *Progress in Obstetrics and Gynaecology*, Vol. 4, pp. 279–89. (Edinburgh, London: Churchill Livingstone)

Shoham, Z., Homburg, R. and Jacobs, H.S. (1990). Induction of ovulation with pulsatile GnRH. In Crosignani, P.G. (ed.) *Induction of Ovulation. Clinical Obstetrics and Gynaecology*, pp. 589–608. (London, Philadelphia: Bailliere Tindall)

Smout, C.F.V., Jacoby, F. and Lillie, E.W. (1969). *Gynaecological and Obstetrical Anatomy*, 4th edn. (Aylesbury, England: H.K. Lewis & Co. Ltd)

Sommerville, I.F. (1964). Methods of hormone assay. In Thompson, R.H.S. and King, E.J. (eds.) *Biochemical Disorders in Human Disease*, 2nd edn. pp. 980–9. (London: J. & A. Churchill Ltd.)

Speert, H. (1973). *Iconographia Gyniatrica. A Pictorial History of Gynaecology and Obstetrics*, p. 190. (Philadelphia: F.A. Davis)

Speroff, L. (1990). *Seminars in Reproductive Endocrinology*, Vol. 8 No. 3. (New York)

Speroff, L., Glass, R.H. and Kase, N.G. (1982). *Clinical Gynecologic Endocrinology & Infertility*, 3rd edn. pp. 307–34. (Baltimore, London: Williams & Wilkins)

Swyer, G.I.M. (ed.) (1970). Control of human fertility. *Br. Med. Bull.*, **26**, no. 1

Tyson, J.E. (ed.) (1978). Neuroendocrinology of reproduction. *Clin. Obstet. Gynecol.*, 5, No. 2

Van Dyke, H.B. (1939). *The Physiology and Pharmacology of the Pituitary Body*, Vol. I, 1936; Vol. II, 1939. (Chicago: University of Chicago Press)

West, E.S., Todd, W.R., Mason, H.S. and Van Bruggen, J.T. (1970). *Textbook of Biochemistry*, 4th edn. (London: Collier-Macmillan Ltd.)

Winfield, A.C. and Wentz, A.C. (1987). *Diagnostic Imaging of Infertility*. (Baltimore, London, Los Angeles, Sydney: Williams and Wilkins)

The menstrual cycle

ANCIENT BELIEFS

The cyclic occurrence of menstruation was noted from earliest times and primitive peoples understood that it recurred at intervals which approximated the lunar month. Women were judged to be 'unclean' during menstruation. They were segregated from the rest of their tribe, and in some instances were subjected to special menstrual rituals. Menstrual blood was viewed as being magical, and as something to be feared, while at the same time its power was captured and used as an ingredient of some medications.

The ancient Hindus were aware that the menstrual flow originated in the uterus which if it was 'wounded' led to cessation of menses and to barrenness. The use of sanitary protection was probably first documented by the Babylonians (recorded in Sumerian as, *tug. nig. dara. ush. a*). They believed that the menstruating woman contaminated and destroyed everything she touched. In ancient Egypt, and among the Hebrews, ritual cleansing baths were mandatory at the end of menstruation. The women were sent to a cleansing bath or *mikveh* which was used to ritually purify a person who had become unclean through discharge from the body or through contact with the dead. The ancient Chinese referred to *Tsang*, which were religious contamination taboos. It was regulated that menstrual blood should not touch the ground for fear of offending the Earth spirit. Misfortune was often blamed on the contaminating female essence. In Arabic the words 'pure' or 'impure' originally referred to menstruation and the term 'taboo' or 'sacred' entered the English language from the Polynesian word *tabu*, or menstruation.

Menstrual regulation was practised by the ancient Egyptians who used douches of honey, sweet beer, garlic, wine, phenol and wonder fruit to regulate the flow. The menstrual cycle was studied by the ancient Greeks who were aware of cycle length and the number of days of menstrual loss.

They observed that the menstrual blood was thinner at the beginning and at the end of menstruation, and that once begun the blood flowed quickly. They measured the blood loss which was said to amount to 'two Attic Cotylae' – about one-sixth of a pint (Graham, 1950). Although menstrual blood was thought to be toxic, it was used to treat various disorders including hydrophobia. It was also an ingredient of abortifacients. The ancient Greeks and Romans venerated a number of deities who protected women throughout life and particularly during menstruation and pregnancy. Juno was the Goddess responsible for menstruation and she also guarded against the possibility of early abortion.

In the Bible, it is written in Leviticus 15:19 that 'when a woman has a discharge of blood which is her regular discharge from her body, she shall be in her impurity for seven days and who ever touches her shall be unclean until the evening... and if any man lie with her at all, and her flowers be upon him, he shall be unclean seven days; and all the bed where on he lieth shall be unclean'.

Pliny in his Natural History (AD first century) considered menstrual loss as 'a fatal poison corrupting and decomposing urine, depriving seeds of their fecundity, blasting garden flowers and grasses, causing fruits to fall from branches, dulling razors ... If the menstrual discharge coincides with an eclipse of the moon or sun, the evils resulting from it are irremediable... congress with a women at such a time being noxious and attended with fatal effects to man'. This notion of the impure nature of the menstrual discharge is reflected in writings from many cultures. Pliny continued, 'Contact with it (menstrual blood) turns new wine sour, crops touched by it become barren, grafts die, seeds in gardens are dried up, the fruit of trees fall off, the edge of steel and the gleam of ivory are dulled, hives of bees die, even bronze and iron are at once seized by rust and a horrible smell fills the air; to taste it drives dogs mad and infects their bites with an incurable poison ... Even that very tiny creature the ant is said to be sensitive to it, and throws away grains of corn that taste of it and does not touch them again ... Over and above there is no limit to woman's power. First of all, they say that hail storms and whirl winds are driven away if menstrual fluid is exposed to the very flashes of lightning; that stormy weather too is thus kept away. It makes a liniment for gout and by her touch a woman in this state relieves scrofula, parotid tumours, superficial abscesses, erysipelas, boils and eye fluxes'.

The male members of the medieval church were fearful of menstruation and it was declared sinful for a menstruating woman to enter a church. The medievial church also forbade sexual intercourse during menstruation as it was judged to be a heinous crime (Eskapa, 1987). In the twelfth century, St Hildegard, abbess of the Rupertsberg convent, wrote about the distinct difference in menstrual flow and quality in virgins compared to those who were 'deflowered'. The virgin was said to have a lighter flow of different colour. St Hildegard declared that menstruation was a punishment for the fall of Eve in the garden of Eden.

DEFINITIONS

Menstruum, was the earliest word used for menstruation and was the neuter form of the latin *menstruus* derived from *menses*, meaning month. The term entered the English language in the late fourteenth century. From the fifteenth to late nineteenth centuries, the term 'flowers' was used to denote the menstrual discharge, and was based on the French word *fleurs* which itself was derived from the Latin *fluor*, meaning flow. The term 'monthly period', (later known as 'period'), appeared in the 1820s and the word 'period' originated from the Greek word denoting going round, or cycle. The adjective 'menstrual', or pertaining to the menses, first entered English use in the fourteenth century. By the mid-eighteenth century the term 'catamenia' (derived from the Greek word for monthly) began to be used but was not as popular as 'menses', the pleural of the Latin *mensis*, which was commonly used from the late sixteenth century. The frequently used euphemism 'the curse' was derived from a nineteenth century expression 'the curse of Eve' which came from the belief that menstruation was the curse God laid upon woman for her sin in Eden. Alternatively the term may have derived from 'course' or 'courses', denoting a flow of liquid (Mills, 1991).

MODERN INVESTIGATIONS

Histology

The investigation of menstruation became possible after Recamier introduced the uterine curette. In his paper Recamier (1850) described the granulations, vegetations and hyperplastic endometrium obtained at curettage. The full significance of his findings, however, was not realized until much later.

The appearance of the endometrium at various stages of the cycle was documented by a number of workers in the late nineteenth century (see Chapter 18), but the definitive work was undertaken by Hitschmann and Adler (1908) of Vienna who first clearly illustrated the histological appearances of the endometrium during the normal menstrual cycle. The histology of the endometrium during the menstrual flow was investigated by Von Bohnen (1927). Endometrial shedding occurred over 3–5 days and most blood flow occurred during the first 3 days.

Haemostasis

Failure of the menstrual blood to clot had been recognized since antiquity, and Schickele (1912) demonstrated that menstrual fluid could be kept for several weeks without evidence of clotting. Much later on it became apparent that both the coagulation and fibrinolytic systems were activated during menstruation. Albrechtsen (1956) discovered that the endometrium had high fibrinolytic activity and Rybo (1966) demonstrated the presence of higher concentrations of endometrial plasminogen activator in patients with excess menstrual blood loss. Further evidence for impairment of clotting at menstruation came from the work of Christiaens *et al.* (1980) who documented reduction in haemostatic plugs during the first 20 hours of menstruation.

Prostaglandins were found to have a role in the haemostatic mechanisms of menstruation. These compounds were isolated by Goldblatt and Von Euler from human semen and the accessory genital glands in males in the early 1930s, and it was Von Euler (1935) who first used the term prostaglandin.

The prostaglandins (which were later found to be derived from arachidonic acid) lead to the production of thromboxane, a powerful vasoconstrictor and platelet proaggregator. Prostacyclin, another compound which is produced from the same precursors, is a potent vasodilator. A complex and delicate interplay maintains normal menstruation but menorrhagia occurs when the relationship between the various components is imbalanced. The regulation of menstruation was eventually determined to be under control of vascular, venostatic and lysomol activity, and also the process of regeneration which begins within 48 hours of the onset of menstrual bleeding (Ferenczy, 1976).

Markee (1940) investigated the role of the endometrial vasculature in menstruation. He observed pieces of transplanted endometrium placed in the anterior chamber of the eye of rhesus monkeys. These implants became vascularized and responded to the hormonal stimulation of the menstrual cycle. He demonstrated stasis, with or without vasodilatation, for 1–5 days before menstrual bleeding. This phase came to an end when vasoconstriction of the spiral arteries occurred 4–24 hours before the onset of menstual blood loss. Although Markee carried out the definitive study on the endometrial vasculature, the presence of spiral arteries had been previously noted by Hunter (1774) and again in the nineteenth century by Leopold (1877). In this century Daron (1936) and others investigated the uterine microvasculature using dye injection techniques.

Calendar records

Arey (1939) analysed 20 000 calendar records from 1500 women and girls and concluded that the menstrual cycle was not perfectly regular. In a study of over 5000 cycles in 485 'normal white women' Arey discovered an average interval of 28.4 days.

Blood loss

The 'normal' blood loss during menstruation was estimated to range from 25 to 60 ml (Barker and Fowler, 1936; Hallberg and Nilsson, 1964; Hallberg et al., 1966). Women could expect to lose 150–400 mg of iron per year due to menstruation. Many methods were used to measure menstrual blood loss but the most popular technique involved the determination of the haemoglobin concentration in menstrual fluid by its conversion to alkaline haematin (Hallberg and Nilsson, 1964). A further technique was introduced by Newton et al. (1977) who used sodium hydroxide in a 15-minute procedure to estimate blood loss in sanitary wear. However, Hallberg's population study of 476 women in Gothenberg and the Cole et al. (1971) study of 348 women in Northumberland formed the basis for our knowledge of the characteristics of menstrual blood loss.

Sanitary protection

Although first documented in ancient Babylonia, sanitary wear of modern design was first marketed in this century. Giscard d'Estaing (1990) told the story thus, – 'Ernest Mahler who was a German chemist working in the United States invented a cotton substitute made from wood pulp, for use as dressings in hospitals. Nursing staff began using the cellulose padded dressings as hygienic menstrual towels ... the Kimberley–Clark Co. learned of this and began marketing them ... under the name Kotex Sanitary Towels in 1921'. Vaginal tampons were designed by an American, Earl Hass ... 'in 1937 he applied for a patent, and founded the Tampax Company ... the use of the tampons spread throughout the world after the Second World War'.

CHRONOLOGY

Antiquity

The Babylonians documented the use of sanitary protection.

The Hindus were aware that menstruation originated in the uterus.

In ancient Egypt and among the Hebrews ritual cleansing baths were mandatory.

The Greeks measured actual blood loss.

Biblical references indicate that menstruating women were 'unclean'.

Pliny (AD 1st C.) wrote on the power of the menstrual discharge.

12th C. St Hildegard subscribed to the popular belief that menstruation was punishment for the fall of Eve in the Garden of Eden.

Alternative terms

menstruum flowers monthly period period
catamenia menses the curse courses

References: Mills (1991); McKay (1901); Graham (1950)

Modern investigations

1850   Recamier introduced the uterine curette.

1908   Hitschmann and Adler defined the histology of the normal menstrual cycle.

1912   Schickele demonstrated failure of menstrual fluid to clot.

1927   Von Bohnen described the histology of endometrium during menstruation.

1935   Von Euler introduced the term prostaglandin.

1936   Barker and Fowler quantified menstrual loss.

1939   Arey analysed the menstrual cycle and discovered an average interval of 28.4 days.

1940   Markee determined the role of endometrial vasculature.

1964   Hallberg and Nilsson determined haemoglobin content, and other parameters of menstrual loss.

1966   Hallberg *et al.* further investigated menstrual loss.

Sanitary protection

1921   The Kimberley-Clark Co. marketed the first commercial sanitary towels based on an invention by Ernst Mahler.

1937   Earl Hass introduced vaginal tampons and founded the Tampax Co.

References: Giscard d'Estaing (1990)

REFERENCES

Albrechtsen, O.K. (1956). The fibrinolytic activity of the human endometrium. *Acta Endocrinol.*, **23**, 219–29

Arey, L.B. (1939). The degree of normal menstrual irregularity. An analysis of 20,000 calendar records from 1,500 individuals. *Am. J. Obstet. Gynecol.*, **37**, 12

Barker, A.P. and Fowler, W.M. (1936). The blood loss during normal menstruation. *Am.J. Obstet. Gynecol.*, **31**, 979

Bohnen, P. von (1927). Wie weit wird das Endometrium bei der Menstruation abgestossen? *Archiv. Gynaekol.*, **129**, 459–72

Christiaens, G.C.M.L., Sixma, J.J. and Haspels, A.A. (1980). Morphology of haemostasis in menstrual endometrium. *Br.J. Obstet. Gynaecol.*, **87**, 425–39

Cole, S.K., Billewicz, W.Z. and Thomson, A.M. (1971). Sources of variation in menstrual blood loss. *J. Obstet. Gynaecol. Br. Commonw,* **78**, 933–9

Daron, G.H. (1936). The arterial pattern of the tunica mucosa of the uterus in macacus rhesus. *Am. J. Anat.*, **58**, 349–85

Eskapa, R. (1987). *Bizarre Sex,* pp. 85–8. (London: Grafton Books)

Ferenczy, A. (1976). Studies on the cytodynamics of human endometrial regeneration. Scanning electron microscopy. *Am. J. Obstet. Gynecol.*, **124**, 64–74

Giscard d'Estaing, V.A. (ed.) (1900). *The Book of Inventions and Discoveries*, p.102. (London: Queen Anne Press Division of MacDonald & Co.)

Graham, H. (1950). *Eternal Eve*, p.42. (London: W. Heinemann)

Hallberg, L. and Nilsson, L. (1964). Determination of menstrual blood loss. *Scand. J. Clin. Labor. Invest.*,**16**, 244–8

Hallberg, L., Hogdahl, A.M., Nilsson, L. and Rybo, G. (1966). Menstrual blood loss – a population study. *Acta Obstet. Gynecol. Scand.*, **45**, 320–51

Hitschmann, F. and Adler, L. (1908). Der Bau der Uterusschleimhaut des geschlechtsreifen Weibes, mit besonderer Berucksichtigung der Menstruation. *Mschr. Geb. Gynaekol.*, **27**, 1–82

Hunter, W. (1774). *Anatomia uteri humani gravidi tabulis illustrata.* (Birmingham; Baskerville)

Leopold, G. (1877). Studien uber die uterusschleimhaut während menstruation, schwangershaft und wochenbett. *Archiv. Gynaekol.*, **11**, 110–30

McKay, W.J.S. (1901). *History of Ancient Gynaecology.* (London: Balliere Tindall Cox)

Markee, J.E. (1940). Menstruation in intraocular endometrial transplants in the rhesus monkey. *Contrib. Embryol.*, **28**, 219

Mills, J. (1991). *Woman Words*, pp. 155–8. (London: Virago Press)

Newton, J., Barnard, G. and Collins, W. (1977). A rapid method for measuring menstrual blood loss using automatic extraction. *Contraception*, **16**, 269

Pliny (The Elder) (1939). *Natural History,* translated by Rackham, H. (Cambridge, Mass.: Harvard University Press)

Recamier, M. (1850). Memoire sur les productions fibreuses et fongueuses intra-uterines. *Union Med. Paris*, **4**, 266

Rybo, G. (1966). Plasminogen activators in the endometrium *Acta Obstet. Gynaecol. Scand.*, **45**, 429–59

Schickele, G. (1912). *Biochem. Z.*, **38**, 169–72

von Euler, V.S. (1935). Uber die spezifische blut drucksende substanz des menslichen prostata und samenblasen secretes. *Klin. W.*, **14**, 1182–7

Menorrhagia

MENORRHAGIA

The term menorrhagia is derived from the Greek: *men*, month: *rhegyai*, to burst forth. In the absence of tumour, inflammation, pregnancy or any other organic disease of the genital tract, abnormal menstrual blood loss is termed dysfunctional uterine bleeding.

ANTIQUITY

One of the earliest references to heavy menstruation is found in the ancient Hindu works on obstetrics and gynaecology. The early Hindu sacred books (the four vedas of Brahma) date from about 1400 BC. A later group of works include the Ayurveda, which contains the oldest Hindu medical and surgical writings. In the first century AD Charaka, a court physician at Peshawar, compiled the *Charaka Ayurveda* of 120 chapters. Another work of importance was that of Sushruta, a disciple of Charaka who is credited with the authorship of *Sushruta Samhita*. It is the works of Charaka and Sushruta which contain references to obstetrics and gynaecology (Graham, 1950). Twenty-four diseases of the female reproductive system are described. Included among them is *prodokoh*, the term used for excessive menstrual blood loss. The condition is said to be accompanied by fever, giddiness, fainting and thirst. Various treatments are advocated, including the application of cold and astringent medicines, the avoidance of venery, and the intake of a diet of cool simple food (McKay, 1901).

The problem of excessive menstrual blood loss was also addressed by the ancient Greeks and Romans. In his Aphorisms, Hippocrates of Cos (c. 460–377 BC) wrote that treatment consisted of cupping, applied to the breasts. Pliny suggested a variety of treatments which included the application of beaver oil and onyx, calves gall, or dried snake. Soranus of Ephesus (AD 98–138), whose teachings had a profound effect on midwifery and gynaecology until the Renaissance, alluded to menorrhagia. He theorized that the debilitated uterus gave rise to menstrual periods which were very profuse, painful, and irregular, with blood flow occurring three to four times per month. In his dissertation he noted that treatment was not necessary in all cases, but where required should be directed to the cause of the condition. Soranus advised that ligatures should be applied to the armpits and groins in an attempt to reduce blood flow to the body and thus to the uterus. He also advocated the intravaginal application of burnt cork and liquid pitch. Pessaries impregnated with the yolks of roasted eggs, or which were made from alum or manna were also applied. These remedies appear to have been copied from the works of Oribasius who also used tight limb bandaging, and the application of sponges soaked in various medications which were inserted both vaginally and rectally.

Paulus of Aegina (AD 625) was a learned physician, surgeon and obstetrician who compiled medical material from the works of Galen, Aetius and others. Towards the end of his third book he concerned himself with normal and abnormal menstruation. He listed a series of emmenagogues and wrote on the problem of menorrhagia. Years later, Avicenna (AD 980–1037) treated excess menstruation in the same way as Oribasius and Soranus, although he added opium to some of his prescriptions.

During the Victorian era, the treatments for menorrhagia included oophorectomy, or the irrigation of the uterine cavity with carbolic acid, silver nitrate, or nitric acid (Atthill, 1883).

EARLY STUDIES

With the development of gynaecology, the introduction of anaesthetics, and the use of the uterine curette from the mid-nineteenth century, the menstrual cycle became the subject of scientific study. Abnormalities of the endometrium were described by Recamier (1850) and by Olshausen (1875), by West and Duncan (1879) and also by

Cullen (1900;1908) all of whom highlighted the histological characteristics of endometrial hyperplasia. Schroder (1914) confirmed that the condition was associated with disturbed ovarian function (see section on Endometrial Hyperplasia, in the chapter on Endometrial Cancer). However, it was not until the 1940s that abnormal menstrual function was investigated in a systematic fashion.

Four separate conditions were discovered which were thought to be related to dysfunctional uterine bleeding. The first of these, *the anovulatory bleeding cycle*, was described in the rhesus monkey by Heape (1897). In this condition heavy bleeding occurred despite anovulation. The first instance of this condition in the human was described by Emil Novak (1927; 1933). A second abnormality (later) termed *luteal phase defect*, in which the development of the secretory phase was impaired, was described by Jones (1949) and a number of other investigators. A third condition termed *irregular shedding of the endometrium*, in which the corpus luteum regressed asynchronously was first recognized in this century by Driessen (1914). The final disorder, that of *endometrial hyperplasia* was thought to occur much more commonly. Although originally described by Recamier (1850) it was mainly in this century that the condition was thoroughly investigated. Cullen (1900) of the United States, in his book on *Cancer of the Uterus*, described a hyperplastic appearance of the endometrium accompanied by uterine bleeding.

However, Robert Schroder is usually credited with the definitive early work on endometrial hyperplasia as a clinical entity. It was mainly Schroder (1914; 1915) who determined its cause and he opined that it was due to persistent follicular action. The hyperplastic state was found to occur in the surface glandular epithelium and could assume a variety of forms. In some areas of the endometrium large glands of irregular shape were found close to glands which were scarcely larger than normal. The histological appearance prompted Novak and Martzloff (1924) to apply the term 'Swiss cheese pattern' to the condition which was later called cystic glandular hyperplasia of the endometrium.

DEFINITIONS AND INVESTIGATIONS

Hallberg *et al.* (1966) in their population study, defined menorrhagia as menstrual blood loss of more than 80 ml per menstruation from a normal secretory endometrium after a normal ovulation. These investigators demonstrated that 39% of women with menstrual blood loss in the range 61–80 ml were anaemic (haemoglobin less than 12 g/dl) compared to 67% if blood loss exceeded 80 ml. Losses in excess of 80 ml were found in 11% of women. Shaw *et al.* (1972) favoured 60 ml as the upper normal limit of menstrual blood loss, and determined that blood loss of that amount had already caused iron deficiency, as reflected in low serum ferritin levels.

Hahn *et al.* (1976) and Rees *et al.* (1985) compared plasma with menstrual fluid clotting factors and found no difference between normal menstruating and menorrhagic women. However, it was thought that locally enhanced fibrinolysis was partially responsible for essential menorrhagia and the beneficial effects of antifibrinolytics supported that hypothesis (Nilsson and Rybo, 1971).

Although the prevalence of menorrhagia is estimated at just over 10%, women were found to be unreliable judges of their menstrual blood loss. Chimbira *et al.* (1980) demonstrated that 34% of patients with blood loss between 80 and 250 ml described their periods as 'light' while 47% of women who lost less than 80 ml thought their periods were 'heavy'. Tampon and sanitary pad usage was found to reflect individual hygiene rather than actual blood loss.

AETIOLOGY

Known causes of menorrhagia include fibroids, endometriosis, malignancies, haemangiomata or following trauma at delivery. Hypothyroidism was implicated by Gardiner-Hill and Forest-Smith (1927) who found that of 23 patients with myxoedema, 78% had menorrhagia (Figures 1 and 2). Worry, fright, fatigue, nervous shock, sexual excesses and perversions were all thought to be causes of uterine haemorrhage (Frank, 1945).

It was known that waitresses in the Swiss Alps had to return to lower levels on account of menorrhagia. Intrauterine contraceptives were noted to increase menstrual blood loss as were some bleeding disorders, haemodialysis and congenital uterine abnormalities. Sterilization was often assumed to be a cause of excess blood loss, although Kasonde and Bonnar (1976) found no significant difference before and after tubal ligation. However, their study referred to one specific type of sterilization only.

In a recent review article, Long and Gast (1990) advocated 'when evaluating the menorrhagic patient, it is important to gear the work up towards the differential diagnosis that includes pregnancy related causes, hormonal problems, iatrogenic aetiologies, mechanical intrauterine disorders, infections of the lower genital tract and gynaecologic cancers (PHIMIC)'.

TREATMENT

Although spontaneous remission of symptoms could occur for up to 10 years from the onset of dysfunctional bleeding (Southam and Richart, 1966) many women who complained of menorrhagia elected to use medical or surgical therapy. Approximately 4% of women in the UK sought medical advice for menstrual disturbances (Charnock,1981) of which the majority were dysfunctional in nature. Despite the fact that women could be unreliable judges of their menstual blood loss, their personal assessment of excessive loss was accepted as fact by most medical personnel, and investigation and/or treatment was instituted.

Medical treatment

Ergometrine

This uterine contracting agent was widely used but did not reduce menstrual blood loss in menorrhagia (Nilsson and Rybo, 1971).

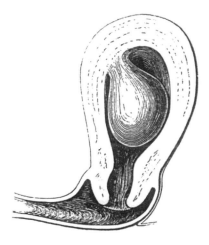

Figure 1 A fibroid polyp causing menorrhagia. The diagnosis was made after dilating the cervix with a sponge tent so that a finger could be inserted. The polyp was removed by passing the chain of an 'ecraseur' around the pedicle. From J. Marion Sims' *Uterine Surgery*, (1866)

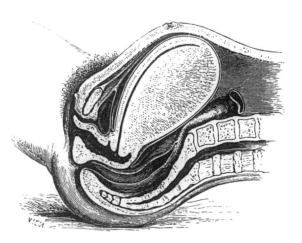

Figure 2 A very large posterior wall uterine fibroid causing menorrhagia while compressing the bladder and the rectum. Also from J. Marion Sims' *Uterine Surgery* (1866)

Antiprostaglandin agents

These were used to treat excess menstrual blood loss from the mid-1970s. Anderson *et al.* (1976) administered mefenamic acid to five women and flufenamic acid to one woman with excessive losses and documented reduced loss from c.119 ml to c.60 ml. The advantage of antiprostaglandins was the need for their administration only during the menstrual flow. Petrusson *et al.* (1977) administered acetylsalicylic acid or paracetamol, but without good effect. In a further study Rybo *et al.* (1981) demonstrated that naproxen reduced excess menstrual blood loss. A study on mefenamic acid therapy was carried out by Fraser *et al.* (1981), who found that 78% of the treated women had reduced loss, with a mean reduction of 28% being observed.

Danazol

Chimbira *et al.* (1979; 1980) studied the effects of danazol on coagulation mechanisms and haematological indices in menorrhagia, and demonstrated a reduced menstrual blood loss of almost 20%, with reduction in menstrual length from 7 to 5 days. Daily medication throughout the cycle proved to be the main disadvantage of this treatment. A further problem was that danazol could only be administered for 6 months due to its metabolic side-effects.

Hormones

Albright (1938) described the action of

progesterone therapy and the 'medical curettage' caused by its withdrawal. Karnaky (1939) devised a method to arrest menstrual flooding by the administration of 10–25 mg of stilboestrol by mouth every 15 minutes until the bleeding stopped, which usually happened within 4–6 hours. Cyclical oestrogen and progesterone therapy was advocated by Hamblen *et al.* (1941).

Scowen (1944) advocated the administration of progesterone until it appeared in the urine, while Hamblen and Davis (1945) advised the use of equine gonadotropin (follicle stimulating hormone). A combination of testosterone propionate and progesterone by injection was advocated by Greenblatt and Kupperman (1946), who claimed that this controlled bleeding on the 1st or 2nd day of treatment. Foss (1960) reported the beneficial effects of progestogens in various dosage regimens. The hormone appeared useful in arresting vaginal haemorrhage but the case for its use was not proven by objective studies. However, Progestasert, a progesterone releasing intrauterine device, was found to be effective in the treatment of intrauterine device-induced menorrhagia (Newton *et al.*, 1976).

The combined oral contraceptive pill was found to be as effective as the antifibrinolytic Cyklokapron (Nilsson and Rybo, 1971). Disadvantages of the combined oral contraceptive pill were that 20% of patients did not respond; daily medication for 3 weeks was necessary; and due to risk factors, many women were unsuitable for long-term treatment. However, menstrual loss was reduced by up to 50% in women who used the oral contraceptive. It was demonstrated that high-dose oestrogen therapy, administered by the intravenous route as 25 mg of conjugated oestrogen 4-hourly, was an effective management for acute excess menstrual blood loss. Bleeding subsided within 12 hours (Devore *et al.*, 1982).

Fibrinolytic inhibitors

Antifibrinolytic agents were found to exert their action by reduction of the enhanced fibrinolytic activity found in association with excessive menstrual blood loss. Nilsson and Rybo (1971) reported their treatment of menorrhagia with tranexamic acid and in a further paper compared the effect of ε-aminocaproic acid in 172 women with tranexamic acid in 85 patients. Women with proven excess blood loss in the two groups showed an average reduction of 47 and 54%, respectively in their menstrual loss. These studies confirmed the

earlier work of Vermylen *et al.* (1968) and Callender *et al.* (1970) who had demonstrated an overall reduction in menstrual blood loss of 35–38%.

Westrom and Bengtsson (1970) investigated the use of Cyklokapron in intrauterine device-induced menorrhagia and found a reduction of almost 12% in menstrual blood loss. Kasonde and Bonnar (1975) compared aminocaproic acid and ethamsylate in a randomized, double-blind, cross-over study. They demonstrated that blood loss was reduced by 50% in women using antifibrinolytic treatment, but ethamsylate was of no value. However, Harrison and Campbell (1976) reported to the *Lancet* their double-blind study of ethamsylate in the treatment of primary and intrauterine device-induced menorrhagia and they determined that the drug (which probably acts by reducing capillary fragility) reduced menstrual blood loss somewhat. A notable advantage of antifibrinolytic agents was that they were administered only during the days of heavy blood loss.

Luteinizing hormone releasing agonists

Shaw and Fraser (1984) reported dramatically reduced excess menstrual blood loss when intranasal luteinizing hormone releasing hormone agonists, such as buserelin were administered. They suggested that such treatment would be of value in the older woman. Their study was carried out in four women and the agonist was used daily for 3 months. Although side-effects were not reported, long-term treatment could cause significant distress.

Surgical treatment

Dilatation and curettage

The procedure was found to have both diagnostic and therapeutic potential. It was generally agreed that during episodes of excess menstrual blood loss uterine curettage had a useful therapeutic effect and Israel (1967) stated that 'it is not only the best therapeutic measure to arrest bleeding but it is also the most informative diagnostically'. However, objective measurements indicated reduced blood loss in only the first cycle following curettage (Nilsson and Rybo, 1971; Haynes *et al.*, 1977). The usual indication for the procedure was to exclude the presence of polyps or malignancy. Polyps were found to occur in about 2% of women (Mackenzie and Bibby, 1978) while endometrial carcinoma was found in 0.7–6.5% of cases (Carey 1968; Mackenzie and Bibby, 1978).

The predicted frequency of endometrial carcinoma in women under the age of 36 was one case per 100 000 per year. Grimes (1982) reported a 20-year experience with Vabra aspiration techniques in which the complication rate was lower, and the detection rate for abnormalities higher, when compared with dilatation and curettage. Although the diagnosis of endometrial pathology was infrequent, patients were reassured by the absence of histological abnormality. Uterine curettage was not without risk however, and Grimes (1982) highlighted occurrences of haemorrhage, sepsis, uterine perforation and resort to laparotomy for unexpected uterine damage.

Endometrial ablation

Writing in the *American Journal of Obstetrics and Gynecology*, Michael Baggish and Pavlos Baltoyannis (1988) of Siracuse, New York, commented that 'since the 1800s attempts have been made to control uterine bleeding by means other than hysterectomy. Alternative methods have included chemicals, ionizing radiation, electrocautery, and cryosurgery. Other treatments included the use of superheated steam, quinacrine or urea injection, and radium packing. The long-term risks of these techniques vary from squamous metaplasia of the endometrium to primary squamous cell carcinoma or mixed mesodermal tumors'.

The technique of endometrial ablation is based on those previous attempts to control menorrhagia and also on the observations by Asherman (1948; 1950) who described amenorrhoea traumatica, a condition which developed as a result of uterine curettage following pregnancy. In his second report he noted partial or complete obliteration of the uterine cavity due to traumatic adhesions. Carmichael (1970) again noted the aetiological factors of endometritis, and of endometrial curettage within 4 weeks of miscarriage or term delivery.

Endometrial ablation was offered as an alternative to hysterectomy in some cases. The technique aimed to ablate permanently all layers of the endometrium, and allow the uterine cavity to become lined with fibrous tissue. Cahan and Brockunier (1967) reported an early experience of cryosurgery to the uterine cavity. Droegemueller *et al.* (1970;1971) also experimented with the technique. Although cryocautery held early

promise, it was an unreliable method of menstrual suppression.

Endometrial electrocautery with resection via a resectoscope was first reported by Neuwirth (1978) who later reviewed the subject (Neuwirth 1983). In the same year DeCherney and Polan (1983) described emergency endometrial electrocoagulation in 11 women. The electrocautery technique was introduced in France by Hamou (1985) and in the UK by Magos *et al.* (1989). The term TransCervical Resection of the Endometrium (TCRE) was coined by an Oxford urologist called Smith (Magos, 1991).

Laser ablation of the endometrium was pioneered by Goldrath *et al.* (1981) who reported the use of hysteroscopic Nd:YAG (neodynium: yttrium-aluminium-garnet) laser photovaporization in a series of 22 cases. This was followed by complete amenorrhoea or light menstruation in 21 of the cases. A further treatment modality was that of radiofrequency-induced thermal endometrial ablation which was introduced by Phipps *et al.* (1990). The radiofrequency-electromagnetic energy was delivered via a probe placed within the uterine cavity. Distension/flushing media were not necessary thus avoiding the fluid overload problems of hysteroscopic techniques.

Hysterectomy

Corscaden *et al.* (1946) indicated that they preferred total hysterectomy to the use of X-rays or radium which were commonly used to treat excess menstrual blood loss. The results of studies on women who were treated by radiation-induced menopause (for benign uterine haemorrhage), showed that they developed endometrial and cervical cancer at a much higher rate than the general population (Corscaden *et al.*, 1946; Browne, 1950; Turnbull, 1956).

Hysterectomy was regarded as the definitive treatment for menorrhagia, and approximately one-third of such operations were performed for menstrual disorders (DHSS, 1985). When assessed at histological examination however, only half of the removed uteri were found to contain a pathological condition (Grant and Hussein, 1984). Studd (1989) noted in a review article that 'the recent literature concerning menorrhagia deals solely with the aetiology and medical treatment. There is hardly a paper to be found in *Index Medicus* over the last 20 years which addresses the issue of hysterectomy for menorrhagia'.

Dicker *et al.* (1982a,b) estimated that there were almost half a million (non-radical) hysterectomies per year carried out in the USA in the 1970s, with an operative morbidity for abdominal hysterectomy as high as 42.8%. Wingo *et al.* (1985) found that there was a low mortality rate for hysterectomy of 6 per 10 000 for benign indications.

Some of the side-effects of hysterectomy included an increased possibility of cardiovascular disease (Centerwall, 1981), premature ovarian failure (Siddle *et al.*, 1987) and intestinal or urinary dysfunction (Taylor *et al.*, 1989). Earlier descriptions of psychosexual problems and a post-hysterectomy syndrome were not borne out by prospective studies (Iles and Gath, 1989). The considerable national and international variations in the incidence of hysterectomy for benign conditions (Coulter *et al.*, 1988) will be further affected by endometrial ablative therapy.

CHRONOLOGY

Antiquity

The ancient Hindus referred to *'prodokoh'*, their term for excessive menstrual blood loss.

c. 400 BC	Hippocrates advocated cupping.
1st C. AD	Pliny offered treatment.
2nd C. AD	Soranus of Ephesus advised limb ligatures and impregnated pessaries.
c. AD 600	Paulus of Aegina offered treatment.
c. AD 1000	Avicenna copied the treatments of Oribasius and Soranus.

References for above: McKay (1901); Graham (1950)

Early studies

1800	Uterine irrigation with various acids was advocated (Athill, 1883).
1850	Recamier documented abnormalities of the endometrium. A similar condition was also described by Olshausen, West and Duncan, and Cullen at later dates.
1897	Heape described the anovulatory bleeding cycle.
1914	Driessen described irregular shedding of the endometrium.
1914/15	Schroder determined that endometrial hyperplasia was a distinct clinical entity.

1924	Novak and Martzloff introduced the term 'Swiss cheese pattern'.
1949	Jones and other investigators described luteal phase defects.

Definition

1966	Hallberg *et al.* defined menorrhagia as menstrual blood loss of more than 80 ml per menstruation.

Aetiology

1927	Gardiner-Hill and Forest-Smith implicated thyroid disorders.
1945	Frank associated 'nervous' causes.

Various reproductive pathology was implicated. Tubal ligation and intrauterine contraceptive devices were also involved.

Treatment

Medical

1938	Albright described progesterone therapy. Soon after various combinations of oestrogen, progesterone and testosterone were used.
1968	Vermylen *et al.* studied the use of fibrinolytic inhibitors.
1976	Anderson *et al.* used antiprostaglandin agents.
1979	Chimbira *et al.* introduced danazol treatment.
1984	Shaw and Fraser administered luteinizing hormone releasing hormone agonists.

Surgical

1940	Investigation of menorrhagia by curettage sometimes improved the condition.
1946	Corscaden *et al.* and others popularized hysterectomy.
1967	Israel stated that curettage was the best therapeutic measure to arrest excess menstrual blood loss. Cahan and Brockunier applied cryosurgery to the endometrium.
1971	Nilsson and Rybo showed that excess blood loss was reduced for the first cycle following curettage.

1981   Goldrath *et al.* pioneered the use of laser ablation.

1983   Amin and Neuwirth introduced endometrial electrocautery.

1990   Phipps *et al.* commenced treatment with radiofrequency induced thermal endometrial ablation.

REFERENCES

Albright, F. (1938). *Maine Med. J.*, **29**, 235, quoted by Bishop (1950) pp. 586–607

Amin, H.K. and Neuwirth, R.S. (1983). Operative hysteroscopy utilizing dextran as distending medium. *Clin. Obstet. Gynecol.*, **26**, 277–84

Anderson, A.B.M., Haynes, P.J., Guillebaud, J. and Turnbull, A.C. (1976). Reduction of menstrual blood loss by prostaglandin synthetase inhibition. *Lancet*, **1**, 774–6

Asherman, J.G. (1948). Amenorrhoea traumatica atretica. *J. Obstet. Gynaecol. Br. Emp.*, **55**, 23–30

Asherman, J.G. (1950). Traumatic intra-uterine adhesions. *J. Obstet. Gynaecol. Br. Emp.*, **57**, 892–6

Atthill, L. (1883). *Clinical Lectures on Diseases Peculiar to Women.* (London: Longman)

Baggish, M.S. and Baltoyannis, P. (1988). New techniques for laser ablation of the endometrium in high risk patients. *Am. J. Obstet. Gynecol.*, **159**, 287–92

Bishop, P.M.F. (1950). Endocrine therapy. In Bowes, K. (ed.) *Modern Trends in Obstetrics and Gynaecology*, Vol. 40, pp. 586–607. (London: Butterworth and Co.)

Browne, F.J. (1950). *Postgraduate Obstetrics and Gynaecology*, pp. 254–62. (London: Butterworth & Co.)

Cahan, W.G. and Brockunier, A. Jr. (1967). Cryosurgery of the uterine cavity. *Am. J. Obstet. Gynecol.*, **99**, 138–53

Callender, S.T., Warner, G.T. and Cope, E. (1970). Treatment of menorrhagia with tranexamic acid. A double-blind trial. *Br. Med. J.*, **4**, 214–16

Carey, E. (1968). In Barter, R.H., Brennan, G., Newman, W. and Merill, K.W. (eds.) The place of curettage in the diagnosis of carcinoma of the endometrium. *Am. J. Obstet. Gynecol.*, **100**, 696–702

Carmichael, D.E. (1970). Asherman's syndrome. *Obstet. Gynecol.*, **36**, 922–8

Centerwall, B.S. (1981). Premenopausal hysterectomy and cardiovascular disease. *Am. J. Obstet. Gynecol.*, **139**, 58–61

Charnock, M. (1981). Major common problems. Dysfunctional uterine bleeding. *Br. J. Hosp. Med.*, Oct., 395–8

Chimbira, T.H., Cope, E., Anderson, A.B.M. and Bolton, F.G. (1979). The effect of danazol on menorrhagia, coagulation mechanisms, haematological indices and body weight. *Br. J. Obstet. Gynaecol.*, **86**, 46–50

Chimbira, T.H., Anderson, A.B.M. and Turnbull, A.C. (1980). Relation between measured menstrual loss and the patient's subjective assessment of loss, duration of bleeding, number of sanitary towels used, uterine weight and endometrial surface area. *Br. J. Obstet. Gynaecol.*, **87**, 603–8

Corscaden, J.A., Hertig, J.W. and Gusberg, S.B. (1946). *Am. J. Obstet. Gynecol.*, **51**, 1, quoted by Browne (1950) p. 262

Coulter, A., McPherson, K. and Vessey, M. (1988). Do British women undergo too many or too few hysterectomies? *Soc. Sci. Med.*, **27**, 987–94

Cullen, T.S. (1900). *Cancer of the Uterus.* (London: Kimpton)

Cullen, T.S. (1908). *Adenomyoma of Uterus.* (Philadelphia: Saunders)

DeCherney, A. and Polan, M.L. (1983). Hysteroscopic management of intrauterine lesions and intractable uterine bleeding. *Obstet. Gynecol.*, **61**, 392–7

Devore, G.R., Owens, O. and Kase, N. (1982). Use of intravenous Premarin in the treatment of dysfunctional uterine bleeding: a double-blind randomized control study. *Obstet. Gynecol.*, **59**, 285

Dewhurst, C.J. (1972). *Integrated Obstetrics and Gynaecology for Postgraduates*, Chap. 35, pp. 511–38. (Oxford, London, Edinburgh, Melbourne: Blackwell Scientific Publications)

DHSS (1985). Department of Health and Social Security and Office of Population Censuses and Surveys. Hospital in-patient enquiry 1985. table p.1. (London: HMSO)

Dicker, R.C., Scally, J.J., Greenspan, J.R., Layde, P.M., Ory, H.W., Maze, J.M. and Smith, J.C. (1982a). Hysterectomy among women of reproductive age. Trends in the United States. *J. Am. Med. Assoc.*, **248**, 323–7

Dicker, R.C., Greenspan, J.R., Strauss, L.T., Cowart, M.R., Scally, J.J., Peterson, H.B., DeStafano, F., Rubin, G.L. and Ory, H.W. (1982b). Complications of abdominal and vaginal hysterectomy among women of reproductive age in the United States. *Am. J. Obstet. Gynecol.*, **144**, 841–8

Driessen, L.F. (1914). Endometritis, Folge abnormaler Menstruation, Ursache profuser Blutungen. *Zentralbl. Gynaekol.*, **38**, 618–22

Droegemueller, W., Greer, B. and Makowski, E. (1970). Preliminary observations of cryocoagulation of the endometrium. *Am. J. Obstet. Gynecol.*, **107**, 958–61

Droegemueller, W., Greer, B. and Makowski, E. (1971). Cryosurgery in patients with dysfunctional uterine bleeding. *Obstet. Gynecol.*, **38**, 256–8

Foss, G.L. (1960). Clinical experience with norethisterone and norethisterone acetate. *Br. Med. J.*, **2**, 1187–91

Frank, I.L. (1945). *Am. J. Med. Sci.*, **210**, 787, quoted by Browne (1950) p. 262

Fraser, I.S., Pearse, L., Shearman, R.P., Elliot, P.M., McIlveen, J. and Markham, R. (1981). Efficacy of mefenamic acid in patients with a complaint of menorrhagia. *Obstet. Gynecol.*, **58**, 543–51

Gardiner-Hill, H. and Forest-Smith, J. (1927). *J. Obstet. Gynaecol. Br. Emp.*, **34**, 701, quoted by Browne (1950) p. 262

Goldrath, M.H., Fuller, T.A. and Segal, S. (1981). Laser photovaporization of endometrium for the treatment of menorrhagia. *Am. J. Obstet. Gynecol.*, **140**, 14–19

Graham, H. (1950). *Eternal Eve*, p. 42. (London: W. Heinemann)

Grant, J.M. and Hussein, I.Y. (1984). An audit of abdominal hysterectomy over a decade in a district hospital. *Br. J. Obstet. Gynaecol.*, **91**, 73–7

Greenblatt, R.B. and Kupperman, H.S. (1946). *J. Clin. Endocrinol.*, **6**, 675, quoted by Bishop (1950) pp. 586–607

Grimes, D.A. (1982). Diagnostic dilation and curettage: a re-appraisal. *Am. J. Obstet. Gynecol.*, **142**, 1–6

Hahn, L., Cederblad, G., Rybo, G. *et al.* (1976). Blood coagulation, fibrinolysis and plasma proteins in women with normal and with excessive menstrual blood loss. *Br. J. Obstet. Gynaecol.*, **83**, 974

Hallberg, L., Hogdahl, A.M., Nilsson, L. and Rybo, G. (1966). Menstrual blood loss – a population study. *Acta Obstet. Gynaecol. Scand.*, **45**, 320–51

Hamblen, E.C. and Davis, C.D. (1945). *Am. J. Obstet. Gynecol.*, **50**, 137, quoted by Browne (1950) p. 262

Hamblen, E.C., Cuyler, W.K., Pattee, C.J. and Axelson, G.J. (1941). *J. Clin. Endocrinol.*, **1**, 211, quoted by Bishop (1950) pp. 586–607

Hamou, J. (1985) quoted by Magos (1991) p. 382

Harrison, R.F. and Campbell, S. (1976). A double blind trial of ethamsylate in the treatment of primary and intrauterine-device menorrhagia. *Lancet*, **2**, 283–5

Haynes, P.J., Hodgson, H., Anderson, A.B.M. and Turnbull, A.C. (1977). Measurement of menstrual blood loss in patients complaining of menorrhagia. *Br. J. Obstet. Gynaecol.*, **84**, 763–8

Heape, W. (1897). The menstruation and ovulation of *Macacus rhesus*, with observations on the changes undergone by the discharged follicle. *Phil. Trans. R. Soc. Lond.*, Part 2 **188**, 135–66

Iles, S. and Gath, D. (1989). Psychological problems and uterine bleeding. *Clin. Obstet. Gynecol.*, **3**, 375–89

Israel, S.L. (1967). *Menstrual Disorders and Sterility*, 5th edn. (New York: Hoeber)

Jones, G.E.S. (1949). Some newer aspects of the management of infertility. *J. Am. Med. Assoc.*, **141**, 1123–8

Karnaky, K.J. (1939). *Bull. Methodist Hosp. Houston, Texas*, quoted by Bishop (1950) pp. 586–607

Kasonde, J.M. and Bonnar, J. (1975). Effect of ethamsylate and aminocaproic acid on menstrual blood loss in women using intrauterine devices. *Br. Med. J.*, **27**, 21–2

Kasonde, J.M. and Bonnar, J. (1976). Effect of sterilization on menstrual blood loss. *Br. J. Obstet. Gynaecol.*, **83**, 572

Long, C.A. and Gast, M.J. (1990). Menorrhagia. *Obstet. Gynecol. Clin. N. Am.*, **17**, 343–50

McKay, W.J.S. (1901). *History of Ancient Gynaecology.* (London: Bailliere Tindall Cox)

Mackenzie, J.Z. and Bibby, J.G. (1978). Critical assessment of dilatation and curettage in 1029 women. *Lancet*, **2**, 566–9

Magos, A.L. (1991). Endometrial ablation for menorrhagia. *Prog. Obstet. Gynaecol.*, **9**, 375–95

Magos, A.L., Baumann, R. and Turnbull, A.C. (1989). Transcervical resection of the endometrium in women with menorrhagia. *Br. Med. J.*, **298**, 1209–12

Mills, J. (1991). *Woman Words*, pp. 155–8. (London: Virago Press)

Neuwirth, R.S. (1978). A new technique for and additional experience with hysteroscopic resection of submucous fibroids. *Am. J. Obstet. Gynecol.*, **131**, 91–4

Neuwirth, R.S. (1983). Hysteroscopic management of symptomatic submucous fibroids. *Obstet. Gynecol.*, **62**, 509–11

Newton, J.R., Snowden, S.A. and Parsons, V. (1976). Control of menstrual bleeding during haemodialysis. *Br. Med. J.*, **1**, 1016–17

Nilsson, L. and Rybo, G. (1971). Treatment of menorrhagia. *Am. J. Obstet. Gynecol.*, **110**, 713–20

Novak, E. (1927). How far can recent studies on the ovarian follicular substance be applied to the human? A brief discussion of the therapeutic aspects of the problem. *Endocrinology*, **11**, 173–94

Novak, E. (1933). Recent advances in the physiology of menstruation. Can menstruation occur without ovulation? *J. Am. Med. Assoc.*, **94**, 833–9

Novak, E. and Martzloff, K.H. (1924). Hyperplasia of the endometrium: a clinical and pathological study. *Am. J. Obstet. Gynecol.*, **8**, 385

Olshausen, R. (1875). Ueber chronische, hyperplasirende Endometritis des Corpus uteri. *Arch. Gynaaekol.*, **8**, 97

Petrussen, B., Hahn, L., Korsan-Bengtsen, K, and Hallberg, L. (1977). Influence of acetylsalicylic acid and paracetamol on menstrual blood loss. *Haemostasis*, **6**, 266–8

Phipps, J.H., Lewis, B.V., Roberts, T., Prior, M.V., Hand, J.N., Elder, M. and Field, S.B. (1990). Treatment of functional menorrhagia by radiofrequency induced thermal endometrial ablation. *Lancet*, **335**, 374–6

Pliny (The Elder) (1939). *Natural History*, translated by Rackham, H. (Cambridge, Mass.: Harvard University Press)

Recamier, M. (1850). Memoire sur les productions fibreuses et fongueuses intra-uterincs. *Union Med. Pais*, **4**, 266

Rees, M.C.P. (1989). Heavy painful periods. In Drife, J.O. (ed.) *Clinics in Obstetrics and Gynaecology: Dysfunctional Uterine Bleeding and Menorrhagia*, Vol. 3, pp. 341–56. (London, Philadelphia, Sydney, Tokyo, Toronto: Bailliere Tindall)

Rees, M.C.P., Cederholm-Williams, S.A. and Turnbull, A.C. (1985). Coagulation factors and fibrinolytic proteins in menstrual fluid collected from normal and menorrhagic women. *Br. J. Obstet. Gynaecol.*, **92**, 1164

Rybo, G., Nilsson, S., Sikstrom, B. and Nygren, K.G. (1981). Naproxen in menorrhagia. *Lancet*, **1**, 608–9

Schroder, R. (1914). Uber das Verhalten der Uterusschleimhaut um die Zeit der Menstruation. *Mschr. Geburtsh. Gynakekol.*, **39**, 3

Schroder, R. (1915). Anatomische Studien zur normalen und pathologischen Physiologie des Menstruationszyklus. *Arch. Gynaekol.*, **104**, 27

Scowen, E.F. (1944). *Proc. R. Soc. Med.*, **37**, 677, quoted by Browne (1950) p. 262

Shaw, S.T., Aaronson, D.E. and Moyer, D.L. (1972). Quantitation of menstrual blood loss – further evaluation of the alkaline hematin method. *Contraception*, **5**, 497

Shaw, W.S. and Fraser, H.M. (1984). Use of a superactive luteinizing hormone releasing hormone (LHRH) agonist in the treatment of menorrhagia. *Br. J. Obstet. Gynaecol.*, **92**, 913–16

Siddle, N., Sarrel, P. and Whitehead, M.I. (1987). The effect of hysterectomy on the age of ovarian failure: identification of a subgroup of women with premature ovarian loss of ovarian function and literature review. *Fertil. Steril.*, **47**, 94–100

Southam, A.L. and Richart, R.M. (1966). *Am. J. Obstet. Gynecol.*, **94**, 637, quoted by Dewhurst (1972) pp. 511–38

Studd, J.W.W. (1989). Hysterectomy and menorrhagia. In Drife, J.O. (ed.) *Dysfunctional Uterine Bleeding and Menorrhagia. Clinics in Obstetrics and Gynaecology*, Vol. 3, No. 2, pp. 415–24. (London, Philadelphia, Sydney: Bailliere Tindall & Co.)

Taylor, T., Smith, A.N. and Fulton, P.M. (1989). Effect of hysterectomy on bowel function. *Br. Med. J.*, **299**, 300–1

Turnbull, A.C. (1956). *J. Obstet. Gynaecol. Br.*

Commonw., **63**, 179, quoted by Dewhurst (1972) p. 538

Vermylen, J., Verhaegen-Declercq, M.L., Verstraete, M. and Fierens, F. (1968). A double blind study of the effect of tranexamic acid in essential menorrhagia. *Thromb. Haemost*, **20**, 583–7

West, C. and Duncan, J.M. (1879). *Disease of Women.* (London: Churchill)

Westrom, L. and Bengtsson, L.P. (1970). Effect of tranexamic acid (AMCA) in menorrhagia with intrauterine contraceptive devices. A double blind study. *J. Reprod. Med.*, **5**, 154–61

Wingo, P.A., Huezo, C.M., Rubin, G.L., Ory, H.W. and Petersen, H.B. (1985). The mortality risk associated with hysterectomy. *Am. J. Obstet. Gynecol.*, **152**, 803–8

FURTHER READING

Bishop, P.M.F. (1950). Endocrine therapy. In Bowes, K. (ed.) *Modern Trends in Obstetrics and Gynaecology*, Vol. 40, pp. 586–607. (London: Butterworth & Co.)

Browne, F.J. (1950). *Postgraduate Obstetrics and Gynaecology*, pp. 254–62. (London: Butterworth & Co.)

Dewhurst, C.J. (1972). *Integrated Obstetrics and Gynaecology for Postgraduates.* (Oxford, London, Edinburgh, Melbourne: Blackwell Scientific Publications)

Dockeray, C.J. (1988). The medical treatment of menorrhagia. In Chamberlain, G. (ed.) *Contemporary Obstetrics and Gynaecology*, chap. 18 pp. 299–314. (London, Boston, Singapore, Sydney, Toronto, Wellington: Butterworths)

Graham, H. (1950). *Eternal Eve.* (London: W. Heinemann)

Gruhn, J.G. and Kazer, R.R. (1989). *Hormonal Regulation of the Menstrual Cycle: The Evolution of Concepts.* (New York, London: Plenum Medical Book Co.)

Haines, M. and Taylor, C.W. (1975). *Gynaecological Pathology*, 2nd edn. (Edinburgh London, New York: Churchill Livingstone)

Hellman, L.M., Pritchard, J.A. and Wynn, R.M. (1971). *Williams Obstetrics*, 14th edn. (London: Butterworths & Co.)

Long, C.A. and Gast, M.J. (1990). Menorrhagia. *Obstet. Gynecol. Clin. N. Am.*, **17**, 343–59

McKay, W.J.S. (1901). *History of Ancient Gynaecology.* (London: Bailliere, Tindall & Cox)

Magos, A.L. (1991). Endometrial ablation for menorrhagia. *Obstet. Gynecol.*, **9**, 375–95

Mills, J. (1991). *Woman Words.* (London: Virago Press)

Rees, M.C.P. and Turnbull, A.C. (1989). Menstrual disorders - an overview. In Drife, J.O. (ed.) *Dysfunctional Uterine Bleeding and Menorrhagia: Clinical Obstetrics and Gynaecology*, Vol. 3 No. 2, pp. 217–26. (London: Balliere Tindall & Co.)

Smith, S.K. (1985). Menorrhagia. *Progr. Obstet. Gynaecol.*, **5**, 293–308

Van Eijkeren, M.A., Christiaens, G.C.M.L., Sixma, J.J. and Haspels, A.A. (1989). Menorrhagia: a review. *Obstet. Gynecol. Surv.*, **44**, 421–9

Chromosomal, hormonal and psychogenic amenorrhoea and oligomenorrhoea

CHROMOSOMES, BARR BODIES AND DRUMSTICKS

The basic laws of inheritance were discovered by Gregor Mendel. His publication (1866) went unrecognized until it was rediscovered in 1900 by de Vries, Correns and Tschermak. Meanwhile the fact that the cell nucleus contained the elements of inheritance became understood by about 1885. The chromatin and non-chromatin structures were well described by the early 1880s and the German anatomist G.Waldyer introduced the term chromosomes in 1888 (Dunn, 1965). However, the knowledge of human chromosomes remained limited because they were held in a complex tangle by the spindle during mitosis.

The correct chromosome number for humans was established by Tjio and Levan (1956) who discovered that the usual number was 46 and not 48 as had been previously thought. The chromosome was found to be split into two identical chromatids which were adherent at the centromere. To conduct chromosome analysis, a preparation of tissue culture of epidermal cells, bone marrow or leukocyte cells was prepared. Mitosis was stopped at a vital stage by adding colchicine which was found to destroy the spindle and thus allow the chromosomes to separate. By the addition of hypotonic solutions, by squashing on a glass slide and by the addition of special materials such as Feulgen stains, the chromosomes then became available for further study. A systematic arrangement of the chromosomes from a single cell was termed a 'karyotype'.

Other developments of the time included the discovery of the nuclear chromatin (Barr body) by Barr and Bertram (1949). These researchers discovered that almost half the animals investigated by them showed chromatin masses beneath the nuclear membrane, and these were all females. Before their discovery it had been assumed that male and female cells were identical. In a further development, Davidson and Smith (1954) demonstrated the presence of a club-shaped appendage to the nuclei of white blood cells and this 'nuclear drumstick' was thought to represent the presence of female (XX) sex chromosome complement. In its absence a male (XY) chromosome complement was inferred. Moore and Barr (1955) introduced the buccal mucosa smear test, a rapid method to determine whether a sex anomaly was present.

In 1950 a group of international cytologists met in Denver, Colorado and devised a system for arranging and naming chromosomes strictly according to their lengths. They numbered the autosomes 1 to 22 in descending order of length, noting that the chromosomes fell into seven groups. The sex chromosomes were signified as X for female and Y for male (Denver Study Group, 1960). By 1959 it was discovered that some patients with congenital malformations had abnormal chromosome numbers (Ford *et al.*, 1959 a,b; Jacobs and Keay, 1959; Jacobs *et al.*, 1959; Lejeune *et al.*, 1959).

INCOMPLETE MASCULINIZATION OF CHROMOSOMAL AND GONADAL MALES

Testicular feminization

It was Morris (1953) who named and outlined this syndrome when reviewing a large number of cases collected from the literature. Prior to that the abnormality was discovered by the detection of gonadal tumours at laparotomy, or by finding normal gonads in the inguinal canals during herniotomy. Cases rarely presented before puberty, but then these patients were noted to have amenorrhoea and on examination had a short 'blind' vagina.

The individuals concerned developed as phenotypic females with large breasts and absent or scanty pubic and axillary hair. Eventually Wilkins (1965) suggested that the syndrome was due to androgen insensitivity, with failure of the sexual organs to respond to circulating testosterone. Most individuals with testicular feminization were found to have chromatin-negative cells and an XY karyotype, but a number were found to have mosaicism. The disorder was also found to occur more frequently in siblings of affected individuals. Testicular adenomas occurred in 25% and malignant change was found in 5–8%.

5α-Reductase syndrome

Although testicular feminization syndrome was the most common form of incomplete masculinization a number of other forms were found. Probably the best known of these was described by Imperato-McGinley et al. (1979) when they described a familial syndrome in which there was a deficiency of 5α-reductase, a defect which affected a number of families in the Dominican Republic. This syndrome was inherited as an autosomal recessive condition. In normal males, testosterone is bound to sex hormone binding globulin, or to albumin, with only 1–3% being active. This free testosterone is converted by 5α-reductase to dihydrotestosterone at cellular level, and then exerts its action by binding with high-affinity receptors which interact with nucleur acceptor sites to produce a cellular response. In the '5α-reductase deficiency syndrome' the male appeared phenotypically female until puberty, when a degree of masculinization of external genitalia occurred. These cases differed from the testicular feminization syndrome in that they had normal virilized Wolffian structures which terminated in the vagina.

CHROMOSOMAL INTERSEX

Turner's syndrome

This condition, also called the 'pterygo-nuchal infantilism syndrome', was described by Turner (1938) whose series of (female) cases was characterized by sexual infantilism, neck webbing, bilateral cubitus valgus, and short stature. Wilkins and Fleischmann (1944) determined that these patients had streak gonads rather than ovaries. While the streak gonads usually contained fibrous tissue, an occasional Turner's syndrome patient menstruated and Bahner et al. (1960) reported one such patient who gave birth to a normal infant.

Although Turner gained eponymic distinction, this form of chromosomal intersex had previously been documented as 'pterygium colli' by Funke (1902) who described a patient with micrognathia, elongated low set ears, high arched palate, retarded growth and sexual immaturity. Further cases were described by Baer (1927) and Ullrich (1930). However, Turner's description of a series

of such individuals established the condition as a syndrome.

Meyer (1931) reported a case of sexual infantilism who was found to have follicle stimulating hormone in the urine, and this finding was substantiated by subsequent investigators. There thus developed a useful test for differentiating between gonadal dysgenesis and pituitary dwarfism. It became apparent that not all of these patients who had female phenotype had a female chromatin pattern (Polani et al., 1954). When sex chromosome analysis became available, Ford et al. (1959b) reported a sex chromosomal anomaly in a case of Turner's syndrome. They observed that the chromosome constitution of the girl was XO. Since then a large number of additional physical features have been observed in true Turner's syndrome cases. These were referred to as 'Turner's stigmata'. It was later found that almost 30% of Turner's cases exhibited chromosomal mosaicism (Race and Sanger, 1969).

A possible male Turner syndrome is depicted in a German woodcut from 1693 and a further male case was again described by Flavell (1943). The karyotype of males with this syndrome was found to be (an apparently normal) 46 XY. (A further form of intersex in the male was described by Klinefelter et al. (1942) who described a syndrome in phenotypic males which was characterized by atrophic testes, azoospermia and gynaecomastia. These were later shown to have a chromosome karyotype of 47 XXY.)

The super female

A form of chromosome abnormality entitled the 'super female' (trisomy X, the triple X syndrome, XXX, triplo X) was reported by Jacobs et al. (1959). Their case was that of a 35-year-old woman who had menstruated irregularly from 14 to 19 years of age and thereafter suffered secondary amenorrhoea. The patient was of average height and weight but her breasts and reproductive tract were underdeveloped, and the ovaries were small and deficient. It was later reported that despite oligomenorrhoea, fertility was possible in some of these patients.

GONADAL INTERSEX

Hermaphroditism

In Greek mythology Hermaphroditus was the son of Aphrodite and Hermes. The child grew to maturity with the nymph Salmacis and bathed in her fountain. She desired never to be separated from him, but Hermaphroditus spurned her love. One day as he swam in her pool Salmacis merged with him physically. He grew long hair and female breasts and thus combined male and female characteristics (Cotterell, 1989). The term 'hermaphrodite' was adopted into the English language in about the fourteenth century and was synonymous with the word 'androgyne' (Mills, 1991). Hermaphroditism was recognized by the ancients. The birth of such an infant was considered an evil omen by the early Romans, and such bisexual children were executed (Warkany, 1971). The Hebrew book *Tosefta* laid down laws for androgynes which prohibited their execution.

Overzier (1963) analysed 171 cases of proven hermaphroditism and Van Niekerk (1974) later described a total of 302 cases and reported on their clinical, morphological and cytogenic aspects. The majority were reared as males but 50% had menstruated. The condition was common among the Bantu tribe in Africa. Spermatogenesis was unusual. Williamson *et al.* (1981) reported to the *American Journal of Obstetrics and Gynecology* their review of true hermaphroditism and noted that term vaginal delivery in such individuals had been reported on at least five occasions.

Pure gonadal dysgenesis

Hoffenberg and Jackson (1957) introduced the term 'pure gonadal dysgenesis', which was applied to women who exhibited gonadal dysgenesis with sexual infantilism, but without other physical stigmata. No chromosomal abnormality was detected, gonads failed to develop, and a female phenotype was usual. In the presence of a 46 XY chromosome constitution the appellation Swyer's syndrome was used (Swyer, 1957). These individuals are predisposed to gonadal malignancy.

PARTIAL MASCULINIZATION OF CHROMOSOMAL AND GONADAL FEMALES

Congenital adrenal hyperplasia (the adrenogenital syndrome).

The name implies that pathology of the adrenal glands affected alterations in the genital organs. In this syndrome masculinization is produced by androgens secreted from the adrenal gland. The condition was described by Pliny the Elder in his *Natural History*. He observed that females could

transform into males, and described such a case observed by him in Africa. Regnier de Graaf illustrated a case report of a female pseudohermaphrodite in 1678 (Panos, 1950). Tilesius in 1803 described the relationship between precocious puberty and adrenal tumours but Marchand, in 1891, was apparently the first to report pseudohermaphroditism in the presence of adreno-cortical hyperplasia (Krabbe, 1921). The condition was eventually found to encompass at least six inherited enzymatic abnormalities which affected steroid synthesis, the most common of which was 21-hydroxylase deficiency. This occurred as a 'salt-losing' or 'non-salt losing type', in both of which there was a build up of 17-hydroxyprogesterone. While the adreno-genital syndrome was usually noted at birth, in some instances its first manifestations were noted at puberty or after. Treatment with cortisol or hydrocortisone suppressed the excessive adrenocorticotrophic hormone levels which were found in the syndrome. Other adrenal causes of amenorrhoea include Cushing's syndrome, Addison's disease and tumours.

The role of sex hormones in the causation of intersexuality was first demonstrated in cattle. In twin bovine pregnancy vascular anastomoses between the two placental plates were observed to occur at the crown–rump length 19 mm stage, prior to external sex differentiation. The female gonads developed in the male direction with formation of medullary cords, rete testes, epididymes and vas deferens while the Müllerian ducts regressed. Although both ovaries assumed testicular structure they were sterile. The external genitalia of the sterile (free martin) cow was almost always of female type.

Female pseudohermaphroditism

In the late 1950s, an increase in the incidence of female pseudohermaphroditism was noticed. It was eventually discovered that this new condition was due to the administration of nortestosterone-derived progestogenic steroids used in the treatment of threatened abortion. Of these compounds, norethisterone (Primolut N) was most commonly associated with masculinizing effects.

PHYSICAL ABNORMALITIES

A well-known congenital Müllerian anomaly was that of imperforate hymen. When the condition was not discovered until after puberty, affected individuals presented with amenorrhoea and lower abdominal pain due to accumulated menstrual blood in the vagina, uterus and tubes. Another intriguing condition was that which was termed congenital absence of the vagina. This became known as the Mayer–Rokitansky–Kuster–Hauser syndrome in which there was a 'blind' shallow vagina, absence of upper vagina, and only rudimentary development of the Müllerian ducts. The ovaries were normal. Chromosome analysis usually showed a 46 XX karyotype. While over 50% of such patients were found to have a solid rudimentary uterus, less than 10% showed evidence of function. The latter developed haematometra which presented with cyclic lower abdominal pain. The aetiology and pathogenesis of the disorder, which was once called *uterus bipartitus solidus rudimentarius cum vagina solida,* were not precisely identified.

A further syndrome described by Asherman (1948; 1950), was accorded the appellation Asherman's syndrome. The condition was secondary to intrauterine adhesions induced by curettage, particularly if performed in the puerperium or after abortions. The awareness of this well-known syndrome later formed the basis of intrauterine therapy to treat menorrhagia.

HYPOTHALAMUS

It became known that amenorrhoea could result from stress, chronic disease, prolonged exercise or poor nutrition. Hermann Zondek (1935) wrote . . . 'menstruation can be arrested by very varied physical influences, such as the fear of becoming pregnant, the intense desire for a child, fright, joy, etc., It is known too that amenorrhoea may follow upon acute or chronic infectious disease . . . it may even result from deficient diet (war amenorrhoea)'. Klinefelter *et al.* (1943) measured follicle stimulating hormone activity in the urine of women with anorexia nervosa and various endocrine disorders and provided early objective evidence of a hypothalamic cause for amenorrhoea. They theorized that there was failure of luteinizing hormone production from the anterior pituitary in such cases. It was later discovered that there was an abnormal pattern of pulsatile gonadotropin releasing hormone release.

A number of syndromes with gonadotropin deficiency combined with systemic disease were described. One such was the Laurence-Moon-Biedl syndrome, an autosomal recessive disease which was characterized by hypogonadotropic (or hypergonadotropic) hypogonadism, mental retardation, retinitis pigmentosa, polydactyly, severe obesity, and occasionally diabetes insipidus or diabetes mellitus (Laurence and Moon, 1866; Biedl, 1922). Another condition was the Prader-Willi syndrome in which there was a hypothalamic defect, partially responsible for hypogonadism and bulimia leading to severe obesity (Prader *et al.*,1956). The patients had characteristic round facies, with small broad hands and feet and also suffered mental retardation, and infantile hypotonia.

Anorexia nervosa

Amenorrhoea occurs when body weight falls to 75% below that which is considered ideal, which in some instances means as little as a 10% weight loss. The condition of anorexia nervosa is accompanied by profound weight loss, psychological changes, food phobias and distortion of body image. In their historical treatise on the subject Dally and Gomez (1979) documented that Simone Porta (1496–1554) was 'sometimes claimed to have given the first description of anorexia nervosa. He described a girl who stopped eating totally when she was 10. For 40 days, apparently under constant observation, she refused all nourishment, claiming that she no longer required food. Simone Porta concluded that she lived on air'. Richard Morton (1694) described two cases of anorexia nervosa which he called 'nervous atrophy'. One case was that of an 18-year-old girl who died 3 months later, and the second was that of an 18-year-old boy who recovered. Morton concluded that the illness was due to 'sadness and anxious cares'.

Sir William Gull (1868) again described the disease, noting that it occurred mostly in young women between 16 and 23 years of age, and called it 'apepsia hysterica'. Six years later however, he introduced the term 'anorexia nervosa' (Gull, 1874) and noted that the condition could affect male or female. Some years later Professor Charles Lasegue (1873) published an account of eight women between 18 and 32 years who suffered from what he called 'anorexie hysterique'. All of his patients recovered. Ten years later the term 'anorexie mentale' was suggested by the Frenchman Huchard (1883) who observed that the hysterical conditions of anaesthesia, blindness and paralysis were not present with the eating disorder. Anorexia nervosa was studied in detail at the beginning of the present century by Pierre Janet

(1903). Soon after this, Dejerine and Gauckler (1913) noted the distinction between eating disorders due to depression or psychotic states, and that of 'anorexie mentale'. Ballet (1907) of France first recorded that amenorrhoea was a frequent presenting symptom of anorexia nervosa. Various studies thereafter have determined an incidence of almost 1% of anorexia in adolescent girls.

Simmonds (1914) a German pathologist, described pituitary lesions which were apparently related to anorexia (cachexia) and death. His observation led to confusion and for some years after that it was mistakenly thought that Simmond's disease and anorexia nervosa were the same condition. However, a number of investigators in England, America and France concluded from early endocrinological investigations that the two conditions were not synonymous. It was Sheehan and Summers (1949) who finally proved that anorexia and Simmond's disease were separate entities.

Although anorexia nervosa was mainly thought to occur in women under 30 years, some investigators related the occurrence of anorexia in older age groups, and even in postmenopausal women (Berkman, 1930). The term 'forma tardive' (or anorexia tardive) was first used by Carrier (1939) to describe these older patients with the condition. While amenorrhoea was a constant finding in anorectic females, Stephens (1941) noted loss of libido and impotence in three male anorectics.

MacGregor (1938) investigated the hormonal basis of anorexia. The results of urinary gonadotropins and oestrogen measurements indicated secondary gonadal insufficiency. The introduction of radioimmunoassay by Berson et al. (1956) revolutionized the study of the field of endocrinology and allowed easier and more detailed appraisal of anorexia and other problems. Marshall and Russell Fraser (1971) used radioimmunoassay techniques to measure serum luteinizing hormone and found reduced levels in anorectic patients. In normal patients, luteinizing hormone was shown to have a pulsatile secretion but in anorectics its pattern equated to that of normal prepubertal girls. Weight gain in these women resulted in the development of normal adult patterns of luteinizing hormone secretion but ovulation and menstruation did not always return despite the women regaining their normal weight. Wiegelmann and Solbach (1972) were the first to determine that luteinizing hormone releasing hormone was effective in releasing both luteinizing hormone and follicle stimulating hormone in anorexia nervosa patients. Marshall and Russell Fraser (1971) demonstrated that they were unresponsive to clomiphene.

Kallman's syndrome

Kallmann, et al. (1944) were the first to describe a syndrome characterized by anosmia and hypogonadisim. Although originally described in males it was later established that women occasionally suffered from complete or relative congenital deficiency of gonadotropin releasing hormone production.

PITUITARY

Persistent galactorrhoea with atrophy of the uterus and ovaries (i.e. hyperprolactinaemia) was described by Chiari et al. (1855) in a 7-year report from the Department of Gynaecology in Vienna. The condition occurred in postnatal women. Frommel (1882) documented a similar state in 1% of postpartum cases. The term 'Chiari-Frommel syndrome' was applied by Mendel (1946) in a further case report and historical review.

A lactation hormone which was produced from the anterior pituitary gland was first discovered by Stricker and Grueter (1929). Three years later Krestin (1932) was the first to describe a relationship between persistent galactorrhoea, amenorrhoea and pituitary hyperfunction. Other medical scientists whose names were associated with hyperprolactinaemia and its investigation were Ahumada and del Castillo of Buenos Aires, and also Argonz, Forbes and Albright. The amino acid sequence of prolactin was first published by Li et al. (1969).

Other pituitary causes of amenorrhoea included Sheehan's syndrome, acromegaly and granulomas. Sheehan and Murdoch (1938) described 128 patients with postpartum haemorrhage or collapse, and clinical evidence of hypopituitarism was evident in almost 50%. These women developed failure of lactation, loss of body hair, cold intolerance with apathy, and infrequent or absent menstruation. In a controlled study none of those features was found in a series of 64 women with a normal last delivery and third stage.

OVARIAN CAUSES

Oligo- or amenorrhoea associated with bilateral polycystic ovaries was described by Irving Stein and Michael Leventhal (1935) when they documented bilateral ovarian wedge resection in 70 amenorrhoeic patients with enlarged ovaries. However a condition of 'sclerocystic' ovaries, or 'microcystic degeneration of the ovary' which may have referred to polycystic ovary syndrome, was first described by Lisfranc in 1830. A similar ovarian disorder was subsequently described by Chereau in 1844, by Tilt in 1850 and by Gallard in 1873. This ovarian condition was reviewed by a number of commentators thereafter. Stein and Leventhal's original observations of 1935 were updated 10 years later when Stein defined their syndrome as consisting of irregular menstruation or amenorrhoea, sterility and hirsutism in the presence of enlarged, polycystic ovaries. While investigating polycystic ovary syndrome patients, elevated androgenic hormone levels were discovered by DeVane *et al.* (1975), and abnormal patterns of luteinizing hormone release were found by Rebar *et al.* (1976). Although wedge resection was used in treatment, its popularity waned in the 1970s due to the introduction of therapy with clomiphene or extracts of human menopausal gonadotropins. Other ovarian disorders including resistant ovary syndrome, ovarian tumours, and premature ovarian failure were documented as causing amenorrhoea.

THYROID

MacGregor (1936) and also Russell and Dean (1942) noted a relationship between thyroid overactivity and oligo or amenorrhoea. A similar situation pertained in hypothyroidism, which was later found to cause amenorrhoea not only by the elevation of thyroid stimulating hormone and hence prolactin levels but possibly also by disrupting oestrogen metabolism. In thyrotoxicosis there were increased sex hormone binding globulin levels which altered both oestradiol and androstenedione metabolism.

CHRONOLOGY

Chromosomes

1866   Gregor Mendel outlined the basic laws of inheritance.

1888   G. Waldyer introduced the term chromosomes (Dunn, 1965).

1949   Barr and Bertram discovered chromatin masses beneath the nuclear membrane in females.

1950   International cytologists met in Denver, and proposed an arrangement and naming of chromosomes.

1954   Davidson and Smith demonstrated the nuclear drumstick in the white cells of females.

1955   Moore and Barr introduced the buccal smear test.

1956   Tjio and Levan deduced the correct chromosome number for humans.

1959   Lejeune *et al.* and others discovered abnormal chromosome numbers in some patients with congenital malformation.

Sex chromosomal disorders

1938   Turner described cases of sexual infantilism with neck webbing and other stigmata (patients of this type were first described by Funke in 1902).

1943   Flavell described a possible male 'Turner syndrome'.

1953   Morris defined the syndrome of 'testicular feminization'.

1959   Jacobs *et al.* described the 'super female'.

Gonadal intersex

Hermaphroditism was recognised since antiquity.

1963   Overzier analysed 171 proven cases.

Pure gonadal dysgenesis

1957   Hoffenberg and Jackson introduced the term 'pure gonadal dysgenesis'.

Congenital adrenal hyperplasia

Observed from antiquity the condition was described by Pliny the Elder.

1678   Regnier de Graaf illustrated a case report (Panos, 1950).

1891   Marchand first reported adreno-corticol hyperplasia associated with pseudohermaphroditism (Krabbe, 1921).

Physical abnormalities

Noted from antiquity.

1948/   Asherman described intrauterine adhe-
50   sions secondary to curettage.

Hypothalamus

16th C. Simone Porta described a possible case of anorexia nervosa (Dally and Gomez, 1979).

1694   Richard Morton documented two cases of anorexia nervosa.

1868   Sir William Gull described its occurrence in women between 16 and 23 years.

1874   The term anorexia was introduced by Gull.

1907   Ballet of France recorded that amenorrhoea was a frequent presenting symptom.

1914   Simmonds described pituitary lesions and anorexia (cachexia).

1939   Carrier introduced the term 'forma tardive' to describe anorexia in older age group women.

1949   Sheehan and Summers proved that anorexia and 'Simmonds disease' were separate entities.

1979   Russell noted that bulimia nervosa was an ominous variant of anorexia.

Others

1866   Laurence and Moon described the syndrome later called the Laurence-Moon-Biedl syndrome.

1956   Prader *et al.* described the syndrome of obesity, cryptorchidism and mental retardation in infants with delayed puberty.

Pituitary

1938   Sheehan and Murdoch described hypopituitarism following obstetric haemorrhage.

Galactorrhoea

1855   Chiari *et al.* described persistent galactorrhoea with atrophy of the reproductive tract.

1882   Frommel documented a similar occurrence in 1% of postpartum women.

1929   Stricker and Grueter isolated a lactation hormone from the pituitary gland.

1932   Krestin described pituitary hyperfunction, persistent galactorrhoea, and amenorrhoea.

1946   Mendel introduced the term Chiari–Frommel syndrome.

1969   Li *et al.* described the amino acid sequence of prolactin.

Ovarian causes

1830   Lisfranc described 'sclerocystic' ovaries. This condition or 'microcystic' degeneration of the ovary was also described by Chereau in 1844, Tilt in 1850 and by Galard in 1873 (Ricci, 1945).

1935   Stein and Leventhal described polycystic ovaries with irregular menstruation or amenorrhoea.

1975   DeVane *et al.* discovered elevated androgenic hormone levels.

1976   Rebar *et al.* documented abnormal patterns of luteinizing hormone release.

REFERENCES

Asherman, J.G. (1948). Amenorrhoea traumatica atretica. *J. Obstet. Gynaecol. Br. Emp.*, **55**, 23–30

Asherman, J.G. (1950). Traumatic intra-uterine adhesions. *J. Obstet. Gynaecol. Br. Emp.*, **57**, 892–6

Baer, W. (1927). Vollkommene angelborene Aplasie beider Ovarien, infantiles Genitale, viriler Habitus. *Zentralbl. Gynaekol.*, **51**, 3241

Bahner, F., Schwarz, G., Harnden, D.G., Jacobs, P.A., Hienz, H.A. and Walter, K. (1960). A fertile female with XO sex chromosome constitution. *Lancet*, **2**, 100–1

Ballet, G. (1907). L'Anorexia mentale. *Rev. Gen. Clin. Therapeut.*, **21**, 293

Barr, M.L. and Bertram, E.G. (1949). A morphological distinction between neurones of the male and female, and the behaviour of the nucleolar satellite during accelerated nucleoprotein synthesis. *Nature (London)*, **163**, 676–8

Berkman, J.M. (1930). Anorexia nervosa, anorexia inanition and low basal metabolic rate. *Am. J. Med. Sci.*, **180**, 411–24

Berson, S.A., Yalow, R.S., Bauman, R., Rothchild, M.A. and Newerly, K. (1956). Insulin (131) metabolism in human subjects; demonstration of insulin binding globulin in the circulation of insulin treated subjects. *J. Clin. Invest.*, **35**, 170–90

Biedl, A. (1922). Ein geschwisterpaar mit adiposogenitaler dystrophie. *Dtsch. Med. Wchschr.*, **48**, 1630

Browne, F.J. (ed.) (1950). Amenorrhoea. *Postgraduate Obstetrics and Gynaecology*, Vol. 20, pp. 244–53. (London: Butterworth & Co)

Carrier, J. (1939). *L'Anorexie Mentale*. (Paris: Libraire E Le Francois)

Chiari, J., Braun, C. and Spaeth, J. (1855). Report of diseases of women observed during the years 1848 to 1855 inclusive in the Department of Gynecology (Municipal Clinic) in Vienna. *Klin. Geburtsh. Gynaekol.*, 371–2

Cotterell, A. (1989). *The Illustrated Encyclopedia of Myths and Legends*, p. 205. (London: Cassell Publishers Ltd)

Dally, P. and Gomez, J. (1979). *Anorexia Nervosa*, pp. 1–11. (London: William Heinemann Medical Books Ltd)

Davidson, W.M. and Smith, D.R. (1954). A morphological sex difference in the polymorphonuclear neutrophil leucocytes. *Br. Med. J.*, **2**, 6–7

Dejerine, J. and Gauckler, E. (1913). *The Psychoneuroses and their Treatment*. (Philadelphia, London: J.D. Lippincott)

Denver Study Group (1960). A proposed standard system of nomenclature of human mitotic chromosomes. *Lancet*, **1**, 1063–5

DeVane, G.W., Czekala, N.M., Judd, H.L. *et al.* (1975). Circulating gonadotropins, estrogens, and androgens in polycystic ovarian diseases. *Am. J. Obstet. Gynecol.*, **121**, 496–500

Dunn, L.C. (1965). *A Short History of Genetics*. (New York: McGraw-Hill Book Co. Inc.)

Flavell, G. (1943). Webbing of neck with Turner's syndrome in a male. *Br. J. Surg.*, **31**, 150

Ford, C.E., Jones, K.W., Miller, O.J., Mittwoch, U., Penrose, L.S., Ridler, M. and Shapiro, A. (1959a). The chromosomes in a patient showing both mongolism and the Klinefelter syndrome. *Lancet*, **1**, 709

Ford, C.E., Jones, K.W., Polani, P.E., deAlmeida, J.C. and Briggs, J.H. (1959b). A sex chromosome anomaly in a case of gonadal dysgenesis (Turner's syndrome) *Lancet*, **1**, 711

Frommel, R. (1882). Ueber puerperale Atrophie des Uterus. *Z. Geburtsh. Gynaekol.*, **7**, 305–13

Funke (1902). Pterygium colli. *Deutsche Z. Chir.*, **63**, 162

Gull, W.W. (1868). The address in medicine. *Lancet*, **2**, 171

Gull, W.W. (1874). Apepsia hysterica: anorexia nervosa. *Trans. Clin. Soc. (London)*, **7**, 2

Hoffenberg, R. and Jackson, W.P.U. (1957). Gonadal dysgenesis in normal looking females. *Br. Med. J.*, **1**, 1281

Huchard, (1883). quoted by Dally and Gomez (1979)

Imperato-McGinley, J., Peterson, R.E., Gautier, T. and Sturla, E. (1979). Male pseudohermaphroditism secondary to a 5a-reductase deficiency – a model for the role of androgens in both the development of the male phenotype and the evolution of a male gender identity. *J. Steroid Biochem.*, **11**, 637–45

Jacobs, P. and Keay, A.J. (1959). Somatic chromosomes in a child with Bonnevie–Ullrich syndrome. *Lancet*, **2**, 732

Jacobs, P.A., Baikie, A.G., Court Brown, W.M., MacGregor, T.N., Maclean, N. and Harnden, D.G. (1959). Evidence for the existence of the human 'super female'. *Lancet*, **2**, 423

Janet, P. (1903). *Les Obsessions et la Psychosthenie*. (Paris: Felix Alcan)

Kallmann, F., Schonfeld, W.A. and Barrera, S.W. (1944). Genetic aspects of primary eunuchoidism. *Am. J. Ment. Defic.*, **48**, 203–36

Klinefelter, H.F. Jr., Albright, F. and Griswold, G.C. (1943). Experience with a quantitative test for normal or decreased amounts of follicle stimulating hormone in the urine in endocrinological diagnosis. *J. Clin. Endocrinol.*, **3**, 529–44

Klinefelter, H.F., Reifenstein, E.C. and Albright, F. (1942). Syndrome characterised by gynecomastia, aspermatogenesis without A-Leydigism, and increased excretion of follicle stimulating hormone. *J. Clin. Endocrinol. Metab.*, **2**, 615–27

Krabbe, K.H. (1921). The relation between the adrenal cortex and sexual development. *N.Y. J. Med.*, **114**, 4

Krestin, D. (1932). Spontaneous lactation associated with enlargement of the pituitary. *Lancet*, **2**, 928–30

Lasegue, C. (1873). De l'anorexie hysterique. *Arch. Gen. Med.*, **2**, 367

Laurence, J.Z. and Moon, R.C. (1866). Four cases of 'retinitis pigmentosa' occurring in the same family, and accompanied by general imperfections of development. *Ophthalm. Rev. (London)*, **2**, 32

Lejeune, J., Gautier, M. and Turpin, R. (1959). Etude des chromosomes somatiques de neuf enfants mongoliens. *C. R. Acad. Sci. (Paris)*, **248**, 1721

Li, C.H., Dixon, J.S., Lo, T.B. *et al.* (1969). Amino-acid sequence of ovine lactogenic hormone. *Nature(London)*, **224**, 695–6

MacGregor, T.N. (1936). *Trans. Edinb. Obstet. Soc.*, **153**, 56, quoted by Browne (1950) pp. 244–53

MacGregor, T.N. (1938). Amenorrhoea: its aetiology and treatment. *Br. Med. J.*, **1**, 717–22

Marshall, J.C. and Russell Fraser, T. (1971). Amenorrhoea in anorexia nervosa: assessment and treatment with clomiphene citrate. *Br. Med. J.*, **4**, 590–2

Mendel, E.B. (1946). Chiari–Frommel syndrome: an historical review with case report. *Am. J. Obstet Gynecol.*, **51**, 889–92

Mendel, G. (1866). Versuche Uber Pflanzhybriden. *Verh. Naturforsch. Verein. Brunn*, **4**, 3

Meyer, R. (1931). Uber gewebliche Anomalien und ihre Beziehung zu einigen Geschwulsten der Ovarien. *Archiv. Gynaekol.*, **145**, 2

Mills, J. (1991). *Woman Words*, pp. 117–18. (London: Virago Press)

Moore, K.L. and Barr, M.L. (1955). Smears from the oral mucosa in the detection of chromosomal sex. *Lancet*, **2**, 57–8

Morris, J.M. (1953). The syndrome of testicular feminisation in male pseudohermaphrodites. *Am. J. Obstet. Gynecol.*, **65**, 1192–211

Morton, R. (1694). *Phthisologia – or a Treatise of Consumptions.* (London: Smith and Walford)

Overzier, C. (1963). True hermaphroditism. In Overzier, C. (ed.) *Intersexuality.* (London, New York: Academic Press)

Panos, T.C. (1950). Female pseudo-hermaphroditism with hypoadrenia. *Pediatrics*, **5**, 972

Pliny (The Elder) (1939). *Natural History*, translated by Rackham, H. Vol. 2. (Cambridge, Mass.: Harvard University Press)

Polani, P.E., Hunter, W.F. and Lennox, B. (1954). Chromosomal sex in Turner's syndrome with coarctation of the aorta. *Lancet*, **2**, 120

Prader, A., Labhart, A. and Willi, H. (1956). Syndrom von Adipositas, Kleinwuchs,

Kryptorchismus and Oligophrenie nach myatonieartigem Zustand im Neugeborenenalter. *Schweiz. Med. Wchnschr.*, **86**, 1260

Race, R.R. and Sanger, R. (1969). Xg and sex-chromsome abnormalities. *Br. Med. Bull.*, **25**, 99–103

Rebar, R.W., Judd., H.L. Yen, S.S.C. *et al.* (1976). Characterization of the inappropriate gonodotropin secretion in polycystic ovary syndrome. *J. Clin. Invest.*, **57**, 1320–9

Ricci, J.V. (1945). *One Hundred Years of Gynaecology 1800–1900*, p. 85. (Philadelphia: The Blakiston Co.)

Russell, P.M.G. and Dean, E.M. (1942). *Lancet*, **2**, 66, quoted by Browne (1950) pp. 244–53

Russell, G.F.M. (1979). Bulimia nervosa: an ominous variant of anorexia nervosa. *Psychol. Med.*, **9**, 429–48

Sheehan, H.L. and Murdoch, R. (1938). Postpartum necrosis of the anterior pituitary; pathological and clinical aspects. *J. Obstet. Gynaecol. Br. Emp.*, **45**, 456–89

Sheehan, H.L. and Summers, V.K. (1949). The syndrome of hypopituitarism. *Q.J. Med.*, **18**, 319

Simmonds, M. (1914). Ueber embolische Prozesse in der Hypophysis. *Arch. Pathol. Anat.*, **217**, 226

Stein, I.F. and Leventhal, M.L. (1935). Amenorrhea associated with bilateral polycystic ovaries. *Am. J. Obstet. Gynecol.*, **29**, 181–91

Stephens, D.J. (1941). Anorexia nervosa. Endocrine factors in undernutrition. *J. Clin. Endocrinol.*, **1**, 257–68

Stricker, P. and Grueter, F. (1929). Action due lobe anterieur de l'hypophyse sur la montee laiteuse. *C.R. Soc. Biol (Paris)*, **99**, 1978–80

Swyer, G.I.M. (1957). Gonadal dysgenesis. *Br. Med. J.*, **1**, 1421

Tjio, J.H. and Levan, A. (1956). The chromosome number of man. *Hereditas*, **42**, 1

Turner, H.H. (1938). A syndrome of infantilism, congenital webbed neck, and cubitus valgus. *Endocrinology*, **23**, 566–74

Ullrich, O. (1930). Uber typische Kombinationsbilder multipler Abartungen. *Z. Kinderh.*, **49**, 271

Van Niekerk, W.A. (1974). *True Hermaphroditism;*

Clinical, Morphologic and Cytogenic Aspects. (Hagerstown: Harper & Row)

Warkany, J. (1971). *Congenital Malformations: Notes and Comments,* pp. 11–12. (Chicago: Year Book Medical Publishers)

Wiegelmann, W. and Solbach, H.G. (1972). Effects of LH-RH on plasma levels of LH and FSH in anorexia nervosa. *Horm. Metab. Res.,* **4,** 404

Wilkins, L. (1965). *The Diagnosis and Treatment of Endocrine Disorders in Childhood and Adolescence,* 3rd Edn. (Springfield, Illinois: Charles C. Thomas)

Wilkins, L. and Fleischman, W. (1944). Ovarian agenesis, pathology, associated clinical symptoms and the bearing on the theories of sex differentiation. *J. Clin. Endocrinol.,* **4,** 357

Williamson, H.O., Phansey, S.A. and Mathur, R.S. (1981). True hermaphroditism with term vaginal delivery and a review. *Am. J. Obstet. Gynecol.,* **141,** 262–5

Zondek, H. (1935). *The Diseases of the Endocrine Glands,* p. 411. (Baltimore: William Wood)

FURTHER READING

Browne, F.J. (ed.) (1950). Amenorrhoea. *Postgraduate Obstetrics and Gynaecology,* Vol. 20, pp. 244–53. (London: Butterworth & Co.)

Dally, P. and Gomez, J. (1979). *Anorexia Nervosa.* (London: William Heinemann Medical Books Ltd)

Gruhn, J.G. and Kazer, R.R. (1989). *Hormonal Regulation of the Menstrual Cycle: The Evolution of Concepts.* (New York, London: Plenum Medical Book Co.)

Scott, J.S. (1985). Intersex and Sex Chromosome Abnormalities. In Macdonald, R. (ed.) *Scientific Basis of Obstetrics and Gynaecology,* 3rd edn., pp. 201–54. (Edinburgh, London, Melbourne, New York: Churchill Livingstone)

Warkany, J, (1971). *Congenital Malformations. Notes and Comments.* (Chicago: Year Book Medical Publishers)

The menopause

DEFINITION

The word menopause is derived from the Greek words *men*, month, and *pausis*, cessation. It is the last menstrual period and marks the end of reproductive life. The term climacteric, derived from the Greek for ladder, was defined by the International Menopause Society in 1976 (during its inaugural meeting in France) as a transitional interval which marked the change from reproductive to non-reproductive status.

OLDEN DAYS

There is reference to the menopause in the Bible, where it was related that Sarah's personality changed when it 'ceased to be with Sarah after the manner of women'. Abraham was aware that older age brought an end to the possibility of childbearing. Among Shakespeare's references to the menopause was his description of Lady Macbeth and the lines he wrote in *Anthony and Cleopatra* about Cleopatra past middle age, 'age cannot wither her, nor custome stale her infinite variety'. In 1845 Colombat de L'Isere wrote in a much more negative fashion 'compelled to yield to the power of time, women now cease to exist for the species . . . their features are stamped with the impress of age, and their genital organs are sealed with the signet of sterility . . . everything is calculated to cause regret for charms that are lost, and enjoyments that are ended forever' (Utian, 1987).

AGE OF ONSET

Aristotle (384–322 BC) considered that menstruation normally ceased at 40 years, but could continue until the 50th year and other writers of the era were in accord. By the sixth century AD Aetius of Amida also agreed and documented that menstruation ceased somewhere between 35 and 50 years. In medieval Europe, similar to the present day, an average age of onset was 50 years (Amudsen and Diers, 1973). However, many women did not live long enough to experience the menopause.

The median age at death (i.e. the age at which 50% of the population had died) in ancient Rome was 34 years for wives and 46.5 for husbands, while in classical Athens it was 35 years for women and 44 for men (Garland, 1990). In the seventeenth century 28% of women lived to experience the menopause, and only 5% survived to the age of 75 (Young, 1971). In modern, developed countries the figures are 95% of women reaching menopause with 50% reaching age 75.

It was estimated in 1986 that there were about ten million postmenopausal women in the UK and West Germany, compared to 40 million in the USA (Schneider, 1986). The average woman could expect to spend almost a third of her life in the postmenopausal state, with 17% of women already in that group. The age of menopause is not related to the menarche, weight, height, race, or socioeconomic factors. Nulliparity was linked with earlier menopause when compared to multiparity. Smokers were also discovered to have an earlier onset of the condition (Jick and Porter, 1977).

AETIOLOGY

Many of the postmenopausal changes are caused, or aggravated, by oestrogen deficiency due to ovarian failure. The ageing of the ovary and consequent drop in oestrogen levels is a slow process which starts during fetal life. When investigating the fetal ovary Bloch (1953) discovered that the number of follicles declined from the 20th week of gestation onwards. A decade later Baker (1963) documented that the maximum count of germ cells was present at the 22nd week of gestation, but from that point on there was a loss of over five million cells, so that at birth only about one million survived (Bloch, 1953; Baker, 1963; Franchi and Baker, 1973). By the age of 7 years about 300 000 oocytes remained but as the woman approached menopause only a few hundred primary oocytes could be detected. Further

317

evidence for declining ovarian activity came from Rossle and Roulet (1941) who showed that the mean weight of the ovary began to decrease from 30 years of age.

For many years the hormonal status was evaluated by vaginal cytology. The method was first introduced to general use by Papanicolaou (1933) and many workers found the technique beneficial. The International Academy of Cytology (1958) published a terminology of cells and indices to be used for classification of hormonal status. A 'karyopyknotic index', an 'eosinophilic index' and also a 'superficial cell index' were popular. Nyklicek (1951) introduced a system which was altered by Frost (1970) into what became 'the maturation index', the most popular method of evaluating hormonal status at cytology. Urinary oestrogen levels were investigated by Pincus et al. (1955) and also Brown et al. (1959), and they documented declining values of the hormone in perimenopausal women. Chakravati et al. (1979) determined that a serum follicle stimulating hormone level greater than 15 U/l was consistent with a peri- or postmenopausal state.

SYMPTOMS

Until the early 1970s symptoms of the menopause were loosely divided into 'autonomic', 'psychological' and 'metabolic'. From that time however they were ascribed to the interactions of three components – decreased ovarian activity with altered hormone profiles; sociocultural or environmental influences; and psychological factors (Utian, 1980).

The sociopsychological symptoms were known to the ancients, and in the late nineteenth century, Edward Tilt commented on the the 'empty nest syndrome' indicating that some symptoms in the age group were aggravated by life events (Wilbush, 1979). Tilt, a London physician, was among the first to address the problems of middle-aged female patients, and also wrote a book on the subject (1887). The lack of menopause symptomatology in animals was alluded to by Currier (1897) who also implied that highly bred civilized women were more likely to complain while the majority of women who were in the lower classes were asymptomatic.

Loss of libido with lethargy, anxiety, irritability and depression, were commonly experienced (Neugarten and Kraines, 1965; Campbell, 1975). Ballinger (1975) investigated the psychiatric morbidity of the menopause and found that

symptoms increased until a year after cessation of menstruation. A decrease in sexual activity was found to occur with increasing age and Bottiglioni (1981) indicated that the menopause accentuated that decline.

The Council of Medical Women's Federation in England (1933) analysed 1000 women at the menopause and found troublesome symptoms in 84.2%, but these were incapacitating in only 10%. Hawkinson (1938) also reviewed 1000 cases and found that 75% suffered from distressing symptoms. About 20% of patients who complained of 'hot flushes' (known as 'flashes' in America) consulted their doctor, and 10% required treatment.

McKinlay and Jeffreys (1974) wrote that 75% of women had hot flushes or night sweats at some time. Molnar (1975) first investigated body temperature changes during hot flushes. No premonitory sign was found to indicate that a hot flush was imminent. The duration of the flush was found to be just under 3 minutes. The temperature estimated at the finger increased 7.5 °F and returned to normal in about 30 minutes. Hot flushes occurred during sleep, and if accompanied by sweating were termed 'night sweats'. Electroencephalographic recordings showed that women wakened just prior to the incident.

In a further study of hot flushes Sturdee et al. (1978a) found peripheral vasodilatation, transient tachycardia, and decreased skin resistance. Tataryn et al. (1979) and Meldrum et al. (1979) recorded similar findings. Casper et al. (1979) demonstrated that the pulse rate increased anything up to 20 beats per minute during a hot flush episode. While Western society has become increasingly aware of and has medicalized the menopause over the last 100 years, other cultures viewed the event in a different fashion. The Japanese concept of 'Konenki' did not correspond to the current Western view of the event (Lock, 1991). Indeed in a recent survey only 9.7% of Japanese women reported hot flushes and just 3.6% complained of night sweats.

OSTEOPOROSIS

Bruns (1882) was the first to point out that fractures of the forearm and hip were more common in women over the age of 50 years compared to men of the same age. Fuller Albright et al. (1940; 1941) (Figure 1) demonstrated the clear relationship between menopause, oestrogen deficiency and osteoporosis. They found that stilboestrol reversed the condition. Alffram and Bauer (1962)

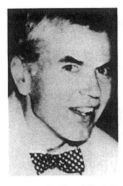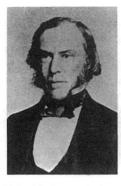

Figure 1 Fuller Albright (left) by kind permission of the Royal Society of Medicine (*see* text)

Figure 2 Charles Edouard Brown-Sequard (1817–1894) (right) was born in Mauritius. He obtained his doctorate in Paris and later became FRCP London, and Physician to the National Hospital, Queen Square, London. He prepared and injected watery solutions of testicular extracts (*see* text). Courtesy of Medvei, V.C. *The History of Clinical Endocrinology* (1993), 2nd edn. pp. 412–13. (UK: Parthenon Publishing)

reported Colles' fractures in 0.5% of women over 70, which was 12 times the incidence for men of the same age. A similar difference was demonstrated for hip fracture (Alhava and Puittinen, 1973). One in three women over the age of 65 developed vertebral fractures, and in older age groups over 30% suffered a fracture of hip.

Nordin *et al.* (1975) estimated that women lose 1% of bone mass each year after cessation of ovarian function. In the following year Heaney (1976) observed that 25% of Caucasian women over the age of 60 years had radiological evidence of vertebral crush fractures. Vertebral crush fractures were usually asymptomatic with less than 1% complaining of pain. Elderly women developed 'dowager's hump' and their height was reduced by probably 2 inches (5 cm). Crilly *et al.* (1978) noted an increased incidence of fractures in White women over the age of 65 years. Gordon (1984) documented that by age 70 a woman had lost 50% of her bone mass while a man had lost only 25% by age 90.

Lindsay and Herrington (1983) estimated that in the years between 1970 and 1980 there was a 40% increase in the annual reported frequency of hip fracture in the USA. Fenton-Lewis (1981) reported similar findings from the UK. In the same year Sweeney and Ashley (1981) reported that fractured neck of femur in postmenopausal women was the third most common cause of bed utilization in National Health hospitals (excluding psychiatric) in England and Wales. Only one-third of the survivors of a hip fracture regained normal activity (Keene and Anderson, 1982). It was estimated that by the end of the decade more than 300 000 hip fractures could be expected per year in the USA with a mortality rate of 10–15% within 6 months of the fracture. The Health Care bill for osteoporosis came to four billion dollars in the USA in 1983 (National Institute of Health Consensus Development Conference, 1984).

TREATMENT

Galen (AD 131–201) advised phlebotomy to allow any 'retained poisons' to be released. In the sixteenth century treatment with purgatives and application of leeches was common. The disturbances suffered by climacteric women were blamed on general debility and anaemia, so in the eighteenth century light exercise and a good diet were advised.

Hormone replacement therapy began when Brown-Sequard (1889) (Figure 2) reported the rejuvenating effects of self-administered injections of testicular extracts, and theorized that ovarian extract would have a beneficial effect in females. The first effective form of hormone replacement therapy was introduced by Murray (1891) who used oral administration of thyroid gland in the treatment of myxoedema. Unfortunately the oral administration of dried ovarian tissue did not prove successful in the postmenopausal female. In 1893 Regas experimented with the injection of ovarian extracts while Chrobak (1896) suggested the use of ovarian grafts. Fraenkel of Berlin described ovarian therapy with a substance obtained from cow or sow ovaries in 1896. Glass grafted ovarian tissue to previously oophorectomized women in 1899. The results were encouraging and led to the technique of implanting ovarian slices under the rectus abdominis muscle (Greenblatt, 1986).

Two decades were to pass before Allen and Doisy (1923) isolated a hormone from pig ovarian follicles (later found to be oestrogen) which induced oestrus in oophorectomized rats. Gruhn and Kazer (1989) stated that 'The first description of the treatment of menopausal symptoms with an oestrogenic compound (a material derived from the amniotic fluid of cattle called Amniotin) was published by Elmer Sevringhaus (1929) of Madison, Wisconsin'. The hormone 'oestrin' was used by Dodds and Robertson (1930) to treat symptomatic women, and 8 years later the synthetic oestrogens stilboestrol and ethinyloestradiol were also used. Bishop (1938) described effective hormone treatment for the first time. Premarin was introduced in 1943 and was derived from pregnant mares' urine (Harding, 1944). Greenblatt and Duran (1949) pioneered the percutaneous implantation of oestradiol implants, which avoided the first-pass liver effect to which oral therapy was subjected.

The publication of *Feminine Forever* by Wilson (1966) brought hormone replacement therapy to the attention of the public, and oestrogens were prescribed in increasing quantities thereafter, particularly for women in the USA. Treatment of the climacteric (in prospective placebo-controlled trials) was investigated by Utian (1972) and Campbell and Whitehead (1977). Utian (1972) noted that oestrogen replacement therapy exerted a mental tonic. The possible danger of hormone replacement therapy was highlighted by Smith *et al.* (1975) who reported an association between the use of cyclical oestrogen therapy and endometrial carcinoma. The report was followed by a massive decline in the number of prescriptions issued for oestrogen products.

Despite that upset, hormone replacement therapy was studied on an ongoing basis. Among other reports Studd (1976) wrote favourably on the use of oestradiol and testosterone implants where there was loss of libido and Campbell and Whitehead (1977) found an average weight increase of 0.5 kg in women on hormone replacement therapy. The conjugated equine oestrogens (Premarin) proved beneficial in the long term for hot flushes, vaginal dryness, insomnia and poor memory. Over the years oestrogens have been administered by mouth, by application of cream, as subcutaneous implants, vaginal rings, or transdermally.

Effects of hormone replacement therapy

Osteoporosis

Christiansen *et al.* (1981) found that women on hormone replacement therapy had significantly more bone mass than non-treated women, and Ettinger *et al.* (1985) noted that the woman in her seventies using hormone replacement therapy had a bone age 10–12 years younger than her chronological age. Women who had more adipose tissue were less affected. Androstenedione which was produced in the adrenal cortex was metabolized to oestrone by the liver, fat, skeletal muscle, kidney, brain and hair follicles. Excess fat led to higher oestrogen levels with some protection against osteoporosis (Siiteri, 1975).

Lindsay *et al.* (1980) first showed that there was a 10-year period of accelerated bone loss after the menopause, but after that, bone loss was not different between men and women. Due to oestrogen replacement therapy bone loss was effectively prevented and vertebral deformities lessened (Lindsay *et al.*, 1980), while fractures of hip and lower forearm were also reduced (Weiss *et al.*, 1980; Kreiger *et al.*, 1982). Although the endocrine status of the individual woman was of great importance other major determinants of bone mass were the genetic endowment of the individual; the amount of mechanical loading imposed on the skeleton; and the nutritional status. Christiansen *et al.* (1981) showed that if hormone replacement therapy was discontinued bone loss commenced again at the same rate as that following a natural menopause.

Breast

Overall statistics show that breast cancer occurs in one of every 11 women in the USA. Its incidence increases throughout a woman's life span and does not peak in any age group. Bittner (1947) first proposed that hormones could increase the incidence of cancer, based on his studies of oestrogens and breast cancer in mice. A cautionary note was sounded when an association between oestrogen replacement therapy and breast cancer in women was reported by Smith *et al.* (1975), Burch *et al.* (1975) and also Hoover *et al.* (1976).

It was decided at the Third International Congress on the Menopause in 1981, that progestogens should be added to hormone replacement therapy for those women who have had a hysterectomy. The additional hormone therapy was to act as a breast protective against the onset of cancer. Some 9 years after the papers which linked hormone therapy with breast cancer, Kaufmann *et al.* (1984) reported from a well-controlled study that oestrogen did not increase the risk of breast cancer. Later in the decade Gambrell (1987) reported a decreased incidence of breast cancer in users of combined oestrogen/progesterone hormonal replacement therapy.

Cardiovascular system

Oliver and Boyd (1959) were among the first to

document the effects of the menopause on plasma lipids and lipoprotein concentrations. It was discovered that women were relatively more immune to coronary heart disease than men. No sex difference pertained however by age 70. Kannel *et al.* (1976) reported that postmenopausal women were three times more likely to suffer coronary heart disease compared with women of the same age who were premenopausal. Heiss *et al.* (1980) determined that low-density lipoprotein (LDL) cholesterol levels were lower in women than men before the age of 50 years. High-density lipoprotein (HDL) concentrations in women exceeded those of men. The LDL/HDL cholesterol ratio remained favourable in women of all ages.

Natural human oestrogens did not affect very low-density lipoprotein (VLDL) levels, but all other oestrogens elevated serum VLDL triglycerides. Natural oestrogens could be used to normalize elevated postmenopausal LDL cholesterol levels (Tikkanan *et al.*, 1978). A reduction in ischaemic heart disease following the use of hormone replacement therapy was demonstrated by Hammond *et al.* (1979). Further evidence of a protective effect was offered by Ross *et al.* (1981) who showed that the administration of conjugated estrogens to postmenopausal women reduced the mortality rate from ischaemic heart disease by a factor of 0.43.

The natural oestrogens, estrone, estradiol, or estriol, were investigated and found not to effect coagulation (Boston Collaborative Drug Surveillance Program, 1974). The possibility of an association between oestrogen replacement therapy and hypertension was first published in 1967, but later reports including that of Hammond *et al.* (1979), failed to find such an association. Coope *et al.* (1975) documented that 'natural oestrogens' were more effective than placebo in reducing hot flushes, and Schiff (1980) found medroxyprogesterone (Provera) to be of benefit.

Endometrium

The annual incidence of endometrial carcinoma in England and Wales (approximately 20 per 100 000) did not alter in response to oestrogen replacement therapy. However, the oestrogen replacement therapy of high dose and prolonged duration was reported to increase the risk of developing the disease (Smith *et al.*, 1975; Ziel and Finkle, 1975; Mack *et al.*, 1976). Cramer and Knapp (1979) determined a risk of 7% for women using oestrogen

replacement therapy (alone) over 15 years compared to 1% for those who did not. Peterson *et al.* (1986) determined that the absolute risk increased from 1 per 1000 in unexposed women to 4 per 1000 per year who were on oestrogen therapy without cyclical progesterones. Jick *et al.* (1979) reported an increased incidence of endometrial carcinoma in New York state during a 14-year period over which the number of women using oestrogen replacement therapy was also increased. A reduced incidence of the disease paralleled the reduction in prescriptions for oestrogen replacement therapy.

Efforts to minimize the risk of endometrial hyperstimulation included routine endometrial biopsy, reducing the oestrogen intake, avoiding oestrone preparations, and prescribing oestriol. Although Albright (1938) had used progesterones to induce withdrawal bleeding, and Greenblatt (1945) suggested cyclic progestogen therapy in oestrogen-treated women the concept of adding progesterone to oestrogen replacement therapy was finally introduced at Wilford Hall USAF Medical Center in 1971 (Gambrell, 1986). Whitehead and Campbell (1978), Paterson *et al.* (1980) and Studd *et al.* (1980) reported that the added progestogens reduced the incidence of cystic and adenomatous hyperplasia (and the risk of endometrial cancer) in patients on hormone replacement therapy. The British Gynaecological Cancer Group (1981) advised that women receiving hormone replacement therapy should have endometrial sampling every 2 years. However, the inclusion of 12 days of progesterone in the oestrogen replacement therapy reduced the incidence of endometrial premalignant change to zero (Whitehead *et al.*, 1982; Studd and Thom, 1981).

Skin

Punnonen (1972) investigated the effects of menopause on the skin. There was gradual thinning with atrophy, and wrinkling attributed to degeneration of elastic and collagenous fibres caused by solar radiation.

Brincat *et al.* (1983) studied the skin in postmenopausal patients and showed that women on hormone replacement therapy had more skin collagen compared to untreated women of the same age. They observed that skin thickness declined after the menopause in a rapid fashion, at a rate similar to the decline in bone mass. In further studies they showed that it was possible to restore skin collagen to premenopausal levels within 6 months of initiating hormone replacement therapy.

Bladder

An association between gynaecological and urological pathology exists, as both the urethra and the vagina develop from the urogenital sinus. Everett (1941) discovered that the vaginal and urethral epithelia were both subject to oestrogenic action. It was later discovered that the sphincteric function of the urethra was also oestrogen dependent and despite previous contradictory studies, a high incidence of urinary incontinence, frequency, nocturia and urgency, was common in climacteric and postmenopausal women (Versi, 1986).

ALTERNATIVE TREATMENTS

In an introduction to non-hormonal medication, Utian (1986) quoted John Leake's statement from 1777 'where the patient is delicate and subject to female weakness, night sweats or an habitual purging, with flushing in the face and a hectic fever: for such; ass's milk, jellies and raw eggs, with cooling fruits will be proper. At meals she may be indulged with half a pint of old, clear London porter, or a glass of Rhenish wine'. Utian also quoted John Burns in 1814 who advised that 'the bowels must be kept open'.

Geist and Mintz (1937) irradiated the pituitary without success and McLaren (1949) used vitamin E but the treatment did not become popular. Appleby (1962) successfully used progesterones in the form of norethisterone to relieve menopausal flushes and later studies showed they were valuable in the prevention of postmenopausal bone loss.

The α-adrenergic agonist clonidine was known to be effective in treating patients with migraine. Menopausal and migraine patients exhibited a similar picture of vasomotor instability and as a result clonidine was assessed as a treatment of 'hot flushes'. Clayden (1972) first observed that clonidine appeared helpful and Clayden et al. (1974) conducted a double-blind cross-over study of the drug. They demonstrated a significant reduction in the number, severity and duration of hot flushes.

Mocquot and Moricard (1936) first drew attention to androgen therapy for menopause symp-toms, and combination treatment with oestrogen and androgen was advocated by Geist and Salmon (1941). Haspels et al. (1978) reported a positive response by the emotional elements of the menopause to the use of vitamin B_6 (pyridoxine). Chesnut et al. (1981) indicated that calcitonin, as a physiological inhibitor of bone resorption, had potential for use in postmenopausal osteoporosis. Veralipride, a benzamide with central antidopaminergic action, was investigated by De Cecco et al. (1981) and found to relieve symptomatic postmenopausal women successfully. It was of particular benefit for hot flushes. Naloxone was also found to decrease the number of hot flushes (Lightman et al., 1981). Ethamsylate, a drug which was principally used for menorrhagia (exerting its action by increasing capillary strength), was reported by Harrison (1981) to reduce hot flushes.

CHRONOLOGY

Age at onset

c. 330 BC	Aristotle suggested 40 years, but possibly 50.
6th C. AD	Aetius suggested between 35 and 50 years.
Medieval Europe	Approximately 50 years.
20th C.	Average age of onset 51 years.

References: Garland (1990) Young (1971)

General

1882	Bruns first documented the increased fracture rate in women over 50 compared to men of the same age.
19th C.	Tilt commented on the 'empty nest syndrome'.
1897	Currier thought menopausal symptoms were mainly found in the upper classes.
1933	A major study (Council of the Medical Women's Federation) discovered troublesome symptoms in 84%.
1938	Hawkinson discovered 75% suffered distressing symptoms.
1940/41	Albright et al. demonstrated the relationship between oestrogen deficiency and osteoporosis.
1959	Oliver and Boyd documented the adverse affects of menopause on plasma lipids.
1962	Alffram and Baeur reported that

Colles' fracture had 12 times the incidence in 70-year-old women compared to men of the same age.

1966   Wilson wrote *Feminine Forever*.

1972   Punnonen investigated the effects of menopause on the skin.

1974   McKinlay and Jeffreys documented 75% of women had hot flushes or night sweats.

1976   Heaney observed that 25% of women over the age of 60 had radiological evidence of vertebral crush fractures.

1981   Sweeney and Ashley reported fracture of femur neck was the third most common cause of bed utilization in the UK.

Treatment

c. 170 AD   Galen advised phlebotomy.

1889   Brown-Sequard pioneered the concept of hormone replacement therapy.

1893   Injected ovarian extract became popular.

1923   Allen and Doisy isolated ovarian hormone (oestrogen).

1929   Sevringhaus treated with amniotin.

1930   Dodds and Robertson used oestrin.

1938   Stilboestrol and ethinyloestradiol were used.
Bishop experimented with oestrin.

1941   Everett documented the effect of oestrogen on the urethra.

1943   Premarin was introduced.

1947   Bittner proposed a link between hormones and breast cancer in mice.

1949   Greenblatt and Duran pioneered oestradiol implants.

1971   Progesterone was added to oestrogen replacement therapy.

1975   Smith *et al.* and others reported an association between oestrogen replacement therapy and breast or endometrial cancer.

1979   Hammond *et al.* reported reduced coronary heart disease when on hormone replacement therapy.

1983   Nevinny-Stickel evaluated the use of a new synthetic steroid Tibolone which displayed weak oestrogenic, androgenic and progestogenic activity and claimed to be without oestrogenic side-effects or withdrawal bleeding.

Alternative treatments

1777   Leake advised ass's milk, fruits and London porter (Utian, 1986).

1814   John Burns advocated an open bowel policy (Utian, 1986).

1936   Mocquot and Moricard advised androgens.

1937   Geist and Mintz used pituitary irradiation.

1972   Clayden found clonidine helpful.

1981   Chesnut *et al.* advised calcitonin.
De Cecco *et al.* advocated the use of Veralipride.
Lightman *et al.* introduced Naloxone.
Harrison pioneered the use of Ethamsylate.

REFERENCES

Aetius of Amida (1950). Translated from the Latin edition of Cornarius (1542) by Ricci, J.V. (Philadelphia: Blakiston)

Albright, F. (1938). Metropathia hemorrhagica. *J. Maine Med. Assoc.*, **29**, 235–8

Albright, F., Bloomberg, E. and Smith, P.H. (1940). Postmenopausal osteoporosis. *Trans. Assoc. Am. Phys.*, **55**, 298–305

Albright, F., Smith, P.H. and Richardon, A.M. (1941). Postmenopausal osteoporosis its clinical features. *J. Am. Med. Assoc.*, **116**, 2465–74

Alffram, P.A. and Bauer, G.C.H. (1962). Epidemiology of fractures of the forearm. *J. Bone Joint Surg.*, **44A**, 105–14

Alhava, E.M. and Puittinen, J. (1973). Fractures of the upper end of the femur as an index of senile osteoporosis in Finland. *Ann. Clin. Res.*, **5**, 398–403

Allen, E. and Doisy, E.A. (1923). An ovarian hormone. A preliminary report on its localization, excretion, and partial purification and action in test animals. *J. Am. Med. Assoc.*, **81**, 819–21

Amudsen, D.W. and Diers, C.J. (1973). The age of the menopause in medieval Europe. *Hum. Biol.*, **45**, 605–8

Appleby, B. (1962). Norethisterone in the control of menopausal symptoms. *Lancet*, **1**, 407–9

Aristotle (1897). *Historia Animalium*, book VII c.350 BC Translated by Creswell, R. (1897) (London: George Bell and Sons)

Baker, T.G. (1963). A quantitative and cytological study of germ cells in human ovaries. *Proc. R. Soc., (London) Ser. B*, **158**, 417–33

Ballinger, C.B. (1975). Psychiatric morbidity and the menopause: screening of general population sample. *Br. Med. J.*, **3**, 344–6

Bishop, P.M.F. (1938). A clinical experiment in oestrin therapy. *Br. Med. J.*, **1**, 939–41

Bishop P.M.F. (1950). Endocrine therapy. In Bowes, K. (ed.) *Modern Trends in Obstetrics and Gynaecology*, Ch. 40, pp. 586–607. (London: Butterworth & Co. Ltd)

Bittner, J.J. (1947). The causes and control of mammary cancer in mice. *Harvey Lecture*, **42**, 221–46

Bloch, E., (1953). Quantitative morphological investigations of the follicular system in newborn female infants. *Acta Anat.*, **17**, 201

Boston Collaborative Drug Surveillance Program (1974). Surgically confirmed gall bladder disease, venous thromboembolism and breast tumours in relation to post-menopausal estrogen therapy. *N. Engl. J. Med.*, **290**, 15–19

Bottiglioni, F. (1981). Sexuality in the menopause. In Van Keep, P.A., Utian, W.H. and Vermeulen, A. (eds.) *The Controversial Climacteric*, pp. 40–1. (Lancaster: MTP Press)

Brincat, M., Moniz, C.E., Studd, J.W.W. *et al.* (1983). Sex hormones and skin collagen content in postmenopausal women. *Br. Med. J.*, **287**, 1337–8

British Gynaecological Cancer Group (1981). Oestrogen replacement and endometrial cancer. Occasional survey. A statement. *Lancet*, **1**, 1359–60

Brown, J.B., Kellar, R. and Matthew, G.D. (1959). Preliminary observations on urinary oestrogen excretion in certain gynaecological disorders. *J. Obstet. Gynaecol. Br. Emp.*, **66**, 177–211

Brown-Sequard, C.E. (1889). Des effets produits chez l'homme par des injections souscutanées d'un liquide retiré des testicules frais de cobaye et de chien. *C.R. Soc. Biol.*, **1**, 415–19

Bruns, P. (1882). Die Allgemaine Lebra von der Knochenbruchen. *Deutsche Chirurgie*, **27**, 1–400

Burch, J.C., Byrd, B.F. and Vaughn, W.K. (1975). The effects of long-term estrogen administration to women following hysterectomy. In Van Keep, P.A. and Lauritzen, C. (eds.) *Estrogens in the Post-Menopause*, pp. 208–14. (Basle: Karger)

Campbell, S. (1975). Psychometric studies on the effect of natural oestrogens in postmenopausal women. In Campbell, S. (ed.) *Management of the Menopause and Postmenopausal Years*, pp. 149–58. (Lancaster: MTP Press)

Campbell, S. and Whitehead, M. (1977). Oestrogen therapy and the menopausal syndrome. In Greenblatt, R.G. and Studd, J.W.W. (eds.) *Clinics in Obstetrics and Gynecology*, Vol. 4, pp. 31–48. (London: W.B. Saunders)

Casper, R.F., Yen, S.S.C. and Wilkes, M.M. (1979). Menopausal flushes: a neuroendocrine link between pulsatile luteinizing hormone secretion. *Science*, **205**, 823–5

Chakravati, S., Collins, W.P. Thom, M.H. and Studd, J.W.W. (1979). Relationship between plasma hormone profiles, symptomatology and response to estrogen in women approaching the menopause. *Br. Med. J.*, **1**, 983–5

Chesnut, C.H., Baylink, D.J., Roos, B.A. *et al.* (1981). In Pecile, A. (ed.) *Calcitonin 1980; Chemistry, Physiology, Pharmacology and Clinical Aspects*, p. 247. (Amsterdam: Excerpta Medica)

Christiansen, C., Christensen, M.S. and Transbol, I. (1981). Bone mass in postmenopausal women after withdrawal of oestrogen/gestagen replacement therapy. *Lancet*, **1**, 459–61

Chrobak, R. (1896). Ueber Einverleibung von Eirstochsgewebe. *Zblatt Gynaekol.*, **20**, 521–4

Clayden, J.R. (1972). Effect of clonidine on menopausal flushing. *Lancet*, **2**, 1361

Clayden, J.R., Bell, J.W. and Pollard, P. (1974). Menopausal flushing: double blind trial of a nonhormonal medication. *Br. J. Med.*, **1**, 409

Coope, J., Thomson, J.M. and Poller, L. (1975). Effects of natural estrogen replacement on menopausal symptoms and blood clotting. *Br. Med. J.*, **4**, 139–43

Council of the Medical Women's Federation (1933). *Lancet*, **1**, 106 quoted by Bishop (1950) p. 602

Cramer, D.W. and Knapp, R.C. (1979). Review of epidemiologic studies of endometrial cancer and exogenous estrogen. *Obstet. Gynecol.*, **54**, 521–6

Crilly, R.G., Horsman, A., Marshall, D.H. and Nordin, B.E.C. (1978). Bone mass in post-menopausal women after withdrawal of oestrogen/gestogen replacement therapy. *Lancet*, **1**, 459–61

Currier, A.F. (1897). *The Menopause*. (New York: Appleton)

De Cecco, L., Venturini, P.L., Alibrandi, M.P. *et al.* (1981). Effet du veralipride sur les taux de LH, FSH et PRL et sur le syndrome climaterique. *Rev. F.R. Gynecol. Obstet*, **76/10**, 691–4

Dodds, E.C. and Robertson, J.D. (1930). Clinical experiments with oestrin. *Lancet*, **1**, 1390–2

Ettinger, B., Genant, H.K. and Cann, C.E. (1985). Long term estrogen replacement therapy prevents bone loss and fractures. *Ann. Intern. Med.*, **102**, 319–24

Everett, H.S. (1941). Urology in the female. *Am. J. Surg.*, **52**, 521

Fenton-Lewis, A. (1981). Fracture of neck of the femur in changing incidence. *Br. Med. J.*, **283**, 1217–20

Franchi, L.L. and Baker, T.G. (1973). Oogenesis and follicular growth. In Hafez, E.S.E. and Evans, T.N. (eds.) *Human Reproduction: Conception and Contraception*, pp. 53–83. (New York, Evanston, San Francisco, London: Harper & Row Hagerstown Md)

Frost, J. (1970). Cytologic evaluation of endocrine status and somatic sex. In *Novak's Textbook of Gynecology*, 8th edn., pp. 666–90. (Baltimore: Williams and Wilkins)

Gambrell, R.D. Jr. (1986). Hormonal replacement therapy and breast cancer. In Greenblatt, R.B. (ed.) *A Modern Approach to the Perimenopausal Years, New Developments in Biosciences*, Vol. 2, pp. 177–88. (Berlin, New York: Walter de Gruyter)

Gambrell, R.D. Jr. (1987). Use of progestogen therapy. *Am. J. Obstet. Gynecol.*, **156**, 1304–13

Garland, R. (1990). *The Greek Way of Life (From Conception to Old Age)*, p. 245. (London: Duckworth & Co. Ltd)

Geist, S.H. and Mintz, M. (1937). Pituitary radiation for the relief of menopause symptoms. *Am. J. Obstet. Gynecol.*, **33**, 643–5

Geist, S.H. and Salmon, U.J. (1941). *J. Am. Med. Assoc.*, **117**, 2207, quoted by Bishop (1950)

Gordon, G.S. (1984). Prevention of bone loss and fractures in women. *Maturitas*, **6**, 225–42

Greenblatt, R.B. (1945). Sexual infantilism in the female. *Western J. Surg. Obstet. Gynecol.*, **53**, 222–6

Greenblatt, R.B. (ed.) (1986). *A Modern Approach to the Perimenopausal Years. New Developments in Biosciences*, Vol. 2 pp. 3–8. (Berlin, New York: Walter de Gruyter)

Greenblatt, R.B. and Duran, R.R. (1949). Indications for hormone pellets in the therapy of endocrine and gynaecological disorders. *J. Obstet. Gynaecol. Br. Emp.*, **51**, 294–301

Gruhn, J.G. and Kazer, R.R. (1989). *Hormonal Regulation of the Menstrual Cycle. The Evolution of Concepts*. p. 187. (New York, London: Plenum Medical Book Co.)

Hammond, C.B., Jelovsek, F.R., Lee, K.C., Creasman, W.T. and Parker, R.J. (1979). Effects of long term estrogen replacement therapy. 1. Metabolic effects *Am. J. Obstet. Gynecol.*, **133**, 525–35

Harding, F.E. (1944). The oral treatment of ovarian deficiency with conjugated estrogens – Equine. *West. J. Surg. Obstet. Gynecol.*, **52**, 31–3

Harkness, R.D. (1962). Historical introduction. In Darson, H. and Grace Eggleton, M. (eds.) *Starling and Lovatt-Evans Principles of Human Physiology*, 13th edn., p. 1387. (London: J. and A. Churchill Ltd.)

Harrison, R.F. (1981). Ethamsylate in the treatment of climacteric flushing. *Maturitas*, **3**, 31–7

Haspels, A.A., Coelingh Bennink, H.J.T. and Schreurs, W.H.P. (1978). Disturbance of tryptophan metabolism and its correction during oestrogen treatment in postmenopausal women. *Maturitas*, **1**, 15

Hawkinson, L.F. (1938). *J. Am. Med. Assoc.*, **111**, 390, quoted by Bishop (1950)

Heaney, R.P. (1976). Estrogens and post-menopausal osteoporosis. *Clin. Obstet. Gynecol.*, **19**, 791–803

Heiss, G., Tamir, I., Davis, C.E., Tyroler, H.A., Rifkind, B.M., Schonfeld, G., Jacobs, D. and Frantz, I.D. (1980). Lipoprotein-cholesterol distributions in selected North American populations: The Lipid Research Clinics Program prevalence study. *Circulation*, **61**, 302–15

Hoover, R., Gray, L.A., Cole, P. and MacMahon, B. (1976). Menopausal estrogens and breast cancer. *N. Engl. J. Med.*, **295**, 401–5

International Academy of Cytology Symposium (1958). Terminology. *Acta Cytologica*, **2**, 63–139

Jick, H. and Porter, J. (1977). Relation between smoking and age of natural menopause. Report from the Boston Collaborative Drug Surveillance

Programe. Boston University Medical Center. *Lancet*, 1, 1354–5

Jick, H., Watkins, R.N., Hunter, J.R., Dinan, B.J., Madsen, S., Rothman, K.J. and Walker, A.M. (1979). Replacement estrogens and endometrial cancer. *N. Engl. J. Med.*, 300, 218–22

Kannel, W.B., Hjortland, M.C., McNamara, P.M. and Gordon, T. (1976). Menopause and risk of cardiovascular disease. The Framingham study. *Ann. Int. Med.*, 85, 447–52

Kaufmann, D.W., Miller, D.R., Rosenburg, L. *et al.* (1984). Noncontraceptive estrogen use and the risk of breast cancer. *J. Am. Med. Assoc.*, 252, 63–7

Keene, J.S. and Anderson, C.A. (1982). *J. Am. Med. Assoc.*, 248, 564, quoted by Notelovitz (1986)

Kreiger, M., Kelsey, J., Holford, T.R. and O'Connor, T. (1982). An epidemiologic study of hip fracture in postmenopausal women. *Am. J. Epidemiol.*, 116, 141–8

Lightman, S.L., Jacobs, H.S. *et al.* (1981). Climacteric flushing: clinical and endocrine response to infusion of naloxone. *Br. J. Obstet. Gynaecol.*, 88, 919–24

Lindsay, R. and Herrington, B.S. (1983). Estrogens and osteoporosis. *Sem. Reprod. Endocrinol.*, 1, 55–67

Lindsay, R., Hart, D.M., Forrest, C. and Baird, C. (1980). Prevention of spinal osteoporosis in oophorectomised women. *Lancet*, 2, 1151–3

Lock, M. (1991). Contested meaning of the menopause. *Lancet*, 337, 1270–2

Mack, T., Pike, M., Henderson, B. *et al.* (1976). Estrogens and endometrial cancer in a retirement community. *N. Engl. J. Med.*, 294, 1262

McKinlay, S.M. and Jeffreys, M. (1974). The menopausal syndrome. *Br. J. Prev. Soc. Med.*, 28, 108–15

McLaren, H.C. (1949). Vitamin E in the menopause. *Br. Med. J.*, 2, 1378–82

Meldrum, D.R., Shamonki, I.M., Frumar, A.M. *et al.* (1979). Elevations of skin temperature of the finger as an objective index of postmenopausal hot flushes: Standardization of the technique. *Am. J. Obstet. Gynecol.*, 135, 713–17

Mocquot, P. and Moricard, R. (1936). *Bull. Soc. Obstet. Gynecol. (Paris)* 25, 787, quoted by Bishop (1950)

Molnar, G.W. (1975). Body temperatures during menopausal hot flushes. *J. Appl. Physiol.*, 38, 499–503

Murray (1891). quoted by Harkness, R.D. (1962).

National Institute of Health Consensus Development Conference (1984). Osteoporosis. *Am. J. Med.*, quoted in Greenblatt (1986) pp. 69–76

Neugarten, B.C. and Kraines, R.J. (1965). "Menopausal symptoms" in women of various ages. *Psychosom. Med.*, 27, 270–84

Nevinny-Stickel, J. (1983). Double-blind cross-over study with Org OD 14 and placebo in postmenopausal patients. *Arch. Gynecol.*, 234, 27–31

Nordin, B.E.C. *et al.* (1975). Post menopausal bone loss. *Curr. Med. Res. Opin.*, 3, Suppl. 28–36

Notelovitz, M. (1986). The influence of nutrition and exercise. In Greenblatt, R.G. (ed.) *A Modern Approach to the Perimenopausal Years, New Developments in Biosciences*, Vol. 2 pp. 109–15. (Berlin, New York: Walter de Gruyer)

Nyklicek, O. (1951). Importance of vaginal cytogram for diagnosis and therapy in the deficiency of estrogenic hormones. *Gynaecologica*, 131, 173–8

Oliver, M.F. and Boyd, G.S. (1959). Effect of bilateral ovariectomy on coronary artery disease and serum lipid levels. *Lancet*, 2, 690–4

Papanicolaou, G. (1933). The sexual cycle in the human as revealed by vaginal smears. *Am. J. Anat.*, 52, Suppl. 3, 519–637

Paterson, M.E.L., Wade-Evans, T., Sturdee, D.W., Thom, M.H. and Studd, J.W.W. (1980). Endometrial disease after treatment with oestrogens and progestogens in the climacteric. *Br. Med. J.*, 1, 822–4

Peterson, H.B., Lee, N.C. and Rubin, G.L. (1986). Genital neoplasia. In Mishell, D.R. (ed.) *Menopause: Physiology and Pharmacology*, pp. 275–98. (Chicago: Year Book Medical Publishers)

Pincus, G., Dorfman, R.I., Romanoff, L.P., Rubin, B.L., Bloch, E., Carlo, J. and Freeman, H. (1955). Steroid metabolosm in aging men and women. *Rec. Progr. Horm. Res.*, 11, 307–41

Punnonen, R. (1972). Effect of castration and peroral estrogen therapy on the skin. *Acta Obstet. Gynecol. Scand.*, Suppl. 21 (5), 1–44

Ross, R.K., Pagnani-Hill, A., Mack, T.M., Arthur,

M. and Henerson, B.E. (1981). Menopausal oestrogen therapy and protection from death from ischaemic heart disease. *Lancet*, **1**, 858–60

Rossle, R. and Roulet, F. (1941). *MaB und Zahl in der Pathologie*. (Berlin: Springer-Verlag)

Schiff, I. (1980). Oral medroxyprogesterone in the treatment of menopausal symptoms. *J. Am. Med. Assoc.*, **244**, 1443–5

Schneider, H.P.G. (1986). The climacteric syndrome. In Greenblatt, R.B. (ed.) *A Modern Approach to the Perimenopausal Years, New Developments in Biosciences*, Vol. 2 pp. 39–55. (Berlin, New York: Walter de Gruyter)

Sevringhaus, E.L. and Evans, J. (1929). Clinical observations on the use of an ovarian hormone: Amniotin. *Am. J. Sci.*, **178**, 638–44

Siiteri, P.K. (1975). Post menopausal oestrogen production. *Frontiers of Hormone Research: Oestrogens in the Post Menopause*, **3**, 40–4

Smith, D.C., Prentice, R., Thompson, D. and Herrman, W. (1975). Association of exogenous estrogens and endometrial cancer. *N. Engl. J. Med.*, **293**, 1164–7, P 202

Studd, J.W.W. (1976). Hormone implants in the climacteric syndrome. In Campbell, S. (ed.) *Management of the Menopause and the Post Menopausal Years*, pp. 383–5. (Lancaster: MTP Press)

Studd, J.W.W. and Thom, M.H. (1981). Oestrogens and endometrial cancer. In Studd, J.W.W. (ed.) *Progress in Obstetrics and Gynaecology*, Vol.1, pp. 182–98. (Edinburgh: Churchill Livingstone)

Studd, J.W.W., Thom, M.H., Paterson, M.E.L. and Wade-Evans, T. (1980). The prevention and treatment of endometrial pathology in postmenopausal women receiving exogenous estrogens. In Pasetto, N., Paoletti, R. and Ambrus, J.L. (eds.) *The Menopause and Postmenopause*, pp. 127–39. (Lancaster: MTP Press)

Sturdee, D.W., Wilson, K.A., Pipili, E. and Crocker, A.D. (1978). Physiological aspects of menopausal hot flush. *Br. Med. J.*, **2**, 79–80

Sweeney, T.K. and Ashley, J.S.A. (1981). Forecasting hospital bed needs. *Br. Med. J.*, **283**, 331–4

Tataryn, I.V., Meldrum, D.R., Lu, K.H. *et al.* (1979). LH, FSH and skin temperature during the menopausal hot flushes. *J. Clin. Endocrinol. Metab.*, **49**, 152–4

Tikkanen, M.J., Nikkila, E.A. and Vartiainen, E. (1978). Natural oestrogen as an effective treatment for type-II hyperlipoproteinaemia in postmenopausal women. *Lancet*, **2**, 490–2

Tilt, E.J. (1887). *The Change of Life in Health and Disease*. (London: Churchill)

Utian, W.H. (1972). The true clinical features of postmenopause and oophorectomy and their response to oestrogen therapy. *S. Afr. Med. J.*, **46**, 732

Utian, W.H. (1980). *Menopause in Modern Perspective*. (New York: Appleton-Century Crofts)

Utian, W.H. (1986). Non-hormonal medication In Greenblatt, R.B. (ed.) *A Modern Approach to the Perimenopausal Years New Developments in Biosciences*, Vol. 2, pp. 117–28. (Berlin, New York: Walter de Gruyter)

Utian, W.H. (1987). Overview on menopause. *Am. J. Obstet. Gynecol.*, **156**, 1280–3

Versi, E. (1986). The bladder in the menopausal woman. In Greenblatt, R.B. (ed.) *A Modern Approach to the Perimenopausal Years New Developments in Biosciences*, Vol. 2, pp. 93–102. (Berlin New York: Walter de Gruyter)

Weiss, N.S., Du, P.H., Ure, C.L., Ballard, J.H., Williams, A.R. and Daling, J.R. (1980). Decreased risk of fractures of the hip and lower forearm with postmenopausal use of estrogen. *N. Engl. J. Med.*, **303**, 1195–9

Whitehead, M.I. and Campbell, S. (1978). In Brush, M.G., King, R.J.B. and Taylor, R.W. (eds.) *Endometrial Cancer*, pp. 65–80. (London: Bailliere Tindall)

Whitehead, M.I., Townsend, P.T., Pryse-Davies, J. *et al.* (1982). Effects of various types and dosages of progestogens on the postmenopausal endometrium. *J. Reprod. Med.*, **27**, 539–48

Wilbush, J. (1979). La Menopausie – the birth of a syndrome. *Maturitas*, **1**, 145–51

Wilson, R.A. (1966). *Feminine Forever*. (London: Mayflower-Dell)

Young, J.Z. (1971). *An Introduction to the Study of Man*. (Oxford: Clarendon Press)

Ziel, H. and Finkle, W. (1975). Increased risk of endometrial carcinoma among users of conjugated estrogens. *N. Engl. J. Med.*, **293**, 1167

FURTHER READING

Bishop, P.M.F. (1950). Endocrine therapy. In Bowes, K. (ed.) *Modern Trends in Obstetrics and Gynaecology*, pp. 586–607. (London: Butterworth & Co. (Publishers) Ltd)

Coissac, P. (ed.) (1985). Postmenopausal Osteoporosis: Prevention and Treatment. *XIth World Congress of Gynecology and Obstetrics Berlin (West)* Sept. 15–20 (Basle: Sandoz)

Greenblatt, R.B. (ed.) (1986). *A Modern Approach to the Perimenopausal Years, new Developments in Biosciences*, Vol. 2. (Berlin, New York: Walter de Gruyter)

Greenblatt, R.B. and Studd, J. (eds.) (1977). *The Menopause, Clinics in Obstetrics and Gynaecology*, Vol. 4/No.1. (London, Philadelphia, Toronto: W.B. Saunders Co. Ltd.)

Judd, H.L. (1987). Oestrogen replacement therapy. In Burger, H.G. (ed.) *Reproductive Endocrinology Baillieres Clinical Endocrinology and Metabolism*, Vol. 1/No.1, pp. 177–206. (London, Philadelphia, Toronto, Mexico City, Sydney, Tokyo, Hong Kong: Bailliere Tindall)

Paterson, M.E.L. (1985). *The Menopause Update Postgraduate Centre Series* (Ayerst International)

Stanton, S.L. (ed.) (1988). *Gynaecology in the Elderly. Clinical Obstetrics and Gynaecology*, Vol. 2, No. 2. (London, Philadelphia, Sydney, Tokyo, Toronto: Bailliere Tindall)

Symposium on Current Perspectives in the Management of the Menopausal and Postmenopausal Patient. (1987). Reprinted from *Am. J. Obstet. Gynecol.*, **156**, 1279–356

Whitehead, M.I. (1985). The climacteric. In Studd, J.W.W. (ed.) *Progress in Obstetrics and Gynaecology*, pp. 332–61. (Edinburgh, London: Churchill Livingstone)

Premenstrual syndrome

Hippocrates of ancient Greece, described how women were subject to 'agitations'. The 'agitated blood' found its way from the head to the uterus whence it escaped the body. He also wrote that 'shivering, lassitude and heaviness of the head' denote the onset and that 'mistiness of vision is resolved by the onset of menstruation' (Bickers and Woods, 1951).

DEFINITIONS

Although premenstrual symptoms were recognized for many years, it was not until 1931 that they were formally identified as a clinical entity, when Robert T. Frank, New York, lectured to his colleagues on the hormonal causes of 'premenstrual tension'. The text was published later in the same year. He referred to women who complained of 'unrest, irritability, a feeling of indescribable tension' and other symptoms, which preceded menstruation by 7–10 days and continued until the menstrual flow occurred. He used roentgen treatment directed at the ovary, with great success.

Morton (1950) of America described 'premenstrual tension' but the term 'premenstrual syndrome' was proposed by Greene and Dalton (1953) as they argued that 'tension' *per se*, was only one of many components of the syndrome. Katherina Dalton (1980) proposed a more strict definition . . . 'the recurrence of symptoms on or after ovulation, increasing during the premenstruum, and subsiding during menstruation, with complete absence of symptoms from the end of menstruation to ovulation'. Four years later, she stated that the symptoms should occur 'exclusively during the second half of the menstrual cycle', and that they should increase in severity as the cycle progressed (Dalton, 1984). They should also always be relieved by the menstrual flow; they should be absent directly after menstruation, and should be present for at least three consecutive menstrual cycles. Many other investigators have also offered definitions.

Taylor (1983) reported from the Premenstrual Syndrome Workshop of the Royal College of Obstetricians and Gynaecologists and they offered the following definition: 'A woman can be said to be suffering from premenstrual syndrome if she complains of regularly recurring psychological or somatic symptoms, or both, which occur specifically during the luteal phase of the cycle. The symptoms must be relieved by the onset of, or during, menstruation; there must be a symptom-free week following menstuation'. In the same year, the National Institute of Mental Health (NIMH) Premenstrual Syndrome Workshop (1983) in the USA specified that there should be a 30% increase in symptom severity in the 5 premenstrual days, compared to the 5 postmenstrual days, in at least two of three cycles.

SYMPTOMS

Frank (1931), Sweeney (1934), Thorn *et al.* (1938) and Israel (1938) were first to describe the symptoms of premenstrual syndrome. Israel reported that women with premenstrual tension suffered 'a cyclic alteration of personality, unreasonable emotional outbursts, headache and nymphomania'. In a report to the *American Journal of Obstetrics and Gynecology*, Moos (1969) noted that over 150 different symptoms of the premenstrual syndrome could be found in the literature. The most commonly reported symptoms were irritability which was sometimes extreme, depression, anxiety, breast swelling and pain, headaches, abdominal bloating, poor concentration, poor co-ordination, food cravings, lethargy, weight gain, and change in libido. Lesser symptoms included acneiform skin eruptions, constipation, mouth ulcers, insomnia, idiopathic bruising, backache and swelling of fingers and ankles. Symptoms could also be divided into physical, psychological, and behavioural changes and were used in symptom clusters for the various menstrual distress questionnaires.

The importance of a strict definition was highlighted by Dalton (1980) (Figure 1) who reported that approximately half of all newly

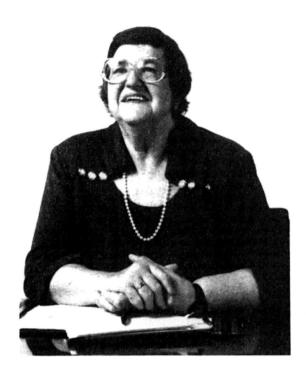

Figure 1   Katharina Dorothea Dalton

referred patients to a premenstrual syndrome clinic were found not to be suffering from premenstrual syndrome. Haskett *et al.* (1980) rejected 80% of the volunteers who claimed severe premenstrual symptoms from their study on the topic.

INCIDENCE

Bickers and Woods (1951) interviewed 1500 factory workers in the USA, and found a 36% incidence of premenstrual syndrome. Figures from 5% to 97% have been reported by Rees (1953a,b) and Sutherland and Stewart (1965). Andersch *et al.* (1986) reported a large study in which 10.8% of sufferers required medical help for their premenstrual syndrome. Brush and Goudsmit (1988) of the Gynaecology Department, St Thomas's Hospital, London, reviewed the literature and reported that 40% of women between the ages of 12 and 50, who were not on the pill, suffered significant premenstrual syndrome symptoms, while 5–10% experienced severe problems. The reported incidence of the premenstrual syndrome varied, depending on the definition, and the sampling procedures used.

AETIOLOGY

Many theories were advanced but putative causes were often refuted by subsequent investigators. Despite this, it was generally held that progesterone levels, and/or their relationship to the oestrogen component in the second half of the cycle were at fault.

Oestrogens

The early report by Frank (1931) indicated that excess oestrogen was to blame, but Israel in 1938 thought that a lack of progesterone was causative. At that time hormonal measurements were indirect, and based on endometrial biopsy. Other workers, including Morton (1950), Greene and Dalton (1953) and Rees (1953a,b), also used indirect assessment, and supported the concept that the progesterone to oestrogen ratio was low in premenstrual syndrome patients.

Progesterones

Plasma estimations of progesterone, and oestrogen or oestradiol, were first carried out in affected women by Bäckström and Carstensen (1974) and Munday (1977). Bäckström and Carstensen compared daily samples from ten women with premenstrual syndrome and eight controls. Low levels of both oestrogen and progesterone were found 4–10 days premenstrually in the premenstrual syndrome group. Munday *et al.*, reported from St Thomas's Hospital, that progesterone levels in premenstrual syndrome women were lower and that the progesterone to oestradiol ratio was higher in controls during the last 8 days of the cycle (Munday *et al.*, 1981).

Vitamins

Vitamins were thought to be implicated from an early stage. Biskind (1943) first suggested vitamin B deficiency, but lack of vitamin B_6 (pyridoxine) was suggested by Brush (1977) as a potential cause of the syndrome, and has continued to be blamed. It was known that in the form of pyridoxal-5-phosphate, vitamin B6 was a co-factor in a number of the body's enzyme reactions, and was a co-enzyme in the production of dopamine from tyrosine, and of serotonin from tryptophan. Rose (1969) and Adams *et al.* (1973) suggested that patients who became depressed on the oral contraceptive pill had a relative deficiency of vitamin B_6 which could be reversed with pyridoxine treatment. This finding was extrapolated to the premenstrual syndrome condition and forms the basis of its treatment with vitamin B_6.

Prolactin

Prolactin was implicated by Friesen et al. (1972), and Horrobin (1973) suggested that prolactin could be responsible for the mental and physical symptoms of the premenstrual syndrome. He further showed that sodium and potassium were retained by the effects of prolactin. Treatment with anti-prolactin agents was found to relieve some symptoms, particularly mastalgia. Magos et al. (1986a) treated postmenopausal women on oestrogen therapy with norethisterone and discovered that a higher dosage of progesterone was related to more intense symptoms.

Aldosterone

Perrini and Pilego (1959) claimed that excess aldosterone was implicated, but premenstrual water retention as measured by weight gain was found to be very slight or absent in a number of studies. No substantial evidence of water retention as a cause of premenstrual syndrome was found.

Prostaglandins

Craig (1980) investigated prostaglandins in the causation of premenstrual syndrome, while Bancroft and Bäckström (1985) reported that a temporal relationship existed in the changes of prostaglandin levels and symptoms.

γ -Linolenic acid

A recent theory to explain premenstrual syndrome related to a deficiency of γ–linolenic acid. Abraham (1983) claimed that premenstrual syndrome was caused by a deficiency of prostaglandin E_1 and could be treated with vegetable oils rich in linolenic acid, thus increasing the synthesis of prostaglandin E_1 at the expense of prostaglandin E_2. Brush (1983) found that γ-linolenic acid, a metabolite of linolenic acid, had significantly lower levels in women with premenstrual syndrome, compared to controls. It was suggested that the women with premenstrual syndrome had a defect in the 6-desaturase enzyme system leading to reduced conversion of cis-linolenic acid to prostaglandin E_1 and that treatment with γ-linolenic acid would help. It was further suggested that women with premenstrual syndrome were abnormally sensitive to normal levels of prolactin. Prostaglandin E_1, which is derived from essential fatty acids, attenuated the biological actions of prolactin; however in the absence of prostaglandin E_1, prolactin had exaggerated effects, including breast tenderness, fluid retention and mood disturbance. Brush (1984) suggested there was a defect in the biosynthetic pathway of essential fatty acids, and Evening Primrose Oil, a rich source of γ-linolenic acid, was used as treatment.

Psychogenic

The psychogenic background to premenstrual syndrome was first explored by Israel in 1938. Clare (1977) pointed out that the symptoms used to score neuroticism overlapped with those of premenstrual syndrome. Takayama (1972) however found that premenstrual syndrome also occurs in mentally retarded women.

Genetic

A genetic tendency was noted by Kantero and Widholm (1971) when they found that 70% of daughters of affected women themselves suffered from premenstrual syndrome, while almost the same percentage of daughters of unaffected mothers were symptom free.

Others

Many other factors have been implicated in premenstrual syndrome including psychological (Israel, 1938), fluid retention (Greenhill and Freed, 1941), hyperinsulinaemia (Billig and Spaulding, 1947), and hypoglycaemia (Morton, 1950).

ASSOCIATED FACTORS

Williams and Weeks (1952) reported on premenstrual syndrome in adolescents. A number of cases may be missed due to a confusion over teenage moodiness or rebellion. Mental symptoms and poor concentration were most common, but sore breasts, headaches and food cravings also occurred. However, abdominal bloating or thickening of fingers or ankles were relatively uncommon (Widholm and Kantero, 1971).

Dalton (1977) noted that the majority of cases started soon after childbirth while Bäckström *et al.* (1981) documented that distressing premenstrual symptoms continued to occur after hysterectomy if the ovaries were conserved.

Premenstrual syndrome was found to have a considerable effect on women in the work place (Lauersen and Stukane, 1983), and in the home (Dalton, 1984). Bancroft *et al.* (1983) reported its effects on sexuality.

ASSESSMENT OF PREMENSTRUAL SYNDROME

Frank in 1931 relied on case histories but Benedek and Rubinstein (1939) analysed patients' dreams, and Silbergeld *et al.* (1971) used a half-hour unstructured interview for their assessment.

Retrospective rating

Moos introduced the menstrual distress questionnaire in 1968 and it became a widely used method. Forty-seven symptoms were rated in severity from 1 to 6, but more recently 116 symptoms were scored 0 to 4. Symptoms were then clustered in eight goups. A premenstrual syndrome self-rating scale was designed and introduced by Steiner *et al.* (1980) which consisted of six symptoms rated on a 'yes' or 'no' response. Halbreich *et al.* (1982) introduced a premenstrual assessment form consisting of 95 items rated 1 to 6.

Prospective rating

The menstrual distress questionnaire and the premenstrual assessment form were used in daily ratings. A daily symptom rating scale was constructed by Taylor (1979a) with 17 symptoms which were rated 0 to 5. A 'profile of mood states' checklist was introduced by McNair *et al.* (1971) which was based on 65 rated items scoring 0 to 4. Visual analogue scales were first used in studies of premenstrual syndrome by O'Brien *et al.* (1979) and the 'prospective record of the impact and severity of menstrual symptomatology' was developed by Reid (1985) which consisted of a 49-day, one page, calendar listing symptoms.

Retrospective versus prospective rating

McCance *et al.* (1937) recognized that there was

poor agreement between mood changes reported retrospectively and prospectively. This finding was confirmed by later workers and it appeared that retrospective rating overestimated the presence and severity of premenstrual syndrome.

DIAGNOSIS

Most physicians based their diagnosis on case history alone, as did Frank in 1931. A distress calendar which related symptoms to a graphic record of the menstrual cycle was evolved by Dalton (1984), and proved most useful. A premenstrual tension 'cator', which allowed women to score their own symptoms throughout the cycle, was introduced by Magos and Studd (1984) and further simplified the diagnostic approach.

TREATMENT

The response to the various forms of active treatment was variable, and there was a high response rate to placebo therapy. Despite that, some forms of treatment were consistently used and remained popular among premenstrual syndrome sufferers.

Progesterones

Gray (1941) reported improvement of symptoms on low-dose progesterone. It was soon found however, that progesterone, if administered orally, was rapidly metabolized and therefore rectal or vaginal suppositories or intramuscular or subcutaneous implants were used. A synthetic oestrogen, dydrogesterone (Duphaston) which was structurally similar to natural progesterone was used to good effect by Taylor (1977), Sampson (1979), Strecker (1980), and Haspels (1981), who showed Duphaston to be significantly more effective than placebo.

Suppression of ovulation

Suppression of ovulation with the oral contraceptive pill was found to reduce the incidence and severity of premenstrual complaints (Moos 1969), although further studies failed to confirm that benefit. Magos *et al.* (1983; 1984) used oestradiol implants with high rates of success, and gonadotropin releasing hormone (GnRH) therapy was used by Muse (1984) and by West *et al.* (1989) with considerable success.

Bromocriptine

Bromocriptine was found to be a useful agent in studies by Cole *et al.* (1975) and by Benedek-Jaszmann and Hearn-Sturtevant (1976). The treatment was particularly valuable for breast pain and discomfort.

Danazol

Danazol was also found to be particularly effective for severe breast discomfort and mood disturbance at a dose of 200 mg daily (Watts *et al.*, 1985). The prostaglandin inhibitor mefenamic acid was found to improve the symptoms of tension, irritability, depression and headaches (Wood and Jakubowicz, 1980).

Diuretics

Diuretics were helpful if the woman's principal symptoms related to swelling, bloatedness, weight gain or fluid retention. O'Brien *et al.* (1979) reported that the aldosterone antagonist spironolactone, at a dose of 25 mg twice daily from days 18–26 of the cycle was effective in relieving fluid retention, and that potassium depletion was avoided.

Pyridoxine and evening primrose oil

Many patients however found that pyridoxine (vitamin B6) and γ-linolenic acid (Evening Primrose Oil) were of major benefit in reducing pre-menstrual symptoms. Both compounds were available without prescription, in pharmacies and health food stores, so self-diagnosis and management became popular. Despite the fact that Stokes and Mendels (1972) found pyridoxine no better than placebo in a double-blind study, it continued to be popular. O'Brien (1987) recommended a dose not higher than 100 mg pyridoxine daily for long-term use as higher doses than that were reported to cause sensory neuropathy by Schaumburg *et al.* (1983) and by Dalton (1985).

Physical symptoms, particularly breast tenderness, were found to respond well to use of Evening Primrose Oil in a study by Brush (1983). A dose of two or three 500-mg capsules of Evening Primrose Oil twice daily after food, from 3 days before the expected start of symptoms until the onset of menstruation was advised. Supplementation of the Evening Primrose Oil with pyridoxine, niacin, ascorbic acid and zinc appeared to increase the efficacy of the product.

Self-help

An article by Diana Sanders (1987) detailed the importance of diet, adequate relaxation, exercise, herbal remedies and 'self-help' groups for the premenstrual syndrome sufferer. She suggested that 'the first step towards health is for the individual to come to terms with premenstrual syndrome and realize that her problems are real and shared by other women. Talking about it is a great help . . . a useful start is advice about what the woman can do to help herself; if problems persist a number of medical treatments can be tried . . . perseverance is often necessary . . . women with severe and persistent problems can be referred on to a specialist premenstrual syndrome clinic'.

MEDICO-LEGAL ASPECTS

In 1890 Icard cited a study by Le Grand Du Saulle, who found that 35 of 56 Parisienne shop lifters committed their offence during menstruation. Icard wrote that the premenstrual woman is subject to kleptomania, pyromania, dipsomania, nymphomania, delusions, acute mania, delirious lying, calumny, illusions, hallucinations and melancholia (O'Brien, 1987). Four years later Lombroso and Ferrero in Italy reported that 71 of 80 women arrested for resistance to public officials were menstruating at the time of their offence. Gudden reported from Germany in 1907 that, in cases investigated for shop lifting, practically all had occurred during a menstrual period.

In 1845 Martha Brixley, a domestic servant, murdered one of her employers' children, but was acquitted as she was suffering from 'obstructed menstruation' and 6 years later Amelia Snoswell was acquitted of murdering her baby niece on the grounds of insanity due to disordered menstruation. In 1980 a 30-year-old bar-maid stabbed and killed a fellow worker, but at the Central Criminal Court was found to have diminished responsibility on the grounds of premenstrual syndrome. In 1981, a 37-year-old woman with a past history of depressive illness and premenstrual tension had a stormy relationship with a man, and when subjected to considerable provocation, drove her car at him. He subsequently died. She pleaded guilty to manslaughter on the grounds of diminished responsibility as the offence was committed shortly before the onset of menstruation (d'Orban, 1983).

In 1980 d'Orban and Dalton investigated females in a remand prison and found that significantly more offences occurred on the 28th, and 1st days of the cycle. It was concluded that women who committed offences of violence were significantly more liable to do so during their paramenstruum. d'Orban (1983) stated that 'it would be unjustifiable to assume that women are generally more liable to commit offences during the paramenstruum; the association may only apply in a sub-group of female offenders who are also prone to psychological or behavioural disturbances at other times of the menstrual cycle. On its own, premenstrual syndrome as a defence to a charge of murder is not likely to succeed . . . '

CHRONOLOGY

Definitions

1931	Frank described 'premenstrual tension' in 15 women. They presented with a variety of complaints including depression, irritability and tension, which occurred 7 to 10 days prior to menstruation and were relieved by the menstrual flow.
1953	Greene and Dalton introduced the term 'premenstrual syndrome'.
1964	Dalton defined the premenstrual syndrome as a variety of cyclical symptoms, usually occurring during the premenstrual or early menstrual phase but occasionally also at ovulation.
1969	Moos reviewed the literature and discovered over 150 different symptoms relating to premenstrual syndrome.
1977	Dalton considered that if even one or two symptoms persisted throughout the cycle, premenstrual syndrome did not exist but a condition of 'menstrual distress' was present.
1980	Dalton further defined premenstrual syndrome – 'The recurrence of symptoms on or after ovulation, increasing during the premenstruum and subsiding during menstruation, with complete absence of symptoms from the end of menstruation to ovulation'.

1981	Reid and Yen included the criterium of 'severity' in their definition.
1983	Abraham defined four sub-groups of premenstrual tension: anxiety and depression; weight gain and bloating; carbohydrate cravings and headaches. Taylor reported a definition adopted at the Royal College of Obstetricians and Gynaecologists. The National Institute of Mental Health (NIMH) in the USA reported their definition.
1984	Dalton stressed that the symptoms should occur exclusively during the second half of the cycle and increase in severity as the cycle progressed. They should be relieved by the onset of full menstrual flow and should be absent directly after the period. They should also be present for at least three cycles.
1987	O'Brien listed 88 common symptoms.

Incidence and prevalencce

1951	Bickers and Woods found a prevalence rate of 36%.
1953	Rees reported a low percentage of women to have premenstrual syndrome.
1979–1984	Brush reported 40% of women not on the pill experienced significant premenstrual symptoms. 5–10% had severe symptoms.
1980	Andersch found that approximately 10% of women would like help, and 3% reported severe symptoms.
1981	Reid and Yen found 70–90% of women reported regular premenstrual symptoms and 20–40% had temporary mental or physical disability.
1982	Hargrove and Abraham estimated an incidence of 50%.

Symptoms

1931	Frank documented the 'indescribable tension and irritability' present from 7 to 10 days preceding menstruation.
1937	McCance et al. found that retrospective recollections of symptoms bore no relationship to the mood changes found on daily recording.

1938   Israel reported 'a cyclic alteration of personality, unreasonable emotional outbursts, headache and nymphomania'.

1964   Dalton defined psychological and physical symptoms.

1980   Haskett *et al.* found that irritability, swelling, depression, painful or tender breasts, tension and mood swings were the most common symptoms.

Dalton documented that almost half of the patients referred to a premenstrual syndrome clinic were not suffering from the condition.

Associated factors

1977   Dalton reported that most cases started soon after childbirth.

1980   Andersch reported that premenstrual symptoms were less in patients using the oral contraceptive pill.

1982   Parlee found that changes in work performance do not occur for most women, as affected women increase their concentration and effort at the time.

1983   Bancroft *et al.* found that sexual activity was more common after menstruation, when the patients general well-being was improved.

Sanders *et al.* reported that women prone to the postnatal blues or who could not tolerate the oral contraceptive, were likely to develop premenstrual syndrome.

1984   Dalton reported many events which were exacerbated in the premenstrual phase of the cycle.

1987   Brush *et al.* observed that in almost 33% of their cases, premenstrual symptoms started at or close to the menarche. The largest number however started soon after childbirth. Tubal ligation, hysterectomy with ovarian conservation, and discontinuing the oral contraceptive pill were all associated with premenstrual syndrome.

Work

1983   Lauersen and Stukane discussed the problems of premenstrual syndrome in relation to work.

Family

1985   Harrison outlined the interfamilial problems due to the condition.

Teenagers

1952   Williams and Weeks reported premenstrual syndrome in teenage years.

1960   Wenzel documented premenstrual syndrome affecting teenagers.

1971   Widholm and Kantero found that premenstrual syndrome symptoms in teenagers were mainly related to the psychological element. They reported an almost 40% incidence of premenstrual syndrome, with irritability, tension and fatigue as main symptoms.

Causation

1981   Bäckström *et al.* noted that premenstrual syndrome could occur posthysterectomy, if the ovaries were conserved.

Oestrogens

1931   Frank proposed that premenstrual syndrome was due to excess oestrogen.

1950   Morton induced premenstrual syndrome by intramuscular injection of oestrogen.

1974   Bäckström and Carstensen showed that plasma oestrogen concentrations were significantly elevated in the premenstrual phase.

1979   Andersch *et al.* found no difference in premenstrual oestrogen levels.

Taylor also found no difference in oestrogen levels.

1981   Munday *et al.* showed increased oestrogen levels premenstrually.

Progesterone deficiency

1938   Israel conjectured that progesterone deficiency, due to inadequate corpus luteum function, was causative.

1974   Bäckström and Carstensen found lower plasma progesterone concentrations premenstrually.

1975   Smith found mean plasma levels of progesterone were lower in the premenstrual phase.

1976   Smith documented low progesterone levels premenstrually.

1977   Munday performed plasma estimations of progesterone and oestrogen and found low progesterone levels.

1979   Andersch et al did not confirm low levels of progesterone.

1980   O'Brien et al found elevated plasma progesterone levels premenstrually in women with premenstrual syndrome vs. controls.

Oestrogen: progesterone ratio

1974   Bäckström and Carstensen documented a high oestrogen: progesterone ratio premenstrually in the condition.

Fluid retention

1941   Greenhill and Freed theorized that abnormal sodium and water metabolism induced the physical symptoms of premenstrual syndrome.

1959   Perrini and Pilego claimed an excess of aldosterone was causative.

1964   Dalton proposed that excessive aldosterone action was involved.

1979   O'Brien et al noted that although some patients complained of bloatedness, no weight gain was found, and this suggested that changes occurred within the extra- and intravascular compartments.

Prolactin

1972   Friesen et al reported higher prolactin levels than in controls.

1973   Horrobin theorized that prolactin, which causes retention of sodium, potassium and water, could have a role to play.

1976   Halbreich et al. found that premenstrual syndrome patients had a higher mean prolactin level in the premenstrual phase.

1979   Brush found raised prolactin and low progesterone levels in premenstrual syndrome.

Vitamin deficiency

1943   Biskind implicated vitamin B.

1969   Rose indicated that a relative deficiency of vitamin B_6 was causative of depression in women on the oral contraceptive pill.

1973   Winston noted that some women on the oral contraceptive pill became depressed. The condition appeared secondary to the development of pyridoxine deficiency due to pill use. Subsequently a deficiency of pyridoxine was implicated in causation of premenstrual syndrome.

1977   Brush suggested that pyridoxine deficiency was a potential cause.

Prostaglandins

1980   Craig suggested that altered prostaglandin metabolism with excess production of prostaglandin E_2 and F_2 was involved.

Wood and Jakubowicz implicated protaglandin activity.

1985   Bancroft and Bäckström found that the change in prostaglandin levels was related to premenstrual syndrome symptomotology.

Deficiency of essential fatty acids

1983   Horrobin noted that in patients with a deficiency of essential fatty acids, prolactin had exaggerated effects and caused premenstrual symptoms.

Abraham postulated that premenstrual syndrome was caused by prostaglandin E_1 deficiency.

1984   Brush et al noted reduction in linolenic acid metabolites which suggested a defect in the biosynthetic pathway of essential fatty acids.

Brush found that metabolites of linolenic acid, e.g. γ-linolenic acid, were significantly lower in level than in controls.

Psychological/psychogenic

1938   Israel considered that there was a large psychological component.

1963   Coppen and Kessel found that neuroticism and severe premenstrual syndrome were positively correlated.

1965   Coppen claimed that premenstrual syndrome sufferers had an underlying primary affective disorder.

1967   Mandell and Mandell noted increased numbers of suicide and suicide attempts in the premenstrual phase.

1972   Takayama found that premenstrual syndrome occurred in the mentally retarded in whom emotional disturbances are not usually seen.

1977   Clare found that the symptoms used to score neuroticism overlap heavily with those used to score premenstrual syndrome.

1989   Stout reviewed the psychiatric diagnoses and personality factors associated with premenstrual syndrome.

Social/genetic

1971   Kantero and Widholm found that 70% of daughters born to women with premenstrual syndrome, suffer the same complaint. Only 37% of those born to non-sufferers develop the syndrome.

1974   Rosseinsky and Hall postulated that the manifested premenstrual symptoms rejected the male, but increased his ardour for the next postmenstrual engagement.

Hyperinsulinaemia/hypoglycaemia

1947   Billig and Spaulding suggested that hyperinsulinism with hypoglycaemia in the premenstrual phase was causative.

1950   Morton proposed reactive hypoglycaemia to be an important factor in premenstrual syndrome.

Allergy

1947   Zondek and Bromberg suggested that an allergic or hypersensitivity reaction to the patients' endogenous hormones or their metabolites could be causative.

Diagnosis

1963   Coppen and Kessel indicated that premenstrual syndrome probably constituted several syndromes, rather than a single identity.

1968   Moos developed the 'Moos Menstrual Distress Questionnaire'. There were 47 symptoms in eight related groups.

1984   Magos and Studd developed a diagnostic disc which they called a 'PMT-Cator'

        Magos et al. found that 40% of premenstrual syndrome patients had suffered postpartum depression compared to a 10% incidence for 'normal' patients.

Assessing premenstrual syndrome

Retrospective rating

1931   Frank relied on case history alone.

1939   Benedek and Rubinstein used dream analysis in their rating.

1968   Moos developed the menstrual distress questionnaire.

1971   Silbergeld et al. used a half hour unstructured interview.

1980   Steiner et al. designed the premenstrual tension self-rating scale.

1982   Halbreich et al. introduced the premenstrual assessment form.

Prospective rating

1971   McNair et al. devised the 'profile of mood states'.

1979   Taylor constructed the 'daily symptom rating scale'.

        O'Brien et al. used the 'visual analogue scale'.

1982   Halbreich et al. introduced a 'premenstrual assessment form'.

1984   Dalton advocated a record chart showing the relationship of symptoms to menstruation.

1985   Reid developed the 'prospective record of the impact and severity of menstrual symptomotology'.

Retrospective versus prospective rating

1937   McCance *et al.* recognized that there was poor agreement between mood rated retrospectively and prospectively.

1985   Metcalf and Hudson showed that retrospective ratings overestimated the presence and severity of premenstrual syndrome.

Treatment

Progesterone

1941   Gray used low-dose progesterone treatment to good effect.

1953   Based on a concept of Greene and Dalton, that progesterone deficiency was causative, progesterone treatment was instituted by vaginal or rectal pessaries, or progesterone injections. Rees reported beneficial effects of progesterone treatment.

1975   Smith carried out a double-blind study comparing placebo and progesterone. Progesterone was not found more effective.

1977   Taylor introduced dydrogesterone, a synthetic, orally active progesterone.

1979   Sampson reported that placebo was as effective as progesterone by suppository.

1980   Kerr *et al.* found that the synthetic progesterone, dydrogesterone (Duphaston) was superior to placebo. Strecker reported that dydrogesterone was of benefit in alleviating premenstrual depression, headaches and oedema.

1981   Haspels carried out a double-blind, placebo-controlled, multicentre study on the efficacy of dydrogesterone (Duphaston). Dydrogesterone was found to be significantly better than placebo. It relieved the depression but not the other symptoms of premenstrual syndrome.

1982   Ylostalo *et al.* found that norethisterone alleviated breast tenderness.

1985   Dennerstein *et al.* used oral progesterone and found it superior to placebo.

Suppression of ovulation

1969   Moos determined that patients on the oral contraceptive pill had a reduced incidence and severity of premenstrual syndrome, especially the psychological symptoms.

1971   Goldzieher *et al.* found that treatment with placebo was as effective as 'the pill'.

1977   Greenblatt *et al.* used oestradiol implants to suppress ovulation, and this technique was later used by Magos *et al.*

1984   Magos *et al.* reported that 97% of women had almost complete relief of premenstrual symptoms, with use of oestradiol implants, while 83% of women were cured of their menstrual migraine (1983).
Muse *et al.* used gonadotropin releasing hormone agonists and symptoms were reduced.

1986   Magos *et al.* used subcutaneous oestradiol implants to good effect.

1989   West *et al.* used the gonadotropin releasing hormone agonist goserelin and showed significant improvement in premenstrual symptoms.

Pyridoxine (vitamin B_6)

1972   Stokes and Mendels reported that pyridoxine was not better than placebo treatment.

1977   Kerr found pyridoxine was helpful to some extent.

1983   Schaumburg *et al.* found that pyridoxine should not be used in doses exceeding 500 mg daily.

1985   Hagen *et al.* did not find any difference between treatment by placebo or pyridoxine.
Dalton noted pyridoxine overdose in a patient with premenstrual syndrome.

1987   O'Brien advised a dose of only 100 mg pyridoxine daily for long-term use.

Bromocriptine

1975   Cole and *et al.* reported beneficial effects when using the dopamine agonist bromocriptine.

1976   Benedek-Jaszmann and Hearn-Sturtevant found an improvement in breast symptoms, oedema, weight gain and mood.

γ-Linolenic acid : Evening Primrose Oil

1983   Brush reported a good response for physical symptoms especially breast tenderness.

1989   Cerin and *et al.* reported no difference between Evening Primrose Oil and placebo.

Diuretics and aldosterone antagonists

1979   O'Brien *et al.* reported that the aldosterone antagonist spironolactone, which was effective for relieving fluid retention, did not cause potassium depletion.

Danazol

1985   Watts *et al.* found that Danazol, at a dose of 200 mg daily, was effective, particularly for severe breast discomfort and excessive mood disturbance.

Prostaglandin inhibitors

1980   Wood and Jakubowicz used mefenamic acid and found significant improvement in mental symptoms.

1984   Jakubowicz *et al.* treated patients with mefenamic acid to good effect.

REFERENCES

Abraham, G.E. (1983). Nutritional factors in the etiology of the premenstrual tension syndromes. *J. Reprod. Med.*, **28**, 446–64

Adams, P.W., Rose, D.P., Folkard, J., Wynn, V., Seed, M. and Strong, R. (1973). Effect of pyridoxine hydrochloride (vitamin B6) upon depression associated with oral contraception. *Lancet*, **1**, 897

Andersch, B. (1980). *Epidemiological, hormonal and water balance studies on premenstrual tension*. Thesis, University of Goteburg, quoted by Hammarbäck (1989)

Andersch, B., Abrahamsson, L., Wendestam, C., Ohman, R. and Hahn, L. (1979). Hormone profile in premenstrual tension: effects of bromocriptine and diuretics. *Clin. Endocrinol.*, **11**, 657–64

Andersch, B., Wendestam, C., Hahn, L. and Ohman, R. (1986). Premenstrual complaints. I. Prevalence of premenstrual symptoms in a Swedish urban population. *J. Psychosom. Obstet. Gynaecol*, **5**, 39–49

Bäckström, T. and Carstensen, H. (1974). Estrogen and progesterone in plasma in relation to premenstrual tension. *J. Steroid Biochem.*, **5**, 257–60

Bäckström, T., Boyle, H. and Baird, D.T. (1981). Persistence of symptoms of premenstrual tension in hysterectomized women. *Br. J. Obstet. Gynaecol.*, **88**, 530–6

Bancroft, J. and Bäckström, T. (1985). Premenstrual syndrome. *Clin. Endocrinol.*, **22**, 313–36

Bancroft, J., Sanders, D., Davidson, D. and Warner, P. (1983). Mood, sexuality, hormones and the menstrual cycle. III. Sexuality and the role of androgens. *Psychosom. Med.*, **45**, 509–16

Benedek, T. and Rubinstein, B.B. (1939). The correlations between ovarian activity and psychodynamic process. *Psychosom. Med.*, **1**, 461–85

Benedek-Jaszmann, L.J. and Hearn-Sturtevant, M.D. (1976). Premenstrual tension and functional infertility *Lancet*, **1**, 1095

Bickers, W. and Woods, M. (1951). Premenstrual tension – rational treatment. *Tex. Rep. Biol. Med.*, **9**, 406–7

Billig, H.E. Jr. and Spaulding, C.A. Jr. (1947). Hyperinsulinism of menses. *Ind. Med.*, **16**, 336

Biskind, M.S. (1943). Nutritional deficiency in the etiology of menorrhagia, metrorrhagia, cystic mastitis and premenstrual tension; treatment with vitamin B complex. *J. Clin. Endocrinol.*, **3**, 227

Brush, M.G. (1977). The possible mechanisms causing the premenstrual tension syndrome. *Curr. Med. Res. Opin.*, **4** (Suppl. 4), 9

Brush, M.G. (1979a). Endocrine and other biochemical factors in the aetiology of the premenstrual syndrome. *Curr. Med. Res. Opin.*, **6** (Suppl. 5), 19

Brush, M.G. (1979b). *Premenstrual Syndrome and Period Pains*. (London: Womens Health Concern)

Brush, M.G. (1983). Efamol (gamma-linolenic acid) in the treatment of the premenstrual syndrome. In Horrobin, D.F. (ed.) *Clinical Uses of Essential Fatty Acids.* (New York: Rowen)

Brush, M.G. (1984). *Understanding Premenstrual Tension.* Book B p.11. (London: Pan)

Brush, M.G. and Goudsmit, E.M. (eds.) (1988). *Functional Disorders of the Menstrual Cycle*, pp. 1–13. (Chichester, New York, Brisbane, Toronto, Singapore: John Wiley & Sons)

Brush, M.G., Watson, S.J., Horrobin, D.F. and Manker, M.S. (1984). Abnormal essential fatty acid levels in plasma of women with premenstrual syndrome. *Am. J. Obstet. Gynecol.*, **150**, 363–6

Brush, M.G., Bennett, T. and Hansen, K. (1987). *A retrospective report on the use of pyridoxine in the treatment of premenstrual syndrome (PMS) at St Thomas's Hospital and Medical School 1976–1983*, quoted by Brush M.G. and Goudsmith E.M. (1988)

Cerin, A., Andersson, L., Collins, A., Landgren, B-M. and Eneroth, P. (1989). Effect of Efamol (gammalinolenic acid) treatment in women with premenstrual tension syndrome. *J. Psychosom. Obstet. Gynaecol.*, **10** (Suppl. 1), 153

Clare, A.W. (1977). Psychological profiles of women complaining of premenstrual symptoms. *Curr. Med. Res. Opin.*, **4** (Suppl. 4), 23

Cole, E.N., Evered, D., Horrobin, D.F., Manku, M.S., Mtabji, J.B. and Nassar, B.A. (1975). Is prolactin a fluid and electrolyte regulating hormone in man? *J. Physiol.*, **252**, 54–5

Coppen, A. (1965). The prevalence of menstrual disorders in psychiatric patients. *Br. J. Psychiatr.*, **111**, 155–67

Coppen, A. and Kessel, N. (1963). Menstruation and personality. *Br. J. Psychiatr.*, **109**, 711–21

Craig, G. (1980). The premenstrual syndrome and prostaglandin metabolism. *Br. J. Fam. Planning*, **6**, 74–7

Dalton, K. (1964). *The Premenstrual Syndrome.* (London: Heinemann)

Dalton, K. (1977). *Premenstrual Syndrome and Progesterone Therapy.* (London: Heinemann)

Dalton, K. (1980). Progesterone, fluid and electrolytes in premenstrual syndrome. *Br. Med. J.*, **281**, 61

Dalton, K. (1984). *The Premenstrual Syndrome and Progesterone Therapy*, 2nd edn. (London: Heinemann)

Dalton, K. (1985). Pyridoxine overdose in premenstual syndrome: letter. *Lancet*, **1**, 1168–9

Dennerstein, L., Spencer-Gardner, C., Gotts, G., Brown, J.B., Smith, M.A. and Burrows, G.D. (1985). Progesterone and the premenstrual syndrome: a double blind crossover trial. *Br. Med. J.*, **290**, 1617–21

d'Orban, P.T. (1983). Medicolegal aspects of the premenstrual syndrome. *Br. J. Hosp. Med.*, **30**, 404–9

Frank, R.H.T. (1931). The hormonal causes of premenstrual tension. *Arch. Neurol. Psychiatr.*, **26**, 1053–7

Friesen, H.G., Hwang, P., Guyda, H., Tolis, G., Tyson, J. and Myers, R. (1972). In Boyes, A.R. and Griffiths, K. (eds.) *Prolactin and Carcinogenesis: Radioimmunoassay for Human Prolactin*, p. 64. (Cardiff: Alpha Omega Alpha Publishing Co.)

Goldzieher, J.W., Moses, L.E., Averkin, E., Scheel, C. and Taber, B.Z. (1971). Nervousness and depression attributed to oral contraceptives: a double-blind, placebo-controlled study. *Am. J. Obstet. Gynecol.*, **111**, 1013–20

Gray, L.A. (1941). The use of progesterone in nervous tension states. *South African Med. J.*, **34**, 1004–6

Greenblatt, R.B., Asch, R.H., Mahesh, V.B. and Bryner, J.R. (1977). Implantation of pure crystalline pellets of estradiol for conception control. *Am. J. Obstet. Gynecol.*, **127**, 520–4

Greene, R. and Dalton, K. (1953). The premenstrual syndrome. *Br. Med. J.*, **1**, 1007–14

Greenhill, J.P. and Freed, S.C. (1941). The electrolyte therapy of premenstrual distress. *J. Am. Med. Assoc.*, **117**, 504–6

Hagen, I., Nesheim, B.I. and Tuntland, T. (1985). No effect of vitamin B-6 against premenstrual tension. A controlled clinical study. *Acta Obstet. Gynaecol. Scand.*, **64**, 667–70

Halbreich, U., Ben-David, M., Assael, M. and Bornstein, R. (1976). Serum prolactin in women with premenstrual syndrome. *Lancet*, **2**, 654

Halbreich, U., Endicott, J., Schacht, S. and Nee, J. (1982). The diversity of premenstrual changes as reflected in the Premenstrual Assessment Form. *Acta Psychiatr. Scand.*, **65**, 46–65

Hammarbäck, S. (1989). The premenstrual syndrome. A study of its diagnosis and pathogenesis. *Acta Obstet. Gynaecol. Scand.*, Suppl. 151, 17

Hargrove, J.T. and Abraham, G.E. (1982). The incidence of premenstrual tension in a gynecologic clinic. *J. Reprod. Med.*, **27**, 721–6

Harrison, M. (1985). *Self-help for Premenstrual Syndrome*, 2nd edn. (New York: Random House)

Haskett, R.F., Steiner, M., Osmun, J.N. and Caroll, B.J. (1980). Severe premenstrual tension: delineation of the syndrome. *Biol. Psychiatr.*, **15**, 121

Haspels, A.A. (1981). A double-blind, placebo-controlled, multi-centre study of the efficacy of dydrogesterone 'Duphaston' In van Keep, P.A. and Utian, W.H. (eds.) *The Premenstrual Syndrome*, pp. 81–92. (Lancaster: MTP Press)

Horrobin, D.F. (1973). *Prolactin: Physiology and Clinical Significance.* (Lancaster: MTP Press)

Horrobin, D.F. (1983). The role of essential fatty acids and prostaglandins in the premenstrual syndrome. *J. Reprod. Med.*, **28**, 465–8

Israel, S.L. (1938). Premenstrual tension. *J. Am. Med. Assoc.*, **110**, 1721–3

Jakubowicz, D.L., Goddard, E. and Dewhurst, J. (1984). The treatment of premenstrual tension with mefenamic acid; analysis of prostaglandin concentrations. *Br. J. Obstet. Gynaecol.*, **91**, 78–84

Kantero, R.L. and Widholm, O. (1971). Correlations of menstrual traits between adolescent girls and their mothers. *Acta Obstet. Gynaecol. Scand.*, **14** (Suppl.14), 30

Kerr, G.D. (1977). The management of the premenstrual syndrome. *Curr. Med. Res. Opin.*, **4** (Suppl. 4), 29

Kerr, G.D., Day, J.B., Munday, M.R., Brush, M.G., Watson, M. and Taylor, R.W. (1980). Dydrogesterone in the treatment of the premenstrual syndrome. *Practitioner*, **224**, 852

Lauersen, N.H. and Stukane, E. (1983). *Premenstrual Syndrome and You.* (New York: Pinnacle)

McCance, R.A., Luff, M.C. and Widdowson, E.E. (1937). Physical and emotional periodicity in women. *J. Hygiene*, **37**, 571–610

McNair, D.M., Lorr, M. and Droppleman, L.F. (1971). *Profile of Mood States Manual.* (San Diego: Educational and Industrial Testing Service)

Magos, A.L. and Studd, J.W.W. (1984) The premenstrual syndrome. In Studd, J. (ed.) *Progress in Obstetrics and Gynaecology*, Vol. 4, pp. 334–50. (Edinburgh, London, Melbourne, New York: Churchill Livingstone)

Magos, A.L., Zilkha, K.J. and Studd, J.W.W. (1983). Treatment of menstrual migraine by oestradiol implants. *J. Neurol. Neurosurg. Psychiatr.*, **46**, 1044–6

Magos, A.L., Collins, W.P. and Studd, J.W.W. (1984). Management of the premenstrual syndrome by subcutaneous implants of oestradiol. *Proceedings of the 3rd International Congress on the Menopause*, Antwerp

Magos, A.L., Brewster, E., Sing, R., O'Dowd, T.M. and Studd, J.W.W. (1986a). The effect of norethisterone in postmenopausal women on oestrogen therapy: a model for the premenstrual syndrome. *Br. J. Obstet. Gynaecol.*, **93**, 1290–6

Magos, A., Brincat, M. and Studd, J.W. (1986b). Treatment of the premenstrual syndrome by subcutaneous estradiol implants and cyclical oral norethisterone: placebo controlled study. *Br. Med. J.*, **292**, 1629–33

Mandell, A.J. and Mandell, M.P. (1967). Suicide and the menstrual cycle. *J. Am. Med. Assoc.*, **200**, 792–3

Metcalf, M.G. and Hudson, S.M. (1985). The premenstrual syndrome: selection of women for treatment trials. *J. Psychosom. Res.*, **29**, 631–8

Moos, R.H. (1968). The development of a menstrual distress questionnaire. *Psychosom. Med.*, **30**, 853–67

Moos, R.H. (1969). Typology of menstrual cycle symptoms. *Am. J. Obstet. Gynecol.*, **103**, 390–402

Morton, J.H. (1950). Premenstrual tension. *Am. J. Obstet. Gynecol.*, **60**, 343–52

Munday, M. (1977). Hormone levels in severe premenstrual tension. *Curr. Med. Res. Opin.*, **4**, 16

Munday, M., Brush, M.G. and Taylor, R.W. (1981). Correlations between progesterone, oestradiol and aldosterone levels in the premenstrual syndrome. *Clin. Endocrinol.*, **14**, 1–9

Muse, K.N., Cetel, N.S., Futterman L.A. and Yen, S.S.C. (1984). The premenstrual syndrome, effects of "medical ovariectomy". *N. Engl. J. Med.*, **311**, 1345–9

National Institute of Mental Health Workshop on Premenstrual Syndrome (1983). Rockville, Maryland, April 14–15

O'Brien, P.M.S. (1987). *Premenstrual Syndrome*, pp.1–4. (Oxford: Blackwell Scientific Publications)

O'Brien, P.M.S., Craven, D., Selby, C. and Symonds, E.M. (1979). Treatment of premenstrual syndrome by spironolactone. *Br. J. Obstet. Gynaecol.*, **86**, 142–7

O'Brien, P.M.S., Selby, C. and Symonds, E.M. (1980). Progesterone, fluid, and electrolytes in premenstrual syndrome. *Br. Med. J.*, **11**, 1161–3

Parlee, M.B. (1982). The psychology of the menstrual cycle: biological and psychological perspective. In Friedman, R.C. (ed.) *Behaviour and the Menstrual Cycle*, pp. 77–99. (New York: Marcel Dekker)

Perrini, A. and Pilego, N. (1959). The increases of aldosterone in premenstrual tension. *Minerva Med.*, **50**, 2897–9

Rees, L. (1953a). Psychosomatic aspects of the premenstrual tension syndrome. *J. Ment. Sci.*, **99**, 62

Rees, L. (1953b). The premenstrual tension syndrome and its treatment. *Br. Med. J.*, **1**, 1014–16

Reid, R.L. (1985). Premenstrual syndrome. *Current Problems in Obstetrics, Gynaecology and Fertility*, Vol. VII, p.2. (Chicago: Year Book Medical Publishers Inc.)

Reid, R.L. and Yen, S.C. (1981). Premenstrual syndrome. *Am J. Obstet. Gynecol.*, **139**, 85–104

Rose, D.P. (1969). Oral contraceptives and depression. *Lancet*, **2**, 321

Rosseinsky, D.R. and Hall, P.G. (1974). An evolutionary theory of premenstrual tension. *Lancet*, **2**, 1024

Sampson, G.A. (1979). Premenstrual syndrome. A double-blind controlled trial of progesterone and placebo *Br. J. Psychiatr.*, **135**, 209–15

Sanders, D. (1987). Premenstrual tension. In McPherson, A. (ed.) *Women's Problems in General Practice*, 2nd edn. pp. 43–64. (Oxford, New York, Tokyo, Melbourne: Oxford University Press)

Sanders, D., Warner, P., Bäckström, T. and Bancroft, J. (1983). Mood, sexuality, hormones and the menstrual cycle. I Changes in mood and physical state: description of subjects and methods. *Psychosom. Med.*, **45**, 487–501

Schaumburg, H., Kaplan, J., Windebank, A., Vick, N., Rasmus, S., Pleasure, D. and Brown, M.J. (1983). Sensory neuropathy from pyridoxine abuse. A new megavitamin syndrome. *N. Engl. J. Med.*, **309**, 445–8

Silbergeld, S., Brast, N. and Noble, E.P. (1971). The menstrual cycle: a double-blind study of symptoms, mood and behaviour, and biochemical variables using Enovid and placebo. *Psychosom. Med.*, **33**, 411–28

Smith, S.L. (1975). Mood and the menstrual cycle. In Sachar, E.J. (ed.) *Topics in Endocrinology*, pp. 19–58. (New York: Grune and Stratton)

Smith, S.L. (1976). The menstrual cycle and mood disturbances. *Clin. Obstet. Gynecol.*, **19**, 391–7

Steiner, M., Haskett, R.F. and Carrol, B.J. (1980). Premenstrual tension syndrome: the development of research diagnostic criteria and new rating scales. *Acta Psychiatr. Scand.*, **62**, 177–90

Stokes, J. and Mendels, J. (1972). Pyridoxine and premenstrual tension. *Lancet*, **1**, 1177–8

Stout, A.L. (1989). Psychiatric diagnoses and personality factors associated with premenstrual syndrome. In van Hall, E.V. and Evered, W. (eds.) *The Free Woman: Women's Health in the 1990s*, pp. 646–58. (Lancaster: The Parthenon Publishing Group)

Strecker, J.R. (1980). An explorative study into the clinical effects of dydrogesterone in the treatment of premenstrual syndrome. In van Keep, P.A. and Utian, W.H. (eds.) *The Premenstrual Syndrome*, Chap. 5, pp. 71–9. (Lancaster: MTP Press Ltd.)

Sutherland, H. and Stewart, I. (1965). A critical analysis of the premenstrual syndrome. *Lancet*, **1**, 1180–3

Sweeney, J.S. (1934). Menstrual oedema. *J. Am. Med Assoc.*, **103**, 234–8

Takayama, T. (1972). A clinical study of premenstrual syndrome. In Morris, N. (ed.) *Psychosomatic Medicine in Obstetrics and Gynaecology*, p. 596. (Basel: Karger)

Taylor, J.W. (1979). The timing of menstruation-related symptoms assessed by a daily symptom rating scale. *Acta Psychiatr. Scand.*, **60**, 87–105

Taylor, R.W. (1977). The treatment of premenstrual tension with dydrogesterone 'Duphaston'. *Curr. Med. Res. Opin.*, Suppl. 4, 35–40

Taylor, R.W. (1983). *Premenstrual Syndrome. Proceedings of a workshop held at the Royal College of Obstetricians and Gynaecologists.* (London: Medical News-Tribune Ltd)

Thorn, G.W., Nelson, K.R. and Thorn, D.W. (1938). The clinicians view of the patient with premenstrual syndrome. *Endocrinology*, **22**, 153–63

Watts, J.F., Logan Edwards, R. and Butt, W.R. (1985). Treatment of premenstrual syndrome using Danazol: preliminary report of a placebo-controlled, double blind, dose-ranging study. *J. Int. Med. Res.*, **13**, 127–8

Wenzel, U. (1960). Periodical twilight states in puberty. *Archiv Psychiatr. Nervenkrankh.*, **201**, 133–50

West, C.P., Lumsden, M.A. and Baird, D.T. (1989). Modification of symptoms of the premenstrual syndrome during ovarian suppression with goserelin (Zoladex) depot – potential for research and clinical investigation. *J. Psychosom. Obstet. Gynaecol.*, **10**, 79–88

Widholm, O. and Kantero, R.L. (1971). Menstrual patterns of adolescent girls according to the chronological and gynecological ages. *Acta Obstet. Gynaecol. Scand.*, Suppl. 14, 19–29

Williams, E.Y. and Weeks, L.R. (1952). Premenstrual tension associated with psychotic episodes: preliminary report. *J. Nerv. Ment. Dis.*, **116**, 321–9

Winston, F. (1973). Oral contraceptives, pyridoxine, and depression. *Am. J. Psychiatr.*, **130**, 1217–21

Wood, C. and Jakubowicz, D.L. (1980). The treatment of premenstrual symptoms with mefenamic acid. *Br. J. Obstet. Gynaecol.*, **87**, 627–30

Ylostalo, P., Kauppila, A., Puolakka, J., Ronnberg, L. and Janne, O. (1982). Bromocriptine and norethisterone in the treatment of the premenstrual syndrome. *Obstet. Gynecol.*, **59**, 292–8

Zondek, B. and Bromberg, Y.M. (1947). Endocrine allergy: clinical reactions of allergy to endogenous hormones and their treatment. *Br. J. Obstet. Gynaecol.*, **54**, 1–19

FURTHER READING

Brush, M.G. and Goudsmit, E.M. (eds.) (1988). General and social considerations in research on menstrual cycle disorders with particular reference to PMS. *Functional Disorders of the Menstrual Cycle*, pp. 1–13. (Chichester, New York, Brisbane, Toronto, Singapore: John Wiley & Sons)

d'Orban, P.T. (1983). Medicolegal aspects of the premenstrual syndrome. *Br. J. Hosp. Med.*, **30**, 404–9

Hammarbäck, S. (1989). The premenstrual syndrome. A study of its diagnosis and pathogenesis. *Acta Obstet. Gynaecol. Scand.*, Suppl. 151

Keep van. P.A. and Utian, W.H. (1981). *The Premenstrual Syndrome.* (Lancaster: MTP Press)

Magos, A. and Studd, J. (1984). The premenstrual syndrome. In Studd, J. (ed.) *Progress in Obstetrics and Gynaecology*, Vol. 4, pp. 334–50. (Edinburgh, London, Melbourne, New York: Churchill Livingstone)

Sanders, D. (1987). Premenstrual tension. In McPherson, A. (ed.) *Women's Problems in General Practice*, Oxford General Practice Series 12, 2nd edn. pp. 43–64. (Oxford, New York, Tokyo, Melbourne: Oxford University Press)

Dysmenorrhoea

INTRODUCTION

Ylikorkola and Dawood (1978) reported that dysmenorrhoea accounted for the loss of 140 million working hours per year in America. The occurrence of difficult or painful menstruation was noted by the ancients. Soranus of Ephesus advised local application of a bladder filled with hot oil and held over the aching lower abdomen. He was also aware that dysmenorrhoea could affect the older parous patient and described what may have been uterine subinvolution as its cause. Thomas Denman described the earliest case of membranous dysmenorrhoea. Denman was admitted as the first Licentiate in midwifery of the College of Physicians of London in 1783, and was the successor of William Hunter, a leading member of the 'man-midwives'. In the early nineteenth century the dysmenorrhoea of old maids and widows was called *colica scortorum*, ovaralgia or hysteralgia and was thought to be caused by an unsatisfied sexual appetite (Graham, 1950). The literature on dysmenorrhoea throughout that century was very extensive (Ricci, 1945).

Clow (1927) reported her experience as a medical officer of a girls' school. She found that over 20% of the girls had developed some form of menstrual disorder within 4 years of puberty. Clow introduced a regimen of healthy living with plenty of open air exercise, thus reducing the incidence of dysmenorrhoea from 46.7% to 10.8%.

Knaus (1929) and also Moir (1933–34) and other investigators studied intrauterine pressures throughout the menstrual cycle. Although early reports were conflicting, it was demonstrated that small and frequent myometrial contractions occurred in the first half of the cycle, but contractions were stronger after the 16th day, increasing in force and frequency during the early part of menstruation. Dysmenorrhoeic patients experienced pain when the pressure reached 80–100 mmHg and it was suggested that muscle ischaemia was causative. Many other theories were advanced to explain the origin of menstrual pain. Sturgis and Albright (1940) proposed the theory that primary dysmenorrhoea occurred only in ovulatory cycles.

Figure 1 illustrates the method devised by Sims, whereby the cervix was incised to improve the outflow of menstrual fluids in cases of dysmenorrhoea.

TREATMENT

In 1830 Charles MacIntosh of Edinburgh treated dysmenorrhoea by the use of graduated sounds to dilate the cervix (Ricci, 1945). The cervical dilators designed by Alfred Hegar (1820–1914) of Germany have been used for the same purpose, right up to the present day. Sponges, laminaria, and tupelo tents which were made from the spongy wood of the roots of the tree *Nyssa uniflora* were inserted in the cervix. The tents expanded as they absorbed fluid. T. Gaillard Thomas of New York advocated intracervical placement of sponge tents to cause uterine congestion with increased nutrition. This in turn was thought to relieve the discomfort (Speert, 1973).

When cervical dilatation was performed it was essential to dilate the cervix 'beyond the size of a

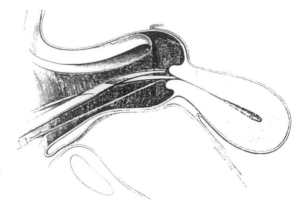

Figure 1 Sims' method of incising the cervix with curved pointed scissors to improve the outflow of menstrual fluids in cases of dysmenorrhoea. From J. Marion Sims' *Uterine Surgery* (1866)

No.11 hegar and it is customary to stop at size No.14 . . . a glass rod with circular phlange at the lower end is now passed into the cervical canal and kept in place with gauze plugged into the vagina. The glass rod should be kept *in situ* for 48 hours and then removed' (Shaw, 1946). Other forms of treatment included open air exercise, treatment of constipation with purges, simple analgesics, atropine, ephedrine and alcohol. Salmon *et al.* (1939) advocated treatment with testosterone propionate. Oestrogens were used in the 1930s without much success but progesterone was found to be helpful. As primary dysmenorrhoea was reported to occur in ovulatory cycles, anovulant therapy became common place. Bilateral oophorectomy was performed in the late nineteenth century, when dysmenorrhoea was accompanied by menorrhagia. Presacral neurectomy was advocated by Cotte of Lyons (1925) who later published optimistic results in 300 patients. O'Donel-Browne (1939) believed that many cases of primary dysmenorrhoea originated in the ovary. He developed an ovarian denervation technique which had no adverse effect either on ovarian function or on pregnancy. Injection of alcohol into the pelvic plexus was also advocated as a remedy. A wide variety of drugs was used to treat the condition. These included iron, ergot, salicylates, belladonna, amyl nitrite, quinine and many others.

Prostaglandins were first isolated by von Euler (1934; 1935) and also by Goldblatt (1933) from the accessory genital glands and human semen. Pickles *et al.*(1965) found higher levels of prostaglandin $F_{2\alpha}$ and prostaglandin E_2 in women with primary dysmenorrhoea compared with those with 'painfree' periods. The recognized involvement of prostaglandins led to the use of prostaglandin synthetase inhibitors as a treatment modality. The prostaglandin synthetase inhibitors included mefenamic acid, ibuprofen and naproxen. Akerlund *et al.* (1979) implicated vasopressin as a cause of the condition. Vasopressin antagonists were manufactured and tested in the mid-1980s but they were short acting, with a half-life of only 17 minutes, and did not realize their potential.

CHRONOLOGY

General

2nd C. AD Soranus of Ephesus described the condition.

1780s Thomas Denman described membranous dysmenorrhoea (Graham, 1950).

19th C. Dysmenorrhoea was termed *collica scortorum*.

1927 Clow detailed the condition in teenage girls.

1929 Knaus studied intrauterine pressure.

Treatment

2nd C. AD Soranus advised local application of a warm, oil-filled bladder.

1830 MacIntosh dilated the cervix with graduated sounds (Cianfrani, 1960).

19th C. Bilateral oophorectomy was performed.

1925 Cotte pioneered presacral neurectomy.

1939 Salmon *et al.* advised testosterone. Oestrogens were also used. Progesterone therapy also began. O'Donel-Browne blocked the ovarian nerve supply.

1965 Pickles implicated prostaglandin as a cause of dysmenorrhoea.

REFERENCES

Akerlund, M., Stromberg, P. and Forsling, M.L. (1979). Primary dysmenorrhoea and vasopressin. *Br. J. Obstet. Gynaecol.*, **86**, 484–87

Bowes, K. (1950). *Modern Trends in Obstetrics and Gynaecology*, pp. 586–607. (London: Butterworth Co.)

Browne, F.J. (1950). *Postgraduate Obstetrics and Gynaecology*, pp. 598–601. (London: Butterworth & Co. Ltd.)

Cianfrani, T. (1960). *A Short History of Obstetrics and Gynecology*, p. 357. (Springfield, Ill.: Charles C. Thomas)

Clow, A.E.S. (1927). quoted by Browne, F.J. (1950). pp. 263–72

Cotte, G. (1925). quoted by Browne, F.J. (1950). pp. 263–72

Euler, V.S. von (1934). Zur kenntnis der pharmakologischem wirkungen von mativeskreten und extrakten mannlicher accessorischer geschlechtsdrusen. *Arch. Exp. Pathol. Pharmakol.*, **175**, 78

Euler, V.S. von (1935). Uber die spezifische blut drucksende substanz des menslichen prostata und samenblasen secretes. *Klinishe Wschr.*, **14**, 1182–7

Goldblatt, M.W. (1933). Depressor substance in seminal fluid. *Chem. Ind.*, **52**, 1056

Graham, H. (1950). *Eternal Eve*, pp. 358; 435. (London: W. Heinemann)

Knaus, H. (1929). quoted by Browne, F.J. (1950), pp. 263–72

Moir, J.C. (1933–34). quoted by Browne, F.J. (1950), pp. 263–72

O'Donel-Browne, T.D. (1939). quoted by Browne, F.J. (1950), pp. 263–72

Pickles, V.R., Hall, W.J., Best, F.A. and Smith, G.N. (1965). Prostaglandins in endomtrium and menstrual fluid from normal and dysmenorrhoeic subjects. *Br. J. Obstet. Gynaecol.*, **72**, 185–95

Ricci, J.V. (1945). *One Hundred Years of Gynecology 1800–1900*, pp. 522–4. (Philadelphia: Blakiston Co.)

Salmon, U.J., Geist, S.H. and Walter, R.I. (1939). Treatment of dysmenorrhoea with testosterone propionate. *Am. J. Obstet. Gynecol.*, **38**, 264

Shaw, W. (1946). *Textbook of Gynaecology*, p. 330. (London: J. & A. Churchill Ltd.)

Speert, H. (1973). *Iconographia Gyniatrica: A Pictorial History of Gynecology and Obstetrics*, p. 460. (Philadelphia: F.A. Davis Co.)

Sturgis, S.H. and Albright, F. (1940). quoted by Bowes, K. (1950), p. 600

Ylikorkola, O. and Dawood, M.Y. (1978). New concepts in dysmenorrhea. *Am. J. Obstet. Gynecol.*, **130**, 833–47

FURTHER READING

Browne, F.J. (1950). *Postgraduate Obstetrics and Gynaecology*, pp. 263–72. (London: Butterworth & Co. Ltd.)

D'Angelo, G.J. (1953). Dilatation and curettage, a developement covering 3,000 years. *Obstet. Gynecol.* **2**, 322–4

Olive, D.L. and Haney, A.F. (1986). Endometriosis – associated fertility: a critical review of therapeutic approaches. *Obstet. Gynecol. Surv.*, **41**, 538–55

Rees, M.C.P. (1989). Heavy, painful periods. In Drife, J.O. (ed.) *Dysfunctional Uterine Bleeding and Menorrhagia: Clinical Obstetrics and Gynaecology*, Vol. 3, No. 2, pp. 341–56. (London, Philadelphia, Sydney, Tokyo, Toronto: Bailliere Tindall)

Infertility

INFERTILITY

The natural urge to procreate assured an interest in fertility, and an admonition from the Omnipotent to 'be fruitful and multiply' (Genesis 1:28) added impetus to our mammalian instincts. So, from earliest times, it was apparent that the human race had an interest in beginning, interrupting or discontinuing the reproductive process. All too soon however, some couples faced what the Talmud describes as 'the living death of barrenness'.

EARLY DISCOVERIES

As is evident from carvings and cave drawings, stone-age people had some knowledge of anatomy and the reproductive process, but the first detailed information comes from Egyptian Papyri, which describe many gynaecological complaints and recipes to increase fertility. Various passages in the Bible confirm the interest of ancient Hebrews in the fertility process, and they were aware that conception was possible 7 days after the cessation of menses.

It was the Greeks who first adequately defined the human form in sculpture and painting and both Hippocrates and Aristotle were aware of the external and internal reproductive organs, although knowledge of the latter was based mainly on observation and dissection of animals. Hippocrates (460–377 BC) held the view that seeds came from all parts of the body of man and woman, flowed together forming a fruit, and then developed. Aristotle (AD 384–322) was the first to record that intercourse was necessary for pregnancy to occur, and he believed that semen and menstrual blood mixed in the uterus and formed a fetus. He did not agree that the ovary was involved in the process (Adams, 1849; Peck, 1943).

In ancient Rome Aurelius Cornelius Celsus (27 BC–AD 50) (q.v. in Biographies) wrote a book on medicine and included remedies for some gynaecological complaints. His *De Medicina* was rediscovered in the fifteenth century and became a standard medical textbook for students and physicians (Spencer, 1938). Another Roman physician, Claudius Galenus (AD 131–201) (q.v. in Biographies) taught that there was a mixing of male and female semen from the ovaries, with the formation of a conception. The heart and liver were formed from the female principle while the brain came from the male. He called the ovary the *testes muliebris*. It was not until 1664 that Stensen introduced the term *ovaria*. Soranus (q.v. in Biographies) (AD 98–138) of Ephesus (a city in Asia Minor) worked in Rome, and became a prolific author. His textbook on gynaecology earned him the title of 'The Father of Gynaecology' (Temkin, 1956).

The Middle Ages, which lasted from the decline of Rome to the beginnings of the Renaissance a thousand years later, was an age of scholasticism, and few advances occurred in medical knowledge. Human dissection was not allowed and anatomy was studied from the pig and other animals. An early University in Salerno Italy, allowed women to join the medical faculty, and around AD 1050 one of them, Trotula, became the first woman to write a text on the subject of obstetrics (Cianfrani, 1960). In 1513 Eucharius Rösslin produced his book on midwifery called the *Rose Garden for Pregnant Women and Midwives*. Written in German it was translated into English and Latin. Most of the material in his book was derived from Moschion of the sixth century AD, who in turn had copied his material from Soranus of Ephesus. Thus the teachings of the ancients were perpetuated, without correction.

During the Renaissance there was a return to scientific investigation, and as a result many new discoveries were made. The works of the ancient authors were found to be inaccurate in many instances, and were refuted.

Leonardo da Vinci (1452–1519) detailed the male and female reproductive anatomy in art. He pictorially represented the act of intercourse, and that anatomical drawing was eventually entitled *de coitu* by Gabriel Peillon in 1891. Da Vinci was the first to depict the human anatomy in a realistic fashion. In 1543, Andreas Vesalius (1514–1564) from the University of Padua, published his *De Humani Corporis Fabrica* (Figure 1). This was the

first anatomical book based on human dissection by the author with illustrations by Jan Stephan van Kalkar. Gabriele Falloppio (1523–1562) described the Fallopian tubes, ovaries, vagina, placenta and clitoris but the earliest definitive description of the ovary with its follicles and corpus

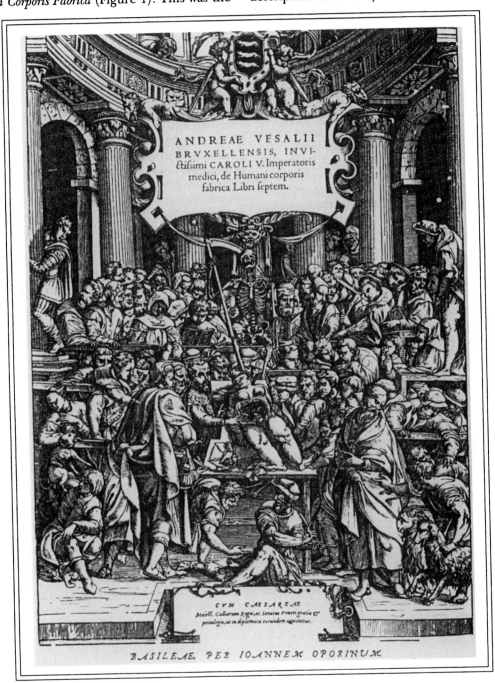

Figure 1 Title page of the revised edition of the *De Humani Corporis Fabrica* (1555)

luteum came from the work of Regnier de Graaf in his *De Mullerium Organis* which was written in 1672. He mistakenly regarded the follicles as eggs, although he had seen but not recognized ova in the Fallopian tubes.

In 1621, Fabricius believed that the fertilizing principle of semen was an emanation which was called the *Aura Seminalis*. He evolved his theory because he knew that in birds, eggs were fertilized far from the site at which semen was deposited. Thirty years later Harvey developed this thinking further, as 'after intercourse there is nothing more to be found in the uterus than was there before the act'. He theorized that the uterus was brought to a stage of ripeness by copulation. It could then proceed to a conception state through the stimulus of the *aura seminalis*, and apparently no physical agent took any part in the process. Many other theories developed as to how conception took place. In the 'theory of evolution' it was believed that the egg contained a fully formed embryo which developed after the stimulus of intercourse. This theory was replaced by that of 'Epigenesis'. For a time a theory of spontaneous generation held sway (Speert, 1973).

Anton van Leeuwenhoek (1632–1723) of Delft, who was a trader and linen draper, became interested in microscopy and he examined various tissues and body fluids. With a Dutch student, Hamen, he described the microscopic appearance of sperm in 1674 and 1677 (van Leeuwenhoek, 1678). Originally spermatozoa were thought to be small parasitic animals until Kolliker in 1841 detailed the development of spermatozoa in the testis (Harkness, 1962).

Caspar (Karl) Friedrich Wolff (1733–1794) published his *Theoria Generationis* in 1759 and is regarded as the 'Father of Embryology' (Graham, 1950). He introduced a new era in embryology and viewed chick embryos through the microscope. Jacobi in 1764 and Lazano Spallanzani (1776) experimented with artificial insemination, and 8 years later John Hunter successfully carried out human artificial insemination, which was followed by the birth of a healthy infant (Cusine, 1988).

William Cumberland Cruikshank of Edinburgh found small spherical bodies (ova) in rabbit Fallopian tubes in 1778 (Cruikshank, 1797) but it was Karl Ernst von Baer (1827) during his research on the embryology of the dog who was credited with the first ever observation of the ovum. A fertilized rabbit egg was first viewed by Martin Barry (1843). Alfred Donne (1844) carried out microscopic examination of vaginal secretions and noted the presence of spermatozoa in some. Percy (1861) reported the presence of living sperm in cervical mucus, although his examination apparently took place 8–9 days after last coitus. Oskar Hertwig, and also Beneden, observed the union of sperm and egg nuclei in 1875 (Gruhn and Kazer, 1989). The first unfertilized living ovum was recovered by Allen *et al.* (1930).

The physiology of erection was founded on the work of Muller in 1838 and also on the studies of Eckhard and others. The fetal circulation was first considered in detail by Sabatier in 1774, and John Mayow had already regarded the placenta as a uterine lung in 1674 (Harkness, 1962).

Advances in the investigation and treatment of infertility gained impetus from scientific research in the fields of embryology, physiology and cellular pathology. In this century gynaecological endocrinology, culdoscopy, laparoscopy, ultrasound and laboratory techniques were developed and helped elucidate the causes and management of infertility. Eventually in the 1980s the assisted conception technologies became available.

CERVICAL MUCUS

Alfred François Donné (1844) investigated the nature of vaginal secretions by microscopy and discovered spermatozoa in the cervical mucus. His work was confirmed by other investigators including Marion Sims (1866; 1868) and Max Huhner (1913).

Meanwhile, Pouchet (1847), Professor of Zoology at Rouen, described cyclic cervical mucus changes during the menstrual cycle. He believed that it would be possible from these to predict ovulation, and it is to him that the concept of a 'rhythm method' of contraception is credited. However, Pouchet erroneously believed that ovulation occurred during menstruation in the human. Almost a hundred years later Viergiver and Pommerenke (1944) found that cervical mucus production increased in quantity throughout the follicular phase, and reached a peak around the time of ovulation. The work of Clift and Hart (1954), and that of subsequent investigators over the following 18 years, led to the publication of three important papers on the topic of the cervix and cervical mucus. Moghissi *et al.* (1972) found that changes in cervical mucus correlated well with peak luteinizing hormone levels in serum. Insler *et al.* (1972) introduced a cervical score based on mucus and the qualities of the cervix, and in Australia, the Billings group (1972) documented their findings on the relationship of cervical mucus to the menstrual cycle. This work was to prove invaluable in both the infertility and family planning areas.

SPERM–MUCUS INTERACTION

James Marion Sims (1813–1883) is credited with the first observation of the presence and motility of sperm in cervical mucus following coitus. He advocated, in a lecture to the New York County Medical Society in 1868, looking for spermatozoa under the microscope in fluid taken from the cervix and the vagina. His lecture was entitled *On the Microscope as an Aid in the Diagnosis and Treatment of Sterility.* He was accused when he first described his postcoital test (later resurrected by Huhner) of 'this dabbling in the vagina with speculum and syringe. . . incompatible with decency and self-respect'. Sims found that spermatozoa lived longer in the cervical mucus than in vaginal fluid, and reported that sperm were active in mucus for up to 40 hours after coitus.

Additional reports appeared in the literature and eventually Max Huhner (1913), a Berlin-born urologist working in New York, reported the results of a large study on postcoital examinations. His name and that of Sims became eponymously related to the postcoital test which became known as the 'Sims-Huhner' test.

Kurzrock and Miller (1928) described an *in vitro* sperm penetration test which because of its simplicity became very popular. Active penetration of mucus by the sperm was taken to indicate cervical mucus and sperm compatibility. Kremer (1965) of the Netherlands, developed an apparatus which was called the sperm penetration meter. A test was devised which imitated the conditions present in the cervical canal, and sperm migration distance, penetration density, with other variables were measured.

A further modification of the postcoital test was introduced by Kroeks and Kremer (1975) and migration rates, velocity, direction and duration were determined. There were many contributors to the debate as to what constituted a poor or negative postcoital test. Ulstein (1973) noted that the ability of sperm to penetrate the cervical mucus was more strongly correlated with fertility than any other seminal parameter and Hull *et al.* confirmed that if the postcoital test was negative

the pregnancy rate was reduced to 20% that of the normal population (Hull *et al.*, 1981; 1982).

PREDICTION OF OVULATION

The ability to predict the process of ovulation depended on the results of investigations involving the cervical mucus, endometrium, morphological aspects of the ovary, and the identification of the many hormones involved in the process. (A full account is given in the chapter on hormones.)

The temperature method became a practicality when Barton *et al.* (1945) showed that the temperature elevation in the second half of the cycle was due to progesterone activity. Previous workers included Squire (1868), van de Velde (1905) and Tompkins (1944).

Ogino (1930) in Japan, and Knaus (1933) in Austria observed a relatively constant relationship between ovulation and the succeeding menstruation. This work gave rise to the calculation or calendar method. The cervical mucus technique popularized by Billings *et al.* (1972), Moghissi *et al.* (1972), and Insler *et al.* (1972) confirmed earlier work by Seguy and Simonnet (1933) and also by Seguy and Vimeux (1933), who had found that the cervical mucus became more fluid in character and more easily penetrable by spermatozoa at the time of ovulation. Mid-cycle or *Mittleschmertz* pain was experienced by some women around the time of ovulation and O'Herlihy *et al.* (1980a,b; 1982) concluded that the pain occurred 24–28 hours prior to the ultra-sonically determined time of ovulation.

Sampling of the endometrium was used to prove that ovulation had occurred. The endometrial curette was introduced in the 1850s by the Parisian, Recamier (Zondek, 1966), and Moricke (1882) was the first investigator to sample endometrium from the living human. Hitschmann and Adler (1907; 1908) clearly demonstrated the histological changes in the endometrial cycle for the first time. Robert Meyer (1911) and Karl Ruge Jr. (1913) correlated cyclical endometrial change with ovarian appearances. Stockard and Papanicolaou (1917) introduced their vaginal cytological method of dating the menstrual cycle but the technique is now seldom used. Markee (1940) and Bartelmez (1931) studied the vascular events of the endometrial cycle and Noyes *et al.* (1950) published their histological technique of dating the endometrium.

Many researchers were involved in the identification of the hormones which influenced the menstrual cycle, but Henry Iscovesco (1912a,b) was the first investigator to discover an active ovarian extract, later recognized as oestrogen. The World Health Organization (1976) reported that the plasma oestradiol peak occurred approximately 37 hours before ovulation. They also noted that the interval between peak serum luteinizing hormone levels and ovulation was 17 hours. The determination of luteinizing hormone levels as a predictor of ovulation proved to be of major benefit, and the technique is now incorporated in a 'dip stick' test for home use.

Ultrasound imaging proved beneficial in the identification of cyclic ovarian, uterine and endometrial changes, but follicular size as determined at scanning did not predict ovulation with great accuracy. Ultrasound-guided techniques for oocyte recovery simplified the problems of ovum 'harvesting' in assisted conception cycles (Wikland et al., 1988).

THE INDUCTION OF OVULATION

Early unsuccessful efforts at ovulation induction included that of Rakoff (1953), who irradiated the pituitary and ovaries of anovulatory women. However, Gemzell et al. (1958) introduced human follicle stimulating hormone and luteinizing hormone for ovulation induction. The gonadotropins were extracted from human pituitaries obtained at autopsy, and soon Lunenfeld et al. (1960) investigated the clinical effects of human postmenopausal gonadotropins obtained from urine which then replaced the pituitary source. The response to gonadotropins was monitored by a rapid method of estimating urinary oestrogen excretion, which was modified from the technique of Brown et al. (1968). Ovarian follicular monitoring by ultrasound was introduced by Hackeloer and his colleagues (Hackeloer and Hansmann, 1976; Hackeloer et al., 1979) and although its use could not help to avoid multiple pregnancy, nor ovarian hyperstimulation, it was found to have a large role to play when combined with oestrogen assay and other monitoring methods (Seibel et al., 1981).

Clomiphene citrate, which is structurally related to diethylstilboestrol, was found to stimulate ovulation and was introduced to clinical practice by Greenblatt et al. (1961). Taymor et al. (1973) combined the use of clomiphene with human menopausal gonadotropins to good effect and with their technique, 45% less gonadotropins were required to induce an ovulatory response.

Gonadotropin releasing hormone was isolated in 1971 by the Schally and Guillemin groups (Matsuo et al., 1971a,b; Schally et al., 1971) and due to the work of Knobil (1980) it was discovered that the drug should be administered in pulsed doses in order to be effective. The first report of a pregnancy in which luteinizing hormone releasing hormone analogues were used to achieve pituitary 'down regulation' came from Porter et al. (1984). With their use, the spontaneous luteinizing hormone surges and high tonic luteinizing hormone levels, which were associated with low rates of implantation and high abortion rates (Howles et al., 1986: Rutherford et al., 1988), were prevented.

Patients with hyperprolactinaemia were readily treatable by bromocriptine (Parlodel) (Lutterback et al., 1971) and this drug gradually replaced the surgical approach of ovarian wedge resection. Pure follicle stimulating hormone was introduced to treat patients with polycystic ovary syndrome in which luteinizing hormone levels are high and follicle stimulating hormone is relatively deficient (Venturoli et al., 1983).

Macrosurgical techniques of wedge resection for polycyctic ovaries induced ovulation but caused a high incidence of postoperative adhesions (Buttram and Vaquero, 1975) and the procedure fell into disfavour. More recently, translaparoscopic laser and cautery to polycystic ovaries has successfully induced ovulation but drug therapy remains the treatment of choice.

SEMEN ANALYSIS

The results of seminal analysis, and those findings which constitute a normal or abnormal result, have been the cause of much debate. Hotchkiss (1941) reviewed the variability of semen samples. Ten years later MacLeod and Gold (1951a,b) determined that if sperm density was less than 20 million per ml, there was an increased incidence of infertility. They also showed that the majority of men have more than 60% normal sperm forms in their semen samples. Testicular biopsy was popular for a time and Howard et al. (1950) reported their experiences and results of testicular biopsy. Not only sperm density, but also motility (MacLeod and Gold, 1951a,b; Rutherford et al., 1963) and anti-sperm antibodies, were found to be important. MacLeod (1969a) developed a motility index and an antibody test was introduced by Jager et al. (1978). The determination of seminal fructose levels was introduced and results were found to correlate positively with androgen levels (Landau and Loughead, 1951) and to vary inversely with sperm count (Phadke *et al.*, 1973). A zona-free hamster egg penetration test was introduced by Yanagimachi *et al.* (1976). The issue of what constituted a normal semen analysis was debated by the American Fertility Society (1971) and they indicated that the lower limit of normal for sperm concentration was 40 million per ml. Eventually the World Health Organization (1980a) published their guidelines on the technique of semen analysis and the interpretation of results.

SEMEN TREATMENT

Efforts to increase male fertility were mainly of magical or mystical character until Charles Eduoard Brown-Sequard (1889) introduced treatment with aqueous extracts of animal testicles which were injected subcutaneously. The extracts were said to invigorate the older man but were also used to increase potency. Ingestion of testicular products was also advocated. These efforts came to fruition when Heller *et al.* (1950) found that oral intake of testosterone for periods of up to 70 days caused an initial reduction in sperm count which was followed by rebound spermatogenesis. The apparent success of testosterone treatment led to later trials of thyroid extract, human chorionic gonadotropin, clomiphene, tamoxifen, luteinizing hormone releasing hormone and other drugs.

Hanley (1955) and MacLeod (1969) reported increased fertility in patients whose varicocoeles were ligated, and proponents of keeping a cool testicle took heart from a report by Zorgniotti *et al.* (1980) who found that a low scrotal temperature resulted in better semen quality. The old technique of intrauterine insemination of prepared semen, and the newer reproductive technologies of gamete intrafallopian transfer (GIFT) and *in vitro* fertilization (IVF) were used as treatment modalities in the 1980s (Yovich *et al.*, 1988).

ARTIFICIAL INSEMINATION

Artificial insemination was used as a treatment for infertility centuries before van Leeuwenhoek and Hamen found sperm in the ejaculate. There are references to artificial insemination from the third century AD, and there was a belief that pregnancy could occur if the unwary female bathed in water contaminated by male ejaculate.

Animal experiments paved the way, and in the fourteenth century Arabs were using insemination techniques to improve breeding quality in their horses. Prior to the identification of sperm in the ejaculate it was theorized that semen gave off 'vapours' which caused pregnancy. De Cherney and Harris (1986) detailed the method by which Spallanzani of Modena disproved the 'vapour' theory. He experimented with frogs by occluding the cloacal area with pieces of cloth and found that frogs with 'pants' on could not fertilize eggs, as semen and eggs did not make contact.

In 1776–1784 Spallanzani (Figure 2) described artificial insemination of donors' sperm, in dogs (Medvei, 1982). The first scientific record was published in 1799 when Everard Home reported that John Hunter in England had, in 1785, inseminated a woman with her husband's semen (Philipp, 1979; Mason, 1990). The need for this procedure was because the husband had hypospadias. The man ejaculated into a jar and Hunter, using a quill, successfully inseminated the wife with her husband's semen. In 1866 Marion Sims performed artificial insemination from the husband in a marriage that had been sterile for 9 years (Figure 3). It was the only success he had, however, in 55 inseminations carried out in six women all with their husbands' semen. By 1890 Dr Robert Dickinson in the USA was performing artificial insemination routinely (Mason, 1990). The first successful donor inseminations were carried out in the USA by Dr Pancoast in 1884 (Joyce and Vassilopoulos, 1981) and Marion Sims reported successes soon afterwards.

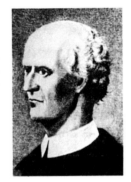

Figure 2 Abate Lazaro Spallanzani. Reproduced with kind permission from the Royal Society of Medicine, London

The technique for collection, dilution and subsequent insemination of equine semen was developed by Ivanov, a Russian scientist, in the early 1900s and his advances were applied to human semen (Kovacs and Burger, 1984). Artificial insemination continued to play its role in infertility, but was not reported in the medical literature as the technique was frowned upon, and many moral and ethical objections to its use were raised. In 1948 a committee set up by the

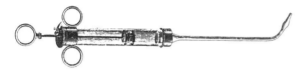

Figure 3 The syringe used by J. Marion Sims to inject half a drop of semen with which he managed to fertilize one patient. Altogether he had carried out 55 intra-uterine injections giving different quantities of semen, and warming the syringe with its glass applicator in hot water to different temperatures. From J. Marion Sims' *Uterine Surgery* (1866)

Archbishop of Canterbury, found that donor semination was wrong in principle and in 1949 Pope Pius the XII rejected donor insemination on moral grounds (Matthews, 1980). With these and other objections it was not surprising that the technique was not reported.

Lazzaro Spallanzani had already, in 1776, noted the effects on human sperm when they were exposed to a freezing temperature and Paolo Mantegazza (1886) made the first proposal for a sperm bank. Jahnel (1938) and also Polge *et al.* (1949) described cryopreservation using glycerol as a sperm cryoprotective agent in animals. Their technique led to successful cryopreservation of human semen. Bunge and co-workers (Bunge and Sherman, 1953; Bunge *et al.*, 1954) reported successful pregnancies from the use of stored frozen spermatozoa. Thereafter, sperm were stored in straws, tubes, or pellets and sperm banking became feasible.

Sherman in 1964 introduced liquid nitrogen as a freezing agent (Sherman, 1973), and Perloff *et al.* (1964) reported four births using sperm which had been stored in nitrogen vapour. Smith and Steinberger (1973) compared the outcome of using either fresh or frozen semen, and found that the live birth rate was better with fresh semen. The problem of oligospermia was investigated by Barwin (1974) who reported a 67% conception rate using intrauterine insemination of husbands' semen. The qualities and health of sperm donors gave rise to concern over the years, particularly with regards to the acquired immune deficiency syndrome and the other sexually transmitted diseases and also the possibility of chromosomal abnormalities. The American Fertility Society (1986) published their guidelines and 2 years later made a further recommendation that a quarantine period of 180 days, from donation to use, should be observed (American Fertility Society, 1988).

Despite the initial objections, donor insemination became widely used. The techniques of semen 'enhancement' by sperm feeding, washing, and swim-up techniques, were of major benefit for both donor insemination and the assisted conception programme. The newer technologies of gamete intrafallopian transfer, direct intraperitoneal insemination and *in vitro* fertilization have increased the oligospermic male's chance of making his partner pregnant.

TUBAL PATENCY

Tyler Smith's method of treating tubal obstruction by transcervical passage of a bougie (1849a,b,c) was reviewed by the *Revue Medico-Chirurgicale de Paris* in 1849, and it was suggested that tubal patency could be investigated by transcervical injection of water or air (Malgaigne, 1849). The technique of hysterosalpingography was first described by Rindfleisch (1910) soon after the development of X-ray techniques by Wilhelm Conrad Röntgen (1845–1923). Rubin (1914) and Carey (1914) independently reported testing for Fallopian tube patency using the radio-opaque silver colloid, collargol.

Isidor Clinton Rubin (1883–1958) a German born gynaecologist working in New York, first used tubal insufflation with oxygen on 3 November 1919 (Rubin, 1920). The gas was insufflated until visible abdominal distension occurred, and the presence of gas in the peritoneal cavity was confirmed by X-ray. The patient became pregnant within 2 months and was later delivered of a full-term infant. Variations of the Rubin's Test have remained popular until recent times (Figure 4). Decker and Cherry (1944) introduced culdoscopic examination of the pelvic organs and this diagnostic method was particularly popular in the USA. Although laparoscopy was introduced in the early 1900s, the technique was not popularized until the 1960s when carbon fibre optics and wide angle lenses were introduced, thus allowing easy visualization of the pelvic and abdominal organs. Steptoe and Edwards (1970) described laparoscopic recovery of preovulatory human oocytes and thus the laparoscope, which was a favoured surgical tool in the investigation of infertility, also became involved in its treatment.

SURGERY OF TUBES AND UTERUS

The surgical treatment of infertility antedated the investigation of tubal and uterine function. Tyler

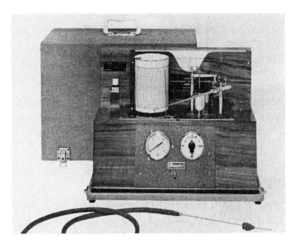

Figure 4 Sharman kymographic tubal insufflation apparatus, Mark III

Smith (1848; 1849a,b,c) was the first to attempt an operation for blocked Fallopian tubes. He also attempted to recanalize blocked Fallopian tubes using a bougie introduced within a curved catheter through the cervix. Further surgical techniques were introduced, and one operation involved the interposition of ovarian tissue between the blocked segment of tube and the uterus (Morris, 1895; Frank, 1898). The ovarian grafts did not survive well, but the problem was overcome when Dudley (1901) and Estes (1909) introduced their operation in which the blood supply to the ovarian graft was retained.

Schroeder was the first to attempt salpingoplasty in 1881 (Schroeder, 1884), and Skutsch (1989) introduced the term 'salpingostomy'. A 'cuff' technique was advocated by Ferguson (1903). John Rock of Boston was the leading American proponent of tubal surgery (see Kistner and Patton, 1975 for a review). As macrosurgical techniques were devised, Hellman (1951) was the first to publish a report detailing use of polyethylene tubing to maintain postoperative tubal patency (in eight patients). Two years later, Mulligan et al. (1953) advocated the use of a polyethylene prosthesis to cover the outer end of repaired tubes (Rock-Mulligan or Mulligan's Hood).

Microsurgical techniques became popular in the 1970s. However, with the advent of in vitro fertilization the popularity of tubal surgery waned somewhat. The newer techniques of minimally invasive surgery using laser laparoscopy for salpingolysis and treatment of endometriosis, have partly reversed the trend.

Abnormalities of the uterus and cervix were found to be associated with infertility. Strassman (1907) and others devised operations for the abnormal uterine body. Douay (1948) of France, and also Palmer and Lacomme (1948) devised operations for the repair of incompetence of the internal cervical os. Further operations were devised by McDonald (1957), Shirodkar (1963) and also by Baden and Baden (1960), Barter et al. (1963) and Lash (1964). Anussat of Paris removed fibroids in 1840 and myomectomy was popularized by Martin (1890), Kelly and Cullen (1909), and Victor Bonney (q.v. in Biographies) (1925). Endoscopic treatment of Asherman's Syndrome further enhanced the surgical repertoire for infertility treatment.

IN VITRO FERTILIZATION

Early attempts at in vitro fertilization took place in the nineteenth century. At that time Schenk (1878) was experimenting with rabbits and guinea-pigs and attempted to fertilize their ova in vitro. These initial attempts failed in their objective but Onanoff (1893) reported fertilization of rabbit and guinea-pig ova. The first attempts at embryo transfer were by Walter Heape (1890) who flushed fertilized ova from the tubes of angora doe rabbits and later transferred them to a foster mother.

In the 1930s Gregory Pincus published a series of important papers on in vitro fertilization, starting with his first description of rabbit experiments (1930). His initial work was carried out in Cambridge but he returned to Harvard to continue his work there, and reported with Enzmann in 1934 the in vitro fertilization and subsequent transfer of fertilized eggs to the Fallopian tube of a New Zealand doe who produced seven offspring 33 days later. Pincus and Enzmann (1934) contended that 'this is the first certain demonstration that mammalian eggs can be fertilized in vitro'. They later went on to work with human oocytes but predicted an oocyte maturation period of 12 hours. Their estimate was wrong and workers who used the 12-hour figure attempted to inseminate oocytes too early and failed to obtain fertilization. The work of Edwards (1965) showed that the correct maturation period in humans was 37 hours. Following that breakthrough, human oocytes were successfully fertilized *in vitro*. The duration between the luteinizing hormone surge and ovulation *in vivo* was later found also to be around 37 hours, thus linking oocyte maturation to high levels of luteinizing hormone.

The induction of ovulation was important not only to help women with oligo- or amenorrhoea, but also to induce superovulation for the *in vitro* fertilization programme. Early attempts by Davis and Koff (1938) showed that it was possible to induce ovulation. They used intravenous injections of an extract of pregnant mare's serum but this induced antibody formation and could not be used repeatedly in the human.

Gemzell *et al.* (1958) introduced human pituitary gonadotropin to induce superovulation, while purified human menopausal gonadotropin and human chorionic gonadotropin were introduced for the same purpose by Lunenfeld *et al.* (1960; 1967; 1970).

Steptoe and Edwards (1970) used gonadotropins to 'prime' the ovaries and then proceeded to retrieve ova at laparoscopy. The early attempts to fertilize human oocytes *in vitro* were unsuccessful despite allowing oocytes to mature for 37 hours (Edwards *et al.*, 1966). However, Edwards *et al.* (1969) later refined their techniques and reported successful human fertilization *in vitro*. Fertilized oocytes were grown in Ham's F 10 culture medium (Ham, 1963). Steptoe and Edwards (1976) reported the occurrence of an ectopic pregnancy after embryo replacement. The years of experimentation and scientific research were rewarded when eventually Steptoe (Figure 5) and Edwards (1978) announced the birth of Louise Brown, who was the first child born from an *in vitro* fertilization programme.

Steptoe and Edwards began to use the natural menstrual cycle in their *in vitro* fertilization attempts, as they were unsuccessful when attempting *in vitro* fertilization in stimulated cycles. Trounson *et al.* (1980; 1982) used ovulation stimulating drugs and harvested multiple oocytes. They delayed the addition of sperm to the oocytes for 5–6 hours, and later reported successful pregnancies.

The technique of ovulation induction became established with stimulation of multiple follicles by the use of clomiphene and gonadotropins. Human chorionic gonadotropin was used to induce oocyte maturation, with laparoscopy and collection of maturing oocytes, 35–36 hours later.

Treated spermatozoa were added to the oocytes, and pronucleate eggs transferred to a nutrient medium. A number of embryos were later transferred to the mother's uterus.

Lenz *et al.* (1981; 1982) described recovery of oocytes under ultrasound guidance, and transvaginal techniques which further simplified oocyte retrieval became available soon afterwards (Wikland *et al.*, 1985). Gradually, oocyte aspiration under ultrasound control replaced the majority of laparoscopic interventions for oocyte harvesting. Embryos which were not replaced could be effectively stored using dimethylsulphoxide as a cryopreservative (Trounson and Mohr, 1983) and glycerol was used for blastocysts (Cohen *et al.*, 1985). Successful non-surgical transfer of an *in vivo* fertilized ovum was reported by Buster *et al.* (1983).

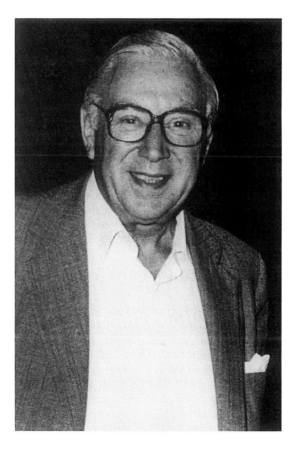

Figure 5 Patrick Steptoe. The birth of Louise Brown, the first *in vitro* fertilization baby delivered near midnight on 25th July 1978 by Patrick Steptoe caused enormous public interest

GAMETE INTRAFALLOPIAN TRANSFER

Tesarik *et al.* (1983) reported successful pregnancy following tubal gamete transfer which they performed at the conclusion of a microsurgical tubal operation. Asch *et al.* (1984) reported the first pregnancy and birth (1985) following translaparoscopic gamete intrafallopian transfer and this was soon seen as an alternative to *in vitro* fertilization in patients whose Fallopian tubes were normal, but where other factors led to infertility. A multicentre study was set up and clinical pregnancy rates of about 35% were reported. Donor oocytes were used by Asch *et al.* (1987) and six clinical pregnancies were achieved. Craft *et al.* (1988) reported an analysis of their first 1071 gamete intrafallopian transfer procedures.

ZYGOTE INTRAFALLOPIAN TRANSFER

Other treatment modalities became available and zygote intrafallopian transfer, which was first described by Devroey *et al.* (1986), allowed replacement into the Fallopian tube of thawed embryos. The first birth following use of the technique was reported by Abdalla and Leonard (1988).

DIRECT INTRAPERITONEAL INSEMINATION OF SPERM

Direct intraperitoneal insemination of sperm was reported by Manhes and Hermabessiere (1985) and Forrler *et al.* (1986) and intrauterine insemination has also proved beneficial in couples where sperm counts and motility were poor.

PERITONEAL OOCYTE AND SPERM TRANSFER

Mason *et al.* (1987) reported on peritoneal oocyte and sperm transfer and 3 years later documented a 24% success rate for the procedure (Mason, 1990). Another innovation was zona drilling, (microinjection of spermatozoa beneath the perivitelline space) and Edwards and Handyside (1990) intimated that the technique would improve treatment options for patients with oligo- or asthenospermia. The acronyms MIST, for microinsemination sperm transfer, and MIMIC for microinsemination microinjection into cytoplasm were proposed by Ng *et al.* (1990).

In an article on the history and development of assisted conception techniques, Edwards and Craft (1990) concluded that 'The overall chance of an embryo implanting in a cross-section of patients still remains at 15% even in the best clinics, yet it was 12.5% in the original Oldham series. It is essential to note that these rates compare reasonably with the reported 25% rate occurring in the normal menstrual cycle at the age of 25, and it is important to stress that lower estimates have been given'. In their review of the literature, they found that 'the risk of anomalies appears to be no greater among an early series of 500 babies, than after conception *in vivo*, except for the sequelae resulting from multiple births'.

Despite the many advances in assisted reproductive technology there was a significant failure rate and many patients did not become pregnant. Not all were affected by 'the living death of barreness' as some became pregnant *au naturel.* Those who failed in their quest, required not only medical help, but the expert back-up of trained counsellors (Appleton, 1990). Despite the high level of successful unplanned pregnancies, in those who do not seek fertility, few infants are now referred for institutional care, so that adoption as a treatment for the infertile couple is a haven for relatively few 'would-be' parents.

CHRONOLOGY

Ovarian activity and ovulation

1883   Edouard van Beneden discovered that both ovum and sperm reduced their chromosome count by one half so that the fertilized ovum had a full complement of genetic material.

1905   Van de Velde first demonstrated the fact that body temperature shows a biphasic pattern during ovulatory cycles (with a difference of circa 0.5 °C between the follicular and luteal phases).

1906   Rowe stated that ovulation occurred at the end of a period of quiescence and directly caused the period of hypertrophy which occurred prior to menstruation.

1917   Stockard and Papanicolaou documented vaginal cytological changes during the oestrous cycle in guinea-pigs.

1923   Edgar Allen and Edward Doisy 'discovered' oestrogen.

1927   Zondek and Aschheim discovered gonadotropic hormones.

1929	George Corner and Willard Allen isolated progesterone.
1931	Fevold *et al.* were the first to extract follicle stimulating hormone and luteinizing hormone from the pituitary.
1933	Papanicolaou documented the characteristic changes in vaginal cytology which occurred throughout the menstrual cycle.
1937	Rock and Bartlett studied changes in the human endometrium and presented a method for dating the endometrial biopsy.
1950	Noyes *et al.* reported their technique of dating the endometrium at various stages of the cycle.
1951	Rubenstein *et al.* noted that the ovum is only fertilizable over a 6-hour period.
1959	McArthur was the first to show a consistent mid-cycle surge in luteinizing hormone.
	Taymor correlated luteinizing hormone assay with corpus luteum biopsy.
1968	Brown *et al.* reported a rapid method for estimating oestrogens in urine.
1970	Yen *et al.* performed longitudinal hormonal profiles by radioimmunoassay on groups of apparently normal women.
1971	Johansson *et al.* used the postovulatory rise in progesterone to prove that ovulation had occurred.
1972	Johansson *et al.* showed that monophasic basal temperature patterns may sometimes occur in ovulatory cycles.
	Abraham *et al.* showed that in women with normal cycles, there is a mid-cycle luteinizing hormone peak, the luteal phase lasting 12–16 days, with progesterone values greater than 5 ng/ml 5–8 days after this luteinizing hormone surge.
1972/73	Kratochwil *et al.* first reported their observations of follicle-like structures in the ovaries at ultrasound examination of the pelvis.
1974	Edwards and Steptoe found that, if adequate follicular development was present, ovulation occurred 36–38 hours after the administration of human chorionic gonadotropin.
	Black *et al.* introduced plasma oestrogen assessment to monitor the response to ovulation induction agents.

1976	The World Health Organization Report noted a time relationship between the serum luteinizing hormone peak and ovulation to have a median figure of 17 hours. The plasma oestradiol peak occurred, on average, 37 hours before ovulation.
1980	The World Health Organization Task Force related onset of serum luteinizing hormone surge to time of ovulation – 32 hours (23.6–38.2) and luteinizing hormone peak – 16.5 hours (9.5–23) (1980b).
	Renaud *et al.* recorded the preovulatory follicle size to be 27 mm.
	O'Herlihy *et al.* monitored follicular development with ultrasound.
1982	O'Herlihy *et al.* found preovulatory follicle size of 20 mm at ultrasound.
1986	Corson reported self-prediction of ovulation utilizing urinary luteinizing hormone kits and found that the luteinizing hormone surge began on the day of the thermal nadir.

Luteal phase deficiency

1949	Jones documented evidence of defective luteal phases in a group of infertile women.
1951	Jones was one of the earliest to prescribe progesterone for luteal phase deficiency.
1956	Noyes proposed that a diagnosis of luteal phase inadequacy should be made when endometrial development was at least 2 days behind that expected according to the dates of ovulation and onset of menses.
1976	Seppala *et al.* and del Pozo *et al.* used bromocriptine to suppress prolactin secretion in women with short luteal phases associated with hyperprolactinaemia. Treatment led to normalized corpus luteum function and normoprolactinaemia.
1978	Marik and Hulka evaluated their patients with laparoscopy. They found that 31% of patients had luteinized unruptured follicles.

The endometrium

1950	Noyes *et al.* demonstrated that the

endometrium could be dated accurately at histopathology.

1963 Hughes *et al.* detailed pathways of carbohydrate metabolism production in the endometrium.

1967 Wynn and Harris carried out electron microscopy of the endometrial surface.

1968 Gorski *et al.* found evidence of oestrogen binding sites in the endometrium.

Krishnan and Daniel had discovered a protein in endometrial secretion in the rabbit which they called blastokinin in 1967 (later termed 'uteroglobin'). One year later, they determined that it was a glycopeptide with a molecular weight of about 30 kDa.

Polycystic ovaries

1830 J. Lisfranc briefly described the condition (Ricci, 1945).

1844 Chereau introduced the term 'sclerotic or sclero-cystic disease of the ovary' (Ricci, 1945).

1895 Waldo advised wedge biopsy as an alternative to oophorectomy which was being performed for sclerocystic ovaries.

1904 Findlay described the use of wedge resection for cystic degeneration of the ovaries (Katz, 1981).

1935 Stein and Leventhal described a series of infertile patients with amenorrhoea and polycystic ovaries. Ovulation returned following ovarian tissue biopsy.

1949 J.V. Meigs first used the appellation Stein–Leventhal syndrome (Katz, 1981).

1950 Lewis *et al.* suggested a relationship between androgens and glucose or insulin secretion.

1969 Hammerstein and Cupceancu first used cyproterone acetate, originally developed as a progestagen, in the treatment of hirsutism.

1971 Crooke *et al.* used an almost pure follicle stimulating hormone preparation with a luteinizing hormone content of less than 20%, in the management of polycystic ovaries.

1975 Buttram and Vaquero reported a high incidence of postoperative adhesions following wedge resection.

1977 Raj *et al.* used follicle stimulating hormone in the treatment of polycystic ovaries.

1984 Rojanasakul and Nillus found that there was mild hyperprolactinaemia in about 30% of patients with polycystic ovaries. Adams *et al.* (1984; 1986) evaluated ultrasound assessment of ovarian change during luteinizing hormone releasing hormone therapy, and went on to describe the ultrasound appearances of polycystic ovary syndrome and multicystic ovaries the following year (Adams *et al.*, 1985).

1985 Chang and Geffner reviewed the available evidence and stated that women with polycystic ovaries exhibit hyperinsulinaemia and are insulin resistant.

Weight loss/anorexia nervosa

1868 Sir William Gull first used the term anorexia nervosa.

1970 Crisp noted a central theme to all cases – as the body configuration feminizes, the patient develops a phobia of becoming fat.

1976 Crisp *et al.* found a prevalence for anorexia of 1 per 200 school girls.

1978 Stein and Susser demonstrated a fall in conception rates when they investigated the Dutch hunger winter from October 1944 to May 1945 at a time when daily calorie intake fell to below 1000 calories.

Exercise

1978 Feicht *et al.* showed that the intensity and duration of training for sports, correlates with the prevalence of amenorrhoea.

1980/83 Warren reported a longitudinal study of 15 ballet dancers. There was a significant delay in onset of menarche.

1983 Frisch noted that intensive training caused increased calorific demands. Nutrition could be relatively inadequate and cause secondary amenorrhoea.

Ovulation induction

1909 Crowe *et al.* showed that the male and female reproductive systems were under the functional control of the anterior hypophysis.

1927 Zondek and Aschheim in Europe discovered gonadotropic hormones.

Smith and Engle first described superovulation after intramuscular implantation of anterior pituitary tissues in mice and rats.

1930 Cole and Hart demonstrated the ability of the serum of pregnant mares to cause superovulation in immature rats.

1953 Rakoff used low-dose irradiation of pituitaries and ovaries in an effort to stimulate ovulation in anovulatory women.

1958 Figueroa Chases documented the potentially life-threatening complications of hormone treatments.

1965 Igarashi *et al.* used cyclic oestrogen and progesterone in an effort to achieve rebound ovulation.

Persson found that cyclofenil was capable of inducing ovulation.

1968 Taymor noted the close relationship between total oestrogen excretion and ovarian enlargement and multiple pregnancy.

1969 Butler, and also Brown *et al.*, developed gonadotropin treatment scheduled at intervals, rather than using the daily regimen of Gemzell *et al.* (1958).

1972 Butler reported a pregnancy rate of 33%, and a multiple pregnancy rate of 20–30%, while using gonadotropin treatment.

Engel *et al.* reviewed the theoretical causes of hyperstimulation with gonadotropins.

1973 Williamson and Ellis detailed their experience of ovulation induction with tamoxifen.

Rakoff *et al.* used small doses of oestrogen in an effort to stimulate ovulation.

Menopausal urine

1949 Donini and Montezemolo prepared gonadotropins from the urine of menopausal women.

1954 Borth *et al.* demonstrated that menopausal urine contained follicle stimulating and luteinizing hormone activity in comparable amounts and predicted that human menopausal gonadoptropins could be used therapeutically.

1960 Lunenfeld successfully extracted and purified human gonadotropins from menopausal urine, and used them for induction of ovulation and pregnancy.

1961 Borth *et al.* reported on the effect of menopausal gonadotropins.

Pregnant mares' serum/urine

1945 Hamblen and Davis successfully induced ovulation which resulted in conception, using pregnant mares' serum gonadotropin and sequential human chorionic gonadotropin.

1964 Shearman proposed the use of pregnant mares serum for testing ovarian responsiveness to follicle stimulating hormone. It was found that this treatment could not be used repeatedly in humans because of antibody formation.

Pituitary

1958 Gemzell *et al.* were the first to report the successful use of follicle stimulating hormone for ovulation induction. The follicle stimulating hormone was produced from human pituitaries obtained at post-mortem and was called human pituitary gonadotropin. Pituitary extracts contained both follicle stimulating and luteinizing hormones.

1959 The first pregnancy following human pituitary gonadotropin treatment was recorded.

1962 Bettendorf *et al.* used preparations of human pituitaries.

1969 Brown *et al.* found that approximately 20% of cycles induced with human pituitary gonadotropin were associated with a shortened luteal phase.

Pure follicle stimulating hormone

1983 Venturoli *et al.* used pure follicle

1985 stimulating hormone, derived from human urine, to induce ovulation. Jones *et al.* reported results of its use for superovulation.

1990 Bettendorf reviewed the available literature of use of follicle stimulating hormone therapy.

Gonadotropin releasing hormone

1971 Burgus *et al.* (and also Matsuo *et al.* and Schally *et al.*) reported the isolation of gonadotropin releasing hormone.

1978 Guillemin and also Schally *et al.* described the biochemical sequence of luteinizing hormone releasing factor.

1980 Knobil demonstrated that pulsatile administration of gonadotropin releasing hormone could restore ovarian function.

Leyendecker *et al.* reported the first successful application of exogenous pulsatile gonadotropin releasing hormone therapy for restoration of ovulatory function in humans with hypothalamic amenorrhoea.

1982 Elkind-Hirsch *et al.* found that luteinizing hormone releasing hormone was released with cyclical frequency of approximately one pulse per hour.

1988 Breckwoldt *et al.* reported ovarian hyperstimulation when using gonadotropin releasing hormone.

Gonadotropin releasing hormone analogues

1982 Fleming *et al.* clinically evaluated the use of down-regulation using luteinizing hormone releasing hormone analogues.

1983 Cetel *et al.* induced a temporary reversible medical hypophysectomy by 'chronic' use of gonadotropin releasing hormone.

1984 The first report of a pregnancy following down-regulation with luteinizing hormone releasing hormone analogues was reported by Porter *et al.* in the *Lancet*.

1985 Hedon *et al.* used gonadotropin releasing hormone agonists with human menopausal gonadotropin to stimulate ovulation (Hedon *et al.*, 1990).

1988 Lewinthal created medical hypophysectomy using leuprolide acetate and then induced ovulation with human menopausal gonadotropin.

Clomiphene citrate and related drugs

1937 Robson and Schonberg reported that triphenylethylene and triphenylchloroethylene were oestrogen agonists of low potency and long duration of action.

1953 Shelton *et al.* demonstrated that the biological potency of oestrogen agonists could be augmented by alkoxy substitution.

1959 Allen *et al.* patented clomiphene citrate, a triphenylethylene derivative substitued with a chloride anion and an amino-alkoxyl.

1960 Tyler *et al.* induced ovulation with MER-25 (a product related to clomiphene citrate).

1961 Kistner and Smith carried out the first clinical trials of ovulation induction using a close structural analogue of clomiphene.

Robert Greenblatt *et al.* reported results of clinical testing with clomiphene, then known as MRL-41. They were the first to report successful induction of ovulation and pregnancy following clomiphene therapy.

1968 Kato *et al.* showed that clomiphene competed with oestrogen for binding sites in the hypothalamus and possibly the pituitary.

1969 Scommegna and Lash reported ovarian hyperstimulation following clomiphene treatment.

1971 Graff noted that treatment with clomiphene 'suppressed' cervical mucus.

1973 Taymor *et al.* reported the use of clomiphene in conjunction with gonadotropins.

1976 Asch and Greenblatt reported that the cis form of clomiphene which was an anti-oestrogen produced ovulation in 78% of patients, while the trans form was mildly oestrogenic with a 51% ovulation rate. The drug most commonly used for therapy contained both forms and had an ovulation rate between 40 and 70%.

Prolactin inhibiting agents/hyperprolactinaemia

1970   Lunenfeld *et al* showed that human menopausal gonadotropin could treat patients with the amenorrhoea-galactorrhoea syndrome.

1971   Lewis *et al* characterized prolactin.
Lutterback *et al* reported treatment of non-puerperal galactorrhoea with ergot alkaloid.

1972   Besser *et al.* reported successful treatment of high plasma prolactin levels by brom-ergocriptine (bromocriptine).
Hwang *et al.* purified prolactin and developed radioimmunoassay techniques for measurement of the hormone.

1975   Bohnet *et al* reported that only half their patients with hyperprolactinaemia had galactorrhoea.

1977   Pepperell *et al* used bromocriptine to suppress elevated prolactin levels, and achieved ovulation rates of up to 96%, and a pregnancy rate of 83%.

1978   De Cecco *et al* reported the effect of the dopamine agonist, lisuride.
Magyar and Marshall reported on women with untreated hyperprolactinaemia who became pregnant.

1980   Leyendecker *et al.* reported that ovulation could be induced in hyperprolactinaemia by pulsatile administration of luteinizing hormone releasing hormone.

1981   Franks *et al.* treated cases of hyperprolactinaemia with pergolide mesylate, another dopamine agonist.

1982   Nyboe Anderson *et al* showed that hyperprolactinaemia suppresses the positive feedback effect of oestrogen on luteinizing hormone secretion.

1983   Franks and Jacobs noted that bromocriptine was the primary treatment for hyperprolactinaemic amenorrhoea.

1986   Ferrari *et al* investigated the use of the long acting cabergoline.

Tubal factors

Investigation

1910   Rindfleisch first described hysterosalpingography.

1914   Rubin, and also Carey, reported the use of hysterosalpingography.

1920   Rubin described the test of tubal insufflation, thereafter called Rubin's Test.

1950   Speck introduced a test involving injection of phenolsulphonophthalene through a cannula, which if it reached the urine proved that tubal patency was present.

1965   Doyle described a grasping action of the fimbrae as it picks up the ovum.

1971   Kremer and Blickman showed that drops of radiological contrast agents were transported through the uterus and tubes by muscle contraction and ciliary action.

1973   Leeton and Talbot found false negative results of 15–25% when testing tubal patency at hysterosalpingography.
Hafez observed that the transport of gametes through the tubes depended on muscular contractions, ciliary action and fluid flow.

1974   Newton *et al* reported that 18% of their patients investigated for infertility had blocked tubes and adhesions.

1975   Cox reported tubal infertility in 11% of their patients.

1976   Pauerstein and Hodgson studied the rate of transport of radioactive particulate models of the ova through the oviducts of animals.

Treatment

1884   Schroeder reported salpingoplasty carried out 3 years previously.

1889   Skutsch used the term salpingostomy.

1894   Mackenrodt reported successful tubal surgery (Greenhill, 1937).

1897   Ries reported that Watkins of Chicago had performed the first cornual excision, and implanted an oviduct.

1900   Goullioud first illustrated a salpingoplastic operation – linear salpingostomy.

1903   Martin reported 24 cases of tubal surgery.
Ferguson illustrated a cuff technique.

1923   Bourne first described total linear salpingostomy.

1953   William J. Mulligan *et al* designed and used a silastic hood prosthesis.

1959 Wolfgang Walz may have been the first surgeon to use an operating microscope in infertility surgery.

1973 Williams reported that most experience with reversal of tubal sterilization procedures involved previous Madlener or Pomeroy operations.

1975 Siegler and Perez reviewed the literature concerning tubal anastomosis in sterilized patients using macro-surgical techniques, and found a pregnancy rate of 22%.

Swolin reported long-term results of electromicrosurgery and salpingos-tomy.

1977 Winston and also Gomel published results for microsurgical treatment of sterilized patients and found almost 70% became pregnant.

1982 Chamberlain and Winston summarized results of tubal surgery (mainly macrosurgical) from the literature. Operations performed on the lateral end of the tube later produced between 3 and 47% viable pregnancies; in the middle tube, 12 to 43% viable pregnancies; and those carried out at the medial end of the tube, 10 to 48%. Ectopic pregnancies overall ranged between 2 and 25%.

1983 Winston documented the available microsurgical techniques.

The male and reproduction

1678 van Leeuwenhoek first described spermatozoa in semen.

1810 Rudolph von Koelleker demonstrated that sperm originated in the testes.

1843 Barry observed fertilization of the rabbit egg.

1865 Franz Schweiger-Scidel showed that sperm cells possess both a nucleus and cytoplasm.

1928 Duran-Reynals first described the action of hyaluronidase, or spreading factor, which was later found in sperm.

1931 Butenandt first isolated male hormone from urine and called it androsterone.

1941 MacCleod and Hotchkiss showed that excess heat adversely affected spermatogenesis.

1944 Hotchkiss noted, that of the approximately 300 million spermatozoa

deposited in the vagina, only one meets the ovum in the upper portion of the Fallopian tube.

1948 Harrison and Weiner showed that the temperature in the testes is lower than that in the interior of the animal.

1951 Chang first suggested the concept of capacitation.

Cohen and Stein noted that sperm retain motility and fertilizing ability for at least 50 hours in the female genital system.

1952 LeBlond and Clermont defined the stages of the cycle of development of sperm in rats.

Tulloch drew attention to the association between varicocoele and disordered spermatogenesis.

Austin introduced the term 'capacitation'.

1953 Barer et al. noted that while most cells contain approximately 70% of water, sperm contain only about 50%. Their high solid content gives them high density, and a high refractive index which can be used to estimate their solid content.

1955 Harvey and Jackson discovered that the first part of the ejaculate contains approximately 80% of the sperm.

1959 Chang documented the in vitro fertilization of rabbit ova and concluded that a ripening process called 'capacitation' is necessary before sperm can fertilize ova.

1961 Noyes reviewed the subject of 'capacitation' of spermatozoa prior to fertilization.

Scott associated varicocoele with subfertility.

1963 Clermont outlined the development of spermatozoa in man.

1965 Bedford demonstrated changes in the surface electrical charge on sperm during their passage along the epididymal duct.

1970 Rowley et al. estimated that it takes 12 days from time of release in the seminiferous tubules to ejaculation.

Johnson et al. doubted the significance of varicocoele in infertility.

1973 Settlage et al. found spermatozoa in the Fallopian tubes within 5 minutes of insemination.

1974	Hoskins *et al.* demonstrated a rise in cyclic AMP content which is associated with an increase in sperm motility during epididymal transit.
1975	Albert *et al.* noted that Furadantin caused degenerative changes in the spermatic tubules that were apparently reversible.
1976	Farbas and Rosens demonstrated decreased sperm production in chronic alcohol intake.
1977	Bibbo *et al.* noted an increased incidence of congenital anomalies of the epididymis in male offspring of mothers who had been treated with diethylstilboestrol.
1981	Evans *et al.* found evidence for increased sperm abnormalities in cigarette smokers.

Semen analysis

1931	Moench and Holt analysed sperm morphology.
1941	Hotchkiss reviewed factors in stability and variability of semen specimens.
1948	Mann found that sperm density in ejaculates fell as a consequence of repeated ejaculations over a short time.
1951	MacLeod and Gold evaluated semen and found that when the sperm count and motility were satisfactory, morphology was usually normal. They showed that 90% of fertile men have more than 60% normal sperm forms.
1954	Frank *et al.* found that the presence of more than one million immature forms per ml was associated with a bad prognosis.
1962	MacLeod and Gold studied the relationship between frequency of ejaculation and sperm count.
1963	Rutherford *et al.* evaluated semen quality and its relationship to normal unplanned pregnancy. Sperm motility appeared to be a more important parameter than sperm density.
1965	Murphy and Torrano reported pregnancies in partners of men whose sperm count was as low as one million.
1966	Lampe and Masters noted that the relatively infertile male suffers marked deterioration in sperm count by too frequent ejaculation.

1969	MacLeod developed a motility index (1969a).
1975	Eliasson endeavoured to standardize seminal fluid analysis.
1977	Smith *et al.* observed that pregnancy rates of up to 50% were possible even when the male had moderately severe abnormalities of semen quality.
	Sherins *et al.* showed that the volume of the ejaculate did not change significantly over a 6–month period.
	Sherins *et al.* also indicated that if sperm motility was poor at the time of first analysis it remained poor.
1980	Makler developed a new technique for human sperm motility determination, using a microcomputer.
	The World Health Organization attempted to standardize sperm morphology (1980a).
1981	Katz *et al.* showed that abnormal sperm progressed less rapidly through mucus than normal sperm from the same ejaculate.

Counts and fertility

1951	MacLeod and Gold showed that the incidence of infertility increased when the sperm density was less than 20 million.
1953	MacLeod and Gold showed that fertile men with sperm concentrations of 20 million per ml or less took significantly longer to produce conception when compared to men with higher sperm concentrations.
1971	The American Fertility Society indicated that a sperm concentration of 40 million per ml was the lower limit of normal.
1979	Schwartz *et al.* found that for each day of abstinence there was an increased sperm count of 13 million and increased volume of 0.4 ml.

Sperm–mucus interactions

1844	Alfred François Donné discovered spermatozoa in vaginal secretions.
1866/68	Marion Sims, father of American Gynaecology, first described the postcoital test.

365

1913   Huhner introduced the postcoital test as a standard part of the investigation of the infertile couple.

1932   Miller and Kurzrock introduced the *in vitro* mucus penetration test.

1965   Kremer suggested an *in vitro* modification of the postcoital test in which the ability of sperm to penetrate ovulatory cervical mucus was tested.

1980   Katz *et al.* found that less than 50% of sperm in contact with cervical mucus actually enter the mucus.

1981/82   Hull *et al.* found the pregnancy rate of couples with a positive postcoital test approximated the normal population but if the test was negative the pregnancy rate was reduced to a fifth.

Immune factors/antibodies

1899   Landsteiner and Metchnikoff working independently, described the presence of antibodies to sperm.

1954   Wilson described the discovery of spermagglutinins in human semen and blood.

1964   Franklin and Dukes first reported spermagglutinating activity in the serum of a high percentage of women with unexplained infertility. They first recommended condom therapy to reduce antibody levels.

1968   Ishojima introduced a test for the detection of sperm antibodies.
Fjallbrant assessed male autoimmunity and found the mechanism of action was severe clumping of sperm.

1974   Rumke *et al.* found a higher incidence of antisperm antibodies in infertile couples when compared to those who were fertile.

1977   Shreiber advocated corticosteroid therapy in an effort to reduce the immune response.

1978   Jager *et al.* developed the mixed erythrocyte-spermatozoal antiglobulin reaction (MAR test) to detect antibody problems.

1979   Schumacher found that although sperm antibodies were present, serum antibodies might not be found.

1980   Mathur *et al.* (and again in 1984) provided evidence that sperm antibodies may exist in cervical mucus and that the titre correlated with results of postcoital tests and with pregnancy outcome.

1981   Ansbacher reviewed the available tests for sperm antibodies.

Special tests in the male

1950   Howard *et al.* detailed their experience of testicular biopsy in cases of semen deficiency.

1951   Landau and Loughead discovered that fructose levels correlate positively with androgen levels.

1966   Amelar found that it was rare for oligospermic men to have obstructive lesions.

1973   Phadke *et al.* found that fructose production varied inversely with sperm count.

1976   Yanagimachi *et al.* reported a test in which the ability of human sperm to penetrate zona-free hamster eggs was assessed.

Treatment of semen

Drugs

1950   Heller *et al.* used testosterone for periods of up to 70 days, in an effort to increase sperm concentration. Treatment with testosterone initially reduced sperm counts and was followed by a rebound of spermatogenesis levels to significantly higher than those before treatment.

1958   Taymor and Selenkow indicated that thyroid treatment was of some empiric value for patients with lowered sperm motility but normal sperm counts.

1964   Turner *et al.* showed that treatment with human chorionic gonadotropin improved spermatogenesis in individuals with hypogonadotropic hypogonadism.

1966   Mellinger and Thompson reported that following treatment with clomiphene, sperm counts improved.

1967   Lunenfeld *et al.* used treatment with follicle stimulating hormone for low sperm counts.
Danezis and Batrinos recorded that five of 11 cases treated with human

menopausal gonadotropin showed improvement in sperm count.

1968 Futterweit and Sobrero used human chorionic gonadotropin alone for patients with persistently low sperm motility. A pregnancy rate of 50% was achieved. Human chorionic gonadotropin appeared to cause a fall in sperm production.

1972 Rowley and Heller reported that testosterone treatment resulted in a rise in sperm concentration.

1973 Zarate *et al.* used luteinizing hormone releasing hormone and showed an increase in sperm count in half their treatment group.

1974 Reyes and Faiman used low doses of clomiphene. They were successful in stimulating sperm production but the pregnancy rate was poor.

1975 Rowley and Heller reported that human chorionic gonadotropin treatment did not stimulate spermatogenesis in normal men.

1976 Segal *et al.* recorded their treatment of men who had oligospermia and hyperprolactinaemia with bromocriptine, and normal semen quality was restored.

1977 Mortimer detailed treatment with gonadotropin releasing hormone for patients with Kallman's syndrome.

1978 Vermeulen and Comhaire used tamoxifen in a dose of 20 mg a day for patients with idiopathic oligospermia, but results were disappointing.

1979 Charny reported that clomiphene treatment had a negative effect on sperm production.

Surgery

1955 Hanley reported optimistically on the results of varicocoele ligation.

1966 Amelar described a technique for repair of epididymal obstruction.

1973 Amelar and Dubin performed vasovasostomy for men with vasectomy.

1976 Schmidt *et al.* reviewed the surgical techniques used for the relief of epididymal obstruction.

Other

1974 Barwin used intrauterine insemination.

1977 Scott *et al.* used cervical cup insemination techniques where the male had mild oligospermia or low semen volume.

1980 Zorgniotti *et al.* found that keeping the scrotum cool resulted in significant improvement of seminal characteristics.

1984 Zavos and Wilson increased the effectivness of treatment for retrograde ejaculation by using specialized buffers and intrauterine insemination.

1987 Arny and Quaglianello, Matson *et al.*, and others applied intrauterine insemination and gamete intrafallopian transfer respectively in the treatment of oligospermic infertility.

Artificial insemination by donor and husband

3rd C. AD Artificial insemination was mentioned in the Babylonian Talmud (Epstein, 1938). It was also felt possible that a woman could conceive as a result of bathing in water into which a man had ejaculated (Rosner, 1972; Kardiman, 1950). Women were advised against lying on bed sheets recently vacated by a man other than their husband, in case the man had deposited semen in the bedding and the woman became pregnant (Schellen, 1957). It was also thought that the daughter of the prophet Jeremiah became pregnant having bathed in water containing ejaculate (Ginzberg, 1968).

14th C. Arabs used artificial insemination with horses (Roehleder, 1934).

15th C. Fish eggs were artifically impregnated (Cusine, 1988).

1764 Ludwick Jacobi is said to have performed the first successful experiments with artifical impregnation of fish (Harkness, 1962).

1776 Spallanzani used artificial insemination.

1780 Spallanzani used artificial insemination to impregnate a dog (Spallanzani, 1789).

1785 John Hunter used artificial insemination in a woman which resulted in the birth of a child (Mason, 1990).

1866 Sims performed artificial insemination.

1868 Marion Sims again reported successful artificial insemination by husband in the USA.

1884   Dr Pancoast performed the first successful donor insemination in America (Joyce and Vassilopoulos, 1981).

1890   Robert Dickenson began using donor semen in the USA (Mason, 1990).

1909   A.D. Hard reported that the first successful donor insemination was carried out in the USA by Dr Pancoast in 1884.

1930s   Dr Margaret Jackson began a donor insemination service in the UK.

Between 50 and 150 babies were born per year from artificial conception of donated sperm in the USA.

1941   Seymour and Koerner surveyed results of artificial insemination in the USA and claimed a success rate of 97%.

1945   Barton *et al.* were the first to report their experience in the UK.

1948   A committee established by the Archbishop of Canterbury found that donor insemination was wrong in principle and contrary to Christian standards (Matthews, 1980).

1949   Pope Pius XII rejected the concept of artificial insemination on moral grounds (Matthews, 1980).

1957   Schellen reviewed artificial insemination techniques and results in humans and animals.

1958   The House of Lords in the UK debated donor insemination (Cusine, 1988).

1959   Haman reported fewer parental problems for 216 insemination babies, when compared with adopted infants.

1960   Lord Feversham produced his report on human artificial insemination.

1968   Behrman showed that couples who were successful with donor insemination have a low incidence of marriage breakdown.

Iizuka *et al.* concluded that children born following donor insemination showed normal physical and mental development.

1970   Hill reported experiences with treatment of 16 patients in Australia.

1972   Jacobs *et al.* indicated that the risk of detecting a serious abnormal autosomal constitution in a phenotypically normal donor was in the order of 3.3 per 1000.

1973   Sherman suggested that only use of fresh semen from very carefully selected sources should be used in an effort to avoid venereal disease.

The Peel Committee established by the British Medical Association produced their report on human artificial insemination (BMA, 1973; Mason, 1990).

1974   Barwin reported intrauterine insemination of husband's semen and found a 67% conception rate for patients with oligospermia.

1976   Matthews found there was an eightfold increase in the demand for donor insemination in Australia between 1971 and 1976.

Jacobsen found a fourfold increased demand in the USA during the same period.

1977   Klaus and Quinn indicated that 'a uniform parentage act' which would allow the law to treat a consenting husband as the natural father of donor insemination children was proposed for legislation in the USA.

1978   Whelan noted that a husband was prevented from bringing forth evidence at a later date to dispute his paternity, and the wife was prevented from re-opening an issue of the child's legitimacy by invoking a doctrine of 'estoppel' – being precluded from a course of action by one's previous behaviour.

1979   Joyce estimated that there are about 20 000 births per year attributable to donor insemination, with about half those occurring in the USA.

1980   A donor insemination programme was set up in France (David and Lansac, 1980).

1986   The American Fertility Society published guidelines for donor screening in a donor insemination programme.

1987   Andrews reported an extensive summary of legislation regarding *in vitro* fertilization and donor insemination in the USA.

1990   Taymor reviewed results of donor insemination from the literature and found pregnancy rates of 4–56%.

Storage of semen

1776	Spallanzani noted the effect of freezing temperature on human spermatozoa.
1886	Mantegazza suggested 'frozen' sperm banking.
1938	Jahnel stored freezing sperm in liquified gas.
1940	Shettles stored sperm by freezing in capillary tubes, but motility was poor on thawing.
1949	Polge *et al.* reported successful cryopreservation of human semen, and used glycerol as a cryoprotective agent to improve sperm motility.
1953	Bunge and Sherman reported the first human pregnancy from frozen stored sperm.
1954	Bunge *et al.* reported successful pregnancy from use of stored frozen spermatozoa.
1964	Sherman used nitrogen vapour to freeze sperm (Sherman, 1973). Perloff *et al.* reported four births with sperm which had been stored in nitrogen vapour.
1969	Fjallbrant and Ackerman reported the deleterious effects of preservation of human spermatozoa, reflected in a reduced ability to penetrate cervical mucus *in vitro*. Matheson *et al.* used plastic straws in which to store sperm.
1973	Sherman used human semen stored for a long period of up to 10 years and several conceptions were recorded. Frozen sperm was effective, with low anomaly and abortion rates. Steinberger and Smith compared fresh with frozen semen. There was a higher pregnancy and live birth rate with fresh semen. Two sperm banks were established in Paris (Cusine, 1988)
1974	Barkay *et al.* used sperm pellets for storage.
1979	Fifteen sperm banks were available in France.
1984	Richter *et al.* compared fresh with frozen sperm and found that frozen sperm were less effective.
1988	The American Fertility Society recommended that frozen sperm be used for donor insemination and that

a quarantine period of 180 days should be observed.

Cervical factors

1844	Alfred Donné discovered spermatozoa in vaginal secretions.
1847	Pouchet was the first to describe the cervical mucus changes during the menstrual cycle.
1866	Marion Sims first described the presence and motility of spermatozoa within cervical mucus following coitus.
1913	Huhner introduced the postcoital test which was used to evaluate the adequacy of coitus and the possible presence of hostile cervical factors which could affect sperm migration.
1928	Kurzrok and Miller described their *in vitro* sperm penetration test.
1944	Viergiver and Pommerenke showed that cervical mucus production increased during the follicular phase to reach a peak just before ovulation.
1954	Clift and Hart collected cervical mucus using a pipette or cannula combined with balloon or syringe, or also with use of forceps.
1960	Harvey found the maximum velocity of spermatozoa in cervical mucus was 3.54 mm per minute. Doyle *et al.* introduced a testing tape to determine mucus glucose levels in an effort to predict ovulation.
1962	Danezis *et al.* found that the higher the cervical mucus sperm count the higher the conception rate.
1963	Marcus and Marcus assessed mucus stretchability *Spinnbarkeit*, as a method of ovulation prediction.
1964	A cervical mucus chloride test, called the 'spot test', was introduced and the chloride content found to be highest at the time of ovulation (McSweeney and Sbarra, 1964).
1965	Kremer developed the sperm penetration metre which was further modified in later years.
1967	Lubke considered the percentage motility of sperm in the mucus to be important.
1970	Gibor *et al.* found no difference in the cervical mucus score between patients

who conceived and those who were infertile.

1972 Moghissi *et al* found that changes in cervical mucus symptoms or score correlated well with a preovulatory peak of luteinizing hormone in serum.

Billings *et al* documented the changes which take place in the cervical mucus at the time of ovulation.

Insler *et al* introduced the concept of a total 'cervical score' based on the amount and quality of mucus and dilatation of the cervical canal.

1973 Odebad observed that under the influence of oestrogen the microfibres of cervical mucus were arranged in longitudinal factions thus aiding sperm migration.

1974 Barwin used intrauterine insemination of husband's semen where there was inadequate cervical mucus.

1975 Kroeks and Kremer performed a sperm mucus penetration test using square capillary tubes.

1976 Kerin *et al* demonstrated that cervical mucus is most receptive to spermatozoa on the day before, and the day of, the preovulatory luteinizing hormone peak. They also found that the maximum 'cervical score' coincided with the day prior to and the day of the plasma luteinizing hormone surge.

1977 Scott *et al* used diethylstilboestrol to improve the quality of inadequate cervical mucus.

Kosasky introduced a 'tackimeter' to detect ovulatory change in cervical mucus.

1978 McBain reported a large series of intrauterine inseminations. The procedure was used in an attempt to bypass apparently hostile cervical mucus.

Telang *et al* found good correlation between poor postcoital tests and the presence of an immune factor.

Cervical operations

1938 Douay in France was the first operator to attempt repair of the internal os (Kistner and Patton, 1975).

1948 Palmer and Lacomme are credited with the first case report of operations for the incompetent cervix.

1953 Rabovits *et al.* demonstrated a radiographic technique to determine incompetent internal os of the cervix.

1957 McDonald reported his suture for cervical incompetence.

1963 Shirodkar introduced his method of incompetent cervix suture.

1964 Lash reviewed 20 years experience with the incompetent os and applied his surgical technique.

Uterine factors

Fibroids

1840 Anussat of Paris removed a pedunculated uterine fibroid (Kistner and Patton, 1975).

1843 Atley of Lancaster also removed a fibroid (Kistner and Patton, 1975).

1890 Martin reported a series of 96 myomectomy patients–18 died postoperatively.

1898 Alexander of Liverpool carried out multiple myomectomy (25) from a single uterus.

1909 Kelly and Cullen carried out myomectomy on 296 patients – 16 died.

1925 Victor Bonney advised myomectomy as elective treatment for fibroids.

1947 Bonney described the operative principles of myomectomy.

1958 Rubin found a 40% infertility rate in the presence of uterine myomata.

1963 Ingersoll reported a 50% conception rate in his series of myomectomies associated with infertility.

1987 West *et al* used gonadotropin releasing hormone treatment to shrink fibroid tumours.

Congenital abnormalities

1884 Ruge reported that Schroeder had removed a uterine septum *per vaginam* in a patient with previous miscarriages, who then carried to term.

1907 Strassman performed unification of a bicornuate uterus through a vaginal colpotomy incision (Strassman, 1952).

1953	Woolf and Allen found that unilateral renal defects were present in all their cases of unilateral Mullerian duct development.
1959	Jones introduced a transabdominal operation for surgical treatment of congenital uterine anomalies.
1961	Strassman described operations for double uterus and endometrial atresia.
1962	Tompkins introduced surgical treatment of uterine abnormalities.
1968	Jones and Baramki reported a miscarriage incidence of between 25 and 53% in association with uterine abnormalities.
1978	Goldstein reported an increased incidence of cervical incompetence in offspring exposed to diethylstilboestrol *in utero*.
1984	Muasher *et al* reported a doubling in the miscarriage rate for women who had been exposed to diethylstilboestrol *in utero*.

Asherman's syndrome

1948	Asherman described amenorrhoea traumatica.
1973	Klein and Garcia reviewed Asherman's syndrome and demonstrated that the diagnosis could be confirmed by hysteroscopy.

Infection

Pelvic inflammatory disease caused by tuberculosis, sexually transmitted disease or from other origins, was found to decrease fertility by its effects on the Fallopian tubes, and also by causing pelvic adhesions.

1972	Gnarpe and Friberg first suggested that *Mycoplasma* infection played a role in human infertility.
1984	Kane *et al.* described evidence of chlamydial infection in infertile women.

Psychosocial factors and counselling

1943	Loeser described women who developed amenorrhoea due to stress following bomb attacks during the war. It was later discovered that other forms

of stress could affect ovulation and the menstrual cycle.

1951	Kroger and Freed attempted to define the emotional element of infertility.
1962	Friedman reported a series of 100 cases of vaginismus in 'virgin wives'.
1968	Ellison, writing on psychosomatic factors, presented a series of 100 cases of non-consummation – vaginismus.
1969	Sandler treated three groups of sterile patients – an organic, an emotional, and a group seeking adoption. The emotional and adoption groups had a 50% pregnancy rate within 16 months. Sandler believed in a 'relief of emotional tension', which could be followed by pregnancy.
1969	Cooper found a subconscious collusion between couples which perpetuated sexual dysfunction.
1970	Masters and Johnson stated that there was no such thing as an uninvolved partner in a coital problem.
1984	The Warnock Report recommended that counselling, preferably by a qualified counsellor, should be available for infertile couples (Report of the Committee of Inquiry into Human Fertilization and Embryology).
1990	Appleton quoted a letter from an infertile couple to a newspaper, 'The sorrow of infertility... can be compared with ... bereavement. Sorrow is private, real, . . . taboo, and failure . . . is always very painful'.
	Fagan and Ponticas reviewed the psychological issues of the *in vitro* fertilization programme.

Unexplained infertility

1925	Kahn noted the beneficial effects of tubal insufflation.
1954	Fischer proposed a condition of 'psychogenic' infertility.
1962	Warner highlighted the significantly reduced pregnancy rates in patients where infertility was 'unexplained' compared to those in whom identified abnormalities were treated.
1974	Greenblatt *et al.* reported a 40% conception rate in patients with 'unexplained' infertility following a 3-month course of danazol.

1975   Behrman and Kistner reviewed pregnancy rates calculated by other workers. They found that 80% of couples had achieved pregnancy within 1 year and 90% within 18 months.

1976   Sher and Katz quoted an incidence of 10% 'unexplained' infertility.

1977   Drake et al. found 'unexplained' infertility in 3.5% of their population. Shivers and Dunbar noted that a small number of patients with 'unexplained' infertility also had antibodies to the zona pellucidae of their oocytes. Koninckx and Brosens reported significant delay in rise of the basal body temperature in a group of patients with 'unexplained' infertility.

1978   Sobowale et al. found a significant reduction in progesterone levels in the early part of the luteal phase, in patients with 'unexplained' infertility.

1980   Templeton and Mortimer found that in 'unexplained' infertility where the tubes were patent, there was a 45% failure rate of sperms to reach the Pouch of Douglas.

In vitro fertilization (IVF)

1878   Schenk first attempted in vitro fertilization, using rabbits and guinea-pigs as subjects.

1890   Walter Heape flushed fertilized rabbit ova from the Fallopian tubes and reimplanted them in a foster mother.

1893   Onanoff may have fertilized rabbit and guinea-pig eggs.

1930   Gregory Pincus described in vitro fertilization in the rabbit.

1946   Rock and Menkin fertilized human eggs in vitro.

1948   Menkin and Rock further reported fertilization of human ova.

1953   Shettles studied in vitro fertilization of the human ovum.

1955   Chang examined fertilizability of rabbit oocytes in vivo. Oocytes which had matured in the Graafian follicle were more likely to be fertilizable.

1965   Edwards reported his observations on maturation of the human ovum.

1969   Edwards et al. in England reported in vitro fertilization of human oocytes which were themselves matured in vitro.

1970   Edwards et al. used a Tyrode's solution containing pyruvate, albumin and antibiotics as their fertilization medium.

1974   Lopata et al. described an apparatus for aspirating follicles.

1975   Edwards and Steptoe treated patients with either human menopausal and human chorionic gonadotropins or clomiphene citrate and human chorionic gonadotropin and collected preovulatory eggs for in vitro fertilization. They used 3000–10 000 IU of human chorionic gonadotropin and collected mature oocytes via follicular aspiration 32–38 hours later.

1976   Steptoe and Edwards reported the placement of a human embryo and formation of an ectopic pregnancy.

1978   Wood considered that tubal transplant, if used as an alternative to in vitro fertilization would pose major technical problems and there would be considerable hazards from immunosuppressive therapy. Steptoe and Edwards reported successful in vitro fertilization, embryo transfer, and birth of the first in vitro fertilization baby, Louise Brown.

1979   Steptoe and Edwards found that children born as a result of in vitro fertilization and embryo replacement were healthy. They reported success rates for in vitro fertilization of preovulatory eggs of 70–80% and approximately 90% of fertilized eggs yielded embryos which cleaved normally in tissue culture. They also pointed out that steroid levels in follicular fluid of hyperstimulated cycles were different from those from normal menstrual cycles, and this could have a bearing on failure rates in in vitro fertilization cycles. They reported that best results were obtained in natural cycles, if eggs were collected via laparoscopy, 15–27 hours after the luteinizing hormone rise was detected.

1980   Trounson et al. found the presence of three or more pronucleui could be indicative of polyspermia. Edwards presented the morphological appearance of human embryo development in vitro. Edwards et al. found greater success rates with the natural cycle.

Ovulation was found to occur approximately 36 hours after onset of the luteinizing hormone surge in the serum or 28 hours after the onset of luteinizing hormone surge in urine in natural cycles.

1981   Edwards monitored follicular events by estimating oestrogen levels in urine.

1982   Craft *et al.* placed oocytes and sperm in the uterine cavity in an effort to simplify *in vitro* fertilization. There was a low success rate.

Carson *et al.* showed that correct levels of 17β-oestradiol and progesterone were critical for fertilization and further development.

Trounson *et al.* used washed sperm – this produced bacteria-free sperm with increased capacitation potential. They also used fertility enhancing drugs, harvested oocytes, and delayed 5–6 hours to allow full maturation of oocytes prior to adding sperm.

1983   Buster *et al.* introduced embryo donation.

Trounson and Mohr established that human pregnancy could follow cryopreservation and thawing of eight-cell embryos.

The Royal College of Obstetricians and Gynaecologists report on *in vitro* fertilization and embryo transfer (replacement) was published.

1984   Yovich and Stranger noted that fertilization and cleavage rates were poor if the motile sperm count fell below 5 million per ml.

Lutjen *et al.* reported embryo donation for *in vitro* fertilization in a patient with primary ovarian failure.

1985   Wilkes *et al.* noted that women over 40 years had low success rates.

Buster reported retrieval of donated embryos by uterine flushing and subsequently transferred the embryo.

1986   Ben Rafael *et al.* reported that those oocytes considered mature by cumulus cell criteria were preincubated for 6–8 hours, and immature oocytes were preincubated for 24–26 hours prior to insemination.

Kruger *et al.* noted an adverse outcome if there was a high incidence of abnormal sperm forms.

Testart *et al.* transferred frozen embryos on day 1 to 4 after the luteinizing hormone surge.

Gamete intrafallopian transfer (GIFT)

1984   Asch *et al.* reported pregnancy following translaparoscopic gamete intrafallopian transfer.

1985   Asch *et al.* added the indications of low sperm count or low sperm motility to their original indication of unexplained infertility, as reasons for gamete intrafallopian transfer. They reported birth following gamete intrafallopian transfer.

1986   A multicentre study was initiated to investigate the use of a common gamete intrafallopian transfer protocol in ten centres world-wide (Dooley *et al.*, 1989).

1987   Asch *et al.* reported on gamete intrafallopian transfer procedures using donated oocytes.

In the *Report on IVF and GIFT Pregnancies in Australia and New Zealand 1986*, figures indicated that there were 261 pregnancies notified after gamete intrafallopian transfer, and live births occurred in 62.8% (National Perinatal Statistics Unit, 1987).

Direct intraperitoneal sperm transfer (DIPI)

1985   Manhes and Hermabessiere reported on direct intraperitoneal sperm transfer.

1986   Forrler *et al.* reported pregnancies in three out of ten patients after this procedure and used the technique in unexplained infertility and cervical infertility.

Zygote intrafallopian transfer (ZIFT)

1986   Devroey *et al.* first described zygote intraperitoneal transfer.

1988   Abdalla and Leonard described a birth following this procedure.

Peritoneal oocyte and sperm transfer (POST)

1987   Mason *et al.* reported on peritoneal oocyte and sperm transfer under ultrasound guidance.

| 1990 | Mason reported that peritoneal oocyte and sperm transfer had a 24% success rate. |

Transuterine Fallopian transfer

1987	Jansen and Anderson reported catheterization of the Fallopian tubes via the vagina. It was thought that the methodology could simplify gamete transfer.
1988	Jansen *et al.* reported installation of cryostored donor semen and embryos via the same route.
1989	Anderson and Jansen placed husband's semen via catheter into the Fallopian tubes.

Ultrasound

1972	Holm described ultrasonically guided puncture techniques for abdominal tumour biopsy (Holm, 1980). Kratochwil *et al.* described ultrasonic tomography of the ovaries.
1976	Hackeloer and Hansmann showed that the number and size of follicles in patients undergoing ovulation stimulation could be successfully monitored using ultrasound.
1979	Hackeloer *et al.* introduced follicular monitoring by ultrasound.
1980	Renaud *et al.* recorded a preovulatory follicle size of 27 mm.
1981	Lenz *et al.* first reported successful collection of human oocytes under ultrasonic guidance.
1982	O'Herlihy *et al.* determined a preovulatory follicle size of 20 mm.
1984	Dellenbach *et al.* described transvaginal-sonography controlled ovarian puncture for oocyte retrieval.
1985	Parsons *et al.* retrieved oocytes by ultrasonically guided needle aspiration via the urethra. Wikland *et al.* reported transvaginal ultrasound.

Laparoscopy

| 1944 | Decker and Cherry described the use of culdoscopy in infertility diagnosis. |
| 1967 | Steptoe re-introduced improved |

laparoscopic techniques and the method went on to replace culdoscopy.

1970	Steptoe and Edwards reported laparoscopic recovery of preovulatory human oocytes.
1972	Parekh and Arronet documented the advantages and disadvantages of culdoscopy and laparoscopy.
1975	Peterson and Behrman noted adequate tubal patency with laparoscopy in up to 25% of patients who were shown to have blocked tubes at X-ray. They also showed that the incidence of unsuspected lesions was high at laparoscopy.
1978	A report of a working party of the Royal College of Obstetricians and Gynaecologists compared complication rates for the procedure in the UK and USA (Chamberlain and Brown, 1978).

Outcome of assisted conception

1983	Collins *et al.* found that pregnancy occurred in 41% of treated and 35% of untreated infertile couples.
1984	The Warnock report was produced for the Department of Health and Social Services in the UK (Report of the Committee of Inquiry into Human Fertilization and Embryology, 1984).
1985	Seppala reported from the World Collaborative Study and noted a preclinical abortion rate of 17% (preclinical – when menstrual period is delayed no more than 14 days). The incidence of clinical abortion was 24%.
1986	Steptoe *et al.* noted a high rate of caesarean section for delivery of babies resulting from *in vitro* fertilization and observed that the overall malformation rate in *in vitro* fertilization and gamete intrafallopian transfer babies was similar to population-based figures. Also the sex ratio of the infants was similar to non-assisted conception infants. Preterm and low birth weight infants were more common after assisted conception.
1988	Results of assisted conception in 2536 children were released by the National Perinatal Statistics Unit in Sydney (National Perinatal Statistics Unit, 1988).

Lancaster found that women over 40 were three times more likely to have a miscarriage when compared to women under 25 years of age.

1989   Steer *et al.* noted that ectopic pregnancy rates were higher in assisted conception.

1990   Births in Great Britain resulting from assisted conception were reported on. (Report of the MRC Working Party, 1990).

Figures from the Medical Research Council *In Vitro* Fertilization Register showed that the risk of multiple order birth increases with the number of embryos or ova transferred at *in vitro* fertilization or gamete intrafallopian transfer (Beral *et al.*, 1990).

REFERENCES

Abdalla, H.I. and Leonard, T. (1988). Cryopreserved zygote intrafallopian transfer for anonymous oocyte donation. *Lancet*, **1**, 835

Abraham, G.E., Odell, W.D., Swerdloff, R.S. and Hopper, K. (1972). Simultaneous radioimmunoassay of FSH, LH, progesterone, 17-hydroxyprogesterone and estradiol-17, during the menstrual cycle. *J. Clin. Endocrinol. Metab.*, **34**, 312–18

Adams, F. (translator) (1849). *The Genuine Works of Hippocrates.* (New York: William Wood)

Adams, J., Mason, W.P., Tucker, M., Morris, P.V. and Jacobs, H.S. (1984). Ultrasound assessment of changes in the ovary and the uterus during LH-RH. *Uppsala J. Med. Sci.*, **89**, 39–41

Adams, J., Franks, S., Polson, D.W. *et al.* (1985). Multifollicular ovaries: clinical and endocrine features and responses to pulsatile gonadotrophin releasing hormone. *Lancet*, **2**, 1375–8

Adams, J., Polson, D.W. and Franks, S. (1986). Prevalence of polycystic ovaries in women with anovulation and idiopathic hirsutism. *Br. Med. J.*, **293**, 355–9

Albert, P.S., Salerno, R.G., Kapoor, S.N. *et al.* (1975). The nitrofurans as sperm-immobilizing agents, their tissue toxicity and their clinical application in vasectomy. *Fertil. Steril.*, **26**, 485

Alexander, W. (1898). quoted by Ricci, J.V. (1945), p. 172

Allen, E. and Doisy, E.A. (1923). An ovarian hormone. Preliminary report on its localization, extraction and partial purification and action in test animals. *J. Am. Med. Assoc.*, **81**, 819–21

Allen, E., Pratt, J.P., Newell, Q.U. and Blandl, J. (1930). Human tubal ova; related corpora lutea and uterine tubes. *Contrib. Embryol.*, **22**, 45

Allen, R.E., Palopoli, F.P., Schumann, E.L. *et al.* (1959). *U.S. Patent*, **2**, 561, 914

Amelar, R. (1966). *Infertility in Men*, p. 83. (Philadelphia: F.A.Davis)

Amelar, R.D. and Dubin, L. (1973). Male infertility, current diagnosis and treatment. *Urology*, **1**, 1

American Fertility Society (1971). *How to Organize a Basic Study of the Infertile Couple.* (Birmingham: American Fertility Society)

American Fertility Society (1986). New guidelines for the use of semen donor insemination. *Fertil. Steril.*, **46**, suppl. 2

American Fertility Society (1988). Revised new guidelines for the use of semen-donor insemination. *Fertil. Steril.*, **49**, 211

Anderson, J.C. and Jansen, R.P.S. (1989). Ultrasound guided catheterization of the Fallopian tube for the non-operative transfer of gametes and embryos. *Proceedings of the World Congress of IVF and ET*, Jerusalem, quoted by Mason (1990)

Andrews, L.B. (1987). Ethical and legal aspects of *in vitro* fertilization and artificial insemination by donor. *Urol. Clin. N. Am.*, **14**, 633

Ansbacher, R. (1981). Sperm antibodies and infertility. *Fertil. Steril.*, **36**, 446

Anussat, (1840). quoted by Kistner, R.W. and Patton, G.W. Jr. (1975) p. 88

Appleton, T. (1990). Counselling, care in infertility: the ethic of care. *Br. Med. Bull.*, **46**, 842–9

Arny, M. and Quaglianello, J. (1987). Semen quality before and after processing by a swim-up method: relationship to outcome of intrauterine insemination. *Fertil. Steril.*, **48**, 643

Asch, R.H. and Greenblatt, R.B. (1976). Update on the safety and efficacy of clomiphene citrate as a therapeutic agent. *J. Reprod. Med.*, **17**, 175

Asch, R.H., Ellsworth, L.R., Balmaceda, J.P. and Wong, P.C. (1984). Pregnancy following translaparoscopic gamete intrafallopian transfer (GIFT). *Lancet*, **2**, 1034–5

Asch, R.H., Ellsworth, L.R., Balmaceda, J.P. and Wong, P.C. (1985). Birth following gamete intrafallopian transfer. *Lancet*, **2**, 163

Asch, R.H., Balmaceda, J., Ord, T. *et al.* (1987). Oocyte donation and gamete intrafallopian transfer as treatment for premature ovarian failure. *Lancet*, **1**, 687

Asherman, J.G. (1948). Amenorrhea traumatica (atretica) *J. Obstet. Gynaecol. Br. Commonw.*, **55**, 23

Austin, C.R. (1952). The "capacitation" of the mammalian sperm. *Nature (London)*, **170**, 326

Baden, W.F. and Baden, E.E. (1960). Cervical incompetence. Current therapy. *Am. J. Obstet. Gynecol.*, **79**, 545

Barer, R., Ross, K.F.A. and Tkaczyk, S. (1953). Refractometry of living cells. *Nature (London)*, **171**, 720–4

Barkay, J., Zuckerman, H. and Heiman, M. (1974). *Fertil. Steril.*, **25**, 399, quoted by Richardson (1976)

Barry, M. (1843). Spermatozoa observed within the mammiferous ovum. *Philos. Trans. R. Soc. Lond.*, **133**, 33

Bartelmez, G.W. (1931). The human uterine mucous membrane during menstruation. *Am. J. Obstet. Gynecol.*, **21**, 623–43

Barter, R.H., Dusbabek, J.A., Tyndal, C.M. and Erkenbach, R.V. (1963). Further experiences with the Shirodkar operation. *Am. J. Obstet. Gynecol.*, **85**, 792

Barton, M., Walker, K. and Wiesner, B.P. (1945). "Artificial Insemination". *Br. Med. J.*, **1**, 40–3

Barwin, B.N. (1974). Intrauterine insemination of husband semen. *J. Reprod. Fertil.*, **36**, 101

Bedford, J.M. (1965). Changes in the fine structure of the rabbit sperm head during passage through the epididymis. *J. Anat.*, **99**, 891

Behrman, S.J. (1968). In Behrman, S.J. and Kistner, R.W. (eds.) *Progress in Infertility*, p. 720. (Boston: Little, Brown & Co.)

Behrman, S.J. and Kistner, R.W. (1975). A rational approach to the evaluation of infertility. In Behrman, S.J. and Kistner, R.W. (eds.) *Progress in Infertility*, pp. 1–14. (Boston: Little, Brown and Co.)

Ben Rafael, Z., Kopf, G., Blasco, L., Tureck, R.W. and Mastroianni, L. Jr. (1986). Fertilization and cleavage after reinsemination of human oocytes *in vitro*. *Fertil. Steril.*, **45**, 58

Beral, V., Doyle, P., Tan, S.L., Mason, B.A. and Campbell, S. (1990). Outcome of pregnancies resulting from assisted conception. *Br. Med. Bull.*, **46**, 753–68

Besser, G.M., Parke, L., Edwards, C.R.W. *et al.* (1972). Galactorrhea-successful treatment of plasma prolactin levels by brom-ergocriptine. *Br. Med. J.*, **3**, 669

Bettendorf, G. (1990). Special preparations: pure FSH and desialo-hCG. In Crosignani, P.G. (ed.) *Clinical Obstetrics and Gynaecology: Induction of Ovulation*, pp. 519–34. (London, Philadelphia, Sydney, Tokyo, Toronto: Bailliere Tindall)

Bettendorf, G., Apostolakis, M. and Voigt, K.D. (1962). Darstellung von Gonadotropin aus menschlichen Hypophysen. *Acta Endocrinol.*, **41**, 1–13

Bibbo, M., Gill, W.B., Azizi, F. *et al.* (1977). Follow-up study of male and female offspring of DES-exposed mothers. *Obstet. Gynecol.*, **49**, 1

Billings, E.L., Billings, J.J., Brown, J.B. and Burger, H.G. (1972). Symptoms and hormonal changes accompanying ovulation. *Lancet*, **1**, 282–4

Black, W.P., Coutts, J.R.T., Codson, K.S. *et al.* (1974.) An assessment of urinary and plasma steroid estimations for monitoring treatment of anovulation with gonadotropins. *J. Obstet. Gynaecol. Br. Commonw.*, **81**, 667

BMA (1973). Report of Panel on Human Artificial Insemination. *Br. Med. J.*, **2**, Suppl. 3, 3

Bohnet, H.G., Dahlen, H.G., Wuttke, W. *et al.* (1975). Hyperprolactinemia anovulatory syndrome. *J. Clin. Endocrinol. Metab.*, **42**, 132

Bonney, V. (1925). Myomectomy as the treatment of election for uterine fibroids. *Lancet*, **2**, 1060

Bonney, V. (1947). *A Textbook of Gynaecological Surgery*, pp. 392–428. (London: Cassell)

Borth, R., Lunenfeld, B. and de Watteville, H. (1954). Activite gonadotrope d'un extrait d'urines de femmes en menopause. *Experientia*, **10**, 266

Borth, R., Lunenfeld, B. and Menzi, A. (1961). Pharmacologic and clinical effects of a gonadotropin preparation from human postmenopausal urine. In Albert, A. (ed.) *Human Pituitary Gonadotropins*, pp. 266–71. (Spring, Ill.: Charles C. Thomas)

Bourne, A. (1923). Discussion of the treatment of acute salpingitis. *Br. Med. J.*, **2**, 399

Bowes, K. (ed.) (1950). *Modern Trends in Obstetrics and Gynaecology*. (London: Butterworth & Co.)

Breckwoldt, F., Geisthovel, F., Neuler, J. and Schillinger, H. (1988). Management of multiple conception after GnRH/analogue human menopausal gonadotropin/human chorionic gonadotropin therapy. *Fertil. Steril.*, **49**, 713

Brown, J.B., Macleod, S.C., MacNaughtan, C. *et al.* (1968). A rapid method for estimating oestrogens in urine using a semiautomatic extractor. *J. Endocrinol.*, **42**, 5

Brown, J.B., Evans, J.H., Adey, F.D., Taft, H.P. and Townsend, L. (1969). Factors involved in clinical induction of fertile ovulation with human gonadotrophins. *J. Obstet. Gynaecol. Br. Commonw.*, **76**, 289–307

Brown-Sequard, C.E. (1889). Des effets produits chez l'homme par des injections sous-cutanees d'un liquide retiré des testicules frais de cobaye de chien. *C.R. Soc. Biol.*, **1**, 415–19

Bunge, R.G. and Sherman, J.K. (1953). Fertilizing capacity of frozen human spermatozoa. *Nature (London)*, **172**, 767–9

Bunge, R.G., Keettel, W.C. and Sherman, J.K. (1954). Clinical use of frozen sperm. *Fertil. Steril.*, **5**, 520

Burgus, R., Butcher, M., Ling, N., Monahan, M., Rivier, J., Fellows, R., Amass, M., Blackwell, R., Vale, R. and Guillemin, W. (1971). Structure moleculaire du facteur hypothalamique (LRF) d'origine ovine controlant la secretion de l'hormone gonadotrope hypophysaire du luteinisation (LH). *C.R. Acad. Sci. (Paris)*, **273**, 1611

Buster, J.E. (1985). Embryo donation by uterine flushing and embryo transfer. *Clin. Obstet. Gynecol.*, **12**, 815–24

Buster, J.E., Bustillo, M., Thorneycroft, I.H. *et al.* (1983). Nonsurgical transfer of *in vivo* fertilised donated ova to five infertile women: report of two pregnancies. *Lancet*, **1**, 816–17

Butenandt, A. (1931). Uber die chemische Untersuchung der Sexualhormone. *Z. angew. Chem.*, **44**, 905–8

Butler, J.K. (1969). Time course of urinary oestrogen estimation after various schemes of therapy with human follicle stimulating hormone (Pergonal). *Proc. R. S. Med.*, **62**, 34

Butler, J.K. (1972). Clinical results with human gonadotrophins in anovulation using two alternative dosage schemes. *Postgrad. Med. J.*, **48**, 23

Buttram, V.C. and Vaquero, C. (1975). Post-ovarian wedge resection adhesive disease. *Fertil. Steril.*, **26**, 874

Carey, W.H. (1914). Note on determination of patency of Fallopian tubes by the use of collargol and X-ray shadow. *Am. J. Obstet. Gynecol.*, **69**, 462–4

Carson, R.S., Trounson, A.O. and Findlay, J.K. (1982). Successful fertilization of human oocytes *in vitro*: concentration of oestradiol-17beta, progesterone and androstenedione in the antral fluid of donor follicles. *J. Clin. Endocrinol. Metab.*, **55**, 798–800

Cetel, N.S., Rivier, J., Valwe, W. and Yen, S.S.C. (1983). The dynamics of gonadotropin inhibition in women induced by an antagonistic analog of gonadotropin-releasing hormone. *J. Clin. Endocrinol. Metab.*, **57**, 62

Chamberlain, G. and Brown, J.C. (1978). *Gynaecological Laparoscopy: the report of the Working Party of the Confidential Enquiry into Gynaecological Laparoscopy*. (London: RCOG)

Chamberlain, G. and Winston, R. (1982). *Tubal Infertility. Diagnosis and Treatment*. (Oxford, London, Edinburgh, Boston, and Melbourne: Blackwell Scientific Publications)

Chang, M.C. (1951). Fertilising capacity of spermatozoa deposited on the Fallopian tubes. *Nature (London)*, **168**, 697

Chang, M.C. (1955). Fertilization and normal development of follicular oocytes in the rabbit. *Science*, **121**, 867–9

Chang, M.C. (1959). Fertilizing capacity of spermatozoa. In Lloyd, C.W. (ed.) *Recent Progress in the Endocrinology of Reproduction*, pp. 131–65. (New York: Academic Press)

Chang, R.J. and Geffner, M.E. (1985). Associated non-ovarian problems of polycystic ovarian disease:

insulin resistance. In Jacobs, H.S. (ed.) *Clinics in Obstetrics and Gynaecology, Reproductive Endocrinology*, Vol. 12, No. 3, pp. 675–85. (London, Philadelphia, Toronto: W.B. Saunders Co.)

Charny, C.W. (1979). Clomiphene therapy in male infertility: a negative report. *Fertil. Steril.*, **32**, 551

Cianfrani, T. (1960). *A Short History of Obstetrics and Gynaecology*, pp. 93–6. (Springfield Ill.: Charles C. Thomas)

Clermont, Y. (1963). The cycle of the seminiferous epithelium in man. *Am. J. Anat.*, **112**, 35

Clift, A. and Hart, J. (1954). Postcoital tests on a statistical basis. *Fertil. Steril.*, **5**, 544.

Cohen, J., Simons, R.F., Edwards, R.G., Fehilly, C.B. and Fishel, S.B. (1985). Pregnancies following the frozen storage of expanding human blastocytes. *J. In Vitro Fertil. Embryo Transfer*, **2**, 59

Cohen, W.R. and Stein, I.F. (1951). Sperm survival at estimated ovulation time. *Fertil. Steril.*, **2**, 20

Cole, H.H. and Hart, G.H. (1930). The potency of blood serum of mares in progressive stages of pregnancy in effecting the sexual maturity of the immature rat. *Am. J. Physiol.*, **93**, 57–68

Collins, J.A., Wrixon, W., James, L.B. and Wilson, E.H. (1983). Treatment independent pregnancy among infertile couples. *N. Engl. J. Med.*, **309**, 1201–6

Committee of Inquiry into Human Fertilization and Embryology (1984). *Report*, Chairman Dame Mary Warnock D.B.E. (London: HMSO)

Cooper, A.J. (1969). An innovation in the behavioural treatment of a case of non-consummation due to vaginismus. *Br. J. Psychiatr.*, **115**, 721–2

Corner, G.W. and Allen, W.M. (1929). Normal growth and implantation of embryos after very early ablation of the ovaries, under the influence of extracts of the corpus luteum. *Am. J. Physiol.*, **88**, 340–6

Corson, S.L. (1986). Self prediction of ovulation using a urinary luteinizing hormone test. *J. Reprod. Med.*, **31** (suppl. 8), 761

Cox, L.W. (1975). Infertility: a comprehensive programme. *Br. J. Obstet. Gynaecol.*, **82**, 2

Craft, I., Djahanbakhch, O., McLeod, F. *et al.* (1982). Human pregnancy following oocyte and sperm transfer to the uterus. *Lancet*, **1**, 1031–3

Craft, I., Ah-Moye, M., Al-Shawaf, T. *et al.* (1988). Analysis of 1071 GIFT procedures – the case for a flexible approach to treatment. *Lancet*, **1**, 1094–8

Crisp, A.H. (1970). Anorexia nervosa "feeding disorder" "nervous malnutrition" or "weight phobia". *World Rev. Nutri. Dietet.*, **12**, 452–504

Crisp, A.H., Palmer, R.L. and Kalucy, R.S. (1976). How common is anorexia nervosa? A prevalence study. *Br. J. Psychiatr.*, **128**, 549–54

Crooke, A.C., Sutaria, U.D. and Bertrand, P.V. (1971). Comparison of daily and twice weekly injections of follicle stimulating hormone for treatment of failure of ovulation. *Am. J. Obstet. Gynecol.*, **111**, 405

Crowe, S.J, Cushing, H. and Homans, J. (1909). quoted in Lunenfeld B. and Donini, P. (1966)

Cruikshank, W.C. (1797). Experiments in which, on the third day after impregnation, the ova of rabbits were found in the Fallopian tubes; and on the fourth day after impregnation in the uterus itself; with the first appearances of the foetus. *Phil. Trans. R. Soc. (Lond).*, **87**, 129–37

Cusine, D.J. (1988). *New Reproductive Techniques. A Legal Perspective*, pp. 11–19. (Aldershot (USA), Hong Kong, Singapore, Sydney: Gower)

Danezis, J. and Batrinos, M. (1967). The effect of human postmenopausal gonadotropins on infertile men with severe oligospermia. *Fertil. Steril.*, **18**, 788

Danezis, J., Sujan, S. and Sobrero, A. (1962). Evaluation of the post-coital test. *Fertil. Steril.*, **13**, 559

David, G. and Lansac, J. (1980). The organisation of centres for the study and preservation of semen in France. In David, G. and Price, W. (eds.) *Human Artificial Insemination and Semen Preservation*, pp. 15–26. (New York: Plenum)

Davis, M.E. and Koff, A.K. (1938). The experimental production of ovulation in the human subject. *Am. J. Obstet. Gynecol.*, **36**, 183

De Cecco, L., Foglia, G., Ragni, N., Rossato, P. and Venturini, P.L. (1978). The effect of lisuride hydrogen maleate in the hyperprolactinaemia-amenorrhoea syndrome: clinical and hormonal responses. *Clin. Endocrinol.*, **9**, 491–8

De Cherney, A.H. and Harris, T.C. (1986). The barren woman through history. In De Cherney,

A.H. (ed.) *Reproductive Failure*, p. 12. (New York, Edinburgh, London: Churchill Livingstone).

Decker, A. and Cherry, T.H. (1944). Culdoscopy, new methods in diagnosis for pelvic disease. *Am. J. Surg.*, **64**, 40

del Pozo, E., Wyss, H., Lancranjan, I., Obolensky, W. and Varga, L. (1976). Prolactin-induced luteal insufficiency and its treatment with bromocriptine: preliminary results. In Crosignani, P.G. and Mishell, D.R. (eds.) *Ovulation in the Human*, pp. 297–9. (London: Academic Press)

Dellenbach, P., Nisand, I., Moreau, L. *et al.* (1984). Transvaginal, sonographically controlled ovarian follicle puncture for egg retrieval. *Lancet*, **1**, 1467

Devreoy, P., Braeckmans P., Smitz, J. *et al.* (1986). Pregnancy after trans-laparoscopic zygote intrafallopian transfer in a patient with serum antibodies. *Lancet*, **1**, 1329

Donini, P. and Montezemolo, R. (1949). Gonadotropina preipofisaria e gonadotropina preipofisosimile umana. *La Rassegna di Clinica Terapia e Scienze Affine*, **48**, 143–63

Donne, A. (1844). *Cours de Microscopique et Physiologie des Fluides de l'Economie*, pp. 291–305. (Paris: Balliere)

Dooley, M., Abdalla, H. and Studd, J. G (1989). Gamete intrafallopian transfer. In Chamberlain, G. and Drife, J. (eds.) *Contemporary Reviews in Obstetrics and Gynaecology*, Vol. 1, No. 2, pp. 152–8. (London: Butterworths)

Douay, M.E. (1948). quoted by Kistner, R.W. and Patton, G.W. Jr. (1975), p. 53

Doyle, J.B., Ewers, F.J. and Sapit, D. (1960). A new fertility testing tape. *J. Am. Med. Assoc.*, **172**, 1744

Doyle, J.J. (1965). Tubo-ovarian mechanisms, observation at laparotomy. *Obstet. Gynecol.*, **8**, 696

Drake, T., Tredway, D., Buchanan, G., Lakaki, N. and Daane, T. (1977). Unexplained infertility – a reappraisal. *Obstet. Gynecol.*, **50**, 644

Dudley, A.P. (1901). Results of ovarian surgery, with further report upon intrauterine implantation of ovarian tissue. *J. Am. Med. Assoc.*, **37**, 357–60

Duran-Reynals, F. (1928). Exaltation de l'activité du virus vaccinal par les extrais de certains organes. *C.R. Soc. Biol.*, **99**, 6–7

Edwards, R.G. (1965). Maturation *in vitro* of human ovarian oocytes. *Lancet*, **2**, 926–9

Edwards, R.G. (1980). *Conception in the Human Female*. (London: Academic Press)

Edwards, R.G. (1981). Test-tube babies. *Nature, (London)*, **293**, 253–6

Edwards, R.G. and Craft, I. (1990). Development of assisted conception. *Br. Med. Bull.*, **46**, 565–79

Edwards, R.G. and Handyside, A.H. (1990). Future developments in IVF. *Br. Med. Bull.*, **46**, 823–41

Edwards, R.G. and Steptoe, P.C. (1974). Control of human ovulation, fertilization and implantation. *Proc. R. Soc. Med.*, **67**, 932

Edwards, R.G. and Steptoe, P.C. (1975). Induction of follicular growth, ovulation and luteinization in the human ovary. *J. Reprod. Fertil.*, **22**, 121

Edwards, R.G., Donaghue, R., Baramki, T. and Jones, H. (1966). Preliminary attempts to fertilize human oocytes matured *in vitro*. *Am. J. Obstet. Gynecol.*, **96**, 192

Edwards, R.G., Bavister, B.D. and Steptoe, P.C. (1969). Early stages of fertilization *in vitro* of human oocytes matured *in vitro*. *Nature (London)*, **221**, 632

Edwards, R.G., Steptoe, P.C. and Purdy, J.M. (1970). Fertilization and cleavage *in vitro* of pre-ovulatory human oocytes. *Nature (London)*, **227**, 1307

Edwards, R.G., Steptoe, P.C. and Purdy, J.M. (1980). Establishing full term human pregnancies using cleaving embryos grown *in vitro*. *Br. J. Obstet. Gynaecol.*, **87**, 757–68

Eliasson, R. (1975). Analysis of semen. In Behrman, S.J. and Kistner, R.W. (eds.) *Progress in Infertility*, 2nd edn., pp. 691–713. (New York: Little, Brown)

Elkind-Hirsch, K., Schiff, I., Ravnikar, V. *et al.* (1982). Determinations of endogenous immunoreactive luteinizing hormone releasing hormone in human plasma. *J. Clin. Endocrinol. Metab.*, **54**, 602

Ellison, C. (1968). Psychosomatic factors in the unconsummated marriage. *J. Psychosom. Res.*, **12**, 61–5

Engel, T., Jewelewicz, R.M. and Dyrenfurth, I. (1972). Ovarian hyperstimulation syndrome.

Report of a case with notes on pathogenesis and treatment. *Am. J. Obstet. Gynecol.*, **112**, 1052

Epstein, I. (ed.) (1938). *The Babylonian Talmud.* (London: Soncino Press)

Estes, W.L. (1909). A method of implanting ovarian tissue in order to maintain ovarian function. *Pennsylvania Med. J.*, **13**, 610–13

Evans, J.H., Fletcher, J., Torrance, M. and Hargreave, T.B. (1981). Sperm abnormalities and cigarette smoking. *Lancet*, **1**, 627

Fagan, P.J. and Ponticas, Y. (1990). Psychological issues in IVF: evaluation and care. In Damewood, M.D. (ed.) *The John Hopkins Handbook of In Vitro Fertilization and Assisted Reproductive Technologies*, pp. 27–38. (Boston, Toronto, London: Little Brown and Co.)

Farbas, M. and Rosens, R. C. (1976). Effect of alcohol on elicited male sexual response. *J. Stud. Alcohol*, **37**, 265

Feicht, C.B., Johnson, T.S., Martin, B.J., Sparkes, K.E. and Wagner, W.W. (1978). Secondary amenorrhoea in athletes. *Lancet*, **2**, 1145–6

Ferguson, A.H. (1903). President's Address. *Med. Fortnight*, **24**, 527

Ferrari, C., Barbieri, C., Caldara, R. *et al.* (1986). Long-lasting prolactin-lowering effect of cabergoline, a new dopamine agonist, in hyperprolactinemic patients. *J. Clin. Endocrinol. Metab.*, **63**, 941–5

Feversham, Lord (1960). *Report of the Departmental Committee on Human Artificial Insemination*, Cmnd 1105. (London: HMSO)

Fevold, H.L., Hisaw, F.C. and Leonard, S.L. (1931). The gonad stimulating and luteinizing hormones of the anterior lobe of the hypophysis. *Am. J. Physiol.*, **97**, 291

Figueroa Chases, P. (1958). Reaccion ovarica monstruosa a las gonadotrofinas: a proposito de un caso fatal. *Anal. Cirug.*, **23**, 116

Finn, W.F. and Muller, P.F. (1950). Abdominal myomectomy. *Am. J Obstet Gynecol.*, **60**, 109

Fischer, I.C. (1954). Psychogenic aspects of sterility. *Fertil. Steril.*, **4**, 466

Fjallbrant, B. (1968). Interaction between high levels of sperm antibodies, reduced penetration of cervical mucus by spermatozoa and sterility in man. *Acta Obstet. Gynaecol. Scand.*, **47**, 102

Fjallbrant, B. and Ackerman, D.R. (1969). Cervical mucus penetration *in vitro* by fresh and frozen preserved human semen specimens. *J. Reprod. Fertil.*, **20**, 515

Fleming, R., Adam, A.H., Barlow, D.H., Black, W.P., McNorton, M.C. and Coutts, J.R.T. (1982). A new systematic treatment for infertile women with abnormal hormone profiles. *Br. J. Obstet. Gynaecol.*, **89**, 80–3

Forrler, A., Deltenbach, P., Nisand, I *et al.* (1986). Direct intraperitoneal insemination in unexplained and cervical infertility. *Lancet*, **1**, 916

Frank, H. (1898). Uber transplantation der Ovarien. *Zentralbl. Gynaekologie*, **22**, 444–7

Frank, I.N., Benjamin, J.A. and Sergerson, J.E. (1954). Cytologic examination of semen. *Fertil. Steril.*, **5**, 217

Franklin, R.R. and Dukes, C.I. (1964). Antispermatozoal antibody and unexplained infertility. *Am. J. Obstet. Gynecol.*, **89**, 6

Franks, S. and Jacobs, H.S. (1983). Hyperprolactinaemia. *Clin. Endocrinol. Metab.*, **12**, 641–68

Franks, S., Horrocks, P.M., Lynch, S.S., Butt, W.R. and London, D.R. (1981). Treatment of hyperprolactinaemia with pergolide mesylate: acute effects and preliminary evaluation of long term treatment. *Lancet*, **2**, 659–61

Friedman, L.J. (1962). *Virgin Wives.* (London: Tavistock)

Frisch, R.E. (1983). Fatness and reproduction: delayed menarche and amenorrhea of ballet dancers and college athletes. In Darby, P.L. *et al.* (eds.) *Anorexia Nervosa: Recent Developments in Research*, pp. 343–63. (New York: Alan R. Liss Inc.)

Futterweit, N. and Sobrero, A.J. (1968). Treatment of normogonadotropic oligospermia with large doses of chorionic gonadotropin. *Fertil. Steril.*, **19**, 971

Gemzell, C.A., Diczfalusy, E. and Tillinger, K.G. (1958). Clinical effect of human pituitary follicle stimulating hormone (FSH) *J. Clin. Endocrinol. Metab.*, **18**, 1333

Gibor, Y., Garcia, C.J., Cohen, M.R. and

Scommegna, A. (1970). The cyclical changes in the physical properties of the cervical mucus and the results of the post-coital test. *Fertil. Steril.*, **21**, 20

Ginzberg, L. (1968). *The Legends of the Jews.*, VI, 400–1. (Philadelphia: Jewish Publication Society of America)

Gnarpe, H. and Friberg, J. (1972). Mycoplasma and human reproductive failure:I. The occurrence of different mycoplasmas in couples with reproductive failure. *Obstet. Gynecol.*, **114**, 727

Goldstein, D.P. (1978). Incompetent cervix in offspring exposed to diethylstilbestrol *in utero*. *Obstet. Gynecol.*, **52**, 738

Gomel, V. (1977). Tubal reanastomosis by microsurgery. *Fertil. Steril.*, **28**, 59

Gorski, J., Toft, D., Shyamala, G., Smith, D. and Notides, A. (1968). Hormone receptors: studies on the interaction of estrogen with the uterus. *Rec. Progr. Horm. Res.*, **24**, 45–80

Gouillioud, P. (1900). De la salpingostomie. *Lyons Med.*, **53**, 13

Graff, G. (1971). Suppression of cervical mucus during clomiphene therapy. *Fertil. Steril.*, **22**, 209

Graham, H. (1950). *Eternal Eve*, p. 313. (London: W. Heinemann)

Greenblatt, R.B., Barfield, W.E., and Jungck, E.C. *et al.* (1961). Induction of ovulation with MRL-41: preliminary report. *J. Am. Med. Assoc.*, **178**, 101

Greenblatt, R.B., Borenstein, R. and Hernandez-Ayup, S. (1974). Experience with Danazol (an antigonadotrophin) in the treatment of infertility. *Am J. Obstet. Gynecol.*, **118**, 783

Greenhill, J.P. (1937). Evaluation of salpingostomy and tubal implantation for the treatment of sterility. *Am. J. Obstet. Gynecol.*, **33**, 39

Gruhn, J.G. and Kazer, R.R. (1989). *Hormonal Regulation of the Menstrual Cycle: The Evolution of Concepts*, p. 33. (New York, London: Plenum Medical Book Co.)

Guillemin, R. (1978). Peptides in the brain; the new endocrinology of the neuron. *Science*, **202**, 390

Gull, W.W. (1868). The address in medicine delivered before the annual meeting of the BMA at Oxford. *Lancet*, **2**, 171–6

Hackeloer, B.J. and Hansmann, M. (1976). Ultraschalldiagnostik in der Fruhschwangerschaft. *Gynaekologie*, **9**, 108

Hackeloer, B.J., Fleming, R., Robinson, H.P., Adams, A.J. and Coutts, A.J. (1979). Correlation of ultrasonic and endocrinologic assessment of human follicular development. *Am. J. Obstet. Gynecol.*, **135**, 122–8

Hafez, E.S.E. (1973). *Female Reproductive System, Handbook of physiology*, section 7, Vol. 11, part 2, p. 113. (Washington: American Physiological Society)

Ham, R.G. (1963). An improved nutrient solution for diploid Chinese hamster and human cell lines. *Exp. Cell. Res.*, **29**, 47

Haman, J.O. (1959). Therapeutic donor insemination. *Calif. Med.*, **90**, 130

Hamblen, E.C. and Davis, C.D. (1945). Treatment of hypoovarianism by sequential and cyclic administration of equine and chorionic gonadotrophins – so called one-two cyclic gonadotropic therapy – summary of 5 years results. *Am. J. Obstet. Gynecol.*, **50**, 137–46

Hammerstein, J. and Cupceancu, B. (1969). The treatment of hirsutism with cyproterone acetate. *Deutsche Med. Wchschr.*, **94**, 829–33

Hanley, H.G. (1955). The surgery of male subfertility. *Ann. R. Coll. Surg. Engl.*, **17**, 159

Hard, A.D. (1909). "Artificial impregnation". *Medical World*, **27**, 163–5

Harkness, R.D. (1962). The provision of special chemical stimulants, and of measures for continuance of the species. Historical Note. In Davson, H. and Grace Eggleton, M. (eds.) *Starling and Lovatt Evans Principles of Human Physiology*, pp. 1387–9. (London: J. & A. Churchill Ltd.)

Harrison, R.G. and Weiner, J.S. (1948). Abdomino-testicular temperature gradients. *J. Physiol.*, **107**, 48–9

Harvey, C. (1960). The speed of human spermatozoa and the effect on it of various diluents, with some preliminary observations on clinical material. *J. Reprod. Fertil.*, **1**, 84

Harvey, C. and Jackson, M.J. (1955). A method of concentrating spermatozoa in human semen. *J. Clin. Pathol.*, **8**, 341

Heape, W. (1890). Preliminary note on the transplantation and growth of mammalian ova within a uterine foster mother. *Proc. R. Soc. Lond.*, **48**, 457–9

Hedon, B., Bringer, J., Arnal, F., Humeau, C., Boulot, P., Audibert, F., Benos, P., Neveu, S., Mares, P., Laffargue, F. and Viala, J.L. ((1990). The use of GnRH agonists with hMG for induction or stimulation of ovulation. In Crosignani, P.G. (ed.) *Clinical Obstetrics and Gynaecology. Induction of Ovulation*, pp. 575–87. (London, Philadelphia, Sydney, Tokyo, Toronto: Balliere Tindall)

Heller, C.G., Nelson, W.O., Hill, I.B., Henderson, E., Maddock, W.O., Jungck, E.C., Paulsen, C.A. and Mortimore, G.E. (1950). Improvement in spermatogenesis following depression of human testes with testosterone. *Fertil. Steril.*, **1**, 415

Hellman, L.M. (1951). The use of polyethylene in human tubal plastic operations. *Fertil. Steril.*, **2**, 498

Hill, A.M. (1970). "Experiences with artificial insemination". *Aust. N.Z. J. Obstet. Gynaecol.*, **10**, 112–14

Hitschmann, F. and Adler, L. (1907). Die Lehre von der Endometritis. *Z. Geburt. Gynaekol.*, **60**, 63–86

Hitschmann, F. and Adler, L. (1908). The structure of the endometrium of sexually mature women with special reference to menstruation. *Mschr. Geburtsh. Gynaekol.*, **27**, 1–82

Holm, H.H. (1980). Procedure of ultrasonically guided puncture. In Holm, H.H. and Kristensen, J.K. (eds.) *Ultrasonically Guided Puncture Technique*, p. 29. (Copenhagen: Munksgaard)

Hoskins, D.D., Stephens, D.T. and Hall, M.L. (1974). Cyclic adenosine 3',5' monophosphate and protein kinase levels in developing bovine spermatozoa. *J. Reprod. Fertil.*, **37**, 131

Hotchkiss, R.S. (1941). Factors in stability and variability of semen specimens. *J. Urol.*, **45**, 875–88

Hotchkiss, R.S. (1944). *Fertility in Men*. (Philadelphia: J.B. Lippincott Co.)

Howard, R.R., Shiffren, R.C., Simmons, F.A. and Albright, F. (1950). Testicular deficiency: A clinical and pathologic study. *J. Clin. Endocrinol. Metab.*, **10**, 121

Howles, C.M., Macnamee, M.C., Edwards, R.G., Goswamy, R.K. and Steptoe, P.C. (1986). Effect of high tonic levels of lutenizing hormone on incidence of *in vitro* fertilization. *Lancet*, **2**, 521–2

Hughes, E.C., Jacobs, R.D., Rubulis, A. and Husney, R.M. (1963). Carbohydrate pathways of the endometrium. *Am. J. Obstet. Gynecol.*, **85**, 594–609

Huhner, M. (1913). *Sterility in the Male and Female and its Treatment*. (New York: Robman)

Hull, M.G.R. *et al.* (1981) quoted by Joyce and Vassilopoulos (1981) p. 587

Hull, M.G.R., Savage, P.E. and Bromham, D.R. (1982). Prognostic value of the postcoital test: a prospective study based on time-specific conception rates. *Br. J. Obstet. Gynaecol.*, **89**, 299–305

Hwang, P., Guyda, H. and Friesen, H.G. (1972). Purification of human prolactin. *J. Biochem.*, **247**, 1955

Igarashi, M., Matsumoto, S. and Hosaka, H. (1965). Further studies on the rebound phenomenon of ovarian function. *Fertil. Steril.*, **16**, 257

Iizuka, R., Sawada, Y. and Nishina, N. (1968). The physical and mental development of children born following artificial insemination. *Int. J. Fertil.*, **13**, 24–32

Ingersoll, F.M. (1963). Fertility following myomectomy. *Fertil. Steril.*, **14**, 596

Insler, V., Melamed, H., Eichenbrenner, I., Serr, D. and Lunenfeld, B. (1972). The cervical score. A simple semi-quantitative method for monitoring of the menstrual cycle. *Int. J. Gynecol. Obstet.*, **10**, 223

Iscovesco, H. (1912a). Le lipoide uterostimulant de l'ovaire. Propriétés physiologiques. *C.R. Soc. Biol. (Paris)*, **63**, 104–6

Iscovesco, H. (1912b). Les lipoides de l'ovaire. *C.R. Soc. Biol. (Paris)*, **63**, 16–18

Ishojima, S., Li, T.S. and Ashitaka, Y. (1968). Immunologic analysis of sperm immobilizing factor found in the serum of women with unexplained sterility. *Am. J. Obstet. Gynecol.*, **101**, 677

Jacobs, P.A., Fackiewicz, A. and Law, P. (1972). Incidence and mutation rates of structural rearrangements of the autosomes in man. *Ann. Hum. Genet.*, **35**, 301

Jacobsen, E. (1976). Up 400%: artificial insemination. *Sex. Med. Today*, December 6

Jager, S., Kremer, J. and van Slochteren-Draaisma, T. (1978). A simple method of screening for antisperm antibodies in the human body. *Int. J. Fertil.*, **23**, 12–21

Jahnel, F. (1938). *Klin. Wchschr.*, **17**, 1273, quoted by Newton (1976) p. 25

Jansen, R.P.S. and Andeson, J.C. (1987). Catheterization of the Fallopian tubes from the vagina. *Lancet*, **2**, 309–10

Jansen, R.P.S., Anderson, J.C. and Sutherland, P.D. (1988a). Nonoperative embryo transfer to the Fallopian tube. *N. Engl. J. Med.*, **319**, 288

Jansen, R.P.S., Anderson, J.C., Radonic, I., Smit, J. and Sutherland, P.D. (1988b). Pregnancies after ultrasound guided Fallopian insemination with cryostored donor semen. *Fertil. Steril.*, **49**, 920–2

Johansson, E.D.B., Wide, L and Gemzell, C. (1971). Luteinizing hormone and progesterone in plasma and LH and oestrogens in urine during 42 normal menstrual cycles. *Acta Endocrinol. (Kbn)*, **68**, 502

Johannson, E.D.B., Larsson-Cohn, V. and Gemzell, C. (1972). Monophasic basal body temperature in ovulatory menstrual cycles. *Am. J. Obstet. Gynecol.*, **113**, 933

Johnson, D.E., Puhl, D.R. and Rivera-Correa, H. (1970). Varicocele: An innocuous condition? *South Med. J.*, **63**, 34

Jones, G.E.S. (1949). Some newer aspects of the management of infertility. J. Am. Med. Assoc., **141**, 1123–8

Jones, G.E.S. (1951). Some newer aspects of management of infertility. *J. Am. Med. Assoc.*, **146**, 212

Jones, G.S., Acosta, A.A., Garcia, J.E., Bernardus, R.E. and Rosenwaks, Z. (1985). The effect of follicle-stimulating hormone without additional luteinizing hormone on follicular stimulation and oocyte development in normal ovulatory women. *Fertil. Steril.*, **43**, 696–702

Jones, H.W. Jr. (1959). Operations for congenital anomalies of the uterus and vagina. *Clin. Obstet. Gynecol.*, **2**, 1053

Jones, H.W. and Baramki, T.A. (1968). Congenital anomalies. In Behrman, S.J. and Kistner, R.W. (eds.) *Progress in Infertility*, 1st edn. p. 63. (Boston: Little, Brown)

Joyce, D.N. (1979). Artificial insemination by donor. *IPPF Med. Bull.*, **13**, 1–2

Joyce, D.N. and Vassilopoulos, D. (1981) Sperm–mucus interaction and artificial insemination. In Hull, M.G.R. (ed.) *Clinics in Obstetrics and Gynaecology*, Vol. 8, No. 3, pp. 587–610. (London, Philadelphia, Toronto: W.B. Saunders Co.)

Kahn, I.W. (1925). The role of the cervix in sterility. *Am. J. Obstet.*, **10**, 254

Kane, J.L., Woodland, R.M., Forsey, T. and Darougay Elder, M.G. (1984). Evidence of chlamydial infection in infertile women and without Fallopian tube obstruction. *Fertil. Steril.*, **42**, 843

Kardiman, S. (1950). Artificial insemination in the Talmud. *Harofe Haivri: Hebrew Medical Journal*, **2**, 164 ff

Kato, J., Kiobayashi, T. and Villee, C.A. (1968). Effect of clomiphene on the uptake of estradiol by the anterior hypothalamus and hypophysis. *Endocrinology*, **82**, 1049

Katz, D.F., Overstreet, J.W. and Hanson, F.W. (1980). A new quantitative test for sperm penetration into cervical mucus. *Fertil. Steril.*, **33**, 179–86

Katz, D.F., Diel, L. and Overstreet, J.W. (1981). Differences in the movement of morphologically normal and abnormal human seminal spermatozoa. *Fertil. Steril.*, **35**, 256–7

Katz, M. (1981). Polycystic ovaries. In Hull, M.G.R. (ed.) *Clinics in Obstetrics and Gynaecology*, Vol. 8, No. 3, *Developments in Infertility Practice*, pp. 715–31. (London, Philadelphia, Toronto: W.B. Saunders Co. Ltd.)

Kelly, H.A. and Cullen, T.S. (1909). *Myomata of Uterus*. (Philadelphia: Saunders)

Kerin, J.F., Matthews, C.D., Svigas, J.M., Makin, A.E., Symons, R.G. and Smeaton, T.C. (1976). Linear and quantitative migration of stored sperm through cervical mucus during the periovular period. *Fertil. Steril.*, **27**, 1054

Kistner, R.W. and Patton, G.W. Jr. (1975). *Atlas of Infertility Surgery*, pp. 51; 95. (Boston: Little, Brown & Co.)

Kistner, R.W. and Smith, O.W. (1961). Observations on the use of nonsteroidal estrogen antagonist MER-25: effects in endometrial hyperplasia and Stein–Leventhal syndrome. *Fertil. Steril.*, **12**, 121

Klaus, J. and Quinn, P.E. (1977). Human artificial insemination. Some social and legal issues. *Med J. Aust.*, **1**, 710

Klein, S. and Garcia, C.R. (1973). Asherman's syndrome: a critique and review. *Fertil. Steril.*, **24**, 905

Knaus, H. (1933). "Die periodische Frucht-und Unfruchtbarkeit des Eribes" *Zentralbl. Gynaekol.*, **57**, 24–33

Knobil, E. (1980). Neuroendocrine control of the menstrual cycle. *Rec. Prog. Horm. Res.*, **36**, 53

Koninckx, P. and Brosens, I.A. (1977). Delayed onset of luteinisation as a cause of infertility. *Fertil. Steril.*, **28**, 292

Kosasky, J.J. (1977). A tackimeter for the determination of tackiness of cervical mucus. *Fertil. Steril.*, **28**, 354

Kovacs, G.T. and Burger, H.G. (1984). Artificial insemination. In Studd, J. (ed.) *Progress in Obstetrics and Gynaecology*, Vol. 4, pp. 322–33. (Edinburgh, London: Churchill Livingstone)

Kratochwil, A., Urban, G. and Freidrich, F. (1972). Ultrasonic tomography of the ovaries. *Ann. Chirur. Gynaecol. Fenn.*, **61**, 211–14

Kratochwil, A., Jentsch, K. and Bressina, K. (1973). Ultraschallanatomie des weiblichen beckens und ihre klinische bedentung. *Archiv. Gynaekol.*, **214**, 273

Kremer, J. (1965). A simple sperm penetration test. *Int. J. Fertil.*, **10**, 209

Kremer, J. and Blickman, J. (1971). Demonstratie met film over het intra-uterine transport van kleine hoeveelheden roentgenocontrastyloeistof. *Nederlands Tijdschrift voor Geneeskunde*, **115**, 860

Krishnan, R.S. and Daniel, J.C. Jr. (1968). Composition of "blastokinin" from rabbit uterus. *Biochim. Biophys. Acta*, **168**, 579–82

Kroeks, M.V.A.M. and Kremer, J. (1975). The fractional postcoital test performed in a square capillary tube. *Acta Europ. Fertil.*, **6**, 371

Kroger, W.S. and Freed, S.C. (1951). *Psychosomatic Gynecology.* (Philadelphia: W.B. Saunders)

Kruger, T.F., Monkveld, R., Stander, F.S.H., Lombard, C.J., Van der Mercwe, J.P., Van Zyl, J.A. and Smith, K. (1986). Sperm morphologic features as a prognostic factor in *in vitro* fertilization. *Fertil. Steril.*, **46**, 1118

Kurzrok, R. and Miller, E.G. (1928). Biochemical studies of human semen and its relation to mucus of the cervix uteri. *Am. J. Obstet. Gynecol.*, **15**, 56

Lampe, E. and Masters, W. (1966). Problems of male fertility: II. Effects of frequent ejaculation. *Fertil. Steril.*, **7**, 123

Lancaster, P.A.L. (1988). Outcome of pregnancy. In Wood, C. and Trounson, A. (eds.) *Clinical In Vitro Fertilization*, pp. 81–94. (Berlin: Springer Verlag)

Landau, R.L. and Loughead, R. (1951). Seminal factors as index of androgenic activity in man. *J. Clin. Endocrinol. Metab.*, **11**, 1411

Landsteiner, K. (1899). Zur kenntnis der spezifisch auf blutkörperchen wirkenden sera. *Zentralbl. Bakteriol.*, **25**, 546

Lash, A.F. (1964). Review of more than 20 years experience with the incompetent internal os of the cervix. *Fertil. Steril.*, **15**, 254

LeBlond, C.P. and Clermont, Y. (1952). Definition of the stages of the cycle of the seminiferous epithelium of the rat. *Ann. N. Y. Acad. Sci.*, **55**, 548

Leeton, J. and Talbot, J. Mc. (1973). A comparative study of laparoscopy with hysterosalpingography in 100 infertility patients. *Aust. N. Z. J. Obstet. Gynaecol.*, **13**, 169

Lenz, S. and Lauritsen, J.G. (1982). Ultrasonically guided percutaneous aspiration of human follicles under local anesthesia: a new method of collecting oocytes for *in vitro* fertilisation. *Fertil. Steril.*, **38**, 673–7

Lenz, S., Lauritsen, J.G. and Kjellow, M. (1981). Collection of human oocytes for *in vitro* fertilization by ultrasonically guided follicular puncture. *Lancet*, **1**, 1163–4

Lewinthal, D. (1988). Induction of ovulation with luprolide acetate and HMG. *Fertil. Steril.*, **49**, 585

Lewis, J.T., Foglia, V.G. and Rodriquez, R.R. (1950). The effect of steroids on the incidence of diabetes in rats after subtotal pancreatectomy. *Endocrinology*, **46**, 111–21

Lewis, U.J., Singh, R.N.P., Sinha, Y.N. *et al.* (1971). Electrophoretic evidence for human prolactin. *J. Clin. Endocrinol.*, **32**, 153

Leyendecker, G., Struve, T. and Plotz, E.J. (1980). Induction of ovulation with chronic intermittent (pulsatile) administration of LHRH in women with hypothalamic and hyperprolactinemic amenorrhea. *Archiv. Gynecol.*, **229**, 177

Loeser, A. (1943). *Lancet*, **2**, 518, quoted by Sandler (1969) p. 51

Lopata, A., Johnston, W.I.H., Leeton, J.F., Muchnicki, D., Talbot, J. Mc., and Wood, C. (1974). Collection of human oocytes at laparoscopy and laparotomy. *Fertil. Steril.*, **25**, 1030

Lubke, F. (1967). Correlation between cervical penetration and seminal tests. *Proceedings of the 5th World Congress Fertility and Sterility*, International Congress Series, No. 133, p. 739. (Stockholm: Excerpta Medica Foundation)

Lunenfeld, B. and Donini, P. (1966) Historic aspects of gonadotropins. In Greenblatt, B. (ed.) *Ovulation*, pp. 9–34. (Toronto: Lippincott)

Lunenfeld, B., Menzi, A. and Volet, B. (1960). Clinical effects of human postmenopausal gonadotrophins. *Acta Endocrinol. (Kbh)*, **51** (Suppl.), 587

Lunenfeld, B., Mor, A. and Mani, M. (1967). Treatment of male infertility. I. Human gonadotrophins. *Fertil. Steril.*, **18**, 581

Lunenfeld, B., Insler, V. and Rabau, E. (1970). Die Prinzipien der Gonadotropintherapie. *Acta Endocrinol.*, **148**, 52–101

Lutjen, P., Trounson, A., Leeton, J., Findlay, J., Wood, C. and Renou, P. (1984). The establishment and maintenance of pregnancy using *in vitro* fertilization and embryo donation in a patient with primary ovarian failure. *Nature (London)*, **307**, 174–5

Lutterback, P.M., Pryor, J.S., Varga, L. *et al.* (1971). Treatment of non-puerperal galactorrhea with an ergot alkaloid. *Br. Med. J.*, **3**, 228

McArthur, J.W. (1959). Midcycle changes in urinary gonadotropin excretion. In Lloyd, C.W. (ed.) *Recent Progress in the Endocrinology of Reproduction*, p. 67. (New York: Academic Press)

McBain, J.C. (1978). Report on the practice of AID in Australia. *Proceedings of the 2nd National Workshop on Aid*, Sydney, quoted by McBain and Pepperell (1980)

McBain, C.H. and Pepperell, R.J. (1980). Unexplained infertility. In Pepperell, R.J., Hudson, B. and Woods, C. (eds.) *The Infertile Couple*, pp. 165–81. (Edinburgh: Churchill Livingstone)

McDonald, I.A. (1957). Suture of the cervix for inevitable miscarriage. *J. Obstet. Gynaecol Br. Emp.*, **64**, 346

MacLeod, J. (1969). Further observations on the role of varicocele in human male infertility. *Fertil. Steril.*, **20**, 545

MacLeod, J. (1969). quoted by Pepperell, R.J., Hudson, B. and Wood, C. (1980), p. 85

MacLeod, J. and Gold, R.Z (1951a). The male factor in fertility and infertility. II Spermatozoa counts in 1000 men of known fertility and 1000 men of infertile marriage. *J. Urol.*, **66**, 436–49

MacLeod, J. and Gold, R.Z. (1951b). The male factor in infertility and fertility: IV. Sperm morphology in fertile and infertile marriage. *Fertil. Steril.*, **2**, 394

MacLeod, J. and Gold, R.Z. (1953). The male factor in fertility and infertility. VI. Semen quality and certain other factors in relation to ease of conception. *Fertil. Steril.*, **4**, 10

MacLeod, J. and Gold, R. (1962). The male factor in fertility and infertility: effects of continence on semen quality *Fertil. Steril.*, **3**, 297

MacLeod, J. and Hotchkiss, R.S. (1941). The effects of hyperpyrexia upon spermatozoa counts in men. *Endocrinology*, **28**, 780

McSweeney, D.J. and Sbarra, A.J. (1964). A new cervical mucus test for hormonal appraisal. *Am. J. Obstet. Gynecol.*, **88**, 705

Magyar, D.M. and Marshall, J.R. (1978). Pituitary tumors and pregnancy. *Am. J. Obstet. Gynecol.*, **132**, 739–51

Makler, A. (1980). Use of a microcomputer in combination with the MEP technique for human sperm motility determination. *J. Urol.*, **124**, 372

Makler, A. (1980). Use of the elaborated multiple exposure photography (MEP) method in routine sperm motility analysis and for research purposes. *Fertil. Steril.*, **33**, 160–6

Malgaigne, J.F. (1849). Du catheterisme de la trompe de Fallope pour remedier a la sterilité, par le docteur Tyler Smyth. *Rev. Med. Chir.*, **6**, 113

Manhes, H. and Hermabessiere, J. (1985). Fecondation. Intra-peritoneale. Premiere grossesse obtenu sur indication du masculin. *Oral presentation. 3rd International Forum in Andrology,* June, Paris, quoted by Mason (1990) pp. 783–95

Mann, T. (1948). Fructose content and fructolysis in semen. Practical application in the evaluation of semen quality. *J. Agric. Sci.*, **38**, 323–31

Mantegazza, J. (1886). Fisiologia sullo sperma umans, *Rendic, Reale Instit. Lomb.*, **3**, 183

Marcus, L.S. and Marcus, C.C. (1963). Cervical mucus and its relation to infertility. *Obstet. Gynecol. Surv.*, **18**, 749

Marik, J. and Hulka, J. (1978). Luteinised unruptured follicle syndrome: a subtle cause of infertility. *Fertil. Steril.*, **28**, 292

Markee, J.E. (1940). Menstruation in intraocular endometrial transplants in the rhesus monkey. *Contrib. Embryol. Carneg. Instn. Wash.*, **28**, 219–308

Martin, A. (1890). quoted by W.F. Finn and P.F. Muller (1950)

Martin, F.H. (1903). Ovarian transplantation and reconstruction of fallopian tubes. *Chic. Med. Recorder*, **25**, 1

Mason, B.A. (1990). Simple techniques past and present as an alternative to *in vitro* fertilization and GIFT. *Br. Med. Bull.*, **46**, 783–95

Mason, B.A., Sharma, V., Riddle, A.F. and Campbell, S. (1987). Ultrasound guided peritoneal oocyte and sperm transfer (POST). *Lancet*, **1**, 386

Masters, W.H. and Johnson, V.E. (1970). *Human Sexual Inadequacy*. (Boston: Little Brown)

Matheson, G.W., Carlborg, L. and Gemzell, C. (1969). *Am. J. Obstet. Gynecol.*, **104**, 495, quoted by Richardson (1976)

Mathur, S., Baker, E.R. Williamson, H.O., Derrick, F.C., Teague, K.S. and Fudenberg, H.H.(1980). Clinical significance of sperm antibodies in infertility. *Fertil. Steril.*, **33**, 239

Mathur, S., Williamson, H.O., Baker, M.E. *et al.* (1984). Sperm motility on postcoital testing correlates with male autoimmunity to sperm. *Fertil. Steril.*, **41**, 81

Matson, P.L., Blackledge, D.G., Richardson, P.A., Turner, S.R., Yovich, J.M. and Yovich, J.L. (1987). The role of gamete intrafallopian transfer (GIFT) on the treatment of oligospermic infertility. *Fertil. Steril.*, **46**, 608

Matsuo, H.L., Baba, Y., Nair, R.M.G., Arimura, A. and Schally, A.V. (1971a). Synthesis of the porcine LH and FSH releasing hormone by the solid phase method. Biochem. *Biophys Res. Commun.*, **25**, 992

Matsuo, H., Baba, Y., Nair, R.M.G., Arimura, A. and Schally, A.V. (1971b). Structure of porcine LH and FSH releasing hormone. 1. The proposed amino acid sequence. *Biochem. Biophys. Res. Commun.*, **43**, 1334–9

Matthews, C.D. (1976). Current status of A.I. in clinical practice. In Brudenell, M., McLaren, A., Short, R.V. and Symonds, E.M. (eds.) *Artificial Insemination*, pp. 42–3. (London: Royal College of Obstetricians and Gynaecologists)

Matthews, C.D. (1980). Artificial insemination – donor and husband. In Pepperell., R.J., Hudson, B. and Wood, C. (eds.) *The Infertile Couple*, pp. 182–208. (Edinburgh, London, New York: Churchill Livingstone)

Medvei, V.C. (1982). *A History of Endocrinology.* (Lancaster, MTP Press)

Mellinger, R. and Thompson, R. (1966). The effect of clomiphene citrate in male infertility *Fertil Steril.*, **17**, 94

Menkin, M.F. and Rock, J. (1948). *In vitro* fertilization and cleavage of human ovarian eggs. *Am. J. Obstet. Gynecol.*, **55**, 440

Metchnikoff, S. (1899). Etudes sur la resorption des cellules. *Ann. Inst. Pasteur. Lille*, **13**, 737

Meyer, R. (1911). Uber Corpus Luteumbildung bei Menschen. *Zentralb. Gynaekol.*, **35**, 1206–8

Miller, E.G. and Kurzrock, R. (1932). Biochemical studies of human semen:III. Factors affecting migration of sperm through the cervix. *Am. J. Obstet. Gynecol.*, **24**, 19–26

Moench, G.L. and Holt, H. (1931). Sperm morphology in relation to fertility. *Am. J. Obstet. Gynecol.*, **22**, 199

Moghissi, K.S., Syner, F.N. and Evans, T. (1972). "A composite picture of the menstrual cycle". *Am. J. Obstet. Gynecol.*, **114**, 405–18

Moricke, R. (1882). Die Uterusschleimhaut in verschiedenen Altersperioden und zur Zeit der Menstruation. *Z. Gynaekol.*, **7**, 84–137

Morris, R.T. (1895). The ovarian graft. *N. Y. Med. J.*, **62**, 436–7

Mortimer, C.H. (1977). Clinical applications of the gonadotropin releasing hormone. *Clin. Endocrinol. Metab.*, **6**, 167–80

MRC (1990). Report of the MRC Working Party on: Children conceived by in-vitro fertilization. Births in Great Britain resulting from assisted conception. *Br. Med. J.*, 1978–87

Muasher, S.T., Garcia, J.E. and Jones, H.W. Jr (1984). Experience with diethylstilbestrol-exposed infertile women in a program of *in vitro* fertilization. *Fertil. Steril.*, **42**, 20

Mulligan, W.J., Rock, J. and Easterday, C.L. (1953). Use of polyethylene in tuboplasty. *Fertil. Steril.*, **4**, 5

Murphy, D. and Torrano, E. (1965). Male fertility in 3620 childless couples. *Fertil. Steril.*, **16**, 337

National Perinatal Statistics Unit. (1987). *IVF and GIFT Pregnancies in Australia and New Zealand 1986.* (Sydney: National Perinatal Statistics Unit)

National Perinatal Statistics Unit. (1988). *IVF and GIFT pregnancies, Australia and New Zealand 1987.* (Sydney: National Perinatal Statistics Unit)

Newton, J. J. (1976). Current status of A.I. in clinical practice. In Brudenell, M., McLaren, A., Short, R., and Symonds, M. (eds.) *Artificial Insemination, Proceedings of the 4th Study of the RCOG*, pp. 25–41. (London: RCOG)

Newton, J.J., Craig, S. and Joyce, D. (1974). The changing pattern of a comprehensive infertility clinic. *J. Biosoc. Sci.*, **6**, 477

Ng, S.C., Bongso, T.A., Sathananthan, A.H. and Ratnam, S.S. (1990). Micro-manipulation; its relevance to human IVF. *Fertil. Steril.*, **53**, 203–19

Noyes, R.W. (1956). Uniformity of secretory endometrium. *Obstet. Gynecol.*, **7**, 221

Noyes, R.W. (1961). The capacitation of spermatozoa. A Review. *Obstet. Gynecol. Surv.*, **14**, 785

Noyes, R.W., Hertig, A.T. and Rock, J. (1950). Dating the endometrial biopsy. *Fertil. Steril.*, **1**, 3–25

Nyboe Andersen, A., Schioler, V., Hertz, J. *et al.* (1982). Effect of metoclopramide induced hyperprolactinemia on the gonadotrophic response to estradiol and LRH. *Acta Endocrinol.*, **100**, 1

Odebad, E. (1973). Biophysical techniques of assessing cervical mucus and microstructure of cervical epithelium on cervical mucus. In Elstein, M., Moghissi, K.S. and Barth, R. (eds.) *Human Reproduction*, pp. 58–74. (Copenhagen: Scriptor)

Ogino, K. (1930). Ovulationstermin und konzeptionstermin. *Zentralb. Gynaekol.*, **54**, 464–79

O'Herlihy, C., Robinson, H.P. and De Crespigny, L.J. Ch. (1980a). Mittelschmerz is a preovulatory symptom. *Br. Med. J.*, **280**, 986

O'Herlihy, C., de Crespigny, L.J.Ch. and Robinson, H.P. (1980b). Monitoring ovarian follicular development with real time ultrasound. *Br. J. Obstet. Gynaecol.*, **87**, 613–18

O'Herlihy, C., Pepperell, R.J. and Robinson, H.P. (1982). Ultrasound timing of human chorionic gonadotropin administration in clomiphene stimulated cycle. *Obstet. Gynecol.*, **59**, 40

Onanoff, M.J. (1893). Recherches sur la fecondation et la gestation des mammiferes. *C. R. Seances Soc. Biol.*, **45**, 719

Palmer, R. and Lacomme, M. (1948). La beance de l'orifice interne, cause d'avortements a la repetition? Une observation de dechirure cervical isthmique reparee chirugicalment, avec gestation a terme consecutive. *Gynecol. Obstet.*, **47**, 905

Papanicolaou, G.N. (1933). The sexual cycle of the human female as revealed by vaginal smears. *Am. J. Anat.*, **52**, 519

Parekh, M.C. and Arronet, G.H. (1972). Diagnostic procedures and methods in the assessment of female pelvic organs, with special reference to infertility. *Clin. Obstet. Gynecol.*, **15**, 1

Parsons, J., Riddle, A. and Booker, M. (1985). Oocyte retrieval for *in vitro* fertilization by ultrasonically guided needle aspiration via the urethra. *Lancet*, **1**, 1076

Pauerstein, C.J. and Hodgson, B.J. (1976). Rate of transport of radioactive ovum models through the oviducts of individual rabbits. *Am. J. Obstet. Gynecol.*, **124**, 840

Peck, A.L. (translator) (1943). *Aristotle, Generation of Animals.* (Cambridge, Mass: Harvard University Press)

Pepperell, R.J., McBain, J.C. and Healy, D.L. (1977). Ovulation induction with bromocriptine in patients with hyperprolactinaemia. *Aust. N. Z. J. Obstet. Gynaecol.*, **17**, 181

Pepperell, R.J., Hudson, B. and Wood, C. (eds.) (1980). *The Infertile Couple.* (Edinburgh, London, New York: Churchill Livingstone)

Percy, S.R. (1861). A fact for medico-legal science. *Am. M. Times,* **2**, 160

Perloff, W.H., Steinberger, E. and Sherman, J.K. (1964). *Fertil. Steril.,* **15**, 501, quoted by Richardson (1976) p. 97

Persson, B.H. (1965a). The effect of Bis (*p*-acetoxyphenyl) cyclohexylidenemethane (compound F6066) on hormone secretion in post menopausal women. *Acta Soc. Medic. Upsal.,* **70**, 1–16

Persson, B.H. (1965b). The effect of Bis (*p*-acetoxyphenyl) cyclohexylidenemethane (compound F6066) on menstrual disorders. *Acta Soc. Medic. Upsal.,* **70**, 71–81

Peterson, E.P. and Behrman, S.J. (1975). Laparoscopy and hysteroscopy. In Behrman, S.J. and Kistner, R.W. (eds.) *Progress in Infertility,* 2nd edn., pp. 865–87. (Boston: Little, Brown)

Phadke, A.M., Samant, N.R. and Shubbada, D.D. (1973). Significance of seminal fructose studies in male infertility. *Fertil. Steril.,* **24**, 894

Philipp, E. (1979). Investigations of the infertile couple. *Med. Soc. Lond. Trans.,* **96**, 23–6

Pincus, G. (1930). Observations on the living eggs of the rabbit. *Proc. Royal Soc. Lond., Series B,* **107**, 132–67

Pincus, G. and Enzmann, E.V. (1934). Can mammalian eggs undergo normal development *in vitro? Proc. Natl. Acad. Sci. USA,* **20**, 121–2

Polge, C., Smith, A.V. and Parkes, A.S. (1949). Revival of spermatozoa after vitrification and dehydration at low temperature. *Nature (London),* **164**, 666

Porter, R., Smith, W., Craft, I.L., Abdulwahid, N. and Jacobs, H. (1984). Induction of ovulation for *in vitro* fertilization using buserelin and gonadotrophins. *Lancet,* **2**, 1284–5

Pouchet, F.A. (1847). *Theorie positive de l'ovulation spontanée et de la fecondation des mammiferes et de l'espece humaine, basée sur l'observation de toute la serie animale.* (Paris: Bailiere)

Rabovits, F.E., Cooperman, N.R. and Lash, A.F. (1953). Habitual abortion: a radiographic technique to demonstrate the incompetent internal os of the cervix. *Am. J. Obstet. Gynecol.,* **66**, 269

Raj, S.G., Berger, M.J., Grimes, E.M. and Taymor, M.L. (1977). The use of gonadotrophins for the induction of ovulation in women with polycystic ovarian disease. *Fertil. Steril.,* **28**, 1280–4

Rakoff, A.E. (1953). Hormonal changes following low dosage irradiation of pituitaries and ovaries in anovulatory women. *Fertil. Steril.,* **4**, 263

Rakoff, A.E., Plaster, E.L. and Goldfarb, A.F. (1973). Comparison of various therapies for treatment of anovulation. In Rosenberg, E. (ed.) *Gonadotropin Therapy in Female Infertility,* p. 128. (Amsterdam: Excerpta Medica)

RCOG (1983). *Report of the RCOG Ethics Committee on In Vitro Fertilization and Embryo Replacement or Transfer.* (London: Chameleon Press Ltd.)

Renaud, R.L., Macier, S., Dervain, I. *et al.* (1980). Echographic study of follicle maturation and ovulation during the normal menstrual cycle. *Fertil. Steril.,* **33**, 272

Report of the Committee of Enquiry in Human Fertilization and Embryology (1984). CMND 9314. (London: HMSO)

Reyes, F.I. and Faiman, C. (1974). Long-term therapy with low-dose *cis*-clomiphene in male infertility: effects on semen, serum FSH, LH, testosterone and estradiol and carbohydrate tolerance. *Int. J. Fertil.,* **19**, 49

Ricci, J.V. (1945). *One Hundred Years of Gynaecology 1800–1900,* p. 85. (Philadelphia: The Blakiston Co.)

Richardson, D.W. (1976). Techniques of sperm storage. In Brudenell, M., McLaren, A., Short, R. and Symonds, M. (eds.) *Artificial Insemination Proceedings of the 4th Study of RCOG,* pp. 97–125. (London: RCOG)

Richter, M., Haning, R.V. and Shapiro, S.S. (1984). Artificial donor insemination: fresh versus frozen semen: the patient as her own control. *Fertil. Steril,* **41**, 277

Ries, E. (1897). Nodular forms of tubal disease. *J. Exp. Med.,* **11**, 26

Rindfleisch, W. (1910). Darstellung des cavum uteri. *Berlin Klin. Wchschr.,* 780

Robertson, W.H. (1990). *An Illustrated History of*

Contraception. (Carnforth: Parthenon Publishing Group)

Robson, J.M. and Schonberg, A. (1937). Oestrous reactions, including mating, produced by triphenylethylene. *Nature (London)*, **140**, 196

Rock, J. and Bartlett, M. (1937). Biopsy studies of human endometrium; criteria of dating and information about amenorrhoea, menorrhagia and time of ovulation. *J. Am. Med. Assoc.*, **108**, 2022

Rock, J. and Menkin, M.F. (1946). *In vitro* fertilization and cleavage of human ovarian eggs. *Science*, **100**, 105–7

Roehleder, H. (1934). *Test Tube Babies.* (New York: Vantage)

Rojanasakul, A. and Nillus, S.J. (1984). Use of bromocriptine in normoprolactinaemic gynaecological disorders. *Gynecol. Endocrinol.*, **2**, 11–22

Rosner, F. (1972). *Studies in Torah Judaism: Modern Medicine and Jewish Law*, p. 91. (New York: Yeshiva University)

Rösslin, E. (1513). *Der Swangern Frawen und Hebammen Roszgarten* (Hagenau), English translation (1540) *The Byrth of Mankynde* (London: Raynold)

Rowe, J.W. (1906). The time of ovulation. *Am. J. Obstet.*, **53**, 662

Rowley, J.J. and Heller, C.G. (1975). Inhibition and stimulation of human spermatogenesis. In Behrman, S.J. and Kistner, W.W. (eds.) *Progress in Infertility*, 2nd edn., p. 719. (Boston: Little, Brown)

Rowley, M.G., Teshima, F. and Heller, C.G. (1970). Duration of transit of spermatozoa through the human male ductular system. *Fertil. Steril.*, **21**, 390

Rowley, M.J. and Heller, C.G. (1972). The testosterone rebound phenomenon in the treatment of male infertility. *Fertil. Steril.*, **23**, 498

Rubenstein, B.B., Strauss, H., Lazarus, M. and Hankin, H. (1951). Sperm survival in women. *Fertil. Steril.*, **2**, 15

Rubin, I.C. (1914). Rontgendiagnostik der Uterustumoren mit Hilfe von intrauterinen Collargolinjektionen. *Zentralbl. f. Gynaekol.*, **38**, 658–60

Rubin, I.C. (1920). Nonoperative determination of patency of Fallopian tubes in sterility. Intra-uterine inflation with oxygen, and production of an artificial pneumoperitoneum. Preliminary report. *J. Am. Med. Assoc.*, **74**, 1017

Rubin, I.C. (1958). Uterine fibromyomas and sterility. *Clin. Obstet. Gynecol.*, **1**, 501

Ruge, C. (1913). Uber Ovulation, Corpus Luteum und Menstruation. *Arch. Gynaekol.*, **100**, 20–48

Ruge, P. (1884). *Geburts. Gynaekol.*, **10**, 141, quoted by Kistner and Patton (1975) p. 65

Rumke, P., Van Amstel, N., Messer, E.M. and Bezomer, P.D. (1974). Prognosis of fertility of men with sperm agglutinins in the semen. *Fertil. Steril.*, **25**, 393

Rutherford, A.J., Subak-Sharpe, R., Dawson, K., Magara, R.A., Franks, S. and Winston, R.M.L. (1988). Dramatic improvement in IVF success following treatment with LH-RH agonist. *Br. Med. J.*, **296**, 1765–8

Rutherford, R., Banks, A., Coburn, W. *et al* (1963). Sperm evaluation as it relates to normal, unplanned parenthood. *Fertil. Steril.*, **14**, 521

Sandler, B. (1969). Emotional stress and infertility. *J. Psychosom. Res.*, **12**, 51–9

Schally, A.V., Arimura, A., Kastin, A.J. *et al* (1971). Gonadotropin-releasing hormone: one polypeptide regulates secretion of luteinizing and follicle stimulating hormones. *Science*, **173**, 1036–7

Schally, A.V., Coy, D.H. and Meyers, C.A. (1978). Hypothalamic regulatory hormones. *Ann. Rev. Biochem.*, **47**, 89–128

Schellen, A.M.C.M. (1957). *Artifical Insemination in the Human.* (New York: Elsevier)

Schenk, S.L. (1878). Das Sagethieri künstlich befruchtet ausserhalb des Mutterthieres. *Mitteilungen aus dem Embryologischen Institut der K.K. Universitat Wein*, **2**, 107–18

Schmidt, S.S., Schoysman, R. and Steward, B.H. (1976). Surgical approaches to male infertility. In Hafez, E.S.E. (ed.) *Human Semen and Fertility Regulation in Men*, pp. 476–93. (St. Louis: C.V. Mosby)

Schwartz, D., Laplanche, A., Jouannet, P. and David, G. (1979). Within subject variability of human semen in regard to sperm count, volume, total number of spermatozoa and length of abstinence. *J. Reprod. Fertil.*, **57**, 391–5

Schweiger-Scidel (1865). quoted by Robertson (1990), p. 57

Schroeder, C. (1884). Die excision von ovarian Tumoren mit Erhaltung des Ovarium. *Zentralb. Gynaekol.*, **8**, 716

Schumacher, G.F.B. (1979). Immunologic factors in infertility: antibodies against spermatozoa. *J. Reprod. Med.*, **23**, 272

Scommegna, L. and Lash, S.R. (1969). Ovarian overstimulation, massive ascites and singleton pregnancy after clomiphene. *J. Am. Med. Assoc.*, **207**, 753

Scott, J.Z., Nakamura, R.M., Mutch, J. and Davajan, V. (1977). The cervical factor in infertility: diagnosis and treatment. *Fertil. Steril.*, **28**, 1289

Scott, L.S. (1961). Varicocele: treatable cause of subfertility. *Br. Med. J.*, **1**, 788

Segal, S., Polishuk, W.Z. and Ben David, M. (1976). Hyperprolactinemic male infertility. *Fertil. Steril.*, **27**, 1425

Seguy, J. and Simmonet, H. (1933). Recherches des signes directs d'ovulation chez la femme. *Gynecol. Obstet.*, **28**, 657

Seguy, J. and Vimeux, J. (1933). Contribution a l'etude des sterilités inexpliquées: etude de l'ascension des spermatozoides dans les voies genitales basses de la femme. *Gynecol. Obstet.*, **27**, 346

Seibel, M.M., McArdle, C.R., Thompson, I.E., Berger, M.J. and Taymor, M.L. (1981). The role of ultrasound in ovulation induction: a critical appraisal. *Fertil. Steril.*, **36**, 573

Seppala, M. (1985). The world collaborative report on *in vitro* fertilization and embryo replacement: current state of the art in January 1984. *Ann. N.Y. Acad. Sci. USA*, **442**, 558–63

Seppala, M., Hirvonen, E. and Ranta, T. (1976). Hyperprolactinaemia and luteal insufficiency. *Lancet*, **1**, 229–30

Settlage, D.S.F., Motoshima, M. and Tredway, D.R. (1973). Sperm transport from the external cervical os to the Fallopian tubes in women: a time and quantitation study. *Fertil. Steril.*, **24**, 655

Seymour, F.I. and Koerner, A. (1941). "Artificial insemination, present status in the USA as shown by a recent survey". *J. Am. Med. Assoc.*, **116**, 2747–9

Shearman, R.P. (1964). Diagnostic ovarian stimulation with heterologous gonadotrophins. *Br. Med. J.*, **2**, 1115

Shelton, R.S., van Campen, M.G. Jr., Meisner, D.F. *et al.* (1953). Synthetic estrogens: halotriphenylethylene derivatives. *J. Am. Chem. Soc.*, **75**, 5491

Sher, G. and Katz M. (1976). Inadequate cervical mucus – a cause of "idiopathic" infertility. *Fertil. Steril.*, **27**, 886

Sherins, R.J., Brightwell, D. and Sternthal, P.M. (1977). Longitudinal analysis of semen of fertile and infertile men. In Troen, P. and Nankin, H.R. (eds.) *The Testis in Normal and Infertile Men*, pp. 473–88. (New York: Raven Press)

Sherman, J.K. (1973). Synopsis of the use of frozen human semen since 1964: state of the art human semen banking. *Fertil. Steril.*, **24**, 397

Shettles, L.B. (1940). *Am. J. Physiol.*, **128**, 408, quoted by Newton (1976)

Shettles, L. B. (1953). Observations on human follicular ova. *Fed. Proc.*, **12**, 131

Shirodkar, V.N. (1963). *Progress in Gynecology*, p. 260. (New York: Grune & Stratton)

Shivers, C.A. and Dunbar, B.S. (1977). Autoantibodies to zona pellucida: a possible cause of infertility in women. *Science*, **197**, 1082

Shreiber, A.D. (1977). Clinical immunology of corticosteroid. *Prog. Clin. Immunol.*, **3**, 103

Siegler, A. and Perez, R.J. (1975). Reconstruction of Fallopian tubes in previously sterilized patients. *Fertil. Steril.*, **26**, 383

Sims, J.M. (1866). *Clinical notes on Uterine Surgery with Special Reference to the Management of the Sterile Condition*. (London: Robert Hardwicke)

Sims, J.M. (1868). Illustrations of the value of the microscope in the treatment of the sterile condition. *Br. Med. J.*, **11**, 465–6

Skutsch, F. (1889). Beitrag sur operativen Therapie der Tubenerkrankum. *Zentralb. Gynaekol.*, **13**, 565

Smith, K.D. and Steinberger, E. (1973). Survival of spermatozoa in a human sperm bank: effects of a long term storage in liquid nitrogen. *J. Am. Med. Assoc.*, **223**, 774

Smith, K.D., Rodriguez-Rigau, L.J. and Steinberger, E. (1977). Relation between indices of semen analysis and pregnancy rate in infertile couples. *Fertil. Steril.*, **28**, 1314

Smith, P.E. and Engle, E.T. (1927). Experimental evidence regarding role of anterior pituitary in development and regulation of genital system. *Am. J. Anat.*, **40**, 159

Smith, W.T. (1848). Lectures on parturition and the principles and practice of obstetrics. *Lancet*, **2**, 308–9

Smith, W.T. (1849a). On a new method of treating sterility, by the removal of obstructions of the Fallopian tubes. *Lancet*, **1**, 529–31

Smith, W.T. (1849b). On a new method of treating sterility by the removal of obstructions of the Fallopian tubes. *Lancet*, **1**, 603–5

Smith, W.T. (1849c). Further observations on the method of treating sterility by the removal of obstructions from the Fallopian tubes. *Lancet*, **2**, 116–19

Sobowale, O., Lenton, E.A., Francis, R. and Cooke, I.D. (1978). Comparison of plasma steroid and gonadotrophin profiles in spontaneous cycles in which conception did and did not occur. *Br. J. Obstet. Gynaecol.*, **85**, 460

Spallanzani, L. (1776). *Opuscoli di Fisca. Animale e Vegetabile Opuscolo II. Osservazioni e Sperienze intorno ai Vermicelli Spermatici deli Vomo e degli Aminali.* Modena. Quoted by Newton (1976)

Spallanzani, L. (1789). *Dissertations Relative to the National History of Animals and Vegetables.* Translated from the Italian of the Abbe Spallanzani, Vol. 11

Speck, G. (1950). Revision of the PSP (Speck) test for tubal patency. *Fertil. Steril.*, **1**, 328

Speert, H. (1973). *Iconographia Gyniatrica: A Pictorial History of Gynecology and Obstetrics*, p. 194. (Philadelphia: F.A. Davis Co.)

Spencer, W.G. (1938). *Celsus De Medicina.* (Cambridge, Mass: Harvard University Press)

Squire, W. (1868). Puerperal temperatures. *Trans. Obstet. Soc. (Lond).*, **9**, 129

Steer, C., Campbell, S., Davies, M., Mason, B.A. and Collins, W. (1989). Spontaneous abortion rates following natural and assisted conception. *Br. Med. J.*, **299**, 1317–18

Stein, I.F. and Leventhal, M.L. (1935). Amenorrhea associated with bilateral polycystic ovaries. *Am. J. Obstet. Gynecol.*, **29**, 181–91

Stein, Z. and Susser, M. (1978). Famine and fertility. In Mosley, W.H. (ed.) *Nutrition and Human Reproduction*, pp. 123–45. (New York: Plenum Press)

Steinberger, E. and Smith, K.D. (1973). Artificial insemination with fresh or frozen semen: a comparative study. *J. Am. Med. Assoc.*, **223**, 778

Steptoe, P.C. (1967). *Laparoscopy in Gynaecology.* (Edinburgh: Livingstone)

Steptoe, P.C. and Edwards, R.G. (1970). Laparoscopic recovery of pre-ovulatory human oocytes after priming of ovaries with gonadotrophins. *Lancet*, **1**, 683–9

Steptoe, P.C. and Edwards, R.G. (1976). Reimplantation of a human embryo with subsequent tubal pregnancy. *Lancet*, **1**, 880

Steptoe, P.C. and Edwards, R.G. (1978). Birth after reimplantation of a human embryo. *Lancet*, **2**, 366

Steptoe, P.C. and Edwards, R.G. (1979). Pregnancies following implantation of human embryos grown in culture. *Scientific Meeting, RCOG,* London quoted by Lopata *et al.* (1980) p. 209

Steptoe, P.C., Edwards, R.G. and Walters, D.E. (1986). Observations on 767 clinical pregnancies and 500 births after human *in vitro* fertilization. *Hum. Reprod.*, **1**, 89–94

Stockard, C.R. and Papanicolaou, G. N. (1917). The existence of a typical oestrus cycle in the guinea pig, with a study of its histological and physiological changes. *Am. J. Anat.*, **22**, 225–84

Strassman, E.O. (1952). Plastic unification of double uterus. *Am. J. Obstet. Gynecol.*, **64**, 25

Strassman, E.O. (1961). Operations for double uterus and endometrial atresia. *Clin. Obstet. Gynecol.*, **4**, 210

Strassman (1907). quoted by Strassman, E.O. (1952)

Swolin, K. (1975). Electromicrosurgery and salpingostomy: long-term results. *Am. J. Obstet. Gynecol.*, **121**, 418

Taymor, M.L. (1959). Timing of ovulation by LH assay. *Fertil. Steril.*, **10**, 212

Taymor, M.L. (1968). Gonadotropin therapy. *J. Am. Med. Assoc.*, **203**, 362

Taymor, M.L. (1990). *Infertility: A Clinician's Guide to Diagnosis and Treatment*, p. 189. (New York, London: Plenum Medical Book Co.)

Taymor, M.L. and Selenkow, H.A. (1958). Clinical experience with L-triiodothyronine in male infertility. *Fertil. Steril.*, **9**, 560

Taymor, M.L., Berger, M.J. and Nudemberg, F. (1973). The combined use of clomiphene citrate and human menopausal gonadotropin in ovulation induction. In Hasegawa, T. (ed.) *Fertil. Steril. Excerpta Medica Int. Cong. Ser.*, **278**, 628

Telang, M., Rayniak, J.V. and Shulman, S. (1978). Antibodies to spermatozoa: VIII. Correlations of sperm antibody activity with post-coital tests in infertile couples. *Int. J. Fertil.*, **23**, 200

Temkin, O. (translator) (1956). *Soranus Gynecology.* (Baltimore: Johns Hopkins Press)

Templeton, A.A. and Mortimer, D. (1980). Laparoscopic sperm recovery in infertile women. *Br. J. Obstet. Gynaecol.*, **87**, 1128–31

Tesarik, J., Pilka, L., Dvorak, M. and Travnik, P. (1983). Oocyte recovery, *in vitro* insemination, and transfer into the oviduct after its microsurgical repair at a single laparotomy. *Fertil. Steril.*, **39**, 472–5

Testart, J., Lassall, B., Blaish-Allant, J. *et al.* (1986). High pregnancy rate after early human embryo freezing. *Fertil. Steril.*, **42**, 268

Tompkins, P. (1944). Use of basal temperature graphs in determining date of ovulation. *J. Am. Med. Assoc.*, **124**, 698

Tompkins, P. (1962). Comments on the bicornuate uterus and twinning. *Surg. Clin. N. Am.*, **42**, 1049

Trounson, A.O., Mohr, L.R., Wood, C. and Leeton, J.F. (1982). Effect of delayed insemination on *in vitro* fertilization culture and transfer of human embryos. *J. Reprod. Fertil.*, **64**, 285

Trounson, A.O. and Mohr, L.R. (1983). Human pregnancy following cryopreservation, thawing and transfer of an 8-cell embryo. *Nature (London)*, **305**, 707–9

Trounson, A.O., Leeton, J.F., Wood, C., Webb, J. and Kovacs, G. (1980). The investigation of idiopathic infertility by *in vitro* fertilization. *Fertil. Steril.*, **34**, 431–8

Tulloch, W.S. (1952). Consideration of sterility: subfertility in the male. *Edinburgh Med. J.*, March

Turner, H., Zanartu, J. and Nelson, W. (1964). Effect of chorionic gonadotropin therapy on fertility in males with scrotal testes. *Fertil. Steril.*, **15**, 24

Tyler, E.T., Olsen, H.J. and Gotlieb, M.H. (1960). Induction of ovulation with an antiestrogen. *Int. J. Fertil.*, **5**, 429

Ulstein, M. (1973). Fertility of donors at heterologous insemination. *Acta Obstet. Gynaecol. Scand.*, **52**, 97–101

van Beneden (1883). quoted by Robertson (1990), p. 57

van de Velde, T.H. (1905). *Uber den zusammenhang zwischen ovarialfunction, wellenbewegung und menstrualblutung und uber die enstenhung des sogenannten mittelschmerzes.* (On the relationship between ovarian function, periodicity and menstrual flow, and of the origins of the so called mittelschmerz), p. 39. (Haarlem: F. Bohn)

van Leeuwenhoek, A. (1678). De natis e semine genitali animalculis. *Philos. Trans. R. Soc. Lond.*, **XII**, 1040

Venturoli, S., Fabbri, R., Paradisi, R., Magrini, O., Porcu, E., Orsini, L.F. and Flamigni, C. (1983). Induction of ovulation with human urinary follicle stimulating hormone: endocrine pattern and ultrasound monitoring. *Eur. J. Obstet. Gynaecol. Reprod. Biol.*, **16**, 135–45

Vermeulen, A. and Comhaire, F. (1978). Hormonal effects of an anti-estrogen, tamoxifen, in normal and oligospermic men. *Fertil. Steril.*, **29**, 320

Viergiver, E. and Pommerenke, W.T. (1944). Measurement of the "cyclic" variations in the quantity of cervical mucus and its correlation with basal temperature. *Am. J. Obstet. Gynecol.*, **48**, 321

von Baer, C.E. (1827). *De ovi mammalium et hominis genesi.* (Lipsiae, L. Vossius)

von Koelleker, R. (1810). quoted by Robertson (1990), p. 57

Waldo, R. (1895). Cyst of the distal end of the left Fallopian tube and cystic degeneration of the right ovary removed one year after the removal of a portion of the left Fallopian tube and small cysts from the right ovary. *Am. J. Obstet. Gynecol.*, **32**, 444

Walz, W. (1959). Fertilitats operationen mit hilfe eines operationenmikroskopes. *Geburts. Gynaekol.*, **153**, 49

Warner, M.P. (1962). Results of a twenty-five year study of 1,553 infertile couples. *N. Y. State J. Med.*, **62**, 2663

Warren, M. (1980). The effects of exercise on pubertal progression and reproductive function in girls. *J. Clin. Endocrinol. Metab.*, **51**, 1050–7

Warren, M.P. (1983). Effects of undernutrition on reproductive function in the human. *Endocr. Rev.*, **4**, 363–77

West, C.P., Lumsden, W.A., Lawson, S., Williamson, J. and Baird, D.T. (1987). Shrinkage of uterine fibroid during therapy with goserelin (Zoladex): a luteinizing hormone-releasing hormone agonist administered as a monthly subcutaneous depot. *Fertil. Steril.*, **48**, 45

Whelan, D. (1978). The law and artificial insemination with donor semen (AID). *Med. J. Aust.*, **1**, 56

Wikland, M., Enk, L. and Hamberger, L. (1985). Transvesical and transvaginal approaches for the aspiration of follicles by use of ultrasound. *Ann. N. Y. Acad. Sci.*, **442**, 182

Wikland, M., Hamberger, L., Enk, L. and Nilsson, L. (1988). Sonographic techniques in human *in vitro* fertilization. *Hum. Reprod.*, **3**, 65–8

Wilkes, C.A., Rosenwaks, Z., Jones, D.C. and Jones, H.W. Jr (1985). Pregnancy related to infertility diagnosis, number of attempts and age in a program of *in vitro* fertilization. *Obstet. Gynecol.*, **66**, 350

Williams, G.F.J. (1973). Fallopian tube surgery for reversal of sterilization. *Br. Med. J.*, **1**, 599

Williamson, J.G. and Ellis, J.D. (1973). Induction of ovulation by Tamoxifen. *J. Obstet. Gynaecol. Br. Commonw.*, **80**, 844–7

Wilson, L. (1954). Sperm agglutinins in human semen and blood. *Proc. Soc. Exp. Biol. Med.*, **85**, 652

Winston, R.M.L. (1977). Microsurgical tubocornual anastomosis for reversal of sterilization. *Lancet*, **1**, 284

Winston, R.W. (1983). Microsurgery of the Fallopian tubes. In Taymor, M.L. and Nelson, J.H. Jr. (eds.) *Progress in Gynecology*, p. 399. (New York: Grune and Stratton)

Wood, C. (1978). New aspects of the treatment of tubal infertility. *Aust. N. Z. J. Obstet. Gynaecol.*, **8**, 67

Woolf, R.B. and Allen, W.M. (1953). Concomitant malformations. *Obstet. Gynecol.*, **2**, 236

World Health Organization (1976). Expanded programme of research, development and research training in human reproduction. *Fifth Annual Report*, p. 47. (Geneva: WHO)

World Health Organization (1980a). *Laboratory manual for the examination of human semen and sperm-cervical mucus interaction.* (Singapore: Press Concern)

World Health Organization (1980b). Task force on methods for determination of the fertile period. *Am. J. Obstet. Gynecol.*, **138**, 838

Wynn, R.M. and Harris, J.A. (1967). Ultrastructural cyclic changes in the human endometrium. I. Normal preovulatory phase. *Fertil. Steril.*, **18**, 632–48

Yanagimachi, R.J., Yanagimachi, H. and Rogers, B.J. (1976). The use of zona-free animal ova is a test for the assessment of fertilizing capacity of human spermatozoa. *Biol. Reprod.*, **15**, 471

Yen, S.S.C., Vela, P., Rankin, J. and Littell, A.S. (1970). Hormonal relationships during the menstrual cycle. *J. Am. Med. Assoc.*, **211**, 1513–17

Yovich, J.L. and Stranger, J.D. (1984). The limitations of *in vitro* fertilization from males with severe oligospermia and abnormal male morphology. *J. In Vitro Fert. Embryo Transfer.*, **1**, 172

Yovich, J.L., Matson, P., Blackledge, D.G. *et al.* (1988). The treatment of normospermic infertility by gamete intrafallopian transfer (GIFT). *Br. J. Obstet. Gynaecol.*, **95**, 361–6

Zarate, A., Valdes-Vallina, F., Gonzalez, A. *et al.* (1973). Therapeutic effect of synthetic luteinizing hormone-releasing hormone (LH-RH) in male infertility due to idiopathic azoospermia and oligospermia. *Fertil. Steril.*, **14**, 485

Zavos, P.M. and Wilson, E.A. (1984). Retrograde ejaculation: etiology and treatment via the use of a new non-invasive method. *Fertil. Steril.*, **42**, 627

Zondek, B. (1966). Foreword. In Greenblatt, R.B. (ed.) *Ovulation*, p. vii. (Philadelphia: J.B. Lippincott)

Zondek, B. and Aschheim, S. (1927). Das Hormon des Hypophysenvorderlappens; Testobject zum Nachweis des Hormons. *Klin. Wochenschr.*, **6**, 248

Zorgniotti, A.W., Cohen, M.S. and Sealfon, A.I. (1980). Chronic scrotal hypothermia: Results in 90 infertile couples. *J. Urol.*, **135**, 944

FURTHER READING

Brudenell, M., McLaren, A., Short, R. and Symonds, M. (eds.) (1976). Artificial Insemination *Proc. R.C.O.G.*

Chamberlain, G. and Drife, D. (1989). *Contemporary Reviews in Obstetrics and Gynaecology*, Vol. 1, No. 2. (London: Butterworth-Heinemann Ltd.)

Chamberlain, G. and Drife, D. (1990). *Contemporary Reviews in Obstetrics and Gynaecology.*, Vol. 2, No. 2. (London: Butterworth-Heinemann Ltd.)

Chamberlain, G. and Winston, R. (eds.) (1982). *Tubal Infertility. Diagnosis & Treatment.* (Oxford, London, Edinburgh, Boston, Melbourne: Blackwell Scientific Publications)

Cooke, I.D. (ed.) (1974). *The Management of Infertility, Clinics in Obstetrics and Gynecology*, Vol. 1 No. 2 (London, Philadelphia, Toronto: W.B. Saunders Co.)

Crosignani, P.G. (ed.) (1990). *Induction of Ovulation, Clinics in Obstetrics and Gynecology*, Vol. 4 No. 3. (London, Philadelphia, Toronto: W.B. Saunders Co.)

Cusine, D.J. (1988). *New Reproductive Techniques A Legal Perspective*, Chap. 3, pp. 11–19. (Aldershot, Brookfield USA, Hong Kong, Singapore, Sydney: Gower)

Damewood, M.D. (ed.) (1990). *The Johns Hopkins Handbook of In Vitro Fertilization and Assisted Reproductive Technologies.* (Boston, Toronto, London: Little, Brown and Co.)

DeCherney, A.H. (ed.) (1986). *Reproductive Failure.* (New York, Edinburgh, London, Melbourne: Churchill Livingstone)

Edwards, R.G. (ed.) (1990). *Assisted Human Conception. Br. Med. Bull.*, **46**, (3) (Edinburgh, London: Churchill Livingstone)

Finegold, W.J. (1976). *Artificial Insemination*, 2nd edn., p. 5. (Springfield Ill: Thomas)

Gamete Intrafallopian Transfer (Conference). (1986) *Lancet*, **2**, 1228

Golden, J. (translator) (1957). *The Living Talmud: The Wisdom of the Fathers.* (New York: New American Library of World Literature)

Huhner, M. (1937). *The Diagnosis and Treatment of Sexual Disorders in the Male and Female.* (Philadelphia: Davis)

Hull, M.G.R. (ed.) (1981) *Developments in Infertility Practice, Clinics in Obstetrics and Gynecology*, Vol. 8, No. 3 (London, Philadelphia, Toronto: W.B. Saunders Co.)

Jacobs, H.S. (ed.) (1985). *Reproductive Endocrinology, Clinics in Obstetrics and Gynecology*, Vol. 12, No. 3 (London. Philadelphia, Toronto: W.B. Saunders Co.)

Kistner, R.W. and Patton, G.W. Jr. (eds.) (1985). *Atlas of Infertility Surgery.* (Boston: Little, Brown and Co.)

Lopata, A., Johnston, W.I.H., Leeton, S. and McBain, F.C. (1980). Use of *in vitro* fertilization. In Pepperell, R.J., Hudson, B. and Wood, C. (eds.) *The Infertile Couple*, p. 209. (Edinburgh, London, New York: Churchill Livingstone)

Lunenfeld, B. and Donini, P. (1966). Historic aspects of gonadotropins. In Greenblatt, B. (ed.) *Ovulation*, pp. 9–34. (Toronto: Lippincott)

Maguiness, S.D., Djahanbakhch, O. and Grudzinskas, J.G. (1992). Assessment of the Fallopian tube. *Obstet. Gynecol. Surv.*, **47**, 587–603

Moghissi, K.S. (1977). Significance and prognostic value of post-coital test. In Insler, V. and Bettendorf, G. (eds.) *The Uterine Cervix in Reproduction*, p. 231. (Stuttgart: Thieme)

Pepperell, R.J., Hudson, B. and Wood C. (1980). *The Infertile Couple.* (Edinburgh: Churchill Livingstone)

Robertson, W.H. (1990). *An Illustrated History of Contraception.* (New Jersey: Parthenon Publishing Group)

Rosenfeld, D.L. (1984). The infertile female: hysterosalpingography. In Garcia, C.S., Mastroianni, L., Amelar, R.D. and Dubin, L. (eds.) *Current Therapy of Infertility 1984–1985*, p. 1.

(Philadelphia, Toronto, London: B.C. Decker Inc. and the C.V. Mosby Co.)

Schellen, A.M.C.M. and Roehleder, H. (1934). *Test-Tube Babies: a History of the Artificial Impregnation of Human Beings*, p. 35. (New York: Panurge Press)

Secretary of State for Social Services (1987). *Human Fertilization and Embryology: a framework for legislation*, Cmnd 259. (London: HMSO)

Studd, J. (ed.) (1989). *Progress in Obstetrics and Gynaecology*, p. 233. (Edinburgh, London, Melbourne, New York: Churchill Livingstone)

Taymor, M.L. (1990). *Infertility A Clinician's Guide to Diagnosis and Treatment.* (New York, London: Plenum Medical Book Company)

Trounson, A. and Wood, C. (eds.) (1984). In vitro *Fertilization and Embryo Transfer.* (Edinburgh, London, Melbourne, New York: Churchill Livingstone)

Tyson, J.E. (ed.) (1978). *Neuroendocrinology of Reproduction, Clinics in Obstetrics and Gynecology*, Vol. 5, No. 2 (London, Philadelphia, Toronto: W.B. Saunders Co.)

The speculum

The word speculum is derived from the Latin (*speculum* – a mirror; *specere* – to look at), and is defined as a funnel- or tube-shaped instrument which is introduced into a body orifice to allow visualization of the cavity beyond. Many different specula were designed and used throughout the ages. Ricci (1948–49) published a list of 614 models, and of the physicians and instrument makers who had devised, reproduced, or illustrated vaginal specula during the years AD 79 to 1940.

The earliest recorded gynaecological history comes from Egyptian times, and although their physicians were aware of, and treated, many gynaecological conditions, their examinations did not include the use of the speculum.

The ancient Greeks used the speculum to investigate rectal disorders and it was theorized by Ligeros (1937) that the *speculum uteri* or *mitroscope* was used for observation of the vagina and cervix during Hippocrates' (460–377 BC) lifetime. Ulcerations of the cervix were described by Hippocrates but Schapiro and Deneffe (1901) claimed that they were detected by touch, and not by speculum examination.

The only definite reference to the speculum in ancient texts comes from the Hebrew Talmud. The Hebrews used a bamboo internode or the stem of a gourd as a speculum (Thompson, 1938), and at a later date, metal tubes were used. Use of the speculum may therefore date back to 1300 BC (Cianfrani, 1960), or over 800 years before the birth of Hippocrates. The ancient Hindus also used the speculum, and McKay (1901) reported that the 'Naru-Juntra consists of 20 varieties of tubular instruments...for examining deep seated parts ...'.

The Roman physician Cornelius Celsus (27 BC–AD 50) is known to have used the speculum, and Galen (AD 131–201) recorded his use of the instrument to dilate and view the female genitalia in his 'Linguarum Explanatio' (Leonard, 1881). He was aware of leukorrhoea and 'ulceration of the womb'.

Soranus of Ephesus (AD 98–138) wrote a book on gynaecology and devoted a chapter to the use of the speculum. He documented that in cases of haemorrhage from the vulva the site of blood loss could be distinguished more accurately by using the speculum (McKay, 1901). Leonides of Alexandria (c.AD 200) was a contemporary of Soranus who practised in Alexandria, Egypt. He described the use of a rectal speculum to observe fistulae, and also mentioned the use of the instrument to dilate and view the vagina.

The speculum was in use during the second century AD, and Arateus, who studied at the medical school in Alexandria, was familiar with the instrument. He described 'ulcers' of the cervix and their treatment. In the same century Archingenes found that cervical 'ulcers' could be brought to light by means of the *dioptra*, and Aspasia mentioned the use of the *dioptra* to demonstrate 'haemorrhoids' at the orifice of the uterus.

In the year AD 79 Pompeii was buried by lava following a major volcanic eruption. Excavations were carried out at the site in 1818 and 1882 during which vaginal specula were recovered from the house of a physician. The instruments were fashioned in bronze and included three- and four-bladed specula, each mounted on a frame. There was a central screw which, when turned, caused the blades to diverge. The specula were of the type used by Galen and Celsus and similar designs were popular until the Middle Ages.

In the sixth century Aetius referred to the vaginal speculum in his work on gynaecology entitled *Tetrabiblion*, and he also described the lithotomy postion. In the following century Paulus of Aegina used several forms of cylindrical and conical vaginal specula whose valves could be separated by means of a screw following insertion. The bronze specula were opened by twisting the simple screw attachment. The length of the vagina was measured prior to application of the instrument.

In 1085 Albucasis described ebony and boxwood specula, and his text on surgery was the first to contain illustrations of the vaginal speculum.

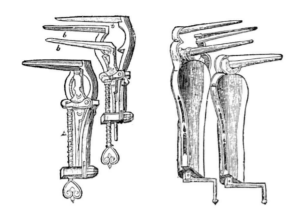

Figure 1 Specula, open and closed, as used in the time of Ambroise Paré. From Marion Sims' *Uterine Surgery*, New York (1866)

He also referred to a type of speculum 'mentioned by the Ancients' (Leonardo, 1944). After his death little was written on the topic of gynaecology until the sixteenth century.

In 1561 Pierre Franco described a speculum similar to the one described in the work of Paulus of Aegina, (Ricci, 1950) and soon afterwards, in 1575, Ambroise Paré used the speculum to observe cancer of the cervix (Figure 1). The speculum was used to dilate the vaginal passage and allow ample exposure, so that cautery could be applied to the diseased cervix.

Jacob Rueffus described a speculum in 1554, and his published work *De Conceptu et Generatione Hominis* (1587) contained a description of a three bladed speculum which was used to dilate the vagina and aid delivery of a child in difficult parturition.

Johann Scultetus described bi-valved and tri-valved specula in his *Armamentarium Chirurgicum* in 1653 and mentioned examination of ' the sheath of the matrix'. The design of his instruments may have been based on those of Paulus of Aegina.

Jacobus Primrose, a Scotsman who practised at Hull in England, wrote a treatise on gynaecology in 1655. He had studied in France and was aware of the value of speculum examination in the diagnosis and treatment of uterine disease (Leonardo, 1944). Henrick van Roonhuyze (1663) wrote the first text on operative gynaecology. Included therein was his description of operative repair for vesico-vaginal fistula, during which a *speculum vaginae* was used to 'widen the body' to plainly see the 'rupture'.

The instrument continued to be popular in France and Pierre Dionis, a French physician, wrote of the *speculum matricis* in 1724. Astruc of the Medical Faculty of Paris described vaginal examination and said that a finger may suffice, alternatively a *speculum uteri* could be used. He 'reinvented' the speculum around 1761. The eighth edition of Laurentius Heister's *Surgery* was published in 1768, and contained both a description and an illustration of a *speculum ani*, which was used to inspect the anus and vagina 'in disorders of those parts'. The speculum used was of the bi-valve variety.

Osiander used a speculum during amputation of the cervix in the years 1801–1808 (Ricci, 1950), but it was Joseph C.A. Recamier (1842) who popularized its use in the early 1800s (Figure 2). He used a steel tube with polished walls which he gradually modified during the years 1801–1818. Recamier's original cylindrical speculum only allowed observation of a section equivalent to its calibre. He later designed an instrument of two half cylinders which could be separated after insertion to increase the visual field. However, his speculum was large and uncomfortable so Guillaume Dupuytren introduced modifications in 1820. He reduced the size, narrowed the external end and equipped it with a handle (Cianfrani, 1960). A vaginal speculum with glass blades was introduced early in the nineteenth century, and in another modification Palfrey introduced a

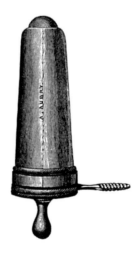

Figure 2 Recamier's speculum in wood, designed according to him, to protect the walls of the vagina when removing material from the uterus with sharp instruments. From J. Marion Sims' *Uterine Surgery* (1866)

skeleton-bladed instrument which allowed an extensive view of the vagina and cervix.

In 1845 James Marion Sims (q.v. in Biographies) introduced a double-ended speculum which was fashioned from a pewter spoon (Figure 3). He reported his new speculum design in a paper on the treatment of vesico-vaginal fistula (1852). Application of the Sim's speculum with the patient in the knee–chest postion allowed entrance of air to the vagina, which caused ballooning with consequent increased visualization. The instrument 'when introduced and held properly, causes no pain whatever ...'. His modified speculum was made of German silver, and when inserted a reflected light was thrown

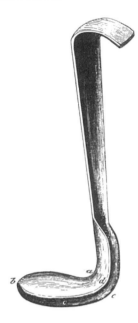

Figure 3 Sims' original lever speculum. From J. Marion Sims' *Uterine Surgery* (1866)

onto 'the concave surface of the bright speculum ... making everything perfectly distinct'. Munde modified Sims' speculum by the addition of a flange which supported the buttock and Cleveland devised a self-retaining type which was held in place by a piece of rubber tubing. The Sims' speculum was attached to a standard on the operating table by J.B. Hunter, and this created a 'mechanical assistant' (Leonardo, 1944) (Figure 4).

Charles D. Meigs, professor of Midwifery and Diseases of Women and Children at Jefferson Medical College, stated in 1848 that examination by vaginal speculum was 'not always necessary'. His conservative attitude was common at that time. Treatment of 'inflammatory congestion of the cervix' by application of leeches was also common, and in 1849 T.R. Mitchell described a method of applying leeches to the cervix through a conical glass speculum (Ricci, 1950). The blood sucking leeches, eight or ten in number, were allowed to stay in the vagina for up to 30 minutes, when it was judged that they were full. The odd leech had to be persuaded to detach by applying a salt solution to its head. Some entered the uterine cavity and caused 'severe distress'.

Edward Cusco invented his bi-valve vaginal speculum about 1859. This design was virtually the same as that which is commonly used today and is often termed the 'duck bill speculum'. Sir William Fergusson of London, modified Recamier's tubular speculum about 1870 and with the addition of a water cooling device it was later used in the 'Percy' treatment of cancer of the cervix. The instrument was a glass tube coated with mercury, covered by India rubber and varnished, and was considered the finest speculum of its day. A 'tel-escopic vaginal speculum was invented by Thomas (1878) and consisted of two cylindrical metal tubes, one sliding into the other, with an adjustable length to suit that of the vagina. Also in the nineteenth century Franz Neugebauer of Warsaw invented a speculum with two separate and freely sliding blades or valves. A single blade was inserted into the vagina, and the second was slid along it and into place. The instrument was popular among gynaecologists in England.

Various modifications of the speculum were advanced by Collins, Goodell and Hirst, and were illustrated in Hirst's *Textbook of Obstetrics* (1918). Arthur Bowen (1938) devised a weighted speculum with a detachable metal cup, which could be used to collect samples obtained at uterine curettage.

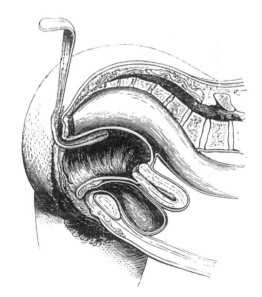

Figure 4 The lever speculum in use. 'The assistant on the right side of the patient introduces into the vagina the lever speculum and then, by lifting the perineum, stretching the sphincter and raising up the recto-vaginal septum, it is easy to view the whole vaginal canal.' From J. Marion Sims' *Uterine Surgery* (1866)

Arthur W. Erskine (1939) introduced an expanding speculum for transvaginal X-ray therapy in 1938. The instrument was a multibladed variety with a wrench mechanism which was used to expand the blades. An X-ray tube was attached and treatment applied to the upper vagina and cervix.

John Stallworthy described a modified Graves speculum (1941) which had illumination applied to the lower blade, thus allowing an excellent view of the cervix and vaginal walls. Walters also introduced an 'Illuminated Sims speculum' in 1942.

Recent innovations included the disposable plastic speculum with a screw or ratchet device in the handle, and also a matt black speculum for use with laser therapy to the cervix.

CHRONOLOGY

1300 BC	Reference to the speculum in the Talmud.
460–377 BC	Hippocrates described 'ulcerations of the cervix', but it is uncertain if they were viewed via speculum.
AD 30	Celsus described a speculum quite similar to modern instruments.
AD 79	Pompeii was buried by lava. Excavations in 1818 and 1882 revealed the house of a doctor, in which vaginal specula were found.
AD 98–138	Soranus of Ephesus wrote a text on gynaecology and included a chapter on the speculum.
AD 113–201	Galen viewed the female genitalia and recognized leukorrhoea and ulcerations of the cervix.
2nd C.	Arateus, Aspasia, Archingenes and Leonides of Alexandria were familiar with the use of vaginal and anal specula.
6th C.	Aetius used a cylindrical form.
7th C.	Paulus of Aegina used a two-bladed variety.
1085	Albucasis used ebony and boxwood specula.
1517	Hans van Gersdorff used a speculum.
1561	Pierre Franco described an instrument similar to that of Paulus of Aegina.
1575	Ambroise Paré cauterized cancer of the cervix and used a speculum.
1587	Jacobus Rueffus illustrated a three-bladed variety in his text.
1653	Johann Scultetus described the speculum in his *Armamentarium Chirurgicum.*
1761	Astruc of Paris 're-invented' the instrument.
1768	Heister described the instrument in his *Surgery.*
1801–18	Recamier 're-introduced' and popularized the speculum.
1820	Dupuytren modified Recamier's version.
1845	James Marion Sims introduced his pewter spoon.
1849	T.R. Mitchell described a conical glass speculum.
1859	Edward Cusco invented a highly efficient bi-valve type.
1870	Sir William Fergusson introduced his cylindrical speculum.
1872	Theodore Thomas used a telescopic variety.
1875	Martin introduced a 'bath speculum' to allow vaginal bathing.
1866	Bozeman's speculum was illustrated in *Brown's Surgical Diseases of Women.*
1889	Cusco's speculum, and a cylindrical variety, were illustrated by Ashurst in his *Principles and Practice of Surgery.*
1896	Franz Neugebauer of Warsaw used a speculum with freely sliding blades.
1918	The Collins, Goodell's, and Hirst specula, were illustrated in Hirst's *Textbook of Obstetrics.*
1938	Arthur Bowen devised a cup to attach to a weighted speculum.
1939	Arthur W. Erskine introduced an expanding variety for transvaginal Roentgen therapy.
1941	John Stallworthy added illumination to the lower blade of a modified Graves speculum.
1942	Walters introduced the 'Illuminated Sims Vaginal Speculum'.
1970–80s	Plastic and black specula introduced.

References: Leonardo (1881); McKay (1901); Schapiro and Deneffe(1901); Ricci (1948–49); Ricci (1950); Speert (1958) and Cianfrani (1960).

REFERENCES

Bowen, A. (1938). Bowen speculum cup. *Am. J. Surg.*, **42**, 435–36

Cianfrani, T. (1960). *A Short History of Obstetrics and Gynecology*. (Springfield Ill.: Charles C. Thomas)

Erskine, A.W. (1939). Expanding speculum for transvaginal Roentgen therapy. *Am. J. Roentgenol.*, **5**, 42

Hirst, B.C. (1918). *Textbook of Obstetrics*. (Philadelphia: Saunders)

Leonard, C.H. (1881). Ancient gynecology. *Obstet. Gaz. Ancinn.*, **3**, 505–10

Leonardo, R.A. (1944). *History of Gynaecology* (New York: Froben)

Ligeros, K.A. (1937). *How Ancient Healing Governs Modern Therapeutics*. (New York: G.P. Putman)

McKay, W.J.S. (1901). *The History of Ancient Gynaecology*. (London: Bailliere Tindall Cox)

Recamier, J. (1842). Invention du speculum plein et brise. *Bull. Acad. Med. Paris.*, **8**, 661–8

Ricci, J.V. (1948–49). The vaginal speculum and its modifications throughout the ages. *Trans. Gynaecol. Dept. City Hosp (N.Y.)*, 1–55

Ricci, J.V. (1950). *Genealogy of Gynecology*, p350. (Philadelphia: Blakiston)

Roonhuyze, H. van (1663). *Heel-konstige Aanmerkkingern Betreffende de Gebreekken der Vrouwen*. (Amsterdam: T. Jacobsz) [English translation (1676) *Medico-Chirurgical Observations. Englished out of Dutch by a careful hand*, pp.125–36. (London: M. Pitt)]

Rueffus, J. (1587). *De Conceptu et Generatione Hominis*, p.24. (Tiguri, C. Froschoverus)

Schapiro, I. and Deneffe, V. (1901). L'antiquité du speculum. *Chronique Med. Par.*, **6**, 553–8

Sims, J.M. (1852). On the treatment of vesico-vaginal fistula. *Am. J. Med. Sci.*, **23**, (n.s.) 59–82

Speert, H. (1958). *Essays in Eponymy*. (New York: MacMillan Co.)

Stallworthy, J. (1941). Useful speculum. *Br. Med. J.*, **26**, 696–7

Thomas, T.G. (1878). *Practical Treatise on the Diseases of Women*, 4th edn., p.67. (Philadelphia: Lea)

Thompson, C.J.S. (1938). The evolution and development of surgical instruments. *Br. J. Surg.*, **26**, 232

Surgery

SURGICAL OPERATIONS

'We are in an era of stupendous advance' – this was Edward A. Schumann's phrase when he wrote the introduction to James V. Ricci's *Genealogy of Gynaecology*. Nobody who writes a history of gynaecological surgery can do so without expressing his indebtedness to Ricci's great works on the subject. These are *Development of Gynaecological Surgery and Instruments* published by Blakiston and Company in Philadelphia in 1949 and *One Hundred Years of Gynaecology (1800–1900)*, published by the same firm in 1945, and a third book *The Genealogy of Gynaecology*, again published by Blakiston in 1950. These three masterly works do contain some overlapping material. They are full of lengthy footnotes and of wonderful and most extensive lists of references. There is little point in repeating these references because for serious scholars they are available in all medical libraries in Ricci's three books.

It is however, over 40 years since the last book was published during which time there have been further 'stupendous' advances in gynaecological surgery, and in particular in laparoscopy and ultrasound which are the subjects of separate chapters in this book. Here it is appropriate to do honour to Professor Raoul Palmer of Paris (q.v.), one of the originators of laparoscopy and Professor Ian Donald (q.v.), the great obstetrician of Glasgow, for his discovery of the uses of ultrasound in obstetrics and gynaecology (Figure 1). These techniques have helped diagnosis immensely; and laparoscopic surgery has also come into its own, not only in gynaecology, but also in general surgery – e.g. in the performance of laparoscopic cholecystectomy. Lasers are used in conjunction with laparoscopy particularly in the treatment of endometriosis. The gonadotropic releasing hormone analogues are now used to lessen the size of fibroids and sometimes of endometrial cysts before surgery is attempted. This, together with the improvement of anaesthetic techniques, has made gynaecological surgery much less disturbing for patients with the result that patients can leave hospital much earlier than after the large major operations that in the past used to be performed.

In view of Ricci's great contribution to the history of the subject, it is sensible for us to concentrate on the great discoveries made since 1945, after just outlining some of the earlier discoveries. Most of the recent work is dealt with in the appropriate sections, e.g. endoscopy.

HISTORY OF OPERATIVE GYNAECOLOGY

It seems likely that the very first operations of a gynaecological nature were female circumcisions or ceremonial infibulations. It equally seems likely that the next most widely practised operation was

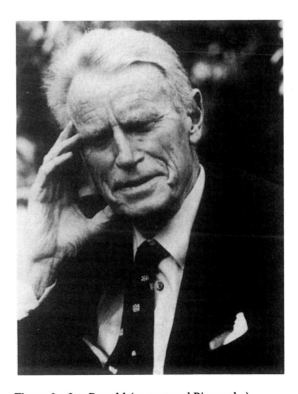

Figure 1 Ian Donald (*see* text and Biography)

abortion. The instruments used in very early history were crude in the extreme and we have no accurate record of what they were like.

DILATATION AND CURETTAGE

In an article in the *Journal of the Royal Society of Medicine* in 1991 Dr John Forrester has poured scorn on some of Ricci's claims about the development of gynaecological surgery and instruments. In his book Ricci (1949) states that Hippocrates frequently mentioned and adequately described specially graduated sets of dilators corresponding to the Hegar or Hanks dilators of today. He claims they were made of tin, lead or wood; and Ricci gives seven lengthy references in his footnotes in the chapter. But Forrester states 'No expert commentator seems to believe that this is a genuine work of the historic Hippocrates who flourished at the end of the fifth century BC but rather of some successor of his'. Forrester also pours scorn on Ricci's implication that Celsus probably wrote about AD 30 that he used hollow lead probes.

It does seem to be very doubtful whether dilatation of the cervix was a regular practice in antiquity, and Forrester seems to think that one of Hippocrates successors may have created a twentieth century myth! It would seem, according to Forrester, that John Mackintosh of Edinburgh may have been the first to take up instrumental dilatation. He did it for dysmenorrhoea in 1826 and claimed originality (Forrester, 1991). Ricci does reproduce in his book photographs of various instruments that he claims come from the Hippocratic period (Ricci, 1949). A photograph is taken from Carl Sudhoff, Mutterrohr and Verwandts' *in Medizinischen Instrumentarium der Antike*. In this photograph there are tubes illustrated, which are said to be cervical (uterine) drainage tubes (Sudhoff *et al.*, 1926).

Of course it is not possible safely to dilate the cervix if one cannot see it and visualization of the cervix had to follow the invention of the vaginal speculum, which could have been in antiquity.

It may well be that the first man who regularly used a *modern* speculum was the Frenchman, Joseph Claude Anthelme Recamier, who started to use it in 1801 when he was 27 years old. His first speculum was a 5-inch-long tin tube. James Young Simpson was one of the first to use Recamier's speculum which was made a little shorter by Dupuytren who attached a handle to his speculum. It was a Frenchwoman, Madame Boivin, who added

a handle, split the cylinder to make it into a bi-valve speculum, and made its screw attachment so it could be opened wider. The modern ones that we use today were devised and adapted by Edward Gabriel Cusco from the Dupuytren and Boivin specula, which are all illustrated in Ricci's book. They all date from the early nineteenth century.

All new inventions have their advocates and detractors. It is not surprising to read that in the middle of the nineteenth century there were as many doctors who opposed the use of the speculum, because it was 'indelicate', as there were who advocated it. Today it is hardly possible to conduct a gynaecological clinic without using a speculum on at least half of the women who attend. In Maygrier's famous textbook (Maygrier, 1822) there are two illustrations of the obstetrician examining his patient vaginally, she being completely covered by a sheet in one illustration and in the other, completely dressed in a long flowing dress. In the first the doctor stands by the patient's bedside, in the second, he kneels in front of his patient. It was common apparently, to examine patients vaginally when they were standing, but when they were lying they were in the left lateral position, although not in Maygrier's illustration where the lady is on her back in the dorsal position. In neither figure nor elsewhere in this beautiful book is there any mention of the vaginal speculum.

OVARIOTOMY

Ephraim McDowell (q.v.) who was the 'father of ovariotomy' was also the real founder of abdominal surgery (Schachaer, 1921) (Figure 2). In Edinburgh, where McDowell was a student in 1793, discussions had already been going on about the feasibility of carrying out operations to remove ovarian tumours, but they had been thought to be too dangerous because the peritoneum was held in such awe and respect.

On the 13 December 1809 however, Ephraim McDowell, now in America since 1796, was called to see a Mrs Jane Todd Crawford, in her home in Motley's Glen, 9 miles to the east of Greensburgh and 60 miles from Danville, Kentucky, where McDowell lived. He and Mrs Crawford, an immensely brave, courageous and determined 47-year-old woman, decided that he would carry out an operation to remove the tumour, which was embarrassing her enormously, making it somewhat difficult for her to breathe and making life a complete misery. She rode to Danville on a

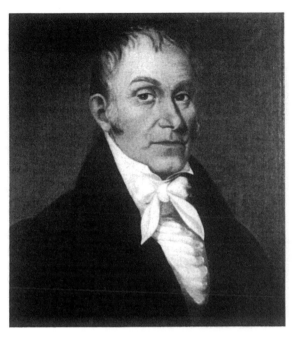

Figure 2 Ephraim McDowell (1771–1830) (*see* text). A founder of abdominal surgery. From a contemporary portrait in oils in the possession of the Department of Obstetrics and Gynecology, in Kansas City, USA. Reproduced with kind permission from Professor K. Krantz (q.v.)

horse resting the tumour on the horn of her saddle.

The day after she arrived in Danville and on a Sunday (Christmas Day to boot), because that was an appropriate day for surgery, McDowell opened the abdomen by an incision 9 inches (23cm) long and 3 inches (8cm) away from the rectus abdominis muscle on the left side. There was, of course, no anaesthesia then, no antisepsis, no antibiotics and only one assistant to help, and throughout the operation Mrs Crawford recited psalms.

This was the procedure. Once he had found the pedicle McDowell ligated the left tube and the ovarian pedicle close to the uterus. He then emptied the 'dirty' gelatinous-looking substance, and then delivered the tumour, which was partly solid even after the substance had been removed. The cystic part weighed 15 lb (6.8 kg) and the solid part weighed 7.5 lb (3.4 kg). He put the bowels, which had come out through the wound, back and tilted the patient further on to her side so that any blood in her peritoneal cavity could drain out. He then sewed the pedicle to the lower end of the wound, which he closed with interrupted sutures. The operation took just 25 minutes.

Five days after the operation Mrs Crawford was found making her bed. She rode home in good health some 20 days after the operation. It is a famous story. There is some doubt as to which part of McDowell's house was used for the operation. The house has now been very well restored. McDowell carried out 13 ovariotomies in all and only one patient died. His was a far more important step than simply starting a branch of gynaecological surgery. It was the first successful major abdominal operation through the peritoneum. Others tried to emulate him. In Edinburgh John Lizars, who was also a pupil of Bell as McDowell had been, vacillated but attempted the operation in October 1823, and failed, and then made three more attempts in 1825.

McDowell was possibly more able to succeed by virtue of the fact that he was living in a frontier town, where people were willing to push at physical boundaries and also where the population was not so thick on the ground nor so imbued with an academic approach as in a large university city. It was a great advantage, in fact, to be away from the centre of things. It may well be that this kind of advantage was reflected in the work of Steptoe and Edwards who 160 years later started *in vitro* fertilization, not in a university hospital department where people could talk and criticize what they were doing, but in an isolated hospital in a small town, Oldham in north England.

Of course there were people who were willing to criticize what McDowell had done, but it may have been an advantage that the operation was not made public until 9 years or so after it had been performed, by which time McDowell had carried out further surgery.

McDowell died on the 25 June 1830. Mrs Crawford, who is the real heroine of the story, lived for more than 30 years after this epoch-making operation.

There is very much chauvinism in surgery, particularly among the French who claim that they were the first to operate on ovarian cysts, but in fact it was almost certainly Robert Houstoun of Glasgow, who lived from 1678 to 1734 who first operated on an ovarian cyst. Unlike McDowell, he did not remove the whole cyst but merely punctured it. Robert Houstoun is hardly famous in the history of gynaecology, but it was almost a hundred years before McDowell's operation that in 1701 he performed the first recorded operation on a large ovarian cyst in Glasgow.

Robert Houstoun was born in Glasgow in 1678 at the time when Glasgow had just 12 000 inhabitants. His father was a surgeon who taught him surgery; and Robert became his father's apothecary. His father advised him to go to France, so he went to study at the Hotel Dieu et la Charité, Paris between 1699 and 1700. It was Louis XIV himself who paid for Houstoun to work as an assistant surgeon and obstetrician at the Hotel Dieu. Having completed his apprenticeship Houstoun set up in practice in Glasgow in 1701. In the very same year, when he was 23 years of age, he operated at a farm in the neighbourhood of Glasgow on Margaret Millar, who was then 58 years of age. She had a very rapidly growing ovarian tumour that was pressing on her abdominal organs and raising up her diaphragm so that she had great difficulty in breathing.

Houstoun opened the abdominal wall and it may well be that this was the first time that the abdomen had been opened on purpose in this way. Using a sharpened trocar made of pinewood and covered at the end that he held in his hand with a cloth, he bored through the thick wall of the cyst and evacuated, after turning the instrument round in the cyst 'a jelly-like substance, like glue, which contained steatoceous and atheromatous tissue with hydatids filled with a yellow serum' (Houston, 1726).

After he had evacuated the fluid by pressing on the cyst and getting out as much as he possibly could, he stitched up the abdomen and using a roll of paper coated with a balm, covered this with compresses and a cloth soaked in French brandy.

Margaret Millar declared on the following day that she had slept better the night following the operation than throughout the previous 3 months. She made a complete recovery from the operation, and died after a short illness 13 years later in October 1714.

It was only 11 years after performing the operation that Houstoun became a Doctor of Medicine of his university, Glasgow, in 1712. In 1717 he moved to London and then published the first case of an ectopic pregnancy that he had diagnosed in a live woman. This paper caused a lot of controversy among his colleagues but all the same he was elected a Fellow of the Royal Society in 1724 under the presidency of Isaac Newton (1642–1727).

Houstoun died at the age of 56 on 15 May 1734. He had not carried out oophorectomy, as McDowell was to do later, but his operation had been important enough for William Smellie to mention it in his book *Cases and Observations in Midwifery* which was published in 1779 and to state that it was a new procedure.

Of course the French, and indeed others, claimed they had carried out the first ovariectomies; among these were Eugene Koeberlé (1828–1915) who operated in Strasbourg in 1862, and Jules Pean (1830–1898) who operated in 1864 in Paris. There were several others who claimed that they had done the first operations but McDowell certainly, with his Christmas day operation, led the way (Journal de Gynecologie, 1987).

The operation by Ephraim McDowell on 25 December 1809, the first fully recorded description of the removal of a whole cystic ovary was rapidly followed by others, in other countries. In Germany it was first performed by a Doctor Chrysman in 1819, 10 years after McDowell in America, but it may not have been performed in France until 1847 by Woyeikowski and in 1848 by Vaullegard.

John Lizars (1794–1860) a teacher of Anatomy and Surgery in Edinburgh, later Professor of Surgery in the College of Surgeons of Edinburgh, and a life-long enemy of the great Syme, carried out four cases of ovariotomy (Lizars, 1825). Although Lizars did not do many operations he was probably the first in Scotland to remove an ovarian cyst successfully. It was in 1836 that William Jeaffreson (1790–1865) of Framlingham, carried out the first successful removal of an ovary in England. This was reported in the *Lancet* in 1837 by King who did another similar operation with Jeaffreson's help.

Charles Clay (1801–1893), however, was the pioneer ovariotomist in Great Britain and he introduced the word ovariotomy (Morton, 1842). In all, he performed 395 ovariotomies with a mortality of about 25. Obviously he was an extremely competent abdominal surgeon. He carried out his first operation in September 1842. He removed a huge tumour through a 24-inch (60-cm) incision – probably the record for the date. His long incision was carried out on purpose as a contrast to Jeaffreson's very short incisions of about 6 inches (15cm).

It was 1857 when the first attempt was made by Thomas Spencer Wells to carry out ovariotomy (Figure 3). At that time no decision had been made whether the 4-inch (10cm) or the 9-inch (23cm) incision should be made in order to enter the abdomen. Similarly there was no decision as

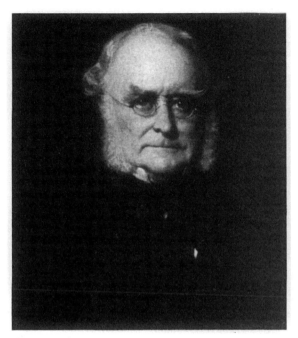

Figure 3 Thomas Spencer Wells (1818–1895). Reproduced with the kind permission from the Royal College of Surgeons of England

had not closed the peritoneum. The technique of dealing with the pedicle was either to tie ligatures long and leave them out of the abdominal wall, or else put a clamp on and leave this on the closed surface of the abdominal wall with the pedicle extruding through the cut in the abdominal wall. The clamp usually dropped off 7–10 days after the operation. The abdominal wall was closed around the stump and the closure was carried out very carefully.

By 1864 ovariotomy was firmly established as a legitimate operation thanks to the work of Spencer Wells and Charles Clay. It was the work of Lister and Pasteur that eventually made operating in the peritoneal cavity safer, as antisepsis had done for obstetrics.

It must have been very difficult for Spencer Wells (q.v. in Biographies) to go on operating with a fairly high mortality rate among his patients and strong criticism from his colleagues. By the end of 1862 he had had 33 recoveries out of the 50 cases he had operated on. At least he was held in high esteem because he was so honest in publishing his results. In 1864 he published his

to whether ligatures to tie the pedicles of the ovaries should be long or short strips. Infection was very common particularly when long strips were used and were left outside the abdominal wall. Sinuses would form if the patient survived long enough; otherwise she was likely to die of peritonitis. (John Atlee in America published a series of 30 cases in 1855; of 26 ovariotomies he completed, 16 recovered.) Spencer Well's first attempt at ovariotomy in December 1857 seems to have been the first abdominal exploration he had ever done. He was assisted by Baker Brown in this and in other surgical procedures (Figure 4). He had read about the other surgeons' work and especially those operations done in the United States. The 1857 operation seems to have been an 'open and shut' matter because Spencer Wells thought that as the tumour was behind the intestines it could not be removed. However, the patient died and at the autopsy it was shown that it could have been removed. In February 1858, again assisted by Baker Brown of St. Mary's Hospital (Figure 5), he operated on a woman of 38 and was successful. He tied the pedicle with silk and left the ends long. The ligature came away on the 12th day and the patient recovered very well. Two more cases were successful but a fourth died; he

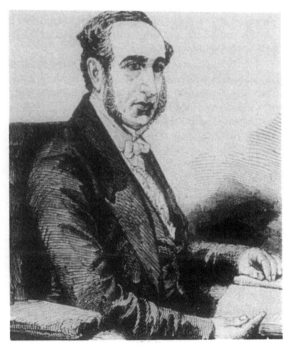

Figure 4 Isaac Baker Brown (died 1873). President of the Medical Society of London 1865. A founder of St. Mary's Hospital, London. Unjustly expelled from the Obstetrical Society of London for performing and publishing a series of clitoridectomies for the cure of hysteria

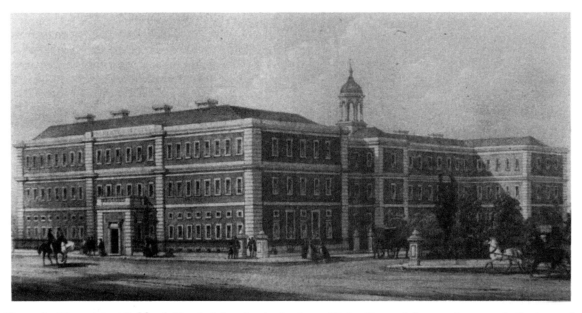

Figure 5 The original St. Mary's Hospital, London in the time of Baker Brown (nineteenth century). Courtesy of the Archivist of St. Mary's Hospital

Notebook for Cases of Ovarian and Other Abdominal Tumours and a copy of 2 pages of this notebook can be found in the biography of Spencer Wells by J.A. Shepherd (1965).

The Samaritan Hospital where Wells did most of his operations was small and built in such a way that the operated patient was kept away from other patients; and therefore the risk of infection was lessened. He often operated in private homes where he kept the temperature of the room at about 75°F. His operations were performed under a general anaesthetic. Originally this was chloroform and later 'Bichloride of Methynene'. Spencer Wells very often operated in front of quite large audiences. The operations were not always carried out at the Samaritan Hospital. For instance in the case note illustrated in Shepherd's book, the operation was performed in Daventry, the patient having been referred by a Daventry general practitioner. He was invited to operate not only in various provincial cities in England but also on the continent in cities such as Zurich and Brussels. The surgery was by no means always successful and many of the patients died. By 1872 Spencer Wells had carried out 500 ovariotomies. He used a clamp that he left on the pedicle outside the abdominal wall, and always published his failures just as he did his successes. The unfortunate Baker Brown, who had done much

operating with Wells and had done much to popularize ovariotomy, came unstuck when he started to remove the clitoris from patients who were psychologically disturbed (Figure 6). He was heavily criticized by his colleagues and was eventually made to stop operating. He died after having been certified insane.

Thomas Spencer Wells wrote that during the preceding century 'surgeons stood and trembled on the brink of ovarian waters'. He invented a clamp as described, to place across the pedicles, but the forceps with the narrow tips only gradually evolved. It was only after Lister had learnt successfully to sterilize ligatures that they became used in the way they are still today. Originally the instruments used to stop bleeding from vessels were sharp tipped, but gradually Spencer Wells realized that it

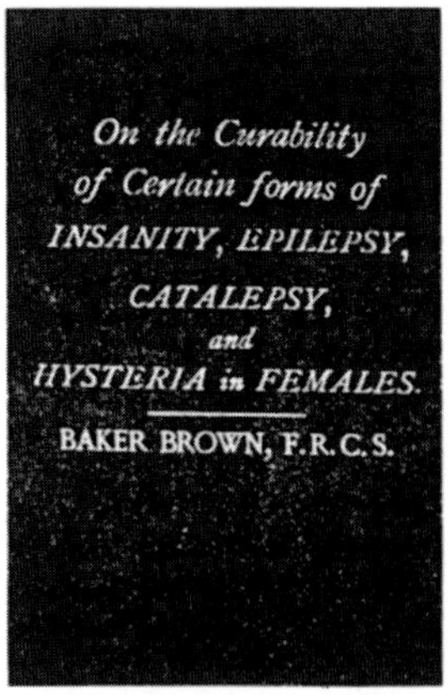

Figure 6 Title page of Isaac Baker Brown's book on clitoridectomy

On the Curability of Certain forms of INSANITY, EPILEPSY, CATALEPSY, and HYSTERIA in FEMALES.

BAKER BROWN, F.R.C.S.

would be easier to tie ligatures round the instruments if the tips were curved. They were originally developed from Liston's cat forceps. Liston was a great amputator of limbs and is recorded as having done one of the first operations under anaesthesia in the United Kingdom. Spencer Wells' improved forceps were developed from the French forceps invented by Pean. In 1868 Spencer Wells treated small bleeding vessels by compression with his forceps that he left on only for a short time although he sometimes placed a temporary ligature on the vessels. At that time his newly developed forceps were called pressure forceps and he advocated 'forci-pressure'. By 1880 Spencer Wells had performed 1000 ovariotomies and by 1890 he had carried out 1230 ovariotomies and his mortality rate had dropped to 4.4%.

The award that Spencer Wells received by being elected President of the Royal College of Surgeons of England was matched by the financial rewards. There is in London a beautiful park near Hampstead Heath called Golders Hill Park. Until it was destroyed in World War II there was a large Victorian house on the edge of this park next to the house in which the late Anna Pavlova the dancer lived. The Victorian house was Thomas Spencer Wells' and the park was his farm with gardens possibly designed by the great Capability Brown (see also Biographies).

AMPUTATION OF THE CERVIX

In 1833 Boivin (1773–1841) and Duges (1798–1835) reported amputation of the cervix for chronic ulceration. They also in the same work recorded for the first time cancer of the female urethra (Boivin and Duges, 1833). Figure 7 illustrates Sims' adaption of an 'ecraseur' to which a blade was added to amputate the cervix.

HYSTERECTOMY

It seems very likely that the first hysterectomy was performed by accident! A Dr G. B. Paletta of Milan carried out the operation on 13 April 1812. He apparently intended to amputate what he thought was a malignant cervix, but to his great surprise he found that he had removed the entire uterus vaginally. The patient is reported to have died after 40 hours, or maybe 3 days following the operation. Her death was from peritonitis. Paletta was assisted by a Dr D. B. Montéggia, an eminent surgeon in Milan. J. N. Sauter Barden was probably the first to perform a properly planned

hysterectomy deliberately. He did this on 22 January 1822. The operation was performed vaginally. The intestines came down and were maintained in position by a pack of dry lint. A vesico-vaginal fistula resulted.

It is believed that Charles Clay carried out the first successful subtotal hysterectomy deliberately in January 1863 having made an unsuccessful attempt in 1843, although Koeberlé of Strasbourg has often been credited with the first successful hysterectomy. Clay later carried out a total removal of the uterus and its appendages (Clay, 1863). He quarrelled hugely with Spencer Wells in public in 1863 about priority and success rates.

On 1 September 1853 Gilman Kimball (1804–

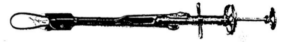

Figure 7 Sims' adaptation of an 'ecraseur' to which a blade was added to amputate the cervix in the same way as tonsils were guillotined using a similar instrument. From J. Marion Sims' *Uterine Surgery* (1866)

1892) reported his first successful total abdominal hysterectomy for fibroids, carried out in Boston, USA (Kimball, 1855). In Leslie T. Morton's book of medical bibliography (1965) there are references to several cases of removal of the ovaries successfully treated by the large incision from the sternum to the pubis (Clay, 1842). The only way out of an otherwise insoluble dilemma for the early 20th century surgeon confronted by a woman in the seventh month of her pregnancy with ruptured membranes and the arm of her fetus prolapsed through the cervix of her uterus, which itself contained multiple fibroids, was to remove the uterus and cervix together with the fetus (Figure 8).

The operation of abdominal hysterectomy was made much easier by the introduction by Friederich Trendelenburg (1844–1924) of the elevated pelvic position. In other words the position of the operating table where the patient's shoulders are much lower than her buttocks as the title of his first paper in 1890 makes clear. His student W. Mayer had already in 1885 given the first description of the elevated pelvic position (Mayer, 1885; Trendelenburg, 1890). Apparently Trendelenburg himself attempted vesico-vaginal repairs as reported in his 1890 publication and used his Trendelenburg position to facilitate the operation.

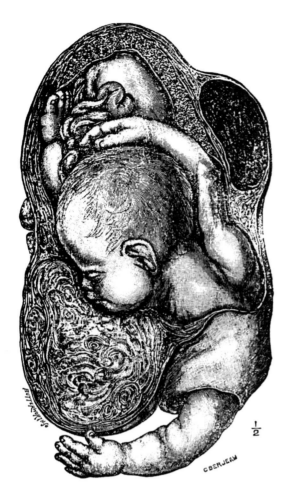

Figure 8 The arm of the fetus prolapsed through the cervix of the uterus of a woman in her seventh month of pregnancy. Hysterectomy specimen held in the Museum of the Royal College of Surgeons

Extended hysterectomy

When it became clear that part of the secret of obtaining a cure in cancer was to remove as much tissue as possible from around the neoplastic lesion and as many lymph nodes as possible, the extended operation was invented. The great master for the performance of this operation was Ernst Wertheim (1864–1920) (q.v.). The first really radical abdominal hysterectomy was carried out by Wertheim on 16 November 1898. The purpose of the operation was to remove the uterus including the cervix and the top part of the vagina, both ovaries and Fallopian tubes, parametrial tissue, the obturator lymph nodes as well as the other lymph nodes of the pelvis, and in fact to make as neat a dissection as possible of the structures of the floor of the pelvis, while maintaining the integrity of the ureters, the bladder and the rectum.

Wertheim obviously had to spare the vascularity of the ureter. He did this by avoiding isolating the ureter all round. He divided the infundibulo-pelvic and round ligaments, dissected the bladder, took the roof off the ureteric tunnel and ligated the uterine vessels. He separated the rectum and isolated the parametrium. He used newly devised clamps on the utero-sacral ligaments and the vagina working outwards as near as possible to the lateral walls of the pelvis. He left the vagina open for drainage, putting a suture around the top and he removed all lymph nodes from the division of the aorta to the obturator fossa by exploring the great iliac vessels and then removed the nodes near them and over them. The peritoneum was closed over a gauze pack, and this remained the procedure even until 1960 at the Chelsea Hospital for Women. His survival rate in his last 50 cases was 98%. He had operated on one case every 10 days over 8 years. The time of his operation at the beginning of his experience was two and a half hours, but later he reduced it to an hour or maybe an hour and a quarter.

Wertheim's first patient died on the 8th day after the operation from severe anaemia. The second patient, who was 29 years of age, was operated on on 13 December 1898, and was alive 6 years later, although his third patient also died postoperatively on the 4th day. His fourth lived, and his fifth, eighth, eleventh and twelfth died after the operations. As he became more experienced so the death rate dropped. Some of the deaths were from the effects of chloroform and others from peritonitis. Half of his first 50 deaths were from this. He advocated lumbar or spinal anaesthesia with Stovain synthesized by Fourneau in France in 1904. He himself examined all his specimens and in all made 50 000 sections and showed that 28% of the regional lymph nodes were affected by cancer. These were all enlarged, but there were enlarged glands that had no cancer in them. He eventually managed to have 60% of his patients free of the disease after 5 years.

MAKING SUTURE MATERIALS SAFE FOR SURGICAL OPERATIONS

Lord Lister (Baron Joseph Lister FRCS 1827–1912) (Figure 9) not only invented the antiseptic techniques, including the carbolic acid

In a lecture in 1881 (Lister, 1909) Lister stated that he tried chromic acid 'on account of its well-known effect on hardening tissues'. Of course operations are now conducted under aseptic rather than antiseptic conditions, as Lister foresaw. It is still desirable that the catgut should last more than 3 or 4 days so surgeons still today use chromatized threads. Lister was well aware of the work of Pasteur on bacteria, and of Calvert on phenol (Calvert, 1863) for controlling bacterial action as well as of Quekett on chemicals to harden tissues. Lister's research was initially derived from his use of the microscope to study the blood flow in the webbed feet of frogs. From this he went on to show how the movement of the blood was reactivated by using chemical agents. From 1863 onwards he used the microscope to find micro-organisms in pus and in water from stagnant pools. He saw that phenol cleaned wounds of the pus. It was in 1867 that he started using chemicals, that he had originally used to fix tissues for microscope work, in order to treat suture materials (Godlee, 1917).

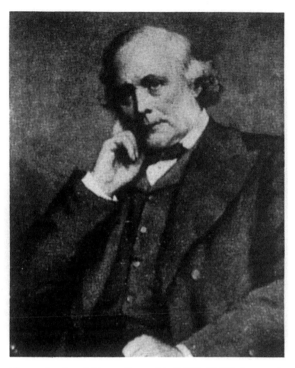

Figure 9 Lord Lister (Joseph) (1827–1912) (*see* text)

spray, in order to avoid infection in surgery, but also between the years 1860 and 1880 concentrated on trying to make suture materials safer and less liable to become infected. He utilized various available chemicals that had been used in the antiseptic treatment of wounds. Lister initially soaked the silk he was going to use to suture wounds in phenol and in similar substances. He checked the results of what he was doing by observations down the microscope. His father Joseph Jackson Lister FRS (1786–1869), who invented the achromatic compound microscope, gave his son the most modern one available at the time. Lister should have been doing most of his research in University College Hospital, London in the Department of Physiology under the directorship of Professor William Sharpey, but found it easier to work in a laboratory at home.

After silk Lister treated catgut, which is made from sheep's intestines, by soaking it in phenol. This however, had the effect of softening it and, since soft catgut disintegrated rapidly, it in turn, by dissolving, had the effect of encouraging secondary haemorrhage to occur. The idea of using catgut as a suture material was derived from its use in musical instruments.

MYOMECTOMY (REMOVAL OF FIBROIDS)

The operation of myomectomy dates from 1840. The first such operation was carried out by Amussat and it was a deliberate removal of a tumour thought at the time to be an ovary because it was on a pedicle (Noble, 1906). W. L. Atlee was the next surgeon to perform a myomectomy and it was the first successful one on record. It was carried out through the vaginal route in 1845. According to Victor Bonney (Bonney, 1931) myomectomy in the early stages of the operation consisted for the most part in removing pedunculated tumours. It was only later experience that gave gynaecologists the courage to remove fibroids having 'shorter and shorter pedicles until at last they assayed to cope with those having none at all'. Bonney referred to W. Alexander of Liverpool who reported in 1898 on a technique by which he had been able to remove as many as 25 tumours from a single uterus. Alexander's work met with hostility and nobody referred to it again until 1922 when Bonney looked up the literature on the subject. Howard A. Kelly (Kelly, 1907), C. P. Noble and the Mayos in America as well as Victor Bonney in England popularized the operation. By 1925 Bonney was able to report the results of 220 consecutive myomectomies. Bonney had done 403 myomectomies by 1930. In spite of his successful results surgeons were hesitant to carry out the operation, preferring hysterectomy to myomectomy because of the haemorrhage that occurs in myomectomy, and which could not be controlled without the use of blood transfusions. Furthermore, postoperative intestinal distension and vomiting were common after the operation. On the other hand, it was no use removing a uterus for fibroids if the woman wanted to become pregnant. It was William J. Mayo, one of the two brothers who founded the famous Mayo Institute, who strongly urged gynaecologists to carry out myomectomy (Mayo, 1922).

There was little reason for carrying out myomectomy except to aid childbearing, but all the same some women were very attached to their uteri and even in 1942 Rubin reported that five women between the ages of 60 and 69 and 14 women aged between 50 and 59 had had myomectomy rather than hysterectomy, out of a total of 481 myomectomies performed by him (Rubin, 1942).

It is quite clear that the postoperative mortality and morbidity were much greater in patients undergoing myomectomy than hysterectomy. The invention by Bonney of a myomectomy clamp to lessen the blood flow through the uterine arteries was an advance because it not only lessened the blood flow, but also helped to hold the uterus up into the wound to make the operation easier.

By 1990 the operation had been rendered much easier and less bloody by administering gonadotropin releasing hormone analogues for a few months preoperatively.

OPERATIONS FOR STRESS INCONTINENCE

For a long time the main procedure for stress incontinence was an anterior colporrhaphy. This was variously known as the Fothergill operation, the Manchester repair operation, or anonymously, anterior colpo-perineorrhaphy. The purpose of the operation was to raise the upper urethra and the neck of the bladder and incidentally to lengthen the urethra. It was believed by authorities such as Jeffcoate (1957) that it was important that there should be an acute angle between the neck of the bladder and the upper end of the urethra.

Krantz (q.v. in Biographies) (Figure 10) published many papers on the anatomy of the urethra and the anterior vaginal wall, as well as on the innervation of the human vulva and vagina and of the uterus and made brilliant dissections from 1949 onwards (Marshall *et al.*, 1949). It was his and Marshall and Marchetti's knowledge that led to the development of the operation to suspend

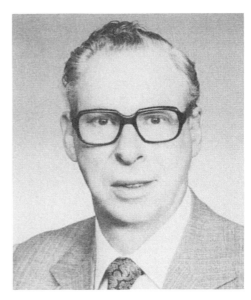

Figure 10 Professor Kermit E. Krantz (born 1923 in Illinois), Chairman of the Department of Gynecology and Professor of Anatomy in the University of Kansas, College of Health Sciences, Kansas City, USA. Published his operations for suspension of the upper urethra and neck of the bladder together with Dr Andrew A. Marchetti and Dr Victor F. Marshall

from above the upper urethra and neck of the bladder by stitches inserted just above the middle third of the urethra into the musculosa of the vagina at the urethro-vesical junction, beside the symphysis pubis.

The retropubic space of Retzius is approached from above by a low suprapubic incision through the skin, the rectus sheath and by a separation between the pyramidalis muscles. The stitches used to support the bladder structures are inserted beside the bladder neck and not into it for fear of making a fistula. They are of non-absorbable material which is also passed into the periosteum of the pubic bones on either side.

A REVIEW OF EARLIER OPERATIONS

Since, as mentioned at the outset of this chapter, James V. Ricci, who was Clinical Professor of Gynaecology and Obstetrics in the New York Medical College and worked in several other hospitals in New York, has written so very fully and with many notes on gynaecological operations, it has seemed to us sensible to quote a little from what he wrote about operations in the second half of the nineteenth century.

Vaginal hysterectomy (Figure 11) was proposed for simple uncomplicated prolapse as early as 1861, and although there was much opposition to it, S. Choppin on 2 January 1861 did perform the operation in New Orleans, without injury to bladder or rectum. This certainly was a considerable feat. The operation seems to have been repeated for prolapse in 1876 by A. Patterson in Glasgow, and Ricci gives a very long list of other operators who followed on after 1876, performing vaginal hysterectomy for prolapse.

Ricci also quoted many authorities who had to deal with cases of inversion of the uterus where attempts to replace it failed. Sometimes ovoid or ball-shaped rods were kept in place with a T-binder, and this idea was mooted as early as 1674 by C. Viardel. If the worst came to the worst, the inverted uterus was amputated in order to avoid the patient bleeding to death, but the operation was very hazardous indeed.

It does seem that the first successful abdominal hysterectomy was performed by mistake by Walter Burnham of Lowell, Massachusetts in June 1853. The patient had had her abdomen opened for the removal of a supposed ovarian cyst. She

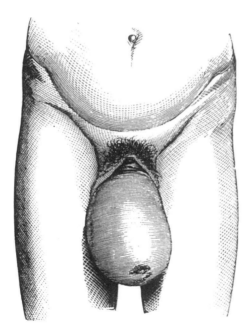

Figure 11 A huge complete procidentia with elongation and ulceration of the cervix. The procidentia contained most of the bladder as well as the lower part of the uterus and several loops of intestine. Sims did not attempt to operate on this case. From J. Marion Sims', *Uterine Surgery* (1866)

vomited, the tumour mass extruded and it could not be replaced. Burnham was forced to remove it although he had had no intention of doing so. He said that he would not repeat the operation but he did 15 times and only three of his patients survived. Others died from shock, peritonitis, sepsis and pyaemia. Apparently the first deliberate hysterectomy for fibroids, with success, was performed by Gilman Kimball, also of Lowell Massachusetts, on 1 September 1853. Of his first four hysterectomies three died, and there is a series of 42 hysterectomies carried out in the following 23 years, of which only nine were successful. One of the first successful abdominal hysterectomies, leaving the cervix behind, was accompanied involuntarily by the removal of both tubes and ovaries. The operation was performed by William Baker of Knoxville, Tennessee. The most important figure in uterine surgery in Europe was E. Koeberlé, of Strasbourg, who operated at about the same time in Europe as Gilman Kimball was working in the USA and the Frenchman Jules Pean was in Paris, France. Koeberlé wrote a history of the operation in 1864. He certainly seems to have been a great innovator.

It is difficult to know who was more heroic, the surgeons who attempted these operations with enormous mortality, or the patients who submitted to them.

It seems that abdominal hysterectomy for fibroids and vaginal hysterectomy for fibroids were being performed with equal enthusiasm in the last quarter of the nineteenth century in many countries of the world, and Ricci quotes a very large literature not only of those who performed the operation, but also those who wrote about the history of it.

The name of Fothergill of Manchester, England, later dominated operations for prolapse of the vagina, the bladder, the rectum and the uterus. He assisted his young chief A. Donald in 1888, to begin to combine repair of the anterior and posterior walls of the vagina and the perineum with high amputation of the cervix. They used silver wire but after visiting Berlin changed for some of the their cases to the use of catgut sutures. The standard operation for prolapse first designed by Donald and Fothergill is still being performed with or without hysterectomy 100 years after its first description. If the cervix was removed then the cardinal ligaments were apposed to form a firm support.

Not only did the operation serve to repair prolapses caused by difficult labours, excessive pulling with forceps and the stretching of tissues that had become thin and aged, but also was used with more or less success for the treatment of incontinence of urine without fistula formation. It was only when Marshall, Marchetti and Krantz advocated the abdominal approach that this became more popular for the treatment for stress incontinence. Over and above the vaginal approaches of W. E. Fothergill with many modifications, performed and described by a whole series of surgeons and the Marshall-Marchetti-Krantz operation, there is a third set of procedures namely the 'sling' operations. The name most associated with this operation has been Aldridge of the USA. Some of the difficulties of his operation lay in setting the sling at the proper tension so that the incontinence was cured but the patient was still able to pass urine and did not suffer retention of urine for too long. Among popular sling operations has been the so-called cruciate bladder sling operation, in which fascial straps prepared from the fascia covering the rectus abdominus muscles, are used.

Other important gynaecological operations are for refashioning of vaginas that either are congenitally absent, have congenital constrictions, or have been damaged. Various materials have been used including skin grafts, segments of bowel, and amnion to line the newly formed vagina, made by boring a tunnel between the urethra and the rectum. These plastic procedures have been carried out by gynaecologists, urologists and plastic surgeons, sometimes working individually, though often by two specialists working together.

CHRONOLOGY

The first gynaecological operations were probably female circumcision or infibulation.

Hippocrates – it is doubtful whether he knew about cervical dilators although they have been mentioned in his non-authenticated works and have been reported by Ricci.

1701	Houston evacuated an ovarian cyst.
1801	Recamier invented the modern speculum.
1809	On Christmas day Ephraim McDowell performed the first ovariotomy and was the first to open the peritoneum and remove the organ successfully.
1812	Paletta performed the first vaginal hysterectomy.

1826	John Mackintosh of Edinburgh used cervical dilators and may have been the first to use modern dilators.
1832	Boivin and Duges carried out the first amputation of the cervix.
1840	The first myomectomy was performed by Amussat who thought he was removing a pedunculated ovarian cyst.
1845	The first successful intentional myomectomy was performed vaginally.
1853	Gilman and Kimball carried out the first successful abdominal hysterectomy.
1862	Koeberlé removed an ovary in Strasbourg.
1863	Charles Clay carried out the first successful hysterectomy and removal of appendages.
1881	Lister made the first chromic catgut.
1885	The Trendelenburg position was first described.
1898	Alexander of Liverpool removed 25 fibroids from one uterus against much opposition.
	Wertheim performed the first radical abdominal hysterectomy.
1922	Mayo, in the USA, urged gynaecologists to perform myomectomy and gave the operation respectability.
1949	The Marshall–Marchetti–Krantz operation was described.
1990	Gonadotropin releasing hormone analogues were administered to render myomectomy and hysterectomy less bloody.

Suture materials

The authors are indebted to Msrs Davis and Geck for help.

3000–1750 BC	The Edwin Smith papyrus gives details of the use of linen thread and animal sinew to suture battle wounds.
350 BC	Susrata (q.v. in Biographies) used cotton strips, plaited horse hair, sinew and fibre.
AD 50	Celsus from Greece referred to ligation of blood vessels.
AD 200	Galen described the use of catgut for ligating aneurysms.

AD 850	Rhazes from Persia, used harp strings made of twisted sheep intestines as sutures as well as using catgut.
AD 1500	Ambroise Paré ligated divided blood vessels after amputating limbs.
1750	John Hunter ligated for aneurysm.
1806	Philip Syng Physik, Hunter's pupil, experimented in Pennsylvania USA, with dissolvable sutures.
1867	Joseph Lister (q.v. in Biographies) carbolized catgut sutures and then chromacised them.
1900	Sterilized catgut was placed into glass tubes.
1930	Atraumatic needles were made which avoided having to thread more old-fashioned needles.
1930–1940	Steel wire was first used as a suture material. It had strength and low potential for infection.
1950s	Braided polyester was introduced. Polyamide sutures – nylon had been used for making parachutes in World War Two – was introduced.
1960s	Polyethylene and polypropylene non-absorbable sutures were introduced as were siliconed silk sutures. Glass was replaced by other packing material.
1970s	Polyglycolic acid was introduced. This was a synthetic absorbable suture material to replace gut in many operations.
1980s	New wholly absorbable materials were made and subcuticular sutures were being used giving less scarring of the skin.

Staples

1000 BC	Hindus used giant ant and beetle heads to clip wound margins together.
1908	The first purpose-made skin stapler was introduced in Hungary.
1980s	Skin staplers and staple removers were introduced as were staples for ligating blood vessels.

REFERENCES

Boivin, M.-V. (née Gillan) and Duges, A. (1833). *Traite Pratique des Maladies de l'uterus et des ses Annexes*, Two Volumes and Atlas, (Paris: J.B. Baillière) (English translation, 1834)

Bonney, V. (1931). *Lancet*, 1, 171

Calvert, C. (1863). The therapeutic properties of carbolic acid. *Lancet*, 2, 362–3

Clay, C. (1842). Cases of peritoneal section, for the exterapation of diseased ovaria, by the large incision from sternum to pubis, successfully treated. *Med. Times*, 7, 43, 59, 67, 83, 99, 139, 153 and 270

Clay, C. (1863). Observations on Ovariotomy Statistical and Practical. *Trans. Obstet. Soc. London*, 5, 58–74

Davis and Geck (1993). *Educational Fact Sheets for Theatre Nursing Staff.* (Gosport, Hampshire)

Forrester, J. (1991). Instrumental dilation of the uterine cervix in antiquity – a myth or not? *J. R. Soc. Med.*, 84, 67

Godlee, R.J. (1917). *Lord Lister.* (London: MacMillan and Co Ltd)

Houstoun, R. (1726). *Philosophical Transactions*, 33, 3

Jeffcoate, T.N.A. (1957). *Principles of Gynaecology*, pp. 256–66. (London: Butterworth & Co.)

Kelly, H.A. (1907). *Am. Med. Assoc. Press*, pp. 1–2

Kimball, G. (1855). Successful case of extirpation of the uterus. *Boston Med. Surg. J.*, 52, 249–55

Lister, J. (1909). An address on the catgut ligature. *The Collected Papers of Joseph Baron Lister*, Vol. 2, pp. 101–18. (Oxford: Clarendon Press)

Lizars, J. (1825). *Observations on Extraction of Diseases Ovaria; illustrated by plates coloured after nature.* (Edinburgh: Daniel Lizars)

Mackintosh, J. (1828). *Elements of Pathology and Practice of Physic*, Vol. II, p. 353. (Edinburgh: John Carfrae)

Marshall, V.F., Marchetti, A.A. and Krantz, K.E. (1949). The correction of stress incontinence by simple vesico-urethral suspension. *Surg. Gynecol. Obstet.*, 88, 509

Mayer, W. (1885). *Arch. Klin. Chir.*, 131, 494–525

Maygrier, J.P. (1822). *Nouvelles Demonstration d'Accouchement.* (Paris: Béchet)

Mayo, W.J. (1922). Myomectomy, Editorial. *Surg. Gynecol. Obstet.*, **34**, 548–50

Morton, L.T. (1965). *Garrison and Morton's Medical Bibliography*, 2nd edn. pp. 527–37. (London: André Deutsch)

Noble, C.P. (1906). *Myomectomy.* (New York: A.R. Elliot Publishing Company)

Ricci, J.V. (1945). *One hundred Years of Gynaecology (1800–1900)*, pp. 163–183 and 285. (Philadelphia: Blakiston Co.)

Ricci, J.V. (1949). *The Development of Gynaecological Surgery and Instruments*, pp. 13, 297, 299, 300 and 301. (Philadelphia: Blakiston Co.)

Ricci, J.V. (1950). *The Genealogy of Gynaecology.* (Philadelphia: Blakiston Co.)

Rubin, I.C. (1942). Paper read to the Brooklyn Gynecological Society. March 6th 1942, Page 5.

Schachaer, A. (1921). *Ephraim McDowell.* (Philadelphia, London: J.B. Lippincott & Co.)

Shepherd, J.A. (1965). *Spencer Wells, The Life and Work of a Victorian Surgeon.* (Edinburgh and London: E. & S. Livingstone Ltd.)

Sudhoff, C., Mutterrohr and Verwandtes (1926). Medizinischen Instrumentarium der Antike. *Arch. G. gesch. d. Med.*, **18**, 51–71

Trendelenburg, F. (1890). Ueber lasenscheidenfisteloperationen und uber Beckenhochlagerung bei Operationen in der Bauchhohle. *Samml. Klin. Vort. R.*, No. **355** (chir) No. **109**, 3372–92

Laparoscopy

Although laparoscopy is a modern technique, it has its foundations in advances made many years ago. The desire to visualize the internal anatomy led to the first description of an invasive procedure. Hippocrates of Kos (460–377 BC) described the use of a rectal speculum which was later adapted for use *per vaginam*. There is evidence from Mesopotamia that the vagina and cervix were visualized directly through a lead tube called a *siphopherot*. Vaginal specula and other instruments were discovered in the ruins of Pompeii which was buried by lava in the year AD 70. Many physicians and artisans refined the shape, blades, handles and screw mechanisms of the speculum over subsequent centuries.

Direct daylight, or candle light reflected by mirrors, were the only methods of illumination available until 1587 when Aranzi used the camera obscura to illuminate the nasal cavities. Peter Borell introduced a concave mirror in the seventeenth century and later Arnaud adapted a small lantern as a light source. In 1806 Bozzini developed an illuminated endoscope to observe the cervix. Meanwhile, the development of the cystoscope was taking place, and Segal in 1826, and Desormeaux (1865) observed the bladder through a tube without lenses, using candle light illumination.

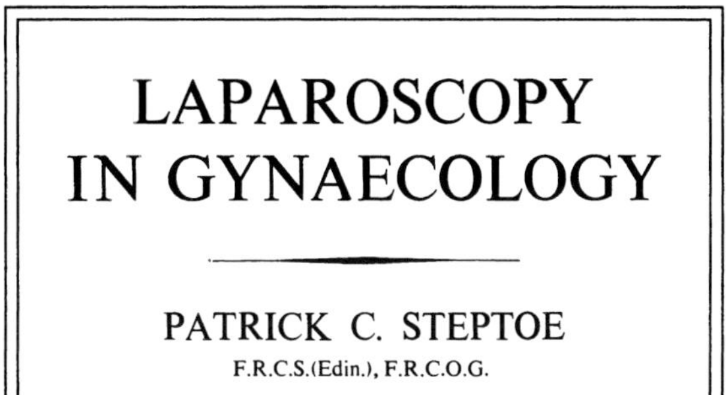

The optical system which converted a hollow tube into a telescope was developed in the nineteenth century and Nitze (1879a,b;1893) (in conjunction with the Berlin optician Reinecke and a Viennese instrument maker Leiter), is credited with the development of the forerunner of optical instrumentation. Initially the light source was an overheated platinum wire loop and later Edison's electric light bulb was used. Then a small electric light bulb was placed at the distal end of the scope.

In September 1901 Dr Georg Kelling reported 'celioscopic' examinations at the German Biological and Medical Society meeting in Hamburg (Kelling, 1902). Having first created a pneumoperitoneum with filtered air, he inserted a cystoscope into the abdomen of a living dog and viewed the viscera. He published a report the following year. Ventroscopy, which is a method whereby the abdominal cavity of pregnant women can be inspected via a culdoscopic opening, was described by von Ott (1901).

LAPAROSCOPY IN GYNAECOLOGY

PATRICK C. STEPTOE
F.R.C.S.(Edin.), F.R.C.O.G.
Consultant Gynaecologist to the Oldham Hospital Group, Lancashire

With a foreword by
W. I. C. MORRIS
M.B., Ch.B., F.R.C.S.(Edin.), F.R.C.O.G.
Professor of Obstetrics and Gynaecology, The University of Manchester

DR. H. FRANGENHEIM, M.D.
of the Rheinischen Landesfrauenklinik, Wuppertal,
W. Germany, contributes a section on Sterility

E. & S. LIVINGSTONE LTD.
EDINBURGH & LONDON
1967

Figure 1 Title page of Patrick Steptoe's book on Laparoscopy 1967. This was the first English publication on what became known as 'key-hole surgery' or 'minimally invasive surgery'. First used by gynaecologists and later by general surgeons

417

H.C. Jacobaeus of Stockholm (1910; 1911; 1912), detailed his inspection of body cavities by means of endoscopy. It was he who also introduced the term 'laparoscopy'. Bertram M. Bernheim (1911) first used laparoscopy in the USA. Orndoff (1920) also of the USA, coined the term 'peritoneoscopy'.

For a time there were many developments in instrumentation, including the use of a trocar by Nordentoeft (1912), the introduction of insufflation needles by Goetze (1918), and the use of carbon dioxide for insufflation by Zollikofer (1924). Janos Veress of Budapest (1938) introduced a new needle for inducing pneumothorax in the treatment of tuberculosis, and that needle was the equivalent of the modern insufflating instrument. Initially laparoscopy was carried out under local anaesthesia for patients with hepatic disease. However, its use was soon extended to gynaecology where until recently it has found its main indication and applications.

Early innovators included Kalk (1929) who developed a new oblique viewing lens system and popularized laparoscopy in Germany. John C. Ruddock (1934) developed a good optical system and introduced a built-in biopsy forceps with electrocoagulation capacity. Both Ruddock (1934) and an American surgeon, E.T. Anderson (1937), suggested laparoscopic sterilization and Power and Barnes (1941) reported such a technique. For a time in the 1940s, due to technical problems with light sources and optical systems, laparoscopy was overtaken by culdoscopy in America. Richard W. Te Linde attempted, but later abandoned, the technique from 1939 (Te Linde and Rutledge, 1948). However, in 1944, Albert Decker introduced the 'knee chest position' to culdoscopy and the technique became standard in the USA until the 1970s (Decker, 1946;1949).

Meanwhile, in Europe Fourestiere et al. (1943) of Paris introduced a cold light illumination source and Hopkins (1953) of Reading introduced an improved lens system in 1953. Both of these developments radically altered the efficiency and worth of the laparoscope. Raoul Palmer of Paris, Frangenheim of Konstanz, Semm of Germany, and others developed and modified the instrumentation and techniques so that laparoscopy became a safe and desirable procedure (Palmer, 1946; 1947; 1950; 1960; 1962; Frangenheim, 1964; 1972; Semm, 1973; 1976; 1977; 1978; 1987; 1988; Semm and Mettler, 1980). Patrick Steptoe (1967) of England (q.v. in Biographies) published the first book in English on laparoscopy

in gynaecology (Figure 1). In this book he described the complete instrumentation and techniques based on his experience in the 1960s. He also described laparoscopic sterilization and it was the use of this technique which caused a resurgence of interest in laparoscopy. The use of unipolar circuitry to coagulate the Fallopian tubes caused major problems with bowel burns and infection. This led on to the development of bipolar coagulation by Rioux and Cloutier (1974), and also by Kleppinger (1977). At the same time, non-electric techniques were explored and various clips and tubal occlusion devices were designed for use via laparoscopy. Gradually laparoscopy developed from being only for diagnostic and sterilizing procedures to a method enabling complex operations to be performed without recourse to laparotomy. Now laparoscopic procedures are classified as basic, intermediate and extensive, and even hysterectomy has been carried out via this route.

Laparoscopy has been of major benefit in the investigation, and treatment of infertility and in newer methods of assisted reproduction, particularly for ovum harvesting (Steptoe and Edwards, 1970) (q.v. in Biographies) (Figure 2) and for gamete intrafallopian transfer procedures (Asch et al., 1984). The introduction of laser laparoscopic surgery by Bruhat et al. (1979) has allowed extensive adhesiolysis and destruction of endometriotic foci to be performed. Brosens and colleagues (Brosens et al., 1987; Brosens and Puttemans, 1989) introduced double optic laparoscopy and the technique was initially used for salpingoscopy.

The development of efficient photographic methods and video technology have increased the facility for record keeping, and have also involved the operator's assistants in laparoscopic

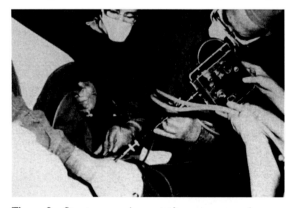

Figure 2 Steptoe carrying out a laparoscopy, using one of the very early cameras to record the operation

procedures. Although laparoscopy has mainly been used by gynaecologists, general surgeons are now rediscovering the technique and there is a revival of interest in its many applications.

CHRONOLOGY

Foundations

460–377 BC Hippocrates of Kos wrote on the use of rectal specula and gynaecological instruments.

AD 70 A three-bladed vaginal speculum was found in the ruins of Pompeii, which was destroyed by volcanic eruption in this year.

95 Archigenes, who practised in Rome at this time, spoke of illumination for endoscopic purposes and mentioned 'by that good bright light from the South'.

95 Vaginal specula were described by physicians from Rome.

108 Soranus of Ephesus, a Roman 'obstetrician', described the vaginal speculum.

500 The Babylonian Talmud refers to a leaden tube called a *siphopherot*, a tube made of lead with a wooden mandrin or *mechul*, through which the vagina and cervix could be observed.

1000 The Arabs introduced mirrors to illuminate body cavities at, or before, this time.

1010 Abulkasim reflected light from a glass mirror into the vaginal cavity.

1587 The first endoscopic light source was the camera obscura which was described by Tulio Caesare Aranzi. In 1590 Leonardo da Vinci attributed its invention to a Benedictine Monk, Don Panuce.

17th C. Peter Borell of Castres introduced the concave mirror.

18th C. The gynaecologist Arnaud introduced the endoscopic lamp which was adapted from small lanterns used by burglars.

1805/06 Bozzini developed a system of illumination through a tube to observe the vagina and cervix.

1826 A cystoscope without lens, and using light from a candle, was developed by Segal.

1843 Desormeaux introduced the first effective endoscope.

1865 Desormeaux further developed cystoscopic instrumentation.

1874 Stein of Frankfurt recommended the use of a photoendoscope.

1879/97 Nitze, with Reinecke (a Berlin optician), and Leiter (a Viennese instrument maker) produced optical instruments with a water cooled platinum wire light source.

1890s Roder introduced the slip knot for paediatric tonsillectomy. The slip knot was later incorporated into laparoscopic surgery for loop ligation (Semm and O'Neill Freys, 1989).

1900 Edison invented the electric light bulb and this was combined later with a cystoscope.

(References for above: Semm 1977; Baggish *et al.*, 1989; Gordon and Magos, 1989)

Development

1901 Laparoscopy was first reported by Kelling in Hamburg, at the German Biological and Medical Society Meeting. He filled the abdominal cavity of a dog with filtered air, and used a Nitze cystoscope to view the viscera.
von Ott from Petersburg reported the first ventroscopy, which was equivalent to a culdoscopic laparoscopy.

1902 Kelling published his report of 1901.

1910 Jacobaeus from Sweden conceived the term 'laparoscopy' and is credited with the first use of the technique in humans when he carried out laparoscopy on 17 patients with ascites.

1912 Nordentoeft (Copenhagen) invented the laparoscope with trocar and combined laparoscopy with the Trendelenburg position.

1918 Goetze developed his automatic needle for safe puncturing and gas insufflation of the abdomen.

1924 Steiner (America) 'rediscovered' laparoscopy as abdominoscopy.
Zollikofer (Switzerland) was the first to use carbon dioxide to insufflate and produce a pneumoperitoneum and examined patients with liver disease.

1925	The Italian Redi called his laparoscopic technique 'splanchnoscopy' (Semm, 1977).
1927	Korbsch (Munich) produced the first textbook of laparo- and thoracoscopy (Semm, 1977).
1929	Kalk (Germany) developed instrumentation for transabdominal endoscopic exploration.
1933	Fervers was first to sever intra-abdominal adhesions by means of the coagulation probe of a ureterocystoscope.
1936	Bosch, in Aarau, Switzerland, viewed the normal internal female genital organs via laparoscopy and mentioned the possibilty of tubal sterilization.
1938	Veress (Budapest) introduced his insufflating needle.
1943	Cold light illumination was invented by Fourestiere *et al.* in Paris.
1944/46	Palmer was the first gynaecologist to make clinical use of gynaecologic laparoscopy (Palmer, 1946).
1946	Due to technical difficulties with the performance of laparoscopy, Decker suggested a transvaginal procedure, later known as culdoscopy, which was popular until the 1970s in America.
1950s	Frangenheim modified and introduced new instruments for laparoscopic surgery, and the first prototype for modern carbon dioxide insufflation techniques (Frangen-heim, 1988). Monopolar electrocoagulation was introduced.
1953	Hopkins of Reading introduced an improved lens system and fibre optics.
1959	Graff *et al.* showed that one litre of carbon dioxide would have to be insufflated before any noticeable cardiovascular effects occurred in the patient under examination.
1960/62	Raoul Palmer wrote extensively on laparoscopy. He introduced the Palmer forceps and other instrumentation in France.
1972	Bipolar coagulation was introduced by Frangenheim (Germany).
1974	Rioux and Cloutier (Canada) further developed bipolar coagulation. The Veress needle was passed through the cervix and the uterine fundus as a new method of insufflation (Sanders and Filshie).

1976	Hopkins introduced the rod lens system, which was incorporated into the laparoscope. Semm described endocoagulation and advised that monopolar diathermy be discontinued.
1982	Gas embolism may occur following uterine trauma or even in the absence of obvious injury (Yacoub *et al.*). Postoperative shoulder tip pain was common despite use of carbon dioxide or nitrous oxide (Sharp *et al.*).
1983	Van Lith *et al.* placed the Veress needle through the posterior fornix to introduce insufflatory gas.
1986	Berci and Cushieri reported that pulmonary aspiration of the gastric contents was one of the commonest lung complications of laparoscopy.

Culdoscopy

1948	Culdoscopy became popular for a time and Te Linde and Rutledge reported 10 years' experience.
1949	The knee chest position was originally introduced by Decker in 1944 and culdoscopy remained popular in the USA until the late 1970s.

Laparoscopic surgery

1933	Fervers, who was a general surgeon, first performed operative laparoscopy – for adhesiolysis.
1950	Robinson and Brown introduced the 'Robinson drain' for use following pelviscopic procedures.
1967	Steptoe described laparoscopic ventrosuspension.
1972	Frangenheim noted that aspiration of cysts was unsatisfactory, as recurrences were not uncommon and the nature of the lesion could only be confirmed by histology and not by cytology.
1978	Kleppinger described fenestration of the ovarian cyst wall to allow for histology and also continuing drainage from the ovarian cyst. The risk of cyst recurrence was estimated at just over 1%. Semm pioneered the use of endoscopic suturing.
1980	Semm and Mettler reported using loop ligature and a tissue punch morcellator

to achieve laparoscopic oophorectomies.

1985   Cornier developed the flexible salpingoscope.

1987   Brosens *et al.* developed a rigid salpingoscope.
Semm listed over 50 indications for laparoscopic surgery in his textbook.

1988   Semm encouraged the use of a classic Z-puncture technique and visually controlled peritoneal perforation for introduction of the laparoscope in patients suspected of having abdominal adhesions.

1989   Reich performed laparoscopic hysterectomy.

Infertility

1970   Steptoe and Edwards primed the ovaries with gonadotropins and used the laparoscope to recover preovulatory oocytes.

1972   Maathius *et al.* reported that laparoscopic investigation was preferable to hysterosalpingography.
Swolin and Rosenkrantz compared laparoscopy and hysterosalpingography.

1975   Moghissi and Sim found that 19% of patients with normal hysterosalpingography had pathology at laparoscopy.

1984   Asch *et al.* reported pregnancy following translaparoscopic gamete intrafallopian transfer.

Tubal surgery and ectopic pregnancy

1937   In the USA Hope described use of the laparoscope in the diagnosis of extrauterine pregnancy.

1973   Shapiro and Adler reported laparoscopic salpingectomy using electrocoagulation followed by excision, for ectopic pregnancy.

1977   Gomel introduced laparoscopic treatment of hydrosalpinges.

1981   Soderstrom used the snare technique for salpingectomy (Meyer and DeCherney, 1989).

1981/82   Linear salpingostomy with a cutting current was described by deCherney *et al.*

Sterilization

1934/37   Use of the laparoscope to facilitate female sterilization was first recorded by Ruddock.

1936   Bosch, in Switzerland, suggested that sterilization could be performed via laparoscopy.

1937   Anderson of the USA advocated tubal coagulation at laparoscopy to achieve sterilization.

1941   Power and Barnes wrote on laparoscopic female sterilization by tubal fulguration.

1964   Hans Frangenheim popularized laparoscopy and tubal cautery in Germany.

1972   The Hulka–Clemens ring was perfected (Hulka *et al.*, 1973; 1975; Filshie, 1989).

1973   Thompson and Wheeless wrote on the dangers of tubal cautery.
Semm developed his thermal coagulation technique (endocoagulation).
The Bleier clip was developed by Bleier.

1974   The Weck clip was perfected (Wheeless, 1974).
Local anaesthetic was used for insertion of the laparoscope in sterilization by Fishburne *et al.*
Hirsch and Roos of Germany developed forceps for tubal sterilization.
Rioux and Cloutier from Quebec developed a bipolar cautery system.

1975   Yoon and King developed the Yoon ring for tubal sterilization.

1977   Lieberman *et al.* further popularized sterilization by application of spring-loaded clips.
Richard Kleppinger developed forceps for tubal sterilization.
In mass sterilization programmes the Veress needle was omitted and insufflation performed down the gas channel of the cannula (Dingfelder).

1978   The Tupla clip came into use (Babenerd and Flehr).

1981   Filshie *et al.* performed tubal occlusion via laparoscopy using titanium silicone rubber clips.

1986   Riedel *et al.* reported pregnancy rates per 1000 for three occlusive devices: 1.1 for endocoagulation, 1.8 for monopolar diathermy, 3.9 for bipolar diathermy.

Laser surgery

1973 The laser was introduced to gynaecology by Kaplan *et al.*, and was used initially for treatment of cervical lesions.

1979 Laser laparoscopy was developed by Bruhat, and the Polyclinique team, Clermont-Ferrand, France.

1981 Tadir *et al.* (Israel) worked with laser laparoscopy.

1982 Daniell and Daniell and Brown in the USA documented their work on laser laparoscopy.

1983 The argon laser was first evaluated at laparoscopy by Keye and Dixon, and Keye *et al.* at the University of Utah.
Lomano introduced the Neodymium-Yttrium aluminium garnet (Nd-YAG) laser at laparoscopy.

1986 Daniell carried out initial investigation on the use of the potassium titanyl phosphate (KTP) laser in North America.

Polycystic ovary syndrome

1935 Polycystic ovarian disease was described by Stein and Leventhal.

1975 Buttram and Vaquero found that patients who had wedge resection developed periovarian adhesions.
Ovarian biopsy via laparoscopy was carried out by Yuzpe and Rioux.

1983 Campo *et al.* introduced ovarian biopsy via laparoscopy as a treatment modality for polycystic ovaries.

1984 Laparoscopic ovarian cautery for treatment of polycystic ovaries was carried out by Gjonnaess.

1988 Keckstein *et al.* used Nd-YAG laser coagulation, and Grochmal used laser vaporization.
Following carbon dioxide laser vaporization 12–15% of patients develop adhesions and only 3% after Nd-YAG contact application (Grochmal, 1988).

1989 Daniell and Miller used carbon dioxide laser vaporization and also KTP–532 laser treatment of polycystic ovaries.

Huber *et al.* used Nd-YAG laser incision for polycystic ovaries.

Endometriosis

1983 Keye and Dixon used argon lasers in treatment of endometriosis.

1986 Carbon dioxide lasers were used to treat endometriosis by Davis.
Nezhat *et al.* reported encouraging conception rates when treatment was for infertility as well as pain.

1987 Lomano used the Nd-YAG laser.

Dysmenorrhoea

1955 Doyle was the first to report successful relief from dysmenorrhoea by dividing the uterosacral ligaments.

1984 Feste suggested that nerve transection with laser, via laparoscopy, could be successful therapy for dysmenorrhoea.

Documentation

1950 The first gynaecological text on laparoscopy was published by Palmer.

1965 Patrick Steptoe pioneered laparoscopy in England and in 1967 wrote the first textbook on laparoscopy in English.

1978 The Royal College of Obstetricians and Gynaecologists (London) confidential enquiry into gynaecological laparoscopy was carried out. There was an overall complication rate of 34 per 1000 (Chamberlain and Brown).

1979 The American Association of Gynaecological Laparoscopists produced their report on gynaecological laparoscopy and its complications (Phillips *et al.*).

1986 Riedel *et al.* reported a large survey from West Germany of both diagnostic and operative laparoscopies.

REFERENCES

Anderson, E.T. (1937). Peritoneoscopy. *Am. J. Surg.*, **35**, 136–9

Asch, R.H., Ellsworth, L.R., Balmaceda, J.P. and Wong, P.C. (1984). Pregnancy after translaparoscopic gamete intrafallopian transfer. *Lancet*, **2**, 1034–5

Babenerd, J. and Flehr, I. (1978). Erfahrungen mit dem Tupla-Clip zur Tubensterilisation per laparoscopiam. *Geburts. Frauenheilk.*, **38**, 299

Baggish, M.S., Barbot, J. and Valle, R.F. (1989). *Diagnostic and Operative Hysteroscopy: a Text and Atlas*, p. 1 (Chicago; London: Year Book Publishers Inc.)

Berci, G. and Cushieri, A. (1986). *Practical Laparoscopy*. (London: Bailliere Tindall)

Bernheim, B.M. (1911). Organoscopy: cystoscopy of the abdominal cavity. *Ann. Surg.*, **53**, 764–9

Bleier, W. (1973). *Tubensterilisation mit einem Polyacetalclip*. (London: Planned Parenthood Foundation)

Bosch, P.F. (1936). Laparoskopische sterilization. *Schweiz. Z. Kranken. Anstaltswesen*, quoted by Gordon and Magos (1989) p. 429

Brosens I.A. and Puttemans P.J. (1989). Double-optic laparoscopy, salpingoscopy, ovarian cystoscopy and endo-ovarian surgery with the argon laser. In Sutton, C.J.G. (ed.) *Clinical Obstetrics and Gynaecology Laparoscopic Surgery*, pp. 595–608. (London, Philadelphia, Sydney, Tokyo, Toronto: Baillière Tindall)

Brosens, I., Boeckx, W., Delattin, P.H., Puttemans, P. and Vasquez, G. (1987). Salpingoscopy: a new preoperative diagnostic tool in tubal infertility? *Br. J. Obstet. Gynaecol.*, **94**, 722–8

Bruhat, M.A., Mage, G. and Manhes, M. (1979). Use of the CO_2 laser by laparoscopy. In Kaplan, I. (ed.) *Laser Surgery 111. Proceedings of the Third International Congress on Laser Surgery*, pp. 275. (Tel Aviv: Jerusalem Press)

Buttram, V.J. and Vaquero, C. (1975). Post-ovarian wedge resection adhesive disease. *Fertil. Steril.*, **26**, 874–6

Campo, S., Garcea, N, Caruso, A. and Siccardi, P. (1983). Effect of coelioscopic ovarian resection in patients with polycystic ovaries. *Gynecol. Obstet. Invest.*, **15**, 213–22

Chamberlain, G. and Brown, J.C. (1978). *Gynaecological laparoscopy. The Report of the Working Party of the Confidential Enquiry into Gynaecological Laparoscopy*. (London: RCOG)

Cornier, E. (1985). l'Ampulloscopic per-coelioscopique. *J. Gynecol. Obstet. Biol. Reprod.*, **14**, 459–66

Daniell, J.F. (1986). Laparoscopic evaluation of the KTP/532 laser for treating endometriosis – Initial report. *Fertil. Steril.*, **46**, 373–7

Daniell, J.F. (1989). Fibreoptic laser laparoscopy. In Sutton, C.J.G. (ed.) *Clinical Obstetrics and Gynaecology. Laparoscopic Surgery*, pp. 545–62. (London Philadelphia Sydney Tokyo Toronto: Baillière Tindall)

Daniell, J.F. and Brown, D.H. (1982). Carbon dioxide laser laparoscopy: initial experience in experimental animals and humans. *Obstet. Gynecol.*, **59**, 761–4

Daniell, J.F. and Miller, W. (1989). Polycystic ovaries treated by laparoscopic laser vaporization. *Fertil. Steril.*, **51**, 232–6

Davis, G.D. (1986). Management of endometriosis and its associated adhesions with the CO_2 laser laparoscope. *Obstet. Gynecol.*, **68**, 422–5

DeCherney, A.H., Romero, R. and Naftolin, F. (1981). Surgical management of unruptured ectopic pregnancy. *Fertil. Steril.*, **35**, 21–4

DeCherney, A.H., Maheaux, R. and Naftolin, F. (1982). Salpingostomy for ectopic pregnancy in the sole patent oviduct: reproductive outcome. *Fertil. Steril.*, **37**, 619–22

Decker, A. (1946). Pelvic culdoscopy. In: Meigs, J.V., Sturgis, S.H. (eds.) *Progress in Gynecology*, pp. 95. (New York: Grune & Stratton)

Decker, A. (1949). Culdoscopy: its diagnostic value in pelvic disease. *J. Am. Med. Assoc.*, **140**, 378–85

Desormeaux A.J. (1865). *De l'endoscope et de ses applications au diagnostic et au traitement des affectations de l'uretre et de la vessie.* (Paris: Bailliere)

Dingfelder, J.R. (1977). Direct trocar insertion without prior pneumoperitoneum. In Phillips, J.M. and Downey, C.A. (eds.) *Endoscopy in Gynecology*, pp. 49–53. (American Association of Gynecologic Laparoscopists)

Doyle, J.B. (1955). Paracervical uterine denervation by transection of the cervical plexus for the relief of dysmenorrhoea. *Am. J. Obstet. Gynecol.*, **70**, 1–16

Fervers, C. (1933). Die Laparoskopie mit dem Cystoskope.. Ein Beitrag zur Vereinfachung der Technik und zur endoskopischen Strangdurchtrennung in der Bauchole. *Med. Klin.*, **29**, 1042–5

Feste, J.R. (1984). CO_2 laser neurectomy for dysmenorrhoea. *Lasers Surg. Med.*, **3**, 327–31

Filshie G.M. (1989). Laparoscopic female sterilization. In Sutton, C.J.G. (ed.) *Clinical Obstetrics and Gynaecology. Laparoscopic Surgery*, Vol.3, No.3, pp. 609–24. (London, Philadelphia, Sydney, Tokyo, Toronto: Baillière Tindall)

Filshie, G.M. Casey, D., Pogmore, J.R. *et al* (1981). The titanium/silicone rubber clip for female sterilization. *Br. J. Obstet. Gynaecol.*, **88**, 655–62

Fishburne, J.I., Omran, H.K., Hulka, J.F., Mercer, J.P. and Edelman, D.A. (1974). Laparoscopic clip tubal sterilisation under local anaesthetic. *Fertil. Steril.*, **25**, 762

Fourestiere M., Gladu, A. and Vulmiere, J. (1943). La peritoneoscope. *Presse Medicale*, **5**, 46–7

Frangenheim, H. (1964). Die tuben sterilisation unter sicht mit dem laparoscope. *Gerbutsh. Frauenheilk.*, **24**, 470–3

Frangenheim, H. (1972). *Laparoscopy and Culdoscopy in Gynecology.* (London: Butterworth)

Frangenheim H. (1988). History of endoscopy. In Gordon, A.G. and Lewis, B.V. (eds.). *Gynaecological Endoscopy*, pp. 1–5. (London: Chapman & Hall)

Gjonnaess, H. (1984). Polycystic ovarian syndrome treated by ovarian electrocautery through the laparosope. *Fertil. Steril.*, **41**, 20–4

Goetze, O. (1918). Die Rontgendiagnostik bei gasgefullter Bauchhohle; eine neue Methode. *Munch. Med. Wchschr.*, **65**, 1275–80

Gomel, V. (1977). Salpingostomy by laparoscopy *J. Reprod. Med.*, **18**, 265–8

Gordon, A.G. and Magos, A.L. (1989). The development of laparoscopic surgery. In Sutton, C.J.G. (ed.) *Clinical Obstetrics and Gynaecology. Laparoscopic Surgery*, Vol. 3, No. 3, Chapter 1 pp. 429–49. (London: Ballière Tindall).

Graff, T.D., Arbgast, N.R., Phillips, O.C. *et al* (1959). Gas embolism. A comparative study of air and carbon dioxide as embolic agents in the systemic venous system. *Am. J. Obstet. Gynecol.*, **78**, 259–65

Grochmal, S. (1988). Contact Nd:YAG superior to CO_2 for treatment of ovarian disease. *Laser Practice Rep.*, **3**, 1S–2S

Hirsch, H.A. and Roos, E. (1974). Laparoskopische Tubensterilisation mit einer neuen Bikoagulationszange. *Geburtsh. Frauenheilk.*, **34**, 340

Hope, R. (1937). The differential diagnosis of ectopic pregnancy by peritoneoscopy. *Surg. Gynecol. Obstet.*, **64**, 229–34

Hopkins, H.H. (1953). On the diffraction theory of optical images. *Proc. R. Soc.*, **A217**, 408

Hopkins, H.H. (1976). Optical principles of the endoscope. In Berci, G. (ed.) *Endoscopy*, pp. 3–27. (New York: Appleton-Century-Crofts)

Huber, J., Hosman, J. and Spona, J. (1989). Endoskopisch vorgenommene Laserincision des polycystischen Ovars. *Geburs. Frauenheilk.*, **49**, 37–40

Hulka, J.F., Fishburne, J.I., Mercer, J.P. *et al* (1973). Laparoscopic sterilization with a spring clip: a report on the first fifty cases. *Am. J. Obstet. Gynecol.*, **116**, 715

Hulka, J.F., Omran, K., Phillips, J.M. *et al* (1975). Sterilization by spring clip. *Fertil. Steril.*, **26**, 1122–31

Jacobaeus, H.C. (1910). Uber die Möglichkeit, die Zystoskopie bei Untersuchung Seroser Hohlungen Anzuwend. *Munch. Med. Wchschr.*, **57**, 2090–2

Jacobaeus, H.C. (1911). Kurze Ubersicht uber meine Erfahrungen mit der Laparoskopie. *Munch. Med. Wchschr.*, **58**, 2017–19

Jacobaeus, H. (1912). Uber Laparo-und Thoracoskopie. *Beitr. Klin. Tuberk.*, **25**, 183–254

Kalk, H. (1929). Erfahrungen mit der Laparoskopie (zugleich mit Beschreibung eines neuen Instrumentes). *Z. klin. Med.*, **111**, 303–48

Kaplan, I., Goldman, J.M. and Ger, R. (1973). The treatment of erosions of the uterine cervix by CO_2 laser. *Obstet. Gynecol.*, **41**, 795–6

Keckstein, J., Finger, A. and Steiner, R. (1988). Laser application in contact and noncontact procedures; sapphire tips in comparison to 'bare-fiber', argon laser in comparison to Nd:YAG laser (in German). *Laser Med. Surg.*, **4**, 158–62

Kelling, G. (1902). Uber Oesophagoskopie, Gastroskopie und Koelioskopie. *Munch. Med. Wochenschr.*, **49**, 21–4

Keye, W.R. Jr. and Dixon, J. (1983). Photocoagulation of endometriosis by the argon laser through the laparoscope. *Obstet. Gynecol.*, **62**, 383–6

Keye, W.R., Matson, G.A. and Dixon, J. (1983). The use of the argon laser in the treatment of experimental endometriosis. *Fertil. Steril.* **39**, 26–9

Kleppinger, R.K. (1977). Ancillary uses of bipolar forceps. *J. Reprod. Med.*, **18**, 254

Kleppinger, R.K. (1978). Ovarian cyst fenestration via laparoscopy *J. Reprod. Med.*, **21**, 16–19

Lieberman, B.A., Gordon, A.G., Bostock, J.F. *et al.* (1977). Laparoscopic sterilisation with spring loaded clips: a double puncture technique. *J. Reprod. Med.*, **18**, 241–5

Lomano, J.M. (1983). Laparoscopic ablation of endometriosis with the YAG laser. *Lasers Surg. Med.*, **3**, 179–83

Lomano, J.M. (1987). Nd:YAG laser ablation of early pelvic endometriosis: a report of 61 cases. *Lasers Surg. Med.*, **7**, 56–60

Maathius, J.B., Horbach, J.G.M. and Van Hall, E.V. (1972). A comparison of the results of hysterosalpingography and laparoscopy in the diagnosis of Fallopian tube discomfort. *Fertil. Steril.*, **22**, 428

Meyer, W.R. and DeCherney, A.H. (1989). Laparoscopic treatment of ectopic pregnancy. In Sutton, C.J.G. (ed.) *Clinical Obstetrics and Gynaecology. Laparoscopic Surgery*, pp. 583–94. (London, Philadelphia, Sydney, Tokyo, Toronto: Ballière Tindall)

Moghissi, K.S. and Sim, G.S. (1975). Correlation between hysterosalpingography and pelvic endoscopy for the evaluation of tubal factor. *Fertil. Steril.*, **26**, 1178

Nezhat, C., Crowgey, S.R. and Garrison, C.P. (1986). Surgical treatment of endometriosis via laser laparoscopy. *Fertil. Steril.*, **45**, 778–83

Nitze, M. (1879a). Uber eine neue behandlungs – methode de hohlen des menslichen korpers. *Med. Press Wien*, **26**, 851

Nitze, M. (1879b). Beobachtung – und untersuchungsmethode fur harnrohe, Harnblase und rectum. *Wein. Med. Wchschr.*, **29**, 649–52

Nitze, M. (1893). Zur Photography der menschlichen Harnrohre. *Berl. Med Wchschr.*, **31**, 744

Nordentoeft, S. (1912). Uber Endoskopie geschlossener Cavitaten mittels meines Trokar-Endoskopes. *Verhandl. Deutch. Gesellsch. Gynakol,* **41**, 78–81

Orndoff, B.H. (1920). The peritoneoscope in the diagnosis of diseases of the abdomen. *J. Radiol. (Iowa City)*, **1**, 307–25

Palmer, R. (1946). La coelioscopie gynecologique. Rapport du Professeur Mocquot. *Acad. de Chir.*, **72**, 363–8

Palmer, R. (1947). Abdominal coelioscopy in the diagnosis and treatment of sterility. *International Congress of Obstetrics and Gynaecology*, Dublin, p. 214, quoted by Semm (1977)

Palmer, R. (1950). *La Sterilité Involuntaire.* (Paris: Masson)

Palmer, R. (1960). Discussion of modern methods of salpingostomy. *Proc. R. Soc. Med.*, **53**, 357–9

Palmer, R. (1962). Essaie de sterilisation tubaire coelioscopique par electrocoagulation isthmique. *R.C. Soc. Franc. Gynecol.*, **5**, 3

Phillips, J.M., Hulka, J., Hulka, B., Keith, D.M. and Keith, L. (1979). American Association of Gynecologic Laparoscopists 1977 Membership Survey. *J. Reprod. Med.*, **23**, 61–4

Power, F.H. and Barnes, A.C. (1941). Sterilization by means of peritoneoscopic fulguration: a preliminary report. *Am. J. Obstet. Gynecol.*, **41**, 1038–43

Reich, H. (1989). New techniques in advanced laparoscopic surgery. In Sutton, C.J.G. (ed.). *Clinical Obstetrics and Gynaecology. Laparoscopic Surgery*, Vol. 3, No. 3, pp. 655–81. (London, Philadelphia, Sydney, Tokyo, Toronto: Baillière Tindall)

Riedel, H.H., Lehmann-Willenbrock, E., Conrad, P. and Semm, K. (1986). German pelviscopic statistics for the years 1978–1982. *Endoscopy*, **18**, 219–22

Rioux, J.E. and Cloutier, D. (1974). Bipolar cautery for sterilization by laparoscopy. *J. Reprod. Med.*, **13**, 6–10

Robinson, J.O. and Brown, A.A. (1950). A new closed drainage system. *Br. J. Surg.*, **67**, 229–30

Ruddock, J.C. (1934). Peritoneoscopy. *West. J. Surg. Obstet. Gynecol.*, **42**, 392–405

Ruddock, J.C. (1937). Peritoneoscopy. *Surg. Gynecol. Obstet.*, **65**, 523–39

Sanders, R.R. and Filshie, G.M. (1974). Transfundal induction of pneumoperitoneum prior to laparoscopy *J. Obstet. Gynaecol. Br. Commonw.*, **8**, 829–30

Semm, K. (1973). Thermal coagulation for sterilization. *Endoscopy*, **5**, 218

Semm, K. (1976). Endocoagulation: a new field of endoscopic surgery. *J. Reprod. Med.*, **16**, 195–203

Semm, K. (1977). *Atlas of Gynecologic Laparoscopy and Hysteroscopy*, translated by Allan Lake Rice. Borrow, L.S. (ed.) pp. 3–14. (Philadelphia, London, Toronto: W.B. Saunders Co.)

Semm, K. (1978). Tissue-puncher and loop-ligation-new aids for surgical therapeutic pelviscopy (laparoscopy) endoscopic intraabdominal surgery. *Endoscopy*, **10**, 119–24

Semm, K. (1987). *Operative Manual for Endoscopic Abdominal Surgery*. (Chicago: Year Book Publishers)

Semm, K. (1988). Sichtkontrollierte Peritoneumperforation zur operativen Pelviskopie. *Geburtsh. Frauenheilk.*, **48**, 436–9

Semm, K. and Mettler, L. (1980). Technical progress in pelvic surgery via operative laparoscopy. *Am. J. Obstet. Gynecol.*, **138**, 121–7

Semm, K. and O'Neill-Freys, I. (1989). Conventional operative laparoscopy (pelviscopy). In Sutton, C.J.G. (ed.) *Clinical Obstetrics and Gynaecology. Laparoscopic Surgery*, Vol. 3, No. 3, pp. 451–83. (London, Philadelphia, Sydney, Tokyo, Toronto: Ballière Tindall)

Shapiro, H.I. and Adler, D.L.N. (1973). Excision of an ectopic pregnancy through the laparoscope. *Am. J. Obstet. Gynecol.*, **117**, 290–1

Sharp, J.R., Pierson, W.P. and Brady III, C.E. (1982). Comparison of CO_2 and N_2O-induced discomfort during peritoneoscopy under local anaesthesia. *Gastroenterology*, **82**, 453–6

Stein, I. and Leventhal, M. (1935). Amenorrhea associated with bilateral polycystic ovaries. *Am. J. Obstet. Gynecol.*, **29**, 181–91

Steiner, O.P. (1924). Abdominoskopie. *Schweiz. Med. Wochenschr.*, **54**, 84–7

Steptoe, P.C. (1965). Gynaecological endoscopy, laparoscopy and culdoscopy. *J. Obstet. Gynaecol. Br. Commonw.*, **72**, 535–43

Steptoe, P.C. (1967). *Laparoscopy and Gynaecology*. (London: Livingstone)

Steptoe, P.C. and Edwards, R.G. (1970). Laparoscopic recovery of preovulatory human oocytes after priming of ovaries with gonadotrophins. *Lancet*, **1**, 683

Swolin, K. and Rosenkrantz, M. (1972). Laparoscopy vs hysterosalpingography in sterility investigations. A comparative study. *Fertil. Steril.*, **23**, 270

Tadir, Y., Ovadia, J., Zuckerman, Z. *et al.* (1981). Laparoscopic applications of the CO_2 laser. In Atsumi, K. and Nimsakul, N. (eds.) *Proceedings of the 4th Congress of the International Society for Laser Surgery*, pp. 25–26. (Tokyo: Japanese Society for Laser Medicine)

Te Linde R.W. and Rutledge F.N. (1948). Culdoscopy, a useful gynecologic procedure. *Am. J. Obstet. Gynecol.*, **55**, 102–15

Thompson, B.H. and Wheeless C.R. Jr. (1973). Gastrointestinal complications of laparoscopic sterilization. *Obstet. Gynecol.*, **41**, 669

Van Lith, D.A.F., Van Schie, K.J., Beetchuizen, W. and Binstock, M. (1983). Coagulation by the Semm and the Wolf techniques. In Van Lith, D.A.F., Keith, L.G. and Van Hall, E.V. (eds.) *New Trends in Female Sterilization*, pp. 61–82. (Chicago, London: Year Book Medical Publishers)

Veress, J. (1938). Ein neues Instrument zur Ausfuhrung von Brust – oder Bauchpunktionen und Pneumothoraxbehandlung. *Deutsch. Med. Wchschr.*, **64**, 1480–1

von Ott, D. (1901). Die direkte Beleuchtung der Bauchhohle, der Harnblase, des Dickdarms und des Uterus zu diagnostischen Zwecken. *Rev. Med. Tcheque (Prague)*, **2**, 27

Wheeless, C.R. (1974). Laparoscopically applied hemoclips for tubal sterilisation. *Obstet. Gynecol.*, **44**, 752–5

Yacoub, O.F., Cardona, I., Coveler, L.A. *et al.* (1982). Carbon dioxide embolism during laparoscopy. *Anesthesiology*, **57**, 533–5

Yoon, I.B. and King, T.M. (1975). A preliminary and intermediate report of a new laparoscopic ring procedure. *J. Reprod. Med.*, **15**, 54–6

Yuzpe, A. and Rioux, J. (1975). The value of laparoscopic ovarian biopsy. *J. Reprod. Med.*, **15**, 432–42

Zollikofer, R. (1924). Uber Laparoskopie. *Schweiz. Med. Wchschr.*, **54**, 264–5

FURTHER READING

Frangenheim, H. (1988). History of endoscopy. In Gordon, A.G. and Lewis, B.V. (eds.). *Gynaecological Endoscopy*. (London: Chapman & Hall)

Gordon, A.G. and Magos, A.L. (1989). The development of laparoscopic surgery. In Sutton, C.J.G.

(ed.) *Clinical Obstetrics and Gynaecology. Laparoscopic Surgery*, Vol. 3, No. 3. (London, Philadelphia, Sydney, Tokyo, Toronto: Bailliere Tindall)

Hulka, J.F. (1985). *Textbook of Laparoscopy*. (New York, London: Grune and Stratton)

Semm, K. (1977). *Atlas of Gynecologic Laparoscopy and Hysteroscopy*, translated by Allan Lake Rice. Borrow, L.S. (ed.) (Philadelphia, London, Toronto: W.B. Saunders Co.)

Soderstrom, R.M. (1978). Foreword. In Phillips, J.M. (ed.). *Endoscopy in Gynecology. Proceedings of the 3rd International Congress on Gynecologic Endoscopy*, pp. viii–ix. (Downey:AAGL)

Sutton, C.J.G. (ed.) (1989). *Laparoscopic Surgery. Clinical Obstetrics and Gynaecology*, Vol. 3 No. 3 (London, Philadelphia, Sydney, Tokyo, Toronto: Baillière Tindall)

Hysteroscopy

Successful hysteroscopy was reported by Pantaleoni (1869) when he described his examination of a 60-year-old woman with postmenopausal bleeding. He found and destroyed, an endometrial polyp. In 1893 Blondel utilized two tubes, one fitting within the other, to achieve a panoramic view of the uterus. The outer tube was opened to separate the uterine walls and the inner tube was reserved for vision. However, the field of vision was narrow and illumination was poor. The developments of Maximilian Nitze in the area of cystoscopy were later applied to hysteroscopy, and his 'energized platinum loop' and optical system were built into the tube (1879). Clado, a French surgeon, described several new hysteroscopy models in 1898 and also used the incandescent lamps invented by Edison in 1879. Charles David (1907) introduced the innovations of Nitze to hysteroscopy and improved illumination by placing a bulb at the intrauterine end of his hysteroscope. He also sealed the distal end of the tube with a piece of glass. The examination carried out by David was a contact hysteroscopy.

In order to increase the view, more complex devices were necessary. Rubin (1920), who described tubal insufflation, combined a cystoscope with carbon dioxide insufflation, of the uterine cavity in 1925. Some patients were adversely affected by the pneumoperitoneum which was caused and he abandoned the method. In Germany, Gauss (1928) used water to distend the uterus. Due to the pressure necessary to separate the uterine walls the distending medium passed through the oviducts into the peritoneal cavity. Silander (1962) introduced a transparent rubber balloon mounted on an endoscope and inflated it within the uterine cavity. Several distending media are now available (e.g. dextran (32%), dextrose (5%) in water, and carbon dioxide).

Until recently, hysteroscopy was available only at specialist centres. It was mainly used in the investigation of abnormal uterine bleeding, sterility, and in suspected intrauterine pathologies such as polyps and fibroids. It became clear that the technique offered an alternative to dilatation and curettage (D & C) when Stock and Kanbour (1975) showed that at curettage less than half the endometrium was sampled. Gimpelson (1984) found that hysteroscopic examination was more accurate than dilatation and curettage in reaching a diagnosis. Hamou *et al.* (1985) and Raju and Taylor (1986) reported very high correlations between hysteroscopic findings and curettage samples.

It was in the treatment of menorrhagia however, that hysteroscopy really came into its own. Goldrath (1989) reported on his 10-year experience with endometrial laser ablation techniques, and obtained an overall success rate of 96%, noting that recurrence of menorrhagia was rare. It would appear that hysteroscopic endometrial ablation is an alternative to hysterectomy for many women. If a hysteroscope is not available, endometrial ablation may be carried out using a urological resectoscope, as described by DeCherney *et al.* (1987).

CHRONOLOGY

Development

1805   Bozzini invented a hollow tube through which natural human cavities could be observed. Illumination was via the light of a candle reflected by a mirror.

1853   Desormeaux presented the first satisfactory endoscope to the Imperial Academy of Medicine in Paris. His instrument was mainly for examination of the urethra and bladder but he recommended its use to inspect the interior of the uterus (Desormeaux, 1865).

1864   Aubinais endeavoured to inspect the human uterine cavity with the naked eye.

1869   Pantaleoni reported the first successful hysteroscopy in the *Medical Press and Circular*. He used Desormeaux's endoscope to cure a 60-year-old woman of an endometrial polyp.

1879　Nitze introduced an electric current via a platinum loop for illumination of cystoscopes and urethroscopes.

1893　Blondel utilized a 'double tube' hysteroscope to separate the uterine walls.

1898　Clado, a French surgeon, wrote on hysteroscopy describing several models of hysteroscope and also introduced the incandescent lamp (invented by Edison in 1879) as a means of illumination.

1907　Charles David wrote on hysteroscopy. He improved illumination by placing an electric bulb at the intrauterine end of the endoscope, and he sealed the distal end with a piece of glass. David's technique was contact hysteroscopy.

1920　Rubin described tubal insufflation with gas.

1925　Rubin combined a cystoscope with carbon dioxide insufflation of the uterine cavity.

1928　Gauss investigated the use of water as a distending medium.

1943　Fourestiere, a French optical engineer, introduced the cold light process of illumination for endoscopy (Fourestiere *et al.*).
Maddi *et al.* documented adverse effects of high molecular weight dextran.
Emmett *et al.* showed that dilutional hyponatraemia may occur due to fluid absorption during transurethral resection.

1970　Edstrom and Fernstrom used a highly viscous dextran solution (Hyskon) to distend the uterine cavity.

1972　Lindemann in Germany and Porto in France renewed interest in carbon dioxide insufflation of the uterine cavity, but the techique did not remain popular.

1973　Parent and Barbot began to use a rigid mineral glass guide for contact hysteroscopy (Parent *et al.*, 1976).

1979　Baggish reported contact hysteroscopy in the USA.

1981　Hamou described contact microcolpohysteroscopy.

1983　Taylor and Hamou described a large series of cases of microhysteroscopy performed as an office procedure without any anaesthetic.
Taylor and Hamou were able to distinguish between flimsy intrauterine adhesions and more solid thick bands of tissue.
Van de Pas designed a single-handed hysteroscope for outpatient use.

1985　Parent *et al.* developed a completely self-contained unit which provided illumination and also gas for distending the uterine cavity.
Gomar *et al.* reported that gas embolism may occur when air rather than CO_2 is used for inflation.
Hamou *et al.* distinguished three types of intrauterine synechiae (Asherman's syndrome).

1986　Goldrath documented fluid absorption complications of operative hysteroscopy.
Hamou described nucleocytoplasmic examination of one cell layer at high magnification (x 150).
Stevens and Van Herendael dated the endometrium by its appearance and this opinion correlated with histology.

1987　Baggish invented a focusing panoramic hysteroscope which could be used for Neodymium: Yttrium–Aluminium–Garnet (Nd: YAG) laser hysteroscopic procedures.
Perino *et al.* operated on congenital abnormalities of the uterus.

1988　Siegler and Valle recommended central venous pressure monitoring if more that 500 ml of Hyskon was used for distension.

Uterine bleeding

1975　Stock and Kanbour showed that at dilatation and curettage less than half the endometrium is sampled in 60% of patients.

1984　Gimpelson compared hysteroscopy with dilatation and curettage and the former was more accurate.

1986　Raju and Taylor reported 100% correlation between hysteroscopic findings and curettage samples in 70 patients.

1987　Fayez *et al.* stated that lesions identified at hysterosalpingography should be confirmed at hysteroscopy.
March and Israel suggest hysteroscopy for women with recurrent miscarriage to exclude congenital or acquired uterine abnormality.

1988　Brooks and Serden identified abnormalities at hysteroscopy which were missed at dilatation and curettage.

1989　At the International Society for Gynecologic Endoscopy it was agreed that hysteroscopy could replace dilatation and curettage in the investigation of the postmenopausal patient with uterine bleeding (Grainger and deCherney).

Endometrial ablation

1971 Droegemueller *et al.* used nitrous oxide cryosurgery to ablate the endometrium.

1972 Schenker and Polishuk demonstrated the ability of rabbit endometrium to regenerate following cryosurgery.

1981 Goldrath *et al.* first reported the use of the Nd: YAG laser to vaporize the endometrium.

1983 Electrosurgical resection techniques were first described by DeCherney and Polan.

1984 DeCherney *et al.* used the resectoscope to ablate the endometrium.

1985 Goldrath showed that fluid overload and pulmonary oedema may occur. Uterine perforation was reported in one case.
Goldrath and Fuller showed the amazing capacity of the endometrium to regenerate following ablation.

1986 Cornier described Nd: YAG laser ablation of the endometrium.

1987 DeCherney *et al.* recommended resection in women not fit for hysterectomy, and used the urological resectoscope to remove endometrium.

1988 Gimpelson used the 'touch' or 'dragging' technique of laser ablation of the endometrium.
Lomono used a 'non-touch' technique with fewer complications than the 'touch' method.

1989 Goldrath reported on his 10-year experience with laser ablation techniques and had an overall success rate of 96%.
Vancaille used 'roller ball' endometrial ablation.

Sterilization and intrauterine devices

1975 Neuwirth noted that if a piece of an intrauterine contraceptive device is missing, hysteroscopy allows confirmation of a fragment in the uterus.

1976 Lindemann and Mohr developed transuterine electrocoagulation of the cornua. The method was later abandoned due to the risks involved and the unacceptably high pregnancy rate post-treatment.

1983 De Maeyer inserted a liquid silicone mixture which solidified in the tubal lumen.
Brundin inserted preformed solid plugs into the cornua.
Loffer injected liquid silicone into the cornual end of the Fallopian tube to form an in-place plug.

Malignancy

1984 Lewis showed that hysteroscopy without biopsy is unreliable in differentiating between premalignant and malignant disease.

1985 Hamou *et al.* found the effect of dilute acetic acid on malignant endometrium was to turn it white.
Parent *et al.* performed hysteroscopy in patients prior to hysterectomy for endometrial cancer. The dissemination risk appeared to be negligible as malignant cells were not recovered from fluid in the Pouch of Douglas.
Hamou *et al.* showed a high correlation between histology and hysteroscopy findings for carcinoma or postmenopausal endometrial atrophy, but poor correlation for endometrial hyperplasia.

1986 Walton and MacPhail noted that hysteroscopy was a useful technique in staging endometrial carcinoma.

Hyperplasia, adenomyosis and myomas

1985 Parent *et al.* wrote on the hysteroscopic findings of cystic glandular hyperplasia, atypical hyperplasia and adenomyosis as viewed at hysteroscopy.

1989 Donnez *et al.* advised the use of gonadotropin releasing hormone agonists to shrink large submucous myomas prior to hysteroscopic treatment.

Outpatient hysteroscopy

1976 Lindemann and Mohr described outpatient hysteroscopy and noted that the examination, which was performed without anaesthetic or paracervical block, was a low-risk procedure.

1983 The method of panoramic hysteroscopy was outlined by Taylor and Hamou.

1986 Mencaglia and Perino showed that outpatient diagnostic hysteroscopy under local anaesthesia was an acceptable alternative to procedures under general anaesthesia.

REFERENCES

Aubinais (1864). *Union Med.*, No.152, quoted by Semm (1977) p. 11

Baggish, M.S. (1979). Contact hysteroscopy: a new technique to explore the uterine cavity. *Obstet. Gynecol.*, **54**, 350

Baggish, M.S. (1987), quoted by Barbot (1989) p. 9

Barbot, J. (1989). The history of hysteroscopy. In Baggish, M.S., Barbot, J. and Valle, R.F. (eds.) *Diagnostic and Operative Hysteroscopy. A Text and Atlas*, pp. 1–10. (Chicago: Year Book Medical Publisher Inc.)

Blondel (1893). quoted by Barbot (1989) p.2

Bozzini (1805). quoted by Barbot (1989) p.1

Brooks, P.G. and Serden, S.P. (1988). Hysteroscopic findings after unsuccessful dilatation and curettage for abnormal uterine bleeding. *Am. J. Obstet. Gynecol.*, **158**, 1354–7

Brundin, J. (1983). P-block as a contraceptive method. In Van de Pas, H. (ed.) *Hysteroscopy*, pp. 137–1. (Boston: MTP Press)

Clado (1898). quoted by Barbot (1989) p.3

Cornier, E. (1986). Traitment hysterofibroscopique ambulatoire des metrorragies rebelles par laser Nd. YAG *J. Gynecol. Obstet. Biol. Reprod.*, **15**, 661–4

David, C. (1907). De l'endoscopie de l'uterus apres avortement et dans les suites de couches a l'etat normal et a l'etat pathologigue. *Bull. Soc. Obstet. Paris*, December

DeCherney, A.H. and Polan, M. L. (1983). Hysteroscopic management of intrauterine lesions and intractable uterine bleeding. *Obstet. Gynecol.*, **61**, 392–7

DeCherney, A.H., Cholst, I. and Naftolin, F. (1984). The management of intractable uterine bleeding utilizing the cystoscopic resectoscope. In Siegler, A.M. and Lindeman, H.J. (eds). *Hysteroscopy: Principles and Practice*, pp. 140–2. (Philadelphia: Lippencott)

DeCherney, A.H., Diamond, M.P., Lavey, G. and Polan, M.L. (1987). Endometrial ablation for intractable uterine bleeding: hysteroscopic resection. *Obstet. Gynecol.*, **70**, 668–70

de Jong, P., Doel, F. and Falconer, A. (1990). Outpatient diagnostic hysteroscopy. *Br. J. Obstet. Gynaecol.*, **4**, 299–303

De Maeyer, J.F.D.E. (1983). Trancervical hysteroscopic sterilisation. In Van de Pas, H. (ed.) *Hysteroscopy*, pp. 191–9. (Boston: MTP Press)

Desormeaux, A.J. (1865). De l'endoscope et de ses applications au diagnostic et au traitement des affections de l'uretre et de la vessie. (Paris: Bailliere)

Donnez, J., Nisolle, M., Gillerot, S. and Clerck, F. (1989) Combined therapy GnRH agonist and Nd:YAG laser hysteroscopy in the treatment of submucous leiomyoma. Presented at the *International Society for Gynecologic Endoscopy First Biennial Meeting*, January, Orlando, FL.

Droegemueller, W., Greer B. and Makowski, E. (1971a). Cryosurgery in patients with dysfunctional uterine bleeding. *Obstet. Gynecol.*, **38**, 256–8

Droegemueller, W., Makowski, E. and Macsalka, R. (1971b). Destruction of the endometrium by cryosurgery. *Am. J. Obstet. Gynecol.*, **110**, 467–9

Edstrom, K. and Fernstrom, I. (1970). The diagnostic possibilities of a modified hysteroscopic technique. *Acta Obstet. Gynaecol. Scand.*, **49**, 327

Emmett, J.L., Gilbaugh, J.H. and McLean, P. (1969). Fluid absorption during transurethral resection. Comparison of mortality and morbidity after irrigation with water and non-haemolytic solutions. *J. Urol.*, **101**, 884–9

Fayez, J.A., Mutie, G. and Schneider, P.J. (1987). The diagnostic value of hysterosalpingography and hysteroscopy in infertility investigation. *Am. J. Obstet. Gynecol.*, **156**, 558–60

Fourestiere, M., Gladu, A. and Vulmiere, J. (1943). La peritoneoscope. *Press Med.*, **5**, 46–7

Gauss, C.J. (1928). Hysteroskopie. *Arch. Gynaekol.*, **133**, 18

Gimpelson, R.J. (1984). Panoramic hysteroscopy with directed biopsies vs. dilatation and curettage for accurate diagnosis *J. Reprod. Med.*, **29**, 575–8

Gimpelson, R.J. (1988). Hysteroscopic Nd:YAG laser ablation of the endometrium. *J. Reprod. Med.*, **33**, 872–6

Goldrath, M.H. (1985). Hysteroscopic laser ablation of the endometrium. In Sharp, F. and Jordan, J.A. (eds.) *Gynaecological Laser Surgery*, pp. 253–69. (New York: Perinatology Press)

Goldrath, M.H. and Fuller, T. (1985). Intrauterine laser surgery. In Keye, W.R. (ed.) *Laser Surgery in Gynecology and Obstetrics*, pp. 93–110. (Tunbridge Wells: Castle House Publications)

Goldrath, M.H., Fuller, T.A. and Segal, S. (1981). Laser photovaporization of endometrium for the treatment of menorrhagia *Am. J. Obstet. Gynecol.*, **140**, 14–19

Goldrath, M.H. (1986). Hysteroscopic laser ablation of the endometrium. In Sharp, F. and Jordan, J.A. (eds.) *Gynaecological Laser Surgery. Proceedings of the RCOG 15th Study Group*, pp. 253–65. (New York: Perinatology Press)

Goldrath, M.H. (1989). Laser ablation of the endometrium. *Proceedings of Second World Congress of Gynecologic Endoscopy*, pp. 93, Clermont-Ferrand, France, quoted by Garry (1990) pp. 199–202

Gomar, C., Fernandez, C., Villonga, A. and Nalda, M.A. (1985). Carbon dioxide embolism during laparoscopy and hysteroscopy *Ann. Fr. Anesth. Reanim.* **4**, 380–2

Grainger, D.A. and DeCherney, A.H. (1989). Hysteroscopic management of uterine bleeding. In Drife, J.O. (ed.) *Clinical Obstetrics and Gynaecology. Dysfunctional Uterine Bleeding and Menorrhagia*, Vol. 32, No. 2, pp. 403–14. (London, Philadelphia, Sydney, Tokyo, Toronto: Balliere Tindall)

Hamou, J. (1981). Microhysteroscopy: a new procedure and its original applications in gynecology. *J. Reprod. Med.* **26**, 375–82

Hamou, J. (1986). *Hysteroscopie et microhysteroscopie.* (Paris: Masson)

Hamou, J., Salat-Baroux, J. and Henrion, R. (1985). Hysteroscopie et microcolpohysteroscopie. In *Encyclopedie medico-chirurgicale*, quoted by Lewis (1990)

Lewis, B.V. (1984). Hysteroscopy in gynaecological practice: a review. *J. R. Soc. Med.*, **77**, 235–7

Lewis, B.V. (1989). Hysteroscopy. In Studd, J. (ed.) *Progress in Obstetrics and Gynaecology*, Vol. 7, pp. 305–17. (Edinburgh: Churchill Livingstone)

Lewis, B.V. (1990). Hysteroscopy for the investigation of abnormal uterine bleeding. *Br. J. Obstet. Gynaecol.*, 97, 283–4

Lindemann, H.J. (1972). The use of CO_2 in the uterine cavity for hysteroscopy *Int. J. Fertil.*, **17**, 221

Lindemann, H.J. and Mohr, J. (1976). CO_2 hysteroscopy. *Am J. Obstet. Gynecol.*, **124**, 129–33

Loffer, F.D. (1983). Hysteroscopic sterilisation with the use of formed in-place silicone plugs. *Am. J. Obstet. Gynecol.*, **149**, 261–70

Lomono, J. (1988). Dragging technique versus blanching technique for endometrial ablation with the Nd:YAG laser in the treatment of chronic menorrhagia. *Am. J. Obstet. Gynecol.*, **159**, 152–5

Maddi, V.I., Wyso, E.M. and Zinner, E.N. (1969). Dextran anaphylaxis. *Angiology*, **20**, 243

March, C.H. and Israel, R. (1987). Hysteroscopic management of recurrent abortion caused by septate uterus. *Am. J. Obstet. Gynecol.*, **156**, 834–42

Mencaglia, L. and Perino, A. (1986). Diagnostic hysteroscopy today. *Acta Eur Fertil.*, **17**, 431–9

Neuwirth, R.S. (1975). *Hysteroscopy: Major Problems in Obstetrics and Gynaecology*, Vol. 8. (London: W.B. Saunders)

Nitze, M. (1879). Uber eine neue behandlungs – methode der höhlen des menslichen korpers. *Med. Press Wien*, **26**, 851

Pantaleoni, D. (1869). On endoscopic examination of the cavity of the womb. *Med. Press Circ.*, **8**, 26–7

Parent, B., Barbot, J. and Doerler, B. (1976). L'Hysteroscopie de Contact Paris, *Documentation Scientifique Lab Roland – Marie Diffusion Edition Publicite*

Parent, B., Guedj, H., Barbot, J. and Nordarian, P. (1985). *Hysteroscopie Panoramique.* (Paris: Maloine)

Perino, A., Mencaglia, L., Hamou, J. and Cittadini, E. (1987). Hysteroscopy for metroplasty of uterine septa. *Fertil. Steril.*, **48**, 321–3

Porto, R. (1972). *Une nouvelle methode d'hysteroscopie,*. Thesis, Marseille quoted by Barbot (1989) p. 7

Raju, K.S. and Taylor, R.W. (1986). Routine hysteroscopy for patients with a high risk of uterine malignancy. *Br. J. Obstet. Gynaecol.*, **93**, 1259–61

Rubin, I.C. (1920). Nonoperative determination of patency of Fallopian tubes in sterility. Intrauterine inflation with oxygen, and production of an artificial pneumoperitoneum. Preliminary report. *J. Am. Med. Assoc.*, **74**, 1017

Rubin, I.C. (1925). Uterine endoscopy. Endometroscopy with the aid of uterine insufflation. *Am J. Obstet Gynecol.*, **10**, 313

Schenker, J.G. and Polishuk, W.Z. (1972). Regeneration of rabbit endometrium after cryosurgery. *Obstet. Gynecol.*, **40**, 638–45

Semm, K. (1977). *Atlas of Gynaecologic Laparoscopy and Hysteroscopy*, p. 11. (London, Philadelphia, Toronto: W.B. Saunders)

Siegler, A.M. and Valle, R.F. (1988). Therapeutic hysteroscopic procedures. *Fertil. Steril.* **50**, 685–701

Silander, T. (1962). Hysteroscopy through a transparent rubber balloon. *Surg. Gynecol. Obstet.*, **114** (1), 125

Stevens, M.J. and Van Herendael (1986). Dating of the endometrium by microhysteroscopy. *Proceedings of the 2nd European Congress of Hysteroscopy*, Antwerp, quoted by de Jong (1990) pp. 299–303

Stock, R.J. and Kanbour, A. (1975). Pre-hysterectomy curettage. *Obstet. Gynecol.*, **45**, 537

Taylor, P.J. and Hamou, J.E. (1983). Hysteroscopy: clinical perspectives. *J. Rep. Med.*, **28**, 359–89

Van de Pas, H. (1983). *Hysteroscopy*, pp. 39–48. (Boston: MTP Press)

Vancaille, T.G. (1989). Electrocoagulation of the endometrium with the ball-end resectoscope. *Obstet. Gynecol.*, **74**, 425–7

Walton, S.M. and MacPhail, S. (1986). The value of hysteroscopy in post menopausal bleeding. *Proceedings of the 24th British Congress of Obstetrics and Gynaecology*, Cardiff, quoted by Lewis (1989) p. 305

FURTHER READING

Barbot, J. (1989). The history of hysteroscopy. In Baggish, M.S., Barbot, J. and Valle, R.F. (eds.) *Diagnostic and Operative Hysteroscopy. A Text and Atlas*, pp. 1–10. (Chicago: Year Book Medical Publisher Inc.)

Garry, R. (March 1990). Hysteroscopic alternatives to hysterectomy. *Br. J. Obstet. Gynaecol.*, **97**, 199–202

Hamou, J. and Lewis, V. (1990). Hysteroscopy and microhysteroscopy. In Bonnar, J. (ed). *Recent Advances in Obstetrics and Gynaecology*, Vol. 16, pp. 185–97. (Edinburgh: Churchill Livingstone)

Lewis, B.V. (1989). Hysteroscopy. In Studd, J. (ed.) *Progress in Obstetrics and Gynaecology*, Vol. 7, pp. 305–17. (Edinburgh: Churchill Livingstone)

Lewis, B.V. (1990). Hysteroscopy for the investigation of abnormal uterine bleeding. *Br. J. Obstet. Gynaecol.* **97**, 283–4

Lindemann, H.J. (1973). Historical aspects of hysteroscopy. *Fertil. Steril.*, **24**, 230–42

MacDonald, R. (1990). Modern treatment of menorrhagia. *Br. J. Obstet. Gynaecol.*, **97**, 3–7

Semm, K. (1977). *Atlas of Gynecologic Laparoscopy and Hysteroscopy*. (Philadelphia, London, Toronto: W.B. Saunders Co.)

Anaesthesia and analgesia

The word anaesthesia, derived from the Greek, means 'an absence of feeling', and in classical times this conveyed a moral state rather than a physical one, i.e. a 'boorishness', and Plato uses it in this sense. However, Dioscorides who wrote at the end of the first century AD, used the word in its usual modern sense when discussing mandragora. Dioscorides was a Greek surgeon physician in Nero's army (AD 54–68). His book on botany *De Materia Medica,* is a classic.

Today, 'anaesthetic' is a general noun referring to the many agents which produce cessation of feeling. The foundations for the specialty were laid in the nineteenth century, and systematization of anaesthesia was accomplished in the twentieth century. The anaesthetic profession is a new one – at the beginning of this century for instance, there were only 100 anaesthetists in the USA. Early in this century the spelling was simplified to 'anesthesia' in the New World.

Most of the advances in anaesthesia and analgesia were applied to obstetrics, but some agents had to be discarded due to their serious side-effects which were only discovered when the drugs were in common use. While refining their art, anaesthetists have found that obstetrics is a high-risk area which requires extra training, close supervision and recognition that the drugs or techniques used may have serious adverse effects on the mother and fetus.

The events outlined here relate to the evolution of anaesthesia and analgesia in general, and also to specific applications of anaesthetic advances to obstetric practice.

EARLY ANALGESICS

Mandragora was used by every civilization after the Egyptian era. The plant contained alkaloids such as scopolamine, and could be eaten, drunk, or rubbed into the body to induce analgesia. Dioscorides used the root of the mandragora plant steeped in wine as an analgesic (Figure 1). Opium was the most important agent before the

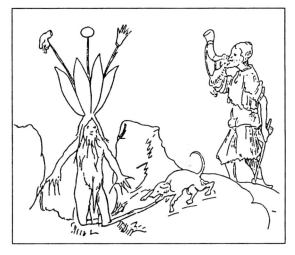

Figure 1 This drawing, dating back to the Middle Ages, shows the removal of the mandrake root. Reproduced with kind permission from the Germanisches National Museum, Nürnberg

discovery of ether. Opium poppy seeds were found in Swiss lake dwellings dating back to the fourth millennium BC and to the second millennium BC in Egypt.

Cannabis was used by some civilizations, especially the Chinese, as early as AD 200. Mixtures of wine, opium and mandragora were also used. Other methods, including occlusion of the carotid arteries, application of a 'memphitic stone' and immersion in cold water, were all used to induce analgesia. In 1562, Ambroise Paré described the use of nerve compression to induce analgesia. The first recorded injection of a drug intravenously was by Sir Christopher Wren. In 1656 he used a bladder and quill to inject alcohol, and his subject was a dog (Armstrong-Davidson, 1970).

In 1591 Eufame MacCalzean (or McAlyane) was executed in Scotland during the reign of James VI for attempting to relieve the pains of childbirth (Moir *et al.,* 1986). She was said to have consulted and sought the help of Annie Samson, a notorious witch, for the relief of pain in labour. Eufame herself was also found guilty on 28 counts concerning witchcraft. The real charge against her however, was for her participation in an attempt to cause the death of the king through her involvement in Satanic rites directed against him. Eufame did not confess to these charges.

EVOLUTION OF THE ANAESTHETIC GASES

The first anaesthetic gas, sweet vitriol (ether), was synthesized around 1540 by Valerius Cordus from a combination of sulphuric acid and alcohol. Paracelsus, who was his contemporary, recognized its sleep-inducing properties. It was not until the eighteenth century, however, that ether was recognized as an effective anaesthetic. Oxygen was discovered simultaneously by Joseph Priestley and Karl Wilhelm Scheele of Sweden in 1771. Priestley also identified carbonic acid and nitrous oxide in 1772. Further investigation of nitrous oxide was carried out by Sir Humphry Davy in 1799 who noted its pleasant effects and called it 'laughing gas' (Lee and Atkinson, 1968).

Davy (1800) wrote on the analgesic effects of nitrous oxide and suggested that it might be used during surgical operations. Eighteen years later Michael Faraday (1818) recorded the anaesthetic effects of sulphuric ether and compared the results with those of inhaling nitrous oxide. In December 1844, the effects of nitrous oxide were demonstrated by G.Q. Colton, a chemist, who was on a visit to Hartford, Connecticut. A dentist called Horace Wells was in the audience and he noted that inhalation of the gas was accompanied by a profound level of analgesia. On the following day Wells had a painless extraction of one of his own teeth while under the effects of nitrous oxide. Wells subsequently demonstrated the use of nitrous oxide at the Massachusetts General Hospital but the anaesthesia was insufficient. The patient cried out during tooth extraction so Wells and nitrous oxide were deemed a failure (Armstrong-Davidson, 1970).

Ether

The intoxicating effects of ether became well known in the 1830s and so-called 'ether frolics' became popular. William E. Clarke of Rochester, New York, became aware of the anaesthetic possibilities of the gas in 1842. Ether was administered by him to a Miss Hobbie and one of her teeth was then painlessly extracted by a dentist named Elijah Pope. In the same year Dr Crawford Williamson Long of Jefferson, Georgia, painlessly removed a tumour from the neck of James Venable under the effects of ether anaesthesia (Long, 1849).

A Boston student and later dentist William T.G. Morton (1846; 1847) however, is the man commonly regarded as the discoverer of anaesthesia. He carried out dental extractions using ether anaesthetic. Following this the use of ether as an anaesthetic quickly spread and, childbirth excepted, medical opposition to its use was virtually non-existent.

It was Oliver Wendell Holmes who suggested the name 'anaesthesia' (which had first been used by Dioscorides) in a letter to Dr Morton, dated Boston, 21 November 1846. Wendell Holmes had predicted in a letter to William Morton that the term 'will be repeated by the tongues of every civilized race of mankind'.

The first effective anaesthetic that William Morton (1819–1868) gave in front of an audience was on 16 October 1846. He had already, on 30 September 1846, removed an ulcerated tooth from a patient by the name of Eben H. Frost and had told him that he would be 'mesmerised'. It was Eben who told the *Boston Journal* of the painless and successful removal of his tooth. Morton designed an inhaler and was invited to use his ether and his inhaler on a patient of Dr John C. Warren. He arrived late because of some adjustments that had to be made by the instrument maker to the inhaler. At this stage Morton was a 2nd year medical student.

Dr John Warren started to get impatient at Morton's late arrival, but fortunately waited long enough for him to administer the anaesthetic. In the operation Dr Warren made an 'incision about 3 inches long through the skin of the neck, and began a dissection among important nerves and blood vessels without any expression of pain on the part of the patient'. Soon after he began to speak incoherently and appeared to be in an agitated state during the remainder of the operation. Being asked immediately afterwards whether he had suffered much, he said he had felt as if his neck had been scratched; 'subsequently when inquired of by me, (Dr Warren) his statement was that he did not experience pain at the time although he was aware that the operation was proceeding'.

At the end of this first operation Dr Warren had told his audience 'Gentlemen, this is no humbug'. The speed with which the discovery became known in Scotland was amazing; Dr James Young Simpson administered ether for the first obstetric case less than 2 months later, on 19 January 1847. The operation was for the delivery of a dead fetus to a woman with a severely contracted pelvis. Simpson (1847a,b), who became Professor of Midwifery in Edinburgh at 29 years of age, evaluated a large number of chemicals in the quest for a better form of anaesthetic and was helped by his assistants J. Matthews Duncan and George Keith.

Chloroform

The first challenge to ether came from chloroform which had been discovered almost simultaneously by Samuel Guthrie of the USA, Eugene Soubeiran in France and Justus Von Liebig in Germany in 1831 (Coleman, 1984). On the suggestion of David Waldy, a Scottish chemist, Simpson tried the effects of chloroform. The first chloroform administered to an obstetric patient was on 8 November 1847.

There was strong public reaction against the use of anaesthesia in childbirth, mainly on moral grounds. The opposition waned however, when Queen Victoria chose to have chloroform administered to her during the birth of her son Prince Leopold on 7 April 1853. The obstetrician was Charles Locock, accoucheur to her Majesty. The first stage of labour was nearly over when the chloroform was commenced. The anaesthetic was administered with each contraction by pouring about 15 minims by measure in a folded handkerchief. The Queen inhaled but did not become unconscious. Treatment commenced at 12.20 and the infant was born at 13.13. The Queen appeared very cheerful after the birth and expressed herself much gratified with the effect of the chloroform.

Four years later she again chose chloroform for the birth of Princess Beatrice. In both cases the anaesthetic was administered by John Snow (q.v. in Biographies) (Figure 2), who by the time of his death in 1858, was England's leading specialist on anaesthetics. The 'Simpson technique' of intermittent inhalational analgesia used by Snow (1848) thereafter became known as 'Chloroform a la Reine'.

Nitrous oxide

Nitrous oxide combined with oxygen delivered from separate cylinders was first used in obstetric practice by the Russian obstetrician S. Klikowitch

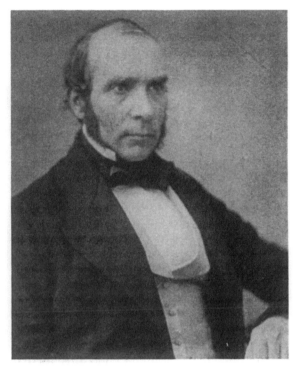

Figure 2 John Snow

of St Petersburg (1881). The technique of self-administration of nitrous oxide in obstetrics was first reported on by A.E. Guedel in 1911. A nitrous oxide and air apparatus was designed by R.J. Minnitt of Liverpool with Charles King of London for self-administration in labour in 1933 (Minnitt, 1938) (Figure 3). Tunstall of Aberdeen (1961) reported on the use of premixed nitrous oxide and oxygen from a single cylinder for use in obstetric analgesia. This was approved in 1965 by the Central Midwifery Board in England. Its obvious advantages over nitrous oxide and air were appreciated and the latter was discontinued around 1970.

Although many anaesthetic agents were available at the end of the nineteenth century, ether, chloroform and nitrous oxide were the most commonly used. It became apparent that nitrous oxide was safe, but chloroform was responsible for many maternal deaths. Chloroform gradually became unpopular and has rarely been used since the 1950s.

Other gases

Trichloroethylene (Trilene) was introduced by Dennis Jackson (1934) and by Striker (1935).

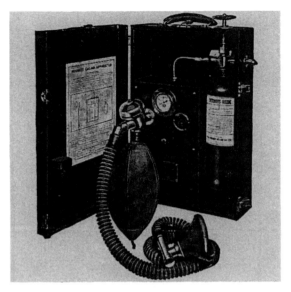

Figure 3 Minnitt gas-air apparatus. Portable model, showing the addition of a reservoir bag of pure nitrous oxide to give a quick start to the analgesia

Methoxyflurane (Penthrane) was first used in 1959. Both anaesthetics were popular for a while, as was cyclopropane.

Halothane (Fluothane) was synthesized by C.W. Suckling in 1951 and studied pharmacologically by J. Raventos (1956) in the succeeding years. It was introduced clinically by M. Johnstone of Manchester and also by Bryce Smith (1964) and O'Brien of Oxford. It was found to be more potent than chloroform or ether (Lee and Atkinson, 1968). However, it was found to have uterine relaxing effects which could induce haemorrhage. Despite that, it has continued to be a popularly used anaesthetic agent. Enflurane (Ethrane) was synthesized by Terrell in 1963 and introduced to clinical practice in 1966. It has been used as a supplement to nitrous oxide–oxygen anaesthesia.

TECHNICAL AND OTHER ADVANCES

Originally the anaesthetic agent was dropped on a handkerchief, which was held to the patient's nose. Over a period of time various cone-shaped appliances were designed to fit over the patient's nose and mouth. The Schimmelbusch mask evolved and remained popular for many years. Endotracheal intubation was first used by Sir William MacEwen in 1878, and Victor Eisenmenger (1893) introduced a rigid endotracheal tube with inflatable cuff and pilot balloon.

The anti-salivary effects of atropine were described by Heidinhane in 1872 and their discovery led to the use of premedication. In 1869 Frederick Trendelenburg, Professor of Surgery at Rostock who later introduced the head down tilt with pelvic elevation for abdominal surgery, used the Trendelenburg Cone for administration of chloroform (Armstrong-Davidson, 1970). The first direct vision laryngoscope was devised by Kirstein (1895). Barbitone (Veronal), the first barbiturate, was synthesized by Emil Fischer and Von Mering in 1903, and heralded the advent of intravenous induction of anaesthesia. The original Boyle's anaesthetic machine, which was a portable nitrous oxide and oxygen apparatus, was described by Henry Edmund Gaskin Boyle in 1917 (Boyle, 1917). The chloroform bottle was later added in 1920. In the same year Magill and Rowbotham developed the modern approach to endotracheal intubation.

MATERNAL MORTALITY

Despite the many advances, maternal deaths related to general anaesthesia were alarmingly high. This was accounted for in part by poor obstetric and anaesthetic training standards, the use of inappropriate anaesthetic agents and the modest facilities available. Most patients were in poor condition prior to surgery and faced the additional hazard of inhalation of gastric contents. Mendelson (1946) demonstrated the often fatal results of acid inhalation. Several methods were devised to overcome this problem, including injection of apomorphine to induce vomiting, or the emptying of stomach contents by nasogastric tube. Antacids were used to decrease gastric acidity but they in turn caused problems if inhaled. Later, histamine type 2 receptor antagonist drugs or those which increased gastric motility and sodium bicarbonate were all used. The introduction of Sellick's manoeuvre of cricoid pressure with oesophageal compression was widely adopted (Sellick, 1961). Today, patients are in better health, their standards of nutrition are improved, obstetric and anaesthetic staff are generally trained to a high level and anaesthetic deaths related to obstetrics are much reduced. A further method of curtailing maternal mortality and morbidity was the introduction and uptake of conduction analgesia.

LOCAL AND CONDUCTION ANALGESIA

Cocaine, a white powder refined from the leaves of the Peruvian coca plant, was discovered by Albert Niemann (1860), although its narcotic power had been known since about the sixteenth century. At Sigmund Freud's suggestion, cocaine was tested by Carl Koller (1884 a,b) an ophthalmologist, and found to be an effective local anaesthetic. This discovery caused acrimony between him and Sigmund Freud, who had been using cocaine in Vienna at the same time, initially to treat a friend of his who had become a morphine addict. He gave this friend, Ernst von Fleischel-Marxow, cocaine as a help to withdraw from morphine (just as methadone is now used in prisons to help morphine addicts withdraw). It may even be that Freud himself perhaps for a short time became an addict.

Koller, like Freud, managed to obtain some cocaine which had been purified by the firm of Merck of Darmstadt, now known as the firm of Merck, Sharpe & Dohme. He used it first on the eye of a frog in Professor Stricker's laboratory. The frog permitted its cornea to be touched. Koller then tried it out on a rabbit and a dog and finally on the eye of a human being. Koller's paper was read for him by a friend, Dr Joseph Brettauer of Trieste at the Ophthalmological Congress in Heidelberg.

Freud's friend Fleischel apparently became an addict to cocaine and morphine, so that cocaine did not do him much good. It is to Koller that credit is due for the discovery of the local anaesthetic properties of cocaine, for its derivatives are now widely used in obstetrics, either for epidural anaesthesia or for local anaesthesia and pudendal block.

William Stewart Halsted experimented with conduction analgesia at Johns Hopkins Hospital in Baltimore and he later became addicted to cocaine. Stiasny (1910) had applied cocaine topically to the vagina and vulva to relieve pain in labour.

J.L. Corning produced analgesia by the accidental subarachnoid injection of cocaine (1885). His technique was refined by Quincke in Germany in 1891. In the same year Giesel isolated tropocaine, the first local anaesthetic alternative to the toxic cocaine. It was August Bier (1899) of Kiel however who first used *spinal analgesia* for surgery. The technique was developed and popularized by Tuffier (1899). Kreis (1900) in Germany was the first to use spinal anaesthesia for operative vaginal delivery. A hyperbaric technique was developed by Pitkin in the USA in 1928.

Caudal analgesia was introduced by Sicard (1901) and Cathelin (1901) in Paris, and Von Stockel (1909) of Marberg reported on the use of caudal block in obstetrics. Pagés (1921) of Spain reported on the use of *extradural lumbar analgesia*. In 1931 Achile Mario Dogliotti (1931; 1933) reintroduced the extradural technique, and it was first used in obstetrics by Graffagnino and Seyler (1938). The 'continuous' technique was pioneered in 1942 by Flowers *et al.* (1949).

The local anaesthetic procaine was synthesized by Alfred Einhorn (1899) while stovaine was introduced by Ernst Fourneau (1904) of Paris. *Pudendal nerve block* with local infiltration was popularized by Muller in 1908, although later investigations questioned its validity. *Paracervical nerve block*, which was first reported by Gellert (1926), was popular for years, but fetal bradycardia and acidosis were reported with its use and the technique fell out of favour. Gellhorn in 1927 described *infiltration of the perineum* with local anaesthetic solutions.

ANALGESICS

Morphine was rarely used in labour until von Steinbuchel combined it with hyoscine in 1902. Due to its depressant effect on fetal breathing it was never as popular as pethidine which was first employed in labour by Benthin (1940). Pentazocine was used for a time but never became popular. Phenothiazine derivatives were used alone or in combination with pethidine, as was diazepam, but most of these combinations are no longer used.

SELF- OR MIDWIFE-ADMINISTERED INHALATIONAL ANALGESIA

It is to Minnitt (1938) that credit must go for popularizing this form of analgesia. The Minnitt apparatus, or intermittent flow machine, was designed to deliver 50% nitrous oxide and 50% air. The concentration of oxygen in the mixture was too low and the apparatus was eventually withdrawn. The use of nitrous oxide and oxygen in one cylinder was initiated by Barach and Rovenstine (1945) and the work leading to a practical method of administration was undertaken by the British Oxygen Company Limited and pioneered in Britain by Tunstall (1961).

The Friedman inhaler was developed in 1943 for administration of analgesic concentrations of Trichloroethylene to labouring women. The Emotril and Tecota mark 6 machines became available for use by midwives in 1955. In 1970 the Cardiff inhaler was introduced for use with 0.35% methoxyflurane. Now however the Entonox apparatus (50% nitrous oxide and 50% oxygen) provides the only inhalational agent available for self- or midwife-administered analgesia, since approval for the other methods was withdrawn.

NATURAL CHILDBIRTH

Effective analgesia in labour is a modern concept. Prior to that unreliable potions were available to some, and a stoic attitude was essential for most in labour. Mesmerism helped to allay anxiety. Fear of labour and the poorly understood process of delivery contributed to the tension which heightened the realization of pain. The importance of a correct mental attitude to pregnancy and pain was advanced in this century by Grantly Dick Read in his books *Natural Childbirth* (1933) and *Childbirth without Fear* (1944; 1960). The technique of psychoprophylaxis was advocated by Vellay (1959). Vellay was Lamaze's assistant and successor in Paris. It reached England in 1960. Lamaze had introduced the method into France after visiting Professor Nicolaiev in Leningrad in 1950. The method used Pavlovian principles (Lamaze, 1972). Leboyer introduced his *Birth without Violence* (1975).

CHRONOLOGY

1591   A woman was executed for seeking medication to relieve labour pains.

Analgesics, hypnotics, dissociative anaesthesia

Morphine is derived from the Greek – *Morpheus,* god of dreams; opium is derived from the Greek word for 'juice' and is obtained from the dried juice of the poppy head.

1806   Serturner isolated morphine from crude opium.

1832   Codeine phosphate (codeine is derived from the Greek name for poppy head) was isolated by Robiquet.

1860   Niemann isolated the alkaloid from the Peruvian coca leaves, and named it Cocaine.

1868   Moreno y Maiz and Bennett (1873) independently showed cocaine to be an anaesthetic.

1869   Liebreich introduced chloral hydrate, a hypnotic which had been synthesized by Liebig in 1822.

1882   The Italian physician Cervello introduced Paraldehyde into medicine. The substance was discovered by Wiedenbusch in 1829. Rowbotham used paraldehyde in oil *per rectum* in 1928 to produce basal narcosis. In 1932 Rosenfield and Davidoff gave it *per rectum* to obstetric patients, particularly those with severe pre-eclampsia or eclampsia (Lee and Atkinson, 1968; Atkinson *et al.*, 1982).

1902   Von Steinbuchel and Gauss (1905) introduced morphine combined with hyoscine as 'twilight sleep' for pain relief in labour.

1909   Sahli introduced papaveretum (Omnopon).

1927   Bromethol (Avertin), discovered by Eicholtz in 1917, was synthesized by Willstaetter and Duisberg in 1923, and was first used by Butzengeiger (Butzengeiger and Eicholtz, 1927; Smith, 1979).

1939   Pethidine hydrochloride was first synthesized by Schaumann and Eisleb.

1940   Pethidine, known also as Dolantin, Dolantal, Meperidine and Demerol, was first employed in labour by Benthin.

1941   Nalorphine Hydrobromide was first described by McCawley *et al.*

1950   Levallorphan was synthesized by Schneider and Hellerbach and was used as an antidote to respiratory depression by Fromherz and Pellmond (1952).

1952   Apgar and Papper noted that although it was the most widely used analgesic in labour pethidine traversed the placenta, and could cause respiratory depression in the fetus.

1957   Morphine was synthesized by Gates and Tschudi. It is one of 25 alkaloids contained in opium but only morphine, codeine and papaverine have had wide clinical use.

1959   Pentazocine (Fortral, Talwin) was described (Lee and Atkinson, 1968).

1960   The application of a subatmospheric pressure to the abdomen (abdominal decompression) was used to relieve pain during the first stage of labour.

Corssen and Domino documented their first clinical experience with phencyclidine.

1961   At this time phenothiazines were used in labour; Moore and Dundee noted that they produced hypotension.

1966   Ketamine was introduced (dissociative anaesthesia), replacing the older phencyclidine.

1967   Beazley et al. found that only 40% of women interviewed postpartum considered pain relief adequate when using parenteral and inhalational analgesia.

1968   Lean et al. recorded the use of Diazepam in the treatment of eclampsia. It was later combined with analgesics, at various stages in labour.

Anaesthetic gases

1540   Valerius Cordus discovered diethyl ether (Coleman, 1984).

1603   Ether was used by Paracelsus.

1771   Priestley and Scheele independently discover oxygen (Lee and Atkinson, 1968).

1775   Nitrous oxide (N_2O) was discovered by Joseph Priestley.

1800   Nitrous oxide was used by Humphry Davy to relieve his own toothache.

1818   Faraday showed that ether caused the same euphoric effects as nitrous oxide. Both chemicals were used for 'frolics'.

1824   Hickman carried out painless operations on animals by using carbon dioxide narcosis. He is recorded as being the first to unite the concept of inhalational anaesthesia and surgical operation.

1842   William Clarke of Rochester New York, administered ether to a Miss Hobbie thereby allowing Elijah Pope to perform a painless tooth extraction for her (Warren and Vandam, 1963).

1845   A Hartford dentist, Horace Wells, demonstrated the use of nitrous oxide for dental extraction to a Harvard Medical School class. The boy concerned cried out during the procedure and Wells was booed from the room (Lee and Atkinson, 1973).

1846   Liston (England), amputated a thigh under ether anaesthesia.

W.T.G. Morton moved from using nitrous oxide to ether at the suggestion of chemistry teacher Charles T. Jackson. Morton demonstrated the use of ether anaesthesia during painless removal of a congenital vascular tumour from a patient's jaw. On observing the painless procedure, the surgeon, John C. Warren said 'Gentlemen, this is no humbug' (Warren and Vandam, 1963 p. 277).

Henry Jacob Bigelow published on the use of ether within 3 weeks of Morton's demonstration.

1847   Chloric ether (Chloroform) was used instead of the diethyl ether of previous workers, by James Y. Simpson in Edinburgh.

1849   Ether was used to eliminate pain during removal of a tumour by Crawford Long.

1853   John Snow of London, now acknowledged as the first obstetric anaesthetist, administered chloroform to Queen Victoria for the delivery of Prince Leopold (Secher, 1989)

1881   Klikowitch introduced nitrous oxide into obstetric practice.

1896   At the golden jubilee of ether, F.W. Hewitt commented that the administration of anaesthesia was too often placed in the hands of unskilled men.

1934/35 Trichloroethylene (Trilene) was evaluated by Dennis Jackson and Striker (Moir et al., 1986).

1941   Trichloroethylene was introduced for clinical use.

1949   Nitrous oxide and oxygen was first used in obstetrics in the UK by Seward.

1951   Halothane was synthesized by C.W. Suckling (Stephen and Fabian, 1989).

1956   Raventos, and also Johnstone, reported on experiences with Fluothane (Halothane).

1957   Fluothane was widely evaluated and soon became the most popular anaesthetic in the world.

1959   Methoxyflurane (Penthrane) was introduced.

1960   Baker noted that all the common gaseous and volatile anaesthetic agents readily crossed the placenta and also found that of the non-depolarizing muscle relaxant drugs in common use,

441

tubocurarine crossed the placenta only in minute amounts but gallamine appeared to cross more readily.

1963 Enfluorane was synthesized by Terrell at Ohio Medical Products and introduced to clinical practice by Virtue *et al.* (1966).

1964 The Bryce-Smith induction unit, using halothane, was introduced.

1965 Crawford suggested that to avoid maternal awareness under general anaesthesia the inspired mixture should contain 50% oxygen and 50% nitrous oxide.

Premedication

Atropine sulphate B.P. (from Atropos, the oldest of the Three Fates who severed the thread of life). Belladonna has been in use for many centuries and Atropine was isolated by Mein (1831).

Hyoscine hydrobromide B.P. (Scopolamine), the name 'scopolamine' is derived from *Scopolia carniolica,* the plant from which it was first isolated. It is derived from *Hyoscyamus niger* (henbane). It was isolated in 1871.

1686 In John Ray's *Historia Plantanum* it was noted that a fresh leaf of deadly nightshade placed on the eye caused pupil enlargement (Adt *et al.*, 1989).

1833 Liebig analysed atropine chemically and deduced its formula (Adt *et al.*, 1989).

1845 Francis Rynd of Dublin developed a primitive syringe (Graham, 1950).

1855 The hollow metallic needle was popularized by Alexander Wood.

1864 Johann N. Nussbaum combined a subcutaneous injection of morphine with chloroform anaesthesia, and this appears to have been the beginning of pre-anaesthetic medication.

1905 Franz von Pitha used atropine with anaesthesia (Adt *et al.*, 1989).

1906 Gauss used hyoscine with morphine to produce amnesia in labour.

1930 Ernst von der Porten recommended atropine and morphine prior to anaesthesia.

Induction agents

1665 Elsholtz injected opiates thus producing

insensibility (Wylie and Churchill-Davidson, 1984).

1872 Chloralhydrate was administered intravenously to induce anaesthesia (Ore).

1927 Pernocton was used to induce anaesthesia (Bumm). Amytal and hexobarbitone soon followed.

1932 Weese and Scharpff introduced the quick acting parenterally administered barbiturate, Hexobarbitone.

1935 Lundy introduced thiopentone to America and it soon replaced the majority of intravenous induction agents.

1939 Weinstein further described the use of thiopentone.

1955 At this time intravenous anaesthetics were used for induction of anaesthesia only, and although a single dose of thiopentone was generally used, the drug traversed the placenta (McKechnie and Converse).

1962 Methohexitone had become popular as an induction agent but crossed the placenta with ease (Sliom *et al.*).

Muscle relaxants

Muscle relaxants were introduced in 1942. Prior to that, rapid smooth induction of anaesthesia and maintenance of a state adequate for surgery was a work of art accomplished regularly by relatively few practitioners. The use of synthetic skeletal muscle relaxants was a significant advance allowing for smoother and safer anaesthesia.

1516 The Italian Peter Martyr d'Anghera wrote the first known account of the use of poison arrows (impregnated with curare) by the South American Indians (Figure 4).

1648 Marggravius first used the word curare.

1812 Benjamin Brodie found that artificial respiration during paralysis by curare in animals, was sufficient to sustain life until spontaneous breathing returned.

1830 Von Martius recognized that a number of plants including strychnos were the chief components of some curare preparations.

1850/ The physiologist Claude Bernard
56/64 found that the action of curare was

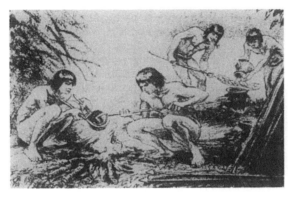

Figure 4 Preparation of the arrow poison by the South American Indians. Reproduced with kind permission from Hughes, R. (1987). *The History of Anaesthesia*, p.258. (Carnforth: Parthenon Publishing)

	localized at some point between nerve and muscle.
1868	Crum-Brown and Fraser recognized the relationship between the quaternary ammonium groups of curare and neuromuscular block.
1879	Charles Waterton, an explorer, described in his *Wanderings in South America* 'the poisoned darts, arrows and spears used by local natives'.
1895	Rudolph Boehm described the three types of curare commonly available: tube curare, pot curare, and calabash curare.
1935	Tubocurarine was first isolated by Harold King from a sample of tube curare.
1942	Harold Griffith and Enid Johnson (Montreal) were advised by Dr Lewis Wright, to use the drug as a skeletal muscle relaxant in anaesthesia and 33 years after Meltzer and Auer's (1909) description of curarized dogs, wrote on their use of curare in general anaesthesia. Muscle relaxants made surgical procedures possible at a much lighter plane of anaesthesia and enhanced post-operative recovery. Griffith was the first to use tubocurarine as an adjunct to anaesthesia.
1947/49	Bovet *et al.* synthesized Gallamine.
1949	Phillips synthesized suxamethonium. Decamethonium was used by Organe and proved a satisfactory substitute for D-tubocurarine, but tachyphylaxis became a serious problem.

1950	Scurr wrote on the use of the short acting relaxant suxamethonium.
1955	Wylie used a cuffed endotracheal tube after suxamethonium induction to reduce regurgitation.
1960	Baker noted that all the common gaseous and volatile anaesthetic agents readily crossed the placenta and the non-depolarizing muscle relaxant drug in common use, tubocurarine, crossed the placenta only in minute amounts but gallamine appeared to cross more readily.
1961	The depolarizing agent suxamethonium crossed the placenta only when very large doses were used. Alcuronium was derived from calabash curare by Frey and Seeger.
1967	Pancuronium was synthesized by Savage *et al.* and described clinically by Baird and Reid.
1973	Vecuronium was described by Buckett *et al.*
1978	Stenlake synthesized atrarcurium.

Regurgitation and aspiration

1848	James Young Simpson reported death under anaesthesia caused by aspiration of gastric contents (Cotton and Smith, 1982; 1984).
1946	Mendelson described the clinical course of 66 patients who aspirated acid gastric contents during labour and delivery (Mendelson's Syndrome).
1957	Dinnick administered oral antacids to reduce the risk of Mendelson's Syndrome. Intravenous apomorphine was used to induce vomiting to effect gastric emptying prior to general anaesthesia. (Holmes).
1961	Sellick proposed cricoid pressure to prevent aspiration of gastric contents at induction of general anaesthesia.
1962	Bannister and Sattilaro suggested that there was a critical pH of 2.5, below which aspirated gastric content caused severe lung reactions.
1972	The first histamine (H2) receptor blocker was synthesized by Black *et al.*
1974	Roberts and Shirley found that the volume of gastric aspirate was important for the production of widespread

1978 pulmonary damage. Volumes of over 25 ml could cause severe lung damage. Cimetidine was used as a single oral dose for prophylaxis against Mendelson's Syndrome by Husemeyer *et al.*

1979 Gibbs *et al.* while experimenting with sodium citrate, found that aspiration produced only transient hypoxia and minimal tissue changes. Sodium citrate was found to be superior in use to magnesium trisilicate.

Masks/inhalers/vaporizers

From Westhorpe (1989)

1847 Simpson placed chloroform on a handkerchief to facilitate inhalation and anaesthesia.

1862 Thomas Skinner, a Liverpool obstetrician, introduced the first wire frame mask which antedated the better known Schimmelbusch mask by almost 30 years.

1869 Friedrich Trendelenburg of Berlin introduced his cone for use of chloroform via a tracheostomy (Armstrong-Davidson, 1970).

1879 Esmarch designed a face mask which was popular until the 1940s.

1885 Carter introduced the so-called 'open' inhaler.

1890 Lawrie devised the Hyderabad cone. Kurt Schimmelbusch designed a mask consisting of a spiral wire tower covered with a waxed cloth.

1890 Sudeck introduced his inhaler with addition of primitive valves.

1910 Dunkley and Gwathmey designed wire masks.

1911 Sir Thomas Dunhill designed an inhaler which included early inspiratory and expiratory valves.

The following workers introduced vaporizers which were commonly used:
1867 Ferdinand Albert-Junker.
1890 Dudley Buxton.
1903 Augustus Vernon-Harcourt.
1914 Carter-Braine.

Intubation/laryngoscopes

Before the discovery of inhalational anaesthesia, tracheostomies or endotracheal tubes were employed in experiments, or during resuscitation, by Galen, Avicenna, Paracelsus, Vesalius, Hook, Desault, Chaussier and others.

1880 MacEwen was the first to employ oral endotracheal intubation electively.

1885 Joseph O'Dwyer, physician to the New York Foundling Hospital introduced blind intubation of the larynx.

1893 Victor Eisenmenger created a rigid endotracheal tube with inflatable cuff and pilot balloon.

1895 Alfred Kirstein introduced the first direct vision laryngoscope.

1905 Endotracheal anaesthesia was administered by Kuhn.

1909 Intratracheal insufflation anaesthesia was developed by Meltzer and Auer.

1911 Franz Kuhn wrote on intubation. He was also the first anaesthetist to use topical cocaine to reduce the patient's discomfort during the passage of an endotracheal tube.
Intratracheal insufflation anaesthesia was adapted to human use by Elsberg.

1919 Ivan Magill and Stanley Rowbotham began their professional association. They created several modifications of insufflation techniques and introduced Rowbotham's 'guiding rod' and Magill's 'angulated forceps' (Calverley, 1989).

1928 Arthur Guedel and Ralph Waters introduced the cuff-endotracheal tube.

1941 Miller introduced a predominantly straight-blade laryngoscope.

1943 Robert Macintosh introduced a curved bladed laryngoscope.

Machines and ventilators

1867 F.A. Junker introduced the first 'blow over' apparatus designed for administration of chloroform.

1917 Boyle used a modified version of Gwathmey's breathing apparatus. This gradually evolved to the apparatus familiar to all anaesthetists today.

1952 As curare became more widespread in use, ventilators were developed (Esplen).

Rectal methods

1913 Gwathmey's rectal ether – a mixture of morphine, magnesium sulphate, quinine and rectal ether was introduced.

444

1934   Reynolds recommended the use of paraldehyde, in a dose of 60 minims per stone of body weight.

Local anaesthetics

1784   Prolonged compression over a nerve supplying an area, to achieve analgesia was used by Moore, and may also have been used by John Hunter.

1884   Koller demonstrated the local analgesic properties of cocaine on the cornea, at the suggestion of Sigmund Freud, at an Ophthalmological Congress at Heidelberg.

1885   William Stewart Halsted, in New York, performed the first nerve block with cocaine; the nerve involved was the mandibular.

1886   Corning, a neurologist, wrote the first textbook on local anaesthesia.

1897   Crile also used nerve block.

1899   Einhorn prepared procaine (Novocain).

1901   Crile used cocaine and eucain to achieve local block.

1904   Fourneau introduced stovaine, also used by Braun (1905).

1929   Uhlmann introduced nupercaine (cinchocaine) which was first synthesized in 1925.

1943   Lofgren synthesized lignocaine hydrochloride (Xylocaine) (Wylie and Churchill-Davidson, 1984).

1947   A.C. Beck used local infiltration for Caesarean section.

1963   Teluvio introduced Bupivacine.

Epidural analgesia

1885   J.L. Corning produced analgesia by cocaine placed epidurally.

1921   Fidel Pagés (Spain) described the lumbar approach to extradural analgesia.

1931/33   The Italian surgeon Dogliotti 'rediscovered' epidural anaesthesia, naming it peridural segmentry analgesia.

1933   Cleland wrote 'Regional anaesthesia, so successfully developed in other fields of surgery, should find its ideal application in obstetrics.' However, it was another 10 years before there was widespread use of regional analgesia in the specialty. It was he who first discovered that the pain fibres from the uterus reached the spinal cord, mainly at T11 and T12 levels.

1938   Extradural lumbar block was first used in obstetrics by Graffagnino and Seyler.

1945   Tuohy introduced the technique of placing a plastic catheter through a Tuohy needle, for continuous administration of analgesia.

1948   Gordh substituted lignocaine for procaine, with subsequent increased lability and duration of effect in local analgesia.

1949   The Cuban anaesthetist, M.M. Curbello inserted a ureteric catheter into the extradural space to achieve continuous analgesia.

Continuous extradural lumbar block was also introduced by Flowers et al.

Continuous lumbar epidural techniques were first used in obstetrics by Cleland in the USA.

1950   Brigden et al. and also Flowers, Hellman and Hingson noted that in the latter weeks of pregnancy the supine position may be associated with hypotension of varying severity.

1960   The 'blood patch' method was introduced by Gormley. Removing venous blood from the patient's arm under sterile conditions he injected it into the epidural space at the dural puncture site.

1963   Bupivacine, with its long duration of action, was introduced by Teluvio.

1965   Hellman reported on a large series of patients in which a 'single dose' method was used for epidural block.

1967   The lumbar approach to the epidural space was preferred to the sacral route in the USA.

1968   Moir and Willocks noted that the use of epidural analgesia reduced the need of Caesarean section for maternal distress.

1969   A survey carried out by Dawkins indicated that even in experienced hands, the failure rate for locating the epidural space via the sacral route was about 10%.

1972   Crawford found a fall in systolic blood pressure of over 10 mm of mercury in 1.4% of 6000 epidural top-up doses.

The incidence of backache was no higher after epidural than after pudendal block, in a study by Moir and Davidson.

1973   In a modification of a technique suggested by Hingson, (Rice and Harwell Dabbs, 1950) Crawford suggested that after inadvertent spinal tap an epidural catheter be inserted in the next intervertebral space; that analgesia be achieved for labour and an elective forceps be performed.

1974   Pearson and Davies noted that epidural analgesia avoided the depressing effect on the fetus of potent narcotic and sedative drugs, and reduced maternal acidosis in the first and second stages of labour.

Crawford found that epidural analgesia did not have a depressant effect on uterine tone.

The blood patch technique for dural tap at epidural analgesia produced complete and permanent relief of headache in 182 of 185 patients within 24h when employed by Ostheimer *et al.*

1975   While it was commonly accepted that the level of sympathetic block extended at least two segments higher than the cutaneous analgesic level Mohan and Potter noted that there was some degree of block which could extend considerably higher.

Caudal analgesia

1901   Cathelin and Sicard employed the sacral approach to extradural analgesia.

1909   von Stoekel used caudal block in gynaecology.

1943   Continuous caudal block was used by Hingson and Edwards.

1965   Perforation of the fetal skull by a caudal needle was described by Finster *et al.*

1971   Stallworthy pointed out the considerable benefit to patients of caudal blocks carried out by obstetricians.

Spinal analgesia

1855   Alexander Wood popularized the hollow needle and a conveniently sized glass syringe.

1884   Koller demonstrated the local analgesic properties of cocaine.

1885   Corning was the first to inject cocaine into the subarachnoid space.

1887   Ephedrine was isolated in pure state and named by Nagai, and put into use in 1927 to combat 'spinal' hypotension.

1899   Bier, and also Tuffier, introduced and developed spinal analgesia.

Procaine was introduced by Einhorn.

1900   Soon after it was employed in general surgery Kreis reported on the use of spinal analgesia for Caesarean section.

1904   Fourneau introduced the local anaesthetic agent Stovaine.

1907   Barker introduced heavy solutions of local anaesthetic for use in spinal blocks.

1927   Ephedrine was used to combat the hypotension of spinal analgesia, by Ockerblad and Dillon and also by Rudolf and Graham.

1929   Uhlmann introduced the long acting analgesic percaine (Nupercaine).

1940   Lemmon wrote on the continuous administration of spinal anaesthesia.

1959   Watt *et al.* reported 2475 cases of low spinal anaesthesia in obstetrics with no maternal mortality due to the anaesthetic.

1961   Headache was the most frequent complication of spinal anaesthesia, occurring in 11% of cases (Dripps *et al*). This figure was much reduced by the introduction of fine gauge spinal needles.

1973   Schnider found an 82% incidence of hypotension in a series of patients in whom spinal block was used for Caesarean section.

1979   Crawford documented his experiences with spinal analgesia in an obstetric unit.

Pudendal block

1908   Pudendal nerve block and local infiltration of the perineum was first performed by Muller (Bonica, 1967).

1916   King wrote on the technique in America.

1953   Klink advocated the transperineal route with local analgesic to block the pudendal nerve, with its three terminal branches.

1956   A transvaginal route to block the pudendal nerve with local analgesic was used by Kobak *et al.*

1966   Scudamore and Yates found that only 36% of pudendal blocks gave effective bilateral analgesia of the perineum and vulva and concluded that much of the efficacy attributed to pudendal blocks was due to the associated local infiltration.

Saddle block/paracervical/paravertebral blocks

1926   Gellert in Germany first used paracervical block for surgical anaesthesia.

1933   Paravertebral block was used by Cleland but did not relieve pain of cervical or perineal stretching.

1945   Rosenfeld introduced paracervical block for obstetric pain relief in the USA.

1946   Saddle block was a term proposed by Adriani and Roma-Vega and involved a zone of analgesia of the perineum and perianal region without leg involvement.

1972   Paracervical block was associated with fetal bradycardia.

Perineal infiltration

1910   Stiasny applied topical cocaine.

1927   Gellhorn described infiltration of the perineum with local anaesthetic solutions.

1928   Brown used local anaesthetics for repair of perineal tears (Bloom *et al.*, 1972).

Self-administered gases

1912   Guedel devised the first machine for self-administration of nitrous oxide in obstetrics.

1934   Ralph Minnitt (and A. Charles King) introduced a prototype apparatus for gas and air analgesia in labour. This was illustrated in Minnitt's book (1938).

1945   The use of mixtures of nitrous oxide and oxygen in one cylinder was initiated by Barach and Rovenstine.

1961   Tunstall introduced the practical method of administration of premixed 50% oxygen and 50% nitrous oxide (Entonox) – available from then in a cylinder with a demand valve apparatus.

1962   Cole and Nainby-Luxmore expressed doubts about the use of nitrous oxide in air for patients in labour. The fetus was at risk due to low maternal oxygen levels.

Natural birth

1799   Mesmerism (hypnosis) was introduced by Mesmer.

1843   Elliotson noted that surgical procedures were possible in the hypnotic state.

1933/   Grantly Dick-Read taught that normal
44/60   labour should be practically free from pain; when pain occurs it is due to abnormal and incoordinate uterine action, and that this could be avoided by instruction and training during the antenatal period. This approach to analgesia was called natural childbirth.

1949   Velvoski, a Russian psychiatrist, advocated a 'psychotherapeutic method of obstetricial analgesia' (Lubic and Ernst, 1975).

1950   Nicolaiev suggested the term psychoprophylaxis (Lubic and Ernst, 1975).

1959   Lamaze and later Vellay advocated a psychosomatic approach.

1975   Leboyer wrote on 'birth without violence'.

Combinations

1908   Anaesthetic combinations were first conceived by Crile, where local anaesthesia was used to reduce the requirements of the inhalant.

Ataralgesia

1957   Scott and Gadd popularized the technique of hypoaesthesia or ataralgesia. The technique consists of intravenous injection of an analgesic with a tranquillizing agent and an analgesic antagonist. The term ataralgesia was coined by Hayward-Butt.

Mortality

1848   J.Y. Simpson recorded a death due to

anaesthesia (Cotten and Smith, 1982; 1984).

1952   The confidential inquiries into maternal deaths in England and Wales began after consultation between the Royal College of Obstetricians and Gynaecologists and the Society of Medical Officers of Health. At that time there were 44 maternal deaths for every thousand deliveries. The number of deaths due to anaesthetic complications remained unchanged for almost the following 20 years. This stimulated an interest in conduction analgesia, as an alternative form of anaesthesia.

REFERENCES

Adriani, J. and Roma-Vega, D. (1946), quoted by Lee and Atkinson (1973) p. 679

Adt, M., Schmuker, P. and Muller, I. (1989). The role of atropine in antiquity and in anaesthesia. In Atkinson, R.S. and Boulton, T.B. (eds.) *The History of Anaesthesia*, pp.40–5. (London and New York: Royal Society of Medicine Services and The Parthenon Publishing Group)

Anghera P.M. d' (1516). *De Orbe Novo*, translated by MacNutt, F.A. (1912) (New York: Putman's Sons)

Apgar, V. and Papper, E.M. (1952). *Curr. Res. Anesth. Analg.*, **31**, 309, quoted by Utting and Gray (A68) p. 80

Armstrong-Davidson, M.H. (1970). *The Evolution of Anaesthesia*, 2nd edn. pp. 67, 104 and 126. (Altringham: J. Sherratt & Son Ltd.) (1st edn. 1965)

Atkinson, R.S., Rushman, G.B. and Lee, J.A. (1982). *A Synopsis of Anaesthesia. General Anaesthesia. Regional Analgesia. Intensive Therapy*, 9th edn. p. 438. (Bristol, London, Boston: Wright P.S.G.)

Baird, W. and Reid, A.M. (1967). quoted by Lee and Atkinson (1973) p. 287

Baker, J.B.E. (1960). *Pharmacol. Rev.*, **12**, 37, quoted by Utting and Gray (1968) p. 80

Bannister, W.K. and Sattilaro, A.J. (1962). Vomiting and aspiration during anaesthesia. *Anesthesiology*, **23**, 251–64

Barach, A.L. and Rovenstine, E.A. (1945). *Anesthesiology*, **6**, 449, quoted by Utting and Gray (1968) p. 80

Barker, A.E. (1907). A report on clinical experiences with spinal analgesia in 100 cases. *Br. Med. J.*, 665–74

Beazley, J.M., Leaver, E.P., Morewood, J.H.M. and Bircumshaw, J. (1967). Relief of pain in labour. *Lancet*, **1**, 1033–5

Beck, A.C. (1947), quoted by Lee and Atkinson (1968) p. 647

Bennett, A. (1873). An experimental inquiry into the physiological action of theine, caffeine, guaranine, cocaine, and theobromine. *Edin. Med. J.*, **19** (Part 1), 323

Benthin, (1940), quoted in Lee and Atkinson (1968) p. 621

Bernard, C. (1850). Action de curare et de la nicotine sur le systeme nerveux et sur le systeme musculaire. *Cr. Seanc. Soc. Biol.*, **2**, 195

Bernard, C. (1856). Analyse physiologique des proprietés des systemes musculaires et nerveux au moyen du curare. *Cr. hebd. Seanc. Acad. Sci. Paris*, **43**, 825–9

Bernard, C. (1864). Etudes physiologiques sur quelques poisons Americains: le curare. *Rev. d Deux Mondes*, **53**, 164–90

Bier, A. (1899). Ver, uber Cocainisierung des Ruckenmark. *Deutsche Zeitschrift fur Chirurgie*, **51**, 361; translated in *'Classical File' Survey of Anesthesiology* (1962) **6**, 352

Bigelow, H.J. (1846). Insensibility during surgical operations produced by inhalation. *Boston M. & S. J.*, **35**, 309

Black, J.W., Duncan, W.A.M., Durant, C.J., Gannellin, C.R. and Parsons, E.M. (1972). Definition and antagonism of histamine H2 receptors. *Nature (London)*, **236**, 385–90

Bloom, S.L., Horswill, C.W. and Curet, L.G. (1972). Effects of paracervical blocks on the fetus during labor: a prospective study. *Am. J. Obstet. Gynecol.*, **114**, 218–22

Boehm, R. (1895). Das Sudamerikanische Pfeilgift curare in chemischer und pharmakologischer Beziehung. 1 Teil: Das Tubo-curare. *Abh. Sachs. Akad. Wiss.*, **22**, 200–38

Bonica, J.J. (1967). *Principles and Practice of Obstetric Analgesia and Anesthesia*, Vol. 1, pp. 107 and 487. (Philadelphia: F.A. Davis Co.)

Bovet, D., Depierre, F. and de Lestrange, Y. (1947). Proprietes curarisantes des ethers phenoliques a fonctions ammonium quaternaires. *Cr. hebd. Seanc. Acad. Sci. Paris*, **225**, 74–6

Bovet, D., Bovet-Nitti, F., Guarino, S., Longo, V.G. and Marotta, M. (1949). Proprieta farmacodinamiche di alcani derivati della succinilcolina dotati di azione curarica *R. C. 1st sup Sanita*, **12**, 106–37

Boyle, H.E.G. (1917). The use of nitrous oxide and oxygen with rebreathing in military surgery. *Lancet*, **2**, 667–9

Braun, H. (1905). Ueber Einege Neure Ortliche Anesthetica (Stovain Alypin, Novocain) *D. Med. Wchnschr.*, **31**, 1667

Brigden, W., Howarth, S. and Sharpey-Schafer, E.P. (1950). Postural changes in the peripheral blood-flow of normal subjects with observation on vaso-vagal fainting reactions as a result of tilting, the lordotic posture, pregnancy and spinal anaesthesia. *Clin. Sci.*, **9**, 79–91

Brodie, B.C. (1812). Further experiments and observations on the action of poison on the animal system. *Phil. Trans. R. Soc.*, **102**, 205–27

Browne, F.J. (1928), quoted by Browne, F.J. (1950) p. 220

Browne, F.J. (1950). *Postgraduate Obstetrics and Gynaecology.* (London: Butterworth and Co.)

Bryce-Smith, R. (1964). Halothane induction unit. *Anaesthesia*, **19**, 393–8

Bryce-Smith, R. and Williams, E.O. (1955). The treatment of eclampsia (imminent or actual) by continuous conduction analgesia. *Lancet*, **1**, 1241–4

Buckett, W.R., Hewett, C.L. and Savage, D.S. (1973). Pancuronium bromide and other steroidal neuromuscular blocking agents containing acetylcholine fragments. *J. Med. Chem.*, **16**, 1116–24

Bumm. R. (1927). Intravenose Narkosen mit Barbitur-Saurederivaten K. *Lin. Wchnschr.*, **6**, 725–6

Butzengeiger, O. and Eicholtz, F. (1927). *Dt Med. Wchnschr.*, **53**, 712, quoted by Lee and Atkinson (1973) p. 126

Calverley, R.K (1989). Intubation in anaesthesia. In Atkinson, R.S. and Boulton, T.B. (eds.) *The History of Anaesthesia*, pp. 333–41. (New York and London: Royal Society of Medicine Services and The Parthenon Publishing Group)

Carrie, L.E. (1977). Conduction analgesia. In Stallworthy, J. and Bourne, G. (eds.) *Recent Advances in Obstetrics and Gynaecology*, Vol. 12, p. 314. (Edinburgh, London: Churchill Livingstone)

Cathelin, F. (1901). Un mot d'histoire a propos des injections epidurales par le canal sacre et notes anatomique. *C. R. Soc. Biol. (Paris)*, **53**, 597–9

Cervello, C. (1882). *Arch. per le Sc. Med.*, **6**, 177, quoted by Lee and Atkinson (1973) p. 128

Cleland, J.G.P. (1933). Paravertebral anesthesia in obstetrics, experimental and clinical basis. *Surg. Gynecol. Obstet.*, **57**, 51–4

Cleland, J.G.P. (1949). Continuous peridural and caudal analgesic in obstetrics. *Curr. Res. Anesth. Analg.*, **28**, 61–76

Cole, P.V. and Nainby-Luxmore, R.C. (1962). The hazards of gas and air in obstetrics. *Anaesthesia*, **17**, 505

Coleman, A.J. (1984). Inhalational anaesthetic agents. In Churchill-Davidson,H.C. (ed.) *Wylie and Churchill Davidsons 'A Practice of Anaesthesia'*, 5th edn. pp. 181 and 194. (London: Lloyd-Luke Medical Books)

Corning, J.L (1885). Spinal anaesthesia and local medication of the cord. *N.Y. State Med. J.*, **42**, 483

Corning, J.L. (1886). *Local Anesthesia.* (New York: Appleton)

Corssen, G. and Domino, E.F. (1960). Dissociative anesthesia: further pharmacologic studies and first clinical experiences with the phencyclidine derivative CL-581. *Anesth. Analg. Curr. Res.*, **45**, 29–40

Cotton, B.R. and Smith, G. (1982). The lower oesophageal sphincter. In Kaufman, L. (ed.) *Anaesthesia Review*, Vol. 1, pp. 65–75. (London: Churchill Livingstone)

Cotton, B.R. and Smith, G. (1984). Regurgitation and aspiration. In Kaufman, L. (ed.) *Anaesthesia Review*, Vol. 2, pp. 162–76. (Edinburgh: Churchill Livingstone)

Crawford, J.S. (1965). *Principles and Practice of Obstetric Anaesthesia*, 2nd edn. (Oxford: Blackwell Scientific Publications)

Crawford, J.S. (1972). The second thousand epidural blocks in an obstetric hospital practice. *Br. J. Anaesth.*, **44**, 1277–87

Crawford, J.S. (1973). Epidural drip and post-spinal headache.(c) *Br. J. Anaesth.*, **45**, 1177

Crawford, J.S. (1974). An appraisal of lumbar epidural blockade in patients with a singleton fetus presenting by the breech. *J. Obstet. Gynaecol. Br. Cwlth.*, **81**, 867

Crawford, J.S. (1979). Experience with spinal analgesia in a British obstetric unit. *Br. J. Anaesth.*, **51**, 531–5

Crile, G.W. (1897), quoted by Armstrong Davidson, (1970) p. 174

Crile, G.W. (1901). On the physiological action of cocaine and eucain when injected into tissues. *Experimental and Clinical Research into Certain Problems Relating to Surgical Operations*, pp. 88–163. (Philadelphia: J.B. Lippincott Co.)

Crile, G.W. (1908). Surgical aspects of Grave's disease with reference to the physic factor. *Ann. Surg.*, **47**, 864

Crum-Brown, A. and Fraser, T.R. (1868). On the connection between chemical constitution and physiological action. *Trans. R. Soc. Edin.*, **25**, 151

Curbello, M.M. (1949). Continuous peridural segmental anesthesia by means of an ureteral catheter. *Anesth. Analg. Curr. Res.*, **28**, 12

Davy, H. (1800). *Researches, Chemical and Philosophical: Chiefly concerning Nitrous Oxide or Dephlogisticated Nitrous Air and its Respiration*, p. 464. (London: Johnson)

Dawkins, C.J.M. (1969). Analysis of the complications of extradural and caudal block. *Anaesthesia*, **24**, 554–63

Dick-Read, G. (1933). *Natural Childbirth.* (London: Heinemann)

Dick-Read, G. (1944). *Childbirth Without Fear.* (London: Heinemann)

Dick-Read, G. (1960). *Childbirth Without Fear*, 4th edn. (London: Heinemann)

Dinnick, O.P. (1957). *Proc. R. Soc. Med.*, **50**, 547, quoted by Utting and Gray (1968) p. 80

Dogliotti, A.M. (1931). Eine neue methode der regionaren anesthesie 'Die peridurale segmentaire anesthesie'. *Zbl. Chir.*, **58**, 3141–5

Dogliotti, A.M. (1933). A new method of block; segmental peridural spinal anesthesia. *Am. J. Surg.*, **20**, 107

Dripps, R.D., Eckenhoff, J.E. and Vandam, L.D. (1961). *Introduction to Anaesthesia: The Principles of Safe Practice*, 2nd edn. pp. 154. (Philadelphia: W.B. Saunders Co.)

Dundee, J.W. and Wyant, G.M. (1974). *Intravenous Anaesthesia*, p. 1. (Edinburgh: Churchill Livingstone)

Einhorn, A. (1899). Ueber-die chemie der localen anaesthetica. *Munchen Med. Wchnschr.*, **46**, 1219–54

Eisenmenger, V. (1893), quoted by Calverley (1989) pp. 333–41

Elliotson, J. (1843). *Numerous Cases of Surgical Operations without Pain in the Mesmeric State.* (London: H. Bailliere)

Elsberg, C.A. (1911). Anaesthesia by the intratracheal insufflation of air and ether, a description of the technic of the method and of a portable apparatus for use in man. *Ann. Surg.*, **53**, 161–8

Esplen, J.R. (1952). A new apparatus for intermittent positive pressure inflation *Br. J. Anaesth.*, **24**, 303–11

Faraday, M. (1818). Effects of inhaling the vapour of sulfuric ether. *J. Sci. Arts*, **4**, 158

Finster, M., Poppers, P.J., Sinclair, J.C., Morishima, H.O. and Daniel, S.S. (1965). Accidental intoxication of the fetus with local anesthetic drug during caudal anesthesia. *Am. J. Obstet. Gynecol.*, **92**, 922–4

Flowers, C., Hellman, L.M. and Hingson, R.A. (1949). Continuous peridural anesthesia and analgesia for labor, delivery and caesarean section. *Curr. Res. Anesth. Analg.*, **28**, 181–9

Fourneau, E. (1904). Stovaine, anaesthetique locale. *Bull. Soc. Pharm. (Paris)*, **10**, 141

Frey, R. and Seeger, R. (1961). Experimental and clinical experiences with toxiferine (alkaloid of calabash-curare). *Can. Anaesth. Soc. J.*, **8**, 99–117

Fromherz, K. and Pellmond, B. (1952). *Experientia*, **8**, 394, quoted by Lee and Atkinson (1973) p. 116

Garrison, F.H. (1913). *An Introduction to the History of Medicine.* (Philadelphia: W.B. Saunders)

Gates, M. and Tschudi, G. (1957). *J. Am. Chem. Soc.*, **74**, 1109, quoted by Lee and Atkinson (1973) p. 103

Gauss, C.J. (1905). *Zentbl. Gynakol.*, 274, quoted by Lee and Atkinson (1973) p. 123

Gauss, C.J. (1906). *Arch. Gynekol.*, **78**, 579, quoted by Lee and Atkinson (1973) p. 123

Gauss, C.J. (1907). *Munch. Med. Wchnschr.*, (Jan) 23, quoted by Lee and Atkinson (1973) p. 123

Gellert, P. (1926). Aufhebung der Wehenschmerzen und Wehenuberdruck. *Monatschrift fur Wchnschr. Geburts. Gynakol. Berlin*, **73**, 143

Gellhorn (1927), quoted by Moir *et al.* (1986) p. 6

Gibbs, C.P., Hempling, R.E., Wynne, J.W. and Hood, C. I. (1979). Antacid pulmonary aspiration. *Anesthesiology*, **51**, S290

Gormley, J.B. (1960). Treatment of postspinal headache. *Anesthesiology*, **21**, 565

Gordh, T. (1948). Xylocaine; a new local analgesic. *Anaesthesia*, **4**, 4

Graffagnino, P. and Seyler, L.W. (1938). *Surg. Gynecol. Obstet.*, **35**, 597, quoted by Lee and Atkinson (1968) p. 627

Graham, H. (1950). *Eternal Eve*, p. 611. (London: Heinemann)

Griffith, H.R. and Johnson, G.E. (1942). The use of curare in general anaesthesia. *Anesthesiology*, **3**, 418–20

Guedel, A.E. (1912). *N.Y. Med. J.*, **95**, 387, quoted by Lee and Atkinson (1968) p. 627

Guedel, A.E. and Waters, R.M. (1928). A new intratracheal catheter. *Curr. Res. Anesth. Anal.*, **7**, 238–9

Gwathmey, J.T. (1913), quoted by Lee and Atkinson (1968) p. 111

Halsted, W.S. (1885). Practical comments on the use and abuse of cocaine; suggested by its invariably successful employment in more than a thousand minor surgical operations. *N.Y. Med. J.*, **42**, 483

Hayward-Butt, J.T. (1957). *Lancet*, **2**, 972, quoted by Utting and Gray (1968) p. 80

Hellman, K (1965). *Can. Anaesth. Soc. J.*, **12**, 398, quoted by Utting and Gray (1968) p. 80

Hewitt, F.W. (1896). The past, present, and future of anaesthesia. *The Practitioner*, **57**, 347

Hickman, H.H. (1824). *A letter on suspended animation, containing experiments showing that it may be safely employed during operations on animals, with the view of ascertaining its probable utility in surgical operations on the human subject.* (Ironbridge: W. Smith)

Hingson, R.A. and Edwards, W.B. (1943). Continuous caudal anesthesia in obstetrics. *J. Am. Med. Assoc.*, **121**, 225

Holmes, J.M. (1957). *Proc. R. Soc. Med.*, **50**, 556, quoted by Lee and Atkinson (1973) p. 640

Hughes, R. (1989). Neuromuscular blocking agents. In Atkinson, R.S. and Bolton, T.B. (eds.) *The History of Anaesthesia*, pp. 257–67. (London and New York: Royal Society of Medicine Services and The Parthenon Publishing Group)

Husemeyer, R.P., Davenport, H.T. and Rajasekaran, T. (1978). Cimetidine as a single oral dose for prophylaxis against Mendelson's syndrome. *Anaesthesia*, **33**, 775–8

Jackson, D. (1934), quoted by Moir *et al.* (1986) p. 4

Johnstone, M. (1956). The human cardiovascular response to Flouthane anaesthesia. *Br. J. Anaesth.*, **28**, 392–410

Junker, F.A. (1867). Description of a new apparatus for administering narcotic vapours. *Med. Tms. Gaz.*, **2**, 590

King, H. (1935). Curare. *Nature (London)*, **135**, 469

King, H. (1935). Curare alkaloids. 1 Tubocurarine. *J. Chem. Soc.*, 1381–9

King, R. (1916). Perineal anesthesia in labour. *Surg. Gynecol. Obstet.*, **23**, 615–18

Kirstein, A. (1895), quoted by Calverley, R.K (1989) p. 336

Klikowitch, H. (1881). *Arch. Gynaekol.*, **18**, 81 [See also Richards, W., Parbrook, G.D. and Wilson, J.D. (1976). Stanislav Klikowitch (1853–1910) Pioneer of nitrous oxide and oxygen analgesia. *Anaesthesia*, **31**, 933–40]

Klink, E.W. (1953). *Obstet. Gynecol. N.Y.*, **1**, 137, quoted by Utting and Gray (1968) p. 80

Kobak, A.J., Evans, E.F. and Johnson, G.R. (1956). *Am. J. Obstet. Gynecol.*, **71**, 981, quoted by Utting and Gray (1968) p. 80

Koller, C. (1884a). Vorlaeufige Mittheilung Uber Locale anaesthesierung am auge. *Klin. Monatsbl. Augenh.*, **42**, 294

451

Koller, C. (1884b). Ueber die Verwendung des Cocain zur anasthesierung am Auge. *Wien. med. Blatter.*, **7**, 1352–5

Kreis, A. (1900). Uber Medullarnarkose bei Gebärenden. *Zentbl. Gynakol.*, July, 742

Kuhn, F. (1905). Perorale Tubagen mit und ohne *Druck. D. Z. f. Chir.*, **76**,148

Kuhn, F. (1911). *Die Perorale Intubation.* (Berlin: S. Karger)

Lamaze, F. (1972). *Painless Childbirth: The Lamaze Method.* (New York: Pocket Books)

Lean, T.H. *et al.* (1968). *J. Obstet. Gynaecol. Br. Cwlth.*, **75**, 856, quoted by Lee and Atkinson (1973) p. 272

Leboyer, F. (1975). *Birth Without Violence.* (New York: A. Knopf)

Lee, J.A. and Atkinson, R.S. (1968). *A Synopsis of Anaesthesia*, 6th edn. pp. 1, 11, 98, 104 and 196. (Bristol: John Wright & Sons Ltd)

Lee, J.A. and Atkinson, R.S. (1973). *A Synopsis of Anaesthesia*, 7th edn. p. 5. (Bristol: John Wright and Sons Ltd and the English Language Book Society)

Lee, A.J., Atkinson, R.S. and Macintosh, R.R. Sir. (1978). *Lumbar Puncture and Spinal Analgesia Intradural and Extradural*, 4th edn. (Edinburgh, London, New York: Churchill Livingstone)

Lemmon, W.T. (1940). A method of continuous spinal anaesthesia. *Ann. Surg.*, **111**, 141

Liebreich, M.E.O. (1869). *Das Chloralhydrat ein neues Hypnoticum und Anastheticum* Berlin, quoted by Lee and Atkinson (1973) p. 119

Liston, R. (1846) cited in Garrison (1913), p. 452

Long, C.W. (1849). An account of the first use of sulphuric ether by inhalation as an anaesthetic in surgical operations. *South Med. Surg.*, **5**, 705

Lubic, R.W. and Ernst, E.K.M. (1975). Psychological analgesia (natural childbirth and psychoprophylaxis). In Bonica, J.J. (ed.) *Obstetric Analgesia-Anaesthesia, Clinical Obstetrics and Gynaecology*, Vol. 3, p. 533. (Philadelphia: W.B. Saunders)

Lundy, J.S. (1935). Intravenous anesthesia: preliminary report of the use of two new Thiobarbiturates. *Proc. Mayo Clinic*, **10**, 536

McCawley, E.L., Hart, E.H. and Marsh, D.F. (1941). *J. Am. Chem. Soc.*, **63**, 314, quoted by Lee and Atkinson (1973) p. 115

MacEwan, W. (1880). Clinical observations on the introduction of tracheal tubes by the mouth instead of performing tracheotomy or laryngotomy. *Br. Med. J.*, **2**, 122–4, 163–5

Macintosh, R.R. (1943). A new laryngoscope. *Lancet*, **1**, 485

Macintosh, R.R., Sir Lee, A.J. and Atkinson, R.S. (1978). *Lumbar Puncture and Spinal Analgesia Intradural and Extradural*, 4th edn. (Edinburgh, London, New York: Churchill Livingstone)

McKechnie, F.B. and Converse, J.G. (1955). *Am. J. Obstet. Gynecol.*, **70**, 639, quoted by Utting and Gray (1968) p. 80

Marggravius, G. (1648). Historiae rerum naturalium Brasiliae libri octo. In Piso, G. (ed.) *De medicina Brasiliensi libri quatuor*, p. 2. (Leiden: Hackius)

von Martius, C.F. (1830). Ueber die Bereitung des Pfeilgiftes Urari bei den Indianern Juris am Rio Yupura in Nordbrasilien. In Buchner von (ed.) *Repertorium fur die Pharmacie*, Vol. 36, pp. 337–53. (Nuremberg: Schrag)

Meltzer and Auer (1909). Continuous respiration without respiratory movements. *J. Exp. Med.*, **11**, 622–5

Mendelson, C.L. (1946). Aspiration of stomach contents into lungs during obstetric anesthesia. *Am. J. Obstet. Gynecol.*, **52**, 191–204

Mesmer, F.A. (1799). *Memoire sur la Decouverte du Magnetisme Animal.* (Geneve, Paris: P.F. Didot Le Jeune)

Miller, R.A. (1941). A new laryngoscope. *Anesthesiology*, **2**, 317–20

Minnitt, R.J. (1934). Self administered analgesia for the midwifery of general practice. *Proc. Soc. Med.*, **27**, 1313

Minnitt, R.J. (1938). *Gas and Air Analgesia.* (London: Balliere Tindall and Cox)

Mohan, J. and Potter, J.M. (1975). Pupillary constriction and ptosis following caudal epidural analgesia, quoted by Carrie (1977) p. 314

Moir, D.D. and Willocks, J. (1968). Epidural analgesia in British obstetrics. *Br. J. Anaesth.*, **40**, 129

Moir, D.D. and Davidson, S. (1972). Post-partum complications of forceps delivery performed under epidural and pudendal nerve block. *Br. J. Anaesth.*, **44**, 1197–9

Moir, D.D., Thorburn, J. and Whittle, M.J. (1986). *Obstetric Anaesthesia and Analgesia*, pp. 1–8. (London, Philadelphia: Baillière Tindall)

Moore, J. (1784). *Method of Preventing or Diminishing Pain in Several Operations of Surgery.* (London: T. Cadell)

Moore, J. and Dundee, J.W. (1961). *Br. J. Anaesth.*, **33**, 422, quoted by Utting and Gray (1968) p. 80

Moreno y Maiz, T. (1868). *Recherches Chimiques et Physiologiques, sur L'erythroxylum Coca du Prou et la Cocaine.* (Paris: L. Leclerc)

Morton, W.T.G. (1846). Circular. *Mortons Letheon.* (Boston: Dutton & Wentworth)

Morton, W.T.G. (1847). *Remarks on the Proper Mode of Administering Sulphuric Ether by Inhalation.* (Boston: Dalton and Wentworth)

Nagai, N. (1887). Ephedrine. *Pharmazeut. Zeitung*, **32**, 700

Niemann, A. (1860). *Ueber eine Neue Organische Base in den Coca Blaettern* (Goettingen: E.A. Huth)

Nussbaum, J.N. (1884), quoted by Atkinson *et al.* (1982) p.104

Ockerblad, N.F. and Dillon, T.G. (1927). The use of ephedrine in spinal anesthesia. *J. Am. Med. Assoc.*, **88**, 1135

O'Dwyer, J. (1885). Intubation of the larynx. *N. Y. Med. J.*, **42**, 145–7

Ore, P.C. (1872). Des injection intraveineuses de chloral. *Bull. Soc. Chirurgie. Paris*, **1**, 400–12

Organe, G.S.W. (1949). Decamethonium iodide (bistrimethylammonium decane diiodide) in anaesthesia. *Lancet*, **1**, 773

Organe, G.S.W., Paton, W.D.M. and Zaimis, E.J. (1949). Preliminary trials of bistrimethyl ammonium decane and pentane di iodide (C10 and C55) in man. *Lancet*, **1**, 21–3

Ostheimer, G.W., Palahniuk, R.J. and Shnider, S.M. (1974). Epidural blood patch for postlumbar puncture headache (c). *Anesthesiology*, **41**, 307–8

Pagés, F. (1921). Anesthesia matamerica. *Rev. Sandidad. Milit. (Madrid)*, **11**, 351–85

Paracelsus, A.P.T. (1603). Opera medico-chimicorum sive paradoxorum, tomus genuinus primus. Agens de caussis, origine ac curatione moroborum in genere. (Nobili Francofurto)

Pearson, J.F. and Davies, P. (1974). The effect of continuous lumbar epidural analgesia upon fetal acid-base status during the first stage of labour. *J. Obstet. Gynaecol. Br. Cwlth.*, **81**, 971 and 975

Phillips, A.P. (1949). Synthetic curare substitutes from aliphatic dicarboxylic acid aminoethyl esters. *J. Am. Chem. Soc.*, **71**, 3264

Porten, E. von der (1930). Das Narkoseproblem in der Praxis. *Die Medizinische Welt*, **52**, 1855–9

Priestley, J. (1779–86). Experiments and Observations Relating to Various Branches of Natural Philosophy, with a Continuation of the Observations on Air. London and Birmingham, quoted by Warren and Van Dam (1963) p. 276

Raventos, J. (1956). The action of Flouthane – a new volatile anaesthetic. *Br. J. Pharmacol. Chemother.*, **11**, 394–410

Reynolds, F.N. (1934). *The Relief of Pain in Childbirth.* (London: Heinemann)

Rice, G.G. and Harwell Dabbs, C. (1950). The use of peridural and subarachnoid injections of saline solution in the treatment of severe postspinal headache. *Anaesthesiology*, **11**, 17–23

Roberts, R.B. and Shirley, M.A. (1974). Reducing the risk of acid aspiration during caesarean section. *Anesth. Analg. (Cleveland Oh.)*, **53**, 859–68

Robiquet (1832). Codeine phosphate. In Lee, J.A. and Atkinson, R.S. (eds.) *A Synopsis of Anaesthesia*, 7th edn. pp. 107. (Bristol: John Wright & Sons Ltd. and The English Language Book Society)

Rosenfeld, S.S. (1945). Paracervical anesthesia for the relief of labor pain. *Am. J. Obstet. Gynecol.*, **50**, 527–30

Rudolf, R.D. and Graham, J.D. (1927). Notes on the sulfate of ephedrine. *Am. J. Med. Sci.*, **173**, 399

Sahli, H. (1909). *Ther Mh. (Halbruch)*, **23**, 1, quoted by Lee and Atkinson (1973) p. 108

Savage, D.S., Sleight, I. and Carlyle, I. (1967), quoted by Hughes, R. (1989) pp. 257–67

Schaumann, O. and Eisleb, O. (1939). *D. Med. Wchnschr.*, **65**, 967, quoted by Lee and Atkinson (1973) p. 108

Schnider, S.M. (1973), quoted by Carrie (1977) p. 309

Scott, J.S. and Gadd, R.L. (1957). *Br. Med. J.*, 1, 971, quoted by Utting and Gray (1968) p. 80

Scudamore, J.H. and Yates, M.J. (1966). Pudendal block – a misnomer? *Lancet*, 1, 23–4

Scurr, C.F. (1950). Use of suxamethonium iodide in anaesthesia for peroral endoscopy. *Br. Med. J.*, 2, 1311

Secher, O. (1989). Chloroform to a royal family. In Atkinson, R.S. and Boulton, T.B. (eds.) *The History of Anaesthesia*, p. 242. (London and New York: Royal Society of Medicine Services and The Parthenon Publishing Group)

Sellick, B.A. (1961). Cricoid pressure to control regurgitation of stomach contents during induction of anaesthesia. *Lancet*, 2, 404–6

Serturner, F.W.A. (1806). Darstellung der reinen Mohnsaure (Opiumsaure) nebst-einer chemischen untersuchung des opiums. Tromsdorff. *J. Pharm.*, 14, 47, 93

Serturner, F.W. (1817). Ueber das morphium, eine neue salzfaehinge grundlage, und die mekonsaeure als haubtbestandtheil des opiums. *Gilbert's Ann. D. Physik.*, 55, 56

Seward, E.H. (1949). *Proc. R. Soc. Med.*, 42, 745, quoted by Lee and Atkinson (1973) p. 439

Sicard, A. (1901). Sur les injections epidurales sacro-coccygiennes. *C. R. Soc. Biol. (Paris)*, 53, 479–81

Simpson, Sir J.Y. (1847a). Discovery of a new anaesthetic agent, more efficient than sulphuric ether. *Lon. Med. Caz. N.S. 5*, 934 [also in *Lancet*, 2, 549]

Simpson, Sir J.Y. (1847b). *Account of a New Anaesthetic Agent as a Substitute for Sulphuric Ether in Surgery and Midwifery*. (Edinburgh: Sutherland and Knox)

Skinner, T. (1862). Anaesthesia in midwifery with a new apparatus for its safer and more economical induction by chloroform. *Br. Med. J.*, 2, 108–11

Sliom, C.M., Frankel, L. and Holbrook, R.A. (1962). *Br. J. Anaesth.*, 34, 316, quoted by Utting and Gray (1968) p. 80

Smith, S.E. (1979). Sedative and hypnotic drugs and intravenous anaesthetics. In Churchill-Davidson, H.C. (ed.) *Wylie and Churchill-Davidson's*

A Practice of Anaesthesia, p. 751. (London: Lloyd-Luke Medical Books Ltd.)

Snow, J. (1848). On the inhalation of chloroform and ether with description of an apparatus. *Lancet*, 1, 177

Stallworthy, J. (1971). Obstetric anaesthesia (c). *Br. Med. J.*, 1, 287

Stenlake, J.B. (1978). Biodegradable neuromuscular blocking agents. In Stoclet, J.C. (ed.) *Advances in Pharmacology and Therapeutics. Ions-Cyclic Nucleotides-Cholinergy*, Vol. 3, pp. 303–11. (Oxford: Pergamon Press)

Stephen, C.R. and Fabian, L.W. (1989). Introduction of halothane to the USA. In Atkinson, R.S. and Boulton, T.B. (eds.) *The History of Anaesthesia*, p. 221. (London and New York: Royal Society of Medicine Services and The Parthenon Publishing Group)

Stiasny (1910), quoted by Moir *et al.* (1986) p. 6

Stoekel, von W. (1909). Uber Sakrale Anaesthesie. *Zbl. Chirurg.*, 33, 1

Striker (1935), quoted by Moir *et al.* (1986) p. 4

Telivuo, L. (1963). A new long-acting local anaesthetic solution for pain relief after thoracotomy. *Ann. Chir. et Gynnec. Fenniae*, 52, 513

Trendelenburg, F. (1869), quoted by Armstrong Davidson (1965) p. 104

Tuffier, T. (1899). Analgesie chirurgicale par l'injection sous arachnoidienne lombaire de cocaine. *C. R. seanc. Soc. Biol. Paris*, 51, 882

Tunstall, M.E. (1961). Use of a fixed nitrous oxide and oxygen. *Lancet*, 2, 964

Tuohy, E.B. (1945). Continuous spinal anesthesia; a new method utilising a ureteral catheter. *Surg. Clin. N. Am.*, 25, 834

Uhlmann, T. (1929). *Narkose und Anaesthesie*, 6, 168

Utting, J.E. and Gray, T.C. (1968). Obstetric anaesthesia and analgesia. *Br. Med. Bull.*, 24, 80–6

Vellay, P. (1959). *Childbirth without Pain* (English translation). (London: Hutchinson and George Allen and Unwin)

Virtue, R.W., Lund, L.O., Phelphs, M.Jr., Vogel, J., Beckwitt, H. and Heron, M. (1966). Difludromethyl 1, 1,2- Trifluoro-2-chloroethyl ether. As an anaesthetic agent: results with dogs and a preliminary note on observations with man. *(Canad). Anaesth. Soc. J.*, **13**, 233

Von Steinbuchel, N. (1902), quoted in Lee and Atkinson (1968) p. 622

Warren, R. and Vandam, L.D. (1963). Anaesthesia. In Warren, R. (ed.) *Surgery*, pp. 276–313. (Philadelphia, London: W.B. Saunders Co).

Waterton, C. (1879). *Wanderings in South America*, pp. 133–8. (London: Macmillan)

Watt, J.D., Philipp, E.E. and Pateman, M.T. (1959). Low spinal anaesthesia in obstetrics. *J. Obstet. Gynaecol. Br. Emp.*, *LXVI*, 424–33

Weese, H. and Scharpff, W. (1932). Evipan, ein neuartiges Einschlafmittel. *D. med. Wchnschr.*, **58**, 1205

Weinstein, M.L. (1939). *Curr. Res. Anesth.*, **18**, 221, quoted by Lee and Atkinson (1973) p. 129

Wells, H. (1847). *A History of the Discovery of the Application of Nitrous Oxide Gas, Ether, and Other Vapours to Surgical Operations.* (Hartford: J.G. Wells)

Westhorpe, R. (1989). Chloroform inhaler in the Geoffrey Kaye museum. In Atkinson, R.S. and Boulton, T.B. (eds.) *The History of Anaesthesia*, pp. 325–7. (London and New York: Royal Society of Medicine Services and The Parthenon Publishing Group)

Wood, A. (1855). A new method of treating neuralgia by direct application of opiates to the painful points. *Edin. Med. J.*, **82**, 265

Wylie, W.D. and Churchill-Davidson, H.C. (1984). Anaesthetic equipment – a historical perspective. In Churchill-Davidson, H.C. (ed.) *A Practice of Anaesthesia*, 5th edn. pp. 1157–87. (London: Lloyd-Luke Ltd.)

Wylie, W.D. (1955). *Proc. R. Soc. Med.*, **48**, 1089, quoted by Utting and Gray (1968) p. 80

FURTHER READING

Armstrong-Davison, M.H. (1965). *The Evolution of Anaesthesia.* (Altringham: John Sherratt and Son Ltd)

Atkinson, R.S. (1970). The 'lost' diaries of John Snow. *Proceedings of the 4th World Congress of Anaesthesia*, 197–9. (Rotterdam: Excerpta Medica)

Atkinson, R.S. (1985). Spinal intradural analgesia. In Atkinson, R.S. and Adams, A.P. (eds.) *Recent Advances in Anaesthesia and Analgesia.* (Edinburgh, London, Melbourne, New York: Churchill Livingstone)

Atkinson, R.S. and Boulton, T.B. (eds.) (1989). *The History of Anaesthesia.* (London, New York: Royal Society of Medicine Services and Parthenon Publishing)

Brownlee, A. (1911). History of Spinal Anaesthesia. *Practitioner*, Feb. 214

Browne, F.J. (1950). Relief of pain in childbirth. In *Postgraduate Obstetrics and Gynaecology*, p. 211. (London: Butterworth & Co. Ltd)

Calverley, R.K (1989). Intubation in anaesthesia. In Atkinson, R.S. and Boulton, T.B. (eds.) *The History of Anaesthesia*, pp. 333–41. (New York and London: Royal Society of Medicine Services and The Parthenon Publishing Group)

Claye, A.M. (1939). *The Evolution of Obstetric Analgesia.* (New York: Oxford University Press).

Clover, J.T. (1871). Discussion on ether and chloroform as anaesthetics. *Med. Tms. Gaz.*, **1**, 604

Cotton, B.R. and Smith, G. (1984). Regurgitation and aspiration. In Kaufman, L. (ed.) *Anaesthesia Review*, Vol. 2, pp. 162–76. (Edinburgh: Churchill Livingstone)

Keys, T.E. (1945). *The History of Surgical Anesthesia*, pp. 8–9. (New York: Schuman)

Lee, J.A. and Atkinson, R.S. (1973). *A Synopsis of Anaesthesia*, 7th edn. (Bristol: John Wright & Sons Ltd. and The English Language Book Society)

Lundy, S.J. and Tovell, R.M. (1934). Some of the newer local and general anesthetic agents, methods of their administration. *Northw. Med. (Seattle)*, **33**, 308–11

McGrew, R.E. (1985). *Encyclopedia of Medical History.* (London: Macmillan Press)

Macintosh, R., Sir, Lee, A.J. and Atkinson, R.S. (1978). *Lumbar Puncture and Spinal Analgesia Intradural and Extradural.* (Edinburgh, London, New York: Churchill Livingstone)

Moir, D.D., Thorburn, J. and Whittle, M.J. (1986). History of Obstetric Anaesthesia. In *Anaesthesia and Analgesia*, 3rd edn. pp. 1–8. (London, Philadelphia: Balliere Tindall)

Thomas, T.A. (1989). Self administered inhalation analgesia in obstetrics. In Atkinson, R.S. and Boulton, T.B. (eds.) *The History of Anaesthesia*, pp.

295–8. (London and New York: Royal Society of Medicine Services and The Parthenon Publishing Group)

Utting, J.E. and Gray, T.C. (1968). Obstetric anaesthesia and analgesia. *Br. Med. Bull.*, **24**, 80–6

Warren, R. and Vandam, L.D. (1963). Anaesthesia. In Warren, R. (ed.) *Surgery*, pp. 276–313. (Philadelphia, London: W.B. Saunders Co.)

Wells, H.A. (1847). *A History of the Discovery of the Application of Nitrous Oxide Gas, Ether and other Vapours to Surgical Operations.* (Hartford: J Gaylord Wells)

Westhorpe, R. (1989). The chloroform inhalers in the Geoffrey Kaye Museum. In Atkinson, R.S. and Bolton, T.B. (eds.) *History of Anaesthesia*, pp. 325–27. (New York and London: Royal Society of Medicine Services and The Parthenon Publishing Group)

Wilkinson, D.J. (1984). Anaesthetic equipment – A Historical Perspective. In Wylie, W.D. and Churchill-Davidson, H.C. (eds.) A *Practice of Anaesthesia*, 5th edn. p. 1157. (London: Lloyd-Luke Ltd.)

Family planning

Nature has provided its own family planning restraints in that the woman is fertile for a limited period in each cycle; reproductive capacity is restricted to the time span between menarche and the menopause; breast feeding inhibits ovulation; and some couples fail to achieve pregnancy. Until relatively recent times the death rates in pregnancy, infancy, childhood and adulthood were high, so large numbers of children were required to ensure continuance of the race. At various times, in different societies, when the number of survivors imperilled the natural food resources, failed contraceptive measures were complemented by the use of abortion or infanticide to combat overpopulation.

EARLY METHODS

In preliterate times herbs and aqueous extracts of plants were used for their contraceptive properties and it is now known for instance that extracts of the Yam family have progestational properties. The native North American Indian is known to have taken herbal remedies, such as those extracted from roots of spotted cowbane, for contraception. Vaginal douching with lemon juice and extracts of mahogany husk was popular, and the lemon's citric acid plus the astringent action of the husks would have been highly spermicidal (Robertson, 1990). Lactational amenorrhoea provided a natural, if unreliable, source of family planning.

Egypt

In ancient Egypt, various intravaginal preparations were used for both barrier and spermicidal effects. Professor Himes (1963) considered that the oldest prescription for family planing is contained within the Petrie or Kahun Papyrus which was written c.1850 BC. Further information was contained in the Ebers Papyrus c.1550 BC and the Berlin Papyrus c.1300 BC. The contraceptive preparations were fashioned into pessaries, or applied as pastes to the vagina and cervix. The dung of crocodile or elephant was popularly used and pessaries of honey with natron, or tips of the acacia tree which contain gum arabic and release lactic acid when fermented, were used. The addition of honey with its adhesive and barrier properties combined with the spermicidal effect of the lactic acid to produce a contraceptive effect.

Greece

Aristotle was the first Greek writer to mention contraception, and he advised intravaginal use of olive oil. A later Greek physician, Dioscorides, listed herbal preparations mixed with honey and fashioned into a pessary (Greek, small stone). The ancient Greeks practised postcoital contraception by squatting and then increasing intraabdominal pressure in an effort to clear the vagina of seminal deposit. They also used a variety of pastes and local applications including oil, honey, cedar gum, myrtle oil, pine bark, pulverized pomegranate and wool tampons impregnated with wine and other extracts. Coitus interruptus and digital vaginal cleansing were also practised. The observation of Hippocrates that fat women tended to be infertile antedated observations on polycystic ovaries by millennia. Abortion was practised as a method of fertility control by both Greek and Roman civilizations and Hippocrates described insertion of substances through the cervix using a hollow lead tube, while the Romans used duck quills for similar purposes.

Hebrews

The ancient Hebrews practised sexual continence, and also used barrier pessaries such as the cotton tampon *mokh* . They also appeared to have some understanding of the fertile segment of the cycle, as Moses specified a lapse of 7 days from the end of menstruation as the time to achieve fruitfulness.

Islamic culture

During the Middle Ages Europe was dominated by the Roman Catholic Church and knowledge of contraception, medicine and science was restricted. This was not the case however in the Islamic world, where religious law did not forbid contraception. Birth control measures included the expulsion of semen from the vagina by violent body movement; use of various intravaginal fumigations; and vaginal contraceptive suppositories. In the sixth century Aetius of Amida (502–575) recommended washing the penis in vinegar or salt solution prior to intercourse. Both preparations are known to be spermicidal. Condoms of animal membrane were used intravaginally. Rhazes (died circa 923–927) was a famous physician during that time and wrote a text on the history of contraception. He advised coitus interruptus, the prevention of ejaculation, and drugs to block the cervix or expel semen. Fifteen different types of vaginal contraceptive suppositories were described in his text.

'Roman Catholic' Europe

In Europe, the Roman Catholic Church was heavily influenced by the teachings of Saint Augustine (AD 354–430) and Saint Thomas Aquinas (AD 1225–1274) who both argued against birth control. St Augustine condemned contraception for all, including married couples. The Roman Catholic Church adopted this teaching, and through its influence had a profound effect on European customs and belief. During the Middle Ages, Saint Thomas Aquinas re-addressed the problem, and concluded that the marriage act was sinful if the possibility of pregnancy was obstructed in any way. At a later time natural methods of family planning were allowed by the Roman Catholic Church, but the Papal encyclical, *Humanae Vitae* (1968) again condemned artificial contraception.

The strict anti-birth-control view was partially reversed in the eighteenth and nineteenth centuries. During that era the classics of Greece and Rome were rediscovered and the advent of new printing techniques meant that medical and other texts became more readily available. The population became educated about family planning methods of the preAugustine period.

THE BIRTH CONTROL MOVEMENT

With the advent of the industrial revolution in the eighteenth and nineteenth centuries, food supplies increased, diseases were controlled, and death rates began to fall. More children survived and they in turn had children themselves. The introduction of artificial milk formulae disrupted the natural infertility of breast feeding, and alternative methods of family spacing became necessary. The inadequate facilities of the time sometimes led to criminal abortion, with its appalling maternal mortality rate.

The British economist, Thomas Robert Malthus (Figure 1) published his *Essay on the Principle of Population* in 1798, in which he argued that populations tend to increase faster than food supplies. He advocated delayed marriage and strict premarital chastity, which he called 'moral restraint'. Marriage was allowed for 12- and 14-year-olds, and extramarital sex was very common in England at that time. Malthus was one of the first to apply the principle of statistics to population growth, the term for which – 'demography' – was first used in 1880. The birth control movement which followed was heavily influenced by Malthus' theories and writings and met with stiff opposition in Europe and America which continued until recent times.

The strict European approach to contraception was later carried to the New World. Those

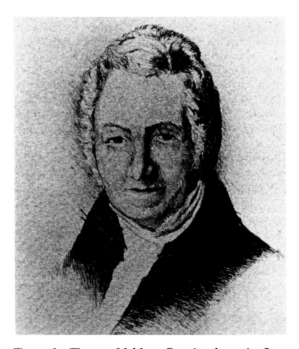

Figure 1 Thomas Malthus. Drawing by artist Scott Fuller, from a portrait by J. Linnell, 1833 (*see* text)

who adopted an anti-birth-control stance, found a champion in Anthony Comstock. One of ten children, he was born in Connecticut in 1844, and was said to have been heavily influenced by his mother who was a strict Puritan. He spent a large part of his life waging war on the emerging birth control movement in America, which he saw as an evil force. Many influential and wealthy people were attracted to his cause, and legislators introduced strict anticontraceptive laws in many of the states. The last of the so called 'Comstock' laws prohibiting contraception was finally struck down in 1973.

An early advocate of the use of contraception in the USA was Robert Dale Owen of Indiana. He had travelled extensively in Europe and discovered that various methods of family planning were in use there, particularly in France. He later became elected to the Indiana Assembly. At that time attitudes were very much of a puritanical nature with a strong anticontraceptive bias. A doctor Charles Knowlton who was influenced by Owen's procontraceptive attitude was prosecuted and spent 3 months in jail for his work on family planning.

During the early part of the twentieth century the birth control movement in America found their champion in Margaret Higgins Sanger. Her father was an Irish agnostic immigrant, and her mother, who gave birth to 11 children, died of tuberculosis at 48. Margaret Sanger blamed excessive childbearing as the cause of her mother's excessive frailty and early death. Sanger worked as a nurse in the tenements of New York, and was deeply disturbed by the misery and suffering she found in the large immigrant families. Having observed the death of a woman due to criminal abortion she resolved to 'do something to change the destiny of mothers' and espoused the birth control cause. Sanger researched the available literature on contraception and soon produced pamphlets, and lectured extensively on the benefits of contraceptive methods and their potential to decrease abortion rates. Her first birth control clinic opened in Brownsville, Brooklyn in 1916.

In general terms the American medical profession was hostile to the cause. Margaret Sanger was fortunate to enlist the help of Dr Robert Dickson, president of the American Gynecologic Society, who, although working within the contraceptive laws of the time, influenced the medical profession to become involved in the whole area of family planning.

On the other side of the Atlantic the birth control movement in Britain had its foundation in the early part of the nineteenth century. Frances Place (1771–1854), who was born to a large family and himself fathered 15 children, became interested in the work of Malthus and later published pamphlets on family limitation using coitus interruptus and an intravaginal sponge method. The work of Place influenced Richard Carlisle who in 1826 published *Everywoman's Book: What is Love?*, the first book in English to discuss the economic, social and medical aspects of family limitation. In 1887 Dr H.A. Allbutt, a physician in Edinburgh, published a pamphlet *The Wife's Handbook* which included a section on contraception. Although the pamphlet was a great success Allbutt had his name removed from the list of Fellows of the Royal College of Physicians of Edinburgh as a consequence of his declared interest in that forbidden topic. Other campaigners included Charles Bradlaugh, Annie Besant and Edward Truelove, who at various stages faced court proceedings due to their writing or publishing of material relating to the subject of contraception. Due to their work however, the distribution of contraceptive material in England became legal from the late nineteenth century. In 1915 Marie Stopes met Margaret Sanger (Figure 2) and later developed a lifelong commitment to the birth control movement. The

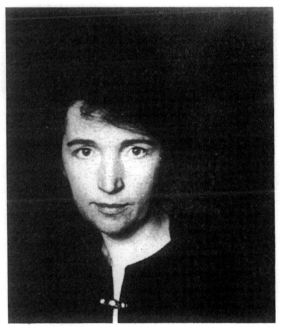

Figure 2 Margaret Sanger. Courtesy of the New Haven Colony Historical Society (*see* text)

Marie Stopes Clinic was opened in the Holloway district of London in 1921 (Figure 3).

Until the early 1960s the provision of family planning services did not fall within the remit of the average general practitioner or gynaecologist. The majority of medical schools did not carry the subject of birth control on their curricula, and when the subject was first introduced students attended in a voluntary capacity. The advent of the oral contraceptive pill in 1962 changed the climate. The 'pill' first became available on private prescription, but the Department of Health and Social Services introduced a 'doctors' charter' which allowed general practitioners a special fee for providing family planning services to women in the National Health Service. As early versions of the pill were soon reported to have dramatic side-effects, the medical profession became involved in health screening of the women who required oral contraceptive prescriptions on a first or repeat basis.

The provision of family planning services in other countries varied markedly. Despite its religious background, France had an ambivalent attitude to religion and sexuality, and family planning methods were widely practised there although they were not available in the UK and America. Japan became the first country to take national action on family planning when in 1948 the government legalized both contraception and abortion. India supported its national birth control programme from the early 1950s, and Pakistan began their birth control programme in 1959. In the early 1960s Korea and Taiwan began birth control programmes and the oral contraceptive became available 'across the counter' without a medical prescription. Similar programmes were developed in many other countries.

In review articles, Malcolm Potts and Alan Rosenfield (1990a;b) assessed the world-wide provision of family planning services in the pre and post-1965 eras. They chose the year 1965 as it was then that Sir Dugald Baird, Professor of Obstetrics and Gynaecology in Aberdeen, coined the term 'the fifth freedom'. The other basic human freedoms were listed by President Roosevelt in the 1940s – freedom of speech and worship, and freedom from want and fear. Baird's fifth freedom was that of 'freedom from the tyranny of excess fertility'. Potts and Rosenfield advocated the use of contraceptive agents to help control family size so that individuals and societies could reach their full potential, and they further indicated that family planning would reduce the number of therapeutic and criminal abortions. Also addressed in their articles were, the development of the various national and international family planning agencies; the support from industrialized nations to 'the cause' and the positive value of effective family planning measures in combating the spread of the human immunodeficiency virus.

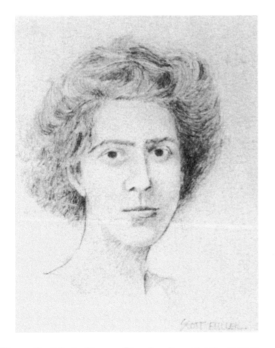

Figure 3 Marie Stopes. Drawing by artist Scott Fuller

NATURAL FAMILY PLANNING

'Natural family planning refers to techniques for planning or preventing pregnancies by observation of the naturally occurring signs and symptoms of the fertile and infertile phases of the menstrual cycle. It is implicit in the definition of natural family planning, when used to avoid pregnancies, that there is abstinence from sexual intercourse during the fertile phase of the menstrual cycle' (WHO, 1979).

A later definition differed slightly ' . . . when used to avoid conception that drugs, devices, and surgical procedures are not used, there is abstinence from sexual intercourse during the fertile phase of the menstrual cycle and the act of intercourse, when it occurs, is complete'.

Despite the clarity of the WHO definition,

some couples also used other forms of family planning, such as coitus interruptus or condoms, during the fertile period, and the mixture of methods used introduced difficulties in the scientific study of natural family planning. Couples who used natural family planning alone had to understand the concept of a fertile period in a current menstrual cycle, and modify their coital activity subsequently. The development of natural family planning educational programmes and training of qualified natural family planning teachers began in the mid-1950s, and Martin in 1975 was a major contributor to the development of educational modules. The World Health Organization became involved in 1975 and developed natural family planning programmes around the world. Comparative analyses of retrospective and prospective studies have been published in detail (Lanctot, 1979; Flynn, 1984). The various methods studied showed method failures of 0.77 – 5%. Three important factors contributed to success or failure – motivation, efficient teaching of the method and the characteristics of the women involved. The following methods of natural family planning have evolved.

The basal body temperature method

The basal body temperature method evolved from research in the nineteenth century by Squire (1868) and also Jacobi. They documented an increase in the basal body temperature in the second half of the cycle. van de Velde (1928) showed the relationship between temperature change and the corpus luteum. In the mid-1930s and early 1940s the 0.3 – 0.5°C rise in temperature was correlated with hormonal and endometrial changes resulting from ovulation. Palmer popularized the basal body temperature method in French-speaking countries (Palmer and Devillers, 1939; Palmer, 1949), and Marshall (1963) helped to promote it in the English-speaking world.

Cervical mucus methods

This form of natural family planning is eponymously associated with Drs John and Evelyn Billings of Australia who proposed their ovulation method or 'Billings Technique' in the early 1970s and introduced an Atlas of the Ovulation Method (Billings and Billings, 1973; Billings et al.,1972; 1977).

The appearance of cervical mucus during the menstrual cycle was probably first described in detail by Pouchet (1847), although Alfred Donne (1836) had documented the presence of sperm in cervical mucus during his microscopic investigations of *Trichomonas vaginalis*. Seguy and Simonnet (1933) and Viergiver and Pommerenke (1944) researched the relationship of cervical mucus to ovulation, and evaluated the technique for both fertility and infertility practice.

Symptothermal methods

This method sought to combine several indices or parameters of ovarian function. The multiple index approach was first described in Canada in the late 1950s, and was popularized by the writings of Baillargeon and Pelletier-Baillargeon (1963). Keefe (1962) described changes in the morphology of the uterine cervix during the fertile phase and in the 1970s the Billings Method (1972; 1973) and the Cervical Score of Insler et al. (1972) were added.

The calendar method

Ogino of Japan (1930) and Knaus of Austria (1933), proved that ovulation occurs between, and not during periods, and they found a relatively constant time span between ovulation and the next menstruation. Ogino noted an 8-day fertile span while Knaus favoured a 5-day interval. From their work, formulae were developed to determine the individual woman's fertile time.

BREASTFEEDING

Lactational amenorrhoea, nature's own contraceptive, has restricted population growth from earliest times and long-term breast feeding is still the norm in most developing countries. In the late nineteenth century artificial milk formulae were produced and the incidence of breast feeding declined. This resulted in earlier ovulation and increased fertility. This in turn acted as an incentive to scientific investigation of contraceptive methods, although they only became widely accepted in the 1960s. Recent investigation by Gray et al. (1990) showed that the risk of ovulation postpartum in exclusively breast feeding mothers was between 1 and 5%. The risk of ovulation rose if the woman continued breast feeding beyond 6 months, or if she menstruated prior to that time.

COITUS INTERRUPTUS AND RESERVATUS

Coitus interruptus is mentioned in the Bible (Genesis 38: 7–10) where Onan 'would spill (semen) on the ground'. This method of contraception was reviled by both Christians and Jews. The revulsion was derived from a possible misinterpretation of the biblical passage in Genesis, Chapter 38, Verses 7–10 'and Er, Judah's first born, was wicked in the sight of the Lord; and the Lord slew him. And Judah said unto Onan: "Go in to thy brother's wife, and perform the duty of the husband's brother unto her, and raise up seed to thy brother!" and Onan knew that the seed would not be his; and it came to pass that whenever he went in unto his brother's wife, that he used to spill it on to the ground, less he should give seed to his brother. The thing that he did was evil in the sight of the Lord; and he slew him also.' The misinterpretation was that Onan's sin was spilling seed i.e. coitus interruptus. Commentators, however, believe that his sin was to refuse to let his sister-in-law have children who might be named after his brother, Er. It seems that both brothers Onan and Er, practised coitus interruptus. Er was said to have been 'flowering in the garden and emptying upon the dung hill' and Onan 'was threshing inside and winnowing outside'.

Coitus reservatus (intercourse without ejaculation) was used by societies such as the ancient Chinese, and was said to benefit both the body and soul. John Humphreys Noyes founded the Oneida Community of New York in 1869 and they lived according to a fundamentalist interpretation of the Bible. The community used coitus reservatus (also called *kerreza*) as their method of family planning.

VAGINAL TAMPONS AND SPONGE

Various forms of material have been moistened and inserted high in the vagina before intercourse, since earliest times. There is reference in the Talmud to the use of *mokh*, a generic term for cotton particularly when used as a tampon. Development of the present day contraceptive sponge began in the mid-1970s at the University of Arizona. At first the sponge was used as a barrier, but Chvapil (1976) and Chvapil *et al.* (1979) suggested the addition of spermicide to increase its efficacy. Due to its absorptive capacity the sponge caused vaginal dryness and in addition, some women were frightened of developing infection from its use. The collatex sponge

(Today) was developed by Bruce Vorhauer and is manufactured from polyurethane impregnated with the spermicide nonoxynol-9. Bounds and Guillebaud (1984) found the failure rate for the sponge contraceptive was more than twice that of the diaphragm.

SPERMICIDALS

Spermicidals act both as a physical barrier and as immobilizing agents. They are the oldest known form of contraception and are also dealt with in the Early Methods section. An English pharmacist Walter Rendell introduced spermicidal pessaries containing quinine sulphate in a soluble cocoa butter base in 1885. Five types of spermicidal agent became available including: lactic acid (which is the oldest), surface-acting agents, enzyme inhibitors, bactericides and membrane-active agents such as local anaesthetics. Spermicidals were also found to protect against sexually transmitted diseases but their effectiveness was poor with a failure rate of 11.9/100 women (Vessey *et al.*, 1982). They eventually became available as foaming or non-foaming suppositories, creams, jellies and pastes, plastic film (C film), spermicidal-releasing vaginal rings, and aerosol foams.

CONDOMS

The origin of the condom is unknown but it is known to be very ancient, dating from prehistoric times. In a cave in Les Combaralles, France, there is a sketch of a man and a woman engaged in intercourse; the male seems to have covered his penis with some form of coat. Another early representation depicts a cover for the glans penis and appears to be from the Egyptian 12th Dynasty (1350–1200 BC). A form of sheath fashioned from goat's bladder is said to have been used in Roman times, and may have served not only as a contraceptive but also to prevent sexually transmitted disease. The ancient Japanese are reputed to have used a tortoise shell for the glans penis, and African women used hollowed out Okra pods as intravaginal condoms. In 1564 Gabrielis Falloppius (Figure 4) described the prophylactic use of the condom in his *De Morbo Gallico* and the chapter which introduced it was entitled 'On Preservation from French Caries (syphilis)'. A letter from Madame de Sévigné to her daughter in 1671 described the condom as 'armour against enjoyment and a spider's web against danger'. Madame

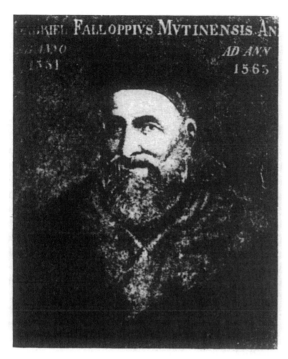

Figure 4 Gabrielis Falloppius, the first to recommend the use of a sheath to protect against disease. Courtesy of the IPPF

la Marquise Marie de Rabutin-Chantal Sévigné (1626–1696) wrote unforgettable letters which are wonderful examples of the art of lively elliptic epistles. Recent researchers claim that such a letter never existed (Youssef, 1993).

In the eighteenth century condoms were made of animals' intestines and a Mrs Phillips advertised their sale from the Phillips warehouse in Bedford Street (late Half Moon Street) seven doors from the strand on the left-hand side. The following lines are taken from the advertising hand bill:

> 'To guard yourself from shame or fear,
> Votaries to Venus, haste here
> none in my wares er found a flaw,
> self preservations natures law'.

Although it is suggested that there may have been a doctor (or Colonel) Condom who 'invented' the sheath as a family planning aid for Charles II (1630–1685) who already had many illegitimate children, it is more likely that the word is derived from Latin – *condus*, or Persian – *kondu*, a receptacle for storing grain. Casanova de Seingalt (1725–1803) and James Boswell both referred to

its use. Boswell referred to dipping his 'armour in the serpentine' (lake) to soften it, prior to use while Casanova bought his stock of 'English riding coats' from a man in Vienna. The condoms originally made from animal intestines were 0.06 mm thick. Their major disadvantages were the hand-sewn seams and also the fact that they were expensive. The thickness of the modern condom was reduced to 0.03 mm in 1974 (Koyama and Oato, 1974).

The vulcanization of rubber was introduced by Goodyear in 1839 and rubber condoms soon became available for use. Their shelf-life was limited however, to about 3 months. The introduction of the latex process in the 1930s improved both the quality and efficacy of condoms. After the Second World War other innovations were to follow. Lubrication and spermicidals were added and eased the application and use of the sheath, while further adding to their safety. The Japanese gained the credit for introducing colour to condoms, and with better packaging and marketing techniques the condom became a family planning success story (Potts, 1984). A recent innovation was the introduction of the 'Femshield' female condom.

As condoms were found to be both air- and water-tight, they were impermeable to micro-organisms and therefore limited the spread of sexually transmitted disease (Mills, 1984). Their effectiveness against contracting gonorrhoea, syphilis, and the human immunodeficiency virus, combined with a protective effect against the onset of uterine cervical dysplasia and their established contraceptive efficacy have confirmed their role as 'armour' or 'implements of safety'.

DIAPHRAGMS

The diaphragm was introduced in 1882 by a German physician, Wilhelm P.J. Mensinga (Himes, 1970), The method quickly became popular and was described in England by H.A. Albutt in 1887. The description of the diaphragm in his *The Wife's Handbook* led to his being struck off the medical register. The diaphragm was the main method of contraception provided by Family Planning Clinics until the early 1960s. Pierce and Rowntree (1961) calculated that 12% of British couples used the method, and in 1965, 10% of American couples used diaphragms (National Fertility Study, 1965). However by the mid-1980s only 2–3% of couples were still using this method (Mills, 1984).

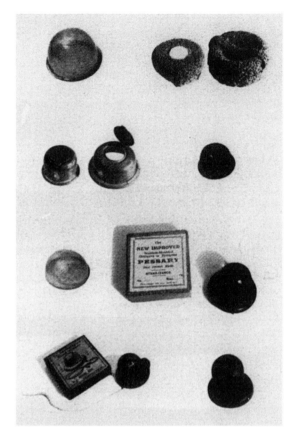

Figure 5 Examples of early contraception devices. Courtesy of the IPPF

The diaphragm was found to be relatively effective, particularly in association with a spermicide, and failure rates varying from 2 to 15% were reported. Few side-effects were noted apart from an increased frequency of urinary tract infections. The diaphragm was found to be protective against sexually transmitted diseases and cervical carcinoma (Vessey *et al.*, 1976) (Figure 5).

THE CAP

The cervical cap was first introduced by Friedrick Adolphe Wilde (1838). The German gynaecologist made wax impressions of his patients' cervices, and then moulded individualized rubber caps which the woman could wear 'to prevent a pregnancy, and remove only during her menstrual period'. Various types became popular including the Dumas, Matrisealus, Mizpah and Dutch cap.

Dr Aletta Jabobs established the first birth control clinic in Amsterdam in 1882, and it was her promotion of the diaphragm/cap which led to it being called the 'Dutch Cap'. Due to difficulty of insertion and removal, the cap was little used (Connell, 1978).

THE INTRAUTERINE DEVICE

A form of intrauterine contraception is said to have been practised by camel drivers in North Africa. The pregnant camels were difficult to manage, and it was discovered that pebbles inserted in the uterus effectively prevented conception. In the nineteenth century collar stud and wishbone pessaries may have been used as experimental intrauterine devices (IUDs). A Dr Richter of Waldenburg in Germany, described a thread pessary for contraceptive use in 1909 and Ernst Gräfenberg (Figure 6), a German gynaecologist, developed a flexible ring for insertion into the uterus in the 1920s (Figure 7). His first IUDs were fashioned from silkworm gut but were frequently expelled. As a further development he introduced a ring made of silver wire – the so called Grafenberg ring (Robertson, 1990). A number of workers

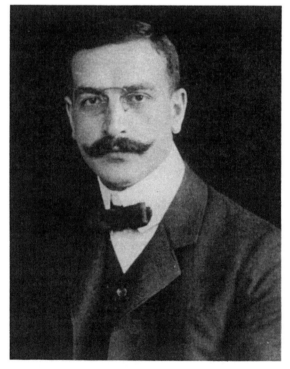

Figure 6 Ernst Gräfenberg

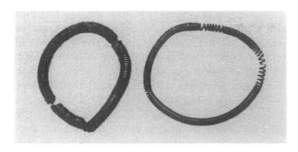

Figure 7 Two Gräfenberg rings which had been left *in utero* of their owners who had forgotten about them for 24 years and 40 years, respectively

devised and developed new IUDs, which were initially fashioned from metal coils (Figure 8). Dr W. Oppenheimer of Israel used the silver ring and silkworm gut IUDs extensively. Teneri Takeo Ota of Japan developed a large selection of Ota rings, made of metal but later replaced by plastic. Atsumi Ishihama, also of Japan, documented his studies on the IUD and their low complication rates. The saf-T coil was invented by Ralph Robinson.

In the 1960s IUDs with a 'memory' first appeared – silastic devices with flexible plastic shapes which returned to their original shape after introduction to the uterine cavity. Copper IUDs were introduced in the 1970s. The devices used from that time to the present include the Gravigard copper 7, the multiload Cu250, copper T, Nova T, Novagaard, and the progestasert. One form of IUD the 'Dalkon Shield' was associated with serious pelvic infection, and fatalities were reported. The popularity of the IUD suffered, but it is estimated that around 8% of women in the UK use the method for contraception.

STERILIZATION

Some ancient societies performed ovariectomy on females and orchidectomy on males for contraceptive, religious, or status motives. The eunuch frequently had power and influence in the Royal Courts. However, sterilization *per se* did not become a reality until much later.

James Blundell recommended bilateral tubal division as a means to prevent pregnancy in women at risk of obstructed labour due to their contracted pelvises. In his *Principles and Practice of Obstetricy* (1834) he wrote 'if the pelvis be contracted . . . delivery could not take place by the natural passage . . . I would advise . . . that a

portion of the tube be removed . . . on either side . . . an operation easily performed, when the women would forever after be sterile'. In May 1880, S.S. Lungren of Toledo, Ohio, performed Caesarean section on a patient with a contracted pelvis (Lungren, 1881). He decided to remove the ovaries as a contraceptive measure, but was afraid of haemorrhage, and instead ligated the Fallopian tubes with a silk ligature about 1 inch (2.5 cm) from their uterine attachment.

Various methods of tubal sterilization were reported over the following years, but there were a large number of failures, and there was a tendency to fistula formation or recanalization of the

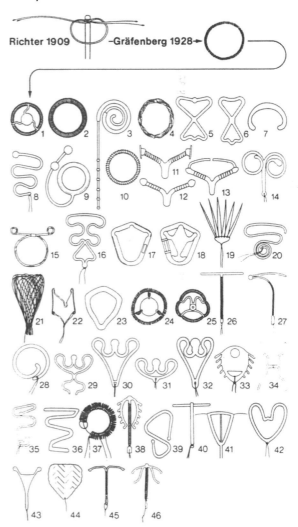

Figure 8 Many varieties of intrauterine device – so called 'children of Gräfenberg's ring'; invented after the rehabilitation of the intrauterine contraceptive device in 1959

tubes. Flatau (1921) reported that 42 different sterilizing procedures had been proposed. Max Madlener (1919) German gynaecologist and surgeon, devised in 1910 one of the most popular forms of sterilization, since known by his name. In his paper of 1919 he described the technique of crushing a loop of Fallopian tube with a forceps and then applying a thread ligature in the groove. Three of the 89 patients who were operated on died, but none of the survivors became pregnant. Thirty-four women had a laparotomy while 55 were operated on through a colpotomy incision. Friedrick Carpenter Irving (1924) proposed his sterilization technique where the tube was divided and the proximal portion buried in a tunnel created in the myometrium. The distal tube was ligated with chromic catgut but not buried. Cooke modified the Irving technique by burying the proximal stump in the round ligament.

The Pomeroy technique was devised by Ralph Pomeroy but was not reported by him. Two of his associates, Bishop and Nelms (1930) reported 100 consecutive cases with no known failures 5 years after Pomeroy's death. In his technique a loop of tube in its mid-portion was ligated with absorbable suture material and the loop was then resected. The operation was feasible *per abdomen* or by the vaginal route. The Kroener fimbriectomy was first described in 1935 (Kroener, 1969). The Uchida (1975) technique was also reported and 20 000 cases were treated without failure.

Laparoscopy was first proposed as an approach to tubal occlusion by the American Anderson (1937), and Power and Barnes (1941) performed sterilization via that method. The instruments and light sources were inadequate and laparoscopy fell into disfavour. Culdoscopic sterilization was developed by Decker (1942) of New York. With the patient in the knee–chest position, the culdoscope was introduced through a puncture wound in the posterior fornix. Each tube was grasped in turn, under direct culdoscopic vision, and was delivered into the vagina where electrical or non-electrical methods of tubal occlusion were applied. Although the procedure could be performed under local anaesthesia and without gas insufflation, laparoscopic techniques became more sophisticated in the 1960s and were reintroduced, and thus culdoscopy was abandoned. Culdotomy allowed access to the tubes via an incision in the posterior fornix but was infrequently used. Hysterectomy, at Caesarean section, or in the non-gravid patient was also used for birth control.

The laparoscopic technique became popular after Palmer of France (1962) and Steptoe of England (1967) documented their cases of laparoscopic sterilization using electrocoagulation. The technique was refined by the addition of transection methods (Wheeless, 1970; Steptoe, 1971), or by tubal resection using a wire snare (Soderstrom and Smith, 1971). Prior to 1970 the unipolar electrocoagulation techniques used resulted in a number of abdominal and bowel burns. Low-voltage high-frequency generators were introduced and virtually eliminated the burns which had previously occurred as a result of sparking. Rioux and Cloutier (1974) of Canada introduced the bipolar forceps for electrical tubal coagulation. A tissue cauterization technique using low-voltage electricity was devised by Semm (1973).

With the advent of mechanical methods of laparoscopic sterilization in the early 1970s, the electrical methods were gradually replaced by tubal occluding devices. The application of hemoclips was popularized by Gutierrez-Najar via a culdoscopic approach but there was a high failure rate as the clips were not sufficiently strong to occlude all Fallopian tubes (Wortman, 1975). The Hulka-Clemens spring loaded clip was developed in 1972 (Hulka and Omran, 1972). The clips were applied under direct laparoscopic vision and slowly occluded the tubes over a number of days with minimal tissue being destroyed. In the same year the Falope ring technique was devised by Yoon, and Yoon and King (1975) reported preliminary testing of it. The ring was fashioned from silicone rubber with 5% barium sulphate, and applied to the mid-portion of the Fallopian tube.

The Filshie clip was introduced in 1974 and early studies were carried out in 1975 (Filshie, 1983). The clip was made of titanium lined with silicone rubber, and became the most commonly used form of laparoscopic tubal occlusion device. Other clips, including that of Bleier, have been described.

Sterilization via a hysteroscopic approach was first used by von Mikulicz-Radecki and Froid in 1927, and by Dickenson 2 years later (Newton, 1984). Various forms of tubal occlusion devices including plugs, chemical agents, and tissue adhesives, were experimented with in the 1970s but the hysteroscopic technique failed to achieve its apparent potential. Puerperal sterilization via a periumbilical incision, laparoscopic approach, or mini-laparotomy (using a uterine elevator) was introduced but has not retained its popularity.

The complications of the various sterilization

operations decreased as techniques were modified and operator skill increased. While side-effects, particularly maternal mortality, are rare, tubal ectopic pregnancy and luteal phase pregnancies were reported, and all methods were found to have a failure rate. Surgical reversal of sterilization proved possible especially for those methods which caused minimal tissue destruction.

VASECTOMY

Sir Astley Cooper (1830) first carried out experimental vasectomy in dogs in 1823, and later in the century Harrison (1899) recommended its use in men, as a 'cure' for prostatic enlargement. Although vasectomy was performed for family planning soon afterwards, it was rarely reported as a procedure in medical publications. Despite that, it became a popular contraceptive method from the 1960s.

Vasectomy became available under the National Health Service in England in 1972 but failed to achieve the popularity of female sterilization there, although commonly used in many countries. The technique of simple interruption of vas continuity, closure of the proximal (testicular) end by fulguration of the mucosal surface (Schmidt, 1966) or compression by Tantalum clip or sutures (Moss, 1972; Leader et al., 1974) followed by fascial interposition, were the techniques found to be most acceptable.

THE ORAL CONTRACEPTIVE PILL (THE PILL)

Although it was known for some time that removal of the ovaries in animals led to uterine atrophy, it was not until the late nineteenth century that the effects of gonadal extracts were experimented with. Sobotta (1896; 1897) had described the process of luteinization which followed ovulation and soon afterwards John Beard (1897) and August Prenant (1898) suggested that the presence of corpus luteum tissue would suppress ovulation. Brown-Sequard (1889) advocated the use of injectable gonadal extracts to act as a rejuvenant, and ovarian extracts were used by Villeneuve of France to treat women with 'hysteria' (Robertson, 1990).

In 1992 Otfried Otto Fellner used extracts of corpus luteum as a contraceptive agent and suggested that ovarian extract which did not contain luteal cells might have the same effect. The isolation of the two main ovarian hormones occurred in the same decade – Edgar Allen and Edward Doisy (1923) reported their work on the extraction of an ovarian hormone, (oestrogen). During 1928–1929 George Corner, Willard Allen and Walter Bluer obtained crude oily extracts of corpora lutea, the active principle of which Corner called progestin (Corner and Allen, 1929; Corner, 1943).

It was the discovery of the steroid skeleton, by German chemist Heinrich Wieland in 1932, which led to the knowledge that cholesterol was the most common sterol in man and other vertebrates. It was demonstrated that if the steroid skeleton was altered, structures with different biological effects were produced, and so the sex hormones, bile salts, and vitamin D were closely related. The difference between one steroid molecule and another was minute but their activity and effects were quite different. In Europe three pharmaceutical companies were active – Schering of Germany, Organon of Holland, and Ciba of Switzerland. Their chemists synthesized testosterone and progesterone from cholesterol. Oestradiol was isolated from the urine of pregnant mares, and thousands of gallons were processed with the production of paltry amounts of hormone. In 1936 four tons of sows' ovaries were used to produce 25 mg of oestrogen. The first artificial oestrogen was synthesized by Cooke et al. (1933), and the first orally active progesterone, 17α-ethinyltestosterone, was synthesized by Hans H. Inhoffen just before the Second World War. The extraction of ovarian hormones proved to be a time consuming, difficult and expensive business. In consequence, researchers investigated plant sources in an effort to synthesize oestrogen and progesterone from cheaper, more available sources. It was already known that sheep who ate certain types of clover became less fertile; and that during the Second World War when a famine occurred in Holland, the Dutch women who ate tulip bulbs became infertile.

The major breakthrough in the evolution of synthetic steroids came about due to the work of Russell Marker, an American chemist and researcher, who had presented his Ph.D. thesis in chemistry to the University of Maryland. He then worked at the Rockefeller Institute and later carried out independently funded research at the Pennsylvania State University. In the early 1940s Russell Marker (Figure 9) was investigating a group

467

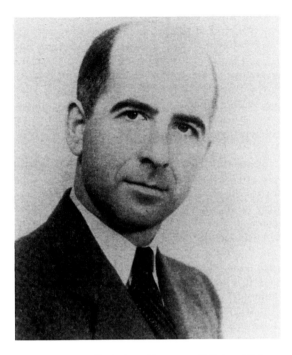

Figure 9 Russell Marker. Courtesy of Richard Edgren and Syntex Laboratory, Palo Alto, California (*see* text)

of steroids called sapogenins (Gunn, 1987) which he discovered were present in 'Lydia Pinkham's Compound', a preparation available in North Carolina which was used to relieve menstrual cramps. These compounds, which were extracted from plants, had soap-like qualities when dissolved in water. Marker discovered that one particular sapogenin, diosgenin, had a steroid nucleus similar to cholesterol but with just one side chain which was different. In a series of investigations he found that it was possible chemically to degrade the side chain and produce a steroid which was pure progesterone. Marker discovered that diosgenin was present in large amounts in the 'black-headed Mexican yam'. He collected over 10 tons of the yam species in the countryside around Vera Cruz and produced the syrupy substance, diosgenin, from them. He extracted 3 kg of progesterone from the diosgenin, and at that time the hormone was worth in excess of $US 80 a gram.

In collaboration with Emeric Somlo and Frederico Lehman, Russell Marker founded a company named Syntex (synthesis + Mexico) which was to manufacture and market the synthetic progesterone. Marker left the company 2 years later, but Somlo and Lehman recruited Dr George Rosenkranz of Switzerland, who went on to synthesize progesterone and also testosterone. In 1949 Carl Djerassi (Figure 10) joined the Syntex team and produced a crystalline '19 nor-progesterone'. The same group eventually synthesized 'norethindrone' (norethisterone), samples of which were sent to a number of clinical researchers who used the product to treat various gynaecological complaints. Soon afterwards, Frank Coulton synthesized 'norethynodrel', which with 'norethindrone' (norethisterone) became commercially available in 1957. Both preparations exerted an intense progesterone effect in small doses when taken orally.

Important research was also undertaken by Sturgis and Albright (USA) in 1940 when they used injections of oestradiol benzoate to inhibit ovulation, and cured dysmenorrhoea. Soon after this, Robert Greenblatt of Atlanta, used stilboesterol suppositories and in the early 1950s introduced a cyclical form of treatment with descending doses of oestrogen, complemented by an oral progesterone for several days, to induce withdrawal bleeding (Greenblatt, 1959).

The next phase in the development of the pill came from the work of research scientists Drs Gregory Pincus and Min Cheuh Chang, and the

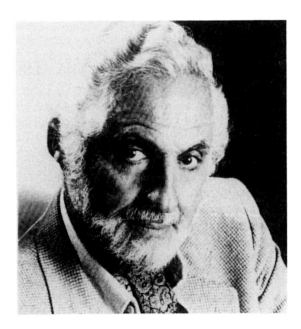

Figure 10 Carl Djerassi (*see* text)

clinicians Drs John Rock and Ramon Garcia (Figures 11–14). Gregory Pincus, known as the 'father of the pill', worked as a biologist at the Worcester Foundation in Shrewsbury, Massachusetts. His main area of interest was reproductive physiology. Pincus received a grant from the Planned Parenthood Federation of America and undertook to carry out research on hormonal birth control. Chang was a collaborator who worked with him at the Worcester Foundation. The third

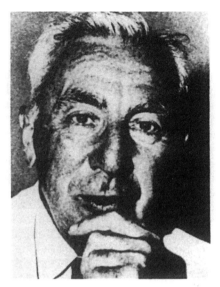

Figure 13 John Rock (*see* text). Courtesy of the IPPF

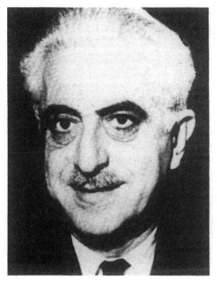

Figure 11 Gregory Pincus – 'the father of the pill' (*see* text). Courtesy of the IPPF

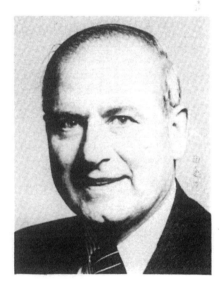

Figure 14 Ramon Garcia (*see* text). Courtesy of the IPPF

member of the team, John Rock, was a Harvard Professor with a major interest in infertility, who had already used progesterone to suppress ovulation and achieve rebound ovarian activity. The first clinical studies on hormonal contraception were carried out on human volunteers in Boston. Due to the Comstock Laws of the nineteenth century (later repealed in 1967) contraception was illegal in Massachusetts. Because of that, and the need for a large clinical trial, Dr Celso Ramon Garcia, who was working in Puerto Rico, was in-

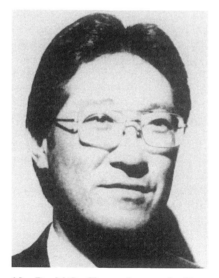

Figure 12 Dr M.C. Chang (*see* text). Courtesy of the IPPF

volved, and the first clinical trials on an oral contraceptive pill were carried out on local women under his supervision.

The hormonal preparation used was norethisterone, and the results were published in 1956 by Rock, Pincus and Garcia (Gunn, 1990). The substance was successfully used to inhibit ovulation, but was later found to be impure and contained small amounts of an oestrogen – later defined as mestranol. The use of a pure progesterone preparation was accompanied by breakthrough bleeding and an unacceptable pregnancy rate. As a result, mestranol was reintroduced to the preparation at a standardized level of 1.5%, and the progesterone/oestrogen pill was born. The first available contraceptive pill, Enovid, was approved for marketing by the Food and Drug Administration board of America in 1960. Conovid was introduced to the UK in 1961.

In its early formulation the pill contained a daily dose of almost 10 mg of progesterone and 150 µg of oestrogen. Many women experienced unwanted side-effects and this provided a stimulus to reduce the dose of both progesterone and oestrogen. By 1961 a pill containing only 50 µg of the oestrogen component was introduced. In 1965 a sequential pill which contained progesterone alone in the latter part of the cycle was introduced. The first progesterone-only pill was marketed in 1965/1966 but the pregnancy rates were found to be higher than with the combined pill. A 30 µg oestrogen pill was introduced in 1972.

By 1979 the progesterone dose had been reduced from 10 mg to 0.15 µg, and the oestrogen from 150 µg to 30 µg. A biphasic pill was introduced in the early 1970s. And a triphasic pill introduced in 1980 contained less than 1% of the daily dose of hormones which had been administered in the pill 20 years previously (Hannse, 1982; Gunn, 1987; Robertson, 1990). Currently, the latest generation of ultra-low-dose combined oral contraceptives are based on the even lower dose of 20 µg oestrogen.

Tausk (1969) noted that the primary mechanism of ovulation inhibition exerted by combined oral contraceptives was a negative feedback on pituitary luteinizing hormone secretion, mediated by progesterone and potentiated by the oestrogen component. Wynants and Ide (1986) compared endometrial morphology between the new triphasic combined oral contraceptive and a monophasic regimen. Drug interaction and reduced efficacy of the oral contraceptive pill was first noted by Reimers and Jeyek (1971) in patients using rifampicin and antituberculous drugs. Interaction with ampicillin, tetracycline and a range of other antibiotics, was reported, while anticonvulsants were also found to reduce oral contraceptive effect. Meanwhile, a number of therapeutic agents, including anticoagulants and insulin, were antagonized by oral contraceptive use.

Bioassays to determine progesterone potency based on the ability of the drug to delay menstruation were introduced by Greenblatt et al. (1958) and Swyer (1982).

Although the pill was a very effective contraceptive, it was soon found that some women experienced major medical complications attributable to either the oestrogen or progesterone components, or both. Most of the side-effects were due to the high dosages in the early pill formulations.

The first major adverse effect of the pill was documented by Dr W. M. Jordan (1962) a Suffolk (UK) family doctor who reported the occurrence of thromboembolism in a patient using Enovid as treatment for endometriosis. Soon afterwards, Boyce et al. (1963) reported the thrombotic effects of Conovid. Other reports which implicated pill use with hypertension and alteration in lipid profiles soon followed. Lipoproteins were found to be affected by both oestrogens and progesterone. Oestrogens were found to increase high-density lipoproteins, which were said to be protective against coronary artery disease, while progesterones increased the low-density lipoproteins which are associated with a high incidence of coronary artery disease. Castelli (1985) reported the Framingham Study and indicated that total plasma cholesterol, triglycerides and very low-density lipoproteins were significantly elevated while high- and low-density lipoproteins were not significantly changed in pill users.

The Royal College of General Practitioners in England began their long-term survey of pill users in 1964. The Committee for the Safety of Medicines related the oestrogen component of the pill to an increased risk of thromboembolic disease (Inman et al. 1970), and the Royal College of General Practitioners (1977) reported similar findings. The Oxford Family Planning Association (UK) and the Centres for Disease Control in the USA, also carried out long-term investigations on the pill's side-effects.

Complications of oral contraceptive pill use were directly related to the quantity of both oestrogen and progesterone, and the low-dose preparations which were produced in response resulted in a pill which is safe in use, with very low complication rates, and high protection against unwanted pregnancy. The results of the Walnut Creek Contraceptive Drug Study (Ramcharan *et al.* 1980) showed that the incidence of thrombosis and embolism, was judged to be negligible in the 'low-dose' pill patient.

The oral contraceptive was also shown to have beneficial side-effects apart from the family planning benefit with a reduction in risk for ovarian and endometrial cancer, and a reduced incidence of benign breast disease, ovarian cysts, ectopic pregnancy and pelvic inflammatory disease. Despite conflicting results it appeared that oral contraceptives were not associated with an increased incidence of breast cancer. The slightly increased risk of cervical neoplasia may have been related to an earlier onset of coitus and increased number of partners, so that doubt is cast upon a direct relationship between oral contraceptive use and cervical cancer. The risks of spontaneous abortion and congenital defects have not increased in pill users. It is estimated that the oral contraceptive is now the most widely used form of contraception, with 60 million women a year using the compounds.

DEPOT PREPARATIONS

Depo-Provera was introduced in 1967. The research workers Junkmann and Wilzel, and Babcock *et al.*, were responsible for the discovery of long-acting hormonal preparations during the years 1953–1958.

NEWER DEVELOPMENTS

Newer developments in hormonal contraception include the provision of ultra-low-dose contraceptive pills; the refining of injectable progesterones; the use of Norplant (implantable contraceptives based on the suggestion of Croxatto and Segal in 1969); vaginal rings containing either oestrogen, progesterone or both; antiprogestins such as mifeprostone; contraceptive vaccines; and the use of Gossypol, antiandrogens, gonadotropin releasing hormone analogues and steroids in males (Drife, 1989).

THE PEARL FORMULA

The number of pregnancies per 100 woman years of exposure, was used to calculate the effective-

ness of the various contraceptive methods. The failure rates were ranked by Tietze (1970). A more recent table of failure rates based on the work of Vessey *et al.* (1982) and the Oxford Family Planning Contraceptive Study, was highlighted by Reid (1985) (Table 1.1).

Table 1.1 Failure rates for different methods of contraception. (Oxford/FPA Contraceptive Study: married women aged 25–30; Vessey *et al.*, 1982)

Method	Failure rate per 100 women years
Combined pills	
50 µg oestrogen	0.16
< 50 µg oestrogen	0.27
Progestogen-only pill	1.2
Intrauterine device	
(average for all types)	1.5
Diaphragm	1.9
Condom	3.6
Chemicals alone	11.9
Rhythm	15.5
Coitus interruptus	6.7
Sterilization	
male	0.02
female	0.13

CHRONOLOGY

Natural family planning

Calendar method

1930	Ogino in Japan, estimated a method of determining the fertile period.
1933	Knaus estimated a 5-day fertile span.
1962	Hartman favoured Ogino's estimate of an 8-day fertile interval.
1967	Treloar *et al.* found menstrual cycle variations of 5–11 days.

Basal body temperature

1868	Squire described an increase in basal body temperature in the second half of the cycle.
1928	Van de Velde noted the relationship between elevated basal body temperature and the presence of the corpus luteum.

1939	Palmer and Devillers established the thermogenic effect of progesterone.
1949	Palmer used temperature recording to monitor the menstrual cycle.
1963	Marshall popularized the basal body temperature method in the English-speaking world.

Cervical mucus

1933	Seguy and Simonnet related mucus changes to ovulation.
1944	Viergiver and Pommerenke measured cervical mucus throughout the cycle and correlated it with the basal body temperature.
1972	John and Evelyn Billings et al. in Australia, found a close association between cervical mucus change and ovarian activity.
1977	Billings et al. produced their Atlas of the Ovulation Method.

Sympto-thermal methods

1938	Ito observed the various symptoms of ovulation.
1962	Keefe documented self-observation of the cervix - dilatation, softening, mucus secretion and inaccessibility to palpation.
1963	Baillargeon and Pelletier-Baillargeon popularized a multiple index approach to determination of the fertile period.
1972	Insler et al. introduced a fertility cervical score.

Barrier methods

Condoms

*References: Himes (1970); Robertson (1990); McLaren (1990)

1350–1200 BC	A penile sheath was depicted on an artifact recovered from the Egyptian 12th dynasty (Robertson, 1990).
Roman times	Goats bladder was used as a condom.*
Renaissance	Caecum and other parts of intestine were used as condoms.*

1564	Gabriele Falloppio first published a description of a linen sheath, forerunner of the condom (Speert, 1973).
1671	Madam de Sévigné described the condom as 'an armour against enjoyment'.*
1725–98	Casanova de Seingalt was known to use the condom.*
1762	James Boswell mentions use of 'armour' (condom).*
1773	Bachaunot's diary contained a couplet, regarding use of the condom.*
1776	Condoms were on sale in London – Mrs Phillips of Half Moon Street.*
1785	The word condom appeared in a dictionary of London's Street Language.*
1834	Vulcanization, a technique which stabilizes the properties of rubber and makes it usable, was invented by the American, Charles Goodyear (d'Estaing, 1990).
Early 1900s	Rubber condoms had a shelf life of 3 months.*
1930s	The latex process improved the quality and efficacy of condoms.*
1970	Tietze reported that the method effectiveness of condoms was 97–98.5%.
1972	Siboulet found a low incidence of infection with gonorrhoea in the male partners of women known to have the disease, if condoms were used.
	Pemberton et al. documented that the risk of contracting syphilis in condom users was lower than in non-users.
1978	Wright et al. concluded that the risk of developing cervical dysplasia was decreased with both condoms and diaphragm use.
1985	Hicks et al. showed that nonoxynol-9, a spermicide used with condoms, inactivated the human immunodeficiency virus.
1986	Conant et al. determined by in vitro studies that condoms prevent the passage of the human immunodeficiency virus.
1988	Mills noted that the spermicide benzalkonium chloride inactivated the human immunodeficiency virus in laboratory studies.

The diaphragm/cap

1725–1803	Casanova used a half squeezed out lemon placed over the cervix as a diaphragm (Robertson, 1990).
1838	Cervical caps were first made by a German gynaecologist F.A. Wilde.
1882	The first diaphragms were described by C. Hasse a German physician who published under the pseudonym, Mensinga.
1887	Allbutt first described the diaphragm in England (Potts and Diggory, 1983).
19th C.	Diaphragms of bees' wax, oil-covered silk paper, and opium were fashioned into receptacles to cover the cervix in Asian women (Wortman, 1976).
1970	Tietze documented method effectiveness of 97–98.5% for diaphragms used with a spermicide.

Spermicidals

1885	Walter Rendell developed spermicidal pessaries containing cocoa butter and quinine sulphate (Robertson, 1990).
1937	Phenylmercuric acetate (PMA) was introduced but its use was later discontinued due to toxicity.
1950s	Surface-acting agents were introduced which interfered with sperm metabolism.

Intrauterine device

Reference: Speert (1973)

1909	Dr Richter of Waldenburg and
1920s	Ernst Grafenberg, described early intrauterine devices.

The following workers are eponymously related to the intrauterine devices listed here.

Jack Lippes of Buffalo – the Lippes Loop
Herbert H. Hall and Martin L. Stone – Hall-Stone Ring
Dr Birnberg – Birnberg Bow
Jaime Zipper – Zipper Ring
Lazar C. Margulies – Margulies Spiral
Teneri Takeo Ota – Ota Ring
Ernst Grafenberg – Grafenberg Ring.

Hormonal contraception

*References: Potts and Diggory (1983); Robertson (1990); Gunn (1987)

1889	Brown-Sequard advocated the use of ovarian extract.
1897	John Beard and August Prenant (1898) suggested that ovulation would be inhibited by corpus luteum extract. Otfried Otto Fellner induced infertility in animals by ovarian transplantation, and ovarian extract administration.*
1923	Edgar Allen and Edward Doisy isolated oestrogen.
1928/29	George Corner, Willard Allen and Walter Bluer isolated progesterone.
1932	Heinrich Wieland discovered the chemical composition of steroids.*
1933	Cooke et al. first synthesized artificial oestrogen.*
1940s	Russell Marker produced progesterone from the Mexican yam.*
1944	The Syntex Company was formed by Marker, Somlo and Lehmann.*
1951	Carl Djerassi and George Rosenkranz produced ethisterone 19-norprogesterone.*
1953	Junkmann discovered a long-lasting progesterone preparation.*
1954	Clinical study on ethisterone 19-norprogesterone started by Roy Hertz, Alexander Lipschutz, Gregory Pincus, Robert Greenblatt and Edward Tyler.*
1956	Frank Coulton patented 'norethynodrel'.* Gregory Pincus, Min Cheuh Chang, John Rock and Celso Garcia used norethisterone successfully to inhibit ovulation. The substance was later found to be impure, and contained small amounts of an oestrogen (mestranol).*
1958	Junkmann and Welzel discovered norethisterone oethanate, and depomedroxyprogesterone acetate was formulated by Babcock et al.*
1960	Enovid was marketed in the USA.
1961	Schering introduced the 50 μg oestrogen pill.
1962	Dr W.M. Jordan, a Suffolk family doctor, reported thromboembolism in a patient using Enovid.

1964	Royal College of General Practitioners (England) began their pill survey.
1965	The 'sequential' pill was invented.
1966	The 'progesterone-only' pill was introduced.
1967	Depo-Provera was introduced.
1969	Morris and Van Wagenen demonstrated the anti-implantation effect of postcoital high-dose oestrogen, thus giving rise to the 'morning after pill'.
1970	The Committee for the Safety of Medicines related oestrogen to increased risk of thromboembolic disease.
1972	The 30 µg oestrogen pill was introduced
1977	The Royal College of General Practitioners implicated oestrogen with thromboembolism.
1979	A 'triphasic' formulation was introduced.
1980	The Walnut Creek Contraceptive Drug Study (USA) found negligible risk in the low-dose pill patient.
1980	The latest generation of ultra-low-dose oral contraceptives were introduced.

Sterilization

Surgical approaches

1834	James Blundell recommended sterilization by bilateral tubal division.
1880	S.S. Lungren carried out tubal sterilization at the time of Caesarean section.
1910	Max Madlener (reported in 1919).
1921	Flateau reported 42 different procedures.
1924	Friedrick Carpenter Irving.
1929	Ralph Pomeroy (Bishop and Nelms, 1930).
1935	The Kroener Technique (Kroener, 1969).
1975	The Uchida Technique.

Laparoscopy (and culdoscopy) – electrical

1941	Power and Barnes – laparoscopic sterilization.
1942	Culdoscopic sterilization developed by Decker.

1962	Palmer (France).
1967	Steptoe (England).

Laparoscopy – Fallopian occlusion devices

1972	Hulka-Clemens Clip. Fallope–Yoon Ring (Yoon and King, 1975).
1974	The Filshie Clip (Filshie, 1983).

Hysteroscopy

1927	Von Mikulicz-Radecki and Froid (Newton, 1984).
1929	Dickenson (Newton, 1984).

Vasectomy

1966	Schmidt – interruption of vas continuity and fulguration.
1972	Tantalum clip introduced.
1974	Compression by sutures.

End piece

1952	International Planned Parenthood Federation (IPPF) founded.
1967	IPPF received its first government support from Sweden. Abortion legislation enacted in England and Wales.
1969	The United Nations Population Fund (UNFPA) was established.
1970	US Congress passed the Family Planning Services and Population Research Act.
1973	Abortion legislation introduced in the USA.
1985	The House of Lords (UK) judged that a doctor may prescribe combined oral contraceptives to girls under 16 years old (within certain guidelines).
1987	The World Bank gave 0.1% in loans to population control and at the same time emphasized the need for lower birth rates.
1988	There were 190 million contraceptive users in the Third World (excluding China).

REFERENCES

Allen, E. and Doisy, E.A. (1923). An ovarian hormone. Preliminary report on its localization, extraction and partial purification and action in test animals. *J. Am. Med. Assoc.*, **81**, 819–21

Anderson, E.T. (1937). Peritoneoscopy. *Am. J. Surg.*, **35**, 136–9

Baillargeon, J. and Pelletier-Baillargeon, H. (1963). *La Regulation des naissances*, p.159. (Montreal: Les Editions du Jour)

Beard, J. (1897). *The Span of Gestation and the Cause of Birth.* (Jena: Fischer)

Billings, E.L. and Billings, I.J. (1973). The idea of the ovulation method. *Austr. Family Physician*, **2**, 81–5

Billings, E.L., Billings, J.J. and Catarinich, M. (1977). *Atlas of the Ovulation Method*, 3rd edn. p.70. (Melbourne: Advocate Press)

Billings, E.L., Billings, J.J., Brown, J.B. and Burger, H.G. (1972). Symptoms and hormonal changes accompanying ovulation. *Lancet*, **1**, 282–4

Bishop, E. and Nelms, W.F. (1930). A simple method of tubal sterilization. *N.Y. State J. Med.*, **30**, 214–16

Blundell, J. (1834). In Castle, T. (ed.) *The Principles and Practices of Obstetricy*, pp. 579–80. (London: E. Cox)

Bounds, W. and Guillebaud, J. (1984). Randomised comparison of the use-effectiveness and patient acceptability of the colltex (Today) contraceptive sponge and the diaphragm. *Br. J. Fam. Plann.* **10**, 69–75

Boyce, J., Fawcett, J.W. and Noall, E.W.O. (1963). Coronary thrombosis and conovid. *Lancet*, **2**, 111

Briggs, M.H. (1977). Combined oral contraceptives. In Diczfalusy, E. (ed.) *Regulation of Human Fertility*, pp. 253–82. (Copenhagen: Scriptor)

Brown-Sequard, C.E. (1889). Des effets produits chez l'homme par des injections souscutanées d'un liquide retiré des testicules frais de cobaye et de chien. *C.R. Soc. Biol.*, **1**, 415–19

Castelli, W.P. (1985). Effects of exogenous steroids: the Framingham experience. In *Lipoproteins, Exogenous Steroids, and Cardiovascular Problems*, p. 53. (Palo Alto, California: Syntex Laboratories Inc.)

Chvapil, M. (1976). An intravaginal contraceptive diaphragm made of collagen sponge: new old principle. *Fertil. Steril.*, **27**, 1387–97

Chvapil, M., Droegemueller, W., Heine, M.W. *et al.* (1979). Collagen sponge as intravaginal barrier method: two years experience. In Zatuchni, G.I., Sobrero, G.J., Speidel, A.J. and Sciarra, J.J. (eds.) *Vaginal Contraception: New Developments*, pp. 110–15. (PARFR Series on Fertility Regulation) (Hagerstown, Maryland: Harper and Row)

Conant, M., Hardy, D., Sernatinger, J., Spicer, D. and Levy, J.A. (1986). Condoms prevent transmission of AIDS-associated retroviruses. *J. Am. Med. Assoc.*, **255**, 1706

Connell, E.B. (1978). Cervical caps. *Medical Aspects of Human Sexuality*, **11**, 81

Cooke, J.W., Dodds, E.C., and Hewett, C.L. (1933). A synthetic oestrus-exciting compound (letter to the editor). *Nature (London)*, **131**, 56–7

Cooper, A. (1830). *Observations on the structure and disease of the testes.* (London: Longman)

Corner, G.W. (1943). Hormones in human reproduction. *Rev. Ed. Princeton*, (N.J: Princeton University Press)

Corner, G.W. and Allen, W.M. (1929). Physiology of the corpus luteum: 11. Production of a special uterine reaction (progestational proliferation) by extracts of the corpus luteum. *Am. J. Physiol.*, **88**, 826

Decker, (1942), quoted by Soderstrom, R.M. and Yuzpe, A.A. (1979)

Donne, A. (1836). Animalcules observés dans les matieres purulentes et le produit des secretions des organes genitaux de l'homme et de la femme. *C. R. hebdom. seances de'Acad. Sci., Paris*, **3**, 385

Drife, J.O. (1989). New developments in contraception. In Studd, J. (ed.) *Progress in Obstetrics and Gynaecology*, Vol. 7, pp. 245–61. (Edinburgh: (Churchill Livingstone)

Filshie, G.M. (1983). The Filshie Clip. In van Lith, D.A.F., Leith, L.G. and Van Hall, E.V. (eds.) *New Trends in Female Sterilisation*, pp. 115–124. (Chicago, London: Year Book Medical)

Flatau, W.S. (1921). Sterilisierung durch Knotung der Tube. *Zentralbl. f. Gynakol.*, **45**, 467–9

Flynn, A. M. (1984). Natural methods of family planning. In Newton, J.R. (ed.) *Clinics in Obstetrics and Gynaecology.* Vol. 11 No. 3. Contraception Update, pp. 661–78. (London, Philadelphia, Toronto: W.B. Saunders Co. Ltd)

Giscard d'Estaing, V.A. (1990). *The Book of Inventions and Discoveries*, p. 69. (London: Queen Anne Press-McDonald & Co Ltd)

Gray, R.H., Campbell, O.M., Apelo R., Eslamis, S., Zacur, H., Ramos, R.M., Gehret, J.C. and Labbok, M.H. (1990). Risk of ovulation during lactation. Clinical Practice. *Lancet*, **335**, 25–9

Greenblatt, R.B. (1959). Hormonal control of functional uterine bleeding. *Clin. Obstet. Gynecol.*, **2**, 232

Greenblatt, R.B., Clark, S.L. and Jungek, E.C. (1958). A new test for efficacy of progestational agents. *Am. N.Y. Acad. Sci.*, **71**, 717

Gruhn, J.G. and Kazer, R.R. (1989). *Hormonal Regulation of the Menstrual Cycle – the Evolution of Concepts*, p. 77. (New York, London: Plenum Medical Book Co.)

Gunn, A.D.G. (1987). *Oral Contraception in Perspective. 30 Years of Clinical Experience with the Pill.* p. 23, 35, 125. (Carnforth: Parthenon Publishing Group)

Hannse, H. (1982). Opening Remarks. In Haspels, A.A. and Rolland, R. (eds.) *Benefits and Risks of Hormonal Contraception. The Proceedings of an International Symposium. Amsterdam.* p. XIII. (Lancaster, Boston, The Hague: MTP Press Ltd)

Harrison, R. (1899). *Selected papers on stone, prostate and other urinary disorders.* (London: Churchill)

Hartman, C. G. (1962). *Science and the Safe Period: a Compendium of Human Reproduction*, p. 294. (Baltimore, Maryland: Williams and Wilkins)

Hicks, D.R., Martin, L.S., Getchell, J.P., Heath, J.L., Francis, D.P., McDougal, J.S., Curran, J.W. and Voeller, B. (1985). Inactivation of HTLV-III/LAV-infected cultures of normal human lymphocytes by nonoxynol-9 *in vitro*. *Lancet*, **2**, 1422

Himes, N.E. (1963). *Medical History of Contraception.* (New York: Gamut Press Inc.)

Himes, N.E. (1970). *Medical history of Contraception.* (New York: Schocken Books)

Hulka, J.F. and Omran, K.F. (1972). Comparative tubal occlusion: rigid and spring loaded clip. *Fertil. Steril.*, **23**, 633–8

Inman, W.H., Vessey, M.P., Westerholm, B. and Engelund, A. (1970). Thromboembolic disease and the steroidal content of oral contraceptives.

A report to the Committee on Safety of Drugs. *Br. Med. J.*, **2**, 203–9

Insler, V., Melmed, H., Eichenbrenner, I., Serr, D.M. and Lunenfeld, B. (1972). The Cervical Score: a simple semiquantitative method for monitoring of the menstrual cycle. *Int. J. Gynaecol. Obstet.*, **10**, 223–8

Irving, F.C. (1924). A new method of insuring sterility following caesarean section. *Am. J. Obstet. Gynecol.*, **8**, 335–7

Ito, H. (1938). On the symptoms of ovulation. *Jpn. J. Obstet. Gynecol.*, **21**, 9

Jordan, W.M. (1962). Pulmonary embolism. *Lancet*, **2**, 1146

Keefe, E.F. (1962). Self-observation of the cervix to distinguish days of possible fertility. *Bulletin of the Sloane Hospital for Women*, **8**, 129–36

Knaus, H. (1933). Die periodische Frucht – und Unfruchtbarkeit des Weibes. *Zbl. Gynakol.*, **57**, 1393

Koyama, I. and Oato, N. (1974). Condom use in Japan. In Redford, M.H., Duncan, G.W. and Prager, D.J. (eds.) *The Condom: Increasing Utilization in the United States.* (San Francisco: San Francisco Press)

Kroener, W.F. Jr. (1969). Surgical sterilization by fimbriectomy. *Am. J. Obstet. Gynecol.*, **104**, 247

Lachnit-Faxson, U. (1980). The rationale for a new triphasic contraceptive. In Greenblatt, R.B. (ed.) *The Development of a New Triphasic Oral Contraceptive*, p. 23. (Lancaster: MTP Press Ltd.)

Lanctot, C.A. (1979). Natural family planning. In Connell, E.B. (ed.) *Clinics in Obstetrics and Gynaecology*, Vol. 6 No. 1, *Contraception*, pp. 109–27. (London, Philadelphia, Toronto: W.B. Saunders Co. Ltd)

Leader, A.J., Alexrod, S.D., Frankowski, R. and Mumford, S.D. (1974). Complications of 2711 vasectomies. *J. Urol.*, **111**, 365–9

Lungren, S.S. (1881). A case of caesarian section twice successfully performed on the same patient. *Am. J. Obstet. Gynecol.*, **14**, 78

McLaren, A. (1990). *A History of Contraception from Antiquity to the Present Day.* (Oxford: Basil Blackwell)

Madlener, M. (1919). Uber sterilisierende Operationen an den Tuben. *Zbl. Gynakol.*, **43**, 380–4

Marshall, J. (1963). *The Infertile Period: Principles and Practice*, p. 118. (Baltimore: Helicon Press)

Mensinga, W.P.J. (1882). Fakultative Sterilate. (Leipzig)

Mills, A. (1984). Barrier contraception. In Newton, J.R. (ed.) *Clinics in Obstetrics and Gynaecology*: Vol. 11, No. 3, *Contraception Update*, pp. 641–60. (London, Philadelphia, Toronto: W.B. Saunders & Co)

Mills, A. (1988). AIDS and barriers. In Hudson, C.N. and Sharp, F. (eds.) *AIDS and Obstetrics and Gynaecology. Proceedings of the 19th Study Group of the RCOG*, London, March 1988

Morris, J.M. and van Wagenen, G. (1969). Post-coital oral contraception. In Sobrero, A.J. and Leweit, S. (eds.) *Advances in Planned Parenthood*. (Amsterdam: Excerpta Medica)

Moss, W.M. (1972). A sutureless technique for bilateral partial vasectomy. *Fertil. Steril.*, **23**, 33

National Fertility Study (1965), reported in Potts, M. and Diggory, P. (1983). *Textbook of Contraceptive Practice*, 2nd edn. p. 122. (Cambridge: Cambridge University Press)

Newton, J.R. (1985). Intrauterine contraceptive devices. In Loudon, N. (ed.) *Handbook of Family Planning*, pp. 152. (Edinburgh, London: Churchill Livingstone)

Ogino, K. (1930). Ovulationstermin und Konzeptionstermin. *Zbl. Gynakol.*, **54**, 464–79

Palmer, A. (1949). The diagnostic use of basal body temperature in gynecology and obstetrics. *Obstet. Gynaecol. Surg.*, **4**, 1–26

Palmer, R. (1962). Essais de sterilisation tubaire coelioscopique par electrocoagulation isthmique. *Bull. Federat. Soc. Gynecol. Obstet.*, **14**, 298

Palmer, R. and Devillers, J. (1939). Action thermique des hormones sexuelles chez la femme. *C. R. Seanc. Soc. Biol.* **130**, 895–6

Pemberton, J., McCann, J.S. and Mahony, J.P.H. (1972). Sociomedical characteristics of patients attending a VD clinic and the circumstances of infection. *Br. J. Venereal Dis.*, **48**, 391–6

Pierce, R.M. and Rowntree, G. (1961). Birth control in Britain part 2. *Pop. Stud.*, **15**, 121

Potts, M (1984). Cabbages and condoms: packaging and channels of distribution. In Newton, J.R. (ed.) *Clinics in Obstetrics and Gynaecology*, Vol. 11, No. 3, *Contraception Update*, pp.799–809. (London, Philadeiphia, Toronto: W.B. Saunders & Co.)

Potts, M. and Diggory, P. (1983). *Textbook of Contraceptive Practice*, 2nd edn. pp. 121;136. (London, New York: Cambridge University Press)

Potts, M. and Rosenfield, A. (1990a). The fifth freedom revisited. *Lancet*, **336**, 1227

Potts, M. and Rosenfield, A. (1990b). The fifth freedom revisited: 11, the way forward. *Lancet*, **336**, 1293–5

Pouchet, F.A. (1847). Theorie positive de l'ovulation spontanée et de la fecondation des mammiferes et de l'espece humaine, basée sur l'observation de toute la serie animale. Paris.

Power, F.H. and Barnes A.C. (1941). Sterilization by means of peritoneoscopic tubal fulguration. *Am. J. Obstet. Gynecol.*, **41**, 1038–43

Prenant, A. (1898). La valeur morphologique du corps jaune. Son action physiologique et therapeutique possible. *Rev. Gen. Sci. Pure. Appl.*, **9**, 646–50

Ramcharan, S., Pellegrin, F.A., Ray, R.M. *et al.* (1980). The Walnut Creek Contraceptive Drug Study: a prospective study of the side effects of oral contraceptives: a comparison of disease occurrence leading to hospitalization or death in users and non-users of oral contraceptives. *J. Reprod. Med.*, **25**, (Suppl.), 345

Reid, K.M. (1985). Choice of method. In Loudon, N. (ed.) *Handbook of Family Planning*, pp. 25–39. (Edinburgh, London, Melbourne, New York: Churchill Livingstone)

Reimers, D. and Jeyek, A. (1971). Simultaneous use of rifampin and other antituberculous agents with oral contraceptions. *Prax. Pneumol.*, **25**, 255–62

Rioux, J.E. and Cloutier, D. (1974). Bipolar cautery for sterilization by laparoscopy. *J. Reprod. Med.*, **13**, 6–10

Robertson, W.H. (1990). *An Illustrated History of Contraception*, pp. 116;121. (Carnforth: Parthenon Publishing Group)

Royal College of General Practitioners Oral Contraception Study (1977). Mortality among oral contraceptive users. *Lancet*, **2**, 727

Schmidt, S.S. (1966). Technics and complications of elective vasectomy: the role of spermatic granuloma in spontaneous recanalization. *Fertil. Steril.*, **17**, 467

Seguy, J. and Simonnet, H. (1933). Recherche de signes directs d'ovulation chez la femme. *Gynecologie et Obstetrique*, **28**, 656–63

Semm, K. (1973). Sterilisierung durch thermokoagulation der pars intramuralis tubae per hysteroscopian. *Endoscopy*, **5**, 218–20

Siboulet, A. (1972). Maladies sexuelles transmissibles: interet des traitements prophylactiques. *Prophylaxie Sanitaire et Morale*, **44**, 155–9

Sobotta, J. (1896). Ueber die bildung des Corpus Luteum bei der maus. *Arch. Mikr. Anat.*, **47**, 261

Sobotta, J. (1897). Uber die bildung des Corpus Luteum beim Kaninchen *Anat. Hefte.*, **8**, 469–524

Soderstrom, R.M. and Smith, M.R. (1971). Tubal sterilization: a new laparoscopic method. *Obstet. Gynecol.*, **3**, 152

Soderstrom, R.M. and Yuzpe, A.A. (1979). Female Sterilization. In Connell, E.B. (cd.) *Clinics in Obstetrics and Gynaecology* Vol. 6/No. 1, April, Contraception, pp. 77–95. (London, Philadelphia, Toronto: W.B. Saunders Co. Ltd.)

Speert, H. (1973). *Iconographia Gyniatrica: A Pictorial History of Gynecology and Obstetrics*, p. 450. (Philadelphia: F.A. Davis Co)

Squire, W. (1868). Puerperal temperatures. *Trans. Obstet. Soc., London*, **9**, 129

Steptoe, P.C. (1967). *Laparoscopy in Gynaecology*. (Edinburgh, London: E. & S. Livingstone)

Steptoe, P.C. (1971). Recent advances in surgical methods of control of fertility and infertility. *Br. Med. Bull.*, **26**, 152

Swyer, G.I.M. (1982). Potency of progestogens in oral contraceptives – further delay of menses data. *Contraception*, **26**, 23

Tausk, M. (1969). The mechanism of action of oral contraceptives. *Acta Obstet. Gynecol. Scand.*, **48** (Suppl. 1), 41

Tietze, C. (1970). Ranking of contraceptive methods by levels of effectiveness. *Advances in Planned Parentage*, **6**, 117–26

Treloar, A.E., Boynton, R.E., Behn, B.G. and Brown, B.W. (1967). Variation of the human menstrual cycle through reproductive life. *Int. J. Fertil.*, **12**, 77–126

Uchida, H. (1975). Uchida tubal sterilization. *Am. J. Obstet. Gynecol.*, **121**, 153

van de Velde, T.H. (1928). *Die Vollkommene Ehe: Eine Studie uber ihre Physiologie und Technik*, 21st edn. (Leipzig and Stuttgart: Medizinischer Verlag)

Vessey, M., Doll, R., Peto, R., Johnson, B. and Wiggins, P. (1976). A long-term follow-up study of women using different methods of contraception: an interim report. *J. Biosoc. Sci.*, **8**, 375–427

Vessey, M., Lawless, M. and Yeates, D. (1982). Efficiency of different contraceptive methods. *Lancet*, **1**, 841–2

Viergiver, E. and Pommerenke, T. (1944). Measurement of the cyclic variations in the quantity of cervical mucus and its correlation with basal temperature. *Am. J. Obstet. Gynecol.*, **48**, 321–8

Wheeless, C.R. Jr. (1970). Instrument and method – elimination of second incision in laparoscopic sterilization. *Obstet. Gynecol.*, **36**, 208

Wilde, F.A. (1838). Das Weibliche Gebar-Unvermogen: Eine Medicinisch-Juridische Abhandlung Zum Gebrauch fur Practische Geburtshelfer, Aerzte, und Juristen.

World Health Organization (1979). Family Planning based on periodic abstinence: a preliminary glossary (draft) *Annexe in Proceedings of an International Conference on the State of the Art in NFP., Washington D.C.* Quoted by Lanctot, C.A. (1979) Natural Family Planning. In Connell, E.B. (ed.) *Contraception. Clinics in Obstetrics and Gynaecology*, Vol. 6 No. 1 p. 109. (London, Philadelphia, Toronto: W.B. Saunders & Co.)

Wortman, J. (1975). Female sterilization using the culdoscope. *Population Reports*, Series C, No. 6

Wortman, J. (1976). The diaphragm and other intravaginal barriers – a review. *Population Reports*, Series H, No. 4

Wright, N.H., Vessey, M.P., Kenward, B., McPherson, K. and Doll, R. (1978). Neoplasia and dysplasia of the cervix uteri and contraception: a possible protective effect of the diaphragm. *Br. J. Cancer*, **38**, 273–9

Wynants, P. and Ide, P. (1986). Endometrial morphology during a normophasic and a triphasic regimen: a comparison. *Contraception*, **33**, 149

Yoon, I.B. and King, T.M. (1975). A preliminary and intermediate report on a new laparoscopic tubal ring procedure. *J. Reprod. Med.*, **15**, 54

Youssef, H. (1993). The history of the condom. *J. R. Soc. Med.*, **86**, 226–8

FURTHER READING

Connel, E.B. (ed.) (1979). *Contraception. Clinics in Obstetrics and Gynaecology*, Vol. 6 No. 1. (London, Philadelphia, Toronto: W.B. Saunders Co. Ltd.)

Derman, R. (1989). Oral contraceptives: a reassessment. *Obstet. Gynaecol. Surv.*, **44**, 662–8

Drife, J.O. (1989). New developments in contraception. In Studd, J. (ed.) *Progress in Obstetrics and Gynaecology*, Vol. 7 pp. 245–61. (Edinburgh, London, Melbourne, New York: Churchill Livingstone)

Flynn, A.M. (1985). Natural family planning. In Loudon, N. and Newton, J. (eds.) *Handbook of Family Planning*, pp. 189–202. (Edinburgh, London, Melbourne, New York: Churchill Livingstone)

Gunn, A.D.G. (1987). *Oral Contraception in Perspective. 30 Years of Clinical Experience with the Pill.* (Carnforth: Parthenon Publishing Group)

Haspels, A.A. and Rolland, R. (eds.) (1982). *Benefits and Risks of Hormonal Contraception. Proceedings of an International Symposium*, Amsterdam, March 1982. (Lancaster: MTP Press)

Himes, N.E. (1970). *Medical History of Contraception.* (New York: Schocken Books)

Loudon, N. and Newton J. (1985). *Handbook of Family Planning.* (Edinburgh, London, Melbourne, New York: Churchill Livingstone)

McLaren, A. (1990). *A History of Contraception from Antiquity to the Present Day.* (Oxford: Basil Blackwell)

Newton, J.R. (ed.) (1984). *Contraception Update. Clinics in Obstetrics and Gynaecology*, Vol. 11 No. 3 (London, Philadelphia, Toronto: W.B. Saunders Co. Ltd.)

Potts, M. and Diggory, P. (1983). *Textbook of Contraceptive Practice*, 2nd edn. (London, New York: Cambridge University Press)

Robertson, W.H. (1990). *An Illustrated History of Contraception.* (Carnforth: Parthenon Publishing Group)

Speert, H. (1958). *Essays in Eponymy: Obstetric and Gynecologic Milestones.* (New York: The MacMillan Co.)

Speert, H. (1973). *Iconographia Gyniatrica: A Pictorial History of Gynecology and Obstetrics.* Philadelphia: F.A. Davis Co.)

Speroff, L. (1989). *Seminars in Reproductive Endocrinology*, Vol. 7, No. 3 *Oral Contraception.* Zacur, H.A. (guest ed.) (New York, Stuttgart: Thieme Medical Publishers, Inc.)

Stewart Taylor, E. (ed.) (1989). *Obstet. Gynecol. Surv.*, **44** (9)

Tayob, Y. and Guillebaud, J. (1990). Barrier methods of contraception. In Studd, J. (ed.) *Progress in Obstetrics and Gynaecology*, Vol. 8 pp. 371–90. (Edinburgh, London, Melbourne, New York: Churchill Livingstone)

Zacur, H.A. (ed.) (1989). *Seminars in Reproductive Endocrinology*, Vol. 7 No. 3. (New York, Stuttgart: Thieme Medical Publishers)

Sexuality

The term 'sex' was adopted from the old French, sexe, and from the Latin sexus (masculine) and secus (neuter). The word was first used in the English language in the late fourteenth century to distinguish between male or female. It passed into common usage in the sixteenth century and became linked with either femininity or masculinity. The concept of stronger, better or sterner sex denoting males, and gentle, weaker, fairer, softer or second sex for females, was introduced in the sixteenth and seventeenth centuries (Mills, 1991). The scientific study of sex and sexuality is relatively modern, with most research into the topic taking place in the last 75 years.

ANTIQUITY

Initially civilization used sexuality as a means of propagating the human species. However, religious practices, tribal customs and laws were soon developed to foster and control the reproductive process. In their historical perspective on sexuality, Masters *et al.* (1992) recorded that 'although written history goes back almost 5000 years, only limited information is available describing sexual behaviour and attitudes in various societies prior to 1000 BC'. They quoted Tannahill (1980) in noting that a prominent taboo against incest developed early in human history.

In ancient Egypt the gods of earth and sky were depicted with erect phalluses. Closely linked with phallus worship was vulvic symbolism and the 'divine triangle' was displayed on artefacts from 4000 BC onwards. In Egypt the mother goddess Mut had both male and female genitalia.

Isis and Osiris were both sister and brother and also husband and wife. Khepera gave birth to a second stage of existence by 'union with my hand, and I embraced my shadow in a love embrace, I poured seed into my own mouth and sent forth from myself issue in the forms of the god's Shu and Tefnut'. The courtesans of ancient Egypt were renowned for their beauty, and prostitution became common. Men were allowed many sexual partners but women's sexuality was repressed and they were considered as property with sexual and reproductive value (Bullough, 1976). Intermarriage was allowed for religious reasons but was not the general rule. Contraceptives were used and they included pessaries (a term derived from the Greek, pessos) of camel dung and other materials. Circumcision of both male and female (Pharaonic mutilation) was practised (Figure 1), and necrophilia was not unknown.

The ancient Greeks considered sexual enjoyment to be the greatest happiness of mankind. Sexual practices which are referred to as perversions in this century, were viewed in a different light at that time, and were equated with love. High class prostitutes or *hetaera* worked in brothels and paid taxes to the state. Those courtesans whose trade was connected with temples were termed *hierodules*, or sacred servants. Homosexual relationships between adult males and adolescents were tolerated (but prohibited

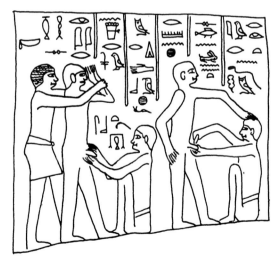

Figure 1 Egyptian scene depicting circumcision from about 2200 BC. Drawing of a carving from Sakkara Cemetery in Memphis. Reproduced with kind permission from Nunn, J.F. (1989). The *History of Anaesthesia*, p. 22. (Carnforth: Parthenon Publishing)

481

for boys under the age of puberty). Similar associations between adults were frowned upon. Although there was a strong emphasis on marriage, women were second class citizens without political or legal rights. Women were regarded as *gyne*, the bearer of children (Tannahill, 1980). Dramatic and orgiastic festivals were held in honour of Dionysis (Bacchus to the Romans) the god of wine, in which female devotees carried a gigantic model of an erect phallus. The fertility gods Hermes and Priapos were depicted in proud state.

In Roman culture it was reasoned that lack of orgasm in the male or female led to psychic imbalance and anxiety. Body oils were used prior to coitus and the Roman orgies of food, drink and sexuality (Bacchanalia) were oft described. The Romans referred to diseases of the sex organs as *morbus indecens* thus giving rise to the idea of sexual indecency. Galen, a respected teacher of medicine, had great curiosity concerning sexual activity and contraceptives, and may well have been the first proponent of sex education for physicians (Farber, 1985). The Romans alleged that oysters were aphrodisiacs and Roman legionnaires transported oysters packed in ice from Britain to Rome to keep the inhabitants in erotic mood. Juvenal (AD 60–140) wrote that oysters were the favourite food of 'lascivious women'.

There are rules about sexual conduct in the Old Testament and adultery was forbidden. Sex was not considered evil but was depicted as a creative or pleasurable force. However, the development of Christianity saw the introduction of a more restrictive attitude towards sexuality. St Augustine of the fourth century spoke of 'hell's black river of lust', and himself 'tormented' by sexual thoughts, was instrumental in the formation of a strong negative attitude to sex in the Christian religion.

MIDDLE AGES

The teachings of the Roman Catholic church which forbade all forms of sexual expression other than direct attempts at procreation within marriage had a major influence on sexuality in Europe. New ideals of love and virtue were promulgated while asceticism and chastity were encouraged. Sex was devalued and the teachings of prominent church members, including those of St Augustine and St Paul, argued for the suppression of the sexual drive while equating it with evil. The clergy were celibate but sexual activity among its members was not unheard of. Physicians were forbidden to provide contraceptives.

Meanwhile in the East, sex was regarded as an act of worship; a path towards immortality, and was generally viewed in a much more positive way. The *Kama Sutra*, an Indian sex manual, was compiled, and similar books which glorified sexual pleasure were available. Sir Richard Burton's translation of the *Kama Sutra* appeared as a small edition in 1883. He dedicated the translation to 'that small portion of the British public which takes enlightened interest in studying the manners and customs of the older east'.

In Hindu belief semen was the basis of health, strength and long life. As such it was taught that the sex fluid should be conserved as far as possible. The early Chinese believed that ejaculation diminished the 'yang' or male life force and therefore threatened man's strength and could even shorten life. The early Tantric tribes, who worshipped the vulva, used various techniques to regulate seminal emission so that an unshed portion of it could ascend and nourish the brain.

THE RENAISSANCE, REFORMATION AND PURITAN PERIODS

Christian traditions continued to regard sexuality in a satanic light and the official attitude was one of repression. Despite that, religious houses themselves were often 'hot beds of sexuality' (Taylor, 1954). Syphilis first appeared during the Renaissance and had a profound effect upon sexual practice. Various methods of treatment for the disease evolved, and Gabriel Fallopius introduced a linen condom to prevent transmission of the infection. A new chaste style of living emerged and courtly love in which women were elevated to an immaculate plane, was introduced. Love and romanticism were celebrated in literature and music. Chastity belts which prevented penetration but allowed for waste elimination were introduced . Although originally designed to prevent rape they were used by many husbands to lock up their wives. By the seventeenth century however, sexual restrictions were loosened and Protestant reformers advocated a more positive attitude towards sexual matters.

THE EIGHTEENTH AND NINETEENTH CENTURIES

Attitudes to sexuality varied in different countries and between different religious groups and levels of society. While American attitudes were puritanical there was a broad tolerance of sexuality both in England and France. However, with the development of large cities in America more tolerant attitudes to sex developed there and soon prostitution became commonplace.

Various groups evolved in the 1820s and 1830s whose primary mission was to combat the social evils of prostitution and rescue 'fallen women' (Masters *et al.*, 1992). As brothels were closed down there was a corresponding rise in 'massage clinics' and 'escort services'.

The Victorian era began in the mid-1800s and once again sexual repression was the order of the day. Physicians advocated the control of sexual activity and it was theorized that the loss of semen through masturbation caused physical debilitation. Despite the Victorian prudery, the poverty of the lower classes forced many women into prostitution at a time when clothing styles did not allow a glimpse of ankle or bare neck, and when pornography was banned by law for the first time. Women were regarded as inferior to men and were thought to have almost no sexual response. Clitoridectomy was advocated for women with an interest in sexual matters (Lowndes Sevely,1987). In the last decades of the nineteenth century there was a spectacular new preoccupation with the scientific study of sexuality, giving rise to a new medical sub-discipline, that of 'sexology' (Weeks, 1985).

TWENTIETH CENTURY

The interest in sexuality increased throughout the twentieth century. Survey research became popular and the Kinsey data of the 1940s and 1950s, the work of Masters and Johnson, the Hunt report of 1974, the Shere Hite surveys and many magazine surveys, pushed sexuality to best seller status and provoked considerable controversy in sex research.

The advent of the oral contraceptive pill and of treatment for sexually transmitted diseases had a major impact on sexual function, as did increased liberalism in books, cinema, television and video films. Interest in marital and sexual counselling developed and technical books about sex were published. The practice of non-marital cohabitation began and assumed importance as a stage preceding marriage. Major strides were made in the treatment of sexual victimization, and the sexual abuse of children and of wives within marriage was highlighted. The permissive

society allowed promiscuous sexual behaviour which induced a backlash from the 'moral majority', who called for an end to non-marital sex. Despite the increased availability of knowledge, some forms of sexual outlet were still viewed as perversions. Many parents and school authorities failed to apply sex education with the result that unwanted pregnancy, and sexually transmitted disease, became commonplace. The recent affliction with the human immuno-deficiency virus has altered sexual behaviour towards 'safe practice' but only among informed homosexuals and in some interested groups.

Although society now treats sexuality with openness and curiosity, this attitude will change. Masters *et al.* (1982) stated that 'we cannot know of course if the changes in trends we see as significant today will have any lasting impact on our sexual behaviour over time . . . the only thing we can be sure of is that our attitudes and behaviours will continue to change – what directions those changes will take, however, is impossible to predict with any accuracy'.

SEXOLOGISTS

Richard von Krafft-Ebing

One of the founding fathers of sexology was Richard von Krafft-Ebing, a German psychiatrist whose *Psychopathia Sexualis* (1886) contained a detailed classification of sexual disorders. His writings had a profound effect on public, medical and legal attitudes. Due to his work as a forensic psychiatrist most of his case histories were taken from criminals and he condemned almost all forms of sexual activity. Although he advocated sympathetic medical concern in dealing with sex criminals, he appeared to equate sex with crime and violence. Krafft-Ebing derived some of his descriptive terms for sexual behaviour from names in literature. He coined the term 'sadism' after the Marquis de Sade and also introduced the term 'masochism' after Sacher Masoch who described sexual relief from self-inflicted pain. In his *Psychopathia Sexualis*, which went through 12 editions, he described details of sexual activities in Latin to ensure that they would be read by doctors only (Figure 2). Although Krafft-Ebing is often considered the founder of modern sexology, he viewed any sexual practice other than a clearly procreative one as a perversion, and ultimately did a disservice to the development of psychosexual medicine.

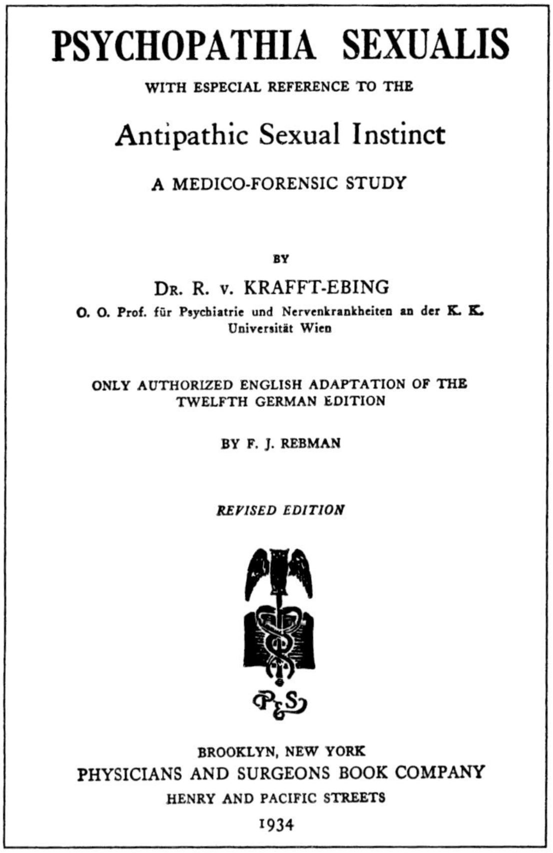

PSYCHOPATHIA SEXUALIS

WITH ESPECIAL REFERENCE TO THE

Antipathic Sexual Instinct

A MEDICO-FORENSIC STUDY

BY

DR. R. v. KRAFFT-EBING

O. O. Prof. für Psychiatrie und Nervenkrankheiten an der K. K.
Universität Wien

ONLY AUTHORIZED ENGLISH ADAPTATION OF THE
TWELFTH GERMAN EDITION

BY F. J. REBMAN

REVISED EDITION

BROOKLYN, NEW YORK
PHYSICIANS AND SURGEONS BOOK COMPANY
HENRY AND PACIFIC STREETS
1934

Figure 2 Title page from the 1934 English edition of R. v. Krafft-Ebing's famous book which was first published in German in Stuttgart in 1886 and went into many editions in many languages

Magnus Hirschfeld

Magnus Hirschfeld (1868–1935) was a German psychiatrist who specialized in homosexuality. He founded the first scientific journal of sexual pathology in 1899. He was the first to make a proper distinction between homosexuality and transvestism. Hirschfeld advocated the reform of laws that penalized homosexuals.

He preceded Alfred Kinsey in compiling data on sexual behaviour, but unfortunately most of his pioneering work was destroyed by the Nazis. His major work was entitled *Sex Anomalies and Perversions*.

Albert von Schrenck-Notzing

Albert von Schrenck-Notzing (1862–1929) was a Viennese psychiatrist whose pioneering work

helped to create the climate in which Sigmund Freud's major discoveries became acceptable. He attempted to modify the sexual orientation of homosexuals with the help of hypnotic suggestion and visits to brothels where he endeavoured to achieve their reconditioning to heterosexual relationships. His book on modifying sexual orientation foreshadowed Pavlov's achievements on conditioned reflexes.

Havelock Ellis

Havelock Ellis (1859–1939) was a man of wide interests who was a prolific writer. He studied medicine at St Thomas's Hospital London, and is famous for his six-volume series called *Studies in the Psychology of Sex*, which was written between 1897 and 1910. Ellis had remarkably modern views for his time and wrote on the recognition of erotic love as art; the importance of touch, smell, sight and hearing in lovemaking; the nature of erotic dreams and other aspects of 'normal sexuality'. He also wrote with open-mindedness on premarital relations, birth control, elimination of criminal laws against homosexual acts between consenting adults, and changes in the divorce laws. He investigated almost every sexual idiosyncracy and he invented the terms 'auto-eroticism' and 'narcissism'. Ellis was widely admired for his compassionate views on sexuality.

Sigmund Freud

Sigmund Freud (1856–1939) (Figure 3) was a Viennese physician whose main discovery was the great influence of sexuality on the development of human personality. Freud brought a new dimension to psychosexual medicine. He described the oral, anal and genital stages of sexual development in the first years of life. Freud introduced the theory that sexuality was the motivating force of human behaviour and a cause of neuroses. He introduced the concepts of the Oedipus complex, castration anxiety, and penis envy. Freud devised the clinical method of psychoanalysis to assess and treat psychological problems.

Marie Stopes

Marie Carmichael Stopes (1880–1958) proclaimed women's rights to personal fulfilment and sexual satisfaction in marriage. Her first marriage was

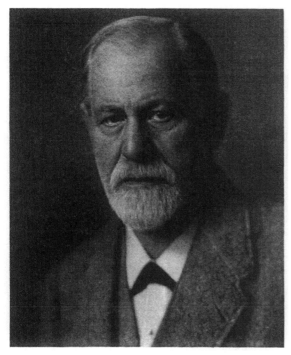

Figure 3 Sigmund Freud (1856–1939). The father of psychoanalysis (*see* text)

sexually unhappy and she sought annulment in 1916. During marriage to her second husband, Vernon Roe, she wrote books on Married Love and Wise Parenthood. Stopes opened the first British birth control clinic in 1921 and advocated the use of the diaphragm. In 1922 she founded the Society for Constructive Birth Control which became the precursor of the Family Planning Association.

Alfred Kinsey

Alfred Charles Kinsey (1894–1956) a zoologist at Indiana university USA, made major contributions to the study of human sexual behaviour. His interest in human sexuality began in the late 1930s when he was asked to participate in teaching a college course on marriage. He found that the existing knowledge of sexual behaviour was lacking in scientific validity.

In 1941 Kinsey established an institute for sexual research at the University of Indiana and was joined by Clyde E. Martin, Wardell B. Pomeroy and Dr Paul Gebbard. Kinsey developed data-gathering methods, mainly in the form of interviews, and analysed statistical information

about the sexual behaviour of thousands of ordinary men and women. With his colleagues Pomeroy and Martin, Kinsey published *Sexual Behaviour in the Human Male* (1948) and then wrote a companion volume on *Sexual Behaviour in the Human Female* (1953).

Masters and Johnson

William H. Masters an American gynaecologist and Virginia E. Johnson of St Louis, Missouri formed a research and therapy team who studied and treated sexuality and its abnormalities. They concentrated on the development of sex therapy for couples and applied specific behavioural techniques in treatment. Masters had begun his work with prostitutes of both sexes but realized that they were not typical of average American citizens. He advertised for an assistant and found Mrs Johnson of the Missouri Ozarks, a separated woman with two children. They formed a formidable research partnership and later they married. The reports of their research in *Human Sexual Response* (1966) and a further book *Human Sexual Inadequacy* (1970) became standard works for sex therapists in the treatment of sexual dysfunction. Further texts added to the stature of their pioneering work in the field of human sexuality (Masters *et al.*, 1982; 1992).

REFERENCES

Bullough, V.L. (1976). *Sexual Variance in Society and History.* (New York: Wiley)

Farber, M. (1985). *Human Sexuality: Psychosexual Effects of Disease*, pp. 3–9. (New York, London: MacMillan Publishing Co.)

Kinsey, A.C., Pomeroy, W.B. and Martin, C.E. (1948). *Sexual Behavior in the Human Male.* (Philadelphia: Saunders)

Kinsey, A.C., Pomeroy, W.B., Martin, C.E. and Gebhard, P.H. (1953). *Sexual Behavior in the Human Female.* (Philadelphia: Saunders)

Krafft-Ebbing von, R. (1906). (English adaptation of the 12th German edition) *Psychopathia Sexualis. Medico Forensic Study with especial reference to the antipathic sexual instinct.* (Brooklyn, New York)

Lowndes Sevely, J. (1987). *Eves Secrets. A New Perspective on Human Sexuality*, p. XV of Introduction. (London, Glasgow: Paladin Grafton Books)

Masters, W.H. and Johnson, V.E. (1966). *Human Sexual Response*, p. 711. (Boston: Little Brown & Co.)

Masters, W.H. and Johnson, V.E. (1970). *Human Sexual Inadequacy*. (Boston: Little Brown & Co.)

Masters, W.H., Johnson, V.E. and Kolodny, R.C. (1982). *Masters and Johnson on Sex and Human Loving*, p. 25. (Boston, London: Little Brown & Co., & MacMillan London Ltd.)

Masters, W.H., Johnson, V.E. and Kolodny, R.C. (1992). *Human Sexuality*, 4th edn. pp. 8–17. (New York: Harper Collins)

Mills, J. (1991). *Woman Words: A Vocabulary of Culture and Patriarchal Society*, pp. 213–14. (London: Virago Press)

Tannahill, R. (1980). *Sex in History*, pp. 94–5. (New York: Stein & Day)

Taylor, G.R. (1954). *Sex and History*, p. 19. (New York: Vanguard)

Weeks (1985). *Sexuality and its Discontents, Meanings, Myths and Modern Sexualities*, pp. 15–32. (London, New York: Routledge)

FURTHER READING

Masters, W.H., Johnson, V.E. and Kolodny, R.C. (1992). *Human Sexuality*, 4th edn. (New York: Harper Collins Publishers)

Sussman, N. (1976). Sex and sexuality in history. In Sadock, B.J., Kaplan, H. and Freedman, A.M. (eds.) *The Sexual Experience*, 1st edn. pp. 7–70. (Baltimore: Williams and Wilkins)

Information technology

The collection, analysis and storage of data have become an important function of medical practice in the second half of the twentieth century. The development of the computer played a major role in the ever-expanding information technology market.

THE COMPUTER

The computer is an electronic device that performs calculations and processes information. It can handle vast amounts of facts and figures and solve complicated problems at incredibly high speeds. The fastest computers are able to process millions of pieces of information in seconds. A recent definition notes that a computer is 'a device designed primarily for doing arithmetic and one which is capable of doing its sums at very high speed. It must further be capable of storing a program (an ordered set of human commands) and of obeying that program under its own control. The ability to handle data, with a capacity and a processing speed commensurate with the current technology, will also be a necessary requirement' (Richards, 1990).

HISTORY OF COMPUTING

The development of the computer owes much to the inventions and ideas of many mathematicians and scientists over the years. The story starts with the introduction of the *abacus*. This was the 'ancestor' of the calculator and was originally used in Babylonia c. 3000 BC. In its original form it was a slab of wood covered with fine sand on which figures were written with a stylus. The abacus later evolved to the form of a bead frame, which aided mathematical operations and on which the result was recorded.

The Scotsman John Napier (1550–1617) invented *logarithms* in 1614 while researching a method of numerical calculation. His system allowed replacement of multiplication by addition, and of division by subtraction. A Frenchman Joseph-Marie Jacquard (1752–1834) devised a *mechanical loom* in 1805. This machine used a card with punched out holes to control weaving patterns. In 1886 an American by the name of Herman Hollerith (1860–1929) combined the Jacquard (and Babbage) *punched card system*, with an electromagnetic invention. His system was first used in 1886 and subsequently played a major role in the analysis of the 1890 census figures. Hollerith later developed *punching and sorting machines* which were the precursors of modern computer peripherals.

Further developments of note included the invention of an *analogue slide rule* device by William Oughtred of England, and the digital mechanical calculator produced by Wilhelm Schickard of Germany in 1623. Schickard was a professor at the University of Heidelberg and he called his arithmetical machine a *calculator clock*. It was capable of performing the four basic operations of addition, subtraction, multiplication and division.

Charles Babbage (1792–1871), Professor of Mathematics at Cambridge University, produced his first calculator in 1823. This machine, which he called an *analytical engine*, was the world's first digital computer. It used a system of 50 cog-wheels and data were entered by means of punched cards (Giscard d'Estaing, 1990). The first programs for this primitive computer were written by Ada, The Countess Lovelace (Figure 1).

The French mathematician and scientist Blaise Pascal constructed a calculating machine which was the ancestor of a modern pocket calculator. Pascal invented his machine (when he was aged 19) to assist his father with tax collection. A further important contribution was made by George Boole an English logician who in the mid-1800s devised a system of logic (*Boolian algebra*) which later helped scientists to design switching circuits for the arithmetic unit of electronic computers. In this system logical statements were formulated symbolically so that they could be written and proved in a way similar to that of ordinary algebra.

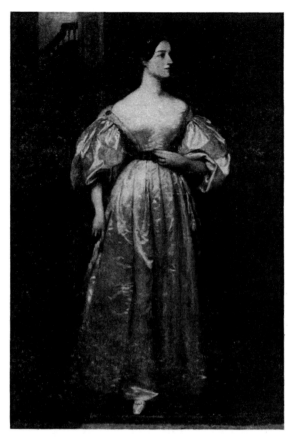

Figure 1 Ada, Countess Lovelace wrote the first computer programs for Babbage's machine (*see* text). Reproduced with kind permission from the Central Photographic Section, National Physical Laboratory, Teddington, Middlesex

The first reliable *analogue computer* was developed by an American electrical engineer Vannevar Bush in 1930. His machine, which was called a 'differential analyser', was developed to solve differential equations. In the 1930s a German engineer Conrad Zuse built a computer, which he named the Z1, based on mechanical principles. Later versions of the machine used electro-mechanical and then electronic relay systems. A further advance included the introduction of a *binary computer* by an American mathematician George R. Stibitz in 1939. The first fully automatic calculator was devised by Howard Aitken of Harvard University in 1943. In the same year *semi-electronic digital computing* was devised by John V. Atanasoff, an American physicist and mathematician.

The *ENIAC* (electronic numerical integrator and computor) project was devised in 1946 by Presper Eckert Jr. with the aid of John W. Mauchly in 1946. These two University of Pennsylvania engineers used vacuum tubes for controlling computing operations. The ENIAC machine worked about 1000 times as fast as the previous best computer. It could perform approximately 5000 arithmetic operations per second. The Hungarian born American mathematician John Von Neumann devised programs which could be coded as numbers and stored in the computer's memory. His machine the *EDVAC* (electronic discrete variable automatic computor) was completed in 1949 and was the first stored-program digital computer.

Meanwhile in Europe, Dr Alan Mathison Turing worked with a group of British numbers' theorists who decoded German military messages. Turing adapted the notion of algorithms to calculate certain functions and postulated the *Turing machine*, which would be capable of calculating any calculable function. In 1943 Professor H.A. Newman formulated the *Colossus* which could process 5000 characters per second. Eventually in 1948 Turing, Newman, F.C. Williams and Tom Kilburn developed a *stored program computer* whose program was a sequence of numbers stored in the computer's memory. Their work was based on the ideas of John Von Neumann of Princeton, New Jersey.

The invention of the *transistor* in 1947 by three physicists at the Bell Laboratories, USA (William Shockley, John Bardeen and Walter Brattain), and of solid-state devices during the 1950s and 1960s resulted in the production of faster and more reliable electronic computers. Various operating systems were introduced from 1954 when Jean Amdahl first designed a system for International Business Machines (IBM). The first computers for general use became available in 1957 and they and their successors were termed *main frame computers*. The *microchip* was invented in 1958 by Jacques St Clair Kilby of the University of Illinois.

The first *integrated circuit* was patented in 1964, 5 years after application. Miniaturization of electronic equipment continued from the late 1960s and led to further advances in computer technology. The first *microprocessor* was developed by Marcian E. Hoff in 1971.

Data storage facilities were upgraded when floppy discs were invented in 1950 by Dr Yashiro Nakamats of the University of Tokyo, who granted the sales licence for the disc to IBM. Hard disc cards were invented in 1985, the same year in which *CD/ROM* (compact disc/read only memory) was also first introduced. The *WORM* (write once read many times) was introduced by IBM in 1987 and offered the capability of storing video and television frames such as histology slides, or various aspects of medical illustration. Although the main function of microprocessors was calculation, the increasing demand for graphics processors led to the introduction of *graphics manipulation* by computer, by Texas Instruments and Intel in 1986.

COMPUTERS IN MEDICINE

Interest in the medical applications of microcomputers developed from the end of the 1970s as clinicians and other health workers realized that considerable benefit could be derived from the application of this new technology to existing clinical problems (Corbett, 1987). It was realized that the microcomputer could be used for the storage and retrieval of patient information; for processing to enable audit application; to aid computer learning and decision support, and could also be tailored to solve specific clinical problems.

During the mid-1960s the only source of maternity statistics available in the UK was a 10% sample of hospital discharges (maternity hospital inpatient enquiry – HIPE). Originally the collection and production of vital statistics for England and Wales was pioneered by William Farr in the late 1830s while in the USA Herman Hollerith invented a punch card system and mechanical sorter which was used in the USA census. The registration of births and deaths began in 1837 in England and Wales, 1855 in Scotland and in 1864 in Ireland. Stillbirth registration became the law in 1927 for England and Wales, in 1939 for Scotland and in 1961 for Northern Ireland (Barron and MacFarlane, 1990). In the UK there were national surveys of births and perinatal mortality statistics in 1946,1958 and 1970. The combination of the statistics for stillbirth with early neonatal death was suggested by Peller (1948) who coined the term 'perinatal'. Dougal Baird of Scotland is also credited with introduction of the term. The hospital inpatient enquiry (HIPE) began during 1949 in England and Wales.

The Royal College of Obstetricians, in collaboration with the Department of Health, introduced a maternity version of hospital activity analysis which provided the government with improved information and offered the possibility of a detailed annual report produced by a main frame computer.

In the mid-1970s discussions began about replacing that system with a modified version to produce a standard maternity information system (SMIS). In 1980 Edith Korner chaired a steering group on health services, known as the Korner Committee, which produced a number of reports later implemented by the health services. The Korner maternity data set was derived mainly from work already carried out for SMIS (Barron, 1987). By the mid-1980s microprocessors were used in gynaecology, for monitoring the expectant mother and fetus in labour, and for use in obstetric data systems.

Information systems were developed for administration – a basic data set for patient identification with social and other data, including the name of family doctor and hospital consultant and hospital identification number. Maternal and fetal risk factors were addressed and special requirements identified.

As time went by computerized literature searches became feasible with 'online access' to biomedical databases such as MEDLINE (Index Medicus online). A BLAISE – LINK service was developed between the British Library and the Northern Library of Medicine in Bethesda, Maryland, USA. Although computerized literature searches were found to have limitations they were thought to be an excellent way to begin planning a clinical trial.

REFERENCES

Barron, S.L. (1987). The impact of information technology on obstetrics and gynaecology. In Dalton, K.J. and Fawdry, R.D.S. (eds.) *The Computer in Obstetrics and Gynaecology*, pp. 1–4. (Oxford: Irl Press Ltd.)

Barron, S.L. and MacFarlane, A.J. (1990). Collection and use of routine maternity data. In Lilford, R.J. (ed.) *Computing and Decision Support in Obstetrics and Gynaecology. Clin. Obstet. Gynaecol.*, **4**, pp. 681–97. (London, Philadelphia, Sydney, Tokyo, Toronto: Bailliere Tindall)

Corbett, W.A. (1987). Introductory remarks. In Corbett, W.A. (ed.) *Medical Applications of Microcomputers*, pp. 1–4. (Chichester, New York, Brisbane, Toronto, Singapore: John Wiley & Sons)

Giscard d'Estaing, V.A. (1990). *The Book of Inventions and Discoveries*, pp. 113–27. (London: Queen

Anne Press Division of MacDonald & Co. Publishers Ltd.)

Peller, S. (1948). Mortality: past and future. *Population Studies*, 1, 405–24

Richards, B. (1990). The technical aspects of computers. In Lilford, R.J. (ed.) *Computing and Decision Support in Obstetrics and Gynaecology: Clin. Obstet. Gynaecol.*, **4**, pp. 655–80. (London, Philadelphia, Sydney, Tokyo, Toronto: Bailliere Tindall)

FURTHER READING

Corbett, W.A. (1987). *Medical Applications of Microcomputers*. (Chichester, New York, Brisbane, Toronto, Singapore: John Wiley & Sons)

Dalton, K.J. and Fawdry, R.D.S. (1987). *The Computer in Obstetrics and Gynaecology*. (Oxford, Washington, D.C.: Irl Press)

Urology

VESICO-VAGINAL FISTULA

The problem of vesico-vaginal fistula dates from antiquity with Mahfouz Bey (1929) reporting the existence of a large vesico-vaginal fistula found at post-mortem examination of the mummified remains of the Egyptian Queen Henhenit, the wife of King Mentuhotep (c.2050 BC). The Greeks were also aware of the problem and Hippocrates referred to the condition (Lower, 1930). The first to associate prolonged labour with urinary incontinence and fistula formation was Avicenna in 1037. The first attempt at a cure was by Heindrik van Roonhuyse of Amsterdam (1663) who dissected the bladder free from the vaginal wall, fastened the fistula edges together with quills, and tied them with silk threads.

Fabricius Hildanus (1560-1634) was a German surgeon who developed methods of breast amputation for cancer. He also described three cases of imperforate hymen. His cure for vesico-vaginal fistula was by frequent vaginal injections of barley water mixed with fenugreek and the mucilage of quince seeds. Treatment continued for 8 months, and was said to have cured one case.

William Smellie (1697–1763) rarely suggested operation, but preferred instead the use of indwelling catheters. The treatment of vesico-vaginal fistula in the eighteenth century consisted of cautery, or abraiding the edges and then approximating the raw surfaces with pins or sharp goose quills. In the early nineteenth century many forms of treatment were experimented with (Falk and Tanger, 1954). Catheters, pessaries, and truss fittings were used by Desault. Nitrates of silver of mercury were applied to the fistula by Lallemand and also by Roux. Various types of sutures, pins and wires, were used by Naegele of Heidelberg. Vaginal obliteration was tried by DeCassls, and edge excision with closure using special twisted sutures was pioneered by Malagodl of Bologne (Ricci, 1943; 1945).

Other operators were Wutzer of Bonn, who availed of suprapubic drainage; Samuel Hobart of Cork who used the knee–elbow position and reported postoperative cure in one case in 1825; Gossett of London also implemented the knee–elbow position and used gilt silver wire for his sutures achieving, 18 years before Sims, a single success which he did not follow up, nor did he appreciate its importance. Lead wire sutures were employed by John Peter Mettauer (1840) of Virginia who reported successful operations for vesico-vaginal fistula in 1838–1847. The first plastic repair was attempted by Jobert De Lamballe (1852) who used flaps of fresh skin from the labia majora or buttocks. George Hayward of Massachusetts General Hospital recorded his operations on nine patients in 1851 (Cianfrani, 1960).

Chassar Moir (1940) graphically described James Marion Sims (q.v. in Biographies) history-making approach to the cure of vesico-vaginal fistula in an address to the Oxford University Medical Society. Sims used a (spoon) speculum with a patient in the knee–chest position to allow adequate visualization of the fistula. During the operation silver wire sutures were used to close the defect. The operative details were reported in the *American Journal of Medical Sciences* (Sims,1852). Sims built a small hospital which housed seven women in the town of Montgomery, Alabama. The occupants were Negro slaves suffering from urinary incontinence due to fistula formation. Sims experimented on three of them – Lucy, Betsy and Anarcha. Multiple attempts were necessary before Sims realized that his silk sutures may have caused the inflammation which in turn led to break down of the vesico-vaginal fistula repair.

Success occurred after Sims designed new suture material. While walking around his house one day, he picked up a small section of brass wire and later wrote 'It was very fine and such as was formerly used as springs in suspenders before the days of Indiarubber. I took it round to Mister Swan who was then my jeweller, and asked him if he could make me a little silver wire about the size of the piece of brass wire. He said yes, and made it. He made it of all pure silver. Anarcha was the subject of this experiment . . . this was the 30th

491

operation performed on Anarcha . . . it seemed to me that the time would never come for the removal of the sutures . . . with a palpating heart and an anxious mind I turned her on her side, introduced the speculum, and there lay the suture apparatus just exactly as I had placed it. There was no inflammation, there was no tumefaction, nothing unnatural, and a very perfect union of the little fistula.' The date was 21 June 1849, and Sims was 36 years of age.

Some years later Sims moved to New York where he established a small hospital which was devoted to the treatment of vesico-vaginal fistula and similar birth injuries. His first success was on a Mary Smith who had recently arrived from Ireland. Eventually, after many operations, her bladder function was partly restored. She later became an assistant at the hospital. Sims was joined by Dr Thomas Addis Emmet and as more work was undertaken, the hospital facilities became inadequate. A new hospital, 'The Womens Hospital in the State of New York' was constructed and was the first proper hospital dedicated to diseases of women.

Emmet adapted Sims' methods to good effect and other operators soon took up the challenge. Colles of Dublin employed a flap dissection of the vaginal wall from the bladder and this approach became popular. Other techniques included the Martius flap operation devised in 1940; the Ingelman-Sundburg technique introduced in 1954 by the Stockholm gynaecologist; the Bastiaanse operation and the Lasko procedure. Alfred Hegar of Germany was another well-known gynaecologist who carried out vesico-vaginal fistula repair. The suprapubic approach to what had previously been a vaginal operation was popularized by O'Connor in 1957 and Dorsey in 1960 (Chassar Moir, 1961).

Mahfouz recorded experience with 758 operations and 210 others of which he kept no records and Lawson from Ibadan reported on 377 fistulae of obstetric origin.

STRESS INCONTINENCE

In 1922 Sir Eardley Holland (Figure 1) introduced the term 'stress incontinence' to refer to the involuntary loss of a small amount of urine through the intact urethra on straining, coughing, sneezing, or laughing (Kohorn 1989). In this condition it was demonstrated that there was urethral sphincter incompetence caused by bladder neck descent through the pelvic floor, or

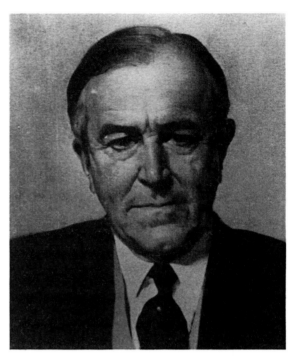

Figure 1 Sir Eardley Holland, 1879–1967. Reproduced with kind permission from the Royal College of Obstetricians and Gynaecologists

less commonly, due to reduced intraurethral pressure which resulted in loss of the positive pressure gradient between urethra and bladder.

Investigation of stress incontinence

Muellner (1949) studied the control of micturition in normal women and those with stress incontinence, by means of fluoroscopic observations of the bladder filled with contrast medium.

Radiographic studies of the urethra and bladder were carried out by Millin and Read (1948). Jeffcoate and Roberts (1952) used lateral cystourethrography on 132 patients and discovered that the urethro-vesical angle was of great importance. Roberts (1953) documented that the normal intravesical pressure was less than 10 cm of water. Bladder pressure remained constant with filling but a desire to micturate usually occurred when the volume of intravesical fluid reached 200 ml. During micturition, the bladder pressure rose to 30–50 cmH_2O, but could reach 70–100 cmH_2O during coughing or violent straining. Hodgkinson (1963) introduced a technique of bead chain cystourethrography with pressure measurements, in his investigations of incontinence.

Continence was achieved when the intra-urethral pressure exceeded that in the bladder at all times except during voiding. Enhorning (1961) discovered that increased intra-abdominal pressure affected both bladder and proximal urethra and thus maintained the pressure differential between the two, thereby allowing continence. Jeffcoate and Roberts (1952) first described the posterior urethro-vesical angle. Loss of that angle, due to tissue laxity, secondary to childbirth or advancing age, was thought to underlie the condition of stress incontinence. McGuire (1977) reported incontinence associated with a low urethral resistance.

Treatment of stress incontinence

Baker-Brown (1864) was the first to document a surgical approach to the problem of stress incontinence. His description of a suprapubic cystotomy procedure was followed by over 150 other operative techniques.

Anterior repair

This procedure was described by Donald (1888). Both he and Fothergill (1908) of Manchester repaired the utero-vaginal prolapse during which the bladder neck was elevated at anterior colporrhaphy. This approach cured many cases of stress incontinence. Howard A. Kelly (1913) of Baltimore reported his operative technique in which he plicated the paraurethral tissues, in an attempt to tighten the bladder neck. Kennedy (1937) refined the technique further. Cure rates of 38–90% were reported for anterior repair in the treatment of stress incontinence. Other operators who used the vaginal approach included Pacey in 1949, TeLinde in 1951 and Ingelman-Sundberg in 1952, each of whom introduced modifications which were found helpful (Lewis, 1964). The anterior repair exerted its effect by supporting the urethra and bladder neck by elevating the bladder neck and possibly by introducing kinking in the urethra.

The abdominal approach

Victor Marshall pioneered a suprapubic approach in 1946, which was later developed into the Marshall–Marchetti–Krantz (1949) procedure. These workers believed that stress incontinence could be cured by elevation and fixation of the urethro-vesical junction high in the pelvis. Pereyra (1959) introduced a simplified 'needle' technique which became very popular. Initially stainless steel wire was looped around the urethra (from an abdominal approach) but was soon replaced by other non-absorbable sutures. Stamey (1973) modified the technique and monitored surgery by endoscopy in an effort to avoid bladder neck or urethral penetration by needles or sutures. Stamey also introduced a 'bolster' to prevent sutures cutting through the paraurethral tissue. Other operators who became known for their modified suprapubic techniques included Burch, Perrin, Baily, Lapides *et al.* and Williams.

Green (1962) introduced a classification based on an original observation by Bailey. Using Hodgkinson's technique he classified two types of incontinence. In Type 1, there was slight posterior and inferior descent of the urethrovesical junction, for which Green advocated transvaginal cystourethropexy. In Type 2, the degree of descent was greater with more posterior and inferior rotational descent of the urethrovesical junction. There was loss of the posterior urethrovesical angle at radiology and also loss of axis of the urethra. For this Type 2 classification, Green encouraged the Marshall–Marchetti–Kranz procedure. In that procedure, the bladder neck is elevated with restoration of normal urethro-trigonal anatomy and a valvular effect is created at the bladder neck.

Sling

Goebell (1910) devised the first successful urethrovesical sling operation using the pyramidalis muscle. The sling increased outflow resistance. Frangenheim (1914) used a strip of rectus muscle fascia with pyramidalis muscle attached, while Stoeckel (1917) combined a vaginal plastic operation with the Goebell–Frangenheim procedure. Aldridge (1942) used fascial transplantation from the abdominal wall in a combined vaginal–transabdominal sling operation, and Millin and Read (1948) used a suprapubic approach to the sling technique. Various synthetic materials were used for sling operations with Marlex, nylon, plastic materials and Gortex being the most popular.

There was concern however, that urethral erosion and infection were more common with synthetic slings. Ingelman-Sundberg (1950) used ischiocavernosus muscle to buttress the urethrovesical junction. Operators whose names were associated with this technique in the 1940s included Aldridge and Studdiford, Millin and Read, Marshall, and Shaw; in the 1950s Millin, and Ingelman-Sundburg; and in the 1960s Sloane and Gordon, and Narik and Palmrich (Lewis,1964). The results of the various procedures were good with successful restoration of continence in up to 90% of cases. Sling procedures increased outflow resistance.

The Burch colposuspension

Burch (1961) first described a technique in which the paraurethral sutures were fixed to Cooper's ligament. By means of this approach Burch increased the outflow resistance which resulted in significant improvement of continence in up to 90% of cases.

Periurethral injections

Politano *et al.* (1974) pioneered the use of perineal Teflon injections for men with postprostatectomy incontinence and Politano extended the technique to stress incontinence in the female (1982) with cure rates of 40–81% being reported.

Artificial sphincter

Scott *et al.* (1974) introduced an artificial sphincter with an inflatable cuff positioned around the bladder neck, and a deflating pump with a pressure-regulating balloon, a fluid resistor and connecting tubes set in the labia majora.

Urethral reconstruction

Tanagho (1980) made a neo-urethra by sectioning the bladder from the urethra at the bladder neck, and fashioning a new urethra from a flap of bladder muscle.

Physiotherapy

Stacey Wilson of Birmingham advocated the use of pelvic exercises in the early 1900s and Green-Armytage (1948) wrote an article on the value of physiotherapy in obstetrics and gynaecology. Arnold Kegel concluded that only 60–70% of women could contract their pelvic floor muscles and he later developed a perineometer (1949a;b). The role of physiotherapy was recognized slowly but has grown in popularity in recent times.

THE UNSTABLE BLADDER

The International Continence Society established a committee for the standardization of terminology of lower urinary tract function in 1973. The unstable bladder was defined by the International Continence Society as one that 'has been shown objectively to contract, spontaneously or on provocation, during its filling phase, while the patient is attempting to inhibit micturition'. Six committee reports were produced from 1976 and provided the common foundation on terminology.

Dudley (1905) reported to the American Gynecological Society on patients who showed 'active incontinence' as opposed to patients with 'passive incontinence' as demonstrated by stress incontinence. Unstable bladder contractions were reported in men (Lappenen, 1962) following prostatectomy. Hodgkinson (1963) investigated women with symptoms of urgency and urge incontinence, and described a condition termed 'detrusor dyssynergia'. A number of terms were used for the condition following that report and Bates (1971) first used the term 'unstable bladder'. Jeffcoate (Figure 2) and Francis (1966) noted that 'two out of every three women referred by their family doctor with a provisional diagnosis of

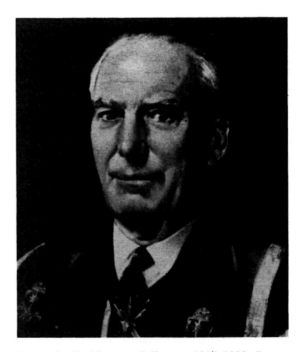

Figure 2 Sir Norman Jeffcoate, 1907–1992. Reproduced with kind permission from the Royal College of Obstetricians and Gynaecologists

stress incontinence, were proved to suffer from urgency incontinence'. Frewen (1970) pointed out that urge incontinence was a psychosomatic disorder and that its treatment should be oriented with that in mind.

Aetiology

Mosso and Pellacani (1882) implicated psychological factors when they reported that strong emotion or the sound of running water led to bladder contraction, and there were a number of reports relating urination to aggressive or erotic components (Menninger, 1941). Disturbances of bladder function associated with emotional states were confirmed by Straub *et al.* (1949). It was reported by Rees and Farhoumand (1977) that women with detrusor instability were likely to have hysterical personality traits.

Investigation

While the symptoms of frequency, urgency, urge incontinence, nocturia and sometimes stress incontinence were attributed to detrusor instability, cystometry became the best technique to diagnose the condition. Mosso and Pellacani (1882) introduced the technique of cystometry, and used incremental filling while measuring bladder pressure with a manometer. The technique was later modified for continuous filling, and a separate channel was used to measure pressure. Victor Bonney (1923) first attempted the measurement of maximum urethral pressure using a technique of retrograde sphincterometry. Simons (1936) introduced the use of the balloon catheter for cystometry and Karlson (1953) simultaneously measured intraurethral and intravesical pressure. Eventually, Asmussen and Ulmsten (1976) introduced the microtip transducer technique which became widely used for urethral pressure profilometry with simultaneous urethrocystometry.

The technique of transvaginal endosonography (Quinn *et al.*, 1988) complemented the radiographic techniques of bead chain cystourethrography (Green, 1962) and video cystourethrography (Enhorning *et al.*, 1964; Bates *et al.*, 1970). The International Continence Society (1976) advocated the use of cystometry in the diagnosis of detrusor instability. The modern urodynamic technique evolved in the late 1960s. Hodgkinson *et al.* (1963) first recognized the clinical significance of

uninhibited detrusor activity. It then became widely accepted that surgery was not indicated in those patients.

Treatment

Drug therapy

Drugs which inhibited bladder contractibility or increased outlet resistance proved to be of value.

Anticholinergic drugs Belladonna was first used by Langworthy (1936) who measured its effect on bladder tone by using a primitive water manometer attached to a kymograph. Propantheline bromide, was introduced by Riskind and Zide (1952) and Detar *et al.*, (1954). Propantheline remained the drug of choice for years and was the standard against which new drugs were judged. Emepromium bromide was found to have poor absorption but had a satisfactory response when administered intramuscularly (Carodozo and Stanton, 1979). The compound was not only poorly absorbed but also caused serious mucosal ulceration of the mouth and oesophagus.

Antispasmodic and spasmolytic agents The main drug in this group was oxybutynin chloride. Paulson (1979) found the drug to be dramatically effective in restoring normal bladder function. Moisey *et al.* (1980) investigated the drug in a placebo-controlled study. Symptomatic improvement was achieved in 69% of the oxybutinin group, compared to only 8% of the placebo group.

Tricyclic antidepressants Imipramine and the newer related compounds were found to have a marked positive symptomatic effect on nocturnal enuresis. The drugs were successfully used for the unstable bladder by Castleden *et al.* (1986).

Calcium antagonists Terodiline was initially developed in Scandinavia as an anti-anginal drug. Ulmsten *et al.* (1985) of Scandinavia investigated its use in detrusor instability and found improvement in all their cases. Due to reported side-effects in older patients this drug was taken off the market in 1991.

Prostaglandin synthetase inhibitors Cardozo *et al.* (1980) evaluated the anti-inflammatory drug flurbiprofen and found that urge incontinence was significantly reduced following its use.

Bladder drill

Jeffcoate and Francis (1966) pioneered the technique of bladder drill. Best results occurred when patients were admitted to hospital, and 80–90% showed resolution of symptoms. This treatment was also found valuable for nocturnal enuresis and Jarvis (1982) reported a 65% cure rate in such cases. Frewen (1970) also reported his experience.

Biofeedback

Biofeedback originally developed in the 1950s, and was successfully used by Stanton (1976) for women with psychogenic urinary retention. Cardozo *et al.* (1978) found the technique helpful in idiopathic detrusor instability.

Hypnotherapy

Hypnotherapy was advocated by Freeman and Baxby (1982) for the incontinent patient with detrusor instability. Subsequent studies showed that the technique had benefits.

Acupuncture

Acupuncture was used with success by Pigne *et al.* (1985).

Electrical stimulation

Electrical stimulation was proposed by Caldwell (1963) and first used for bladder inhibition by Godec *et al.* (1975).

Psychotherapy

A study of 26 patients was reported by Hafner *et al.* (1977) and one-third benefited considerably.

Surgery

Thiermann (1953) and Marshall (1954) described their technique of sacral parasympathectomy and soon afterwards a number of different techniques of interrupting the detrusor nerve supply were documented. Ewing *et al.* (1982) described transvesical phenolization of the pelvic plexus for patients with neuropathic detrusor hyperreflexia and achieved an almost 70% subjective response for their pioneering venture. Clam augmentation ileocystoplasty was first subjected to trial by Bramble (1982) with a reported 87% success rate.

Hormone replacement therapy

Oestrogen replacement therapy was suggested by Roberts and Smith (1968) for the postmenopausal patient with atrophic vaginal and urethral change.

URINARY INFECTION

The bladder is usually resistant to infection. Cox and Hinman (1961) noted that its main defence mechanism was the constant washing effect of urine. Further protection was offered by a glycosaminoglycan which lined the bladder and reduced bacterial adherence to its mucosa (Parsons *et al.*, 1977). Despite the natural defence mechanisms, infections occur commonly in pregnancy, or following surgery and catheterization or after intercourse. Kass (1955) defined 'significant bacteriuria' - that is where greater or equal to 100 000 colony forming units per ml from a clean catch mid-stream urine were present at microscopy. However, not all patients with infection showed significant bacteriuria. *Escherichia coli* was cultured from 60 to 85% of infected urines, while *Proteus, Pseudomonas, Staphylococcus, Klebsiella, Enterobacter* and *Streptococcus* made up the remainder.

OLIGURIA AND ANURIA

These life-threatening disorders were common until the 1950s. In obstetric practice oliguria or anuria could result from accidental haemorrhage, and Young (1949) who noted an incidence of 25% cortical necrosis in women after concealed accidental haemorrhage theorized that red infarcts of the placenta released a toxin which affected the kidney. The iatrogenic causes included the injection of vasopressin (Byrom, 1938). Much more common causes were incompatible blood transfusion, eclampsia, and puerperal or postabortal sepsis. Ureteric blockage due to sulphonamides crystallizing in urine was also reported as a cause.

Abel *et al.* (1913) were the first to describe a type of artificial kidney. Its modern form was introduced by Kolff (1947) and described in his book *'New Ways of Treating Uraemia'*. Peritoneal dialysis and intestinal lavage were complementary forms of therapy.

CYSTOSCOPY

Endoscopy began in the early nineteenth century when Bozzini in 1805 invented a hollow tube which could be used to observe the various human cavities. Desormeaux (1865) perfected the first satisfactory endoscope with illumination provided by a lamp which burned a mixture of turpentine and alcohol. Maximilian Nitze (1879) described a cystoscopic instrument quite similar to the modern variety. Edison's incandescent lamp was also invented in that year and a modified version of it was used for illumination at endoscopy.

The cystoscopic technique was used to investigate urinary incontinence and some authors noted trabeculations in patients with detrusor instability. Endoscopy with bladder dilatation was sometimes used to treat the condition. Cystoscopy was indicated in haematuria or when bladder stones or neoplasia were suspected.

INNERVATION OF THE BLADDER

The bladder is supplied by both sympathetic and parasympathetic afferent and efferent innervation although its activity is mainly under the control of the parasympathetic system. The neurotransmitter is acetylcholine. Cholinergic parasympathetic innervation is present throughout the detrusor muscle and urethra. The hypogastric nerve contains a few efferent fibres which arise from T11 to L3 which pass to the bladder base and urethra. Adrenergic sympathetic innervation is virtually absent from the dome of the bladder. The sympathetic nervous system plays a major role in the storage phase. The profuse distribution of motor nerves explains the importance of the parasympathetic supply in initiating and sustaining bladder contraction at micturition.

VESICOURETERIC REFLUX

Primary vesicoureteric reflux in children can be due to congenital absence or deficiency of longitudinal muscle in the submucosal layer of the ureter. This results in upward and lateral displacement of the ureteric orifice with consequent reduction in the length of obliquity of the submucosal ureter which results in vesicoureteric junction incompetence. O'Donnell and Puri began to treat vesicoureteric reflux endoscopically in March 1984. In their procedure, they described endoscopic injection of Polytef paste into the lamina propria behind the submucosal ureter.

Their results for 94 ureters thus treated were documented in the *British Medical Journal* (1986).

CHRONOLOGY

Vesico-vaginal fistula

c.2050 BC	The Egyptian queen Henhenit suffered from vesico-vaginal fistula (Mahfouz Bey, 1929).
c. 400 BC	Hippocrates referred to incontinence in this condition (Lower, 1930).
AD 980-1037	Avicenna associated prolonged labour with fistula formation.
1663	Van Roonhuyse attempted repair.
18th C.	Cautery or approximation was used.
19th C.	Catheters, cautery, and sutures were used.
1825	Samuel Hobart of Cork reported cure in a case.
1840	Mettauer used lead sutures.
1852	Sims introduced silver wire sutures. DeLamballe attempted plastic repair.
1928	Martius used a flap operation.
1954	The Ingelman-Sundberg technique was introduced.
1957	O'Connor popularized the suprapubic approach (Chassar Moir, 1961).

Stress incontinence

1922	Eardley Holland introduced the term (Kohorn, 1989).
1948	Millin and Read studied the urethra and bladder at radiography.
1949	Muellner used fluoroscopic techniques to investigate the condition.
1952	Jeffcoate and Roberts documented the importance of the urethrovesical angle.
1961	Enhorning advanced his theory on maintenance of continence.
1963	Hodgkinson introduced bead chain cystourethrography.
1977	McGuire reported the condition of low urethral resistance.

Treatment of stress incontinence

1864	Baker-Brown first used a surgical approach to stress incontinence.

1888	Donald described anterior repair.
1900s	Wilson advocated pelvic exercises (Green-Armytage, 1948).
1908	Fothergill elevated the bladder neck at anterior colporrhaphy.
1910	Goebell devised the urethrovesical sling operation.
1913	Kelly plicated the paraurethral tissues.
1949	Marshall–Marchetti–Krantz procedure introduced.
1959	Pereyra introduced a needle technique.
1961	Burch introduced a colposuspension technique.
1973	Stamey modified the abdominal approach.
1974	Scott *et al.* introduced an artificial sphincter.
1980	Tanagho pioneered urethral reconstruction.
1982	Politano injected Teflon.

The unstable bladder

1882	Mosso and Pellacani implicated psychological factors in urinary incontinence.
1905	Dudley reported on 'active incontinence'.
1963	Hodgkinson described detrusor dyssynergia.
1971	Bates introduced the term 'unstable bladder'.

Investigation

1882	Mosso and Pellacani pioneered cystometric techniques.
1923	Bonney measured urethral pressure.
1936	Simons introduced balloon catheters.
1953	Karlson measured urethral and bladder pressure simultaneously.
1976	Asmussen and Ulmsten introduced microtip transducers.
1988	Quinn *et al.* introduced transvaginal endosonography.

Treatment

1936	Langworthy used belladonna.
1952	Riskind and Zide introduced propantheline bromide.

1953	Thiermann described sacral parasympathectomy.
1966	Jeffcoate and Francis advocated 'bladder drill'.
1968	Roberts and Smith suggested oestrogen replacement therapy.
1976	Stanton advised biofeedback.
1979	Paulson pioneered the use of oxybutynin chloride.
1980	Cardozo *et al.* used prostaglandin synthetase inhibitors.
1982	Freeman and Baxby advocated hypnotherapy.
1985	Ulmsten *et al.* investigated treatment with terodiline.

Cystoscopy

1805	Bozzini introduced endoscopy (Baggish *et al.*, 1989).
1865	Desormeaux perfected endoscopy and introduced illumination.
1879	Nitze further modified the technique.

REFERENCES

Abel, J.J., Rowntree, L.G. and Turner, B.B. (1913). *J. Pharmacol.*, **5**, 275, quoted by Browne (1950) p. 434

Aldridge, A.H. (1942). Transplantation of fascia for relief of urinary stress incontinence. *Am. J. Obstet. Gynecol.*, **44**, 398

Asmussen, M. and Ulmsten, U. (1976). Simultaneous urethrocystometry with a user technique. *Scand. J. Urol. Nephrol.*, **10**, 7–11

Avicenna (1037), quoted by Cianfrani (1960) p.323

Baggish, M.S., Barbot, J. and Valle, R.F. (1989). *Diagnostic and Operative Hysteroscopy: A Text and Atlas*, pp. 1–10. (Chicago, London, Boca Raton: Year Book Medical Publishers Inc.)

Baker-Brown, I. (1864). On diseases of women remediable by operation. *Lancet*, **1**, 263–6

Bates, C.P. (1971). Continence and incontinence. *Ann. R. Coll. Surgeons of England*, **49**, 18–34

Bates, C.P., Whiteside, C.G. and Turner-Warwick, R. (1970). Synchronous cine/pressure/flow/cystourethrography with special reference to stress incontinence. *Br. J. Urol.*, **42**, 714–23

Bonney, V. (1923). On diurnal incontinence of urine in women. *J. Obstet. Gynaecol. Br. Emp.*, **30**, 358–65

Bramble, F.J. (1982). The treatment of adult enuresis and urge incontinence by enterocystoplasty. *Br. J. Urol.*, **54**, 693–6

Browne, F.J. (1950). *Postgraduate Obstetrics and Gynaecology*, pp. 420–35. (London: Butterworth & Co.)

Burch, J.C. (1961). Urethrovaginal fixation to Cooper's ligament for correction of stress incontinence, cystocele and prolapse. *Am. J. Obstet. Gynecol.*, **81**, 281

Byrom, F.B. (1938), quoted by Browne (1950) p. 420–35

Caldwell, K.P. (1963). The electrical control of sphincter incompetence. *Lancet*, **2**, 174

Cardozo, L.D. and Stanton, S.L. (1979). An objective comparison of the effects of parenterally administered drugs in patients suffering from detrusor instability. *J. Urol.*, **122**, 58

Cardozo, L.D., Stanton, S.L., Hafner, J. and Allen, V. (1978). Biofeedback in the treatment of detrusor instability. *Br. J. Urol.*, **50**, 250–4

Cardozo, L.D., Stanton, S.L., Robinson, H. and Hole, D. (1980). Evaluation of flurbiprofen in detrusor instability. *Br. Med. J.*, **280**, 281–2

Castleden, C.M., Duffin, C.M. and Gulati, R.S. (1986). Double-blind study of imipramine and placebo for incontinence due to bladder instability. *Age Aging*, **15**, 299

Chassar Moir, J. (1940), quoted by Chassar Moir, J. (1961) pp. 1–16

Chassar Moir, J. (1961). *The Vesico-Vaginal Fistula*, pp.127–133. (London: Bailliere Tindall & Cox)

Cianfrani, T. (1960). *A Short History of Obstetrics and Gynecology*, p.321. (Springfield: C.C. Thomas)

Cox, C.E. and Hinman, F. Jr. (1961). Experiments with induced bacteriuria, vesical emptying and bacterial growth on the mechanism of bladder defense to infection. *J. Urol.*, **86**, 739

De Lamballe, J. (1852). *Traites des Fistules Vesico-uterines*. (Paris: Balliere)

Desormeaux, A.J. (1865). *De l'Endoscope et de ses Applications au Diagnostic et au Traitement des Affections de l'Uretre et de la Vessie*. (Paris: Balliere)

Detar, J.H., Graham, S.D. and Corey, E.L. (1954). Banthine as a urologic drug: a clinical and electromyographic study. *J. Urol.*, **72**, 45

Donald, A. (1888). Plastic vaginal surgery. In Munro Kerr, J., Johnstone, R.W. and Phillips, M.H. (eds.) *Historical Review of British Obstetrics and Gynaecology*, (1954) p.373. (Edinburgh: Churchill Livingstone)

Dudley, E.C. (1905). The expansion of gynecology, and a suggestion for the surgical treatment of incontinence of urine in women. *Trans. Am. Gynecol. Soc.*, **30**, 4–14

Enhorning, G. (1961). Simultaneous recording of intravesical and intraurethral pressure: a study of urethral closure pressures in normal and incontinent women. *Acta Chir. Scand.*, **276**, (suppl.) 1

Enhorning, G., Miller, E.R. and Hinman, F. Jr. (1964). Urethral closure studied with cine roentgenography and simultaneous bladder-urethra pressure recording. *Surg. Gynecol. Obstet.*, **118**, 507–16

Ewing, R., Bultitude, M.E. and Shuttleworth, K.E.D. (1982). Subtrigonal phenol injection for urge incontinence secondary to detrusor instability in females. *Br. J. Urol.*, **54**, 689–92

Falk, H.C. and Tanger, M.L. (1954). Vesico-vaginal fistula; historical survey. *Obstet. Gynecol.*, **3**, 337–41

Fothergill, W.E. (1908). On the pathology and the operative treatment of displacements of the pelvic viscera. *J. Obstet. Gynaecol. Br. Emp.*, **13**, 410

Frangenheim, P. (1914), quoted by Browne (1950) p.427

Freeman, R.M. and Baxby, K. (1982). Hypnotherapy for incontinence caused by the unstable detrusor. *Br. Med. J.*, **284**, 1831–4

Freeman, R.M. and Malvern, J. (1989). *The Unstable Bladder*, p. 80. (London, Boston, Sydney: Wright)

Frewen, W.K. (1970). Urge and stress incontinence: fact and fiction. *Br. J. Obstet. Gynaecol.*, **77**, 932

Godec, C., Cass, A.S. and Ayala, G. (1975). Bladder inhibition with functional electrical stimulation. *Urology*, **6**, 663

Goebell, R. (1910). Zur operativen Beseitigung der angeborenen Incontinentia vesicae. *Z. Gynak. Urol.*, **2**, 187

Gossett, M. (1834). Advantages of the gilt wire suture. *Lancet*, **1**, 345

Graham, H. (1950). *Eternal Eve.* (London: Heinemann)

Green, T.H. (1962). Development of a plan for the diagnosis and treatment of urinary stress incontinence. *Am. J. Obstet. Gynecol.*, **83**, 632–48

Green-Armytage, V.B. (1948). The role of physiotherapy in obstetrics and gynaecology. *J. Obstet. Gynaecol. Br. Emp.*, **52**, 21–3

Hafner, R.J., Stanton, S.L. and Guy, J. (1977). A psychiatric study of women with urgency and urgency incontinence. *Br. J. Urol*, **49**, 211

Hayward, G. (1839). Case of vesico-vaginal fistula successfully treated by an operation. *Am. J. Med. Sci.*, **24**, 283–8

Hayward, G. (1851). Cases of vesico-vaginal fistula treated by operation. *Boston Med. Surg. J.*, **XLVI**, 209

Hildanus, F. (1646). Opera observationum et curationum medico-chirurgicarum quae extantomnia. *Centuria*, **III**, Obs 69

Hobart, S. (1825), quoted by Graham (1950) p.441.

Hobart, S. (1836). In *De Fistula Urethro et Vesicovaginali Commentatio*, p. 64: plate 1, fig. 15–17. (Havniae: J.C. Bendz)

Hodgkinson, C.P. (1963). Urinary stress incontinence in the female; a program for preoperative investigation. *Clin. Obstet. Gynecol.*, **6**, 154

Hodgkinson, C.P., Ayers, M.A. and Drukker, B.H. (1963). Dyssynergic detrusor dysfunction in the apparently normal female. *Am. J. Obstet. Gynecol.*, **87**, 717–30

Ingelman-Sundberg, A. (1950). Plastic repair of the pelvic floor with a report of 31 cases of stress incontinence. *Acta Obstet. Gynecol. Scand.*, **30**, 319

International Continence Society (C.P. Bates *et al.*) (1981). Fourth report on the standardization of terminology of lower urinary tract function. Standardization Committee. *Br. J. Urol*, **53**, 333–5

International Continence Society (C.P. Bates *et al.*) (1976). First report on the standardization of terminology of the lower urinary tract function. *Br. J. Urol.*, **48**, 39–42

Jarvis, G.J. (1982). Bladder drill for the treatment of enuresis in adults. *Br. J. Urol.*, **54**, 118–19

Jeffcoate, T.N.A. and Roberts, H. (1952). Stress incontinence of urine. *J. Obstet. Gynaecol. Br. Emp.*, **59**, 685

Jeffcoate, T.N.A. and Francis, W.J.A. (1966). Urgency incontinence in the female. *Am. J. Obstet. Gynecol.*, **94**, 604–18

Karlson, S. (1953). Experimental studies in the functioning of the female urinary bladder and urethra. *Acta Obstet. Gynecol. Scand.*, **32**, 285–307

Kass, E.H. (1955). Chemotherapeutic and antibiotic drugs in the management of infections of the urinary tract. *Am. J. Med.*, **18**, 764

Kegel, A.H. (1949a). The physiologic treatment of tone and function of the genital muscles and of urinary incontinence. *West. J. Surg.*, **57**, 527–35

Kegel, A.H. (1949b). Progressive resistance exercises in functional restoration of the perineal muscles. *Am. J. Obstet. Gynecol.*, **56**, 238–48

Kelly, H.A. (1913). Incontinence of urine in women. *Urol. Cutan. Rev.*, **17**, 291–3

Kennedy, W.T. (1937). Incontinence of urine in the female: the urethral sphincter mechanism, damage of function, and restoration of control. *Am. J. Obstet. Gynecol.*, **34**, 576

Kohorn, E.I. (1989). The surgery of stress urinary incontinence. In Thiede, H.A. (ed.) *Urogynecology*, Vol. 16.4, p.841 *Obstetrics and Gynecology Clinics of North America.* (Philadelphia, London: W.B. Saunders Co.)

Kolff, W.J. (1947). *New Ways of Treating Uraemia.* (London: Churchill)

Langworthy, O.R. (1936). A new approach to the diagnosis and treatment of disorders of micturition in diseases of the nervous system. *Int. Clin.*, **3**, 98

Lappenen, M.K. (1962). A cystometric study of the function of the urinary bladder in prostatic patients. *Urologia Internationalis*, **14**, 226–38

Lewis, T.L.T. (1964). *Stress Incontinence. Progress in Clinical Obstetrics and Gynaecology.* 2nd edn. pp. 418–41. (London: J. & A. Churchill Ltd.)

Lower, W.E. (1930). Vesico-vaginal fistula. *Ann. Surg.*, **92**, 774–8

McGuire, E.J. (1977). Combined radiographic and manometric assessment of urethral sphincter function. *J. Urol.*, **118**, 632

Mahfouz Bey, N. (1929). Urinary and rectovaginal fistulae in women. *J. Obstet. Gynaecol. Br. Emp.*, **36**, 581–9

Marshall, C.J. (1954). Persistent adult bed-wetting treated by sacral neurotomy. Br. Med. J., 1, 308–11

Marshall, V.F., Marchetti, A.A. and Krantz, K.E. (1949). The correction of stress incontinence by simple vesicourethral suspension. Surg. Gynecol. Obstet., 88, 509

Martius, H. (1928). Zlb. Gynakol., 18, 180

Menninger, K.A. (1941). Some observations on the psychological factors in urination and genitourinary afflictions. Psychoanal. Rev., 28, 117–29

Mettauer, J.P. (1840). Vesico-vaginal fistula. Boston M. and S.J., 22, 154

Millin, T. and Read, C.D. (1948). Stress incontinence of urine in females. Postgrad. Med. J., 24, 51

Moisey, C.U., Stephenson, T.P. and Brendler, C.B. (1980). The urodynamic and subjective results of treatment of detrusor instability with oxybutynin chloride. Br. J. Urol., 52, 472–5

Mosso, A. and Pellacani, P. (1882). Sur les fonctions de la vessie. Arch. Ital. Biol., 1, 97–127

Muellner, S.R. (1949), quoted by Lewis (1964) p.418

Nitze, M. (1879). Uber eine neue behandlungs – methode de hohlen des menslichen korpers. Med. Press. Wien., 26, 851

O'Donnell, B. and Puri, P. (1986). Endoscopic correction of primary vesicoureteric reflux: results in 94 ureters. Br. Med. J., 293, 1404–6

Parsons, C.L., Greenspan, C., Moore, S.W. et al. (1977). Role of surface mucin in primary antibacterial defense of bladder. Urology, 9, 48

Paulson, D.F. (1979). Oxybutynin chloride in the management of idiopathic detrusor instability. South. Med. J., 72, 374

Pereyra, A.J. (1959). A simplified surgical procedure for the correction of stress incontinence in women. West. J. Obstet. Gynecol., 67, 223

Pigne, A., DeGoursac, C., Nyssen, C. and Barrat, J. (1985). Acupuncture and unstable bladder. In Proceedings 15th Annual Meeting International Continence Society, London, pp.186–7, quoted by Freeman and Malvern (1989) p. 80

Politano, V.A. (1982). Periurethral polytetrafluorethylene injection for urinary incontinence. J. Urol., 127, 439–42

Politano, V.A., Small, M.P., Harper, J.M. and Lynne, C.M. (1974). Periurethral Teflon injection for urinary incontinence. J. Urol., 111, 180–3

Quinn, M.J., Beynon, J., Mortensen, N.J.McC. and Smith, P.J.B. (1988). Transvaginal endosonography: a new method to study the anatomy of the lower urinary tract in urinary stress incontinence. Br. J. Urol., 62, 414–18

Rees, D.L.P. and Farhoumand, N. (1977). Psychiatric aspects of recurrent cystitis in women. Br. J. Urol., 49, 651–8

Ricci, J.V. (1943). The Genealogy of Gynaecology: History of Development of Gynaecology throughout the Ages 2000 BC–AD 1800, pp. 521–5. (Philadelphia: The Blakiston Co.)

Ricci, J.V. (1945). One Hundred Years of Gynaecology 1800–1900, pp. 111–40. (Philadelphia: The Blakiston Co.)

Riskind, L.A. and Zide, H.A. (1952). Banthine in urologic disorders. J. Urol., 68, 636

Roberts, H. (1953), quoted by Lewis (1964) p.419

Roberts, M. and Smith, P. (1968). Non malignant obstruction of the female urethra. Br. J. Urol., 40, 694–702

Roonhuyse, H. van (1663). Heel-konstige Aanmerkkingern Betreffende de Gebreekken der Vrouwen. (Amsterdam: T. Jacobsz) English translation: Medico-Chirurgical Observations. [Englished out of Dutch by a careful hand. M. Pitt, London (1676) pp. 125–36]

Scott, F.B., Bradley, W.E. and Timm, G. (1974). Treatment of urinary incontinence by an implant or prosthetic urinary sphincter. J. Urol., 112, 7S

Simons, I. (1936). Studies on bladder function. The Sphincterometer. Urology, 35, 96–102

Sims, J.M. (1852). On the treatment of vesico-vaginal fistula. Am. J. M. Sci., 23 (n.s.), 59–82

Smellie, W. (1752). Treatise on the Theory and Practice of Midwifery, 2nd edn. pp. 160–1. (London: Wilson: Wilson, D. & Durham, T.)

Stamey, T.A. (1973). Endoscopic suspension of the vesical neck for urinary incontinence. Surg. Gynecol. Obstet., 136, 547

Stanton, S.L. (1976). Communication to the 6th International Continence Society Meeting, Antwerp reported (1978) in Urologica Int. J., 33, 1–204, quoted by Freeman and Stanton (1989) p. 71

Stoeckel, W. (1917), quoted by Browne (1950) p.427

Straub, L.R., Ripley, H.S. and Wolf, S. (1949). Disturbances of bladder function associated with emotional states. *J. Am. Med. Assoc.*, **141**, 1139–43

Tanagho, E. (1980). Neo-urethra: rationale, surgical technique and indications. In Stanton, S.L. and Tanagho, E. (eds.) *Surgery of Female Incontinence,* p. 111. (Heidelberg: Springer-Verlag)

Thiermann, E. (1953). Der sakrale Zugang in der Urologie. *Z. Urol.*, **46**, 777–801

Ulmsten, U., Ekman, G. and Andersson, K.E. (1985). The effect of terodiline treatment in women with motor urge incontinence. *Am. J. Obstet. Gynecol.*, **193**, 619–22

Wutzer, C.W. (1843). Ueber Heilung der Blasenscheiden – Fistel mit Hülfe der Punction der Blase. *Organ f. die gesammte Heilk. Bonn*, II, 481

Young, J. (1949). *Proc. R. Soc. Med.*, **42**, 375, quoted by Browne (1950) p. 429

FURTHER READING

Baggish, M.S., Barbot, J. and Valle, R.F. (1989). *Diagnostic and Operative Hysteroscopy: A Text and Atlas.* (Chicago, London, Boca Raton: Year Book Medical Publishers Inc.)

Browne, F.J. (1950). *Stress Incontinence. Postgraduate Obstetrics and Gynaecology*, pp.420–28. (London: Butterworth & Co.)

Chassar Moir, J. (1961). *The Vesico-Vaginal Fistula.* (London: Bailliere Tindall & Cox)

Cianfrani, T. (1960). *A Short History of Obstetrics and Gynecology.* (Springfield: C.C. Thomas)

Drife, J.O., Hilton, P. and Stanton, S.L. (eds.) (1990). *Micturition.* (London, Berlin, Heidelberg, New York, Paris, Tokyo, Hong Kong: Springer-Verlag)

Freeman, R.M. and Malvern, J. (1989). *The Unstable Bladder.* (London, Boston, Singapore, Sydney, Toronto, Wellington: Wright)

Hoey, H.M.C.V. and Puri, P. (eds.) (1990). *Paediatric Nephrourology. Progress in Research and Practice.* (Chichester, New York, Brisbane, Toronto, Singapore: J. Wiley & Sons)

Jordan, J.A. and Stanton, S.L. (eds.) (1981). *The Incontinent Woman. Proceedings of a Scientific Meeting of the RCOG*, 13 February

Lewis, T.L.T. (1964). *Stress Incontinence. Progress in Clinical Obstetrics and Gynaecology*, 2nd edn. pp. 418–41. (London: J.& A. Churchill Ltd.)

Raz, S. (ed.) (1985). *Gynaecological urology. Clin. Obstet. Gynaecol.*, **12**, no. 2

Thiede, H.A. (ed.) (1989). *Urogynecology. Obstet. Gynecol. Clin. N. Am.*, **16**, no. 4

Wall, L.L. (1990). Diagnosis and management of urinary incontinence due to detrusor instability. *Obstet. Gynecol. Surv.*, **45**, 11 (suppl.)

Immunology

INTRODUCTION

Immunology, the scientific study of the way living bodies protect themselves against invasion, developed in the second half of the nineteenth century. The concept of a body defence mechanism dates to antiquity. In ancient India and China the practice of 'variolation' was practised, in which protection against smallpox was obtained by inoculating live organisms from disease pustules (Roitt, 1971).

An early experimenter in the immunological field was Edward Jenner (1749–1823) (Figure 1) who qualified from London University and settled down as a country doctor in Berkeley. Jenner inoculated men and maid servants against smallpox, using the time honoured method. The pus of variola was allowed to dry on threads and this 'weakened' smallpox residue was introduced into scratches made on the skin. Later, Jenner observed that a previous attack of 'cow pox' (a pustular disease of the cow udder) which caused a

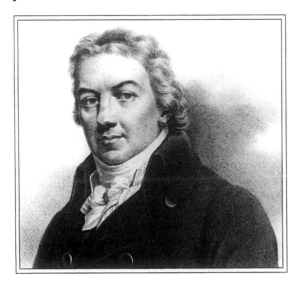

Figure 1 Edward Jenner (*see* text). Reproduced with kind permission from The Wellcome Institute Library, London

milder illness protected against subsequent smallpox. He began inoculating cowpox as a protective against smallpox, in 1796–1798. Although Jenner gains the credit, a teacher from Holstein called Plett may have used a similar technique in 1791 (Venzmer, 1968). The term variolation was replaced by vaccination (Latin *vacca*, cow).

The scientific approach to the study of immunology began with the work of Louis Pasteur (1822–1895). Pasteur experimented with chicken cholera, anthrax and rabies. In 1888 he developed a *live attenuated vaccine* for anthrax which he used to protect sheep and cattle against infection. In 1884 Elie Metchnikoff developed the *cellular defence theory* in which he stated that cells which he called phagocytes (cell eaters) attacked foreign matter. He found that their number increased when infection occurred (Grabar, 1984). Soon after, the *toxin–antitoxin* reaction in diphtheria and tetanus was discovered, by Pierre Paul Emile Roux and A.E.J. Yersin in 1888. Karl Fraenkel demonstrated that heat-killed organisms could be injected into susceptible animals who in turn could resist diphtheria infections (McGrew, 1985). Emile Behring and the Japanese Shibasaburo Kitazato, who were both pupils of Robert Koch, used the term *antitoxin* and are credited with the discovery of antitoxic immunity. Robert Koch (1843–1910), who carried out pioneering work in the discovery of the cholera and tubercle bacilli, also discovered *lymphocytes*, thus contributing to the already identified cellular and immune responses.

Paul Ehrlich (1854–1915) (q.v. in Biographies) made major contributions to the theory of immunology between the years 1891 and 1903. He noted variability in the effectiveness of antitoxins. Ehrlich developed the theory of combining a modified toxin with antitoxin, thereby producing *toxoid*. This substance offered immunity, and also protected against a possible inoculation infection. It won him the Nobel Prize for medicine in 1908.

In 1895 Denies and Leclef discovered that phagocytosis was greatly enhanced by immunization. Four years later Bordet discovered that lysis of cells by antibody required the presence of a serum factor or factors now known as *complement*. A further advance was the discovery in 1900 of human ABO blood groups and natural *isohaemagglutinins* by Karl Landsteiner.

Theobald Smith of Harvard and Charles Richet of Paris carried out important work in 1902. Smith had noticed that guinea-pigs used for testing diphtheria antitoxin, became ill if there were long periods between injections. Meanwhile in 1905 von Pirquet and Schuk discovered that the injection of foreign protein into an animal produced a *hypersensitivity* reaction and a second injection killed the animal through a reaction called *anaphylaxis*. Von Pirquet advocated the term *allergy* for a modified immune reaction.

Hans Zinsser demonstrated that infection mobilized the entire defence system and that the various elements within it were complementary. *Antibodies* were discovered in the late 1930s. Their production by plasma cells in bone marrow and lymph nodes was established by Astrid E. Fagraeus in 1948. Robert Goode later showed that lymphocytes (which were originally derived from the primitive cells lining the embryonic yolk sac) travelled at high speed to an area of infection, and triggered a protective response against antigens in foreign cell walls (Parish, 1968; Roitt, 1971; Graber, 1984; McGrew, 1985).

INFERTILITY

The relationship of the immune process to infertility was first demonstrated independently by Landsteiner (1899) and Metchnikoff (1899) who described the presence of antisperm antibodies. In this century, Wilson (1954) and Rumke (1954) described the discovery of spermagglutinins in blood and semen. Sperm agglutinating activity in female serum was first reported by Franklin and Dukes (1964), although the high incidence quoted by them was not confirmed by other workers.

A further indication of immunological activity was documented by Halpern *et al.* (1967) who reported a case of hypersensitivity reaction induced at coitus by seminal plasma. The responsible antigen was a low molecular weight glyco-protein and the patient was discovered to be unduly sensitive to foreign protein. Fjallabrant (1969) demonstrated reduced penetration of cervical mucus by sperms in the presence of sperm antibodies and Roberts and Boettcher (1969) identified human sperm-coating antigens.

A number of investigations were introduced to detect antisperm antibodies in the 1970s. The tests were relatively inaccurate due to high false-positive and false-negative rates. Using more precise methods Mathur and associates (1984) demonstrated the presence of sperm antibodies in the cervical mucus of infertile women, and also documented their association with the results of postcoital tests and subsequent pregnancy. Sperm antibodies produced their effect by immobilizing sperm, by interfering with the process of capacitation, by causing sperm agglutination, or by directly affecting the fertilizing process.

The cervix was discovered to be the major site of immunological activity, with some participation by the endometrium and Fallopian tubes. Cervical mucus immunoglobulins contained the serum components immunoglobulins A and G and the secretory immunoglobulin A. Lippes *et al.* (1970;1972) demonstrated antibodies in both tubal and follicular fluids. Autoimmunization in the male occurred following surgery, trauma, or infection, as a result of which, the blood–testis barrier was compromised and autoimmunity to testicular and or seminal antigens developed (Rumke and Hekamn, 1975).

The postcoital test was a guide to the presence of sperm antibodies in seminal plasma or cervical mucus. A sperm cervical mucus contact test was used by Kremer and Jager (1976). If local antibodies were present the sperm was noted to have a characteristic shaking movement when in contact with cervical mucus. Crossed hostility testing was developed by Morgan *et al.* (1977). Combinations of sperm or cervical mucus were tested against donor sperm and mucus, to determine whether one or both partners had antibodies.

Franklin and Dukes (1964) recommended the use of condoms to avoid contact of semen and cervix thereby reducing the production of cervical antibodies. Occlusive therapy continued for up to 12 months and over 50% of treated couples achieved fertilizing capability within the year. Condom therapy was not found useful in patients with circulating antisperm antibodies. Corticosteroid therapy was suggested for the male (Hendry *et al.*, 1981) and the female (Mathur *et al.*, 1980) but was not always helpful and sometimes carried risks of complications. Ackerman *et al.* (1984) reported good results for *in vitro* fertilization in antibody cases. Intrauterine insemination was successfully used for some women with cervical antisperm antibodies. Other techniques included the temporary suppression of spermatogenesis, and a sperm washing technique.

OVARIAN FAILURE

The existence of autoimmune ovarian failure, similar in character to Hashimoto's thyroiditis and the autoimmune diseases of other endocrine glands, was reported in the 1970s. Several organs can be affected in the same woman, who after ovarian failure may develop diabetes, myxoedema or adrenal failure (Addison's disease).

CONTRACEPTION

In the 1920s and 1930s infertility was induced by immunizing women against crude sperm extracts (Jones, 1982). From the 1970s onwards researchers targeted potential antigens in spermatozoa, seminal fluid, or the zona pellucida. Trophoblastic hormones and other feto–maternal antigens could be affected by an immunological attack. Realizing the seriousness of potential complications from immunological contraception a steering Committee of the World Health Organization issued a set of safety guidelines (Task Force on Immunological Methods of Fertility Regulation WHO, 1978).

PREGNANCY

In a review article, Nicholas (1989) stated that 'the question of human fetal allograft survival and growth in a potentially hostile immunological environment constitutes the greatest paradox of all the laws of tissue transplantation'. Medawar (1953) proposed five main theories for the survival of the fetal allograft, and Nicholas addressed each of these in turn. Medawar's theories were, that the conceptus was antigenically immature; the intrauterine site was immunologically privileged; the placenta was a barrier; the pregnant mother became immunologically incompetent; or a serum blocking factor was present. Each theory was disproven.

Recurrent spontaneous abortion

When other factors were excluded, some evidence accrued that immunological disorders could cause miscarriage. Mowbray and Underwood (1985) and Mowbray et al. (1985) described treatment with paternal or third party leukocytes in such cases and reported successful pregnancies thereafter.

Pre-eclamptic toxaemia

The clinical picture of pre-eclamptic toxaemia was thought to bear the hallmarks of an immune response. The placenta was known to be of central importance, and a familial role was advocated but immunological data were inconclusive.

Gestational trophoblastic disease

It was discovered that complete hydatidiform moles had a diploid nuclear genome of paternal genetic origin. Partial mole had an extra haploid component which was also paternal. Chorion carcinoma was the only naturally occurring example of a genetically foreign (allogeneic) tumour.

Rhesus isoimmunization

The isoimmunization which involved fetal red cell antigens in the rhesus and ABO blood groups comprised a problem which was only combated in this century. The administration of high titre anti-D immunoglobulin to non-sensitized rhesus-negative women who delivered rhesus-positive infants, afforded over 95% protection against classic rhesus disease. Isoimmunization in the ABO system mainly affected group O women. The antibodies involved were in the immunoglobulin M class which did not cross the placenta, and the clinical effects of treatment were usually mild.

Existing autoimmune diseases and pregnancy

A number of women with autoimmune disease become pregnant, or develop the disease during pregnancy. One such disorder is autoimmune thrombocytopaenic purpura. This condition is characterized by platelet-associated immunoglobulin G autoantibodies bound to cell surface antigens and platelets. As maternal antiplatelet autoantibody can cross the placenta, the fetus is at risk of intrauterine or neonatal thrombocytopenia.

CHRONOLOGY

General immunology

Variolation was practised in ancient India and China.

1796–98   Edward Jenner inoculated cowpox to protect against smallpox.

1880	Louis Pasteur developed attenuated vaccines.
1884	Elie Metchnikoff developed the cellular defence theory.
1888	Roux and Yersin developed the bacterial toxin theory.
1890	Von Behring and Kitasato developed antitoxins, the foundation of serotherapy.
1890s	Paul Ehrlich developed toxoid.
1899	Bordet proposed the existence of complement.
1900	Karl Landsteiner discovered isohaemagglutinins.
1905	Von Pirquet and Schick observed hypersensitivity reaction.
1906	Von Pirquet proposed the term 'allergy'.
1930s	Antibodies were discovered.
1948	Fagraeus determined that antibodies were formed in plasma cells.

References: McGrew (1985); Roitt (1971); Crabar (1984); Parish (1968)

Infertility

1899	Landsteiner and also Metchnikoff discovered antisperm antibodies.
1954	Wilson and also Rumke described spermagglutinins in semen and blood.
1964	Franklin and Dukes reported antibodies to sperm in females and recommended occlusive therapy with condoms.
1969	Fjallabrant demonstrated reduced sperm penetration of cervical mucus containing antibodies.
1976	Kremer and Jager used the cervical mucus contact test.
1977	Morgan et al. developed crossed hostility testing.
1981	Hendry et al. suggested corticosteroid therapy in the male.
1984	Ackerman et al. reported good results for in vitro fertilization.

Contraception

1920s	Infertility was induced by immunization against sperm extract (Jones, 1982).
1953	Medawar proposed theories for survival of the fetal allograft.

1970	Contraception by immunization against antigens in spermatazoa, seminal fluid, or zona pellucida was mooted.

REFERENCES

Ackerman, S.B., Graff, D., Van Clem, J., Swanson, R.J., Veeck, L.L., Acosta, A.A. and Garcia, J.E. (1984). Immunologic infertility and in vitro fertilization. Fertil. Steril., 42, 474

Fjallbrant, B. (1969). Cervical mucus penetration by human spermatozoa treated with antispermatozoal antibodies from rabbit and man. Acta Obstet. Gynecol. Scand., 48, 71

Franklin, R.R. and Dukes, C.I. (1964). Antispermatozoal antibody and unexplained infertility. Am. J. Obstet. Gynecol., 89, 6

Grabar, P. (1984). The historical background of immunology. In Stites, D.P., Stobo, J.D., Fudenberg, H.H. and Wells, J.V. (eds.). Basic and Clinical Immunology, 5th edn. pp. 1–12. (Los Altos California: Lange Medical Publications)

Halpern, B.M., Ky, I. and Roberts, B. (1967). Clinical and immunological study of an exceptional case of reaginic type sensitisation to human seminal fluid. Immunology, 12, 247–58

Hendry, W.R., Stedronska, J., Parslow, J. and Hughes, L. (1981). The results of intermittent high dose steroid therapy for male infertility due to antisperm antibodies. Fertil. Steril., 36, 351

Jones, W.R. (1982). Immunological approach to contraception. In Studd, J. (ed.) Progress in Obstetrics and Gynaecology, Vol. 2, pp. 184–97. (Edinburgh, London, Melbourne, New York: Churchill Livingstone)

Kremer, J. and Jager, S. (1976). The sperm cervical mucus contact test: a preliminary report. Fertil. Steril., 27, 335

Landsteiner, K. (1899). Zur kenntnis der spezifisch auf blütkorperchen wirkenden sera. Zbl. Bakteriol., 25, 546

Lippes, J., Ogra, S.S., Tomasi, T.B. and Tourville, D.R. (1970). Immunohistochemical localisation of IgG, IgA, IgM, secretory piece and lactoferrin in the human female genital tract. Contraception, 1, 163

Lippes, J., Enders, R.G., Pragay, D.A. and Bartholomew, W.R. (1972). The collection and analysis of human Fallopian tube fluid. *Contraception*, **5**, 85

McGrew, R. (1985). *Encyclopedia of Medical History*, pp. 147. (London: MacMillan Press)

Mathur, S., Baker, E.R., Williamson, H.O., Derrick, F.C., Teague, K.S. and Fudenberg, H.H. (1980). Clinical significance of sperm antibodies in infertility. *Fertil. Steril.*, **33**, 239

Mathur, S., Williamson, H.O., Baker, M.E., Rust, P.F., Holtz, G.L. and Fudenberg, H.H. (1984). Sperm motility on postcoital testing correlates with male autoimmunity to sperm. *Fertil. Steril.*, **41**, 81

Medawar, P.D. (1953). Some immunological and endocrinological problems raised by the evolution of viviparity in vertebrates. In Danielli, J.F. and Brown, R. (eds.) *Symposia of the Society for Experimental Biology*, Vol. VII, pp. 320–38. (Oxford: Oxford University Press)

Metchnikoff, S. (1899). Etudes sur la resorption des cellules. *Ann. Inst. Pasteur Lille*, **13**, 737

Morgan, H., Stedronska, J., Hendry, W.F., Chamberlain, G.V.P. and Dewhurst, C.J. (1977). Sperm/cervical-mucus crossed hostility testing and anti-sperm antibodies in the husband. *Lancet*, **1**, 1228

Mowbray, J.F. and Underwood, J.L. (1985). Immunology of abortion. *Clin. Exp. Immunol.*, **60**, 1–7

Mowbray, J.F., Gibbings, C., Liddell, H., Reginald, P.W., Underwood, J.L. and Beard, R.W. (1985). Controlled trial of treatment of recurrent spontaneous abortion by immunisation with paternal cells. *Lancet*, **1**, 941–3

Nicholas, N.S. (1989). Human fetal allograft survival. In Studd, J. (ed.) *Progress in Obstetrics and Gynaecology*, Vol. 7, pp. 1–25. (Edinburgh, London, Melbourne, New York: Churchill Livingstone)

Parish, H.J. (1968). *Victory with Vaccines*. (Edinburgh: Livingstone)

Roberts, T.K. and Boettcher, B. (1969). Identification of human sperm-coating antigens. *J. Reprod. Fertil.*, **18**, 347–50

Roitt, I. (1971). *Essential Immunology*, 2nd edn., pp. 1–18. (Oxford, London, Edinburgh, Melbourne: Blackwell Scientific Publications)

Rumke, P. (1954). The presence of sperm antibodies in the serum of two patients with oligozoospermia. *Vox Sang.*, **4**, 135

Rumke, P. and Hekman, A. (1975). Auto- and isoimmunity to sperm in infertility. *Clin. Endocrinol. Metab.*, **4**, 473

Task Force on Immunological Methods for Fertility Regulation, WHO (1978). Evaluating the safety and efficacy of placental antigen vaccines for fertility regulation. *Clin. Exp. Immunol.*, **33**, 360–75

Venzmer, G. (1968). *5000 Years of Medicine*, translated by Marion Koenig, p. 229–31. (London: MacDonald)

Wilson, L. (1954). Sperm agglutinins in human semen and blood. *Proc. Soc. Exp. Biol. Med.*, **85**, 652

FURTHER READING

Centaro, A. and Carretti, N. (eds.) (1974). *Immunology in Obstetrics and Gynaecology*. (Amsterdam, New York: Excerpta Medica Elsevier)

De Cherney, A.H. (1986). *Reproductive Failure*. (New York, Edinburgh, London, Melbourne: Churchill Livingstone)

Grabar, P. (1984). The historical background of immunology. In Stites, D.P., Stobo, J.D., Fudenberg, H.H. and Wells, J.V. (eds.) *Basic and Clinical Immunology*, 5th edn., pp. 1–12. (Los Altos California: Lange Medical Publications)

Hull, M.G.R. (ed.) (1981). *Developments in Infertility Practice. Clinics in Obstetrics and Gynaecology*, Vol. 8 no. 3. (London, Philadelphia, Toronto: W.B. Saunders & Co.)

Johnson, P.M. (1989). Immunology of pregnancy. In Turnbull, Sir A. and Chamberlain, G. (eds.) *Obstetrics*, pp. 173–87. (Edinburgh, London, Melbourne, New York: Churchill Livingstone)

Jones, W.R. (ed.) (1979). Tissue-specific autoimmune disease in pregnancy. In *Immunological Aspects of Reproduction. Clinics in Obstetrics and Gynaecology*, Vol. 6 no. 3, pp. 473–91. (London, Philadelphia, Toronto: W.B. Saunders & Co.)

Jones, W.R. (1982). Immunological approach to contraception. In Studd, J. (ed.) *Progress in Obstetrics and Gynaecology*, Vol. 2, pp. 184–97. (Edinburgh, London, Melbourne, New York: Churchill Livingstone)

Nicholas, N.S. (1989). Human fetal allograft survival. In Studd, J. (ed.) *Progress in Obstetrics and Gynaecology*, Vol. 7, pp. 1–25. (Edinburgh, London, Melbourne, New York: Churchill Livingstone)

Parish, H.J. (1968). *Victory with Vaccines.* (Edinburgh: Livingstone)

Pepperell, R.J., Hudson, B. and Wood, C. (1980). *The Infertile Couple.* (Edinburgh, London, New York: Churchill Livingstone)

Roitt, I. (1971). *Essential Immunology,* 2nd edn. (Oxford, London, Edinburgh, Melbourne: Blackwell Scientific Publication)

Taymor, M.L. (1990). *Infertility: A Clinicians Guide to Diagnosis and Treatment.* (New York, London: Plenum Medical Book Co.)

Radiology and imaging in obstetrics and gynaecology

RADIOLOGY

The discovery of X-rays for diagnostic and later for therapeutic purposes is one of the great milestones in medical history (Grigg, 1965). Wilhelm Conrad Roentgen (1845–1923) was the discoverer. He was born in Remscheid-Lennep in Germany. On 29 December 1895 he submitted his first *Provisoral* communication to the Wurzburg Physico-Medical Society. He entitled this *Ueber die Neue Art von Strahlen* (on a new kind of rays). On 23 January 1896 he demonstrated the bones of A. P. von Kolliker's (1817–1905) hand (Röntgen, 1895).

This was not the first time somebody had postulated that there were waves that could not be seen. Roger Bacon (1220–1292) a Franciscan monk known as 'Doctor Mirabilis' affected . . . 'there are many dense bodies that . . . interfere with the visual and other sensitive (organs) of man so that rays cannot pass . . . yet . . . rays do really pass through without our being aware of it'.

Sir William Crookes (1832–1919), a great chemist and physicist, came very near to discovering X-rays when carrying out his cathode-ray studies. Roentgen used the light emitted from one of Crookes' vacuum tubes (a cathode-ray tube) through which an electric current was passed to act on an ordinary photographic plate. Wood and other substances were transparent, whilst metal and bones were opaque to this invisible light. Roentgen had observed while experimenting with the electric current in the cathode ray tube that a nearby piece of barium platinocyanide gave off light when the tube was in operation. He propounded the theory that when the cathode rays (electrons) struck the glass wall of the tube irradiation was formed that struck the chemical and caused it to fluoresce, and he found that it affected photographic plates. He called the phenomenon X-radiation because he did not know what it was!

People started to experiment with the newly discovered X-rays. Already by 1896 it was possible to guess that the so-called 'fluoroscopists', who were those using the X-ray apparatus, could be damaged by Roentgen irradiation.

The use of radiotherapy

Already in 1903 a Dr G.P. Gerdwood of Montreal in Canada, reported to the Third Annual Meeting of the American Roentgen Ray Society held in Chicago, three cases of cancer of the breast treated with X-rays with the relief of pain. At that time he also reported a case of pyosalpinx treated by him with X-rays, but without any improvement. At the end of 30 days of exposure the patient was operated on. The abscess burst, and she died of acute peritonitis a few days later. He thought that the peritonitis had to be tubercular in origin. So, one of the very first cases of gynaecological treatment with X-rays was reported in 1903 and was probably a tuberculous peritonitis and certainly ended fatally.

Margaret Cleaves (1903) wrote on the use of radium rays for cancer and the first mention in a book of the use of radiotherapy, was by Dr Leopold Freund of Iena who wrote that radiotherapy had been used in gynaecology to treat prurigo (Freund, 1904). Freund also pointed out that the surgeons S.J.O. Gren and Sederholm had found decidedly beneficial results in pruritis ani and vulvae after a very few exposures. No explanation was given as to why X-rays were effective except 'it should be borne in mind that the presence of the high-tension electricity accumulated on the surface of a roentgen-tube connection is quite sufficient in itself to explain the relief afforded in the cases of pruritis'. In the same book there is an extract of a paper by Auset, and Bedard, (Auset, 1898) who reported treatment of a case of chronic tuberculosis before the turn of the century. Fifty daily sittings of half an hour were given; and it was reported that the general condition of the patient improved.

There is no mention of the treatment of any other gynaecological conditions by X-rays or radium at that time.

(Antoine-) Henri Becqerel (1852–1908), having learnt of the discovery of X-rays by Roentgen, thought that X-rays could be produced by stimulating crystals with ultraviolet light. He investigated uranium salts and discovered the emission of radioactive substances similar to X-rays and given out by radium.

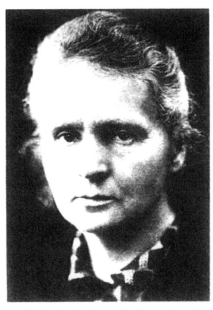

Figure 1 Marie Curie (*see* text). Reproduced with kind permission from the Wellcome Institute Library, London

He communicated his discoveries to Pierre Curie (1859–1906) and his wife Marie (née Sklodowska) (1867–1934) (Figure 1). The Curies isolated a radioactive element in pitchblende. Radium was discovered in 1898 by the Curies and an assistant G. Bemont after Mme Curie had observed that the radioactivity of pitchblende was four or five times greater than that of the uranium it contained. The story of how they isolated radium after working with several tons of pitchblende residues is utterly fascinating, but not directly concerned with obstetrics and gynaecology.

Early theories as to the way X-rays worked to cure conditions such as lupus, acne and glandular tuberculosis, postulated that there was an 'opsonic factor'. This factor was said to lead to the formation of certain antibodies in the serum, which so injured germs that they became an easy prey to white blood cells. By this time (1904) it was realized that X-rays when given to hair-bearing skin areas could cause loss of hair.

Dr David Arthur and Dr John Muir (1909) stated 'where cancer is superficial the effects of X-ray exposure is marked and a cure for it in most cases, but where the process is deep seated we fear that revised diagnosis would dismiss most of the so-called cures by X-rays', although Arthur and Muir did advocate its use for palliation when surgery was impossible. They were still of the same opinion in 1917 in the second edition of their book published by Heinemann.

Robert Knox, radiographer to King's College London, in his textbook (Knox, 1915) wrote 100 pages devoted to the treatment of gynaecological conditions, of which only three described treatment by radium.

Radium was used to treat chronic inflammatory conditions of the cervix, chronic endometritis, leucoplakia vulvae, and cancer of the cervix as well as fibromata. The textbook interestingly states 'continental writers who have been using radium and mesothorium claim that the operative treatment of cancer of the cervix is no longer necessary'. Knox, however, doubted that this was so, because 'the tendency to recurrence exists whether either radiotherapy or operative treatment are used'. Once more Knox's book recommends the use of radiation to treat pruritis.

Albert Franklin Tyler was reporting in his book (Tyler, 1919) that he had used radiotherapy for haemorrhage and pain in the recurrence of carcinoma in the vault of the vagina in a woman of 35 years of age who had had a hysterectomy a year previously for cancer of the uterus. No details were given of the way the radiotherapy was applied. Drs Bythell and Barclay (1912) reported in their book that continental doctors had used X-rays for the treatment of fibroids very enthusiastically, and had reported that haemorrhage was arrested, general health was improved and the fibroids were reduced in size.

Among these were Antoine Beclere, endocrinologist, virologist and immunologist, who pioneered French radiology (Beclere, 1973).

Radiotherapy vs. surgery

Already by 1926 a dispute had started between those who advocated surgery for cancer of the cervix, and those who advocated radiotherapy.

This dispute still continues in the 1990s. The early arguments were encapsulated in an article by Heymann on 'Radiological treatment of uterine cancer versus surgical intervention' (Heymann, 1925). This article stated that radiological therapy carried out in the Radium-Hemmett in Stockholm was greatly superior to surgical intervention because it could be given to women in poorer medical condition than those who were submitted to surgery. The recurrence rate was about 20% and was the same for each group of women.

Radiotherapy was held to be superior to surgery for vaginal carcinoma (Flemming, 1968).

In 1922 in a large book (Simpson, 1922) Simpson summarized the effect of radium rays on bacteria and various tissues of higher animals. Much of the summary is in the nature of histology. The effects of radiating testes and ovaries of guinea-pigs and rabbits resulting in atrophy of the seminiferous epithelium in the former and the Graafian follicles in the latter are dealt with (Matthews, 1923). Radium was used for the first time in 1905 by Dr Robert Abbe of New York for the treatment of fibromyoma of the uterus, and many others later reported cases. In particular Kelley reported a series of 210 cases that he had treated with radium, particularly for uterine haemorrhage. This same treatment was certainly still given in 1947 in the Middlesex Hospital when the uterus was thought to be too large for safe removal. Of course, even in 1947, blood transfusion was not easy to come by.

I.C. Rubin, interestingly, at a meeting of the New York Obstetrical Society on 9 February 1926 (Rubin, 1926a) reported that between 4 December 1923 and 31 December 1925 he had treated patients with amenorrhoea and oligomenorrhoea using X-rays to the ovaries. He was not the first person to do this – it had originally been done by Van der Velde in 1915 and later by Flatau and Thaler who used small doses in the treatment of amenorrhoea. The dose that Flatau used was equivalent to a third of the castration dose; and after giving this dose menstruation 'set in normally in the course of 3–6 weeks'. Thaler apparently treated quite a large number of cases. H.B. Matthews thought that giving irradiation to a fetus in animal experiments could cause teratogenic changes; and Rubin said that the lethal result of radiation among young embryos was very serious as had been known for a long time. In his paper Rubin explained the details of his treatment to the ovaries in 12 cases with the birth of five children and one late abortion.

The mode of action of X-rays used in therapy was being considered by Dr Robert Lenk (1926) of the University of Vienna. He stated 'each living cell which has absorbed X-rays undergoes a change . . . definite conclusions about this change have not yet been arrived at and X-rays can be used to degenerate and destroy tissues as well as to [according to the translator] stimulate, if given in small doses'.

By the outbreak of the Second World War little was known about the histological changes produced in human cancers by radiation. Research went on, particularly in the USA, on the way tissues reacted to radiotherapy by carrying out serial biopsies of human malignant tumours at intervals of time throughout irradiation. The result was to acquire radiobiological information (Ahnfeldt and Allen, 1966). The majority of the research work was done during the war and immediately after by Dr M. Friedman, but in 1941 Glucksmann reported on the effects of radiology on histology in humans (Glucksmann, 1941). Following the more scientific observation of the way the cervix reacted, it was found that whereas radium treatment had been proposed with supervoltage radiotherapy preliminary to the radium treatment, serial biopsies showed marked radiosensitivity in some tumours so that they were destroyed in about 28 days, obviating the need for subsequent radium therapy. Other carcinomas of the cervix proved extremely radium resistant. Very often they persisted in spite of very large doses of both X-rays and radium leading to the need to remove them surgically. It was found that the laws of radiosensitivity did not apply to carcinoma of the cervix. About 20% of cervical neoplasms are very radio-sensitive and about 20% are very radio-resistant (Ahnfeldt and Allen, 1966).

Radiation treatment of cancer of the cervix

In 1974 Margaret Snelling and T.H.E. Briant were able to describe their new technique for treating carcinoma of the cervix with a Cathetron, a remote-loading high-dose rate unit. The patient is placed under an anaesthetic in the treatment room. The cervix is dilated and catheters are placed in position, both after insertion of a rectal retractor. The position of the applicators is checked by diagnostic X-rays and the patient is treated, after microsources have been inserted to estimate the rectal dose, by two treatments of 1400 rads in 4–10 min each to point A at the same interval, then with 2800 rads for 10 min some days later.

This was considered to be an advance on treatment by radioactive cobalt. The great advantage was that far less dosage to nursing personnel was inevitable than with radium treatment inside the cervix (Snelling and Briant, 1974).

Radiography in gynaecological diagnosis

The first time radiography was used in gynaecological practice was by Lewers in 1903 (Lewers, 1903). He was able to identify a hairpin in the uterine cavity, and in 1909 Ludlow was able to demonstrate calcification within uterine fibroids by X-ray (Ludlow, 1909).

The first clinical injection of a radio-opaque medium into the uterus was made in 1910 by Rindfleisch (Rindfleisch, 1910). He used a thick bismuth suspension.

It would appear that one of the first, if not the first, papers on visualization of the fetus *in utero* came on 8 August 1913 at the 17th International Congress of Medicine when three French doctors Potocki, Delherm and Laquerrière, the first an Accoucheur in the Pitié Hospital and the other two radiologists in that hospital, reported on their technique for visualizing fetal bones. They pointed out that this was not often satisfactory until the fetus was of 6 or 7 months' gestation. Earlier than 5 months the results were all negative.

In 1926 Douay reported on injection of the uterus for diagnosis by Lelorier (Douay, 1926).

There is some confusion as to who first described the use of X-rays for diagnosis of tubal patency. It may well have been W.H. Cary (Cary, 1914) who wrote a 'note on determination of patency of the Fallopian tubes by use of Collargol and X-ray shadows'. He seems to have been the first to perform salpingography although I.C. Rubin of New York City also performed it independently of Cary in 1914. Pride of place however, for the use of Collargol to outline the uterine cavity and its irregularities must almost certainly go to Rubin. He described in 1914 in a German journal the X-ray diagnosis of tumours in the uterus using intrauterine Collargol (Rubin, 1914). He demonstrated the use of this silver preparation to outline the cavity of a rabbit's uterus and of its uterine horns in his first figure, and in his second figure Rubin demonstrated the cavity of the human uterus as well as the Fallopian tubes (although it is not stated that this is what they were in the legend to the figure). Although Rubin

was an American his article appeared in German which was his first language.

He clearly stated that the use of X-rays for diagnostic purposes followed on the use of X-rays as therapy for treatment of uterine growths. The two and a half page article ends with the promise that further publications will deal with the improvements in the technique of injection, because there was considerable spill back from the cervix, resulting in staining tissues with Collargol on the X-ray films. The 'patient' was a corpse; and in this most important paper Rubin suggested that the technique would be adaptable for the living patient.

Rubin was as good as his word and in 1915 he described the uses and limitations of the hysteroscope and his inability to carry out catheterization of the Fallopian tubes (Rubin, 1915). Hence, the need for X-ray visualization. In fact, catheterization of the Fallopian tubes to visualize them had to wait for the development of salpingoscopy (q.v.) in the 1980s. But injection of contrast material into the tubes was reported by Rubin in the 1915 publication in which he outlined the investigation of eight cases and in which he described his technique for carrying out what later became known as hysterosalpingography. He had experimented on rabbits before injecting a 15% solution of Collargol into a patient in the gynaecological service of the Beth Israel Hospital in New York. The procedures were carried out in July, August and September 1914. The quality of the pictures improved as years went by so that by 1926 Rubin could show very clear hystero-salpingography pictures (Rubin, 1926b).

In 1926 Rubin reported that Lipiodol for visualization of the uterus and tubes was introduced by Sicard and Forestier (Sicard, 1922). I. C. Rubin and A. J. Bendick (Rubin, 1926b) were able to demonstrate peristalsis of the Fallopian tubes by using Lipiodol. They pointed out that it might be dangerous for the Lipiodol to stay in blocked tubes, as its presence could be seen in the tubes for several months after its injection. In that paper they stated that when Collargol had been used 'sometimes an appreciable amount of peritoneal irritation was seen'. So, Lipiodol had the disadvantage of not being completely absorbed, or at least not rapidly, and Collargol had the disadvantage of being an irritant.

That started the search, therefore, for water-soluble organic iodide preparations which could not only be diluted in water, but also if necessary be mixed with analgesic watery solutions, or with antibiotics, and with substances to make them more viscous in desired proportions. The very good new preparations were often completely absorbed within half an hour except from large hydrosalpinges; but the trouble with some of these solutions was that they were hypertonic.

By 1951 Pulsford and Palmer had perfected a polyvinyl-pyrrolidone solution with a viscosity of around 100 centipoises. This had the great advantage of a slow flow of the dye with clear-cut uterine, tubal and peritoneal phases. As the chemistry improved di-iodides were replaced by tri-iodides and later hexa-iodides. This lessened the hypertonicity and thus the pain. Still later, substances used for X-raying kidneys such as uroselectan containing 37% iodine were used, as was Vasurix a tri-iodo-acetyl-amino-benzoate of methyl-glucamine. The substance was rapidly absorbed and resulted in the reporting of a few cases of intolerance to iodine (Philipp and Carruthers, 1981).

X-ray pictures were taken not only of the pelvis and abdomen but also of the pituitary fossa, particularly in cases of hyperprolactinaemia where adenomas of the pituitary gland are found and are recognized by deformities of the sella turcica.

In the 1950s X-rays were used in surgery to demonstrate the position of an ectopic ureter going into the vaginal fornix. It is probable that Katzman and Trachtman (1954) were the first to demonstrate this on X-ray.

In 1954 Brody diagnosed, probably for the first time by X-ray, a double uterus with a double pregnancy (Brody, 1954).

Vaginography

In the 1970s and 1980s X-ray pictures were being taken after the vagina had been filled with a water-soluble contrast medium which was injected into the vagina through a Foley catheter in order to demonstrate fistulae between the vagina and the ureter, the vagina and the bladder and the rectum, as well as congenital and acquired abnormalities of the vagina; and to localize the opening in the vagina of an ectopic ureter (Whitehouse and Wright, 1992).

X-rays in obstetric diagnosis

In 1931 Peter Curley in his textbook (Curley, 1931) was able to write 'obstetrical diagnosis has reached such a high degree of accuracy that the

aid of the radiologist is seldom required'. He then went on to describe the technique to demonstrate the presence of a fetus in the uterus after 10 weeks' gestation and said that only the outlines of the bones of the skull could be seen so early, and he described the technique for carrying out the examination. He quoted that at the International Congress of Radiology in 1925 Heuser had suggested diagnosing pregnancy in the 1st and 2nd months by means of an injection of Lipiodol into the uterus and stated that he did not think that this would cause an abortion, but 'the danger of this is so obvious that the method has not been generally adopted'. Curley in his book describes the use of Lipiodol in infertility and using a Sinex synatograph camera he described radiography of the uterus while filling it with Lipiodol. He also described sterilization by means of X-rays, but pointed out 'of considerable value is the use of X-rays for stimulating the ovaries . . . remarkable results have been obtained by delivering minute doses of X-rays on to the ovaries'. He said that it was sometimes helpful to give small doses to the thyroid as well as to the ovaries.

Robert's Pelvis was first described by F. Robert in 1853 (Robert, 1853). As recently as 1933 Julius Jarcho was advocating not only X-ray pelvimetry but combining it with external pelvimetry (Jarcho, 1933). Jarchos' method was an adaptation of Thoms' method described below.

X-rays were used early to diagnose fetal death, and the first report of the most valuable sign, namely over-riding of the skull bones due to the shrinking of the cerebrum, was by A.B. Spalding in 1922 (Spalding, 1922). Roberts in 1944 was the first to show that gas in the fetal circulatory system was a sign of intrauterine fetal death (Roberts, 1944).

Pelvimetry

Until Caesarean section became a safe and very frequently practised operation obstetrics was largely a mechanical art. As A. Rongy (1930) wrote 'every case of labour is an engineering problem. The obstetrician like the engineer must guide himself wholly in accordance with the principles which make a given mechanical problem safe or unsafe, possible or impossible'. It became very important, therefore, to be able to decide on the shape and the size of the pelvis of any and every woman whose fetus was not presenting by the head and did not go into the pelvis before labour started.

Herbert Thoms (1956) was the man who put X-ray pelvimetry on to the map. For the first time he described in detail not only the anatomical differences in structure of different types of pelvis, but also their X-ray appearances. His book classified four types of pelvis in white women as follows:

(1) *Dolichopellic* This is the normal shape of the pelvis in early childhood. It is relatively elongated antero-posteriorly. About 18% of women retain this shape to adult life.

(2) *Mesatipellic* In this type of pelvis the inlet is essentially round. It is found in 45.9% of all women.

(3) *Brachypellic* In this type of pelvis the transverse diameter exceeds the antero-posterior diameter by more than 1 cm and less than 3 cm. It is found in about 32% of all women.

(4) *Platypellic* This type of pelvis is wide and flattened antero-posteriorly with an index of less than 90.

Thoms was able to show, with Greulic, that socially well-favoured women were very unlikely indeed to have a Platypellic type of pelvis, because these were more likely to occur in women who had rickets in childhood. Thoms stated that it was valuable to X-ray the pelvis for its shape and size antenatally. He pointed out, however, that measurement of the bony structures did not constitute 'an entirely complete survey of the birth passage and its passenger'. The rest of his book is devoted to giving the measurements and ascertaining them by X-rays, and to debunking the value of the external measurements of the pelvis that had been standardly described in every textbook. Thoms stated that it was illogical to classify pelves by means of the four external measurements that had commonly been taken until then (Figure 2).

Until Thoms' work, almost every antenatal clinic had been provided with a pair of metal callipers for measuring external diameters. It took until 1948 when Eastman, Professor of Obstetrics pointed out that since 1943 he had had 'the temerity to discontinue the taking of these (external) parameters as well as the external conjugate'. A year later Dr Greenhill, the author of a very successful textbook on obstetrics, deleted external measurement from his book.

In Thoms' book it is pointed out that there are five valuable measurements that can be taken, namely the antero-posterior measured on the

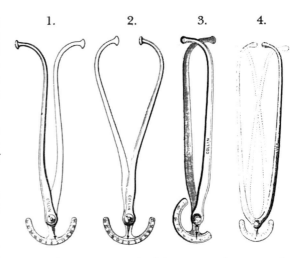

Figure 2 Four types of pelvimeters used to assess the size of the female pelvis. (1) Collin's internal pelvimeter; (2) Collin's external pelvimeter; (3) Collin's internal and external pelvimeter combined; (4) Stanesco's Compass. All these were highly inaccurate in assessing the pelvic diameter through which the fetus had to pass

lateral film, the transverse, measured on the inlet film, the posterior saggital, measured on the inlet film after projecting the antero-posterior on it, the obstetric transverse and the anterior transverse both measured on the inlet film. He described the diameters of his different types of pelvis. The book is interesting, too, because it tells how the female pelvis develops. Thoms discussed the role of nutrition, and particularly of malnutrition leading to rickets, in the development of different types of pelvis.

Caldwell *et al.* (1934) classified pelves into anthropoid, anthropoid–android, gynaecoid and android. The last was supposed to be a male type of pelvis. The anthropoid pelvis was said to be found in apes where the long diameter of the brim is situated antero-posteriorly, the side walls being straight. It was easier for a woman to deliver normally vaginally if she had a large pelvis rather than a small one; certainly easier if the infant was small rather than large. Thoms pointed out the measurements of the inlet alone were inadequate because the pelvis could be narrowed in the mid-section; and in his book he gave details of how the X-rays should be taken. His technique now slightly modified is sometimes still used particularly after a Caesarean section has had to be undertaken for previously undiagnosed disproportion; and in order to make available information for the next delivery.

One of the first mentions in the literature of measuring the fetal head was by Thoms in 1930 (Thoms, 1930). The book also contains a very interesting chapter on the grossly abnormal pelvis that was described in 1839 by Naegele (Naegele F., 1839).

The great Munro Kerr believed that X-ray pelvimetry 'before many years passed could be accepted as an essential detail of the antenatal examination'. In his day the ill-effects of X-rays had not yet been discovered.

It was recognized in 1972 that X-rays could damage the developing fetus (Brent and Gorson, 1972). The damage to the fetus is related to the dose that it receives, and also particularly to the time in the pregnancy when the exposure is made. The most vulnerable time for organs is when they are being laid down and this has now been worked out very accurately. It is unlikely that the usual doses of radiation given to women whose pelves are being assessed, particularly in late pregnancy, can affect the fetus.

Exposing the fetus to radiation while X-raying the placenta

As early as 1933 Munro Kerr used X-rays to diagnose placenta praevia (Kerr and Mackay, 1933), and he was followed soon after by Snow and Powell (1934). From the time of the earliest use of X-rays for the diagnosis of the placental site, a whole series of papers appeared. Of particular historical interest were those of Ude and Weum (1934), as well as of Chassar Moir (1944), McCort *et al.* (1944) followed soon after by Seeley (1945), Hartnett (1948), Stevenson (1949), Reid (1949), Quist (1952), Sutton (1952) and Norman (1953).

The methods for localizing the placenta were reviewed at a symposium held at the Annual Congress of the British Institute of Radiology in December 1952 by J. Chassar Moir (1953), and these in short consisted of

(1) Displacement of the head;

(2) Amniography;

(3) Soft tissue radiography; and

(4) The injection of a radioactive substance into the blood stream.

Amniography, which was also used for the detection of fetal abnormalities, consisted of the injection of water-soluble contrast agents into the amniotic cavity. Fetography took the procedure

one step further by injecting oil-soluble contrast media, in particular Myodil, into the cavity, so that the vernix caseosa and the fetal skin showed up on X-rays. Both amniography and fetography had hazards for the fetus which had not previously been appreciated (Russell, 1973).

It was in about 1960 that the dangers of radiation to both the mother and the fetus became appreciated. Until that time X-rays were used fairly extensively during mid- and late pregnancy to assess how mature the fetus was and to look for fetal abnormalities as well as to localize the placenta. It was fortunate that ultrasonography was able to take over without the risks of teratogenicity or damage to the mother.

COMPUTERIZED TOMOGRAPHY IN GYNAECOLOGICAL DIAGNOSIS

This technique involves carrying out X-ray scans and it is of value in gynaecology in assessing the degree of pelvic malignancy and in particular the presence of enlarged lymph nodes. It is questionable whether it gives much more information than straight X-rays and ultrasound combined, but when there is doubt as to the presence or the extent of malignant disease and in particular of extraperitoneal disease which cannot be reached with a laparoscope, it does have a value. Cuts of 50 mm are made and the patient is scanned in the supine position. The value of the examination for lymph nodes may be increased if lymphangiography using a radio-opaque coloured medium is added. It is possible that magnetic resonance imaging will replace the use of computerized tomography as an adjunct to ultrasound. Wright compared the merits of computerized tomography and ultrasound in gynaecology in a good review article (Wright, 1981).

ULTRASOUND

The diagnosis of pregnancy can be made very rapidly, sometimes as early as 7–9 days after ovulation, by detecting the presence of human chorionic gonadotropin in the serum or in the urine. The hormone is produced by the syncytiotrophoblast. Ultrasound cannot compete in the detection of pregnancy at this time, but 3 weeks after fertilization, i.e. 5–6 weeks after the last period, an intrauterine sac can usually be identified using a vaginal probe, and just 1 week later, at 7 weeks postmenstrual, a fetal pole can be measured and the fetal heart movement may well be diagnosed.

The Doppler effect

Christian Doppler (1803–1853) was the physicist who discovered the effect that velocity has on the observed frequency of light and sound waves. There is an apparent change in the frequency of the wave (as a light wave or sound wave) which results from a change in the distance between the source of the wave and the receiver. Doppler theorized that as the picture/sound from a moving source varies for the stationary observer as the source moves, the colour of the light from a star should alter according to the star's velocity relative to the earth. This may seem to be far from the development of ultrasound in obstetrics and gynaecology, following on the work of Ian Donald (q.v.); but it is not.

Doppler's first paper on the subject was published in 1842. The first medical men to adopt and adapt his techniques were the vascular surgeons. Ian Donald's initial work did not include the Doppler effect (Donald *et al.*, 1958).

Ultrasonic waves exist in frequency ranges over 20 000 Hz (cycles per second) i.e. above the upper limit of human hearing. They have been known about for a very long time, but it took until 1910 for them to be used to detect the presence of submerged submarines. This followed the successful development of the piezoelectric transducer. In these tranducers there is a piezoelectric material such as a quartz crystal which generates an electric voltage in response to mechanical pressures, or oscillates mechanically when an oscillating voltage is applied to it.

The first obstetricians to use Doppler techniques in obstetrics were Irish (Fitzgerald and Drumm, 1977), but later in the 1980s the use of Doppler wave forms started to play an important role particularly in the diagnosis of intrauterine circulatory disturbances of the fetus. It became known then that where there were no recordable frequencies in end-to-end diastole fetuses would be both hypoxic and acidotic.

Colour-flow mapping

Colour-flow mapping can and has been used for outlining the blood flow to the uterus. One of its most dramatic uses is for the detection of vasa praevia, a rare condition but one which can easily jeopardize the life of the fetus because if the blood vessels are compressed in labour or worse still rupture, the infant may die of asphyxia, haemorrhage, or both. It has been possible to diagnose vasa praevia by the usual forms of ultrasonography, but if there is a band discovered in the lower uterine segment using ordinary real-time scanning, it is worth carrying out colour-flow mapping to search for umbilical vessels. This was done by Fon-Jouhsie and colleagues when beautiful pictures were obtained of vasa praevia, i.e. the umbilical artery and the umbilical vein in front of the presenting part (Hsieh, 1991).

By the late 1980s it was possible to carry out colour-flow Doppler imaging of the fetal heart and even of the fetal circle of Willis (Pearce and Malcolm, 1991).

The value of ultrasound in the first trimester of pregnancy

Although ultrasound is not as reliable as human chorionic gonadotropin estimations to diagnose early pregnancy it has been shown to be very useful in the differential diagnosis between an intrauterine pregnancy and an extrauterine (ectopic) pregnancy. In both pregnancies the human chorionic gonadotropin levels are raised. If there is bleeding in early pregnancy and ultrasound shows a gestational sac with a beating fetal heart inside the uterus, the diagnosis must be that of threatened abortion. If the endometrium is shown on ultrasound to be thickened but the sac is not in the uterus, a search must be made for it in one of the Fallopian tubes. If it is found, early diagnosis of tubal pregnancy can be made. This is very important because when an extrauterine ectopic pregnancy in a tube is diagnosed early it can be removed through the laparoscope instead of removing the tube, thus avoiding major abdominal surgery (Nyberg *et al.*, 1986).

Early diagnosis of a pregnancy in the first trimester allows moderately accurate dating of the pregnancy. The vaginal probe in some cases has made this easier (Scheer, 1977). This is of particular use, especially when several tiny embryos have been placed in a uterus in an *in vitro* fertilization or gamete intrafallopian transfer procedure, to detect the number of embryos that are surviving. Furthermore, it is known that sometimes twin or triplet pregnancies may continue with the loss of one fetus. This has been described by Landy *et al.* (1986). In cases where there is a suspicion of congenital fetal abnormality due to chromosomal abnormalities chorionic villus sampling can be carried out. This is made safer if done under ultrasound control (Rhoads *et al.,* 1989)

When multiple intrauterine pregnancies are diagnosed and it is considered that it is unsafe for the woman to carry three or even two fetuses, selective reduction of the number of fetuses in the uterus has been carried out, under ultrasound control (Berkowitz *et al.,* 1988).

Ultrasound in the second trimester (Figure 3)

Ultrasound is used routinely in many hospitals in antenatal clinics in the second trimester for the diagnosis of fetal well-being, the rate of growth of the fetus, information on the estimated duration of pregnancy, and above all, detection of abnormalities in the skeletal, the gastrointestinal, the central nervous, and other systems. It is particularly valuable for dating a pregnancy, although not as accurate as ultrasound taken in the first trimester.

Ultrasound is also very valuable for localization of the placenta. In women with a history of spontaneous second trimester or third trimester abortions it is possible to visualize the cervix and the degree of dilatation. Furthermore, amniocentesis can be safely carried out under ultrasound guidance earlier in the pregnancy (i.e. before the 16th week) since the obstetrician can be sure where he is placing the needle and that it is in the amniotic sac. Furthermore it has often been used when sampling umbilical blood or

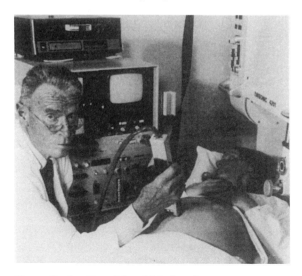

Figure 3   Ian Donald and his daughter

placental blood, particularly in cases of isoimmunization (Nicolaides *et al.,* 1986).

Rodeck and others have carried out fetal surgery under ultrasound guidance in the third trimester of pregnancy for such conditions as drainage of a fetal hydrothorax or the preventive treatment of fetal hydronephrosis, as well as for transfusing the fetus inside the uterus in cases of rhesus immunization (Rodeck *et al.,* 1988).

It must be remembered that amniocentesis was first performed by Bevis for rhesus sensitization but was perfected by Liley in 1961 and it is his early work that led to Rodeck and others treating the fetus by transfusion into the umbilical blood vessels under ultrasound guidance.

The ability to study the anatomical features and the physiological behaviour of the fetal heart has been very important in the early diagnosis of congenital heart disease. The early detection of such abnormalities is not just an academic exercise, particularly since it is now known that many congenital cardiac conditions are associated with chromosome abnormalities such as trisomy 21 (Downs syndrome) (Huhta and Rotondo, 1991).

Intrauterine growth retardation is a very common condition in which the fetus is light in weight for the duration of the pregnancy (at or below the 10th percentile for the duration of the pregnancy) and it is now routinely recognized by ultrasonography. It is important to know whether the fetus is growth retarded. It is no use simply to calculate from measurements such as the circumference of the skull, the length of the long bones, and the circumference of the fetal abdomen, unless one is certain of the dates. Since it is thought that most cases of intrauterine growth retardation are due to the placenta failing to provide adequate nourishment to the fetus (placental insufficiency) the Doppler blood flow studies first used extensively in the 1980s were an important landmark in fetal medicine (Cohen *et al.,* 1990).

Ultrasound in the localization of the placenta

Almost as soon as it became possible to take obstetric polaroid ultrasound pictures and to see good images on the ultrasound screen, ultrasound took over from X-rays as *the* method for localizing the placenta, assessing its size, and looking for textural changes in the placenta (Fleischer *et al.,* 1986). There are two types of scanner used in obstetrics. The first produces 'static' images; these scanners have the transducer mounted on an articulated arm. The second devices are 'real-time' scanners which show only a small area but are very flexible. Localization of the placenta is often done using serial tomographic static images, but the state of the fetal heart is detected using real-time scanning. It is known that fetal organs develop particularly between the 9th and 15th weeks of pregnancy and therefore wise radiologists and scanners restrict exposure from either X-rays or ultrasound to a minimum between those dates. This precaution was advocated in 1978 (Baker and Dalrymple, 1978).

Campbell and Newman (1971) were the first to discuss the growth of the head of the fetus in pregnancy.

The safety of ultrasound in obstetrics

The Food and Drug Administration of the USA has monitored very carefully whether ultrasound is safe or not for the fetus and for the mother. The only apparent risk would be from hyperthermia. As Ziskin (1990) pointed out with ultrasound as a form of energy, when ultrasonic intensities are high, as they are with Doppler instruments, there is a possible risk of hyperthermia which may be teratogenic. It is known that hyperthermia can cause fetal abnormalities, but these are from such conditions as high temperature in infectious diseases or accidental exposure. The Food and Drug Administration concluded on 29 August 1989 that the benefits of ultrasound, including Doppler ultrasound, were far greater than the risks.

MAGNETIC RESONANCE IMAGING

The phenomenon of magnetic resonance imaging was first described quite independently, but at the same time, by Bloch, and Purcell in 1946, and they were both awarded the Nobel Prize for Physics for this discovery in 1952.

Magnetic resonance imaging (which was originally called nuclear magnetic resonance) describes the phenomenon whereby the nuclei of certain atoms, when placed in a magnetic field, can absorb and emit radio-frequency energy of a specific frequency.

The practical application of the technique is to produce detailed cross-sectional images of the body's soft tissues. This is done by placing the patient inside a magnetic field about 50 000 times stronger than the earth's magnetic field. This excites atomic nuclei within the body. These

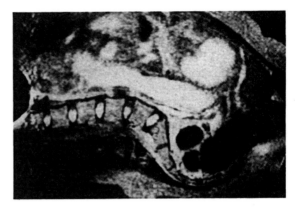

Figure 4 Magnetic resonance imaging showing a cephalic presentation with a low-lying placenta on the posterior wall of the uterus

nuclei, which most often are of hydrogen, give off radio-frequency signals which can be recorded by the imager and can be converted into computerized images (Figure 4).

The magnetic field is measured in teslas. It has been recommended that because of the heating effect pregnant women should not be scanned during the first three months of pregnancy (Godlee, 1991).

During the 1950s and 1960s Erik Odeblat (Odeblat and Lindstrom, 1955), who was both a physicist and gynaecologist working in Sweden, studied the proton magnetic resonance properties of human red blood cells, of cervical mucus, of the muscle of the uterus, and of other fluids.

In 1971 Damadian showed that it was possible to diagnose tumours by detecting differences between the magnetic resonance imaging properties of these tumours and the heart in rats. He used proton magnetic resonance imaging spectroscopy and others confirmed his work, but it was Lauterbur (1973) who first used a method of spatial localization by varying the magnetic field applied to the sample. The first human *in vivo* images were published by Mansfield and Maudsley in 1977.

CHRONOLOGY

1890	Sir William Crookes made the first cathode-ray tubes.
29 December 1895	Wilhelm Conrad Roentgen described 'a new kind of rays'.
23 January 1896	Roentgen demonstrated the bones of the hands as seen by X-rays.

1898	Radium discovered by Pierre Curie and his wife Marie. A hairpin was demonstrated in the uterine cavity by radiography.
1903	Cancer of the breast treated with X-rays to relieve pain.
1904	Radiotherapy used in gynaecology to treat prurigo.
1909	Dr David Arthur recommended radiotherapy for superficial cancers.
1910	Sonar first introduced to detect submarines on the sea bed and from this ultrasound and its use in gynaecology was developed in the 1950s by Ian Donald of Glasgow. A radio-opaque medium was first injected into the uterus by Rindfleisch.
1912	X-rays reported in the treatment of fibroids.
1914 & 1915	Cary and then Rubin used X-rays to determine the patency of Fallopian tubes using Collargol as the contrast medium.
1915	Robert Knox wrote 100 pages on the X-ray treatment of gynaecological conditions.
1926	I.C. Rubin described using X-rays for treating menstrual disorders. Lipiodol introduced by Rubin.
1928	The discussion about radiotherapy vs. surgery was well under way.
1931	X-rays were used in obstetrics.
1933	Munro Kerr used X-rays to diagnose placenta praevia.
1941	The histological changes brought about by radiotherapy were investigated.
1946	Bloch and Purcell discovered magnetic resonance imaging.
1950	Urography introduced into gynaecology.
1956	Herbert Thoms improved X-ray pelvimetry and made a different classification of four types of pelvis from Caldwell and Molloy (1934).
1981	Computerized tomography became established in gynaecology.

REFERENCES

Ahnfeldt, A.L. and Allen, K.D.A. (1966). Radiology in World War II, pp. 212-14. Prepared and published under the direction of Leonard D. Heaton. Editor in Chief: Arnold Lorentz Ahnfeldt, Editor for Radiology: Kenneth D. A. Allen. (Washington, D.C.: Office of the Surgeon General. United States War Department)

Arthur, D. and Muir, J. (1909). *A Manual of Practical X-ray Work*, p. 230. (London: Rebman Ltd. and William Heinemann)

Auset, (1898). *Echo Med. du Nord*, no. 461

Baker, M. and Dalrymple, G. (1978). Biological effects of diagnostic ultrasound: a review. *Radiology*, **126**, 479-83

Beclere, A. (1973). *Antoine Beclere (1856–1939): Pionnier en Endocrinologie: l'un des fondateurs de la virologie et de l'immunologie: fondateur de la radiologie Francaise*. (Antoine Beclere: Pioneer in Endocrinology: one of the founders of virology and immunology; founder of French radiology), in the series of General History of Radiology. (Paris: Publishers J. B. Bailliere)

Berkowitz, R.L., Lynch, L., Chitkara, U. *et al.* (1988). Selective reduction of multifetal pregnancies in the first trimester. *N. Engl. J. Med.*, **318**, 1043–7

Brent, R.L. and Gorson, R.O.(1972). Radiation exposure in pregnancy. *Curr. Prob. Radiol.*, **2**, 1–48

Brody, S. (1954). Double uterus with double pregnancy. *Am. J. Obstet. Gynecol.*, **67**, 161–7

Bythell, W.J.S. and Barclay, A.E. (1912). *X-ray – Diagnosis and Treatment*, p. 128. (London: Henry Frowde and Hodder & Stoughton)

Caldwell, W. E., Moloy, H.C. and D'Esopo, D.A. (1934). A roentgenologic study of the mechanism of engagement of the fetal head. *Am. J. Obstet. Gynecol.*, **28**, 824–41

Campbell, S. and Newman, G. (1971). Growth of fetal biparietal diameter during normal pregnancy. *Br. J. Obstet. Gynaecol.*, **78**, 513–19

Cary, W.H. (1914). Note on determination of patency of Fallopian tubes by the use of Collargol and X-ray shadow. *Am. J. Obstet. Dis. Wom.*, **69**, 462–4

Chassar Moir, J. (1944). Fallacies in soft tissue placentography. *Am. J. Obstet. Gynecol.*, **47**, 198

Chassar Moir, J. (1953). A review of placentography. *Br. J. Radiol.*, **26**, 385

Cleaves, M.A. (1903). Radium: with a preliminary note on radium rays in the treatment of cancer. *Med. Rec.*, **64**, 601–10

Cohen, A.W., Lindenbaum, C.R., Jackson, G.M., Forouzan, I. and Eife, S.B. (1990). The role of ultrasound in the clinical practice of obstetrics. *Seminars in Roentgenology*, pp. 287–93. (Philadelphia: W.B. Saunders)

Curley, P. (1931). *Recent Advances in Radiology*, pp. 286, 289. (London: Churchill Livingstone)

Donald, I., MacVicar, J. and Brown, T.G. (1958). Investigation of abdominal masses by pulsed ultrasound. *Lancet*, **1**, 1188–95

Douay, E. (1926). Insufflation tubaire. *J. Med. Chir. Prat.*, **97**, 709–16

Fitzgerald, D.E. and Drumm, J.E. (1977). Noninvasive measurement of the fetal circrculation using ultrasound: a new method. *Br. J. Obstet. Gynaecol.*, **2**, 1450–1

Fleischer, A.C., Boehm, F.H., Winfield, A.C., Millis, J., Schaff, M.I., James, A.E. and Gibbs, J. (1986). In Grainger, R.G. and Allison D.J. (eds.) *Diagnostic Radiology: an Anglo-American Textbook of Imaging*, Vol. 3, Section 8. pp. 1551–92. (London: Churchill Livingstone)

Flemming, M. (1968). *History and Development of Radiology in Denmark, 1896–1950*, p. 327. (Copenhagen: Nyt Nordisk. Arnold Busck)

Freund, L. (1904). *Elements of General Radio-Therapy for Practitioners*, translated by G. H. Lancashire. (New York: Rebman Company)

Glucksmann, A. (1941). Preliminary observations on the quantitative examination of human biopsy material taken from irradiated carcinomata. *Br. J. Radiol.*, **14**, 187–98

Godlee, F. (1991). Warning over magnetic resonance imaging. *Br. Med. J.*, **303**, 205

Grigg, E.R.N. (1965). *The Trail of the Invisible Light from X-Strahlen to Radio(biol)ogy*. (Springfield, Illinois: Charles C. Thomas)

Hartnett, L.J. (1948). Possible significance of arterial visualisation in the diagnosis of placenta previa. *Am. J. Obstet. Gynecol.*, **55**, 940

Heyman, J. (1925). Final results in the treatment of carcinoma of the uterine cervix at 'Radium Hemmet' Stockholm. *Am. J. Roentg.*, **13**, 158–61

Hsieh, F-J., Chen, H-F., Ko, T-M. Hsieh, C-Y. and Chen, H-Y. (1991). Antenatal diagnosis of vasa previa by color-flow mapping. *J. Ultrasound Med.*, **10**, 397–9

Huhta, J.C. and Rotondo, K.M. (1991). Fetal echocardiography. *Seminars in Roentgenology*, Vol. 26 no. 1 pp. 5–11, 298 and 304. (Philadelphia: W. B. Saunders Co.)

Jarcho, J. (1933). *The Pelvis and Obstetrics*. (New York: Paul B. Hober)

Katzman, P. and Trachtman, D. (1954). Diagnosis of vaginal ectopic ureter by vaginogram. *J. Urol.*, **72**, 808–11

Kerr, J.M.M. and Mackay, W.G. (1933). The diagnosis of placenta praevia with special reference to the use of X-rays for this purpose. *Edin. Med. J.*, **40**, 21

Knox, R. (1915). *Radiography – X-ray Therapeutics and Radium Therapy*. (London: A. & C. Black)

Landy, H.J., Weiner, S., Carson, S.L., *et al.* (1986). The vanishing twin: ultrasonographic assessment of fetal disappearance in the first trimester. *Am. J. Obstet. Gynecol.*, **154**, 14–20

Lauterbur, P.C. (1973). Image formation by induced local interactions: examples employing MRI, *Nature (London)*, **242**, 190–1

Lenk, R. (1926). *Index and Handbook of X-ray Therapy*, p. 1. (Oxford: Humphrey Milford)

Lewers, A.H.N. (1903). A case of hairpin in the uterus discovered by the X-rays. *Br. Med. J.*, **2**, 814–15

Ludlow, I. (1909). Calcification of fibromyomata of the uterus. *Cleveland Med. J.*, **8**, 398–411

McCort, J.J., Davidson, C.N. and Walton, H.J. (1944). Determination of the placental site during bleeding in the third trimester. *Am. J. Roentg.*, **52**, 440

Mansfield, P. and Maudsley, A.A. (1977). Medical imaging by nuclear magnetic resonance. *Br. J. Radiol.*, **50**, 188–94

Matthews, H.B. (1923). The effects of radium rays upon the ovary: an experimental, pathological and clinical study. *Trans. Am. Gynecol. Soc.*, **48**, 39–56

Naegele, F.C. (1839). *Das Schrag Verengte Becken.* (Mainz: von Zabern)

Nicolaides, K., Soothil, R. and Rodeck, C. (1986). Ultrasound guided sampling of the umbilical cord and placental blood to assess fetal well-being. *Lancet*, **1**, 1065–7

Norman, 0. (1953). Localisation of the placenta by means of arteriography and auscultation. *Br. J. Radiol.*, **26**, 393

Nyberg, D.A., Laing, F.C. and Filly, R.A. (1986). Threatened abortion: sonographic distinction of normal and abnormal gestation sacs. *Radiology*, **158**, 397–400

Odeblat, E. and Lindstrom, G. (1955). Some preliminary observations on the proton magnetic resonance in biologic samples. *Acta Radiol.*, **43**, 469–75

Pearce, J.M. (1991). Twenty-five years of obstetrics. *Br. J. Hosp. Med.*, **46**, 247–8

Philipp, E.E. and Carruthers, G.B. (1981). *Infertility*, p. 94. (London: Heinemann Medical Books)

Potocki, M.M., Delherm and Laquerriere (1913). La radiographie du fetus *in utero*. 17th International Congress of Medicine, London. *Radiology*, **XXII**, 157–8

Qvist, C.F. (1952). Soft-tissue radiography of the placenta. *Acta Radiol.*, **37**, 510

Reid, F. (1949). Aluminium filter for use in localisation of placental site. *Br. J. Radiol.*, **22**, 81

Rhoads, G.G., Jackson, L.G., Schlesselman, S.E. *et al.* (1989). The safety and efficacy of chorionic villus sampling for early pre-natal diagnosis of cytogenic abnormalities. *N. Engl. J. Med.*, **320**, 609–17

Rindfleisch, W. (1910). Darstellung des Cavum uteri. *Berlin klin. Wchnschr.*, 780

Robert, F. (1853). *Ein durch Mechanische Verletzung und ihre Folgen Querverengtes Becken.* (Berlin)

Roberts , J. B. (1944). Gas in the fetal circulatory system as a sign of intrauterine fetal death. *Am. J. Roentg.*, **51**, 631

Rodeck, C.H., Fisk, M.N., Fraser, D.I. and Nicolini, U. (1988). Longterm *in utero* drainage of fetal hydrothorax. *N. Engl. J. Med.*, **319**, 1135–8

Rongy, A.L. (1930). Some aspects of the mechanism of labor. *Med. J. Record*, **131**, 420–2

Röntgen, W.C. (1895). Ueber eine neue Art von Strahlen. *S. B. Phys. Med. Ges. Wurzburg*, 132–41. Reproduced in facsimile in *Isis* 1936, 26, 349–69 and in English in 1896, *Nature*, **53**, 274 and 377

Rubin, I.C. (1914). Röntgen Diagnostik der Uterus Tumoren mit Hilfe von Intrauterinen Collargol Injektionen. *Zbl. Gynakol.*, **18**, 1–3

Rubin, I.C. (1914). X-ray diagnosis of tumours of the uterus by means of intrauterine collargol injections: preliminary communications. *Zbl. Gynakol.*, **38**, 658–60

Rubin, I.C. (1915). X-ray diagnosis in gynecology with the aid of intrauterine collargol injection. *Surg. Gynecol. Obstet.* April In Rubin (1954)

Rubin, I.C. (1926a). *Meeting New York Obstetrical Society*, 9 February 1926 In Rubin (1954)

Rubin, I.C. (1926b). *J. Am. Med. Assoc.*, **86**, 648; 657

Rubin, I.C. (1954). *Collected papers* – 132 in total written between 1910 and 1954. (Published privately)

Russell, J.G.B. (1973). *Radiology in Obsterics and Antenatal Paediatrics.* (London: Butterworth)

Scheer, K. (1977). Sonography as a routine obstetrical diagnostic procedure. *J. Clin. Ultrasound*, **5**, 101–2

Seeley, W.F. (1945). A study of 250 cases of placenta previa. *Am. J. Obstet. Gynecol.*, **49**, 85–94

Sicard, J.A. and Forestier, J. (1922). Iodised oil as a contrast medium in radioscopy. *Bull. Mem. Soc. Med.* Paris, **46**, 463–9

Simpson, F.E. (1922). *Radium Therapy.* (London: Henry Kimpton)

Snelling, M. and Briant, T.H.E. (1974). *Cancer of the Cervix.* (Bethesda, MD: Department of Health Education and Welfare. Food & Drug Administration, N.I.H.)

Snow, W. and Powell, C.B. (1934). Roentgen visualization of the placenta. *Am. J. Roentg.*, **31**, 37–40

Spalding, A.B. (1922). Pathognomonic sign of intrauterine death. *Surg. Gynecol. Obstet.*, **34**, 754

Stevenson, C.C. (1949). X-ray visualisation of the placenta; experiences with soft tissue and cystographic technics in the diagnosis of placenta previa. *Am. J. Obstet. Gynecol.*, **58**, 15

Stenstrom, W. (1926). Physics and radiology. *Acta Radiol.*, **7**, 547–58

Sutton, D. (1952). Placental and pelvic angiography by retrograde percutaneous injection of the femoral artery. *Br. J. Radiol.*, **25**, 320

Thoms, H. (1930). Fetal cephalometry *in utero*. *J. Am. Med. Assoc.*, **95**, 21–4

Thoms, H. (1956). *Pelvimetry*. (London: Cassell & Co. Ltd.,)

Tyler, A.F. (1919). *Roentgenotherapy*. (London: Henry Kimpton)

Ude, W.H., Weum, T.W. and Urner, J.A. (1934). Roentgenologic diagnosis of placenta praevia. *Am. J. Roentg.*, **31**, 230–3

Whitehouse, G.H. and Wright, C.H. (1992). Imaging in gynaecology. In Granger, R.G. and Alison, D.J. (eds.) *Diagnostic Radiology*, 2nd edn. Vol. 3, p. 1825. (London: Churchill Livingstone)

Wright, C.H., (1981). In Whitehouse, G.H. (ed.) *Gynaecological Radiology*, pp. 226–34. (Oxford: Blackwell Scientific Publications)

Ziskin, M.C. (1990). Update on the safety of ultrasound in obstetrics. In *Seminars in Roentgenology*, pp. 294–8. (Philadelphia: W.B. Saunders & Co.)

FURTHER READING

Suggested use of nuclear medicine techniques

Browne, J.C.M. (1951). Localisation of the placenta by means of radio-active sodium. *Proc. R. Soc. Med.*, **44**, 715

Ultrasound

Donald, I. and Abdulla, U. (1968). Placentography by sonar. *J. Obstet. Gynaecol. Br. Cwlth.*, **75**, 993

Gottesfeld, K.R. *et al.* (1966). Ultrasonic placentography – a new method. *Am. J. Obstet. Gynecol.*, **96**, 538–47

Brim pelvimetry

Chassard and Lapine, (1923). Etude radiographique de l'arcade pubierine chez la femme enceinte. Une nouvelle methode d'appreciation du diametre bi-ischiatique. *J. Radiol. d'Electrol.*, **7**, 113–24

Hueblein, A.C., Roberts, D.J. and Ogden, R.T. (1928). Roentgen pelvimetry after the Thoms methods with a simplification of technique. *J. Roentg.*, **20**, 64–6

Martius, H. (1915). *Fortschritte*, **22**, Section 6

Roberts, R.E. (1927). Internal pelvimetry by X-rays. *Br. J. Radiol.*, **32**, 11–15

Thoms, H. (1926). *Am. J. Obstet.*, **12**, 543

Benign pathology

ENDOMETRIOSIS

The occurrence of endometriosis was first discovered by Carl Von Rokitansky (1860), a Czech pathologist working in Vienna. In 1861 he further reported the condition of ovarian endometriosis, described by him as *cystosarcoma adenides ovarii uterinum* (Ricci, 1945). Other reports of the condition in the last century came from Von Recklinghausen (1885), Cullen (1896), Iwanhoff (1898) and Russell (1899). Robert Meyer (1903) published an extensive description. Sampson (1921) described perforating haemorrhagic 'chocolate' cysts of the ovary. He termed the condition 'endometriosis' and was also the first to document malignant change in extrauterine endometriotic tissue (1925a). The term 'endometrioma' was first introduced by Blair Bell (1922).

With the advent of culdoscopy, laparoscopy and the more common use of laparotomy in this century, the disorder was diagnosed with increasing frequency. The incidence in White women varied from 10 to 25% but it was less common in Negroes. Henriksen (1955) analysed 1000 cases and showed that 82% of the patients were in the 30–45-year age group. It was shown that endometriotic tissue could involve the pelvic cavity, the recto-vaginal septum, the vaginal vault, the gastrointestinal, genital and urinary tracts, Caesarean section wounds, and other sites. Menorrhagia, dysmenorrhoea, deep dyspareunia, and infertility were reported in association with the condition.

Theories of origin

Von Recklinghausen (1885) described the condition and suggested that it developed from tissue of Wolffian origin. Cullen (1896) described adenomyoma of the round ligaments which he asserted was tissue of Müllerian origin. Iwanhoff (1898) advocated the theory of serosal metaplasia. Further theories of origin were postulated during the late nineteenth century and developed in the early part of this century. Dr J.A. Sampson (1921) Albany, New York, began his series of reports on endometriosis and documented his further observations over the following 25 years. His theory (Sampson, 1922) of retrograde menstruation caused much debate but failed to resolve the issue. Halban (1924; 1925) first proposed a theory of endolymphatic spread, which was supported by Javert (1949) who reported microscopic evidence of endometrial cells in lymphatics and lymph nodes.

Sampson (1925b) also proposed a haematogenous dissemination theory which received support from Javert (1952) who demonstrated the spread of benign and malignant endometrium in the pelvic veins. Robert Meyer was of the opinion that endometriosis developed by metaplasia at the original coelomic epithelium (Meyer, 1930; Haines and Taylor, 1962) but Navrital and Kramer (1936) opted for a vascular embolization theory. McVeigh (1955) proposed that corona radiata (cumulus) cells which escaped at ovulation were later transformed to endometriosis. Gruenwald (1942), in a report to the *American Journal of Obstetrics and Gynecology*, concluded that endometriosis in most locations originated from tissue derived from the primitive coelom (serosa). Despite its frequent diagnosis over many years, no consensus existed as to the aetiology of this enigmatic disease.

Pathology

Histological examination revealed the presence of tissue resembling endometrium but in many instances cyclical activity was not observed. Hertig's observation 'the more advanced the lesion clinically, the poorer the histological detail', described the situation in which no tissue was recognizable as endometrium (Hertig and Sommers, 1949). However, in these instances a layer of haemosiderin laden macrophages and epithelium was found to line the cystic endometriotic cavities (Stewart, 1935).

Staging

As with other complex disease entities, a grading system was found necessary. This allowed for comparison of presenting features, documentation of quantifiable disease, and response to treatment. Classifications were produced by Acosta *et al.* (1973), Kistner *et al.* (1977), Buttram (1978), and the American Fertility Society (1979). Each system was thought to have missed out on some essential element.

Treatment

Surgery

Fraser (1925) suggested ovarian extirpation which not only removed possible endometriotic tissue but also eliminated the main source of oestrogen and progesterone, which were necessary for the maintenance and growth of that tissue. The surgical approach included total abdominal hysterectomy with ovarian conservation, or total abdominal hysterectomy with bilateral salpingo-oophorectomy when the ovaries were involved. Radical surgery was the treatment of choice where fertility was not desired. This approach also treated the adenomyosis which was found to accompany endometriosis in about 10% of cases. Those patients who had bilateral oophorectomy could have hormone replacement therapy which rarely caused recurrence of endometriosis (Hammond *et al.*, 1976).

Lesser forms of surgery included laparotomy with local ablation of endometriotic tissue and conservation of the reproductive organs. The laparoscopic approach became popular and allowed electrocoagulation and laser destruction therapy. Conservative surgery was the procedure of choice for patients who had failed to conceive following 'medical' treatment. The assisted reproduction technologies were successfully applied in the endometriotic infertile patient. A success rate of 8.2% per cycle was reported in the World Collaborative Report on *in vitro* fertilization and embryo transfer (Seppala, 1985).

Medical treatment

Karnaky (1948) introduced a high-dose oestrogen (stilboestrol) regimen which remained the only available hormonal treatment for endometriosis in the early 1950s. Many patients found the treatment unacceptable due to its side- effects.

'Pseudopregnancy' therapy was introduced by Kistner (1958) based on Sampson's observation that pregnancy had a beneficial effect on the endometriotic state. Kistner treated 12 patients with progesterone and oestrogen in graduated fashion. The effects of pseudopregnancy were an initial decidualization, followed after several months by atrophy of the tissue (Andrews *et al.*, 1959). Pseudopregnancy remained popular throughout the 1970s and was effected by oral or injectable progesterones, or with the combined oral contraceptive pill.

The next treatment was that of 'pseudomenopause'. Greenblatt *et al.* (1971) introduced danazol which caused a hormonal state similar to chronic anovulation. There was absence of the follicle stimulating hormone and luteinizing hormone surge, elevated oestrogen levels, increased androgens and altered steroidogenesis in the ovary and adrenal (Guillebaud *et al.*, 1977; Barbieri *et al.*, 1977) and atrophy of endometriosis implants (Floyd 1980). The reduction in serum oestriol and progesterone levels was accompanied by epithelial thinning with glandular and stromal atrophy of endometriosis.

The next approach was that of 'medical oophorectomy' therapy using gonadotropin releasing hormone agonists. Meldrum *et al.* (1982) treated patients with long-acting gonadotropin releasing hormone analogs. The continuous stimulation caused 'down-regulation' with pituitary receptor desensitization. A hypogonadal state resulted in 2–6 weeks. Both the gonadotropin releasing hormone agonists and danazol were found to be quantitatively similar in efficacy but their side-effects differed (Meldrum *et al.*, 1983; Barbieri, 1988).

Another form of therapy in the early years was the use of methyltestosterone, a drug which was found useful for alleviating the pain associated with endometriosis. It did not however, appear to enhance fertility (Hamblen, 1957). Gossypol was an experimental drug mainly used in China, and early reports indicated that the drug relieved endometriotic pain (Han, 1980). The antioestrogen clomiphene citrate was also experimented with. Many investigators combined medical and surgical treatments.

Luteinized unruptured follicle syndrome

Indirect evidence suggested that there was an association between endometriosis and luteinized unruptured follicle syndrome. Stein and Leventhal (1935) first suggested follicle rupture with oocyte entrapment beneath the ovarian cortex (Edes and Coulam, 1988). Jewelewicz (1975) introduced the term 'luteinized unruptured follicle' when he proposed that luteinization of the ovarian stroma and follicles occurred in some instances secondary to the use of clomiphene citrate. The luteinized unruptured follicles were then said to secrete progesterone, causing progestational change without ovulation. Koninckx et al. (1978a,b) demonstrated luteinized unruptured follicle syndrome at laparoscopy. Marik and Hulka (1978) independently presented similar evidence and Coulam et al. (1982) diagnosed the condition at ultrasound examination.

ADENOMYOSIS

Morbid anatomists were aware of this condition for some time, but it was Von Recklinghausen (1896) who brought it to popular attention. In his treatise on the subject, he suggested that adenomyosis arose in mesonephric (Wolffian) remnants. Subsequent workers disagreed with his theory which was later abandoned. Cullen (1897) of America, developed an interest in the topic and later reported his examination of 50 specimens of diffuse adenomyosis of the uterus (Cullen, 1908). He demonstrated that adenomyosis was produced by a downward extension of endometrium into the myometrium. Doran and Lockyer (1908) recorded a rare condition which they called 'peri-endothelioma' or stromal endometriosis. Subsequent workers documented the occurrence of adenomyosis in uterine malformations (Frankl, 1912); the development of tuberculosis in adenomyosis (Stewart and Oldfield, 1932); decidual reaction of the tissue in pregnancy (Sandberg and Cohn, 1962); and response to synthetic progestogens (Molitor, 1971). Atypical hyperplasia and adenocarcinoma of adenomyotic tissue were rarely found.

FIBROIDS

The fibroid, otherwise termed fibromyoma or leiomyoma, is a benign tumour of muscle origin. Fibroids were recognized by the ancients, but they were unaware of their origins. The term 'mole' was applied to both fibroids and cancer. Examination of Egyptian mummy remains has revealed some instances of calcified fibroids. Hippocrates called them 'womb stones' and Galen described them in the second century AD as 'scleroma'. The term 'fibroid' was introduced by J.M. Klob (1863) and Carl Von Rokitansky (1860). Virchow demonstrated their derivation from smooth muscle and introduced the designation 'myoma'. Th. Billroth suggested the name myofibromata while Mallory introduced the term leiomyoma. The distinction between cancer and fibroids was finally made in 1844 by Samuel Ashwell and by James H. Bennett of London in 1845. During operations for ovarian cysts, large fibroid masses were frequently found. At least two of Ephraim McDowell's cases were fibroid growths rather than ovarian cysts (Ricci, 1945; Graham, 1950).

In the early part of this century, Kelly and Cullen (1909) and Lockyer (1918) observed that the tumours were more common in Negroes, and were rare before the age of 20 years. Lockyer opined that fibroids were a familial condition. Mahfouz and Magdi (1941) presented a series of almost 1000 cases of fibromyomas and reviewed the historical aspects of the tumour. Lipschutz (1942) injected guinea-pigs with oestrogens, and produced peritoneal, but not uterine, fibromyomas. Steiner (1939) recorded an unusual case of metastasizing fibroleiomyoma and Novak (1952) documented the recurrence of fibroids postmyomectomy.

The first completed supravaginal hysterectomy for fibroids was performed in 1845 by A.M. Heath of Manchester (Ricci, 1945). Charles Clay, also of Manchester, performed the second such operation soon afterwards. Both patients died. Walther Burnham (Massachusetts) was the first to successfully remove a fibroid uterus in 1853. The first successful myomectomy was performed in 1844 by Washington L. Atlee of America (1853). Charles D. Meigs in 1848, and James Young Simpson in 1863, both rejected the possibility of a surgical approach to fibroids.

Electrical treatment of fibroids was popularized by Ciniselli of Cremona in 1869, and this form of therapy was used until the end of the nineteenth century. Various medications were ingested or applied, including potassium bromide or potassium iodide taken by mouth or administered by vaginal pessary. However, Marion Sims documented in 1866 that he had never seen any effect from medication on such tumours (Graham, 1950). Goodman (1946) used progesterone therapy to control the growth of fibromyomas. Later attempts using luteinizing hormone releasing hormone analogues proved more successful.

HYDATIDIFORM MOLE

Both Hippocrates and Aetius of Amida described molar pregnancy. Oribasius (c. AD 325–403) recounted a case in which the uterus became enlarged but the woman went on to deliver a fleshy mass. Expulsion of a mole weighing 12 lb (5.45 kg) was documented by Christopher de Vigo in 1564. During the sixteenth century the condition was again reported by Francois Valleriola but it was Nikolaas Tulpius (1593–1674) of Amsterdam who gave the first accurate description. In 1664 Mauriceau removed a mole by digital manipulation. In 1690 Marcello Malpighi (1628–1694) deduced that hydatidiform mole developed from placental tissue (Figure 1). The aetiology of hydatidiform mole was eventually clinched in the nineteenth century by Virchow. Chorioepithelioma was first reported by F.I. Meckel in 1795 and Max Sanger in 1888 presented to the Gynaecological Society of Leipzig a case of a very malignant sarcoma-like growth which occurred after an 8-week miscarriage.

CHRONOLOGY

Endometriosis

1860	Carl Von Rokitansky first described this condition.
1921	Sampson coined the term 'endometriosis'.
1922	Blair Bell introduced the term 'endometrioma'.
1973	Acosta *et al.* produced a classification of the disorder.
1979	The American Fertility Society proposed their classification.

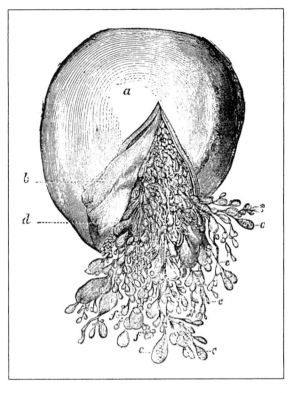

Figure 1 Hydatidiform mole. Uterus opened to reveal the grape-like structure of the mole: (a) uterus; (b) incised muscle wall; (c) a hydatidiform vesicle; (d) general mass from a tumour from an early twentieth century French publication. From Schaeffer-Bouglé, *Atlas-Manuel de Gynécologie*, Paris (1903)

1942	Gruenwald favoured its derivation from the primitive coelom.
1955	McVeigh suggested transformation of corona radiata cells.

Theories of origin

1885	Von Recklinghausen suggested a Wolffian origin.
1896	Cullen favoured Müllerian origin.
1898	Iwanhoff advocated the theory of serosal metaplasia.
1922	Sampson developed the theory of retrograde menstruation.
1924	Halban proposed endolymphatic spread.
1925	Sampson presented a theory of haematogenous dissemination.
1936	Navrital and Kramer evolved the vascular embolization theory.

Treatment

1925	Fraser suggested bilateral oophorectomy.
1948	Karnaky pioneered stilboestrol therapy.
1957	Hamblen used methyltestosterone.
1958	Kistner introduced pseudopregnancy therapy.
1971	Greenblatt *et al.* advocated pseudomenopause therapy with danazol.
1980	Han experimented with gossypol.
1982	Meldrum *et al.* used gonadotropin releasing hormone analogs to achieve medical oophorectomy.

ADENOMYOSIS

1896	Von Recklinghausen brought this previously diagnosed condition to popular attention.
1908	Cullen determined that adenomyosis was a downward extension of endometrium which involved the myometrium.
	Doran and Lockyer recorded stromal endometriosis.

FIBROIDS

2000 BC	Calcified fibroids were discovered in mummies from this era.
c.400 BC	Hippocrates termed them 'womb stones'.
c. AD 170	Galen used the term 'scleroma'.
1844	Ashwell distinguished between fibroids and cancer (Ricci, 1945).
	Atlee introduced myomectomy (Cianfrani, 1960).
1845	Heath first operated on fibroids (Cianfrani, 1960).
1853	Burnham performed a hysterectomy for fibroids (Graham, 1950).
1909	Kelly and Cullen determined that fibroids were more common in Negroes.
1941	Mahfouz and Magdi reviewed 1000 cases.
1946	Bonney described details of how to perform myomectomy.

HYDATIDIFORM MOLE

c.400 BC	Hippocrates described hydatidiform mole.
17th C.	Tulpius first accurately described the condition.
1690	Malpighi discovered its placental origin (Ricci, 1945).
19th C.	Virchow, among others, determined its aetiology.

REFERENCES

Acosta, A.A., Buttram, V.C., Jr., Besch, P.K., Malinak, L.R., Franklin, R.R. and Vanderheyden, J.D. (1973). A proposed classification of endometriosis. *Obstet. Gynecol.*, **42**, 19–25

American Fertility Society (1979). Classification of endometriosis. *Fertil. Steril.*, **32**, 633–4

Andrews, M.C., Andrews, W.C. and Strauss, A.F. (1959). Effects of progestin-induced pseudopregnancy on endometriosis: clinical and microscopic studies. *Am. J. Obstet. Gynecol.*, **78**, 776

Atlee, W.L. (1853). *The Surgical Treatment of Certain Fibrous Tumours of the Uterus.* (Philadelphia: Collins)

Barbieri, R.L. (1988). New therapy for endometriosis. *N. Engl. J. Med.*, **318**, 512

Barbieri, R.L., Canick, J.A., Makris, A., Todd, R.B., Davies, I.J. and Ryan, K.J. (1977). Danazol inhibits steroidogenesis. *Fertil. Steril.*, **28**, 809–13

Bell, W.B. (1922). Endometrioma and endometriomyoma of the ovary. *J. Obstet. Gynaecol. Br. Emp.*, **29**, 443

Bonney, V. (1946). *The Technical Minutiae of Extended Myomectomy and Ovarian Cystectomy.* (London: Cassell)

Buttram, V.C., Jr. (1978). An expanded classification of endometriosis. *Fertil. Steril.*, **30**, 240–2

Cianfrani, T. (1960). *A Short History of Obstetrics and Gynecology*, pp. 345; 391. (Springfield, Illinois: Charles C. Thomas)

Coulam, C.B., Hill, L.M. and Breckle, R. (1982). Ultrasonic evidence for luteinization of unruptured preovulatory follicles. *Fertil. Steril.*, **37**, 524

Cullen, T.S. (1896). Adenomyoma of the round ligament. *Johns Hopkins Hosp. Bull.*, **7**, 112–13

Cullen, T.S. (1897). Adeno-myoma uteri diffusum benignum. *Johns Hopkins Hosp. Rep.*, **6**, 133

Cullen, T.S. (1908). *Adenomyoma of Uterus.* (Philadelphia: Saunders)

Doran, A.H.G. and Lockyer, C. (1908). Two cases of uterine fibroids showing peritheliomatous changes: long immunity from recurrence after operation. *Proc. R. Soc. Med.*, **2**, *Obstet. Gynaecol. Section*, 25

Edes, E.E. and Coulam, C.B. (1988). Relationship between the luteinized unruptured follicle syndrome and endometriosis. In Speroff, L. (ed.) *Seminars in Reproductive Endocrinology, Pathophysiology of the Infertility Associated with Endometriosis*, pp. 273–7. (New York: Thieme Medical Publishers Inc.)

Floyd, W.S. (1980). Danazol: endocrine and endometrial effects. *Int. J. Fertil.*, **25**, 75

Frankl, O. (1912), quoted by Lockyer (1918)

Fraser, J.R. (1925). Progress in gynecology in the last twenty years. *Surg. Gynecol. Obstet. Int. Abst. Surg.*, **40**, 452

Goodman, A.L. (1946). Progesterone therapy in uterine fibromyoma. *J. Clin. Endocrinol.*, **6**, 402

Graham, H. (1950). *Eternal Eve*, p. 523. (London: W. Heinemann)

Greenblatt, R.B., Dmowski, L.P., Mahesh, U. and Scholer, H.F.C. (1971). Clinical studies with an anti-gonadotrophin – danazol. *Fertil. Steril.*, **22**, 102–13

Gruenwald, P. (1942). Origin of endometriosis from the mesenchyme of the celomic walls. *Am. J. Obstet. Gynecol.*, **44**, 470

Guillebaud, J., Fraser, I.S., Thorburn, G.D. and Jenken, G. (1977). Endocrine effects of danazol in menstruating women. *J. Int. Med. Res.*, **5**, (Suppl. 3), 57

Haines, M. and Taylor, C.W. (1962). *Gynaecological Pathology*, p. 503. (London: J. and A. Churchill Ltd.)

Halban, J. (1924). Hysteroadenosis metastatic. *Wien. Klin. Wchnschr.*, **37**, 1205

Halban, J. (1925). Hysteroadenosis metastatica. Die lymphogere Genese der sog. Adenofibromatosis heterotopica. *Arch. Gynaekol.*, **124**, 457

Hamblen, E.C. (1957). Androgen treatment of women. *South. Med. J.*, **50**, 743

Hammond, C.B., Rock, J.A. and Parker, R.T. (1976). Conservative treatment of endometriosis: the effects of limited surgery and hormonal pseudopregnancy. *Fertil. Steril.*, **27**, 756

Han, M. (1980). Preliminary results of the gossypol treatment in the menopausal functional uterine bleeding, myoma, and endometriosis. *Acta Med. Chin. Acad. Med. Sci.*, **2**, 167

Henriksen, E. (1955). Endometriosis. *Am. J. Surg.*, **90**, 331

Hertig, A.T. and Sommers, S.C. (1949). Genesis of endometrial carcinoma. Study of prior biopsies. *Cancer*, **2**, 946 and 964–71

Iwanhoff, N.S. (1898). *Monatts. Geburtsch. Gynakol.*, **7**, 195

Javert, C.T. (1949). Pathogenesis of endometriosis based on endometrial homeoplasia direct extension, exfoliation and implantation, lymphomatic and hematogenous metastasis. *Cancer*, **2**, 399

Javert, C.T. (1952). The spread of benign and malignant endometrium in the lymphatic system with a note of coexisting vascular involvement. *Am. J. Obstet. Gynecol.*, **64**, 780

Jewelewicz, R. (1975). Management of infertility resulting from anovulation. *Am. J. Obstet. Gynecol.*, **122**, 909–20

Karnaky, K.J. (1948). The use of stilbestrol for endometriosis. *South. Med. J.*, **41**, 1109

Kelly, H.A. and Cullen, T.S. (1909). *Myomata of the Uterus.* (Philadelphia: Saunders)

Kistner, R.W. (1958). The use of newer progestins in the treatment of endometriosis. *Am. J. Obstet. Gynecol.*, **75**, 264–78

Kistner, R.W., Siegel, A.M. and Behrman, S.J. (1977). Suggested classification for endometriosis and relationship to infertility. *Fertil. Steril.*, **78**, 1008–10

Klob, J.M. (1863). Myoma. *Wchblt. d. Zeit d K. K. gesellsh. d. Aerzte v. Wien*, **XVIII**, 292

Koninckx, P.R., Brosens, I.A. and Corvelyn, P.A. (1978a). A study of plasma progesterone, oestradiol-17B, prolactin and LH levels and of the luteal phase appearance of the ovaries in patients with endometriosis and infertility. *Br. J. Obstet. Gynaecol.*, **85**, 246

Koninckx, P.R., Heyns, W.J., Corvelyn, P.A. and Brosens, I.A. (1978b). Delayed onset of luteinization as a cause of infertility. *Fertil. Steril.*, **29**, 266

Lipschutz, A. (1942). Experimental fibroids and the antifibromatogenic action of steroid hormones. *J. Am. Med. Assoc.*, **120**, 171

Lockyer, C. (1918). *Fibroids and Allied Tumours.* (London: MacMillan & Co.)

McVeigh, J.S. (1955). An origin of endometriosis theory based on histological morphology. *New Zealand Med. J.*, **54**, 346–9

Mahfouz, N.P. and Magdi, I. (1941). Fibroid tumours of the uterus. *J. Obstet. Gynaecol. Br. Emp.*, **48**, 293

Marik, J. and Hulka, J. (1978). Luteinized unruptured follicle syndrome: a subtle cause of infertility. *Fertil. Steril.*, **29**, 270

Meldrum, D.R., Change, R.J., Lu, J., Vale, W., Rivier, J. and Judd, H.L. (1982). Medical oophorectomy using a long acting GnRH agonist – a possible new approach to the treatment of endometriosis. *J. Clin. Endocrin. Metab.*, **54**, 1081–3

Meldrum, D.R., Pardridge, W.M., Kadow, W.G., Rivier, J., Vale, W. and Judd, H.L. (1983). Hormonal effects of danazol and medical oophorectomy in endometriosis. *Obstet. Gynecol.*, **62**, 480–5

Meyer, R. (1903). Ueber eine Adenomatose. Wuchurng der serosa in einer Bauchnabe. *Z. Geburts. Gynäkol.*, **49**, 32–45

Meyer, R. (1930). *Handbuch der speziellen pathologischen Anatomie und Histologie.* Bd 1 Wiebliche geschlectsorgane Bearbeitet von Frank, I., Kaufmann, Meyer, R. *et al.* Teil 1 uterus und tuben, p. 806.

Molitor, J.J. (1971). Adenomyosis: a clinical and pathologic appraisal. *Am. J. Obstet. Gynecol.*, **110**, 275

Navrital, E. and Kramer, A. (1936). Endometriose in der Armmuskulatur. *Klin. Wchnschr.*, **15**, 1765–70

Novak, E. (1952) Quoted by Haines, M. and Taylor, C.W. (1975). *Gynaecological Pathology*, p. 285. (Edinburgh London New York: Churchill Livingstone)

Ricci, J.V. (1945). *One Hundred Years of Gynecology 1800–1900*, pp. 110; 157; 163; 491. (Philadelphia: The Blakiston Co.)

Russell, W.W. (1899). Aberrant portions of the Mullerian duct found in an ovary. *Johns Hopkins Hosp. Bull.*, **10**, 8

Sampson, J.A. (1921). Perforating hemorrhagic (chocolate) cysts of the ovary. *Arch. Surg.*, **3**, 245

Sampson, J.A. (1922). The life history of ovarian haematomas (haemorrhagic cysts) of endometrial (Mullerian) type. *Am. J. Obstet. Gynecol.*, **4**, 451–6

Sampson, J.A. (1925a). Endometrial carcinoma of the ovary arising in endometrial tissue in that organ. *Arch. Surg.*, **10**, 15

Sampson, J.A. (1925b). Heterotopic or misplaced endometrial tissue. *Am. J. Obstet. Gynecol.*, **10**, 649

Sandberg, E.C. and Cohn, F. (1962). Adenomyosis in the gravid uterus at term. *Am. J. Obstet. Gynecol.*, **84**, 1457

Seppala, M. (1985). The World Collaborative Report on *in vitro* fertilization and embryo replacement: current state of the art in January 1984. In Seppala, M. and Edwards, R.G. (eds.) *In Vitro Fertilization and Embryo Transfer, Ann. N.Y. Acad. Sci.*, **442**, 558

Stein, I.F. and Leventhal, M.L. (1935). Amenorrhoea associated with bilateral polycystic ovaries. *Am. J. Obstet. Gynecol.*, **29**, 181–91

Steiner, P.E. (1939). Metastasizing fibroleiomyoma of the uterus. *Am. J. Pathol.*, **15**, 89

Stewart, M.J. (1935). Endometriosis and adenomyoma. In Teacher, J.H. (ed.) *A Manual of Obstetrical and Gynaecological Pathology*, pp. 229–58. (London: Oxford University Press)

Stewart, M.J. and Oldfield, C. (1932). Endometriosis uteri diffusa with secondary tuberculous infection. *J. Obstet. Gynaecol. Brit. Emp.*, **39**, 759

Von Recklinghausen, F. (1885). Veber die venose embolic und den regrograden transport in den venen und in den lymphgefassen. *Virchows Archives (Pathology: Anatomy)*, **100**, 503

Von Recklinghausen, F. (1896). *Die Adenomyome und Cystadenoma der Uterus und Tubenwandung.* (Berlin: Hirschwald)

Von Rokitansky, C. (1860). Ueber Uterusdrusen-Neubildung in Uterus and Ovarialsarcomen. *Zkk. Gesellsch. d. Aerzte zu Wien*, **37**, 577

FURTHER READING

Cattel, R.B. and Swinton, N.W. (1936). Endometriosis with particular reference to conservative treatment. *N. Engl. J. Med.*, **241**, 341

Cianfrani, T. (1960). *A Short History of Obstetrics and Gynecology.* (Springfield, Illinois: Charles C. Thomas)

Graham, H. (1950). *Eternal Eve.* (London: W. Heinemann)

Haines, M. and Taylor, C.W. (1975). *Gynaecological Pathology*, 2nd edn. (Edinburgh, London, New York: Churchill Livingstone)

Haydon, G.B. (1942). A study of 569 cases of endometriosis. *Am. J. Obstet. Gynecol.*, **43**, 704

Hurst, B.S. and Rock, J.A. (1989). Endometriosis: pathophysiology, diagnosis and treatment. In Taylor, E.S. (ed.) *Obstetrical and Gynecological Survey*, pp. 297–304. (Baltimore: Williams & Wilkins)

O'Connor, D.T. (1987). Endometriosis. In Singer, A. and Jordan, J. (eds.) *Current Reviews in Obstetrics and Gynaecology*, 12. (Edinburgh, London, Melbourne, New York: Churchill Livingstone)

Olive, D.L. and Haney, A.F. (1986). Endometriosis: a critical review of therapeutic approaches. In Taylor, E.S. (ed.) *Obstetrical and Gynecological Survey*, pp. 538–55. (Baltimore: Williams & Wilkins)

Speroff, L. (1988). *Seminars in Reproductive Endocrinology*, Vol. 6, No. 3. (New York, Stuttgart: Thieme Medical Publishers)

Von Rokitansky, C. (1842–46). *Handbuch der pathologischen Anatomie*, 3 Vols. (Vienna: Braumuller)

Cancer

INTRODUCTION

The word cancer is derived from the Greek term for crab. Its first description was based on breast cancer where the exterior surface was compared to the crab's shell, and swollen veins were likened to the legs. The pain of the condition resembled sharp claws penetrating the body.

Evidence of a cancer process dates to the dinosaurs in the cretaceous age. The oldest example of malignant tumour in man is found in the Kanam mandibular fragment from East Africa. The bony remnant, dated as between 500 000 and 2 million years old, was discovered in Kenya by Leakey in 1932, and contains remnants of a tumour which is thought to resemble a (Burkitt's) lymphoma (Stathopoulos, 1975). Traces of cancer were discovered in Egyptian mummies from the third to the fifth dynasties c. 3000–2500 BC. Granville (1826) dissected mummified remains and discovered a diseased right ovary later thought to be a malignant cystadenocarcinoma. The Edwin Smith papyrus c.1700 BC (Figure 1) described eight cases of breast tumour or ulcer (Raven, 1990) and the Ebers Papyrus c.1550 BC documented a tumour which was probably a Kaposi's sarcoma, a neoplastic entity known to be endemic in the Nile region.

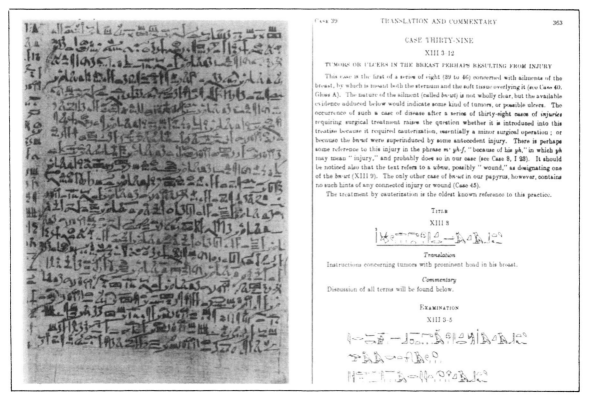

Figure 1   An extract from the Edwin Smith surgical Papyrus and the English translation of case 39

Hippocrates of Cos described a variety of cancer conditions which were cauterized or excised when accessible. Based on their concept of humoral physiology the Greeks believed that cancer was caused by an accumulation of black bile, the melancholic humour. Galen of Pergamus, a physician who worked in Rome during the second century AD, further popularized the humoral theory. According to that doctrine, a flux of black bile mixed with blood was said to produce a scirrhous form of precancer, while black bile alone could produce cancer directly. This humoral theory of disease was to last for almost 1500 years.

Rectal and stomach cancers were described in the fourteenth and fifteenth centuries and Giovanni Filippo Ingrassi published a list of various tumours in 1553. The first book which argued against the humoral doctrine on cancer formation was written by Deshaies Gendron and was published in 1700. In the eighteenth century cancer was considered an unfavourable outcome of inflammation. John Hunter formulated the concept of 'coagulating lymph' (the constituents of blood clot) which he believed was the basis of diseased tissue. Hunter's 'coagulable lymph' was later known as 'blastema' in the early 19th century.

In 1800 the French anatomist Marie Francois Xavier Bichat declared that tumours were due to an overgrowth of cellular tissue. By the 1830s, Mathias Schleiden and Theodor Schwann produced evidence which showed that animal tissues were formed from basic cell units. Johannes Muller of Germany, and also Carl Von Rokitansky and Rudolph Virchow, further developed the cell theory and its relationship to the cancer process.

Wilhelm Waldeyer formulated an approach to cancer in 1867 which is not unlike present concepts. Waldeyer asserted that cancer cells developed from previously normal cells and spread into adjacent tissues. Metastases resulted from carriage of cancerous elements by blood, lymph, or other fluid, to distant sites. Before the twentieth century, cancer was thought to be more common in the female, probably due to its ready diagnosis as breast tumours. Studies in the present century have confirmed that cancer is more common in males. Cancers were reported most commonly in the 40–65-year age group, and were thought to be due in part to declining effectiveness of the immunological system with advancing age.

Carcinogens, chemical or other agents which induced a cancer process, were identified with certainty in the eighteenth century when soot was found to be responsible for the high incidence of scrotal cancer in chimney sweeps (Pott, 1775). Other carcinogenic agents were soon identified. Industrial oils, tars, aniline dyes, radiation exposure, cigarette smoking, nutritional deficiency, alcohol abuse and a large number of other substances were inculpated.

While treatment of cancer was attempted in some cases, effective therapy only evolved in this century. The first cancer institution was built in 1740 at Rheims in France, and some 50 years later a cancer ward was set up at the Middlesex Hospital, London. Various cancer institutes were set up in Europe in the early 1900s (McGrew, 1985).

CHRONOLOGY

The oldest known tumour in man, is contained in the Kanam mandible and dates back 2 million years (Stathopoulos, 1986).

3000 BC	Mummified remains contained a malignant cystadenocarcinoma.
1700 BC	The Edwin Smith papyrus described breast cancer.
c.350 BC	Hippocrates described cancer.
c. AD 170	Galen developed the humoral theory of cancer causation.
1553	Giovanni Ingrassi published a list of tumours.
1700	Deshaies Gendron wrote on cancer.
1775	Percival Potts implicated soot in the causation of scrotal cancer.
1800	Bichat proposed that tumours were overgrowth of cellular tissue.
1830s	Schleiden and Schwann developed the cellular theory of cancer. Further contributions were made by Muller, Von Rokitansky, and Virchow.
1867	Waldeyer concluded that cancer cells developed from previously normal tissue.

REFERENCES

Graham, H. (1950). *Eternal Eve*, p. 54. (London: Heinemann)

Granville (1826), quoted by Ghalioungui, P. (1986) Malignancy in ancient Egypt. In Retsas, S. (ed.) *Palaeo-oncology. The Antiquity of Cancer, from Hippocrates to Galen*, p. 31. (London: Farrand Press)

McGrew, R. (1985). *Encyclopedia of Medical History*, pp. 46–51. (London: MacMillan Press)

Pott, P. (1775). *Chirurgical Observations Relative to the Cataract, the Polypus of the Nose, the Cancer of the Scrotum etc.*, pp. 705–37. (London: Hawes, Clarke and Collins)

Raven, R.W. (1990). *The Theory and Practice of Oncology Historical Evolution and Present Principles*, pp. 1–17. (Carnforth: Parthenon Publishing Group)

Stathopoulos, G.P. (1975). Kanam mandible's tumour. *Lancet*, 1, 165

Stathopoulos, G.P. (1986). Bone tumours in antiquity. In Retsas, S. (ed.) *Palaeo-oncology. The Antiquity of Cancer; from Hippocrates to Galen*, pp. 41–53. (London: Farrand Press)

Cancer of the vulva

INTRODUCTION

The condition of vulval cancer was described by Morgagni (1769) in his *The Seats and Causes of Diseases Investigated by Anatomy,* and he reported that 'in regard to the (cancer of) genital parts of women I have seen many of them, but as yet I have never had any opportunity of dissecting them . . .'. Vulval cancer was redescribed in the nineteenth century, but mainly as single case reports. All of our present knowledge of the epidemiology, surgery, pathology and outcome of the disease, has evolved in the present century.

The first major study on cancer of the vulva was described by Rothschild (1912). However, it was Basset (1912) (Figure 1) who first drew attention to many facets of the disease, and evolved what could be called the modern treatment of it. Although he was of the opinion that the cancer began as a primary epithelioma of the clitoris, this was eventually found not to be a common form of the disease. Basset distinguished between benign and malignant disease; demonstrated the importance of the lymphatic drainage; and developed an operative technique which was the basis of modern radical vulvectomy. In his graduation thesis, Basset described 147 cases of vulval cancer – no mean feat when one considers the low frequency of the condition.

Taussig of St Louis (1941) (Figure 2) adopted the Basset operative procedure and reported a 5-year survival rate of 52.6%, when the inguinal, but not the pelvic nodes were involved. It was Taussig who popularized vulval surgery in the English-speaking world.

AETIOLOGY

A number of agents were found to have a role in the development of the disease. Stacey (1939) implicated the accidental application of toxic sub-

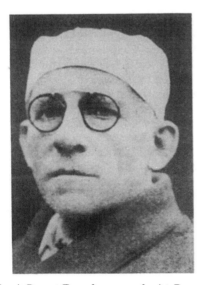

Figure 1   A. Basset, French gynaecologist. Reproduced with kind permission from Way, S. (1982). *Malignant Disease of the Vulva,* opposite the title page. (New York: Churchill Livingstone)

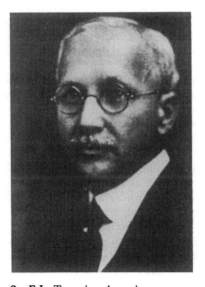

Figure 2   F.J. Taussig, American gynaecologist. Reproduced with kind permission from Way, S. (1982). *Malignant Disease of the Vulva,* opposite the title page. (New York: Churchill Livingstone)

stances to the vulva. The disease was found to be common in the cotton spinning areas and dye works where employees were at high risk due to soilage of clothing with bituminous oils and dyes. Young women in the tobacco plantations of North America developed the disease secondary to contamination with arsenic-based sprays. Dermatologists, who frequently prescribed arsenical compounds for pruritus vulvae during the 1930s, induced iatrogenic neoplasia (Way, 1982). Cancer of the vulva was also found in young women who were known to suffer from granuloma inguinale or lymphogranuloma venereum (Hay and Cole, 1961). Lack of vulval hygiene was also implicated.

Leukoplakia (Greek, white plaques) was found to be a premalignant condition and Berkeley and Bonney (1909) published the original studies on this disease. Four stages were described, the first of which was reddening of the vulval skin. This was followed by fissuring, the development of hyperkeratotic white plaques and eventually the skin became thin and atrophic. Cancer was found to develop from either stage 3 or 4. Taussig (1940) recorded that the condition was present in almost 70% of 155 cases analysed between the years 1911 and 1940. Dickens and Weihl-Malherbe (1943) demonstrated that the metabolic rate of leukoplakic skin was intermediate between normal skin and that which was affected by cancer. Berkeley and Bonney (1909) determined that carcinoma of the vulva spread locally, and then by the lymphatics. Way (1948) described the pathological anatomy of lymphatic metastases and in a further communication (1951) emphasized that apparently unenlarged nodes could contain metastatic tumour.

Preinvasive carcinoma was described as a skin lesion of red appearance which gave rise to severe irritation. The condition is eponymously related to Paget (1874) and also to Queyrat (1911) and Bowen (1912) who each described a precancerous atypical epithelial state. Paget's disease of the vulva was documented by Dubreuilh (1901). The disease was rare, and was later found to have an incidence of just under 2% of vulval carcinomas. The terms 'intraepidermal carcinoma' or 'Bowen's disease' were commonly used but were replaced by carcinoma in situ. A new classification, that of vulvar intraepithelial neoplasia, was introduced at the 7th International Congress of the International Society for the Study of Vulvar Disease in 1983. The condition was further subdivided into a 'squamous type' (with or without koilocytosis), and graded from 1 to 3 depending on severity,

and a 'non-squamous' type was further subdivided into Paget's disease and/or melanoma in situ.

Various forms of treatment, including diathermy, vulvectomy, application of cytotoxics, and laser destruction techniques, were described. The majority of women who contracted the disease were in the 61–80-year age group, were parous, and mainly from social classes 3–5. The majority presented with a lump or ulcer which was preceded by pruritus.

The concept of microcarcinoma, or microinvasive carcinoma, was introduced by Mestwerdt (1947) to describe the smallest invasive carcinoma of the cervix. Wharton et al. (1974) used the term microinvasive carcinoma in relation to the vulva, which was defined as a lesion or lesions, whose depth of stromal invasion did not exceed 5 mm when measured from the basal layer of adjacent epithelium. Of patients with microinvasive disease, 10% were found to have lymph node metastases, although a higher figure was quoted by some authors.

TYPES

Various methods of classification were used, including that of Broders (1925). With the formation of the International Federation of Gynaecology and Obstetrics (FIGO), recommendations were laid down for pathological and clinical staging of gynaecological cancers. The last update came from their meeting in Rio de Janeiro in October 1988.

Another type of vulval cancer was the verrucous carcinoma, a variant of epidermoid carcinoma, first described by Ackerman (1948). Other forms included the basal cell carcinoma, adenoid squamous cell carcinoma of the vulva, and primary adenocarcinoma. Willis defined basal cell carcinomas as those of superficial origin, e.g. rodent ulcer, and those basal cell growths of subepidermal origin (Willis, 1953). Siegler and Greene (1951) reviewed the literature and traced 65 cases. It was later determined that the basal cell carcinomas accounted for 6% of primary carcinomas of the vulva. Sarcoma of the vulva was very rare and Bell (1907) reported one of the first known cases of the condition. Clayton (1946) reviewed the literature and found fewer than 100 reports of vulval malignant melanoma.

The hiradenoma, a rare form of benign tumour of the vulva, was first described by Pick in 1904 (Novak, 1947). The tumour developed from vulvar sweat glands, and was a lesion which could readily be mistaken for adenocarcinoma. Among the various benign ulcerations of the vulva was that first described by Lipschutz in 1895 (Lipschutz, 1927) which was found to be readily amenable to antiseptic treatment. Willis (1934) documented six cases of 'kissing ulcers' with evidence of lymphatic drainage from one to the other. Way (1951) disputed the concept of kissing ulcers being due to lymphatic permeation, but asserted that they were really multiple primaries and not implant tumours.

Secondary tumours of the vulva were uncommon, but chorionepithelioma, or secondaries from cervical carcinoma, cancer of the large bowel, bladder carcinomas, and sarcoma from a primary in a fibroid uterus, were all documented.

SPREAD

Cancer of the vulva spreads by local extension, or by lymphatic involvement. The lymphatics drain to the superficial inguinal nodes, which in turn drain to the external iliac group. The frequency of lymph node involvement was reviewed by Cahen (1933). Clinical assessment of the lymph nodes showed poor correlation with histological diagnosis (Plentl and Friedman, 1971; Way and Benedet, 1973). There was little evidence of remote metastases, even in cases which showed evidence of local recurrence. The predominant histological lesion was of a squamous carcinoma although melanomas, sarcomas and adenocarcinomas of Bartholin's duct were reported.

Stanley Way of Newcastle (1951) documented his experience of the disease and described it as 'a . . . slowly growing tumour . . . its tendency to develop in known premalignant lesions which themselves have a striking symptomatology, makes it exceptional among genital tract tumours . . . its local progress, in many cases, is very slow, yet despite this a high incidence of lymph node involvement is encountered . . . they tend to remain localized to the groin and external iliac group (often in the groin alone) for a very long time . . . these facts explain why cancer of the vulva can be cured'.

TREATMENT

The best form of treatment for vulval cancer is radical vulvectomy, with superficial and deep node dissection. Operators of note who published their findings include Basset, Taussig, Stanley Way, Macafee, Kelly, Green, Collins, Parry-Jones and Amreich (Way, 1982; Parry-Jones, 1976). Until the 1950s radiotherapy was advocated but results were poor and radiation necrosis was a major problem. Results of surgery are good, with two-thirds of the patients being long-term survivors. Of the third who died the majority did so within the 1st year. The risk of dying after 3 years had elapsed was found to be very low.

To be effective, surgery had to be extremely radical with wide removal of the vulva as well as the inguinal and deep nodes. Basset (1912) advocated the surgical approach. Kehrer (1912) and Stoeckel (1930) combined vulval excision with removal of some lymphatic glands. Way (1949) stressed that previous failures were due to limited removal of the vulva, incomplete removal of superficial nodes and failure to remove deep lymphatics.

In Basset's operation (1912) the vulva was first excised. Two weeks afterwards the inguinal, iliac and hypogastric glands were removed by an extraperitoneal approach. Kehrer (1912) devised a method of removing the iliac and hypogastric glands by an extraperitoneal approach. Stoeckel (1930) introduced the method of removal of the iliac and hypogastric glands at the time of complete vulvectomy, with bilateral excision of inguinal glands. Diathermy coagulation was advocated by Berven (1941; 1949) as an alternative to surgery but did not become popular.

COMPLICATIONS OF SURGERY

Wound sepsis was the most serious complication and McKelvey (1947) estimated that it occurred in 90% of his patients. Malpas (1947) advised leaving the wound open to encourage healing by first intention, but this technique and also that of immediate skin grafting were abandoned. Other complications included an operative mortality of almost 15%, haemorrhage and fluid loss, deep venous thrombosis, and at a later date lymphoedema, erysipelas, hernia, prolapse, and stenosis of the vagina. As the disease was relatively uncommon Professor F.J. Browne suggested in 1939 that cases should be referred to selected centres for surgery.

LYMPHATICS OF THE VULVA

The lymphatics of the vulva were first investigated by Sappey (1874) and documented thus: 'From the periphery of this profuse network a large number of trunks arise which take different directions. Those which come from the antero-superior part of the vulva travel more or less vertically before inclining to right or left in long arcs whose concavity is inferior. They terminate in the superior inguinal glands. The others go forward and outwards in the fold between the vulva and the thigh to terminate in one or two glands below the preceding ones. The trunks which arise from the posterior part of the vulval ring travel forwards on the inner aspect of the thigh immediately outside the labio-crural fold to end in the inferior inguinal glands. They are accompanied by the trunks which come from the perineum and the anal region and which terminate in the same group of glands'.

Parry-Jones (1959) reinvestigated the superficial lymphatics of the vulva and demonstrated that there was no lateral spread to the thigh. It was only those superficial lymphatics from the perineum which went to the groin. This was an important concept in planning a surgical procedure. Stanley Way based his incision on the work of Sappey and also Poirier (1903). Marshall (1953) made an abdominal incision higher than that of Stanley Way and also differed in that his medial incision went to the top of the thigh and not below it. The vulval incision was restricted to the vulval boundary.

CHRONOLOGY

General

1769   Morgagni described the condition.
1912   Rothschild and Basset independently drew attention to the disease.

Aetiology

1874   Paget described a red lesion which was preinvasive.
1901   Dubreuilh documented Paget's disease of the vulva.
1909   Berkeley and Bonney determined that leukoplakia was a premalignant condition.
1911   Queyrat described atypical epithelium of precancerous variety.
1912   Bowen described a precancer lesion.
1940   Taussig recorded vulval red lesions in 70% of cancer cases.
1947   Mestwerdt described microcarcinoma in relation to the cervix.

1974   Wharton *et al.* used the term 'microinvasive carcinoma' in relation to the vulva.
1983   The term 'vulvar intraepithelial neoplasia' was introduced.

Treatment

1912   Basset popularized vulvectomy.
      Kehrer combined vulvectomy with removal of lymphatics.
1925   Broders proposed a method of classification.
1930   Stoeckel removed iliac and hypogastric glands at vulvectomy.
1939   Browne suggested selected centres for performance of vulvectomy.
1947   Malpas advocated healing by first intention.
1951   Stanley Way documented his experience.

Lymphatics of the vulva

1874   Sappey first investigated the vulval lymph drainage.

REFERENCES

Ackerman, L.V. (1948). Verrucous carcinoma of the oral cavity. *Surgery*, **23**, 670–8

Basset, A. (1912). *L'epithelioma Primitif du Clitoris: Son retentissment ganglionaire et Son Traitment Operatoire*, no. 180. (Paris: G. Steinheil)

Bell, W.B. (1907). Sarcoma of the vulva including an account of a case of spindle-celled sarcoma of the labium minus. *J. Obstet. Gynaecol. Br. Emp.*, **12**, 275

Berkeley, C. and Bonney, V. (1909). Leucoplakic vulvitis and its relationship to kraurosis and carcinoma of the vulva. *Proc. R. Soc. Med.*, **3**, 29

Berven, E. (1941), quoted by Way (1951) pp. 1–49

Berven, E. (1949), quoted by Way (1951) pp. 1–49

Bowen, J.T. (1912). Precancerous dermatoses: a study of two cases of chronic atypical epithelial proliferation. *J. Cutan. Dis. Syphil.*, **30**, 241

Broders, A.C. (1925). The grading of carcinoma. *Minnesota Med.*, **8**, 726.

Browne, F.J. (1939), quoted by Way (1951) pp. 1–49

Cahen, J. (1933), quoted by Way (1951) pp. 1–49

Clayton, S.G. (1946). Melanoma of the vulva with pregnancy. *Proc. R. Soc. Med.*, **39**, 578

Dickens, F. and Weihl-Malherbe, H. (1943), quoted by Way (1951) pp. 1–49

Dubreuilh, W. (1901). Paget's disease of the vulva. *Br. J. Dermatol.*, **13**, 407–18

Hay, D.M. and Cole, F.M. (1961). Primary invasive carcinoma of the vulva in Jamaica. *J. Obstet. Gynaecol. Br. Cwlth.*, **76**, 821

Kehrer, E. (1912), quoted by Way (1951) pp. 1–49

Lipschutz, B. (1927). Ulcus Vulvae Acutum. *Jadassohns Handb. der Haut- und Geschlechtskrankheiten*, **21**, 392 (Berlin: Julius Springer)

McKelvey, J.L. (1947), quoted by Way (1951) pp. 1–49

Malpas, P. (1947), quoted by Way (1951) pp. 1–49

Marshall, C.M. (1953). The newer gynecology: some surgical and anatomical implications. *Am. J. Obstet. Gynecol.*, **65**, 773–88

Mestwerdt, G. (1947). Die Fruhdiagnose des Kollumkarzinoms. *Zbl. Gynakol.*, **69**, 198–202

Morgagni, J.B. (1769). *The Seats and Causes of Diseases Investigated by Anatomy*, Vol. 3, p. 70. (London: Millar Cadell Johnson and Payne)

Novak, E. (1947). *Gynecological and Obstetrical Pathology: With Clinical and Endocrine Relations*, 2nd Edn. (Philadelphia, London: W.B. Saunders Co)

Paget, J. (1874). On disease of the mammary areola preceding cancer of the mammary gland. *St Bartholomew's Hospital Reports*, **10**, 87

Parry-Jones, E. (1959). *Superficial Lymphoma of the Vulva*, p. 36 *et seq.* M.S. Thesis, University of London

Parry-Jones, E. (1976). The management of premalignant and malignant conditions of the vulva. In Langley, F.A. (ed.) *Clinics in Obstetrics and Gynaecology. Cancer of the Vulva, Vagina and Uterus*, Vol. 3 pp. 217–28. (London, Philadelphia, Toronto: W.B. Saunders Co.)

Pick, (1904), quoted by Novak (1947) p. 39

Plentl, A.A. and Friedman, E.A. (1971). *Lymphatic System of the Genitalia*, pp. 27. (Philadelphia: Saunders)

Poirier, P. (1903), quoted by Delamere, G., Poirier, P. and Cuneo, B. (1903). *The Lymphatics.* pp. 60–158. (London: Constable)

Queyrat, L. (1911). Erythrophasie du gland. *Bull. Soc. Franc. Dermatol. Syphil.*, **28**, 378

Rothschild, F. (1912). Inaugural dissertation. Freiburg, quoted by Taussig, F.J. (1931). *Diseases of the Vulva*, p. 142. (New York: Appleton and Co)

Sappey, C. (1874). *Traité d'Anatomie, Physiologie et Pathologie des Vaisseaux Lymphatiques, Considerés Chez l'Homme et les Vertebres*, p. 54. (Paris: Delahaye)

Siegler, A.M. and Greene, H.J. (1951). Basal-cell carcinoma of the vulva. *Am. J. Obstet. Gynecol.*, **62**, 1219

Stacey, J.E. (1939). Epithelioma of the vulva. *Proc. R. Soc. Med.*, **32**, 304

Stoeckel, W. (1930), quoted by Way (1951) pp. 1–49

Taussig, F.J. (1940). Cancer of the vulva: analysis of 155 cases 1911–40. *Am. J. Obstet. Gynaecol.*, **40**, 764

Taussig, F.J. (1941). Results in treatment of lymph node metastasis in cancer of the cervix and the vulva. *Am. J. Roentg.*, **45**, 813

Way, S. (1948). The anatomy of the lymphatic drainage of the vulva and its influence on the radical operation for carcinoma. *Ann. R. Coll. Surg. Engl.*, **3**, 187

Way, S. (1949), quoted by Way (1951) pp. 1–49

Way, S. (1951). *Malignant Disease of the Female Genital Tract.* (London: J. & A. Churchill)

Way, S. (1982). *Malignant Disease of the Vulva*, p. 4. (Edinburgh, London, Melbourne, New York: Churchill Livingstone)

Way, S. and Benedet, J.L. (1973). Involvement of the inguinal lymph nodes in carcinoma of the vulva: a comparison of clinical assessment with histological examination. *Gynecol. Oncol.*, **1**, 119

Wharton, J.T., Gallager, S. and Rutledge, F.N. (1974). Microinvasive carcinoma of the vulva. *Am. J. Obstet. Gynecol.*, **118**, 159

Willis, R.A. (1934). *The Spread of Tumours in the Human Body*, p. 26. (London: Churchill)

Willis, R.A. (1953). *Pathology of Tumours*, 2nd edn. (London: Butterworth)

FURTHER READING

Burghardt, E. (1984). Microinvasive carcinoma in gynaecological pathology. In Fox, H. (ed.) *Gynaecological Pathology: Advances, Perspectives and Problems: Clinics in Obstetrics and Gynaecology*, Vol. 11, no. 1 pp. 239–57. (London, Philadelphia, Toronto: W.B. Saunders Co.)

Fox, H. (ed.) (1984). *Gynaecological Pathology: Advances, Perspectives and Problems: Clinics in Obstetrics and Gynaecology*, Vol. 11, no. 1. (London, Philadelphia, Toronto: W.B. Saunders Co.)

Fox, H. (ed.) (1987). *Haines and Taylor Obstetrical and Gynaecological Pathology*, 3rd edn. Vol. 1. (Edinburgh, London, Melbourne, New York: Churchill Livingstone)

Haines, M. and Taylor, C.W. (1962). *Gynaecological Pathology*. (London: J. & A. Churchill Ltd.)

Novak, E. (1947). *Gynecological and Obstetrical Pathology: With Clinical and Endocrine Relations*, 2nd edn. (Philadelphia, London: W.B. Saunders Co.)

Way, S. (1951). *Malignant Disease of the Female Genital Tract*. (London: J.& A. Churchill Ltd.)

Way, S. (1982). *Malignant Disease of the Vulva*. (Edinburgh, London, Melbourne, New York: Churchill Livingstone)

Cancer of the vagina

Carcinoma of the vagina is uncommon, occurring in 1.6% of genital cancers and in any age group. There is a frequency of one vaginal for every 22 cervical, or every four vulval carcinomas. The commonest symptom is vaginal bleeding, when ulceration has taken place. The majority of vaginal cancers are of the squamous variety. Bonney and Glendinning described benign 'adenomatosis vaginae' in 1910 (Way, 1951), while primary adenocarcinoma of the vagina was described by Stanley Way in 1948 (Way, 1951). Secondary carcinomas in the vagina from choriocarcinoma, from other pelvic tumours and from distant sites are rarely recorded.

Carcinoma of the vagina was first described by Cruveilhier of Paris in 1827 (Ricci, 1945). Seventy years later, Roberts (1896) advised excision of small vaginal tumours but Stevens (1923) noted that such growths were difficult to treat and the results were poor. The issue was summed up by Taussig (1935) in these words 'we acknowledge our total inability to do anything effective for primary cancer of the vagina'. de Buben (1931) related a 5-year survival rate of 4% for patients with the condition who were treated with radium.

Herbst *et al.* (1971) described the association of vaginal adenocarcinoma in the offspring of mothers treated with diethylstilboestrol. A tumour registry of clear-cell adenocarcinoma was set up at Boston in 1971. Ulfelder (1973) noted some cases of adenocarcinoma in which there was no history of exposure to hormone therapy *in utero*. However, there was a large increase of adolescent vaginal adenocarcinomas in those who were exposed. Most of the cases reported thereafter were associated with diethylstilboestrol therapy. The drug was introduced into clinical practice in 1938.

Another possible mode of ingestion was through eating meat, as since 1954 over 75% of US cattle, and some poultry, had their feed supplemented with diethylstilboestrol in order to increase their weight. In the UK it was estimated that 7500 women were treated with diethylstilboestrol during their pregnancies in the years 1940–1971. Kinlen *et al.* (1974) reported a survey of obstetricians in the UK which failed to unearth a single case of carcinoma among the offspring of diethylstilboestrol-treated women.

The Department of Pathology in Birmingham (UK) analysed the reports of vaginal biopsy specimens for the years 1950–1975. Forty-seven primary malignant tumours of the vagina and 81 secondary tumours were recorded (Wade-Evans, 1976).

Sandberg *et al.* (1965) reviewed all the reports of vaginal adenosis from the first one documented in 1877 by von Preuschen, and presented a classification which placed the lesion into five categories. It became accepted that vaginal adenosis originated *in utero* and was not due to tissue alteration in later life. It is the site from which adenocarcinoma arises.

BOTRYOID SARCOMA

The first case of sarcoma botryoides of the vagina was probably recorded by P. Guersant in 1854 (Ricci, 1945). A number of reports of malignant polypi, and also an unusual lesion described by Spiegelberg (1879) as *sarcoma colli uteri hydropicum papillare*, were later termed sarcoma botryoides. The tumour was described by Pfannenstiel (1892) as a growth with grape-like, or botryoid appearance (Greek *Botrys*, a bunch of grapes, *Eidos*, form). These tumours were found to arise from the vagina and vulva, and less frequently from the cervix. Other sarcomatous tumours of the uterus, and of the Fallopian tube were found to be extremely rare.

CHRONOLOGY

General

1827	Cruveilhier of Paris first described the condition (Ricci, 1945).
1910	Bonney and Glendinning described benign adenomatosis vaginae (Way, 1951).

1923   Stephens noted the condition was difficult to treat.

1931   de Buben documented a 4% 5-year survival postradiotherapy.

1935   Taussig noted lack of proper therapy.

1948   Stanley Way described primary vaginal adenocarcinoma (Way, 1951).

1971   Herbst *et al.* reported the association of vaginal adenocarcinoma in offspring of mothers treated with diethylstilboestrol in pregnancy.

Sarcoma

1854   P. Guersant first recorded the condition (Ricci, 1945).

1879   Spiegelberg described a condition later termed 'sarcoma botryoid'.

1892   Pfannenstiel reported sarcoma of the vagina and cervix.

REFERENCES

de Buben, I. (1931). *Surg. Gynecol. Obstet.*, **52**, 884

Herbst, A.L., Ulfelder, H. and Poskanzer, C.D. (1971). Adenocarcinoma of the vagina: association of maternal stilbestrol therapy with tumor appearance in young women. *N. Engl. J. Med.*, **284**, 878–81

Kinlen, L.J., Badaracco, M.A., Moffett, J. and Vessey, K.P. (1974). A survey of the use of oestrogens during pregnancy in the United Kingdom and of genito-urinary cancer mortality and incidence in young people in England and Wales. *J. Obstet. Gynaecol. Br. Cwlth.*, **81**, 849–55

Pfannenstiel, J. (1892). Das traubige Sarcom der Cervix uteri. *Virchows Arch.*, **127**, 305

Ricci, J.V. (1945). *One Hundred Years of Gynaecology 1800–1900*, p. 448. (Philadelphia: Blakiston Co.)

Roberts, C.H. (1896). *Trans. Obstet. Soc. London*, **38**, 381

Sandberg, E.C., Danielson, R.W., Cauwet, R.W. and Bonar, B.E. (1965). Adenosis vaginae. *Am. J. Obstet. Gynecol.*, **93**, 209–22

Spiegelberg, (1879), quoted by Novak, E. and Woodruff, J.D. (1962). *Novak's Gynecologic and Obstetric Pathology: With Clinical and Endocrine Relations.* (Philadelphia, London: W.B. Saunders Co.)

Stevens, T.G. (1923). *J. Obstet. Gynaecol. Br. Emp.*, **30**, 42

Taussig, F.J. (1935). *Surg. Gynecol. Obstet.*, **60**, 477

Ulfelder, H. (1973). Stilbestrol, adenosis, and adenocarcinoma. *Am. J. Obstet. Gynecol.*, **117**, 794–98

Wade-Evans, T. (1976). The aetiology and pathology of cancer of the vagina. In Langley, F.A. (ed.) *Clinics in Obstetrics and Gynaecology. Cancer of the Vulva, Vagina and Uterus*, Vol. 3 pp. 229–41. (London, Philadelphia, Toronto: W.B. Saunders Co.)

Way, S. (1951). *Malignant Disease of the Female Genital Tract*, pp. 50–62. (London: J. & A. Churchill Ltd.)

FURTHER READING

Haines, M. and Taylor, C.W. (1975). *Gynaecological Pathology.* (Edinburgh, London, New York: Churchill Livingstone)

Langley, F.A. (ed.) (1976). Cancer of the vulva, vagina and uterus. *Clinics in Obstetrics and Gynaecology*, Vol. 3 no. 2. (London, Philadelphia, Toronto: W.B. Saunders Co.)

Novak, E.R. and Woodruff, J.D. (1962). *Gynecologic and Obstetric Pathology: With Clinical and Endocrine Relations*, 5th edn. (Philadelphia, London: W.B. Saunders Co.)

Way, S. (1951). *Malignant Disease of the Female Genital Tract.* (London: J. & A. Churchill Ltd.)

Cancer of the cervix

INTRODUCTION

The first references to cancer of the uterus appear in the Edwin Smith papyrus c.1700 BC. Hippocrates (460–377 BC) was aware of the condition and mentioned that when the disease was well advanced it was incurable (McKay, 1901). The Hindus in about the fifth century BC were known to have had an interest in surgical technique, and a text of the time described tumours of the cervix and vagina.

During the second and first centuries BC surgery developed as a specialty at Alexandria. Philoxenus (c.75 BC) who was a surgeon, was an acknowledged 'expert' on tumours, especially cancers of the womb (Jackson, 1988). The Romans incorporated the teachings of the Greeks into their medical practice and Soranus (AD 98–138), was one of the first authors to mention use of the 'dioptra' or vaginal speculum (Ricci, 1950). The instrument was used in the examination of patients with vaginal bleeding and 'ulcers of the womb'. Galen (AD 131–201) described cancer of the uterus in his *De Morbis Mulierum* and was aware of a bad prognosis.

Aetius of Amida (AD 502–575) was born in Mesopotamia and studied medicine in Alexandria. His gynaecology was based on that of Soranus. His writings summarized the available knowledge of gynaecology and were copied through the centuries. They later formed the basis of Caspar Wolff's *Harmonia Gynaeciorum*. Aetius' writings, the *Medici Graeci Tetra Biblos* were published in four volumes. The chapter *de Cancris Uteri* was written by Archigenes and categorized uterine cancer into ulcerative and non-ulcerative types (Jameson, 1936). A lengthy account of the different forms of cancers affecting the uterus was given but surgical treatment was not mentioned. Aetius advised against operations for 'malignant thymus' or 'polypus' of the womb. He was aware of the structures which were later termed Nabothian follicles, but did not confuse them with cancer. Oribasius (c. 325–403), who was a prolific medical author and compiler, advised the use of cautery in cases of 'malignant thymus'.

Over the years cancer was recognized and mentioned in the available medical literature. Ambroise Paré (1510–1590) of France, used the speculum to examine uterine cancer, and recommended amputation of the cervix in such cases. Nikolaas Tulpius (1593–1674) performed the first such operation in 1652. Jean Astruc (q.v. in biography) (1684–1766) wrote his *Treatise on the Diseases of Women* (1762), a work in six volumes, in which he referred to bimanual examination of the pelvis and the value of the speculum. Astruc described pelvic inflammatory disease and cervical cancer. He was of the opinion that all cancers started in the lymphatics and later developed into 'true' cancer.

Matthew Baillie (1793), nephew of William Hunter, illustrated a pathological specimen showing a cervical tumour eroding into the uterus and upper vagina in his *Engravings of Morbid Anatomy* (Figure 1). Textbooks in the early nineteenth century discussed cervical cancer noting that women of all ages were at risk. Whether treatment was offered or not the 'cauliflower excrescence' soon led to fatality (Burns, 1813; Dewees, 1826). As surgery and anaesthesia had not yet evolved, treatment consisted of bleeding the patient by means of cupping or the application of leeches to the diseased cervix. Pain relief and general measures to treat debility were the only other methods of treatment. The gross and microscopic appearances of cervical cancer were documented by John Clarke, Rudolph Virchow, R. Hooper, and J.H. Bennett. William Byford (1865) introduced a descriptive classification of the disease and in 1872 T. Gaillard Thomas offered a relatively precise light microscopic classification (Shingleton and Orr, 1987; Ricci, 1945). In his classification Byford differentiated between cancerous and simple ulcerations and gave a detailed description of 'cancer in the scirrhous condition'.

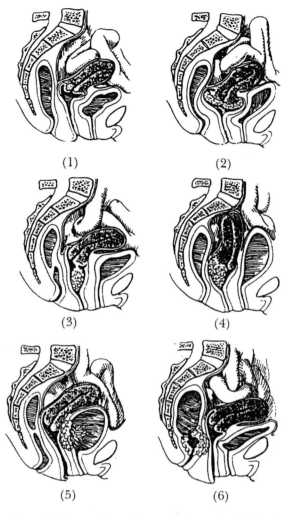

Figure 1 Stages of carcinoma of the cervix. (1) Early carcinoma of the cervix; (2) carcinoma of the cervix affecting the whole ectocervix; (3) papilliferous polypoid carcinoma of the cervix; (4) carcinoma of the cervix involving upper posterior wall of the vagina; (5) carcinoma of the cervix invading the bladder; (6) carcinoma of the lower part of the rectum and the anus invading the recto-vaginal septum. From Schaeffer-Bouglé, *Atlas-Manuel de Gynécologie*, Paris (1903)

INCIDENCE

Cervical cancer was found to be responsible for 4% of all deaths from neoplasia in women and ranged third, after breast and ovarian cancer, in the malignancies of breast and genital tract. In the 1980s approximately 4000 new cases of invasive cervical cancer were reported annually in England and Wales, while the figure in the USA reached 20 000 per year.

EPIDEMIOLOGY

The epidemiological approach to cancer was applied by Percival Pott (1755) during his investigations of scrotal cancer among chimney sweeps. Systematic observational studies were also applied during the major epidemics of acute communicable diseases in the nineteenth century, and John Snow (1855) was one of a number of workers who reported studies on the investigation and isolation of disease sources. The most notable epidemiological study on cervical cancer was reported from Italy. Professor Domenico Rigoni-Stern (1842) of Verona analysed cancer mortality based on deaths in that city from 1760 to 1839. He reported the higher frequency of breast cancer among unmarried women and nuns, relative to married or widowed. He also discovered that cervical cancer was not common in unmarried women and was very rare in nuns. This latter finding was confirmed by Gagnon (1950) in a study of nuns in Quebec, Canada.

Further observations on the relationship of sexual behaviour and the occurrence of cervical neoplasia were suggested by Broussais (1826) and later in the century by Virchow (1863). The theories suggested that the recurrent lacerations, abrasions and infections, associated with multiparity and poor obstetrical care, were aetiological factors. An increased incidence was found in the lower socioeconomic classes, and also among multiparous and non-White women (Weinberg and Gastpar, 1904). An exception to that observation was noted among Jewish women. Vineberg (1906) reviewed his own practice from 1893 to 1906 and reported that cervical cancer was 20 times more common among non-Jewish compared with Jewish patients. The lower risk in Jewish women was variously attributed to their observance of Jewish law on sexual intercourse, to dietary practice, or genetic factors. It was not until 1935 however, that an association between circumcision and cervical cancer was noted. Handley (1936) reported that cervical cancer was less common in native Fijians compared to resident Indians in the Fijian Islands. He suggested that the operation of circumcision afforded protection against mixed bacterial infection of the cervix during intercourse and thus reduced the incidence of cervical neoplasia. However, Kessler and Aurelian (1974) failed to substantiate the circumcision hypothesis.

Further proof of a sexual factor in the aetiology of cervical cancer was offered by Rojel (1953) of

Denmark who found a higher incidence of the disease among prostitutes. Eventually Wynder *et al.* (1954) and Rotkin and King (1962) discovered that the key variable was that of the age of first coitus. Rotkin (1973) evaluated the epidemiological studies in cervical cancer and indicated that a number of characteristics were related to onset of the disease. These included early onset of coitus, multiple sexual partners, coital frequency, age at first marriage, multiple marriage, parity and other variables.

The role of social class was highlighted by Vineberg (1906) and also Weinberg and Gastpar (1904). Further evidence was provided by Theilhaber and Greischer (1908) who noted that wives of journeymen and day labourers were more likely to suffer the disease, compared to wives whose husbands were in professional or the well-to-do classes. Kennaway (1948) again referred to the racial and social incidence of cancer of the uterus while Wakefield *et al.* (1973) found a definite correlation between social class and positive exfoliative cytology smears. The role of tobacco smoking was highlighted by Buckley *et al.* (1981).

The concept of the high-risk male was emphasized by Singer (1973a). Some time previously it was reported that spouses of males with prostate or penile cancer were more likely to develop cervical cancer (Martinez, 1969; Feminella, 1973). A particular male was incriminated by Blythe-Smith and Jenkins (1969) for an 'outbreak' of cervical cancer at a housing estate in Georgia, USA. Kessler (1976) discovered that second and third wives of males whose first wife developed the disease were also at higher risk.

AETIOLOGY

In the early part of the nineteenth century physicians related the onset of cancer to stress. However, F. Von Scanzoni (1861) was the first to observe that city dwellers had a higher incidence of the disease. He considered that excessive sexual excitation was causative. Although other theories abounded, Scanzoni's was the only one of value. The role of sexual practice, already alluded to, offered the most promising avenue in aetiological research.

Semen

A number of possible aetiological factors were studied (including smegma). Coppleson (1970) first proposed a carcinogenic action for sperm DNA incorporated into unstable cervical cells. Some 6 years later it was suggested that protamine, a protein in the sperm head, interfered with the regulatory mechanisms which normally control the cell, and thus induced neoplastic change (Singer *et al.* 1976).

Human papillomavirus

The specific cellular changes induced by human papillomavirus infection were described by Ayre (1949) and he suggested a link with neoplasia. Koss and Durfee (1956) introduced the term 'koilocytotic atypia' and suggested that the cellular pattern induced by human papillomavirus was associated with precancer. The cellular changes ascribed to human papillomavirus infection were further described by Meisels and Fortin (1976) and Syrjanen *et al.* (1981) and an association between the virus and neoplastic change of the cervix was noted. Further evidence for the association between human papillomavirus and cervical cancer was derived from immunochemistry, DNA/DNA hybridization, and serological studies.

Chlamydia and herpes

A role for micro-organisms such as *Chlamydia* and the herpes virus was first proposed by Reid (1962). The herpes simplex virus type 2 was demonstrated by Naib *et al.* (1969) to occur with increased frequency in patients with cytological evidence of cervical dysplasia. Rawls *et al.* (1970) discovered antibodies to genital herpes simplex virus in patients with carcinoma of the cervix. Aurelian *et al.* (1971) isolated a virus identical to herpes simplex virus type 2 in cervical cancer cells grown in tissue culture.

Cytomegalovirus

This virus was isolated from cervical secretions and semen and in the early 1970s was considered to cause a sexually transmitted disease. Albrecht and Rapp (1973) first noted the malignant potential of the virus when they exposed hamster embryo fibroblasts to ultraviolet-irradiated human cytomegalovirus. The sera of tumour-bearing animals were found to contain antibodies to cytomegalovirus antigens.

Diethylstilboestrol

A report which implicated maternal diethylstilboestrol use in early pregnancy with vaginal clear cell adenocarcinoma in their adolescent daughters, stimulated research as to whether vaginal adenosis was a precancerous lesion (Herbst *et al.*, 1971). Some studies showed twice the rate of squamous neoplasia and intraepithelial lesions in diethylstilboestrol-exposed women.

Immunosuppression

Porecco *et al.* (1975) discovered a 14-fold increase of intraepithelial carcinoma in immunosuppressed patients.

Whatever the cause, it was found from colposcopic and histological evidence that the transformation zone contained the majority of pre-invasive and invasive cervical squamous cell carcinomas. The detection of premalignant and malignant conditions of the cervix was based on cervical cytology and colposcopy.

CYTOLOGY

Early discoveries in cytology

Alfred Donné, a former lawyer, changed professions and became a doctor of medicine. While in Paris he developed a major interest in microscopy, and reported his observations on tissues and fluids from many parts of the body. In his thesis *Recherches Physiologiques et Chemico-Microscopiques sur les Globules du Sang, du Pus, du Mucus, et sur Ceux des Humeurs de l'Oeil* (1831) Donne detailed research on mucus, blood and pus. He discovered *Trichomonas vaginalis* in vaginal secretions, and reported his findings in his *Nature of Mucus* (1836). He described the presence of sperm in vaginal fluid; is credited with the first observation of leukaemia; and in 1838 described the cellular content of colostrum. His *Atlas exécuté d'apres Nature au Microscope-Daguerreotype* (1845) contained the first photomicrographs used in medicine.

Johannes Muller, a Berlin physiologist, is regarded as the initiator of clinical cytology, and numbered among his 'disciples' were Schwann, Virchow, Henle, Remak, Haeckel, Waldeyer, Dubois-Reymond and Helmholtz. He wrote a monograph *On the Nature and Structural Characteristics of Cancer and those Morbid Growths that may be confounded with it* (1840). The cellular structures of malignant tumours had previously been mentioned by him in 1836 when addressing an audience at the Friedrich Wilhelm Institute, which was celebrating its 42nd anniversary. Muller's book contained microscopic criteria for the fundamental differentiation of benign and malignant tissues. In his histological groups he defined 'sarcoma' and 'carcinoma' and proved for the first time that all malignant tumours were closely related physiologically.

Dr Julius Vogel of Gottingen, was the first to report (1843) on two diagnoses made by what, a century later became known as exfoliative cytology. The first case was of a tumour close to the mandibular angle. A fistula developed, and microscopy of the expressed fluid revealed pus and malignant cells. The second case was an ulcerating breast lesion. The discharged fluid contained pus and granulation tissue only and Vogel determined that the ulcer was not malignant. The patient made a complete recovery. In the same year Gluge (1843) studied spreads and scrapings from many sources, including cancer tissue, and wrote that 'cancer cells are double the ordinary size or more, and they not infrequently contain several nuclei . . .'.

F.A. Pouchet (1847) who was working in Paris observed the appearances of cells in vaginal secretions in relation to various stages of the menstrual cycle, and thus laid the early foundations of 'hormonal cytology'. Two years later Bennett (1849), an English disciple of Donne, described for the first time the cytological examination of ascitic fluid, obtained from a patient with a probable diagnosis of ovarian cancer.

Donaldson (1853) of the USA described malignant cells in body fluids. His studies were based on smears of fluid obtained from the cut surface of the tissue by gentle pressure or by scraping with a knife. He preferred the cytological method as he found that his attempts to examine small slices of tissue were relatively unsuccessful as 'the lens employed must be much feebler, and the cell is not seen to the same advantage'.

Rudolph Virchow (q.v. in Biographies) (1821–1902) studied medicine in Berlin and graduated in 1843. He became interested in histology through the work of Johannes Muller and in his advance from surgeon's assistant to prosector at the Charité, gathered a vast amount of pathological experience. In 1847 he introduced a new medical journal *Archive of Pathological Anatomy and Physiology and of Clinical Medicine*. He is credited with the concept that the human organism was a cell-state, *omnis cellula e cellula* – every cell comes only from another cell, and his *Cellular Pathology and its Foundation in Physiological and Pathological Histology* (1858) was a landmark publication. Virchow was certain that the process of disease and neoplasia took place in the individual cell.

Lambl (1856) diagnosed a case of uterine carcinoma which had invaded the bladder, from cytological examination of the urine. Some years later L.S. Beale, Professor of Physiology and Morbid Anatomy in London, together with Dr Newham published a case of pharyngeal carcinoma diagnosed by sputum cytology. These cases were early and rare attempts at the use of diagnostic exfoliative cytology in the detection of cancer. Beale (1861) was the first to compare exfoliated cells with cells from autopsy material of the tumour.

J.G. Richardson (1871) of Philadelphia recommended that 'a small portion of the secretion from the os uteri, or from the ulcerated surface of the growth . . .' should be obtained and high power examination of 200 diameters 'will probably disclose at least a few cells on each slide which will indicate with more or less certainty the character of the morbid formation'.

C. Friedlander (1886) also used the cytological method, and indicated that 'In carcinoma uteri, one will find suspended in the liquid, cellular elements originating from the carcinomatous ulceration . . . In doubtful cases . . . the excision of a small piece of tissue has to be performed, and its histological examination will confirm the diagnosis.

Little else was published on the subject in the last century apart from a paper by Amann (1897) which included illustrations of uterine cancer cells. Bruch, Gluge and Leber contributed pictures from imprints of uterine cancers.

Modern cytology

George Nicholas Papanicolaou (Figure 2) was born on 13 May 1883 in the city of Kymi (Coumi) on the Greek island of Euboea (Koss, 1983). He became a medically qualified zoologist and emigrated from Greece to New York in 1913. His research had a profound influence on the development of modern cytology.

The first breakthrough came when Stockard and Papanicolaou (1917) reported their study of the oestrous cycle in animals. They discovered that smears taken from the vagina showed cyclical

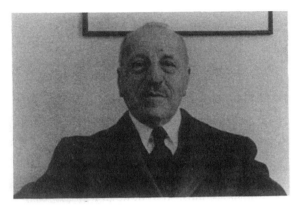

Figure 2   G.N. Papanicolaou

cellular changes which could be used to detect the time of ovulation. Papanicolaou later applied the vaginal smear technique to the human female (1928; 1933) and developed a staining method which carries his name (1942).

Meanwhile, Schiller (1927; 1928a,b) documented that the diagnosis of cervical carcinoma could be made from purely cytological atypia, without evidence of invasive growth, and thus emphasized the concept of the pre-invasive stage of carcinoma.

The cytological diagnosis of cervical cancer by means of cervico-vaginal smears was pioneered not by Papanicolaou, but by Dr Aurel Babes (1886–1962), Professor of Pathology in Bucharest. In his study, samples were taken from the cervix using a platinum loop and after air-drying were stained with Giemsa. The technique was reported by Daniel and Babes (1927) to the Bucharest Gynaecological Society.

Babes (1928) also reported the method in an illustrated article in the *Presse Medicale*. He stated that the diagnosis could be reliably made from smears, and that this was achieved in 18 out of 20 cases studied, some of which were 'incipient'. Babes and Daniel called their technique the Romanian method. The first clinical trial of the technique was conducted by O. Viana of Verona (1928) on 12 cases but he saw no advantage in the method as the cervix was readily accessible to speculum examination and biopsy if required.

Papanicolaou (1928) reported at the 3rd Race Betterment Conference at Battle Creek, Michigan, that he had discovered the tumour cells of cervical cancer in vaginal aspirates, during his work at the Women's Hospital, New York. The paper appeared to have little impact. The next communication on the subject from Papanicolaou was in 1941 when, with the gynaecologist Dr Herbert Traut, he wrote a paper on the diagnostic value of vaginal smears in carcinoma of the uterus. Their paper appeared in the *American Journal of Obstetrics and Gynecology* (Papanicolaou and Traut, 1941). Papanicolaou noted that 'because of its simplicity it may eventually be applied widely, so that the incipient phases of the disease may come more promptly within the range of our modern modes of treatment . . . the method makes the material for examination easily and frequently available at low cost . . .'.

Two years later, Papanicolaou and Traut (1943) produced an illustrated monograph, *Diagnosis of Uterine Cancer by the Vaginal Smear* which was based on a study of over 3000 cases, of whom 127 had carcinoma of the cervix and seven had early intradermal types of squamous carcinoma. Other investigators applied the technique and Meigs *et al.* (1943), Ayre (1944), and Jones *et al.* (1945) reported that their preliminary results confirmed Papanicolaou's findings.

In the beginning, cytology smears were made from vaginal aspirate. Ayre (1946) compared vaginal and cervical cytology in the diagnosis of cervical neoplasia, and found that smears from the cervix gave more accurate information. He designed a wooden spatula (1947) which was specially shaped so as to collect cells from the squamocolumnar junction of the cervix. The sample was taken, spread onto a glass slide, fixed with 95% ethyl alcohol and stained with haematoxylin and eosin, or the Papanicolaou staining method. Papanicolaou and colleagues introduced a grading system for the reporting of cervical smears in 1948. A training course was set up in the New York Cornell Medical Centre in Papanicolaou's laboratory in the late 1940s. Pathologists were slow to accept the technique, and initially gynaecologists carried out their own cytology examinations and reporting.

Cytological terminology

The classification of cytology smears in Papanicolaou's *Atlas of Exfoliative Cytology* (1954) contained five grades; Class 1 or negative; Class 2, atypical/inflammatory; Class 3, suspicious; Class 4, strongly suggestive of malignancy; and Class 5 or conclusive for malignancy. Other classifications and grading systems evolved, and as a result comparisons between different cytology centres became difficult. The various grading systems also led to misinterpretation of cytological results and inappropriate management of women with abnormal cervical cytology reports.

In recent times the British Society for Clinical Cytology (BSCC) published recommendations on terminology (Spriggs *et al*, 1978; Evans *et al*, 1986) which were endorsed by the Intercollegiate Working Party on cervical cytology screening (1987). It was recommended that a cervical cytology report should consist of: a precise description of the cells present in clearly defined and generally accepted terms; a prediction of the histological condition; and a recommendation for the further management of the individual patient.

It was further recommended that the nuclear abnormalities if any, should form the basis of cytological diagnosis. If nuclear abnormalities were absent the smear result was to be termed negative. Those nuclear abnormalities which did exist could range from minor degrees which were usually associated with inflammatory conditions, to the more striking abnormalities associated with either cervical intraepithelial neoplasia or with invasive carcinoma. The term 'dyskaryosis' was used to describe nuclear abnormalities judged to be greater than those encountered in inflammatory conditions, and indicated that a diagnosis of cervical intraepithelial neoplasia (CIN) or invasive carcinoma was likely at histopathology of biopsy samples. The degree of dyskaryosis was thought to correlate approximately with the severity of the histological condition: mild dyskaryosis indicated CIN Grade 1; moderate dyskaryosis, CIN 2; and severe dyskaryosis, either CIN 3 or invasive carcinoma.

The terminology Committees of the American Society of Cytology and the International Academy of Cytology also recommended using descriptive cytological interpretation instead of numerical reports (Noumoff, 1987). An American Bethesda System was advanced as a replacement of the Papanicolaou classification in 1988 (National Cancer Institute Workshop, 1989).

The term 'atypia' was introduced but caused confusion as some investigators used it to signify a benign cytological pattern, while others equated 'atypia' with CIN 1 (Holmquist, 1987). The Intercollegiate Working Party (1987) defined atypical cells as, 'cells which cannot be classified as normal, but which do not fit neatly into any of the abnormal categories'. The preferred term is now 'borderline' or 'doubtful'. Reports in this category were to pose a frequent challenge to the cytologist and gynaecologist (Hudson, 1990).

Cervical cytology screening

When cytology screening began, it was offered on a limited scale to gynaecological patients. Lombard and colleagues, and also McSweeney and McKay of Massachusetts initiated the first cytology screening programmes in 1945 (Lombard et al., 1948; McSweeney and McKay, 1948) for women attending gynaecological outpatient clinics. The first national cytology conference was held in Boston in 1948. Large-scale screening of asymptomatic women was introduced to British Columbia by David Boyes et al. in 1947, and their report to the *British Medical Journal* (1962) detailed the early results. Smears were taken from 146 833 women, of whom 828 were found to have intraepithelial neoplasia, and 87 had invasive carcinoma. The reported series ran from 1949 to 1960. From 1955, the authors indicated that the incidence of clinically invasive carcinoma fell by 30.5%, from 28.4 to 19.7 per 1000 women. Their study was of major importance, and it became generally accepted that cytology screening was an effective method of detecting cervical cancer in all its forms. Detection could lead to cure, and thus if screening were rigorously applied, eradication of cervical cancer was possible. Cervical screening was soon applied on a large scale, and epidemiologists later criticized the lack of controlled studies of the technique, prior to its worldwide adoption.

Cervical cytology was introduced to the UK by Anderson (1950) who used the test on gynaecological patients in Edinburgh. McLaren and Attwood (1961) reported their use of the technique in Birmingham and reported their findings in the *British Medical Journal*. Cervical cytology was launched as a screening programme in the UK in 1966 and women over the age of 35 years of age were invited to take part at 5-yearly intervals. McLaren and Attwood (1961) compared cervical scraping with vaginal aspiration in over 5000 patients, and found that the cervical smear test was better than aspiration in the detection of intraepithelial carcinoma.

Kaiser et al. reported in 1960 that over 3 million US women were being screened for cancer each year. The same author reported a survey of 605 200 women from Memphis. Intraepithelial carcinoma of the cervix was found in 2.45 per 1000, while invasive cancer of the cervix was found in 1.5 per 1000.

Minor degrees of cytological abnormality

As time went by, investigators focused their attention on the lesser degrees of cytological abnormality in an effort to discover the relationship of those abnormalities to invasive cervical cancer, and their possible rates of progression to a cancer state. Kaufmann et al. (1983) noted that infection with human papillomavirus caused a change in cervical smears which was indistinguishable from the mild dyskaryosis of CIN 1. Singer et al. (1984) found that cervical cytology had poor specificity for reports at the lower end of abnormality compared with the higher specificity of reporting severe dyskaryosis. Although the results of studies were varied, many women with mild dyskaryosis at cytology were found to have CIN 3 when investigated further (Kitchener et al., 1987; Chomet, 1987). Jordan (1988) suggested a multicentre prospective study among women with minor degrees of cytological and histological abnormality to settle the problem as to what actually happened in those cases.

Another area of investigation was that of the inflammatory cervical smear and its relationship to cervical cancer. Novak (1929) was one of the first to differentiate between inflammatory, premalignant or malignant conditions of the cervix. In a large group of studies reported in the literature, the inflammatory smear rates varied from a low of 4.2% (Figge et al., 1970) to a high of 70% (Luthra et al., 1987), reflecting the populations sampled, the diagnostic criteria used, and intraobserver variations between laboratories. A number of studies investigated the relationship of inflammatory cervical cytology to CIN. In women with inflammatory cytology CIN was present at rates ranging from a low of 7.6% (Hulka, 1968) to a high of 68% (Benedet and Boyes, 1976). The majority of investigators found CIN rates which varied from 10 to 29% in patients with inflammatory smears, and Singer (1986) wrote that CIN could be present in about one-fifth of women with persistent inflammatory smears. The problem of inflammatory cervical cytology in a 'low-risk' population was investigated and only 4.8% of patients were found to have CIN, with 3.8% in the categories CIN 2 and CIN 3 (O'Dowd, 1990).

False negative and positive cytology

As cytology screening gained momentum, it was soon recognized that false-positive or false-negative tests would impair the predictive value of the technique. False-positive tests were those in which a malignant or suspicious smear was reported but histopathology of cervical biopsy was negative, and the reverse situation pertained for false negatives. Anderson (1956) screened almost 13 000 women and had a false-positive rate of 12%. The false-negative rate was 0.11%.

Reagan and Patten (1962a) demonstrated a 90% correct correlation between gynaecological cytology and histopathology reports, with 10% being either over or under called. MacGregor (1964) introduced a note of caution, as it was observed that a negative smear could be obtained from a clinically invasive cancer of the cervix. Yule (1973) reported that a 12.7% false-negative rate was found in a cohort of women examined at regular intervals.

The effectiveness of cervical screening was thought to be reflected by a declining incidence of cervical cancer. The reduction in mortality was most marked in areas with a comprehensive screening service such as British Columbia (Boyes *et al.*, 1982), Iceland (Johannesson *et al.*, 1982), Denmark (Berget, 1979), Sweden (Petterson *et al.*, 1985) and Finland (Hakama, 1978). However, an editorial in the *Lancet* (1985) expressed disappointment that a greater impact had not been made on death rates in Britain, probably due to the fact that those women most at risk did not appear to have smears taken. Skrabanek and McCormick (1989) in their appraisal of the *Lancet* paper pointed out that 40 000 smears and 200 excision biopsies were performed for each cervical cancer death thought to be prevented by screening.

Abnormal cytology in pregnancy

Marsh and Fitzgerald (1956) summarized the reported cases of carcinoma *in situ* in the literature and added 20 of their own, making a total of 75 reported cases. Almost 30% were discovered to have regressed spontaneously following pregnancy. Rad *et al.* (1966) documented a similar prevalence rate for carcinoma *in situ* in pregnancy compared to the non-pregnant state. Takeuchi and McKay (1960) quantified the area involved by carcinoma *in situ* as 0.25 cm^2 and that of dysplasia as 0.9 cm^2. Jordan (1976) commented that over one-third of Takeuchi and McKay's cases would have been treated by a single biopsy. From that he deduced that 'many of the so-called regressions following pregnancy have actually been a result of the diagnostic procedure being therapeutic'.

COLPOSCOPY

The colposcope was developed by Hans Hinselmann of Hamburg in 1924. He was requested at that time to write a chapter on the aetiology, symptoms and diagnosis of uterine cancer, for the third edition of the *Handbook of Gynaecology* which was edited by Veit and Stockel. Hinselmann was dissatisfied with the available diagnostic methods of palpation and naked eye examination in the early diagnosis of cervical cancer. He wished to view a magnified image of the cervix with binocular vision, and with light provided from an intense light source. This led to the construction of a colposcope which he first used in December 1924, and subsequently reported (1925).

Hinselmann used a Leitz binocular dissecting microscope with an attached light source, and discovered that magnification of 3.5 – 30 times was possible. He attached the optical system to a stand which allowed movement in every direction, and also supplied a screw for fine adjustment. Hinselmann discovered that colposcopy could allow the detection of even dot-sized tumours, where previously the detection of a cervical tumour the size of a pigeon's egg was regarded as early diagnosis.

Hinselmann was aware of the work of his own teacher von Franque (1901;1907) and others who had described the earliest condition of cervical cancer as a 'surface carcinoma' or 'intraepithelial carcinoma', later called 'carcinoma *in situ*' or 'cervical intraepithelial neoplasia' (CIN) 3. By studying areas which he called 'leukoplakia' Hinselmann (1936) discovered patterns of punctation and mosaic which were associated with many cases of intraepithelial neoplasia. In his efforts to coagulate and remove cervical mucus from the visual field Hinselmann experimented with various chemicals. In this way he discovered the effect of acetic acid. The chemical coagulated mucus and Hinselmann (1925) reported that it also stained abnormal epithelium white due to its effects on cell proteins.

As an additional aid to colposcopic study, Hinselmann applied an iodine solution to the cervix, a test first advocated by Schiller (1928a,b). Schiller (1933) also recommended the test as a useful screen for cancer in a busy outpatient setting. Hinselmann also used coloured filters as outlined by Kraatz (1939) and found that use of a green filter during inspection of the cervix, increased the colour contrast so that red appeared as black, and examination of subepithelial capillaries was thereby facilitated. The 'saline technique' was described much later by Koller (1963).

As time went by, Hinselmann compared his colposcopic findings to those from histopathology, and also devised a system of colposcopic terminology (Hinselmann, 1930; 1933; 1934; 1938). His concept of the 'matrix area' in which malignant transformation occurred was later replaced by that of the 'atypical transformation zone'. Colposcopy, cervical cytology, histopathology and the theories on morphogenesis of cervical carcinoma evolved together. Fischer-Wasels (1927) attributed particular importance to the role of metaplasia and Wespi (1949) also stressed its importance.

Schiller (1929) discovered asymptomatic lesions which he described as 'the smallest cervical carcinomas'. He observed that squamous carcinomas of the cervix were lacking in glycogen and described the Schiller Iodine test. Normal squamous cell epithelial cells, which contained glycogen stained dark brown, but columnar epithelium or abnormal epithelium, which contained little or no glycogen, was unstained. Schiller emigrated to Boston, Massachusetts in 1932 and although his test was accepted, colposcopy was rejected for a further 20 years.

Koller (1963) noted that use of acetic acid or Schiller's iodine made interpretation of the angioarchitecture of the cervix difficult. He described a 'saline technique' where the cervix was exposed; its mucus removed; and the epithelium soaked in normal saline. By this means he could make a detailed study of the subepithelial vascular supply. The saline technique was further described by Kolstad and Stafl (1972) who were also working from the Norwegian Radium Hospital in Oslo.

The introduction of cervical cytology by Papanicolaou and Traut (1943) offered a simpler method for the detection of preinvasive cervical lesions, and its use rapidly spread throughout the English-speaking world. Although cytology was found to be a more accurate method of detecting precancer of the cervix, it gave no indication of the site of the lesion and histological clarification was dependent on 'blind' biopsy or conization. Selective colposcopy with the identification of epithelial abnormalities and directed biopsies, in those women with abnormal cervical cytology, proved to be the best method of management.

The colposcope remained popular in Germany and in German-speaking areas of South America, but was little used elsewhere. The introduction of the colposcope to France was recorded by Bret and Coupez (1960). Koller (1963) and Kolstad (1964) of Norway developed photographic methods which allowed detailed studies of the capillary angioarchitecture. Stafl et al. (1963) reported colposcopic histological studies from Czechoslovakia. Although Ries (1932) of America had used the instrument, it was little used there until popularized by Lang (1956) and Bolten and Jacques (1960) who referrred to this 'neglected method of cervical evaluation'.

Colposcopy was first used in England during 1955 at Professor Stallworthy's department in Oxford (Coppleson, 1977), and its further use was popularized by Anderson (1962), Jordan (1969), Singer (1973b; 1975) and Crompton and Langley (1973), in Birmingham, Oxford and Manchester respectively. Coppleson and Reid (1967) and other clinicians popularized its use in Australia.

Wespi (1949) introduced his nomenclature and divided colposcopic findings into four groups. A classification of colposcopic appearances introduced by Hinselmann (1954) included those findings which were judged to be normal, and/or pathological. Other classifications were proposed in Germany, America, and Australia. During the Second Congress of Cervical Pathology and Colposcopy in Graz in 1975 a new colposcopic terminology was evolved which was to be adopted world-wide.

Various grading systems were developed in an effort to forecast the likely significance of lesions found at colposcopy. One such system was developed by Johannison et al. (1966) and relied on vascular patterns and the differences in intercapillary distance to grade atypical colposcopic lesions. They accurately predicted histology results in 96.5% of cases.

In the early 1970s it was reported that the use of colposcopy with directed biopsy obviated the need for cone biopsy in the majority of women, including those pregnant patients with abnormal smears. The use of the colposcopic method dramatically increased from the late 1970s, as more gynaecologists became attracted to the technique, and the increased cytology screening services produced large numbers of women with abnormal smear reports who required the detailed examination offered at colposcopy. During the same period the treatment of cervical precancer by hysterectomy or cone biopsy was largely bypassed as other methods of local tissue destruction became available.

HISTOPATHOLOGY

Premalignancy

The development of histopathology took place in the nineteenth century and was pioneered by Johannes Muller in 1830. The first histological classification of tissues was introduced by Jacob Henle of Zurich and Heidelberg. Rudolph Virchow (q.v. in Biographies) (1858) of Berlin, who is regarded as the founder of cellular pathology, first observed the downward growth of an 'epithelioma' of the cervix into the deeper layers. Sir John Williams (1886a) during his Harveian Lecture described the lesion which became known as carcinoma *in situ*. He stated 'this is the earliest condition of undoubted cancer of the portio vaginalis that I have met with; and it is the earliest condition which is recognizable as cancer. It presented with no distinct symptoms, and was discovered accidentally'.

Cullen (1900) also described the histopathological picture of what was later termed squamous carcinoma *in situ*. Schauenstein (1908) developed the view that invasive cervical cancer was preceded by an intraepithelial phase of growth. Further support for this view was published by Pronai (1909), Rubin (1910), and Schottlander and Kermauner (1912). Rubin (1910) asserted that . . . 'pathological examination . . . may often furnish the first evidence of a latent carcinoma, and the pathological diagnosis of carcinoma of the uterus in the preclinical stage is possible'. The terms 'preinvasive carcinoma' (Schiller, 1928a,b) and 'surface carcinoma' (Meyer, 1930) were replaced by the term 'carcinoma *in situ*' (Schottlander and Kermauner, 1912; Broders, 1932). Reagan *et al.* (1953) introduced the term 'dysplasia' to describe intraepithelial lesions whose disordered growth patterns were less severe than those of carcinoma *in situ*. Reagan reported that the majority of untreated lesions regressed or remained unchanged for many years. Richart (1966;1967;1973) introduced the modern terminology of CIN. He devised this as 'a generic term to designate the spectrum of intraepithelial disease that antedates invasive cancer'. This terminology replaced that of dysplasia and preinvasive carcinoma *in situ*. Three grades of CIN

were recognized (Buckley *et al.*, 1982; Ferenczy, 1982).

Malignancy

Broders introduced a histological classification of cervical cancer based on four grades while Reagan *et al.* (1957) used three groups: keratinizing, large cell non-keratinizing, and small cell non-keratinizing. These categories were later adopted by the World Health Organization. Ashley (1966) proposed that there were two forms of squamous cell carcinoma. One was slow growing while the other was a rapidly developing tumour.

Progression of CIN

Koss *et al.* (1963) noted that 'following a biopsy, even in the presence of histologically demonstrable residual carcinoma *in situ*, the number of abnormal cells in smears often diminished very markedly, occasionally to the point of transient absence of cancer cells'. This problem of biopsy removal of *in situ* lesions meant that the progression rates of CIN were difficult to interpret. The natural history of intraepithelial lesions was studied by Reagan and Patten (1962b).

Progression of dysplasia to CIN, and CIN to invasive cancer

Richart and Barron (1969) assessed patients with cytological evidence of dysplasia by repeat cytology and colpomicroscopy without biopsy. They found that transit times for progression from mild, moderate and severe dysplasia, to carcinoma *in situ*, were 58 months, 38 months, and 12 months respectively. They noted a regression rate of 6%. Galvin *et al.* (1955) documented that where there was severe dysplastic change, 65.7% progressed to carcinoma *in situ*, while only 17.1% regressed.

The relationship of CIN to invasive carcinoma was studied by Petersen (1956) who reported a 26% progression rate to invasive disease, while Kottmeier (1961) reported a 71% rate. Widely ranging results were quoted from other studies. Based on cytological evidence (Richart and Barron, 1969), or epidemiological results (Fidler *et al.*, 1968), there was a 10-year delay before CIN became invasive. More recent reports suggested a delay of 3–10 years. McIndoe *et al.* (1984) followed up 300 women with evidence of untreated carcinoma *in situ* over a 20-year period. At the end of 10 years, 18%, and at 20 years, 36% had developed evidence of invasive cancer.

TREATMENT OF CIN

The first attempts at treatment of intraepithelial neoplasia were by biopsy or hysterectomy, and the latter was standard textbook therapy in the USA until the late 1960s. When biopsy was introduced the intent was to obtain tissue for pathological study. It became obvious however, that biopsy could also remove the suspected disease.

Cervical biopsy

Bennett (1845) described the technique of biopsy and histology in his introductory address on the use of the microscope. Ruge and Veit (1878) used the technique for the preoperative diagnosis of cervical cancer and Williams (1886b) described in biopsy material, the earliest condition of cervical cancer, the condition later termed carcinoma *in situ.*

Schiller (1933) of Vienna used Lugol's iodine to stain the cervix and delineate abnormal areas for biopsy. [It was later recognized that this test was not totally reliable as immature metaplastic epithelium, or atrophic, and glandular epithelium did not contain glycogen and therefore did not stain deep brown with iodine. Richart (1964) showed that 72% of carcinoma *in situ* lesions and 57% of dysplasias overall, failed to take up the stain when iodine was applied to the cervix.]

Cervical conization

Lisfranc (1815) was the first to describe cervical conization. At that time the indications included infection or cancer. Marion Sims (1861) used silver wire sutures to close the coned cervix and Sturmdorf (1916) described the technique of cervical suture and closure. Martzloff (1938) referred to 'cone biopsy' which was used to detect the presence of carcinoma *in situ.* At that time multiple blind punch biopsies and quadrant biopsies were being taken, but were found to be unreliable methods of localizing lesions and were eventually abandoned. Cold knife conization of the cervix was advocated by Thornton *et al.* (1954) and Scott and Reagan (1956).

McLaren (1960) used 'deep ring biopsy' and conization as means of curing carcinoma *in situ,* and later reported that 93% of cases were successfully treated. Local infiltration with physiological saline and adrenaline prior to biopsy was described by Scott *et al.* (1960). Their technique reduced the operative blood loss. Fluhmann (1961) advocated the use of Sturmdorf sutures to cover the cone bed, but McLaren disagreed with this concept as the in-turning of vaginal epithelium might bury residual pathological tissue. Burghardt and Albeggar (1969) advocated the use of diathermy to the cone bed. Following the introduction of colposcopically directed cone biopsies, smaller amounts of tissue were removed with equal benefit (Jordan, 1972).

The first pregnancy to follow cone biopsy was reported by Ayre (1950). McLaren *et al.* (1974) reported 60 pregnancies following cone biopsy and found premature delivery in three cases and cervical dystocia due to fibrosis in two.

In 1960, Parker *et al.* reported treatment by conization and multiple biopsy. In the same year Scott *et al.* (1960) reported a 'cold knife' bloodless cervical conization technique, which was also called ring biopsy. Early reports including that of Wagner (1961) recorded an unacceptably high level of cytological recurrence after the technique but Coppleson (1981) reviewed the world literature and indicated that there was little therapeutic difference between the effects of cone biopsy and simple hysterectomy. Recurrence risk was very low.

Laser

The first ruby medical laser was developed by Theodore H. Maiman in 1960 and was used as early as 1964 by a Doctor Freeman for the treatment of retinal lesions. The carbon dioxide laser was discovered by Platel in 1964. In the following year the Nd–Yag (neodymium–yttrium-aluminium-garnet) laser was first used, and the argon laser was introduced in 1978. Pulsed Yag lasers were developed in 1980 (Giscard d'Estaing, 1990).

The laser (an acronym for light amplification by stimulated emission of radiation) beam is emitted by controlled excitation and decay of electrons in the lasing medium. A beam of energy is generated and may be focused to vaporize tissue precisely.

Kaplan *et al.* (1973) reported their use of the carbon dioxide laser in treatment of cervical erosions. Stafl (1975) used the CO_2 laser, and he and his associates (1977) reported its use for treatment of cervical and vaginal neoplasia in 40 patients. They claimed a 90% success rate. Bellina (1977) reported his treatment of 205 patients, and in later work reported a single treatment success rate of 93%. Toaff (1976) and Dorsey and Diggs (1979) reported cone biopsy by laser. Wetchler (1984) reviewed the 17 published English-language series on CO_2 laser treatment of CIN. An overall cure rate for one or more treatments of 63–99% for all grades of CIN was found, and a 50–99% cure rate for CIN 3. Cure rates improved when the entire transformation zone was vaporized to a depth of 5–7 mm.

Cryocautery

Early experience of cryocautery was reported by Crisp *et al.* (1970) when they applied the technique to treatment of premalignant disease. Crisp (1971) noted that the depth of destruction of properly applied double-freeze cryotherapy was 5–6 mm. The early cure rates for the technique were low, and Creasman *et al.* (1973) reported rates of 27–75%. Townsend and Richart (1983) prospectively compared cryotherapy with laser and found no significant difference in failure rates between the two modalities. Singer and Walker (1985) however, assessed the available literature and suggested that the modality was associated with significant persistence or recurrence of all grades of CIN.

Electrocautery/electrodiathermy

Younge *et al.* (1949) studied 135 cases of carcinoma *in situ* and wrote that 'when the disease is early (surface involvement only) cauterization or sharp shallow conization can be offered as a non-sterilizing treatment to these young women, with an 85% apparent chance of success'. In a further paper Younge (1957) reported a 70% cure rate for carcinoma *in situ*, when electrocautery alone was used. Richart and Sciarra (1968) followed up 170 patients by cytology and colposcopy, and reported a 97% success rate in the eradication of disease. Chanen and Hollyock (1971; 1974) using a more radical approach found the method to be effective in eradicating focal lesions within colposcopic view, and reported a success rate of 90%. Coppleson (1977) reported on the use of electrodiathermy in Sydney, first introduced there in 1966. Chanen and Rome (1983) reviewed their 15 years with electrocoagulation diathermy and reported a 97.3% success rate in 1864 patients.

Semm's cold coagulator

Kurt Semm introduced the instrument in 1966 for the treatment of benign conditions of the cervix and Staland (1978) first described its use for treatment of premalignant lesions. Duncan (1983a,b) of Scotland popularized the use of the instrument so that in the late 1980s most patients in the UK were treated by either cold coagulation or laser therapy. Diathermy and cryotherapy became less popular as diathermy required a general anaesthetic, and cryotherapy success rates were variable. Gordon and Duncan (1991) reported a 14-year experience with cold coagulation therapy, which prompted Giles and Gafar (1991) to write that 'as cold coagulation is technically easier, quicker to use and considerably cheaper, it must be considered the treatment of choice for local destruction of CIN'.

Diathermy loop

Cartier *et al.* (1981) originally described the use of a low-voltage diathermy loop both as a means of investigating and treating CIN. He used a small loop with a diameter of 0.5 cm to remove the transformation zone in strips. Prendiville *et al.* (1986) compared the technique with punch biopsy forceps as a method of obtaining biopsies. Prendiville *et al.* (1989) introduced the technique of 'large loop excision of the transformation zone' (LLETZ) in which a large diathermy loop was used to remove the transformation zone in one or two pieces. Low-voltage diathermy was applied via a Valley Lab generator.

Use of LLETZ allowed outpatient excisional biopsy treatment. The technique was carried out with comfort and speed, with the cervical tissue available for full histological appraisal and diagnosis. Another approach was that of Luesley *et al.* (1990) who advocated loop diathermy for the clinically abnormal cervix at the first visit to a colposcopy clinic. This scheme reduced the number of patient visits, but could result in about 25% of cases being over treated (Giles and Gafar, 1991).

Other treatments

Other treatment modalities included antibiotics which were advocated in the 1950s, and human leukocyte interferon or folic acid supplementation in the 1980s. Contraceptive barrier techniques appeared helpful both in prevention, and regression of CIN. Some cases of CIN regressed following biopsy, and up to 70% regressed spontaneously without treatment.

MICROINVASIVE CARCINOMA

Mestwerdt (1947) introduced the term 'microcarcinoma'. The term described tumours invading not more than 5 mm into the cervical stroma. Conservative treatment by cone biopsy or hysterectomy evolved for this form of disease as it was recognized that involvement of the parametrium and lymphatics was rare. However, great caution was necessary in properly diagnosing the disorder as lesions with deeper stromal involvement were not so readily cured.

Boyes *et al.* (1970) indicated that microinvasive carcinoma behaved in similar fashion to carcinoma *in situ*, and required follow up whether the patient had hysterectomy or not. It was estimated that 2% of patients would develop further disease in 5 years, and over 8% in 10 years.

TREATMENT OF INVASIVE CERVICAL CANCER

The Greeks recorded the use of local fumigation therapy for symptomatic relief. Aetius of Amida (6th century AD) used vaginal irrigation with herbal compounds, and baths or poultices to alleviate pain and discomfort. Various non-surgical techniques including tumour injection with extract of nightshade were described by Astruc in 1762. In the nineteenth century application of leeches, red hot cautery, or caustics was favoured.

Surgery

Ambroise Paré recommended cervical amputation and Nikolaas Tulpius of Amsterdam first recorded its use in 1652. Frederich Benjamin Osiander of Gottingen amputated the carcinomatous vaginal portion of the uterus in eight cases between 1801 and 1808 (Ricci, 1950). Conrad Langenbeck may have been the first to carry out vaginal hysterectomy for the treatment of cervical cancer in 1813, and by the mid-1850s 25 authentic cases had been reported (Shingleton and Orr, 1987).

Prior to 1850, the main form of treatment was by cervical cautery. Electrocautery was introduced later in the century and was popular. Another approach was that of the 'ecraseur' which was used to perform cervical amputations. This was an instrument with a snare device to place around the tumour. By tightening a screw, the snare cut through and eventually amputated the ensnared part. Surgical amputation by dissection was popularized by Dr Marion Sims (1879). He removed all palpable tumour and used cotton wool soaked in sulphate of iron to achieve haemostasis. Four or 5 days later the cotton wool was removed and cotton balls soaked in zinc of chloride were substituted for a further 5 days.

Freund (1878) described treatment by total abdominal hysterectomy. He used anaesthesia and antisepsis, and also attempted adequate haemostasis. McGraw (1879) was aware of the poor outcome of limited surgery and recommended a more extensive procedure. Ries (1895) experimented with the dissection of cadavers and animals, and showed the feasibility of total hysterectomy combined with pelvic lymphadenectomy and excision of the broad ligaments. In the same year, J.G. Clark (1895) reported his radical hysterectomies for cervical cancer in the *Johns Hopkins Hospital Bulletin*. Each of 12 operations performed by him differed slightly. In some the lymph nodes were removed, and in others the parametrium and a vaginal cuff were removed.

Ernst Wertheim (q.v. in Biographies) of Vienna developed a radical procedure of total hysterectomy with removal of pelvic lymph nodes and the parametrium in 1898 (Wertheim, 1900) and reported his first 270 cases 7 years later (Wertheim, 1905). The operative mortality rate exceeded 18% and there were significant surgical complications in 31%. The pelvic lymph nodes were removed if enlarged or suspicious for metastases. Schauta (1902) developed radical vaginal hysterectomy in 1901, and the operation was found to have lower operative mortality, compared to the abdominal approach.

In the late nineteenth century the postoperative mortality in patients treated by hysterectomy was such that Dr Reeves Jackson of Chicago was prompted to state that hysterectomy for cancer of the cervix was 'scarcely more than an ante-mortem examination' (Speert, 1980). Due to the high operative mortality rate for surgical procedures, and the emerging use of radium therapy there was a temporary abandonment of surgical treatment.

Although the surgical approach was out of favour, Victor Bonney (q.v. in Biographies) modified the Wertheim technique and performed 483 radical operations from 1907. During his series the operative mortality rate fell to 9.5%, with a 5-year cure rate of 20%. F.J. Taussig (1943) reported combined therapy with surgery and radiation. He documented an operative mortality rate of 1.7% and a 5-year survival rate of 38.6% which was superior to the use of radiation alone. J.V. Meigs (1944) of the USA was aware of the complications of radiation and described a modified Wertheim's operation with removal of all pelvic nodes. He reported a 5-year survival rate of 75% for stage 1 disease. His figures for survival and postoperative complications compared favourably with radiation therapy.

Brunschwig (1948) pioneered pelvic exenteration for advanced and recurrent carcinoma of the pelvis, an operation which he first performed in 1946. The operation consisted of total removal of the uterus, cervix, vagina and the adjacent pelvic organs, with urinary and faecal diversion. A later development was the addition of hemipelvectomy or removal of some part of the bony pelvis when those structures were affected by disease. Exenterative surgery was used for both advanced primary pelvic carcinoma and recurrent disease but was contraindicated if there was evidence of distant metastases. Buchsbaum and White (1973) devised an omental sling for pelvic floor management following the exenteration and Stanley Way (1974) introduced a 'sac technique' using flaps of peritoneum to form a sac to hold the entire bowel content above the pelvic brim postoperatively. In the years which followed, many improvements were introduced including better preoperative patient assessment; increased awareness of ureteric damage; and improved anaesthetic and postoperative care.

Prior to treatment, all cases required accurate evaluation and from 1971 were classified according to recommendations of the International Federation of Gynaecology and Obstetrics (FIGO) on clinical staging of carcinoma of the cervix.

Radiotherapy

Wilhelm Conrad von Roentgen (q.v. in Chapter 36) discovered 'a new kind of ray' in 1895 which he called X-rays and his discovery earned him the first Nobel Prize 6 years later. X-rays were soon used in the diagnosis of fractures and other complaints, while their first therapeutic benefit was found in dermatology. X-ray therapy was applied to cervical cancer and initial treatment was applied by the use of intravaginal cones. Marie and Pierre Curie discovered radium in 1889. Margaret

Cleaves (1903) and also Danysz first used radium as a treatment modality for cervical cancer (Shingleton and Orr, 1987). Following further work on the radioactive metallic element by Madame Curie at the Sorbonne, in 1910, the use of radium became more widespread. Three main centres developed their own techniques for administering radium. The first Radium Hospital was the Radiumhemmet, Stockholm, which opened in 1910. Their method of intracavitary radium was developed from 1910 to 1914. The Paris method evolved at the Curie Foundation in 1919. The Manchester system began in 1933 and was further developed by Tod and Meredith (1938) and Fletcher et al. (1953). The use of external beam radiotherapy developed in the 1920s and 1930s when X-ray equipment which generated higher energy was introduced. Supervoltage cobalt units became available in the late 1950s and 1960s while linear accelerators were developed thereafter.

The discovery that hypoxic cells were resistant to radiation led to the development of methods for radiosensitization of such cells. Churchill-Davidson et al. (1955) developed a hyperbaric oxygen technique. Promising results were obtained initially, but there was an increase in normal tissue damage due to an overall increase in radiation effect. Adams et al. (1976) investigated the use of chemical agents as hypoxic cell sensitizers. The drug misonidazole was the first to have large-scale clinical testing, but was found to be neurotoxic.

Chemotherapy

Cervical cancer was found to be chemosensitive and remissions were produced in patients with advanced disease. It was believed that chemotherapeutic agents had a role to play in the management of the patient prior to surgery or radiotherapy.

OTHER CANCERS OF THE CERVIX

Adenocarcinoma was found to account for 5–10% of cases. Adenoid cystic carcinoma, sarcomas, mixed mesodermal tumours, lymphomas and malignant melanomas were reported. Secondary tumours were rarely encountered. Adenocarcinoma in situ was recognized in the mid-1950s. It was found to occur in patients who were 15–18 years younger than those with invasive adenocarcinoma. The condition was found to metastasize more quickly to the local lymph nodes and was more resistant to radiotherapy compared to squamous carcinoma.

CHRONOLOGY

Introduction

1700 BC	The Edwin Smith Papyrus mentioned uterine cancer.
400 BC	Hippocrates was aware of the condition.
	The Hindus described tumours of the uterus.
75 BC	Philoxenus wrote on tumours, including those of the womb.
2nd C. AD	Galen signified a bad prognosis for the disease.
6th C. AD	Aetius of Amida with Archigenes categorized ulcerative and non-ulcerative types.
16th C.	Ambroise Paré advised cervical amputation.
1652	Nikolaas Tulpius first performed amputation of the cervix.
1762	Jean Astruc described the disease.
19th C.	Virchow and other workers documented the gross and microscopic appearances of cervical cancer.

References: Shingleton and Orr (1987); Mettler (1947); Jameson (1936)

Epidemiology

1842	Domenico Rigoni-Stern of Verona discovered the rarity of the condition in unmarried women and nuns.
1863	Virchow related sexual behaviour to the onset of the disease.
1904	Weinberg and Gastpar related social class and parity.
1906	Vineberg noted a lower incidence in Jewish women.
1936	Handley proposed that the uncircumcised male was causative.
1962	Rotkin and King implicated early age of first coitus.
1973	Rotkin reviewed the epidemiological studies on cervical cancer.
	Singer proposed the concept of the 'high risk male' (1973a).

Aetiology

1949	Ayre described cellular changes induced by human papillomavirus and suggested a link with neoplasia.
1962	Reid proposed a role for *Chlamydia*.
1969	Naib *et al.* implicated the herpes simplex virus type 2.
1970	Coppleson proposed a carcinogenic action for sperm DNA.
1970s	Cytomegalovirus, diethlystilboestrol, and immunosuppression were blamed.

Cytology

Early discoveries in cytology

1831	Alfred Donné was one of the first to carry out cytological studies.
1838	Johannes Muller was considered the initiator of clinical cytology.
1843	Julius Vogel reported two diagnoses based on exfoliative cytology.
	Gluge studied cytological samples from cancer tissue.
1847	Pouchet studied vaginal secretions.
1849	Bennett examined ascitic fluid.
1853	Donaldson described cancer cells in body fluids.
1856	Lambl diagnosed uterine carcinoma by cytology.
1858	Rudolph Virchow wrote his *Cellular Pathology*....
1861	Beale compared cytology with histology of tumours.
1871	Richardson recommended cytological study of ulcerated growths.
1886	Friedlander recommended cytology in carcinoma of the uterus.
1897	Amann included illustrations of uterine cancer cells in his publication.

Modern cytology

1917	Stockard and Papanicolaou reported studies on the oestrous cycle in animals.
1927	Daniel and Babes reported their study of cervico-vaginal cytology.
1928	Viana reported the first clinical trial of cervical cytology.

	Papanicolaou reported tumour cells in vaginal aspirates.
1941	Papanicolaou and Traut reported on the value of vaginal smears in the diagnosis of carcinoma of the uterus.
1943	Papanicolaou and Traut produced their monograph *Diagnosis of Uterine Cancer by the Vaginal Smear*.
1947	Ayre introduced the cervical scrape using a wooden spatula.
1954	Papanicolaou proposed a cytological classification.

Cervical cytology screening

1948	Lombard *et al.*, and also McSweeney and McKay of Massachusetts, introduced the first (limited) screening programmes.
1947	The British Columbia large-scale screening service was introduced.
1966	Cervical cytology screening was initiated in the UK.

False-negative and false-positive cytology

1956	Anderson found a false-positive rate of 12% and a false-negative of less than 1%.
1962	Reagan and Patten demonstrated that 10% of smears were either under- or overcalled when compared to histopathology results.

Colposcopy

1925	Hans Hinselmann of Hamburg constructed the first colposcope.
	Hinselmann used acetic acid to coagulate cervical mucus.
1928	Schiller introduced the Lugol's iodine technique.
1932	Ries used the colposcope in the USA.
1939	Kraatz pioneered use of the green filter.
1949	Wespi introduced a classification of colposcopic findings.
1954	Hinselmann documented his classification.
1963	Koller described the saline technique.
1966	Johannison *et al.* suggested a grading system based on intercapillary distance.

Histopathology

Premalignancy

1838/40	Johannes Muller pioneered histo-pathology of tumours.
1858	Rudolph Virchow described epithelioma of the cervix.
1886	Sir John Williams described a lesion later known as carcinoma *in situ*.
1900	Cullen described histopathology of intraepithelial neoplasia. Other reports came from Schauenstein (1908), Pronai (1909), Rubin (1910), and Schottlander and Kermauner (1912).
1932	Broders replaced previous terminology with carcinoma *in situ*.
1953	Reagan *et al.* introduced the term 'dysplasia'.
1966–73	Richart introduced the cervical intraepithelial neoplasia (CIN) terminology.

Malignancy

1930s	Broders introduced the histological classification.
1947	Mestwerdt introduced the term 'microcarcinoma'.
1957	The classification of Reagan *et al.* was adopted by the World Health Organization.

Treatment of CIN

Biopsy

1845	Bennett described a cervical biopsy technique.
1878	Ruge and Veit recorded their use of cervical biopsy.
1944	Te Linde and Galvin described a series of cases in which preinvasive carcinoma was diagnosed by biopsy.
1960	Takeuchi and McKay reported that due to their size more than one-third of intraepithelial neoplasia cases could have been cured by a single biopsy. As such the diagnostic procedure was therapeutic, and could also be the cause of many reported spontaneous regressions.

Cone biopsy

1815	Lisfranc first described the technique.

1938	Martzloff referred to cone biopsy.
1960	Scott *et al.* described cold knife conization.
1961	Wagner found a 17% cytological recurrence.
1966	Green advocated conization for 'microinvasive' carcinoma.
1976	Kolstad and Klem reported the long-term follow up of 1120 patients with carcinoma *in situ*, of whom 795 had therapeutic cone biopsy. There was recurrence in 2.3%, and 0.9% developed invasive cancer.
1979	Dorsey and Diggs established the technique of laser excision cone biopsy. Jones *et al.* reported a case–control study of pregnancy outcome after cone biopsy. Women who had previously undergone cone biopsy were five times as likely to have a preterm delivery and twice as likely to have an infant under 2.5 kg.
1981	Coppleson reviewed the world literature.
1982	Singer and Walker advised that due to its complications cone biopsy should not be used to treat all precancer lesions of the cervix.

Laser

1960	The first ruby medical laser was developed by Theodore H. Maiman.
1964	Carbon dioxide laser was introduced by Platel.
1975	Stafl began work with the carbon dioxide laser.
1976	Toaff described laser cone biopsy.
1977	Stafl *et al.*, and also Bellina, used the laser for treatment of CIN.
1979	Dorsey and Diggs described laser conization under colposcopic control.
1982	Jordan and Mylotte reported that the depth of destruction should reach 5–7 mm. With such techniques a cure rate in the region of 96% for selected patients could be expected.

Cryocautery

1970	Crisp *et al.* reported the technique, already in use by them.
1971	Crisp reported a depth of destruction

of 5–6 mm for double freeze cryotherapy.

1973	Creasman *et al.* reported low success rates.
1981	Wright and Davies compared cryotherapy and laser, using historical controls.
1980	Creasman and Wood reported significant vaginal discharge post-treatment.
1982	Singer and Walker advised against the use of cryocautery for CIN 3.
1983	Townsend and Richart found no difference in cure rates between cryocautery and laser therapy.
1983	Figge and Creasman found that an effective double freeze technique produced better results.

Electrocautery/electrodiathermy

1949	Younge *et al.* reported successful use of the technique.
1968	Richart and Sciarra reported early experience with the modality.
1971	Chanen and Hollyock reported their experiences.
1976	Hollyock and Chanen reported radical electrodiathermy – the cervix was coagulated initially by multiple punctures with a needle electrode to a depth of 1.5 cm into the cervical stroma.
1983	Chanen and Rome reported their experience of 1864 patients of whom 64% had CIN 3. Their overall cure rate was 97%.

Semm's cold coagulator

1966	Kurt Semm introduced the instrument.
1978	Staland used cold coagulation for premalignant lesions.
1983	Duncan popularized cold coagulation in the UK (1983a,b).
1991	Gordon and Duncan reported on 14 years of experience of the treatment.

Diathermy loop

1981	Cartier *et al.* pioneered the diathermy loop.
1989	Prendiville popularized large loop excision of the transformation zone.

1990	Luesley *et al.* introduced 'a see and treat' policy.

Treatment of invasive cervical cancer

Surgery

1652	Nikolaas Tulpius used cervical amputation, first recommended by Ambroise Paré (Way, 1951); (Shingleton and Orr, 1987).
1801–1808	Frederich Osiander amputated cervical cancer in eight cases. (Cianfrani, 1960).
1813	Conrad Langenbeck performed vaginal hysterectomy to treat the condition.
1878	Freund documented the use of abdominal hysterectomy.
1879	Dr Marion Sims detailed cases of cervical amputation.
1895	Ries advised hysterectomy with pelvic lymphadenectomy. J.G. Clark reported radical hysterectomy.
1900	Ernst Wertheim developed radical abdominal hysterectomy.
1902	Schauta pioneered radical vaginal hysterectomy.
1907	Victor Bonney began a series of 483 radical abdominal operations. (Bonney, 1941;1949).
1943	Taussig combined surgery and radiation.
1944	J.V. Meigs described radical abdominal hysterectomy with removal of all pelvic lymph nodes.
1948	Brunschwig pioneered pelvic exenteration.
1971	The FIGO clinical staging was introduced.
1973	Buchsbaum and White developed an omental sling for the postexenterative patient.
1974	Stanley Way introduced a sac technique to hold bowel contents above the pelvic brim.

Radiotherapy

1889	Marie and Pierre Curie discovered radium.
1895	Wilhelm Conrad von Roentgen discovered X-rays.
1903	Cleaves, and also Danysz (Shingleton and Orr, 1987) used radium as treatment for cervical cancer.
1910	The Radiumhemmet opened in Stockholm.
1919	The Curie Foundation evolved its treatment method.
1933	The Manchester System began.
1955	Churchill-Davidson *et al.* developed hyperbaric oxygen techniques with radiotherapy.

REFERENCES

Adams, G.E., Fowler, J.F., Dische, S. and Thomlison, R.H. (1976). Hypoxic cell sensitizers in radiotherapy. *Lancet*, **1**, 186–8.

Albrecht, T. and Rapp, F. (1973). Malignant transformation of hamster embryo fibroblasts following exposure to ultraviolet irradiated human cytomegalovirus. *Virology*, **55**, 53–61

Amann, J.A. Jr. (1897). *Kurzgefaßtes Lehrbuch der mikroskopisch-gynakologischen Diagnostik*. (Wiesbaden: J.F. Bergmann Verlag)

Anderson, A.F. (1950). The diagnosis of early carcinoma of the cervix and its implications. *J. Obstet. Gynaecol. Br. Emp.*, **57**, 1–9

Anderson, A.F. (1956). Cytology in the diagnosis of carcinoma of the cervix. *J. Obstet. Gynaecol. Br. Emp.*, **63**, 439–48

Anderson, A.F. (1962). New inventions: the Vann-Watson colposcope. *Lancet*, **2**, 813–14

Ashley, D.J.B. (1966). Evidence for the existence of two forms of cervical carcinoma. *J. Obstet. Gynaecol. Br. Cwlth.*, **73**, 382–9

Astruc, J. (1762). *A treatise on the diseases of Women*. (Translated from the French original and printed in London for J. Nocuse.)

Aurelian, L., Strandberg, J.D., Melendez, L.V. and Johnson, L.A. (1971). Herpesvirus type 2 isolated from cervical tumor cells grown in tissue culture. *Science*, **174**, 704–7

Ayre, J.E. (1944). A simple office test for uterine cancer diagnosis. *Canad. Med. Assoc. J.*, **51**, 17

Ayre, J.E. (1946). Vaginal and cervical cytology in uterine cancer diagnosis. *Am. J. Obstet. Gynecol.*, **51**, 143

Ayre, J.E. (1947). Selective cytology smear for

diagnosis of cancer. *Am. J. Obstet. Gynecol.*, **53/54**, 609

Ayre, J.E. (1949). The vaginal smear: 'precancer' cell studies using a modified technique. *Am. J. Obstet. Gynecol.*, **58**, 1205–19

Ayre, J.E. (1950). Pregnancy following cervical cancer: a report of 2 cases treated in a pre-invasive stage. *Surg. Gynecol. Obstet.*, **90**, 298–304

Babes, A. (1928). Diagnostic du cancer du col uterin par les frottis. *La Presse Medicale*, **36**, 451. (Reprinted in translation in *Acta Cytologica* (1967) **11**, 217)

Baillie, M. (1793). *Engravings of Morbid Anatomy.* (London: W.Bulmer & Co.)

Beale, L.S. (1861). Results of the chemical and microscopical examination of solid organs and secretions. Examination of sputum from a case of cancer of the pharynx and the adjacent parts. *Arch. Med. (London)*, **2**, 44

Bellina, J.H. (1977). Carbon dioxide laser in gynecology. *Obstet. Gynecol. Ann.*, **6**, 371

Benedet, J.L. and Boyes, D.A. (1976). Colposcopic evaluation of patients with abnormal cervical cytology. *Br. J. Obstet. Gynaecol.*, **83**, 177–82

Bennett, J.H. (1845). Introductory address to a course of lectures on histology and the use of the microscope. *Lancet*, **1**, 517–22

Bennett, J.H. (1849). *On Cancerous and Cancroid Growths.* (Edinburgh: Sutherland and Knox)

Berget, A. (1979). Influence of population screening on morbidity and mortality of cancer of the uterine cervix in Maribo Amt (Denmark). *Danish Med. Bull.*, **26**, 91–100

Blythe-Smith, D. and Jenkins, R. (1969). Cervical cancer in a housing project: report of a cluster of cases. *Am. J. Obstet. Gynecol.*, **104**, 603–5

Bolten, K.A. and Jacques, W.E. (1960). *Introduction to Colposcopy.* (New York: Grune and Stratton)

Bonney, V. (1941). The results of 55 cases of Wertheim's operation for carcinoma of the cervix. *J. Obstet. Gynaecol. Br. Emp.*, **48**, 421

Bonney, V. (1949). Wertheim's operation in retrospect. *Lancet*, **1**, 637

Boyes, D.A., Fidler, H.K. and Lock, D.R. (1962). Significance of *in situ* carcinoma of the uterine cervix. *Br. Med. J.*, **1**, 203

Boyes, D.A., Worth, A.J. and Fidler, H.K. (1970). The results of treatment of 4389 cases of preclinical cervical squamous carcinoma. *J. Obstet. Gynaecol. Br. Cwlth.*, **77**, 769–80

Boyes, D.A., Morrison, B., Knox, E.G., Draper, G.J. and Miller, A.B. (1982). A cohort study of cervical cancer screening in British Columbia. *Clin. Invest. Med.*, **5**, 1–29

Bret, A.J. and Coupez, F. (1960). *Colposcopie.* (Paris: Masson)

Broders, A.C. (1932). Carcinoma *in situ* contrasted with benign penetrating epithelium. *J. Am. Med. Assoc.*, **99**, 1670–4

Broussais, F.J.V. (1826). *Histoire des Phlegmasies ou Inflammations Chroniques*, 4th edn. (Paris), quoted by Kessler (1974) p. 173

Brunschwig, A. (1948). Complete excision of pelvic viscera for advanced carcinoma. *Cancer*, **1**, 177–83

Buchsbaum, H.J. and White, A.J. (1973). Omental sling for management of the pelvic floor following exenteration. *Am. J. Obstet. Gynecol.*, **117**, 407–12

Buckley, J.D., Harris, R.W. and Doll, R. (1981). Case control study of the husbands of women with dysplasia and carcinoma of the cervix uteri. *Lancet*, **2**, 1010–12

Buckley, C.H., Butler, E.B. and Fox, M. (1982). Cervical intraepithelial neoplasia. *J. Clin. Pathol.*, **35**, 1–13

Burghardt, E. and Albeggar, H. (1969). Local infiltration for cone biopsy. *Geburts. und Frauenheilkunde*, **29**, 1–8

Burns, J. (1813). *Principles of Midwifery including the Diseases of Women and Children*, (3rd American edn. from 2nd London edn. with improvements and notes by Thomas C. James). (Philadelphia: Mathew Carey *et al.*)

Cartier, R., Sopena, B. and Cartier, I. (1981). Use of the diathermy loop in the diagnosis and treatment of lesions of the uterine cervix. [Abstract] *Proc. Int. Fed. Cervical Pathology and Colposcopy*, London

Chanen, W. and Hollyock, V.E. (1971). Colposcopy and electrocoagulation diathermy for cervical dysplasia and carcinoma *in situ*. *Obstet. Gynecol.*, **37**, 623–8

Chanen, W. and Hollyock, V.E. (1974). Colposcopy and the conservative management of cervical dysplasia and carcinoma *in situ*. *Obstet. Gynecol.*, **43**, 527–34

Chanen, W. and Rome, R.M. (1983). Electrocoagulation diathermy for cervical dysplasia and carcinoma *in situ*: a 15 year survey. *Obstet. Gynecol.*, **61**, 673–9

Chomet, J. (1987). Screening for cervical cancer: a new scope for general practitioners? Results of the first year of colposcopy in general practice. *Br. Med. J.*, **294**, 1326–8

Churchill-Davidson, I., Sanger, C. and Thomlinson, R.H. (1955). High-pressure oxygen and radiotherapy. *Lancet*, **1**, 1091–5

Cianfrani, T. (1960). *A Short History of Obstetrics and Gynecology*, p. 347. (Springfield Illinois: C.C. Thomas)

Clark, J.G. (1895). More radical method of performing hysterectomy for cancer of the uterus. *Johns Hopkins Hosp. Bull.*, **6**, 120

Cleaves, M.A. (1903). Radium: with a preliminary note on radium rays in the treatment of cancer. *Med. Rec.*, **64**, 601–10

Coppleson, M. (1970). The origin and nature of premalignant lesions of the cervix uteri. *Int. J. Gynecol. Obstet.*, **8**, 539

Coppleson, M. (1977). Colposcopy. In Stallworthy, J. and Bourne, G. (eds.) *Recent Advances in Obstetrics and Gynaecology*, no. 12 pp. 155–87. (Edinburgh, London, New York: Churchill Livingstone)

Coppleson, M. (1981). The management of cervical premalignant and malignant disease. *Gynaecological Oncology, Fundamental Principles and Clinical Practice*, p. 453. (Edinburgh: Churchill Livingstone)

Coppleson, M. and Reid, B.L. (1967). *Preclinical Carcinoma of the Cervix: Its Origin, Nature and Management*. (Oxford: Pergamon)

Creasman, W.T. and Wood, J.C. Jr. (1980). Conservative management of CIN. *Clin. Obstet. Gynecol.*, **23**, 281

Creasman, W.T., Weed, J.G. Jr., Curry, S.L., Johnston, W.W. and Parker, R.T. (1973). Efficacy of cryosurgical treatment of severe intraepithelial neoplasia. *Obstet. Gynecol.*, **41**, 501

Crisp, W.E. (1971). Cryosurgery in the treatment of abnormal cervical lesions: an invitational symposium. *J.Reprod. Med.*, **7**, 147

Crisp, W.E., Smith, M.S., Asadourian, L.A. and Warrenburg, C.B. (1970). Cryosurgical treatment of premalignant disease of the uterine cavity. *Am. J. Obstet. Gynecol.*, **107**, 737–42

Crompton, A.C. and Langley, F.A. (1973). *Epithelial Abnormalities of the Cervix Uteri*. (London: Heinemann)

Cullen, T.S. (1900). *Cancer of the Uterus*. (New York: Appleton & Co.)

Daniel, C. and Babes, A. (1927). Posibilitatea diagnosticului cancerului uterin cu ajutorul frotiului. *Proc. Bucharest Gynaecol. Soc.*, January

Dewees, W.P. (1826). *A Treatise on the Diseases of Females*. (Philadelphia: H.C. Carey & I. Lea)

Donaldson, R. (1853). The practical application of the microscope to the diagnosis of cancer. *Am. J. Med. Sci.*, **25**, 43

Donne, A. (1831). *Recherches physiologiques et chimico-microscopiques sur les Globules du Sang, du Pus, du Mucus et sur ceux des Humeurs de l'Oeil*. (Paris: Imprim. Didot le jeune)

Donne, A. (1836). Animalcules observés dans les matieres purulentes et le produit des secretions des organes genitaux de l'homme et de la femme. *C. R. Acad. Sci.*, **3**, 385

Donne, A. (1845). Cours de Microscopie complementaire des Etudes Medicales. Anatomie microscopique et Physiologie des Fluides de l'Economie. *Atlas executé d'apres Nature au Microscope-Daguerroetype*. (Paris: Bailliere)

Dorsey, J.H. (1980). Cervical conization and the CO_2 laser. In Bellina, J.H. (ed.) *Gynecologic Laser Surgery*, pp. 131–43. (New York, London: Plenum Press)

Dorsey, J.H. and Diggs, E.S. (1979). Microsurgical conization of the cervix by carbon dioxide laser. *Obstet. Gynecol.*, **54**, 565

Duncan, I. (1983a). The Semm cold coagulator in the management of cervical intraepithelial neoplasia. *Clin. Obstet. Gynecol.*, **26**, 996–1006

Duncan, I. (1983b). Recent developments in gynaecological oncology. In Morrow, C.P. (ed.) *Progress in Cancer Research and Therapy*, Vol. 24, p. 15. (New York: Raven Press)

Evans, D.M.D., Hudson, E.A., Brown, C.L., Boddington, M.M., Hughes, H.E., Mackenzie, E.F.D. and Marshall, T. (1986). Terminology in gynaecological cytopathology: report of the working party of the British Society for Clinical Cytology. *J. Clin. Pathol.*, **39**, 933–44

Feminella, J. (1973). An apparent increase in genital carcinomas amongst wives of men with prostate cancer: an epidemiological study. *Bull. Clin. Med.*, **20**, 63–7

Ferenczy, A. (1982). Cervical intraepithelial neoplasia. In Blaustein, A. (ed.) *Pathology of the Female Genital Tract*, 2nd edn. pp. 156–77. (New York, Heidelberg, Berlin: Springer–Verlag)

Fidler, F.M., Boyes, D.A. and Worth, A.J. (1968). Cervical cancer detection in British Columbia. *J. Obstet. Gynaecol. Br. Cwlth.*, **75**, 392–404

Figge, D.C. and Creasman, W.T. (1983). Cryotherapy in the treatment of cervical intraepithelial neoplasia. *Obstet. Gynecol.*, **62**, 353

Figge, D.C., Bennington, J.L. and Schweid, A.I. (1970). Cervical cancer after initial negative and atypical vaginal cytology. *Am. J. Obstet. Gynecol.*, **108**, 422–8

Fischer-Wasels, B. (1927). Metaplasie und Gewebsmißbildung. In: *Bethes: Handbuch der normalen und pathologischen Physiologie*, Bd XIV/2. (Berlin: Springer)

Fletcher, G.H., Wall, J.A., Bloedorn, F.G. *et al.* (1953). Direct measurements and isodose calculations in radium therapy of carcinoma of the cervix. *Radiology*, **61**, 885–901

Fluhmann, C.F. (1961). *The Cervix Uteri and its Diseases*, p. 129. (London: W.B. Saunders)

Franque von, O. (1901). Das beginnende Portiokankroid und die Ausbreitungswege des Gebärmutterhalskrebses. *Z. Geburtsh.*, **44**, 173

Franque von, O. (1907). Leukoplakia und Carcinoma vaginae et uteri. *Z. Geburtsh.*, **60**, 237

Freund, W.A. (1878). Eine neue Methode der Exstirpation des ganzen Uterus. *Sammlung klinischer Vortrage*, no. 133. (Gynak. no. 41; 911) Leipzig.

Friedlander, C. (1886). *Microskopische Technik zum Gebrauch bei medicinischen und pathologisch-anatomischen Untersuchungen 3 Aufl.* (Berlin: Fischer)

Gagnon, F. (1950). Contributions to the study of the etiology and prevention of cervical cancer. *Am. J. Obstet. Gynecol.*, **60**, 516–22

Galvin, G.A., Jones, H.W. and TeLinde, R.W. (1955). The significance of basal cell hyperactivity in cervical biopsies. *Am. J. Obstet. Gynecol.*, **70**, 808–21

Giles, J.A. and Gafar, A. (1991). The treatment of CIN: do we need lasers?. *Br. J. Obstet. Gynaecol.*, **98**, 3–6

Giscard d'Estaing, V.A. (1990). *The Book of Inventions and Discoveries*, p. 179. (London: Queen Anne Press, MacDonald & Co.)

Gluge, G. (1843). *Atlas der Pathologischen Anatomie.* (Jena: Mauke)

Gordon, H.K. and Duncan, I.D. (1991). Effective destruction of CIN 111 at 100 degrees C using the Semm cold coagulator: 14 years experience. *Br. J. Obstet. Gynaecol.*, **98**, 14–20

Green, G.H. (1966). The significance of cervical carcinoma *in situ*. *Am. J. Obstet. Gynecol.*, **94**, 1009–22

Hakama, M. (1978). Mass screening for cervical cancer in Finland. In Muller, A.B. (ed.) *Report of a UICC International Workshop, Toronto*, UICC Technical Report Series **40**, 9080–682, pp. 93–107

Handley, W.S. (1936). The prevention of cancer. *Lancet*, **1**, 987–91

Herbst, A.L., Ulfelder, H. and Poskanzer, D.C. (1971). Adenocarcinoma of the vagina: association of maternal stilbestrol therapy with tumor appearance in young woman. *N. Engl. J. Med.*, **284**, 878–81

Hertig, A.T. (1979). Early concepts of dysplasia and carcinoma *in situ* (a backward glance at a forward process): a brief historical review. *Obstet. Gynecol. Surv.*, **34**, 795

Hinselmann, H. (1925). Verbesserung der Inspektionsmöglichkeiten von Vulva, Vagina und Portio. *Munch. Med. Wchnschr.*, 1733

Hinselmann, H. (1930). Die Ätiologie. Symptomatologie und Diagnostik des Uteruscarcinoms. In Veit-Stockel: *Handbuch der Gynakologie Bd 6/1* 854. (Munchen: Bergmann)

Hinselmann, H. (1933). Ausgewahlte Gesichtspunkte zur Beurteilung des Zusammenhanges der Matrixbezirke und des

Karzinoms der sichtbaren Abschnitte des weiblichen Genitaltraktes. *Z. Geburtsh.*, **104**, 228

Hinselmann, H. (1934). Die klinische und mikroskopische Frühdiagnose des Portiokarzinoms. *Arch. Gynakol.*, **156**, 239

Hinselmann, H. (1936). Die Kolposkopie. In *Klinische Fortbildung. Neue Deutsche Klinik 4*, Erganzungsbd 717

Hinselmann, H. (1938). *14 Jahre Kolposkopie. Ein Rueckblick und Ausblick. Hippokrates (D)* 661, quoted by Wespi (1949) p. 91

Hinselmann, H. (1954). *Die Kolposkopie.* (Wuppertal-Elberfeld: Girardet)

Hollyock, V.E. and Chanen, W. (1976). Electrocoagulation diathermy for the treatment of cervical dysplasia and carcinoma *in situ. Obstet. Gynecol.*, **47**, 196

Holmquist, N.D. (1987). Letter: 'Squamous atypia' of the uterine cervix. *Acta Cytol.*, **31**, 201–2

Hudson, E.A. (1990). Cytological terminology. *Br. J. Obstet. Gynaecol.*, **97**, 202–4

Hulka, B.S. (1968). Cytologic and histologic outcome following an atypical cervical smear. *Am. J. Obstet. Gynecol.*, **101**, 190–9

Intercollegiate Working Party (1987). *Report on Cervical Cytology Screening.* (London: RCOG)

Jackson, R. (1988). *Doctors and Diseases in the Roman Empire*, p. 30. (London: British Museum Publications)

Jameson, E. (ed.) (1936). *Clio Medica, Gynecology and Obstetrics.* (New York: Paul B. Heober)

Johannison, E., Kolstad, P. and Soderberg, (1966). Cytologic, vascular and histologic patterns of dysplasia, carcinoma *in situ* and early invasive carcinoma of the cervix. *Acta Radiologica*, Suppl. 258

Johannesson, G., Geirson, G., Day, N. and Tulinius, H. (1982). Screening for cancer of the uterine cervix in Iceland 1965–1978. *Acta Obstet. Gynecol. Scand.*, **61**, 199–203

Jones, C.A., Neustaedter, T. and MacKenzie, L.L. (1945). The value of vaginal smears in the diagnostic of early malignancy. *Am. J. Obstet. Gynecol.*, **49**, 159

Jones, J.M., Sweetman, P. and Hibbard, B.M. (1979). The outcome of pregnancy after cone

biopsy of the cervix: a case control study. *Br. J. Obstet. Gynaecol.*, **86**, 913

Jordan, J.A. (1969). Cancer of the cervix uteri with particular reference to cytology. *Practitioner,* **202**, 351–62

Jordan, J.A. (1972). Colposcopy in gynaecological practice. In Jakob, C.A. and Franco, M.A. (eds.) *Proceedings of the First World Congress of Colposcopy and Cervical Pathology*, pp. 131–7. (Rosario, Argentina: Molachino Establecimiento Grafico)

Jordan, J.A. (1976). The diagnosis and management of premalignant conditions of the cervix. In Langley, F.A. (ed.) *Cancer of the Vulva, Vagina and Uterus. Clinics in Obstetrics and Gynaecology*, Vol. 3 p. 311. (London, Philadelphia, Toronto: W.B. Saunders Co. Ltd)

Jordan, J.A. (1988). Minor degrees of cervical intraepithelial neoplasia. Time to establish a multicentre prospective study to resolve the question. *Br. Med. J.*, **297**, 6

Jordan, J.A. and Mylotte, M.J. (1982). Treatment of CIN by destruction – laser. In Jordan, J.A., Sharp, F. and Singer, A. (eds.) *Preclinical Neoplasia of the Cervix, Proceedings of the 9th Study Group of the RCOG*, October 1981, pp. 205–11. (London: Royal College of Obstetricians and Gynaecologists)

Kaiser, R.F., Bouser, M.M., Ingraham, S.C., II and Hilberg, A.W. (1960). *Public Health Report (Washington)*, **75**, 423, quoted by Lewis (1964) pp. 539–48

Kaplan, I., Goldman, J. and Ger, R. (1973). The treatment of erosion of the uterine cervix by use of the CO_2 laser. *Obstet. Gynecol.*, **41**, 794

Kaufmann, R.H., Koss, L.G., Kurman, R.J. *et al.* (1983). Statement of caution in the interpretation of papillomavirus – associated lesions of the epithelium of the uterine cervix. *Acta Cytol.*, **27**, 107–8

Kennaway, E.L. (1948). The racial and social incidence of cancer of the uterus. *Br. J. Cancer*, **2**, 177–93

Kessler, I.I. (1974). Cervical cancer. Epidemiology in historical perspecive. *J. Reprod. Med.*, **12**(5), 173–85

Kessler, I.I. (1976). Human cervix cancer as a venereal disease. *Cancer Res.*, **36**, 738–40

Kessler, I.I. and Aurelian, L. (1974). *Cervical Cancer:*

Problem, Progress, Prospects. (Berlin, New York: Springer-Verlag)

Kitchener, H.C., Burnett, R.A., Wilson, E.S.B. and Cordiner, J.W. (1987). Colposcopy in a family planning clinic: a future model? *Br. Med. J.*, **294**, 1313–15

Koller, O. (1963). *The Vascular Patterns of the Uterine Cervix.* (Oslo: Universitetsforlaget)

Kolstad, P. (1964). *Vascularisation, Oxygen Tension and Radiocurability in Cancer of the Cervix.* (Oslo: Universitetsforlaget)

Kolstad, P. and Klem, V. (1976). Long term follow-up of 1121 cases of carcinoma *in situ. Obstet. Gynecol.*, **48**, 125

Kolstad, P. and Stafl, A. (1972). *Atlas of Colposcopy.* (Oslo: Universitetsforlaget)

Koss, L.G. (1983). Papanicolaou's 100th Birthday (editorial). *Acta Cytol.*, **27**, 217–19

Koss, L.G. and Durfee, G.R. (1956). Unusual patterns of squamous epithelium of uterine cervix: cytologic and pathologic study of koilocytotic atypia. *Ann. N. Y. Acad. Sci.*, **63**, 1235–61

Koss, L.G., Stewart, F.W., Foote, F.W., Jordan, M.J., Bader, G.M. and Day, E. (1963). Some histological aspects of behaviour of epidermoid carcinoma *in situ* and related lesions of the uterine cervix: a long-term prospective study. *Cancer*, **16**, 1160–211

Kottmeier, H.L. (1961). Evolution et traitment des epitheliomas. *Rev. Franc. Gynecol. d'Obstet.*, **56**, 821–6

Kraatz, H. (1939). Farbfiltervorschaltung zur leichteren Erlernung der Kolposkopie. *Zbl. Gynakol.*, 2307

Lambl, W. Dr. (1856). Uber Harnblasenkrebs *Prager Viertelj. schr. f. Heilkunde*, **49**, 1

Lancet (1985). Cancer of the cervix – death by incompetence, editorial. *Lancet*, **2**, 363–4

Lang, W.R. (1956). Colposcopy and diagnosis of early carcinoma of cervix. C.A. *A Bulletin of Cancer Progress*, **6**, 205–7

Lewis, T.L.T. (1964). *Progress in Clinical Obstetrics and Gynaecology*, 2nd edn. (London: J. & A. Churchill)

Lisfranc, J. (1815). *Gaz. Med. France*, **2**, 835

Lombard, H.L., Middleton, M., Wallren, S. and

Gates, O. (1948). Use of the vaginal smear as a screening test. *N. Engl. J. Med.*, **238**, 867

Luesley, D.M., Cullimore, J., Redman, C.W.E., Lawton, F.G., Emens, J.M., Rollason, T.P. and Williams, D.R. (1990). Loop diathermy excision of the cervical transformation zone in patients with abnormal cervical smears. *Br. Med. J.*, **300**, 1690–3

Luthra, U.K., Prabhaker, A.K., Seth, P., Agarwal, S.S., Murphy, N.S., Bhatnager, P., Das, D.K. and Sharma, B.K. (1987). Natural history of precancerous and early cancerous lesions of the uterine cervix. *Acta Cytol.*, **31**, 226–34

McGraw, T.A. (1879). Cases of operations for cancer of the womb. *Michigan Medical News*, **2**, 98

MacGregor, J.E. (1964). Cancer diagnosis. *Br. Med. J.*, **2**, 754

McIndoe, W.A., McLean, M.R., Jones, R.W. and Mullins, P.R. (1984). The invasive potential of carcinoma *in situ* of the cervix. *Obstet. Gynecol.*, **64**, 451–8

McKay, W.J.S. (1901). *The History of Ancient Gynaecology.* (London: Balliere-Tindall Cox)

McLaren, H.C. (1960). The treatment of carcinoma *in situ. Extrait de Acta Union Internationale Contre le Cancer*, **16**, 385

McLaren, H.C. and Attwood, M.E. (1961). Methods of diagnosing cervical carcinoma *in situ. Br. Med. J.*, **2**, 4

McLaren, H.C., Jordan, J.A., Glover, M. and Attwood, M.E. (1974). Pregnancy after cone biopsy of the cervix. *J. Obstet. Gynaecol. Br. Cwlth.*, **81**, 383–4

McSweeney, D.J. and McKay, D. (1948). Uterine cancer: its detection by simple screening methods. *N. Engl. J. Med.*, **238**, 867–70

Marsh, M. and Fitzgerald, P.J. (1956). Carcinoma *in situ* of the human uterine cervix in pregnancy. *Cancer*, **9**, 1195–207

Martinez, I. (1969). Relationship of squamous cell carcinoma of the cervix to squamous cell carcinoma of the penis. *Cancer*, **24**, 777–80

Martzloff, K.H. (1938). Cancer of the cervix uteri: recognition of early manifestations. *J. Am. Med. Assoc.*, **111**, 1921–4

Meigs, J.V. (1944). Radical hysterectomy with bilateral pelvic lymph node dissection. Report of

100 cases operated on 5 years or more. *Am. J. Obstet. Gynecol.*, **62**, 854

Meigs, J.V., Graham, R.M., Fremont-Smith, M., Kapnick, I. and Rawson, R. (1943). The value of the vaginal smear in the diagnosis of uterine cancer. *Surg. Gynecol. Obstet.*, **77**, 449

Meisels, A. and Fortin, R. (1976). Condylomatous lesions of the cervix and vagina. I. Cytologic patterns. *Acta Cytol. (Baltimore)*, **20**, 505–9

Mestwerdt, C. (1947). Probexcision und kolposkopie in der fruhdiagnose des portiokarcinoms. *Zbl. Gynakol.*, **4**, 326

Mettler, C. (1947). *History of Medicine.* (PA: Blakiston Co.)

Meyer, R. (1930). Die pathologische Anatomie der Gebärmutter. In Henke, F. and Lubarsch, O. (ed.) *Handbuch der Spez. pathol. Anatomie und Histologie*, vol. 7/1, pp. 1–538. (Berlin: Springer)

Muller, J. (1838). *Uber den Feineren Bau und die Formen der krankhaften Geschwülste.* (Berlin: G. Reimer)

Muller, J. (1840). *On the Nature and Structural Characteristics of Cancer and those Morbid Growths which may be Confounded with it.* (Translated by C. West). (London: Sherwood, Gilbert & Piper)

Naib, Z.M., Nahmias, A.J., Josey, W.E. and Kramer, J.H. (1969). Genital herpetic infection: association with cervical dysplasia and carcinoma. *Cancer*, **23**, 940–5

National Cancer Institute Workshop (1989). The 1988 Bethesda System for reporting cervical/vaginal cytologic diagnoses. *J. Am. Med. Assoc.*, **262**, 931–4

Noumoff, J.S. (1987). Atypia in cervical cytology as a risk factor for intraepithelial neoplasia. *Am. J. Obstet. Gynecol.*, **156**, 628–31

Novak, E. (1929). Pathologic diagnosis of early cervical and corporal cancer with special reference to the differentiation from pseudomalignant inflammatory conditions. *Am. J. Obstet. Gynecol.*, **18**, 449

O'Dowd, M.J. (1990). *What is an Inflammatory Cervical Smear?* M.D. Thesis University College, Galway

Papanicolaou, G.N. (1928). New cancer diagnosis. In *Proceedings of the 3rd Race Betterment Conference*, Battle Creek: Race Betterment Fdn., 528

Papanicolaou, G.N. (1933). The sexual cycle in the human female as revealed by vaginal smears. *Am. J. Anat.*, **52**, 519

Papanicolaou, G.N. (1942). A new procedure for staining vaginal smears. *Science*, **95**, 438

Papanicolaou, G.N. (1954). *Atlas of Exfoliative Cytology.* (Cambridge, Mass: Harvard University Press)

Papanicolaou, G. N. and Traut, H.F. (1941). The diagnostic value of vaginal smears in carcinoma of the uterus. *Am. J. Obstet. Gynecol.*, **42**, 193

Papanicolaou, G.N. and Traut, H.F. (1943). *Diagnosis of Uterine Cancer by the Vaginal Smear.* (New York: The Commonwealth Fund)

Parker, R.T., Cuyler, W.K., Kaufmann, L.A., Carter, B., Thomas, W.L., Creadick, R.N., Turner, V.H., Peete, C.H. and Cherney, W.B. (1960). Intraepithelial (stage 0) cancer of the cervix. A 13-year cumulative study of 485 patients. *Am. J. Obstet. Gynecol.*, **80**, 693–710

Peterson, O. (1956). Spontaneous course of cervical precancerous conditions. *Am. J. Obstet. Gynecol.*, **72**, 1063–71

Petterson, F., Bjorkholm, E. and Naslund, I. (1985). Evaluation of screening for cervical cancer in Sweden. Trends in incidence and mortality 1958–1980. *Int. J. Epidemiol.*, **14**, 521–7

Porecco, R., Israel, P., Droegemuller, W., Grar, B. and Makowski, E. (1975). Gynecological malignancies in immunosuppressed organ homograft recipients. *Obstet. Gynecol.*, **45**, 359–64

Pott, P. (1775). *The Chirurgical Works of Percival Pott.* (London: W. Clarke Hawes and R. Collins)

Pouchet, F.A. (1847). *Theorie positive de l'ovulation spontanée et de la fecondation des mammiferes et de l'espece humaine. Basée sur l'observation de toute la serie animale.* (Paris: J.B. Bailliere)

Prendiville, W., Cullimore, J. and Norman, S. (1989). Large loop excision of the transformation zone (LLETZ). A new method of management for women with cervical intraepithelial neoplasia. *Br. J. Obstet. Gynaecol.*, **96**, 1054–60

Prendiville, W., Sheperd, A. and Davies, W.A.R. (1986). A low voltage diathermy loop for taking cervical biopsies. A qualitative comparison with punch biopsy forceps. *Br. J. Obstet. Gynaecol.*, **93**, 773–6

Pronai, K. (1909). Zur Lehre von der Histogenese und dem Wachstum des Uteruscarcinoms. *Archiv. Gynakol.*, **89**, 596–607

Rad, M., Marczinke, I., Boyes, D.A. and Fidler, H.K. (1966). The use of exfoliative vaginal cytology in pregnancy. *Am. J. Obstet. Gynecol.*, **94**, 465–9

Rawls, W.E., Gardner, H.L. and Kaufman, R.L. (1970). Antibodies to genital herpesvirus in patients with carcinoma of the cervix. *Am. J. Obstet. Gynecol.*, **107**, 710–16

Reagan, J.W. and Patten, S.F. (1962a). Cytology and its office application as viewed by the pathologist. *Clin. Obstet. Gynecol.*, **5**, 167

Reagan, J.W. and Patten, S.F. Jr. (1962b). Dysplasia: a basic reaction to injury in the uterine cervix. *Ann. N.Y. Acad. Sci.*, **97**, 662–82

Reagan, J.W., Hamonic, M.J. and Wentz, W.B. (1957). Analytical study of the cells in cervical squamous cell carcinoma. *Lab. Invest.*, **6**, 241–50

Reagan, J.W., Seidemand, I.L. and Saracusa, Y. (1953). The cellular morphology of carcinoma *in situ* and dysplasia or atypical hyperplasia of the uterine cervix. *Cancer*, **6**, 224–35

Reid, B.L. (1962). The role of virus in the origin and progression of epithelial anomalies of the ectocervix. *Proceedings of the First International Congress on Exfoliate Cytology*, p. 62. (Philadelphia: Lippincott)

Ricci, J.V. (1945). *One Hundred Years of Gynecology.* (Philadelphia: Blakiston Co.)

Ricci, J.V. (1950). *The Genealogy of Gynaecology.* (Philadelphia: Blakiston Co.)

Richardson, J.G. (1871). *A Handbook of Medical Microscopy.* (Philadelphia: Lippincott)

Richart, R.M. (1964). The correlation of Schiller positive areas on the exposed portion of the cervix with intraepithelial neoplasia. *Am. J. Obstet. Gynecol.*, **90**, 697–701

Richart, R.M. (1966). Colpomicroscopic studies of cervical intraepithelial neoplasia. *Cancer*, **19**, 395

Richart, R.M. (1967). Natural history of cervical intraepithelial neoplasia. *Clin. Obstet. Gynecol.*, **10**, 748–84

Richart, R.M. (1973). Cervical intraepithelial neoplasia. In Sommers, S.C. (ed.) *Pathology Annual.* (New York: Appleton-Century-Crofts)

Richart, R.M. and Barron, B.A. (1969). A follow-up study of patients with cervical dysplasia. *Am. J. Obstet. Gynecol.*, **105**, 386–93

Richart, R.M. and Sciarra, J.J. (1968). Treatment of cervical dysplasia by outpatient electrocauterisation. *Am. J. Obstet. Gynecol.*, **101**, 200–5

Ries, E. (1895). Eine neue operations Methode des Uterus-Carcinoma. *Z. Geburts. Gynakol.*, **32**, 266

Ries, E. (1932). Erosion, leukoplakia and the colposcope in relation to carcinoma of the cervix. *Am J. Obstet. Gynecol.*, **23**, 393–9

Rigoni-Stern, D. (1842). Fatti Statistici Relativi Alle Malattie Cancerose. *Gior. Servire Progr. Path. Terap.*, **2**, 507–17

Rojel, J. (1953). The interrelation between uterine cancer and syphilis. *Acta Pathol. Microbiol. Scand.*, Suppl. 97

Rotkin, I.D. (1973). A comparison review of key epidemiologic studies in cervical cancer related to current searches for transmissible agents. *Cancer Res.*, **33**, 1353–67

Rotkin, I.D. and King, R.W. (1962). Environmental variables related to cervical cancer. *Am. J. Obstet. Gynecol.*, **83**, 720–8

Rubin, I.C. (1910). The pathological diagnosis of incipient carcinoma of the uterus. *Am. J. Obstet.*, **62**, 668–76

Ruge, C. and Veit, J. (1878). Fur Pathologie der Vaginalportion. *Z. Geburtsch Gynakol.*, **2**, 415

Schauenstein, W. (1908). Histologische Untersuchungen uber atypisches Plattenepithel an der Portio und an der Innenflache der Cervix uteri. *Arch. Gynakol.*, **85**, 576–616

Schauta, F. (1902). Die Operation des Gebärmutterkrebses mittels des Schuchardt'schen Paravaginatschmittes. *Monatsschrift Geburtsch. Gynakol.*, **15**, 133

Schiller, W. (1927). Untersuchungen zur Entstehung der Geschwuelste. Teil Collumcarcinom des Uterus. *Virchows Arch.*, **263**, 279

Schiller, W. (1928a). Uber Fruehstadien des Portiokarzinoms und ihre Diagnose. *Arch. Gynakol.*, **133**, 211

Schiller, W. (1928b). Zur klinischen Fruehdiagnose des Portiokarzinoms. *Zbl. Gynakol.*, 1886

Schiller, W. (1929). Jodpinselung und Abschabung des Portioepithels. *Z. Gynakol.*, **53**, 1056–64

Schiller, W. (1933). Early diagnosis of carcinoma of the cervix. *Surg. Gynecol. Obstet.*, **56**, 210–22

Schottlander, J. and Kermauner, F. (1912). Zur Kenntis des Uterus Karzinoms: Monographische. *Studie uber Morphologie Entwichlung, Waschstum nebst Beitragen zur klinik der Erkrankung.* (Berlin: S. Karger)

Scott, J.W., Welch, W.B. and Blake, T.F. (1960). Bloodless technique of cold knife conisation (ring biopsy). *Am. J. Obstet. Gynecol.*, **79**, 62–6

Scott, R.B. and Reagan, J.W. (1956). Diagnostic cervical biopsy techniques for study of early cancer; value of cold knife conisation procedure. *J. Am. Med. Assoc.*, **160**, 343–7

Shingleton, H.M. and Orr, J.W. (eds.) (1987). *Cancer of the Cervix: Diagnosis and Treatment*, pp. 1–20. (Edinburgh, London: Churchill Livingstone)

Sims, J.M. (1861). *Trans Med. Soc. N.Y.*, **137**, 367

Sims, J.M. (1879) The treatment of epithelioma of the cervix uteri. *Am. J. Obstet.*, **12**, 451–89

Singer, A. (1973a). A male factor in the aetiology of cervical cancer? *Oxford Medical School Gazette*, **25**, 18–19

Singer, A. (1973b). *D.Phil. Thesis* University of Oxford, quoted by Coppleson (1977) p. 155

Singer, A. (1975). The uterine cervix from adolescence to the menopause. *Br. J. Obstet. Gynaecol.*, **82**, 81–99

Singer, A. (1986). The abnormal smear. Clinical algorithms. *Br. Med. J.*, **293**, 1551–6

Singer, A. and Walker, P. (1982). Cone biopsy – complications, which invalidate its use in treating all precancerous lesions. *Br. J. Obstet. Gynaecol.*, **89**, 335–7

Singer, A. and Walker, P. (1985). The treatment of CIN: conservative methods. In Singer, A. (ed.) *Cancer of the Cervix: Diagnosis and Treatment. Clinics in Obstetrics and Gynaecology*, pp. 121–32. (London:W.B. Saunders)

Singer, A., Reid, B.L. and Coppleson, M. (1976). A hypothesis: the role of a high risk male in the etiology of cervical carcinoma. A correlation of epidemiology and molecular biology. *Am. J. Obstet. Gynecol.*, **126**, 110

Singer, A., Walker, P., Tay, S.K. and Dyson, J.

(1984). Impact of introduction of colposcopy to a district general hospital. *Br. Med. J.*, **289**, 1049–51

Skrabanek, P. and McCormick, J. (1989). *Follies and Fallacies in Medicine*, p. 105. (Glasgow: The Targon Press)

Snow, J. (1855). *On the Mode of Communication of Cholera.* 2nd edn. (London: Churchill) (Reproduced in *Snow on Cholera.* Commonwealth Fund, New York, 1936. Reprinted by Hafner, New York, 1965)

Speert, H. (1980). *Obstetrics and Gynecology in America. A History*, p. 57. (Chicago: American College of Obstetricians and Gynecologists)

Spriggs, A.I., Butler, E.B., Evans, D.M.D., Grubb, C., Hussain, O.A.N. and Wachtel, G.E. (1978). Problems of cell nomenclature in cervical cytology smears. *J. Clin. Pathol.*, **31**, 1226–7

Stafl, A. (1975), quoted by Jordan (1976) p. 309

Stafl, A., Dohnal, V. and Linhartova, A. (1963). On colposcopic, histological and vascular findings in the pathologically changed cervix. *Geburtsh. Frauenheilk.*, **23**, 437–45

Stafl, A., Wilkinson, E.J. and Mattingly, R.S. (1977). Laser treatment of cervical and vaginal neoplasia. *Am. J. Obstet. Gynecol.*, **128**, 125

Staland, B. (1978). Treatment of premalignant lesions of the uterine cervix by means of moderate heat thermosurgery using the Semm coagulator. *Ann. Chirurg. Gynaecol.*, **67**, 112

Stockard, C.R. and Papanicolaou, G.N. (1917). The existence of a typical oestrous cycle in the guinea pig: with a study of its histological and physiological changes. *Am. J. Anat.*, **22**, 225

Sturmdorf, A. (1916). *Surg. Gynecol. Obstet.*, **22**, 93

Syrjanen, K.J., Heinonen, U.M. and Kauraniemi, T. (1981). Cytologic evidence of the association of condylomatous lesions with dysplastic and neoplastic changes in the uterine cervix. *Acta Cytol.*, **25**, 17–22

Takeuchi, A. and McKay, D.G. (1960). The area of cervix involved by carcinoma *in situ* and anaplasia (atypical hyperplasia). *Obstet. Gynecol.*, **15**, 134–45

Taussig, F.J. (1943). Iliac lymphadenectomy for group 11 cancer of the cervix. *Am. J. Obstet. Gynecol.*, **45**, 733–58

Te Linde, R.W. and Galvin, G. (1944). Minimum

histological changes in biopsies to justify diagnosis of cervical cancer. *Am. J. Obstet Gynecol.*, **48**, 774

Theilhaber, A. and Greischer, S. (1908). Cited by Kennaway, E.L. (1948). The racial and social incidence of cancer of the uterus. *Br. J. Cancer*, **2**, 177

Thornton, W.N., Waters, L.N., Pearce, L.S., Wilson, L.A. and Nodes, T.M. (1954). Carcinoma *in situ*; value of cold knife cone biopsy. *Obstet. Gynecol.*, **3**, 587–94

Toaff, R. (1976). The carbon dioxide laser in Gynae Surgery. *Laser Surgery*, **1–2**, 64

Tod, M.C. and Meredith, W.J. (1938). A dosage system for use in the treatment of cancer of the uterine cervix. *Br. J. Radiol.*, **11**, 809–24

Townsend, D.E. and Richart, R.M. (1983). Cryotherapy and CO_2 laser management of CIN. *Obstet. Gynecol.*, **61**, 75

Viana, O. (1928). The early diagnosis of uterine cancer by smears. *La Clinica Obstetrica*, **30**, 781 (Reprinted in translation in *Acta Cytologica*, **14**, 544, 1970)

Vineberg, H.N. (1906). The etiology of cancer of the pelvic organs. *Am. J. Obstet.*, **53**, 410–19

Virchow, R. (1858). Die Cellularpathologie in ihrer Begrundung auf die physiologische und pathologische Gewebelehre. *20 Vorlesungen im Pathologischen Institut zu Berlin: Aug Hirschwald* (Berlin: Hirschwald)

Virchow, R. (1863). *Die Krankhaften Geschwulsten*, 3rd edn. (Berlin: Hirschwald)

Vogel, J. (1843). *Erlauterungstafeln zur pathologischen Histologie mit vorzuglicher Rucksicht auf sein Handbuch der pathologischen Anatomie. 26 Tafeln mit 291, Figuren, wovon 270 nach d. Natur gezeichnet sind.* (Leipzig: Leopold VoB)

Von Scanzoni, F. (1861), quoted by Shingleton and Orr (1987) p. 3

Wagner, D. (1961). Die erfassung des rezidiverenden oberflachen karzinomas am collum uteri nach konservativer therapie. *Geburts. Frauenheilk.*, **21**, 944–61

Wakefield, J., Yule, R., Smith, A. and Adelstein, A.M. (1973). Relation of abnormal cytological smears and carcinoma of the cervix uteri to husband's occupations. *Br. Med. J.*, **2**, 142–3

Way, S. (1951). *Malignant Disease of the Female Genital Tract*, p. 109. (London: J.& A. Churchill Ltd.)

Way, S. (1974). The use of the sac technique in pelvic exenteration. *Gynecol. Oncol.*, **2**, 476–81

Weinberg, W. and Gastpar, K. (1904). Die bösartigen Neubildungen in Stuttgart 1873–1902. *Z. Krebsf.*, **2**, 195–260

Wertheim, E. (1900). Zur Frage der Radikaloperation beim Uteruskrebs. *Arch. Gynakol.*, **61**, 627

Wertheim, E. (1905). Discussion on the diagnosis and treatment of carcinoma of the uterus. *Br. Med. J.*, **2**, 689

Wespi, H. (1949). *Early Carcinoma of the Uterine Cervix, Pathogenesis and Detection.* (New York: Grune and Stratton)

Wetchler, S.J. (1984). Treatment of cervical intraepithelial neoplasia with the CO_2 laser: laser versus cryotherapy. A review of effectiveness and cost. *Obstet. Gynecol. Surv.*, **39**(8), 469–73

Williams, Sir J. (1886a). *Cancer of the uterus. Harveian Lectures for 1886.* (London: H.K. Lewis)

Williams, Sir J. (1886b), quoted by Hertig (1979) p. 795

Wright, V.C. and Davies, E.M. (1981). The conservative management of cervical intraepithelial neoplasia: the use of cryosurgery and the carbon dioxide laser. *Br. J. Obstet. Gynaecol.*, **88**, 663

Wynder, E.L., Cornfield, J., Schroff, P.D. and Doraiswami, K.R. (1954). A study of environmental factors in cancer of the cervix. *Am. J. Obstet. Gynecol.*, **68**, 1016–52

Younge, P.A. (1957). The conservative treatment of carcinoma *in situ* of the cervix. *Third National Cancer Conference Proceedings*, pp. 682–92. (Philadelphia: Lippincott)

Younge, P.A., Hertig, A.T. and Armstrong, D. (1949). A study of 135 cases of carcinoma *in situ* of the cervix at the Free Hospital for women. *Am. J. Obstet. Gynecol.*, **58**, 867–95

Yule, R. (1973). The prevention of cancer of the cervix by cytological screening of the population. In Easson, E.C. (ed.) *Cancer of the Uterine Cervix*, p. 11. (London, Philadelphia, Toronto: W.B. Saunders Co.)

FURTHER READING

Burghardt, E. (1984). *Colposcopy Cervical Pathology Textbook and Atlas*, translated by and with the collaboration of Andrew G. Ostor. (Stuttgart, New York: Georg Thieme Verlag)

Cavanagh, D., Ruffolo, E.H. and Marsden, D.E. (1985). *Gynecologic Cancer: a Clinicopathologic Approach.* (Norwalk, Connecticut: Appleton-Century-Crofts)

Codling, B.W., Bigrigg, M.A., Pearson, P., Read, M.D. and Swingler, G.R. (1990). *A description of the development of an effective and economical method of histological interpretation of tissue removed by diathermy loop excision.* (Gloucester, UK: Gloucester Health Authority)

Coleman, D.V. and Evans, D.M.D. (1988). *Biopsy Pathology and Cytology of the Cervix.* (London: Chapman and Hall Medical)

Coppleson, M. (1977). Colposcopy. In Stallworthy, J. and Bourne, G. (eds.) *Recent Advances in Obstetrics and Gynaecology*, no. 12. (Edinburgh, London, New York: Churchill Livingstone)

Dorsey, J.H. (1980). Cervical conization and the CO_2 laser. In Bellina, J.H. (ed.) *Gynecologic Laser Surgery*, pp. 131–43. (New York, London: Plenum Press)

Fox, H. (ed). (1984). *Gynaecological Pathology: Advances, Perspectives and Problems. Clinics in Obstetrics and Gynaecology*, Vol. 11, no. 1. (London, Philadelphia, Toronto: W.B. Saunders Co.)

Fox, H. (1987). Cervical smears: new terminology and new demands. *Br. Med. J.*, **294**, 1307–8

Giles, J.A. and Gafar, A. (1991). The treatment of CIN: do we need lasers? *Br. J. Obstet. Gynaecol.*, **98**, 3–6

Grunze, H. and Spriggs, A.I. (1983). *History of Clinical Cytology. A Selection of Documents*, 2nd edn. G-I-T. Darmstadt: Verlag Ernst Ghebelar)

Kessler, I.I. (1974). Cervical cancer epidemiology in historical perspective. *J. Reprod. Med.*, **12**, no. 5, 173–85

Langley, F.A. (ed.) (1976). Cancer of the vulva, vagina and uterus. *Clinics in Obstetrics and Gynaecology*, vol. 3, no. 2. (London, Philadelphia, Toronto: W.B. Saunders Co.)

Luesley, D.M., Cullimore, J., Redman, C.W.E., Lawton, F.G., Emens, J.M., Rollason, T.P., Williams, D.R. and Buxton, E.J. (1990). Loop diathermy excision of the cervical transformation zone in patients with abnormal cervical smears. *Br. Med. J.*, **300**, 1690–3

Rotkin, I.D. (1973). A comparison review of key epidemiological studies in cervical cancer related to current searches for transmissible agents. *Cancer Res.*, **33**, 1353–67

Retsas, S. (ed.) (1986). *Palaeo-Oncology. The Antiquity of Cancer.* (London: Farrand Press)

Rhodes, P. (1988). *An Outline History of Medicine.* (London, Boston: Butterworths)

Shingleton, H. (1986). Presidential Address, Society of Gynecologic Oncologists. February. Cervical Cancer: A Treatment Evolves. *Gynecol. Oncol.*, **25**, 260–70

Shingleton, H.M. and Orr, J.W. (eds.) (1987). *Cancer of the Cervix: Diagnosis and Treatment.* (Edinburgh, London, Melbourne, New York: Churchill Livingstone)

Singer, A. (ed.) (1985). Cancer of the cervix: diagnosis and treatment. *Clinics in Obstetrics and Gynaecology*, Vol. 12, no. 1. (London, Philadelphia, Toronto: W.B. Saunders Co.)

Wespi, H. (1949). *Early Carcinoma of the Uterine Cervix.* (New York: Grune and Stratton)

Cancer of the uterus

BODY OF THE UTERUS

Although cancer of the uterine body had been described for some time, it was not until hysterectomy was introduced that proper scientific evaluation of the disease became possible. Vaginal hysterectomy was perfected prior to the abdominal operation. Soranus of Ephesus in the second century AD gets the credit for first recording a form of the operation when he amputated a gangrenous inverted uterus (Leonardo, 1944). There are references to the technique during the Middle Ages but it was Osiander of Gottingen who first performed a radical vaginal operation in Germany in 1801, during which he amputated the vaginal portion of a carcinomatous uterus (Ricci, 1950)

DIAGNOSIS OF ENDOMETRIAL CANCER

Cells of endometrial carcinoma were identified on cervical cytology smears, but endometrial curettage as an office or hospital procedure was a much superior diagnostic method. Hysterography and hysteroscopy provided useful information, while ultrasound and computed axial tomography were also found to be of value in the preoperative assessment of these cases.

PREDISPOSING CONDITIONS

There was considerable debate in the early part of this century as to whether endometrial hyperplasia, endometrial polyps, or fibroids were premalignant conditions. Approximately 20% of patients with adenomatous hyperplasia, or over 70% with atypical hyperplasia and carcinoma *in situ*, progressed to invasive adenocarcinoma of the uterus.

Endometrial hyperplasia

Taylor (1932) and Novak (Figure 1) and Yui (1936) proposed that postmenopausal hyperplasia was a precursor of cancer. Endometrial hyperplasia was recognized in the nineteenth century by Recamier

(1850). It was also documented by Olshausen (1875) and by West and Duncan (1879). Brennecke (1882) debated on the aetiology of the condition and considered that it was associated with a disturbance of ovarian function. Cullen (1900a,b,c; 1908) detailed the histological characteristics. Schroder (1914) investigated endometrial hyperplasia in detail. Schroder's publications were the first to recognize its true significance, and he also confirmed that the abnormality was present in conditions of disturbed ovarian function. Novak (1920) and Shaw (1929) noted that hyperplasia was sometimes accompanied by adenomyosis. Endometrial hyperplasia was characterized by an increased quantity of endometrium which retained the features of the follicular phase.

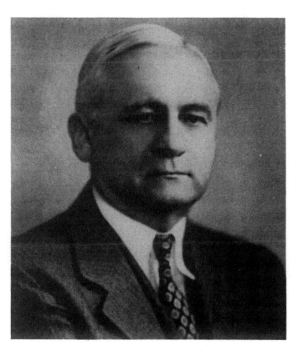

Figure 1 Emil Novak. Reproduced with kind permission from Novak, E.R. and Woodruff, J.D. (1967). *Novak's Gynecologic and Obstetric Pathology*, 6th edn. (Philadelphia: W.B. Saunders Co.)

The term 'Swiss cheese' pattern was introduced by Novak and Martzloff (1924) to describe the large cystic glands found at microscopy. An alternative term 'cystic glandular hyperplasia' was also used.

Although endometrial hyperplasia was documented in all age groups, Shaw (1929) ascertained that the highest incidence was found in patients approaching the menopause. Postmeno-pausal endometrial hyperplasia was rare – Novak and Yui (1936) recorded only 15 out of 804 cases. Hyperplasia was associated with prolonged exposure of the endometrium to oestrogens. Follicular cysts or feminizing tumours of the ovary were sometimes responsible. Gusberg (1947) documented the relationship between prolonged oestrogen administration, obesity, oligomenorrhoea, and dysfunctional uterine bleeding.

Despite the considerable interest in endometrial hyperplasia as a premalignant condition, Hertig and Sommers (1949) and Schroder (1954) determined that an association between endometrial hyperplasia and carcinoma of the endometrium was infrequent. Gusberg *et al.* (1954) reported their study of 100 cases of adenomatous hyperplasia and 10% were found to be associated with adenocarcinoma. The term atypical hyperplasia was introduced by Novak and Rutledge (1948), and the concept of carcinoma *in situ* of the endometrium was advocated by Hertig *et al.* (1949). MacDonald and Siitteri (1974) noted the association between extraglandular production of oestrone from the adrenal prehormone androstenedione in adipose tissue, and its relationship to endometrial hyperplasia.

Polyps

A number of authors noted the association between polyps and carcinoma of the endometrium. Willis (1948) documented that polyps could be precancerous or they might be regarded as localized hyperplasia and thus not have any particular relationship. Peterson and Novak (1956) found polyps to be associated with malignancy in over 15% of postmenopausal cases.

Fibroids

The older writers stressed the importance of a connection between fibroids and endometrial carcinoma. Willis (1948) pointed out that nulliparity, fibroids and carcinoma of the endometrium were frequently associated and had a common aetiology.

Inherited predisposition

In 1912 Sir Halliday Croom reported the occurrence of endometrial cancer in identical twins. Other authors recorded the disease as being more frequent in families.

Associated lesions and hormones

An association was found between diabetes mellitus and the onset of endometrial carcinoma by several authors during the 1940s. Stanley Way (1951) documented that 14% of 68 patients reported by him, were diabetic. Other investigators noted obesity, hypertension, delayed menopause and oestrogenic tumours to be associated. Gusberg (1947) and Gusberg and Hall (1961) reported an association between oestrogen therapy and endometrial cancer.

Oestrogens were implicated in the pathogenesis of endometrial carcinoma from the 1920s on when Allen and Doisy (1923) isolated the oestrogenic hormone. The concept of inducing withdrawal bleeding by administration of progesterone was first introduced by Albright (1938), and Greenblatt (1945) suggested their use in a cyclic fashion for oestrogen-treated women. Fremont-Smith *et al.* (1946) reported an association between long-term oestrogen therapy and endometrial carcinoma. Final confirmation was provided by Smith *et al.* (1975) and Ziel and Finkle (1975) from their controlled studies. It was evident that patients on unopposed oestrogen therapy were three times more likely to develop endometrial carcinoma when compared with non-oestrogen-treated women.

Although Greenblatt advocated the use of cyclic progesterone for patients on oestrogen replacement therapy in 1945, the practice was only introduced on a wide scale in 1971. That treatment was found to be very effective in protecting oestrogen users against endometrial adenocarcinoma. Gambrell (1986) advocated the use of a progesterone challenge test to identify asymptomatic postmenopausal women with endometrial hyperplasia.

CLINICAL GROUPING/STAGING

Various classifications for uterine cancer evolved including that of Healy and Browne (1939) who suggested that patients be placed in three groups. Group 1 included those patients in whom no palpable uterine enlargement or extension of the disease was found beyond the fundus. In group 2 there was uterine enlargement but no fixation, and no evidence of disease elsewhere. In group 3 there were clinical signs of tumours beyond the confines of the uterus. This classification was modified by Taylor and Beckner (1947). Other classifications were suggested by Miller and Henderson (1946) and the American College of Surgeons.

CARCINOMA

Most cases were found to occur between the ages of 50 and 60 years. Miller (1940) noted that 27% of his patients were nulliparous. Various estimates of nulliparity ranged from 19 to 50% in subsequent reports. The primary symptom appeared to be uterine haemorrhage. Most cases presented with postmenopausal bleeding. The majority of tumours were adenocarcinomas but some showed squamous metaplasia (Nicholson, 1923). The term for such a case was adenoacanthoma. Two main types were recognized, the 'diffuse' in which a large area of the endometrium was affected, or the 'circumscribed' when a small area was involved. Four histological groups were recognized and Mahle (1923) showed that patients in groups 1 and 2 had twice the survival rate of patients in grade 3. All those in grade 4 succumbed early. A new histological grading system was introduced by Broders (1925). Almost 6% of cases with surgical stage 1 disease were found to have pelvic lymph metastases. Palmer *et al* (1949) determined that the majority of patients were graded as group 1 or 2 and from this it was surmised that the tumour was a slowly growing type with a relatively good chance of cure.

An agreed system of clinical staging of endometrial cancer was drawn up by the American Joint Committee on Cancer, the International Federation of Gynaecology and Obstetrics (FIGO) and the Union International Contra Cancer. This allowed for clinical, surgical, and pathological staging. The World Health Organization's Classification of uterine tumours is commonly used (Poulson *et al*, 1975), and is as follows: 1, adenocarcinoma; 2, clear cell (mesonephroid adenocarcinoma); 3, squamous cell carcinoma; 4, adenosquamous (mucoepidermoid carcinoma); 5, undifferentiated carcinoma. Adenocarcinoma was the most common of the subtypes comprising over 60% of endometrial carcinomas. The majority

were grade 1, or well-differentiated. The FIGO Group updated the system a number of times, and their last recommendations were published in 1988.

Adenoacanthomas, which contain squamous elements, occur in about 25%, and their prognosis is somewhat worse than endometrial adenocarcinoma. Cullen (1900a,b,c) documented a rare but aggressive form of neoplasm, now known as 'papillary adenocarcinoma'. 'Mixed adenosquamous carcinoma' constituted less than 10% of the subtype and was found to be an aggressive form. 'Clear cell carcinoma', the least common variety, was considered by Schiller (1939) to be of mesonephric origin. The tumours were designated as mesonephromas, but were later thought to be of Müllerian origin.

Endometrial carcinoma is a slowly growing tumour. The lungs and bone are affected by metastatic spread. Vaginal vault recurrence is likely. Suburethral metastases were found in 12% of cases by Meigs (1929). Ovarian metastases were documented in 5-10% by Barns (1941). In 1985 endometrial cancer was the most common genital tract cancer, with almost four times the frequency of cervical cancer (American Cancer Society, 1985), the ratio having changed greatly in the preceding 40 years partly due to earlier treatment of precancerous forms of cervical disease and partly due to decreased childbearing.

AGE

The peak incidence of the disease was in the 58 - 60-year group (Gusberg and Kaplan, 1963), which is 10 years later than the peak of adenomatous hyperplasia. About 10% of endometrial cancers were found to occur before the age of 50.

TREATMENT

Surgery

The first deliberate vaginal hysterectomy in a case of uterine cancer was performed by Conrad Langenbeck in 1813. During the early part of the nineteenth century the operation was attempted by Lauvariol and Baudelocque of France, Paletta of Italy, and J.C. Warren and other operators in the USA. In 1819, Windsor ligatured a uterine inversion, tightened it daily, and eventually amputated the portion distal to the ligature (Mathieu, 1934). Vaginal hysterectomy was abandoned due to its high mortality, and as anaesthesia was not yet available it was a cruel operation. The technique was reintroduced by Vincent Czerny of Heidelberg in 1879. Schauta pioneered a radical vaginal hysterectomy with removal of pelvic glands in 1898.

The technique of abdominal hysterectomy evolved from attempts at myomectomy. Heath of Manchester was the first to perform abdominal hysterectomy for fibroids in 1845 (Ricci, 1945) although he preoperatively diagnosed ovarian cysts. Clay, also of Manchester, carried out hysterectomy within a short time of Heath's case. Abdominal hysterectomy was reported by a number of operators subsequently, but Burnham of Massachusetts was the first to carry out abdominal hysterectomy for cancer when he removed the uterus of a patient who was found to have a sarcoma. There was a strong lobby of opinion which condemned the operation of abdominal hysterectomy due to its high mortality. However, Freund of Strassburg introduced an improved technique in 1878. He placed the patient in head down position, packed off the intestines, ligated vessels and introduced proper abdominal closure. Twenty years later Wertheim (q.v. in Biographies) performed his radical abdominal hysterectomy with removal of lymph nodes. In 1900 Pusey and Pfahler first used X-ray therapy for endometrial carcinoma. In the same year Cullen published what was considered to be a classic monograph on uterine cancer (Cullen, 1900a,b,c).

In the early days subtotal hysterectomy was performed but the results were consistently bad (Way, 1951). Wertheim (1905) pioneered radical hysterectomy but due to the relative lack of lymph node involvement in cancers of the endometrium and the operative mortality for extended hysterectomy being up to 20%, the procedure was abandoned. Total abdominal hysterectomy with removal of both appendages became the standard method of treatment. Masson (1934) declared an almost 50% absolute survival rate, but by the late 1940s a cure rate of 70% was claimed.

Radiotherapy

A role for irradiation was recognized by the 1920s. Healy and Cutler (1930) and Arneson (1936) popularized radiotherapy in the USA while Heyman (1935) developed the Stockholm method and popularized its use in Europe. By the 1940s combined radiation and surgery was the treatment of choice. Heyman et al. (1941) advocated intrauterine radium therapy and claimed a 5-year survival rate of 45% which later improved to almost 65%. Many of the cases referred for radiotherapy were considered too obese for surgery. Interest in combined radiotherapy and surgical treatment led to preoperative or postoperative irradiation but the former was more popular. The vaginal recurrence rate of 7–14% for surgery alone was obtained by either technique.

During the 1960s the dangers to both patients and staff from the technique of live radium packing was recognized and a different approach became inevitable. Underwood et al. (1977) introduced a technique where radiation was focused primarily on the vagina and was followed immediately by surgery. External sources of radiation became popular about the same time. It was demonstrated in the 1980s that external irradiation was not as satisfactory as the intravaginal techniques in preventing vaginal metastases.

Progesterones

Progesterone in oil was used for a patient with pulmonary metastases from endometrial cancer by Rita Kelley and William Baker, at the suggestion of Ira Nathanson in 1950. The patient responded but died later of disease recurrence (Kneale, 1986). By 1955 hydroxyprogesterone caproate was substituted for the progesterone in oil and good results were reported. Kelley and Baker (1961) reported improvement with striking regression of the process in patients treated with large doses of progesterone. Kelley and Baker (1961) documented further successes with progesterone treatment, as did other workers. During the 1970s a number of symposia reported the response rates to treatment with progestogens. When used for advanced disease, approximately one-third of patients showed a clinical response.

Cytotoxic chemotherapy

Thigpen et al. (1979) were the first to report a well-designed prospective study on the use of adriamycin for patients with advanced or recurrent endometrial carcinoma. A number of other cytotoxic agents were used. Cohen et al. (1977) reported the first combination cytotoxic therapy. Response rates of around 30% were recorded.

SECONDARY CARCINOMA

The commonest secondary tumours were those which spread from the cervix. However, tumours of any of the pelvic contents could spread by direct involvement. Blood- and lymph-borne metastases from primaries of kidney, breast, pancreas, lung, and also of malignant melanoma, were described (Willis, 1934).

OTHER CANCERS

Sarcoma of the uterus (Figure 2)

Proper and Simpson (1919) found sarcomatous degeneration in 6% of fibroids while Voght (1923) found the same condition in less than 0.5%.

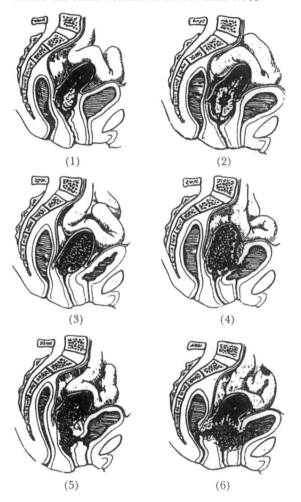

(1) (2)

(3) (4)

(5) (6)

Figure 2 Carcinoma of the body of the uterus and endocervix. (1) Cancer of the endocervix; (2) Cancer of the endocervix and the lower endometrium; (3) Cancer of the uterus filling the cavity; (4) Cancer of the uterus invading the bladder wall; (5) Cancer of the uterus invading the bladder wall and the vagina; (6) Cancer of the uterus invading the bladder wall, the vagina and the rectum. From Schaeffer-Bouglé, *Atlas-Manuel de Gynécologie*, Paris (1903)

This rare neoplasm was found to arise from all uterine constituents and more than half developed in a fibroid. Masson (1923) reviewed earlier publications and estimated a 10% incidence of the development of sarcoma in fibroids. This finding was not borne out in further studies and Persaud and Arjoon (1970) quoted an incidence of 0.5%.

Novak and Anderson (1937) documented a relationship between clinical behaviour and mitotic activity of sarcomas and reported that 66% of their sarcomatous cases arose in a fibroid. Bartsich *et al.* (1968), in their 50-year review on the topic, reported 5-year survival rates for treated patients of 14–46%.

Chorionic carcinoma (chorion epithelioma)

Although described by F.I. Meckel in 1795, by Max Sanger in 1888, and others (Ricci, 1945) chorionic carcinoma, in which there was malignant change of the trophoblast, was a doubtful diagnosis until the work of Marchand (1895) and also of Teacher (1903). The cancer was sometimes accompanied by large ovarian cysts, as described by Rokitansky (1855). Ewing (1910) described the condition of 'chorioadenoma destruens', later known as invasive or malignant mole. Chorion epithelioma was reported by Sanger in 1899.

STEROID RECEPTORS

Brush *et al.* (1968) discovered that 17β-oestradiol became bound to endometrial cancer cells and this initiated the concept of steroid receptors. Oestrogen and progesterone receptors, or binding proteins, were found necessary for the expression of steroid hormonal effects within the individual cell. Receptor content was found to correlate with histological differentiation, and the prognosis of primary endometrial carcinomas. Monoclonal antibodies were used to localize receptors in tissue samples, in the hope that more accurate predictions of tumour behaviour could be made.

CHRONOLOGY

2nd C. AD Soranus of Ephesus amputated the gangrenous portion of an inverted uterus (Leonardo, 1944).

1801 Osiander of Gottingen amputated part of a cancerous uterus (Ricci, 1950).

Endometrial hyperplasia

1850   Recamier recognized the condition.

1914   Schroder associated the condition with abnormalities of ovarian function and spoke of 'metropathia hemorrhagica'.

1920   Novak encountered hyperplasia in association with adenomyosis.

1924   Novak and Martzloff introduced the term 'Swiss cheese' endometrium.

1929   Shaw determined that endometrial hyperplasia was most commonly found in perimenopausal patients.

1948   Novak and Rutledge introduced the term 'atypical hyperplasia'.
Willis noted that polyps could be precancerous.

1949   Hertig *et al.* described adenocarcinoma *in situ.*

Uterine cancer

1900   Cullen documented the rare 'papillary adenocarcinoma'.

1920   Oestrogens were implicated in the pathogenesis of endometrial cancer.

1923   Nicholson documented that some adenocarcinomas showed squamous metaplastic changes.
Histological grading was introduced by Broders (Haines and Taylor, 1975).
Mahle reported survival rates.

1929   Meigs described suburethral metastases in 12%. Vaginal recurrence rates of 7-14% were found.

1946   Fremont-Smith *et al.* associated exogenous oestrogens with endometrial carcinoma.

1949   Palmer *et al.* showed that the majority of patients were in group 1 or 2.

1950   An International classification evolved.

1975   Smith *et al.* and also Ziel and Finkle confirmed an association between unopposed oestrogen therapy and endometrial adenocarcinoma.
Poulsen detailed the World Health Organization classification.

Treatment

* Reference: (Ricci 1945)

1813   Conrad Langenbeck performed vaginal hysterectomy.*

1855   Heath, and later Clay, performed abdominal hysterectomy.*

1878   Freund improved the operative technique.*

1879   Vincent Czerny reintroduced vaginal hysterectomy which had been attempted on other occasions in the early part of the nineteenth century.*

1888   Wertheim began his radical operations (Wertheim, 1905).

1898   Schauta pioneered radical vaginal hysterectomy.*

1900   X-ray therapy was used.

1930   Radiotherapy was popularized in the USA.

1935   Heyman developed the Stockholm method.

1940s   A cure rate of 70% was claimed for surgical intervention.

1941   Heyman *et al.* popularized intrauterine radium therapy.

1950   Progesterone was used by Kelley and Baker (Kneale, 1986).

1960   The dangers of radium therapy were recognized.

1970s   Cytotoxics were used. Response rates of about 30% were reported.

REFERENCES

Albright, F. (1938). Metropathia hemorrhagica. *J. Maine Med. Assoc.*, **29**, 235–8

Allen, E. and Doisy, E.A. (1923). An ovarian hormone. *J. Am. Med. Assoc.*, **81**, 819–21

American Cancer Society (1985). *Cancer Facts and Figures.* (New York: American Cancer Society)

Arneson, A. (1936). Clinical results and histologic changes following the radiation treatment of cancer of the corpus uteri. *Am. J. Roentgenol.*, **36**, 461

Barns, H.H.F. (1941). Early involvement of the ovaries in carcinomas of the body of the uterus. *J. Obstet. Gynaecol. Br. Emp.*, **48**, 443

Bartsich, E.G., Bowe, E.T. and Moore, J.G. (1968). Leiomyosarcoma of the uterus. A 50 year review of 42 cases. *Obstet. Gynecol.*, **32**, 101–6

Brennecke, (1882). Zur Aetiologie der "Endometritis fungosa" speciell der "chronischen hyperplasirenden Endometritis Olshausen's". *Arch. Gynakol.*, **20**, 455

Broders, A.C. (1925). The grading of carcinoma. *Minnesota Med.*, **8**, 726

Brush, M.G., Taylor, R.W. and King, R.B.J. (1968). The uptake of (6, 7x3-H)-oestradiol by the normal human reproductive tract. *J. Endocrinol.*, **39**, 599

Cohen, C.J., Deppe, G. and Bruckner, H.W. (1977). Treatment of advanced adenocarcinoma of the endometrium with melphalan, 5-fluorouracil and medroxyprogesterone acetate. A preliminary study. *Obstet. Gynecol.*, **50** (4), 415–17

Cullen, T.S. (1900a). *Cancer of the Uterus.* (London: Kimpton)

Cullen, T.S. (1900b). *Cancer of the Uterus.* (Philadelphia: W.B. Saunders & Co.)

Cullen, T.S. (1900c). *Cancer of the Uterus: Its Pathology, Symptomatology, Diagnosis and Treatment.* (New York: D. Appleton)

Cullen, T.S. (1908). *Adenomyoma of Uterus.* (Philadelphia: W.B. Saunders & Co.)

Ewing, J. (1910). *Chorioma. Surg. Gynecol. Obstet.*, **10**, 366

Fremont-Smith, M., Meigs, J.V., Graham, R.H. and Gilbert, H.H. (1946). Cancer of the endometrium and prolonged estrogen therapy. *J. Am. Med. Assoc.*, **131**, 805

Gambrell, R.D. Jr. (1986). The role of hormones in the etiology and prevention of endometrial cancer. In Creasman, W.T. (ed.) *Clinics in Obstetrics and Gynaecology, Endometrial Cancer*, Vol. 13 No. 4, pp. 695–723. (London, Philadelphia, Toronto: W.B. Saunders Co.)

Greenblatt, R.B. (1945). Sexual infantilism in the female. *West. J. Surg. Obstet. Gynecol.*, **53**, 222–6

Gusberg, S.B. (1947). Precursors of corpus carcinoma, oestrogens and adenomatous hyperplasia. *Am. J. Obstet. Gynecol.*, **54**, 905

Gusberg, S.B. and Hall, R.E. (1961). Precursors of corpus cancer. The appearance of cancer of the endometrium in estrogenically conditional patients. *Obstet. Gynecol.*, **17**, 397

Gusberg, S.B. and Kaplan, A.L. (1963). Precursors of corpus cancer adenomatous hyperplasia as stage 0. *Am. J. Obstet. Gynecol.*, **87**, 662–76

Gusberg, S.B., Moore, D.B. and Martin, F. (1954). Precursors of corpus cancer. A clinical and pathological study of adenomatous hyperplasia. *Am. J. Obstet. Gynecol.*, **68**, 1472

Haines, M. and Taylor, C.W. (1975). *Gynaecological Pathology*, 2nd edn. p. 260. (Edinburgh, London, New York: Churchill Livingstone)

Halliday Croom, J. (1912), quoted by Way (1951) p.181

Healy, W. and Cutler, M. (1930). Radiation and surgical treatment of carcinoma of body of the uterus. *Am. J. Obstet. Gynecol.*, **19**, 457

Healy, W.P. and Brown, R.L. (1939) Experience with surgical and radiation therapy in carcinoma of the corpus uteri. *Am. J. Obstet. Gynecol.*, **38**, 1–13

Hertig, A.T. and Sommers, S.C. (1949). Genesis of endometrial carcinoma. Study of prior biopsies. *Cancer*, **2**, 946

Hertig, A.T. Sommers, S.C. and Bengloff, H. (1949). Genesis of endometrial carcinoma. Carcinoma *in situ. Cancer*, **2**, 964–71

Heyman, J. (1935). The so-called Stockholm method and the results of treatment of uterine cancer at the Radiumhemmet. *Acta Radiol.*, **15**, 129

Heyman, J., Reuterwall, O. and Benner, S. (1941), quoted by Way (1951) p. 181

Kelley, R.M. and Baker, W.H. (1961). Progesterone for endometrial cancer. *N. Engl. J. Med.*, **264**, 216

Kneale, B.L. (1986). Adjunctive and therapeutic progestins in endometrial cancer. In Creasman, W.T. (ed.) *Clinics in Obstetrics and Gynaecology: Endometrial Cancer*, Vol. 13., No. 4. pp. 789–809. (London, Philadelphia, Toronto: W.B. Saunders Co.)

Leonardo, R.A. (1944) *History of Gynaecology*, p. 313. (New York: Froben)

MacDonald, P.C. and Siiteri, P.K. (1974). Relationship between extraglandular production of estrone and endometrial neoplasia. *Gynecol. Oncol.*, **2**, 259

Mahle, A.E. (1923), quoted by Way (1951) p. 181

Marchand, F. (1895), quoted by Ricci (1945) p. 495

Masson, J.C. (1923). Sarcoma of the uterus. *Am. J. Obstet. Gynecol.*, **5**, 345

Masson, J.C. (1934), quoted by Way (1951) p. 181

Mathieu, A. (1934). History of hysterectomy. *West, J. Surg. Obstet. Gynecol.*, **42**, 2

Meigs, J.V. (1929), quoted by Way (1951) p. 181

Miller, N.F. (1940), quoted by Way (1951) p. 181

Miller, N.F. and Henderson, C.W. (1946), quoted by Way (1951) p. 181

Nicholson, G.W. (1923). Studies in tumour formation. The heterotopic tumours. *Guy's Hosp. Rep.*, **73**, 298

Novak, E. (1920). Relation of hyperplasia of endometrium to so-called functional uterine bleeding. *J. Am. Med. Assoc.*, **75**, 292

Novak, E. and Anderson, D.F. (1937). Sarcoma of the uterus. *Am. J. Obstet. Gynecol.*, **34**, 470

Novak, E. and Martzloff, K.H. (1924). Hyperplasia of the endometrium: a clinical and pathological study. *Am. J. Obstet. Gynecol.*, **8**, 385

Novak, E. and Rutledge, F. (1948). Atypical endometrial hyperplasia simulating adenocarcinoma. *Am. J. Obstet. Gynecol.*, **55**, 46–55

Novak, E. and Yui, E. (1936). Relation of endometrial hyperplasia to adenocarcinoma of the uterus. *Am. J. Obstet. Gynecol.*, **32**, 674

Olshausen, R. (1875). Ueber chronische, hyperplasirende Endometritis des Corpus uteri. *Arch. Gynakol.*, **8**, 97

Palmer, J.P., Reinhard, M.C., Sadugor, M.G. and Goltz, H.L. (1949). A statistical study of cancer of the corpus uteri. *Am. J. Obstet. Gynecol.*, **58**, 457

Persaud, V. and Arjoon, P.D. (1970). Uterine leiomyoma: incidence of degenerative change and a correlation of associated symptoms. *Obstet. Gynecol.*, **35**, 432

Peterson, W.F. and Novak, E.R. (1956). Endometrial polyps. *Obstet. Gynecol.*, **8**, 40

Poulsen, H.E., Taylor, C.W. and Sobin, L.H. (1975). Histological typing of female genital tract tumors. *International Classification of Tumors*, vol. 13, pp. 64–5. (Geneva: World Health Organization)

Proper, M.S. and Simpson, B.T. (1919), quoted by Way (1951) p. 227

Recamier, M. (1850). Memoire sur les productions fibreuses et fongueuses intra-uterines. *Union Med. Paris*, **4**, 266

Ricci, J.V. (1945). *One Hundred Years of Gynecology 1800-1900*, pp. 166, 174–180, 494. (Philadelphia: Blakiston Co.)

Ricci, J.V. (1950). *Genealogy of Gynecology*, p. 350. (Philadelphia: Blakiston Co.)

Rokitansky, C. (1855). Ovarien-cysten. *Wbl. Ges. Artze. Wien.*, **1**, 1. In Selye, H. (ed.) *Encyclopedia of Endocrinology*, Sect. IV Ovary, Vol. VII. (Montreal: Richardson Bond and Wright)

Schiller, W. (1939). Mesonephroma ovarii. *Am J. Cancer*, **35**, 1–21

Schroder, R. (1914). Uber das Verhalten der Uterusschleimhaut um die Zeit der Menstruation. *Mschr. Geburtsh. Gynakol.*, **39**, 3

Schroder, R. (1954). Endometrial hyperplasia in relation to genital function. *Am. J. Obstet. Gynecol.*, **68**, 294

Shaw, W. (1929). Irregular uterine haemorrhage. *J. Obstet. Gynaecol. Br. Emp.*, **36**, 1

Smith, D.C., Prentice, R., Thompson, D.J. and Herrman, W.L. (1975). Association of exogenous estrogen and endometrial carcinoma. *N. Engl. J. Med.*, **293**, 1164–7

Taylor, H.C. Jr. (1932). Endometrial hyperplasia and carcinoma of body of uterus. *Am. J. Obstet. Gynecol.*, **23**, 309

Taylor, H.C. Jr. and Beckner, W.F. (1947), quoted by Way (1951) p. 181

Teacher, J.H. (1903). On chorionepithelioma and the occurrence of chorionepitheliomatous and hydatidiform mole-like structures in teratomata. A pathological and clinical study. *J. Obstet. Gynaecol. Br. Emp.*, **4**, 1

Thigpen, T., Buchsbaum, W.J., Mangan, C. and Blessing, J.A. (1979). Phase II trial of adriamycin in the treatment of advanced or recurrent endometrial carcinoma. A Gynecologic Oncology Group Study. *Cancer Treatment Rep.*, **63**, 21–7

Underwood, P.B. Jr., Lutz, M.H., Kreutner, A., Miller, M.C. and Johnson, R.D. (1977). Carcinoma of the endometrium: radiation followed immediately by operation. *Am. J. Obstet. Gynecol.*, **128**, 86

Voght, M.E. (1923), quoted by Way (1951) p. 227

Way, S. (1951). *Malignant Disease of the Female Genital Tract*, p. 167. (London: J & A Churchill Ltd.)

Wertheim, E. (1905), quoted by Way (1951) p. 153

West, C. and Duncan, J.M. (1879). *Disease of Women.* (London: Churchill)

Willis, R.A. (1934). *Spread of Tumours in the Human Body*, p. 401. (London: Churchill)

Willis, R.A. (1948). *Pathology of Tumours*, p. 539. (London: Butterworth)

Ziel, H.K. and Finkle, W.D. (1975). Increased risk of endometrial carcinoma among users of conjugated oestrogens. *N. Engl. J. Med.*, **293**, 1167–70

FURTHER READING

Christopherson, W.M. (1986). The significance of the pathologic findings in endometrial cancer. In Creasman, W.T. (ed.) *Endometrial Cancer: Clinics in Obstetrics and Gynaecology*, Vol. 13, No. 4 pp. 673–93. (London, Philadelphia, Toronto: W.B. Saunders Co.)

Cianfrani, T. (1960). *A Short History of Obstetrics and Gynaecology.* (Springfield Illinois: Charles C. Thomas)

Don Gambrell, R, Jr. (1986). The role of hormones in the etiology and prevention of endometrial cancer. In Creasman, W.T. (ed.) *Endometrial Cancer: Clinics in Obstetrics and Gynaecology*, Vol. 13 No. 4, pp. 695–723. (London, Philadelphia, Toronto: W.B. Saunders Co.)

Haines, M. and Taylor, C.W. (1962). *Gynaecological Pathology.* (London: J.&A. Churchill Ltd.)

Haines, M. and Taylor, C.W. (1975). *Gynaecological Pathology.* (Edinburgh London New York: Churchill Livingstone)

Norris, H.J., Connor, M.P. and Kurman, R.J. (1986) Preinvasive lesions of the endometrium. In Creasman, W.T. (ed) *Endometrial Cancer: Clinics in Obstetrics and Ganaecology*, Vol. 13, No. 4 pp. 725–38. (London, Philadelphia, Toronto: W.B. Saunders Co.)

Novak, E.R. and Woodruff, J.D. (1962). *Novak's Gynecologic and Obstetric Pathology: With Clinical and Endocrine Relations*, 5th edn. (Philadelphia, London: W.B. Saunders Co.)

Way, S. (1951). *Malignant Disease of the Female Genital Tract.* (London: J.&A. Churchill Ltd.)

Cancer of the ovary

INTRODUCTION

Johann Schenck von Grafenberg reported ovarian malignancy in 1595, and also described a dermoid tumour. In 1686 DeLamzweerde documented the occurrence of both ovarian cysts and fibroids. He speculated that fibroid growths resulted from degeneration of semen. A contemporary, Theodorus Schorkopff wrote the earliest work devoted entirely to ovarian cysts, in 1685. He also gets the credit for first using the term 'annexa' (adnexa); for the observation of ovarian abscess; and was the first to suggest removal of ovaries as a cure for ovarian cyst formation (Cianfrani, 1960).

William Hunter (1718–1783) suggested tapping or removing ovarian cysts in 1775, but did not perform either procedure. Johannes C.A. Theden removed an ovarian cyst in 1771 and a similar operation was carried out by Samuel Hartman d'Escher in 1807. However, Ephraim McDowell (1771–1830) usually gains the credit for the first successful ovariotomy. The patient was a Mrs Jane Todd Crawford, who was 47 years old. McDowell carried out the operation in Danville Kentucky, in 1809. He reported three cases of ovarian extirpation (1817) and was conferred with an honorary M.D. degree by the University of Maryland in 1825. The cyst that McDowell removed contained 15 lb (6.8 kg). of gelatinous material, and the sac itself weighed 7.5 lb (3.2 kg). Ovariotomy was performed by a number of operators in America and Europe soon after McDowell's historic operation. Lawson Tait (1845–1899; q.v. Biographies) of England was one of the most famous ovariotomists of the nineteenth century (Figure 1).

The occurrence of malignant change in benign ovarian cysts was first considered by J.M. Delpech in 1828. Later in the nineteenth century a large number of types of benign cyst were documented. As clinicians and pathologists accepted the various classifications of ovarian cyst, they also discovered that many had the potential for malignant change. Carcinoma arising from ovarian endometriosis was documented by Sampson (1925). A further group of tumours was classified as 'mesonephroma of ovary' by Schiller (1939) which he indicated could be either benign or malignant.

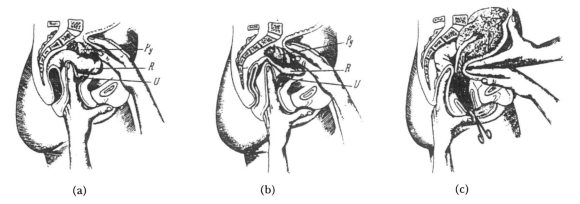

(a)   (b)   (c)

Figure 1 Bimanual palpation of the ovary with the index finger of the left hand in the vagina and the fingers of the right hand pressing in to the lower abdominal wall (a and b). Bimanual examination with the index finger of the left hand in the rectum, with a sponge or tampon on a sponge holder pushed high into the vagina, with the fingers of the right hand pushed deeply into the anterior lower abdominal wall while an assistant using the left hand raises up the tumour to try to estimate its size (c). From Shaeffer-Bouglé, *Atlas-Manuel de Gynécologie*, Paris (1903)

Subsequent investigators however did not agree with his interpretation. Malignant degeneration was found to occur in pseudomucinous cystadenocarcinoma in about 5–12% while Meyer (1915) quoted 1.7% cancerous change in dermoid cysts. The primary solid carcinomas were subdivided originally into six types, with adenocarcinoma being the most common variety.

Joe Vincent Meigs and J.W. Cass (1937) documented the association of hydrothorax, ascites, and ovarian tumour commonly seen in association with ovarian fibromas, but also noted with ovarian cancer. The condition was previously documented by Otto Spiegelberg (1866), Cullingworth (1879), Tait (1892), and others. Meigs, who later became clinical Professor of Gynaecology at Harvard, however, gained the eponymic distinction. Meigs and Somers (1957) recognized a separate group of tumours including dermoid cysts, teratomata, leiomyomata and sarcomata which were associated with symptoms similiar to the original 'Meigs syndrome' but known as 'pseudo-Meigs' syndrome.

When ovarian cancer spread the uterus, tubes (Figure 2), other ovary and peritoneum were most commonly involved. Ascites developed when the peritoneum became involved. Lymphatic spread to the retroperitoneal, inguinal, mediastinal and supraclavicular glands was documented. Distant spread affected the liver, lungs and other sites.

SECONDARY MALIGNANT DISEASE

The ovary was found to be a striking exception to Virchow's dictum which held that organs which were frequently the seat of primary cancer were rarely involved in a secondary malignancy and vice versa (Novak, 1947). In 1874 G. Leopold noted a definite relationship between gastric cancer and ovarian malignancy. By 1893 R. Bucher was able to report nine cases in the literature whose ovarian malignancy was related to either stomach or breast cancer. However, the first clear description was by Friedrich Krukenberg (1893;1896) who described what he thought was a primary ovarian tumour of apparent fibrosarcomatous tissue containing 'signet ring' cells distended with mucus. In his 1896 paper he documented six cases which were collected in Marchand's laboratory at Marburg. At the suggestion of Marchand he termed the tumour 'fibrosarcoma ovarii mucocellulare carcinomatoides'. His error in designating the tumours as

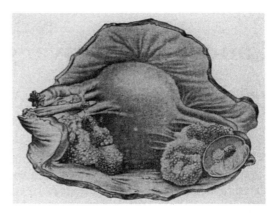

Figure 2 Papilliferous growths in both ovaries (after Howard Kelly) from a postmortem specimen. From Schaeffer-Bouglé, *Atlas – Manuel de Gynécologie*, Paris (1903)

sarcomas was corrected by Schlagenhaufer (1902) who described 79 cases of secondary ovarian cancer; established the epithelial origin of the growths; and also demonstrated that they were most often secondary to carcinoma elsewhere.

Review of autopsy material by Ley (1920) showed that the secondary cancer most commonly came from the gut, breast, or opposite ovary. According to Shaw (1932; 1933) and subsequent investigators, ovarian tumours of metastatic origin accounted for 20% of all malignant ovarian tumours. Primary Krukenberg tumours were described by Woodruff and Novak (1960). They documented ten cases, which were culled from the ovarian tumour registry.

INCIDENCE

Stanley Way (1951) summarized reports from the 1930s and 1940s, and quoted an incidence of 20–28% of all reported malignant tumours in females. In his analysis of age, he found that malignant ovarian tumours most frequently occurred during the decade between the ages of 51 and 60 years. Seventy-five per cent of patients were parous. No early symptoms were related apart from vague abdominal discomfort and mild digestive disturbances. Abdominal swelling and pain were the two symptoms which attracted attention to the disease.

Meyer (1930a) analysed several series of reported cases. He determined that carcinoma of the ovary could present as a solid or cystic structure with the latter being more common. He also noted that almost 15% of all ovarian tumours were cancerous, while 50% of those were bilateral. Nulliparity was found to be a significant risk factor. Hysterectomy or unilateral oophorectomy appeared to place patients at lower risk for subsequent development of ovarian cancer. Cutler *et al.* (1976) reported that between 1945 and 1949 only 27% of ovarian cancers were adequately diagnosed, and during the period 1965–1969 the figure was only 28%.

In the late 1980s, cancer of the ovary was found to be the fifth most common type of cancer of women in America, and the fourth leading cause of cancer death, preceded by cancer of breast, lung, colon and rectum. It was the second most common female pelvic genital malignancy. Creasman and Clarke-Pearson (1983) estimated that one out of every nine females in the USA would die from ovarian malignancy. They further documented that two-thirds of all ovarian cancers were stage 3 or 4 when diagnosed; over 90% with advanced disease would die from their malignancy, and 40% of stage 1 patients would die within 5 years.

PATHOLOGY AND STAGING

Pfannenstiel introduced a classification of ovarian tumours in 1898 which was the accepted standard until the 1920s. Robert Meyer amended that classification in 1915 and went on to describe granulosa cell tumours, arrhenoblastoma and dysgerminoma. In 1923 he demonstrated that some tumours produced masculinizing or feminizing effects (Cianfrani, 1960).

Broders (1926) developed a grading system applicable to various tumours. He emphasized the importance of the number of mitotic figures and the degree of tissue differentiation. Other methods of histological grading were used and Taylor (1929) defined three groups as follows:

(1) Those in which well-differentiated columnar epithelium was present;

(2) Tumours with glandular or papillary structure and actively malignant; and

(3) Tumours showing undifferentiated epithelial cells with marked nuclear changes and little or no glandular or papillary structure.

Meyer (1930a) identified three groups of primary cystic carcinoma of the ovary:

(1) Carcinoma arising in pseudomucinous cystadenoma;

(2) Carcinoma arising in serous cystadenoma; and

(3) Carcinoma arising in dermoid cysts.

More than 30 separate types of ovarian neoplasm were described. The tumours could be classified under three broad categories: epithelial, stromal and germ cell. Almost 60% were found to be of epithelial origin, and of all malignant ovarian tumours 90% came from the epithelial group. Initially the ovarian tumours were classed as either 'benign' or 'malignant' neoplasms, but a third category of 'low malignant potential' was introduced in the 1960s. However, Taylor (1929) was the first to report a group of hyperplastic serous low malignant potential tumours. The prognosis was usually favourable but some patients died. Taylor referred to 'borderline malignancy' in these tumours.

Hart (1977) indicated that the tumours of low malignant potential shared the cytological atypia and histological features of invasive carcinoma. The destructive infiltrative growth of invasive carcinoma was however in the low malignant potential group, which was found to constitute less than 20% of ovarian neoplasms. The World Health Organization classification of ovarian tumours became widely accepted (Serov and Scully, 1973) but was presented in modified versions by many authors.

The stage at laparotomy was found to determine the prognosis. In stage 1 disease the cancer was limited to one ovary while in stage 4 there were metastases beyond the peritoneal cavity. Five-year survival rates for stages 1 and 2 were almost 50% but for stages 3 and 4 they were in single figures. The cancer commission of the League of Nations initiated talks on the formulation of an international classification in the late 1920s. This led to the International Federation of Gynaecology and Obstetrics (FIGO) classification, which was last updated in 1988.

TREATMENT

Accurate staging of the disease was important as it was the primary factor in the selection of appropriate treatment. The staging of ovarian cancer was based on the findings at surgical exploration and the histological grade and type of tumour. Also, the adoption of a team approach including the expertise of the gynaecologist, pathologist, chemotherapist and radiation expert was of extreme importance for the prognosis of the disease.

Surgery

Pemberton (1940) advised that 'it would be wise to remove the omentum, whether or not gross metastases can be seen, because it is so often affected by, and may be a source of, recurrence later'. Hysterectomy with removal of both adnexa, omentectomy, and removal of as much intraperitoneal tumour as possible became the standard method of treatment. Cytoreductive surgery (or debulking) was found to be the mainstay of therapy, and removal of any diseased tissue above 2 cm size was necessary to improve long-term survival.

Chemotherapy

Rundles and Burton (1952) first reported the use of alkylating agents in patients with advanced ovarian cancer, and reported a favourable response in about 30%. The drugs became widely available in 1961. Single alkylating agents were commonly used and produced temporary clinical response (Lebhertz et al., 1965). Other drugs including thiotepa, chlorambucil and other antimitotic drugs were instilled intraperitoneally during surgery.

A combination of methotrexate with thiotepa was introduced about 1961 by Greenspan (1968), but alkylating agents remained the premier chemotherapeutic modality until the 1970s. Wiltshaw and Kroner (1976) demonstrated the activity of cis-dichlorodiamineplatinum (cisplatin) against epithelial ovarian cancer and soon after Young et al. (1978) demonstrated the superiority of combination therapy over single alkylating agent chemotherapy in a prospective comparison.

Triple therapy treatment was first documented by Smith and Rutledge (1975) who studied the effect of vincristine, actinomycin-D, and cyclophosphamide (VAC). Creasman et al. (1979) used a different combination – methotrexate, actinomycin-D, and cyclophosphamide (MAC). Chemotherapy had many disagreeable side-effects including depression of the haematological system, gastrointestinal upset, severe nephrotoxicity and alopecia. Long-term problems included the development of myeloblastic leukaemia. Prior to 1970, the roles of surgery, radiotherapy and chemotherapy in ovarian cancer were poorly defined.

Radiotherapy

In the 1950s external radiation of the pelvis and abdomen was the only treatment available after surgery. Until the 1970s, the evidence for radiation as a therapeutic modality was derived from retrospective studies. Puck et al. (1957) for instance demonstrated that radiation was effective when the ovarian tumour was properly debulked. The Gynecology Oncology Group began a study of adjuvant therapy for stage 1 ovarian carcinoma in 1971.

This study ran for over 7 years and more than 20 institutions were involved. Analysis of results indicated that radiotherapy played a curative role in postoperative treatment, although a number of workers considered that radiation therapy was of doubtful value in advanced disease.

Radioisotopes

The first use of radioisotopes was reported by Muller (1945) who used radioactive zinc as palliative therapy in ovarian cancer. Subsequent workers used a variety of compounds including a colloidal suspension of radiogold or chromic phosphate. Jones et al. (1944) developed a chemically inert colloidal form of phosphate. From 1955 radioactive isotopes of phosphate became the agent of choice for both treatment and palliation.

Immunotherapy

Patients with cancerous tumours were found to have decreased immunological competence. Adjuvant immunotherapy had the potential to partially reverse the immunosuppressed state and improve the patient's own tumour rejection capabilities. There was also a possibility that immunotherapy would play a synergistic role with alkylating agent therapy. Interferon was discovered simultaneously in 1957 by the British virologist Alick Isaacs, and J. Lindenmann of Switzerland. The substance was found to be produced in response to virus infection. Interferon, a multifunctional lymphokine, was discovered to have antitumour effects. Its ability to activate macrophages and increase the number and activity of natural killer lymphocytes was documented. Interferon was scarce and could only be produced in any quantity after genetic engineering made its production possible towards the end of the 1970s. Interferon was first marketed in 1987.

In the late 1980s, Professor Stephen Rosenberg,

a pioneer of immunotherapy, researched the possibility of genetically marking a patient's own cells so that their progress within the diseased organism could be monitored. It appeared that the existing treatments of surgery, chemotherapy and radiotherapy could be complemented by that of immunotherapy as a fourth weapon in the fight against cancer.

SECOND-LOOK PROCEDURES

The concept of 'second-look' exploratory laparotomy was introduced by Wangensteen *et al.* (1951) to identify early recurrent bowel carcinoma. A similar approach was pioneered by Rutledge and Burns (1966) for patients with ovarian cancer. The finding of persistent disease at second-look operations indicated a poor prognosis. Second-look laparotomy was necessary to evaluate the impact of previous debulking operations and subsequent chemo- or radiotherapy. Clinical and imaging techniques compared poorly with this approach.

Laparoscopic investigation was introduced as an intermediate method to determine the optimal duration of chemotherapy and to assist with the timing of second-look laparotomy. Hassan (1971) pioneered the technique of 'open laparoscopy' in an effort to reduce the incidence of bowel injury encountered at 'normal' or closed laparoscopy. As the technique became more popular, laparoscopy was also used in the initial staging of ovarian cancer cases (Bagley *et al.*, 1973). Rosenoff *et al.* (1975) indicated that 39% of patients thought to be in clinical remission had recurrent tumour evident at laparoscopy. The sensitivity of laparoscopy as a 'second-look' procedure was found to be about 70%. Second-look laparotomy however remained the definitive procedure.

TUMOUR 'MARKERS'

In a review of this subject Van Nagell Jr. (1983) defined a tumour marker as . . . 'a substance which is selectively produced by tumour cells and released into the circulation in detectable amounts. Such markers are thought to be neoantigens expressed at the time of neoplastic transformation, or are normal tissue antigens produced in increased concentrations by rapidly proliferating tumour cells'. He went on to say that . . . 'this marker could be used as an adjunct in

diagnosis, as a target for radiolabelled antibodies used in photoscanning studies, and as a biochemical monitor of the response of disease to treatment'.

Oncofetal antigens

These are normal tissue antigens produced in excess amounts by embryonic and neoplastic cells in ovarian tumours. Gold and Friedman (1962) first discovered carcinoembryonic antigen in colonic carcinoma. Khoo and MacKay (1973) found elevated levels in the tumours and plasma of ovarian cancer victims. Plasma carcinoembryonic antigen levels were elevated in almost 50% of patients with ovarian cancer compared to 18% of non-cancer patients, but the antigen was found to lack specificity. It was mainly used in the follow-up of postoperative cases, and in the detection of mucinous cystadenocarcinomas.

α-Fetoprotein, another glycoprotein, was first described by Abelev (1963) and was linked to teratocarcinomas of the ovary by the same author 3 years later. Low concentrations of the substance were found in the sera of patients with epithelial ovarian cancer by Donaldson *et al.* (1980). This antigen was useful in the detection of patients with germ cell tumours.

Carcinoplacental proteins

Human chorionic gonadotropin was first used by Li *et al.* (1958) as a marker for patients with testicular choriocarcinoma and trophoblastic malignancies. The glycoprotein was found to be an effective marker in ovarian choriocarcinoma, embryonal cell carcinoma and trophoblastic malignancies.

Human placental lactogen was originally discovered in placental tissue by Josimovitch and MacClaren (1962). Elevated levels were found in gynaecological patients with ovarian choriocarcinoma and trophoblastic tumours.

Although elevated levels of placental alkaline phosphatase were present in 20% of patients with ovarian cancer, estimation of these levels was of limited value.

Tumour-associated antigens

The search for a tumour-specific marker in ovarian cancer appeared to end when Witebsky *et al.* (1956) reported the isolation of antisera to mucinous ovarian cancer. As a result of that work, Bhattacharya and Barlow (1972; 1975) reported studies of ovarian cystadenocarcinoma antigen. Radioimmunoassay techniques were developed and levels of ovarian cystadenocarcinoma antigen were found to correlate with ovarian tumour mass.

A second antigen, the ovarian cancer antigen, was described by Knauf and Urbach (1974). Both antigens were useful in monitoring postoperative patients.

Ultrasound

Another method of screening for ovarian cancer was by ultrasound examination as pioneered by Campbell *et al.* (1982).

MALIGNANT GERM CELL TUMOURS

Brenner tumours

This tumour was first described by Orthmann (1899) who called it 'fibroma papillare superficiale carcinomatosum ovarii'. Fritz Brenner (1907) described three further cases and used the designation 'oophoroma folliculare'. He intimated that the tumour was related to granulosa cell lesions or arose from Pfluger's tubules. Robert Meyer (1932) noted its association with pseudomucinous cysts and called the lesion a 'Brenner tumour'. Meyer theorized that the tumour arose in islands of squamous or transitional epithelial cells, a group of indifferent cells first described by Walthard in 1903 (Walthard inclusions). Malignant change rarely occurred. In some instances, the tumour was found to exert an oestrogenic influence on the endometrium and Schifferman (1932) was the first to report irregular uterine bleeding accompanying Brenner tumours. Virilism as a result of the tumour was described by Morris and Scully (1958).

Dysgerminoma

Although E.G. Orthmann may have described this condition in 1899, it was M. Chevassu (1906) of Paris who first described it clearly, noting its resemblance to testicular tissue. This tumour originated from germ cells in their undifferentiated stage. Robert Meyer (1931) suggested their origin and termed them 'dysgerminomas of the ovary'. The tumour was malignant, but varied in its intensity in individual cases. Dysgerminoma was predominantly a tumour of early life and at one time

was termed 'carcinoma puellarum'. Germ cell tumours were found to be bilateral in 3–10% of cases. Dysgerminoma quickly spread through the lymphatic system to the pelvic, aortic and supraclavicular lymph nodes. The tumour was found to have a predilection for the right side.

Endodermal sinus tumours

As with other germ cell tumours, adbominal pain was frequently the initial symptom of endodermal sinus tumours. Until the advent of combination chemotherapy 95% of patients died within 2 years of discovery and treatment.

Embryonal carcinoma

Embryonal carcinoma, which was found to be analogous to embryonal carcinoma of the adult testis, was included in the World Health Organization classification of 1973. It was characterized as a separate tumour (distinct from endodermal sinus tumour) by Kurman and Norris (1976) who reported 15 cases of this previously undescribed germ cell tumour of the ovary.

FEMINIZING TUMOURS (GRANULOSA AND THECA CELL)

This tumour was first described by C. von Kahlden in 1895. Further descriptions by F. von Werdt in 1914 and R. Meyer in 1915 led to a clear understanding of the disordered growth in the tumour. Robert Meyer (1931) explained that these tumours arose from rests of redundant granulosa cells, left over from the process of follicle formation. The tumours were solid but contained small cystic cavities.

Von Kahlden (1895) noted a resemblance of the cystic cavities to that of large Graafian follicles, and termed them 'folliculoma malignum'. A rare variety of the tumour was found to contain clear cells rich in lipid. These tumours were termed 'folliculome lipidique' by Lecene in 1910. Granulosa or theca cell tumours were associated with adenocarcinoma of the uterus. They could occur at any age, but were less malignant than other ovarian cancers. While thecoma was generally regarded as non-malignant, Loffler and Priesel (1932) first reported malignancy arising from that form of tumour. Pali (1942) first reported masculinization which developed in a pregnant patient in association with a thecoma.

VIRILIZING OVARIAN TUMOURS

Arrhenoblastoma

This rare group of tumours with masculinizing ability was found to originate in male-directed cells which persisted in the ovary from fetal life. A highly differentiated arrhenoblastoma was originally described by Ludwig Pick (1905) and designated as 'testicular adenoma'. The term 'arrhenoblastoma' was introduced by Meyer (1930a,b). The degree of differentiation determined the level of endocrine function. Affected patients became virilized and a malignancy rate of 26% was noted by Javert and Finn (1951). Brentnall (1945) reported the first case known to occur in pregnancy.

Adrenal tumours

Adrenal tumours of the ovary were very rare. This type of tumour was first reported by F. Marchand in 1883. Due to its macroscopic and microscopic appearance H. Peham termed it hypernephroma in 1899. These neoplasms were also called 'hypernephroid tumours' or 'masculinovoblastoma' as proposed by Rottino and McGrath (1939). They were usually benign, but were capable of producing virilization.

Gynandroblastoma

The term was introduced by Robert Meyer who first reported this group of ovarian tumours in 1930. They were found to have mixed granulosa or theca elements together with microscopic evidence of arrhenoblastoma tissue. Their effect could be masculinizing or oestrogen dominant. Hobbs (1949) described a malignant case of gynandroblastoma. 'Annular tubule tumour' was a rare form described by Scully (1970).

Hilus or Leydig cell tumours

Berger (1923) reported this small group of virilizing tumours with cells similiar to those in the adrenal, arrayed in adenomatous fashion with connective tissue matrix.

OTHER OVARIAN TUMOURS

Dermoid cysts

These tumours were described as long ago as the sixteenth century by Johann Schenck von Grafenberg (1595). About 25% were found to be bilateral and these benign cystic teratomas made up 5–10% of all cystic neoplasms of the ovary, and 25% of all ovarian tumours complicating pregnancy (McKerron, 1903). Blackwell et al. (1946) estimated that about 3% underwent malignant change. Early reports of malignant change in dermoid cysts were unauthenticated and probably the earliest genuine observation came from R. Biermann in 1885. Case reports of malignant teratoma were published by M. Litten and R. Virchow in 1879 (Ricci, 1945a).

Solid teratoma

These were less common than cystic dermoids. A Blastomere Theory (Marchand–Bonnet) was advanced which claimed that the tumours arose from blastomere which was segregated at an early phase of embryonic development. This rare tumour was almost never found in its malignant form.

Carcinoid tumours

These tumours were almost never found as pure ovarian primary neoplasms. Most were found in association with a teratoma, usually a dermoid cyst (Govan, 1976). Nissen (1959) reviewed the eight cases reported in the literature and noted that gastrointestinal or respiratory epithelium was found in each case.

Struma ovarii (thyroid tumour of ovary)

The first reference to this tumour came from R. Boettlin in 1889. This type of teratoma was composed predominantly of thyroid tissue, with hyperthyroidism resulting in some cases. Plaut (1930) determined their iodine content.

Ovarian endometrial cysts

Sampson (1921) described 'chocolate' cysts of the ovary and 4 years later documented a small group of ovarian cancer cases which he believed had their origin in endometriomata.

Polyvesicular vitelline tumour

This type of yolk sac tumour which was similar to

endodermal sinus tumour, was described by Teilum (1965). It was found to contain blastocyst-like yolk sac (endoblast) vesicles scattered through a compact stroma.

Choriocarcinoma

Non-gestational choriocarcinoma was an extremely rare diagnosis.

Lipid cell tumours

The first case of the rare lipid cell tumour was reported by Bovin (1908). Sarcomas and other rare tumours have been documented.

CHILDHOOD

Norris and Jensen (1972) reviewed 350 cases of ovarian neoplasia in patients under the age of 20. Germ cell tumours were commonest at approximately 50–60% of the total. Serous and mucinous cysts formed almost 19%. Gonadal stromal tumours were present in 18%. The commonest germ cell tumour was the simple dermoid. Precocious puberty occurred in association with chorionic elements in solid teratomas, and was also caused by granulosa cell tumours. Tumours which caused masculinizing symptoms were extremely rare.

CHRONOLOGY

General

1595   von Grafenberg described ovarian malignancy.
1685   Schorkopff wrote the earliest work devoted to ovarian cysts.
1775   Hunter suggested tapping or removal.
1817   McDowell reported the first oophorectomies.
1866   Spiegelberg documented ovarian cysts with ascites and hydrothorax.
1893   Krukenberg documented the tumour for which he is known.
1898   Pfannenstiel introduced a classification of ovarian tumours.
1902   Schlagenhaufer described 79 cases of secondary ovarian cancer.
1915   Meyer amended the pathological classification.
1920   Ley documented that secondary cancer came from gut, breast, or the opposite ovary.

1925   Sampson described carcinoma arising from ovarian endometriosis.
1926   Broders developed a grading system.
1929   Taylor first reported low malignant potential tumours.
Late 1920s   The League of Nations initiated talks on a common classification.
1930   Meyer identified three groups of primary cystic carcinoma.
1932   Shaw discovered that 20% of ovarian tumours were of metastatic origin.
1937   Meigs and Kass described 'Meigs Syndrome'.
1951   Way summarized previous reports and documented ovarian cancer as causing 30% of malignant tumours in females.
1957   Meigs and Somers documented the 'pseudo-Meigs syndrome'.
1982   Campbell et al. explored the use of ultrasound examination.

Treatment

Surgery was the mainstay and:

1940   Pemberton advised omentectomy.
1945   Muller advocated the use of radioisotopes
1950s   External radiation was commonly used.
1952   Rundles and Burton used alkylating agents.
1957   Interferon was discovered.
1961   Alkylating agents became widely available.
1966   Rutledge and Burns pioneered 'second-look' laparotomy for ovarian cancer.
1968   Greenspan documented the use of combined methotrexate and thiotepa.
1971   Hassan pioneered 'open' laparoscopy.
1973   Bagley et al. used laparoscopy in the initial staging.
1976   Wiltshaw and Kroner described the use of cisplatin.
1978   Young et al. proved the superiority of combination therapy.
1975   Smith and Rutledge documented triple therapy.

Tumour 'markers'

1956   Witebsky et al. isolated antisera to mucinous cancers.
1958   Li et al. used chorionic gonadotrophin as a marker.

1962   Gold and Friedman discovered carcinoembryonic antigen.

1963   Abelev described α-fetoprotein.

1972–75 Bhattacharya and Barlow studied cystadenocarcinoma antigen.

1974   Knauf and Urbach described ovarian cancer antigen.

Some ovarian tumours

1595   von Grafenberg described dermoid cysts.

1889   Boettlin documented struma ovarii.

1895   von Kahlden described feminizing tumours.

1899   Peham introduced the term hypernephroma.

1905   Ludwick Pick documented the occurrence of arrhenoblastoma.

1906   Chevassu first clearly described dysgerminoma.

1907   Brenner described the 'Brenner Tumour' which was previously documented by Orthmann in 1899.

1908   Bovin described lipid cell tumours.

1915   Meyer amended the pathology gradings and went on to describe granulosa cell, arrhenoblastoma and dysgerminomas (1930;1931;1932).

1921   Sampson described 'chocolate' cysts.

1923   Berger documented hilus or Leydig cell tumours.

1930   Meyer reported gynandroblastoma.

1965   Teilum reported the polyvesicular vitelline tumour.

REFERENCES

Abelev, G.I. (1963). Study of the antigenic structure of tumors. *Acta Unionis Internationalis contra Cancrum*, **19**, 80–92

Bagley, C.M., Young, R.C., Schien, P.S. *et al.* (1973). Ovarian cancer metastatic to the diaphragm frequently undiagnosed at laparotomy. A preliminary report. *Am. J. Obstet. Gynecol.*, **116**, 397–404

Berger, L. (1923). La glande sympathicotrope du hile de l'ovaire; ses homologies avec la gland interstitielle du testicule. Les rapports nerveuses des deux glandes. *Arch. d'anat., d'histol. et d'embryol.*, **2**, 255

Bhattacharya, M. and Barlow, J.J. (1972). Immunologic studies of human serous cystadeno-carcinoma of ovary. *Cancer*, **31**, 588–95

Bhattacharya, M. and Barlow, J.J. (1975). A tumor-associated antigen from cystadenocarcinomas of the ovary. *Nat. Can. Inst. Monographs*, **42**, 25–32

Blackwell, W.J., Dockerty, M.B., Masson, J.C. and Mussey, R.D. (1946). Dermoid cysts of ovary: clinical and pathological significance. *Am. J. Obstet. Gynecol.*, **51**, 151

Boettlin, R. (1889), quoted by Ricci (1945) p.91

Bovin, E. (1908). Primary hypernephroid tumour in the female genitals. *Nord. Med. Archiv*, **41**, 1–5

Brenner, F. (1907). Das Oophoroma folliculare. *Frankf. Ztschr. f. Path.*, **1**, 150

Brentnall, P.P. (1945), quoted by Browne (1950) p. 376

Broders, A.C. (1926). Carcinoma: grading and practical application. *Arch. Pathol.*, **2**, 376–81

Browne, F.J. (1950). *Postgraduate Obstetrics and Gynaecology.* (London: Butterworths & Co.)

Campbell, S., Goessens, L., Goswamy, R. and Whitehead, M. (1982). Realtime ultrasonography for determination of ovarian morphology and volume: a possible early screening test for ovarian cancer? *Lancet*, **1**, 425

Chevassu, M. (1906). *Tumeurs du Testicule.* (Paris: Steinhall)

Cianfrani, T. (1960). *A Short History of Obstetrics and Gynecology.* (Springfield Illinois: C.C. Thomas)

Creasman, W.T. and Clarke-Pearson, D.L. (1983). Immunotherapy of ovarian cancer. In DiSaia, P.J. (ed.) *Clinics in Obstetrics and Gynaecology*, Vol. 10, no. 2, *Ovarian Cancer.* pp. 297–306. (London, Philadelphia, Toronto: W.B. Saunders Co.)

Creasman, W.T., Fetter, B.F., Hammond, C.B. and Parker, R.T. (1979). Germ cell malignancies of the ovary. *Obstet. Gynecol.*, **53**, 226–30

Cullingworth, C.J. (1879). Fibroma of both ovaries. *Trans. Obstet. Soc. Lond.*, **21**, 276

Cutler, S.J., Myers, M.H. and White, P.C. (1976). Who are we missing and why? *Cancer*, **37**, 421

Donaldson, E.S., van Nagell, J.R., Pursell, S. *et al.* (1980). Multiple biochemical markers in patients with gynecologic malignancies. *Cancer*, **45**, 948–53

Gold, P. and Friedman, S.O. (1962). Demonstration of tumor specific antigens in human colonic carcinoma by immunological tolerance and absorption techniques. *J. Exp. Med.*, **121**, 439–62

Govan, A.D.T. (1976). Ovarian tumours: clinical and pathological features. In Macnaughton, M.C. and Govan, A.D.T. (eds.) *Clinics in Obstetrics and Gynaecology*, Vol. 3, no. 1, *The Ovary*, pp.89–158. (London, Philadelphia, Toronto: W.B. Saunders and Co.)

Greenspan, E.M. (1968). Thio-tepa and methotrexate chemotherapy of advanced ovarian carcinoma. *Mount Sinai J. Med.*, **35**, 52–67

Hart, W.R. (1977). Ovarian epithelial tumors of borderline malignancy (carcinomas of low malignant potential). *Hum. Pathol.*, **8**, 541–9

Hassan, H.M. (1971). A modified instrument and method for laparoscopy. *Am. J. Obstet. Gynecol.*, **110**, 886–9

Hobbs, J.E. (1949). Gynandroblastoma of the ovary. *Am. J. Obstet. Gynecol.*, **57**, 85–96

Hunter, W. (1775), quoted by Cianfrani (1960) p. 260

Javert, C.T. and Finn, W.F. (1951). Arrhenoblastoma. *Cancer*, **4**, 60

Jones, H.B., Wrobel, C.J. and Lyons, W.R. (1944). A method of distributing beta-radiation to the reticulo-endothelial system and adjacent tissue. *J. Clin. Invest.*, **28**, 783–8

Josimovitch, J.B. and MacClaren, J.A. (1962). Presence in the human placenta and term serum of a highly lactogenic substance immunologically related to human growth hormone. *Endocrinology*, **71**, 209–15

Khoo, S.K. and MacKay, E.V. (1973). Carcinoembryonic antigen in cancer of the female reproductive system. Sequential levels and effects of treatment. *Aust. N.Z. J. Obstet. Gynaecol.*, **13**, 1–7

Knauf, S. and Urbach, E.I. (1974) Ovarian tumorspecific antigens. *Am. J. Obstet. Gynecol.*, **119**, 966–70

Krukenberg, F. (1893). Fibrosarcoma ovarii mucocellulare. *Arch. Gynakol.*, **1**, 287

Krukenberg, F. (1896). Uber das Fibrosarcoma ovarii mucocellulare (carcinomatodes). *Arch. Gynakol.*, **50**, 287–321

Kurman, R.J. and Norris, H.J. (1976). Embryonal carcinoma of the ovary. A clinicopathologic entity distinct from endodermal sinus tumor and resembling embryonal carcinoma of the adult testis. *Cancer*, **38**, 2420–33

Lebhertz, J.B., Huston, J.W. and Austin, J.A. (1965). Sustained palliation in ovarian carcinoma. *Obstet. Gynecol.*, **25**, 475–8

Ley, G. (1920). *Proc. R. Soc. Med.*, **13**, 95

Li, M.C., Hertz, R. and Bergenstral, D.M. (1958). Therapy of choriocarcinoma and related trophoblastic tumors with folic acid and purine antagonist. *N. Engl. J. Med.*, **259**, 66–70

Loffler, E. and Priesel, A. (1932). Fibroma thecocellulare xanthomatodes ovarii. *Betrage zur Pathologischen Anatomie und zur Allgemeinen Pathologie*, **90**, 199–221

McDowell, E. (1817). Three cases of extirpation of diseased ovarii. *Eclectic Repertory and Analytic Review*, **7**, 242

McKerron, R.G. (1903a). *Pregnancy, Labour and Childbirth with Ovarian Tumour.* (London: Rebman)

Meigs, J.V. and Cass, J.W. (1937). Fibroma of the ovary with ascites and hydrothorax. *Am. J. Obstet. Gynecol.*, **33**, 249–67

Meigs, J.V. and Somers, H.S. (1957). *Progress in Gynaecology*, Vol. 3, pp. 424–31. (New York, London: Grune and Stratton)

Meyer, R. (1915), quoted by Cianfrani (1960) p. 410

Meyer, R. (1930a). In Henke, F. and Lubarsch, O. (eds.) *Hanbuch der spez. path. Anat. u. Hist.* Vol. vii/3. (Berlin: Julius Springer)

Meyer, R. (1930b). Tubulare (testikulare) und solide Formen des Andreioblastoma ovarii. *Beitr. f. path. Anat.*, **84**, 485

Meyer, R. (1931). The pathology of some special ovarian tumors and their relation to sex characteristics. *Am. J. Obstet. Gynecol.*, **22**, 697

Meyer, R. (1932). Der Tumor Ovarii Brenner. *Zbl. Gynakol.*, **56**, 770

Morris, J.M. and Scully, R.E. (1958). *The Endocrine Pathology of the Ovary.* (London: Henry Kimpton)

Muller, J.H. (1945). Uber die verwendung von Kunstlichen radioaktiven isotopen zur erzielung von lokalisierten biologischen strahlenwirkungen. *Experientia*, **1**, 199–200

Nissen, E.D. (1959). Consideration of the malignant carcinoid syndrome primary argentaffin carcinomas arising in benign cystic teratomas of the ovary. *Obstet. Gynecol. Surv.*, **14**, 459–88

Norris, H.J. and Jensen, R.D. (1972). Relative frequency of ovarian neoplasms in children and adolescents. *Cancer*, **30**, 713–19

Novak, E. (1947). *Gynecological and Obstetrical Pathology With Clinical and Endocrine Relations*, 2nd edn. p. 344. (Philadelphia, London: W.B. Saunders Co.)

Orthmann, E.G. (1899). Zur casuistik einiger seltenerer Ovarial und Tuben-Tumoren. *Monatschr. f Geburtsh. u. Gynakol.*, plate VII, **9**, 771–82

Pali, K. (1942). Torsion of the pedicle of an ovarian tumor showing exceptional hormone production. *Zbl. Gynakol.*, **66**, 477–82

Peham, H. (1899), quoted by Ricci (1945) p. 92

Pemberton, F.A. (1940). Carcinoma of the ovary. *Am. J. Obstet. Gynecol.*, **40**, 751–63

Pfannenstiel (1898), quoted by Cianfrani (1960) p. 410

Pick, L. (1905). Adenoma der mannlichen und weiblichen Keimdruse. *Berl. klin. Wchn.*, **42**, 502

Plaut, A. (1930). Struma of ovary. *Arch. Path.*, **10**, 161

Puck, T.T., Morkovin, D., Marcus, P.I. and Cieciura, S.J. (1957). Action of X-rays on mammalian cells. II. Survival curves of cells from normal human tissues. *J. Exp. Med.*, **106**, 485

Ricci, J.V. (1945a) *One Hundred Years of Gynecology, 1800–1900*, p. 88. (Philadelphia: The Blakiston Co.)

Ricci, J.V. (1945b). *The Genealogy of Gynaecology*, p. 327. (New York: The Blakiston Co.)

Rosenoff, S.H., Young, R.C., Anderson, T. *et al.* (1975). Peritoneoscopy: a valuable staging tool in ovarian carcinoma. *Ann. Intern. Med.*, **83**, 37–41

Rottino, A. and McGrath, J.F. (1939). Masculinovoblastoma, primary masculinizing tumor of ovary. *Arch. Int. Med.*, **63**, 686

Rundles, R.W. and Burton, W.B. (1952). Triethylene melamine in the treatment of neoplastic disease. *Blood*, **7**, 483–507

Rutledge, F. and Burns, B. (1966). Chemotherapy for advanced ovarian cancer. *Am. J. Obstet. Gynecol.*, **96**, 761–70

Sampson, J.A. (1921). Perforating hemorrhagic (chocolate) cysts of the ovary, their importance and especially their relation to pelvic adenomas of the endometrial type. *Arch. Surg.*, **3**, 245

Sampson, J.A. (1925). Endometrial carcinoma of ovary arising in endometrial tissue in that organ. *Arch. Surg.*, **10**, 1–72

Schifferman, J. (1932). Post-menopausal bleeding and Brenner tumor of the ovary. *Arch. Gynakol.*, **150**, 159–75

Schiller, W. (1939). Mesonephroma ovarii. *Am. J. Cancer*, **35**, 1

Schlagenhaufer, F. (1902). Uber das metastatische Ovarialkarzinom nach Krebs des Magens, Darmes und anderer Bauchorgane. *Monatschr. f. Geb. u. Gynakol.*, **15**, 485

Schorkopff (1685), quoted by Cianfrani (1960) p. 183

Scully, R.E. (1970). Sex cord tumor with annular tubules. A distinctive ovarian tumor of the Peutz–Jeghers syndrome. *Cancer*, **25**, 1107–21

Serov, S.F. and Scully, R.E. (1973). Histological typing of ovarian tumors. *International Histological Classification of Tumors*, no. 9. (Geneva: World Health Organization)

Shaw, W. (1932). Pathology of ovarian tumours. *J. Obstet. Gynaecol. Br. Emp.*, **39**, 13, 324

Shaw, W. (1933). Pathology of ovarian tumours. *J. Obstet. Gynaecol. Br. Emp.*, **40**, 805, 1125

Smith, J.P. and Rutledge, F. (1975). Advances in chemotherapy for gynecologic cancer. *Cancer*, **36**, 669–74

Speert, H. (1958). *Essays in Eponymy. Obstetric and Gynecologic Milestones*, p.407. (New York: The McMillan Co.)

Spiegelberg, O. (1866). Mittheilungen aus der gynakologischen Klinik von Otto Spiegelberg. I. Fibrom des Eierstockes von enormer Grosse. *Monatschr. f. Geburtsk. u. Frauenk.*, **28**, 415–25

Tait, L. (1892). On the occurrence of pleural effusion associated with disease of the abdomen. *Med-Chir. Tr.*, **75**, 109–18

Taylor, H.C. (1929). Malignant and semimalignant tumors of the ovary. *Surg. Gynecol. Obstet.*, **48**, 204–30

Teilum, G. (1965). Classification of endodermal sinus tumor (mesoblastoma vitellinum) and so called 'embryonal carcinoma' of the ovary. *Acta Pathol. Microbiol. Scand.*, **64**, 407–29

Van Nagell, Jr. J.R. (1983). Tumour markers in ovarian cancer. In DiSaia, P.J. (ed.) *Clinics in Obstetrics and Gynaecology*, Vol. 10, no. 2. *Ovarian Cancer*, pp.197–212. (London, Philadelphia, Toronto: W.B. Saunders Co.)

von Grafenberg, J.S. (1595), quoted by Cianfrani (1960) p. 125

von Kahlden, C. (1895). Uber eine eigentumliche Form des Ovarialkarzinoms. *Zbl. Path.*, **6**, 257

Wangensteen, O.H., Lewis, F.J. and Tongen, L.A. (1951). The 'second look' in the cancer surgery. *Lancet*, **71**, 303–7

Way, S. (1951). *Malignant Disease of the Female Genital Tract.* (London: J. & A. Churchill Ltd.)

Wiltshaw, E. and Kroner, T. (1976). Phase II study of cis-dichlorodiamineplatinum (II) (NSC-119875) in advanced adenocarcinoma of the ovary. *Cancer Treatment Reports*, **60**, 55–60

Witebsky, E., Rose, N.R. and Schulman, S. (1956). Studies of normal and malignant tissue antigens. *Cancer Res.*, **16**, 831–41

Woodruff, J.D. and Novak, E.R. (1960). Krukenberg tumors of the ovary. *Obstet. Gynecol.*, **15**, 351

Young, R.C., Chabner, B.A., Hubbard, S.P. *et al.* (1978). Advanced ovarian adenocarcinoma: a prospective clinical trial of melphalan (L-PAM) versus combination chemotherapy. *N. Engl. J. Med.*, **229**, 1261–6

FURTHER READING

diSaia, P.J. (ed.) (1983). *Ovarian Cancer. Clinics in Obstetrics and Gynaecology*, Vol. 10, no. 2., August. (London, Philadelphia, Toronto: W.B. Saunders Co.)

Govan, A.D.T. (1976). Ovarian tumours: clinical and pathological features. In Macnaughton, M.C. and Govan, A.D.T. (eds.) *The Ovary. Clinics in Obstetrics and Gynaecology*, Vol. 3, no. 1 pp.89–157. (London, Philadelphia, Toronto: W.B. Saunders Co.)

Novak, E. (1947). *Gynecological and Obstetrical Pathology With Clinical and Endocrine Relations*, 2nd Edn. (London, Philadelphia, Toronto: W.B. Saunders Co.)

Novak, E.R. and Woodruff, J.D. (1962). *Novak's Gynecologic and Obstetric Pathology With Clinical and Endocrine Relations*, 5th Edn. (London, Philadelphia, Toronto: W.B. Saunders Co.)

Ricci, J.V. (1945). *One Hundred Years of Gynaecology, 1800–1900.* (Philadelphia: The Blakiston Co.)

Speert, H. (1958). *Essays in Eponymy. Obstetric and Gynaecologic Milestones.* (New York: The MacMillan Co.)

Way, S. (1951). *Malignant Disease of the Female Genital Tract.* (London: J.& A. Churchill Ltd.)

Spreading knowledge

THE UNIVERSITIES

Although much medical education and medical research is, and for long has been, centred on universities, and on university teaching hospitals, it is difficult to find out which university first had a medical school or taught midwifery systematically. The honour may be divided between the University of Paris, which is one of the oldest of European universities and was founded about 1170, and the University of Padua (or Padova) which was founded in 1222. Both Paris and Padua Universities were originally founded mainly for the study of theology. The saintly Albertus Magnus (q.v. Biographies) of Cologne in Germany was a teacher in the University of Paris after having been a student in the University of Padua in 1223. He was basically a theologian and philosopher; but he also made great contributions to science; and although the scientific works he wrote, in particular *De Animalibus*, were based on classical Greek authorities and particularly Aristotle, he made new observations which included some anatomical discoveries. These were important because the basis of gynaecology is anatomical knowledge. Serious study of anatomy started in the fourteenth century, in Italian universities.

The first large practical school of midwifery attached to a university was probably the Hotel de Dieu in Paris, which was a training school for midwives and later for doctors.

The University of Oxford was founded in the twelfth century soon after Paris University, on which it was modelled; and the University of Cambridge was founded in 1209 when a number of students from Oxford migrated there. It was, however, not formally incorporated as a University until 1571, although its first college, Peterhouse which was modelled on Merton College, Oxford, was established in 1284. From the beginning, or at any rate from the fourteenth century, the university had not only faculties of theology and law but also of medicine and of the arts. University College in Oxford is the oldest of the colleges.

The colleges in Oxford and Cambridge Universities were originally just boarding houses for poor students, and still to some extent they are very special boarding houses with the main responsibility for teaching and research being centred on the University itself.

The great Harvey (q.v. Biographies) was one of a galaxy of medical students who have attended Cambridge University in the past 500 years. Harvey was a student at Gonville and Caius College. After graduating from Cambridge he went to Padua University where he probably did most of his research on the circulation of the blood.

There has always been contact between most of the great universities of the world. It is difficult for someone who has not gone through the British college and university system to understand the interrelationship between the colleges and the university. This has developed slowly over the centuries. A student today who goes to Oxford or Cambridge University will first have to be accepted by one of the colleges, in which he will reside for at least part of his several years at university, and to which he will be attached no matter how loosely for the rest of his life. While an undergraduate he will be expected to eat several meals a month in the communal dining hall, and he may well belong to athletic and social, e.g. musical, clubs, connected with his college as well as to university societies. Tutorials in which he receives individual tuition and for which he writes essays will be arranged by his college. The main thrust of the teaching he will receive, however, will be in the larger lecture theatres, the anatomy schools and the science laboratories and hospitals which belong to the university. The Professor of Gynaecology and Obstetrics for instance at Cambridge, is elected to his post by the university department and works in the university hospital (Addenbrooke's), but will almost certainly also hold a Fellowship of one of the university colleges. The college system does not exist in most European universities, nor does it exist in many of the provincial universities in the UK.

University teaching from the very beginning was inevitably more concerned with theory and research than with practice and the treatment of patients, partly because of the distribution of the population. So, patient care was, and still is, carried out much more widely throughout the country in non-university than in university hospitals. But once universities became established for research as well as for teaching, they had great appeal for teachers of medicine who could lecture to large bodies of students in them, while spending some of their time in research. Yet the majority of patients in the UK are treated in District General Hospitals and the majority of postgraduate obstetricians and gynaecologists receive most of their training in non-university hospitals which are, however, supervised by the Royal Colleges, of which more later.

It is not possible to enter university as a medical student without some training in the basic sciences either at school or in a preuniversity training institution. All the undergraduate teaching hospitals throughout the UK are affiliated to a university. For instance University College Hospital in London is affiliated to University College London and to the University of London. King's College Hospital, a most important teaching hospital, is a constituent of the University of London and linked to King's College which is a part of the University of London.

THE ROYAL COLLEGES OF THE VARIOUS BRANCHES OF MEDICINE

Probably the most important element in the training and in the regulation of medicine in England was brought about in 1518 when Thomas Linacre (1460–1524) obtained from Henry VIII letters patent for the institution of a body of regular physicians empowered to decide who should practise medicine in Greater London. This institute, later the *Royal College of Physicians of London*, obtained authority to examine and license physicians and to fine and otherwise punish, if necessary by imprisonment, offenders (with the exception of graduates of Oxford and Cambridge!). It was not the first of the Royal Colleges because the *Royal College of Surgeons of Edinburgh*, which was an organization of Scottish surgeons, received its charter in 1505.

On 6 December 1617 the *Society of Apothecaries* was founded due to the efforts of Gideon de Laune, apothecary to Queen Anne of Denmark,

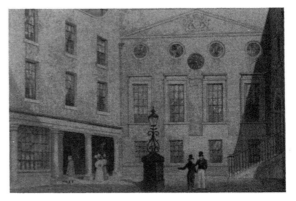

Figure 1 The courtyard of the Worshipful Society of Apothecaries, London. The general appearance of this courtyard is still as in this illustration

wife of King James I and VI. Already by that time the *College of Physicians* and the *Barber-Surgeons' Company* were well established in the City of London (Figure 1).

The Society of Apothecaries was an offshoot of the ancient Grocers' Company. Like other city companies it built a hall for its purposes in 1632 on the site of an old monastery. This hall was rebuilt in 1668–1670 after its destruction in the Great Fire of London in 1666. The Society grants a certificate of registration (LMSSA) to candidates trained in hospitals approved by the General Medical Council enabling the holders to practise medicine. It has a small teaching committment and grants postgraduate diplomas in specialized subjects such as jurisprudence and the history of medicine. The Apothecaries' Act of 1815 extended the authority of the Society of Apothecaries; and it is recorded that in 1827 the Society of Apothecaries wanted candidates for its diploma to have had some training in obstetrics. The other colleges continued to object to the teaching of obstetrics (not a job for nice men!) until 1829 when there was some relaxation of the attitude taken by the court of examiners of the Royal College of Surgeons who for the first time allowed their members to consult with obstetricians. The Society of Apothecaries formerly granted a mastership in obstetrics and gynaecology (MMSA), but as the influence of the Royal College of Obstetricians and Gynaecologists increased, this was abandoned.

The Company of Barber-Surgeons was originally incorporated in 1461. It had no disciplinary powers and it seemed to have lapsed until 1540 when it was reincorporated and given disciplinary powers. Members of the Barber-Surgeons' Company seem also to have kept shops to sell medicines and this is when the term 'apothecary' started to be used.

The Royal College of Surgeons of England was not established until 1800 by members of the Company of Barber-Surgeons. The College of Obstetricians and Gynaecologists became established in 1929, after some opposition from leading gynaecologists such as Victor Bonney (q.v.) who may have been opposed to the establishment of the college on personal grounds because he had hoped to become President of the Royal College of Surgeons of England. Normally a college has to show its worth for some years after its founding before being given a royal charter. For instance the College of Obstetricians and Gynaecologists was only given a Royal Charter some years after its foundation when a member of the royal family became the patron of the college. The process was the acceptance by the Board of Trade in 1929 of registration as a limited company with permission to drop the word 'limited'. The King authorized the use of 'Royal' from December 1938 but because of World War II the application for a charter was suspended and was granted to the College only in March 1947 (Thornton and Want, 1973). All the specialist colleges have developed gradually over decades and even centuries.

The function of specialist colleges such as the Royal College of Obstetricians and Gynaecologists, founded by William Blair-Bell (q.v.) in 1929, is to regulate the practice of the specialist subject. It does this, as do the other Royal Colleges, by examinations and regular inspections of the training hospitals to ensure that the equipment and training methods are adequate. The colleges set syllabuses for examinations in their specialist subjects. The training hospitals do not have to be university teaching hospitals, although a proportion are.

The colleges, do not have sole responsibility for maintaining high standards because the General Medical Council of the United Kingdom supervises the colleges' and the licensing bodies' examinations. So an examiner for one of the degrees at the Royal College may very well find that he is not only sitting opposite the candidate for the degree, but has behind him an inspector from the General Medical Council to make sure that the examination is conducted fairly and to an adequate standard.

The General Medical Council was established by a medical act in 1858. It controls admission to the medical register, and as such supervises preregistration medical education throughout the country in universities and in non-university hospitals. It ensures that the registrable diplomas of the Royal Colleges and of the universities are only awarded after certain standards have been reached.

The basic training before entering universities to study medicine in all countries consists of a preliminary study of physics, chemistry and biology, and thereafter at the university, anatomy, physiology and biochemistry with pharmacology and pathology. There has been a recent development in the UK in that some universities such as Nottingham and Southampton admit medical students to the hospital wards from the very first day of entry to the University. In the USA the regulation of the standard of teaching is controlled by the Council of Medical Education and Hospitals which is part of the American Medical Association. High standards of specialist training are assured in North America where specialist board examinations have to be passed before recognition as a specialist, and more recently as a 'super specialist' in a subsubject such as gynaecological oncology, perinatology or infertility.

The British Medical Association is not a college nor a university nor a teaching centre, but a union of doctors which sets standards by various committees such as its ethical committee. It is totally different from the General Medical Council which not only ensures that standards of education are high enough, but also that all admitted to the register have been properly trained in teaching hospitals somewhere in the world and ensures that they conform to certain standards of behaviour after registration.

The history and functions of the Royal College of Obstetricians and Gynaecologists and how they are carried out

The main purpose of a college is to ensure that the highest possible standards of a specialty are maintained. A Dr Augustus Bozzi Granville (1783–1872) who was a lecturer in midwifery in London together with some of his co-lecturers decided in 1826 to found an Obstetrical Society, in order to 'secure some recognized system of instruction and regulation by putting pressure on the English Medical Corporations, and if necessary, on the Government'. This was because in

England, unlike in Edinburgh and some of the foreign universities, midwifery was not part of the syllabus for qualifying as a doctor (Donnison, 1988). Granville was a graduate of Pavia University and he had gained his obstetric experience, as had so many others, in Paris. The Obstetrical Society led to the formation of the Royal College of Obstetricians and Gynaecologists.

The Society of Apothecaries did include midwifery in their examinations, but the Royal Colleges of Physicians and of Surgeons were both prejudiced against men practising midwifery.

The position of the obstetrician in the formation of the Obstetrical Society in 1826 was viewed with disdain by the President of the Royal College of Physicians, who wrote in 1827 'the practise of midwifery was an act foreign to the habits of gentlemen of a large academic education' (Clark, 1966). In 1836 Sir Anthony Carlisle, a surgeon, said 'It is an imposture to pretend that a medical man is required at a labour' In 1859 the Obstetrical Society of London, then under the presidency of William Tyler Smith (1815–1873), tried to push for more recognition by the Royal Colleges of Physicians and of Surgeons.

In 1884 James Hobson Aveling (q.v. in Biographies) and Robert Barnes founded the British Gynaecological Society to improve the status and recognition of gynaecologists and obstetricians. They were the forerunners of what later became under the impetus of William Blair-Bell (q.v. in Biographies) and Fletcher Shaw, The Royal College of Obstetricians and Gynaecologists (Peel, 1986).

Unlike the Royal Colleges of Physicians and of Surgeons, the Royal College of Obstetricians and Gynaecologists (RCOG) is entirely a postgraduate college and is not concerned with undergraduate teaching. It maintains standards by the institution of examinations, so that a candidate after being examined can be sure that he is fit to work (after obtaining the diploma, the lowest certificate that is granted) as a general practitioner who performs antenatal care, some basic medical gynaecology and some normal obstetrics. If he wishes to specialize in obstetrics and gynaecology a candidate after several years postgraduate hospital training, has to pass the examination for the membership of the Royal College of Obstetricians and Gynaecologists (MRCOG) but he or she is not yet able to take a post as a consultant in charge of hospital beds. To do this he must carry out several years further training in recognized units as a specialist usually at Senior Registrar level

under the supervision of a consultant. He then obtains a certificate of accreditation; after this he can apply for consultant appointments. All training centres where postgraduates can study for the membership of the Royal College of Obstetricians and Gynaecologists and after that be trained for accreditation are regularly inspected by the Royal College. This system evolved gradually on patterns set by the older colleges.

The membership examination of the Royal College of Obstetricians and Gynaecologists, taken after training in basic medicine and surgery as well as several years of specialist training in obstetrics and gynaecology, is in two parts. The first is in the scientific foundations of the subject and the second in the clinical practice of the subject.

There are written papers, multiple choice papers, pathology examinations and, for the second part, clinical examinations. In this last part of the examination, candidates have to examine patients with different pathological conditions and diagnose them. They are watched by their examiners while they are examining the patients to make sure they do so thoroughly but with the necessary gentleness. There are examination committees supervising the examiners to ensure that the examinations are carried out scrupulously and fairly.

The College awards Fellowships some years after membership to those members who have made a contribution to advance the subject, or who have rendered sterling service in hospital for many years.

Perhaps the most important work of the college is to supervise the hospitals in which its future members are being trained. These hospitals apply for recognition as training centres and a team of two and sometimes three experienced members and fellows go to inspect the work of the hospital and to make sure that facilities for teaching are of the necessary high standard. Many hospitals in many countries have been examined for recognition as teaching centres by the Royal College of Obstetricians and Gynaecologists. Recognition once granted can be taken away if the standards fall short of those needed to ensure correct training. Recognition has another good effect and that is that it ensures a certain high standard of treatment for the patients of those hospitals.

The work of a Royal College must not be confused with that of a University. The purpose of the university is primarily to hold classes to teach, and then to hold examinations to prove that a certain standard has been reached. Whilst the college fulfils the second function including examinations, it does far less teaching.

The Royal College of Obstetricians and Gynaecologists does have a research arm known as Birthright. Its function is to collect money for research to be carried out in laboratories and hospital departments spread all over the country and overseas. It finances research in fetal medicine, and pain relief in childbirth as well as many research projects designed to help to solve the manifold subjects still needing elucidation. Birthright's connection with the Royal College of Obstetricians and Gynaecologists is a loose one. Its appeal offices happen to be housed in the College building; and decisions about who should be given research grants are carried out by a committee, many of whose members are Fellows of the College.

No research work is done within the College. In this it differs totally from a university. Cambridge and Oxford Universities for instance both have research departments in obstetrics and gynaecology, and some of their work may be funded by Birthright. The work in these departments has had enormous effects on obstetrics and gynaecology. R.G. Edwards for instance, did most of his scientific work on *in vitro* fertilization in the physiology laboratory of Cambridge University where he later became a Professor; but the clinical work by P.C. Steptoe was carried out in a non-university hospital, which was however recognized by the Royal College of Obstetricians and Gynaecologists for specialist training.

SCIENTIFIC SOCIETIES FOR THE INTERCHANGE OF INFORMATION

The Royal Society was established in 1645 by the meeting of 'Divers worthy persons, inquisitive into natural philosophy, and other parts of human learning, did, by agreement, meet weekly in London, on a certain day, to discourse of such affairs'.

The original Fellows of the Royal Society were medical men, theologians such as Dr Wilkins later a Bishop, a Professor of Astronomy, a mathematician, and some learned foreign scientists. At their early meetings the decision was made to form the Society, one of the most prestigious gatherings of scientists anywhere in the world.

One of the first subjects to be discussed in the Royal Society was Harvey's discovery of the circulation of the blood which he communicated to the fellows; as did Leeuwenhoek with his microscope discoveries, by writing 300 or more

letters to the Secretary of the Royal Society. It is still the most prestigious gathering of scientists in the world and election to the Royal Society is an honour achieved only by recognized 'excellence' in a branch of science. Clubs had previously existed for political, theological and sectarian gatherings, but not for scientific discussions.

At the time of writing this, Sir Anthony Epstein the discoverer of the Epstein–Barr virus by intensive use of electron microscopy, is a very senior Fellow and foreign secretary of the Society. Notable obstetricians elected to the Royal Society in recent years include Mr Patrick Steptoe. The *Philosophical Transactions*, otherwise called proceedings, were among the first publications of a scientific nature to have a wide readership, because they are not circulated only to the Fellows, but are on sale to the general public.

While the Royal Society of London is certainly not an institution for the propagation of knowledge of gynaecological and obstetrical matters, it did fulfil this function in part from its foundation in 1660. One of its founding Fellows Henry Oldenberg (Figure 2) may have obtained the idea

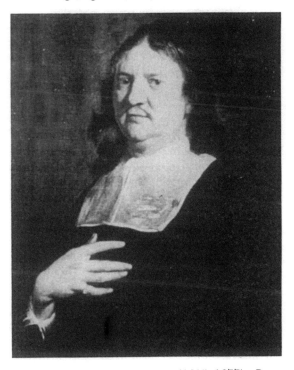

Figure 2 Henry Oldenberg (1615–1677). Born Bremen, Germany, Diplomatic agent first to the Court of Oliver Cromwell – the Lord Protector and then to Charles II. The first Secretary of the Royal Society (*see* text)

of founding this society in Paris where he attended the Académie Française. It was a year after he together with Ranelegh attended the academy in France, that they founded the Royal Society and organized it as a scientific society in 1660. It received its first charter of incorporation through Charles II in 1662. It may very well be that the idea of such a society originated in the mind of Francis Bacon (1561–1626). Certainly Oldenberg's correspondence with scientists all over the world, including his 300 letters exchanged with Leeuwenhoek of Delft had a most important effect in disseminating knowledge of the microscopic work carried out by this man.

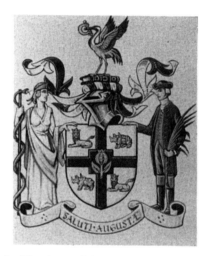

Figure 3   The Arms of the Medical Society of London

In the early eighteenth century, many local societies were founded in London and in the provinces. The oldest of these the Medical Society of London (Figure 3) in the West End was soon followed by the Hunterian Society of London whose meetings were and still are, mainly held in the City of London. There were also a large number of smaller societies which amalgamated to form the Royal Society of Medicine situated in the West End of London. None of these societies specialized in gynaecology, but there is a section of obstetrics and gynaecology at the Royal Society of Medicine which holds regular lecture and discussion meetings throughout the year except in the summer months, and has honorary officers who are all members or fellows of the Royal College of Obstetricians and Gynaecologists.

Thus, there is a loose but very workable connection between the old universities of England,

the more modern Royal Colleges, and the Medical Societies, all with the aim of furthering the subject.

HISTORY AND THE FUNCTION OF THE MEDICAL SOCIETIES

It is all too easy after leaving university and after obtaining a licence to practise either as a general practitioner or a specialist, to become divorced from the acquisition of new ideas and from the interchange of ideas between colleagues of various disciplines. Reading journals and books is one way of avoiding this and attending meetings of various medical societies is another and very important way of exchanging ideas.

Doctors of all disciplines, and in particular general practitioners, have long felt the need for continuing part-time (although not full-time) education and contact with their colleagues. One of the ways this was achieved was by the formation of the medical societies. The first of these was the Medical Society of London in 1773. It was to have a great effect on the development of medicine in the UK and further afield because it brought together for the first time physicians, surgeons and apothecaries who had met in their own colleges and associations but had not met with one another. The doctors who worked in the great teaching hospitals such as St Bartholomew's, the oldest, and St Thomas's, met with one another and did exchange information; but formal meetings where doctors of all disciplines could come together were not held anywhere until 1773 when the Medical Society of London was founded by a Quaker doctor John Coakley Lettsom, born on 22 November 1744 on the Island of Little Van Dyke in the West Indies (Hunt, 1972). His father grew sugar and cotton in Tortola, the largest of the British Virgin Islands. He was educated in England at St Thomas's Hospital and joined the Quaker community in London. He then returned to Tortola and made a great deal of money after which he returned to England. In 1773, after he was elected a Fellow of the Royal Society, he founded the Medical Society of London. This was when he was second physician to the Aldersgate General Dispensary situated near the City of London Maternity Hospital which had been instituted in March 1750 in Shaftesbury House in Aldersgate Street (Figure 4).

The Medical Society of London first met in taverns and then found a suitable meeting place in the City, but by 1850 it was obvious that the City

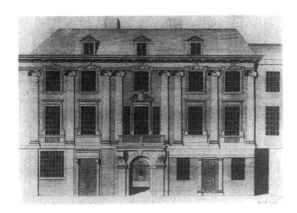

Figure 4 The City of London Maternity Hospital; its first building (*see* text)

was not such a salubrious residential area, and the Medical Society of London merged with a larger medical society that was called the Westminster Society. They moved to their new premises at 11 Chandos Street in 1872.

The Transactions of the Medical Society of London is the only medical journal of the eighteenth century that still survives (Booth, 1982).

If we return to the earlier days of the Society it had fulfilled Lettsom's original purpose for bringing together healers of different disciplines. For instance Lord Lister, when he came to London, chose the Medical Society of London to explain and further his ideas. He addressed the members at least four times and he demonstrated as he operated on a healthy knee joint, and on seven cases to treat fractures of the patella by wiring them with silver wire. He was not always all that well received.

The Royal Society of Medicine

There was a quarrel in 1805 when some members of the Medical Society of London left to form the Medico-Chirurgical Society. The importance of this breakaway society lay in the fact that it linked pathological, obstetrical and epidemiological societies in London to form the Royal Society of Medicine (RSM) in 1905. The Royal Society of Medicine which is now far bigger than the Medical Society of London, consists of many sections, each devoted to a specialist subject; and there is a vigorous and thriving section of Obstetrics and Gynaecology. This section meets once a month and the meetings are attended by obstetricians and gynaecologists both fully trained and in

training (registrars are encouraged to present cases) so that new techniques as well as old theories can be presented and discussed. Very often different sections of the Royal Society of Medicine combine, and it was at a combined meeting of the Sections of Obstetrics and Gynaecology and the Section of Endocrinology that Patrick Steptoe first demonstrated slides of views down the laparoscope and first met Robert Edwards.

The Hunterian Society

The move to the West End of doctors and medical societies left the East End of London without a medical society (Hunt, 1972). Surgeons and general practitioners working at the London Hospital in the East End of London were advised to found a new society in 1893 in the 'Eastern district and metropolis, to concentrate the zeal and experience of a large number of respectable practitioners, whose grand object will be the reception and discussion of communications on professional subjects... 'Sir William Blizard (1753–1845) (Figure 5) FRS, PRCS, was not only the President of the Royal College of Surgeons of England, but also the first President of the

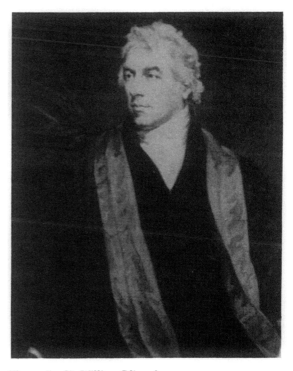

Figure 5 Sir William Blizard

599

Hunterian Society and he held this position from 1819 to 1822. The reason why this new society, founded 25 years after Hunter's death in 1793, was named after him was because the society looked to Hunter as its parent ' . . . it received from him, through those taught by his former pupils, its earliest members, the impulse of existence, the fruitful seed of that character for sound practical observation . . . '. The society not only honoured John Hunter (Figure 6), but also his older brother William Hunter (q.v.), the obstetrician who looked after Queen Charlotte, supervising her many pregnancies and lyings-in. Since the formation of the three important societies the Medical Society of London, The Royal Society of Medicine and the Hunterian Society, there have been many other medical societies.

Other medical societies

The first local society in the world devoted exclusively to obstetrics and gynaecology was the Boston Gynaecological Society which was founded on 22 January 1869; and the first national organization in the world devoted to the specialty was the American Gynaecological Society, founded on 3 June 1876 (Greenhill, 1944).

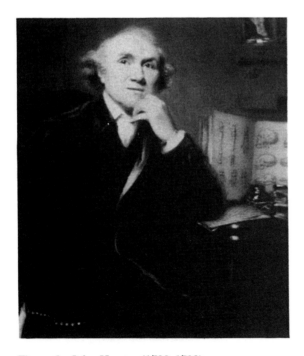

Figure 6 John Hunter (1728–1793)

In France there is a society of Obstetrics and Gynaecology which meets regularly and which has constituent branches in various parts of the country.

Many societies are based on hospitals, and there are others based on geographical areas such as The North of England Obstetric and Gynaecological Society. Such specialist societies exist in many countries. There are vast gynaecological societies in France and America, where apart from the American Gynaecological Society and the American Gynaecological Club there are town-based societies such as the Orleans Obstetric and Gynaecological Society. This is true also for smaller cities such as Edmonton in Alberta, Canada, and many other towns and cities.

SPREAD OF KNOWLEDGE THROUGH CONGRESSES AND JOURNALS

Exchange of ideas between specialists from different countries is achieved in international congresses. Some of these may be small if they deal with a highly specialized subject (such as sperm function), but others may be huge. For instance the meetings of the International Federation of Obstetrics and Gynaecology (FIGO), founded by François De Watteville in Geneva, are held every 3 years in a different country and attended by 10 000 or more participants. Lectures and demonstrations are held in various rooms of the conference centre over several days. More recently the International Federation of Fertility Societies (IFFS), also founded by De Watteville, has instituted huge international tri-annual congresses. These congresses and the small subcommittees formed by some members attending them, serve to standardize international nomenclature, such as for the staging of cancers, and to demonstrate on film and video practices such as microsurgery, to participants who otherwise would not know what is going on in different countries.

Scientific and medical journals

If a great scientist or surgeon wished to publicize the work he had done, he did so by delivering lectures. This is precisely how William Harvey communicated his discoveries when he lectured about them in 1616. Twelve years later he published the lectures in Latin, the *lingua franca* of the time (Booth, 1982), in a badly printed book issued in Frankfurt (Morton, 1990). That lasted until about the second half of the eighteenth century when English took over in England and America and French elsewhere as the common language.

It was in the second half of the seventeenth century that scientific and medical journals first appeared. Until then if a scientist wished to publish his research findings he did it by lectures, publishing books, or writing to other scientists. The main way of spreading knowledge was by letters from one scientist to another. When Henry Oldenburg (?1615–1677) became Secretary of the Royal Society of London, he started to write to scientists all over the world and found that his work was so hard that he had to have a 'committee of correspondent'. Similarly in France in 1663 the original moves were made to publish multiple copies of letters in a scientific periodical. The first of these publications appeared in Paris on 5 January 1665 in the *Journal de Scavans*. In England the Council of the Royal Society ordered 'the philosophical transactions be composed by Mr Oldenberg, to be printed the first Monday of each month', and the first issue appeared on 6 March 1665. At first it was a private venture by Oldenberg which he published at his own expense. He gave it a lengthy title, but the shorter version of this was *The Philosophical Transactions*. It was printed by the printers of the Royal Society and in 1753 the Royal Society became officially responsible for publication of the transactions. *The Philosophical Transactions* has always had items of medical interest including gynaecological matters. There were similar transactions started in the seventeenth and eighteenth centuries in various countries, including one by Thomas Bartholin the Danish anatomist (1616–1680) who described various gynaecological organs and first published his journal in 1660. The quality of journals varies, but refereeing, started by the Royal Society, maintains high standards. All articles are submitted to experts in their fields before publication to ensure as far as possible that they are of a high medical standard. The first medical journal published in Britain was in Edinburgh in 1731 when the *Medical Essays and Observations* appeared. It was only in 1823 that the *Lancet* first appeared. It is still published weekly. Of course now many learned societies have their journals to report scientific matters, and there are papers that also report newsworthy happenings by doctors and scientists (Lefanu, 1938).

CHRONOLOGY

Universities where midwifery is taught

1170	Foundation of the University of Paris. Soon after followed foundation of the University of Oxford.
1209	Foundation of the University of Cambridge.
1222	Foundation of the University of Padua.
1284	Peterhouse, the first College to be founded in Cambridge.

The Royal Colleges of Medicine

1505	Foundation of the Royal College of Surgeons of Edinburgh.
1518	Foundation of the Royal College of Physicians of London.
1540	Re-incorporation of the Company of Barber-Surgeons with powers to discipline.
1617	Society of Apothecaries founded by Charter of King James I as an offshoot of the Grocers' Company.
1800	Royal College of Surgeons of England founded from the members of the Barber-Surgeons' Company.
1929	Royal College of Obstetricians and Gynaecologists founded.

Seventeen Colleges and faculties meet together under the chairmanship of one of the Presidents of the Royal Colleges in the Conference of Medical Royal Colleges and their faculties. It is an important body to co-ordinate their work and policies in order to maintain high standards of clinical practice. This conference was founded in 1976 and meets about six times a year for a whole day. The chairmanship rotates between the presidents of the various member Colleges.

1858	General Medical Council founded to supervise and control medical education and later registration.

Medical Societies

1660	Foundation of the Royal Society of London.
1773	Foundation of the Medical Society of London.
1805	Foundation of the Medico-Chirurgical Society.
1826	Foundation of the Obstetrical Society of London.

1869	Foundation of the Boston Gynaecological Society – the first local society devoted exclusively to obstetrics and gynaecology.
1876	Foundation of the American Gynaecological Society.
1905	The Royal Society of Medicine founded by amalgamation of several societies.

Periodicals

1660	First number of the *Philosophical Transactions* of the Royal Society appeared.
1665	*Journal de Scavans* appeared in France.
1673	Danish anatomist Thomas Bartholin published his journal.

REFERENCES

Booth, C.C. (1982). Medical communication, the old and the new: the development of medical journals in Britain. *Br. Med. J.*, **285**, 105–8

Clark, G. (1966). *A History of the Royal College of Physicians of London.* (Oxford: Clarendon Press)

Donnison, J. (1988). *Midwives and Medical Men, A History of Inter-professional Rivalry and Women's Rights,* pp. 50–60. (London: Historical Publications)

Greenhill, J.P. (1944). Foreward. In Leonardo, R.A. (ed.) *History of Gynaecology*, p. xi. (New York: Froben Press)

Hunt, T. (1972). *The Medical Society of London 1773–1973.* (London: William Heinemann Medical Books Ltd)

Lefanu, W.R. (1938). *British Periodicals of Medicine, A Chronological List, Bulletin of the Institute of the History of Medicine*, Vol. 5, nos. 8 and 9, October and November 1937, and Vol. 6, no. 6, June 1938. (Baltimore: Johns Hopkins)

Morton, L.T. (1990). The Birth of Medical Periodical Literature. In Alainson, A. (ed.) *Thornton's Medical Books, Libraries and Collectors*, 3rd edn. pp. 221–38. (Aldershot: Gower Publishing Co. Ltd.)

Peel, J. (1986). *William Blair-Bell – Father and Founder.* (London: Royal College of Obstetricians and Gynaecologists)

Thornton, J.L. and Want, P.C. (1973). The Royal College of Obstetricians and Gynaecologists. *St. Bartholomew's Hosp.* J., **LXVII**, 36–9

Ethics and the law in obstetrics and gynaecology

INTRODUCTION

The medical profession has a history of ethical behaviour that goes back at least to the time of Hippocrates. Ethics is defined in the *Random House Dictionary of the English Language* as 'the body of moral principles or values governing or distinctive of a particular culture or group'. A second definition is 'in accordance with the rules or standards for right conduct or practice especially the standards of a profession'. Medical Ethics has been defined as 'the obligations of a moral nature which govern the practice of medicine ... they are the common possession of the medical profession and members are expected both by fellow doctors and by the society in which their patients are found to adhere to them' (Duncan *et al*, 1981). In everyday usage the terms 'morals' and 'ethics' are used synonymously. The word 'moral', from the Latin *moralis*, means customs or manners and is taken to mean something right, wrong, good or bad.

THE GREEK INFLUENCE

The three great Greek philosophers Socrates, Plato, and Aristotle not only laid the philosophical foundations of Western culture, but also enunciated the strong ethical principles which for many centuries have influenced the whole of Western ethical behaviour, including medical ethical behaviour. Although ancient Greece led much in medicine, medical ethical behaviour has also been derived from rules formulated from Babylon, Egypt, India and China, and from Jewish teachings.

There is an admixture of human and god-like figuration in the main early Greek physicians of tradition as can be seen from their biographies in the following chapter.

'Ethics', from the Greek word *ethos* or *ethizo* – to be accustomed or used to, means character

and is also used to mean right, wrong, good or bad. Ethics are formal, theoretical statements which intellectualize morals and involve professional values such as those seen in codes, of which there are several in obstetrics and gynaecology, to regulate treatment and research or enquiry. Plato (427/8–347 BC) writing on the professional man, said 'all that is said and done will be said and done with a view to what is good for those on whom he practises his art, so every art sees not its own advantage, but the well-being of the subject on whom it is exercised or, put more bluntly or less eloquently; that the patient takes no harm'. Doctors who follow Plato do not go far wrong. *Primum non nocere.*

A professional man or woman does not meet his patients or clients on equal terms. The word patient is derived from the Latin word *patiens* meaning one who is suffering. The word client is derived from the Latin word *cliens* which originally meant one who listened, and which later acquired the more technical meaning of a plebeian or one under the protection of a patrician, that is a person who is under protection or is dependent. This is to be compared with a customer in a business. A customer is a much more sturdy person and his relationship with the businessman with whom he is having dealings is at least in theory, more equal than a patient in his dealings with his doctor. There should not be a great divorce between ethics and the law.

THE HIPPOCRATIC INFLUENCE
(see also Biographies)

The Hippocratic Oath, only parts of which are now retained at the end of the twentieth century, is particularly appropriate to the practice of obstetrics and gynaecology. It states, according to a modern translation, among other things 'I swear by Apollo, physician and Asclepius and Hygeia and Panaceia and all the gods and goddesses, making them my witnesses that I will fulfil according to my ability and judgement this oath and this covenant . . . I will neither give a deadly drug to anybody if asked for it, nor will I make a suggestion to this effect. Similarly I will not give to any woman an abortive remedy. Impurity and holiness I will guard against with my life and with my heart . . . medical students will look upon their teachers as upon their parents . . . they will teach medicine to their teachers' children if they wish to learn, without fee . . . We will only prescribe to help and not to harm our patients: we will give no drugs, especially not help to procure abortions. Whenever we go into the house for the benefit of the sick, we will do what we can to help and will not seduce male or female, even slaves. Whatever I see or hear concerning the life of men in my attendance on the sick, or even apart therefrom, which ought not to be noised abroad, I will keep silent thereon. Counting such things to be as sacred secrets.'

It is believed that the Hippocratic Oath in turn was partly derived from old Egyptian sources dating from 2000 BC as well as from Hammurabi, the King of Babylon in 1880 BC.

THE CHINESE INFLUENCE

The Chinese systems of medicine and of medical ethics are probably the oldest in the world and may well have commenced about 3000 BC, with Fu Hsi and continued with the emperors Shen Nung and Huang Ti. This last is said to have been the author of the canon of internal medicine named *Nei Ching*, which is still held in respect in China.

Confucius (551–479 BC) founded Confucianism in China as being synonymous with learning. His was a social ethic and he was passionately reformist. Although not particularly a leader in medical ethics his whole philosophy inevitably permeated into Chinese medicine and its influence is still very widespread, particularly in neighbouring countries such as Korea, Japan, and North and South Vietnam. The key to Confucianism is *jen* which Confucius himself defined as 'love men'.

It is difficult for a Western doctor who is not familiar with the history of China to unravel the interplay between Confucianism and Buddhism. One of the basic tenets of Confucianism is for the physician to be mentally calm and of a firm disposition and he should have a commitment and willingness to undertake efforts to save every living creature.

THE INDIAN INFLUENCE

In Hindu medicine physicians were expected to be competent in their craft and although protected against suits from disgruntled patients were nevertheless liable to fines for incompetent or malicious treatments. Although abortion was outlawed as a sin, where the mother's life was at stake it took precedence over the rights of the fetus.

The Buddha (Gautama Siddhārtha, 563–483 BC), the Indian founder of Buddhism, was more liberal in his religious philosophy than that of most religions, in particular Roman Catholicism. Buddhism emphasized the need for physical well-being as a prerequisite to mental health. The Buddha's emphasis on the ethical duty of all towards the ill is illustrated in a famous sermon when he said to his disciples 'Brethren, he who would wait on me, let him wait on the sick'.

THE JUDAEO-CHRISTIAN INFLUENCE

This, following on the previous definitions, is the body of moral principles or values which are distinctive of Jewish culture or groups. Christianity, which originally was an offshoot of Judaism, shares most of these values. For Christians (as for Jews) the relationship between God and human creatures is such that God is regarded as the Lord of life, whereas we humans possess at best not the complete disposal of the gift of life, but only a stewardship of creation in general and of human life in particular (Mahoney, 1990). Since all moral philosophers agree that Christian medical ethics are based on Judaic teachings some of these are detailed.

The particularity of Jewish medical ethics is that historically the teachings of the Old Testament always form the basis of the rules and regulations for everyday good ethical behaviour. These traditions and concepts have been absorbed and, so to speak, filtered through the moral and legislative systems of Judaism, so that a decisive role has been exercised in this process of assimilation by the concept of monotheism which gives the divinity the power of healing. In this way 'Hebrew medicine' differs from that of all other peoples of antiquity.

Christianity has followed in part Judaic teachings and sought to make 'people forget their faith in magic and occult practices, thus returning to the initial Jewish concept where salvation comes from within the faith and that there is no true medication without prayer'. Jewish medical ethics are based on what is called the *Halakhah*. This is the corpus of Jewish law elucidated and transmitted down through the generations, adding on to it the oral law handed down from one generation to the next until it was recorded in the *Mishnah* and amplified in the *Gemara*. These two books together are called the *Talmud*. Since they are large and discursive works they have needed codification. This was done by a great rabbi, doctor and philosopher of the twelfth century, called Maimonides (q.v.), and further codification was carried out by Rabbi Joseph Karo in the sixteenth century in his book the *Shulchan Arukh*, and by others.

As medicine progressed, and as answers to the new problems, and particularly ethical ones set up by such progress, could not be found in the older standard works, rabbis had to give answers when questioned by their congregations, or if they were very important rabbis, by other rabbis or members of other congregations. The answers they gave are called *Responsa*, and they deal with specific cases and so in a way can be compared with English 'case law'. When a modern rabbi is asked questions, as for instance, on the very modern problem of fetal reduction, he goes right back to the Talmud to find the answer as to whether he can advise for fetal reduction. He will argue that if there are five or six embryos in the womb there are too many, both for the health of the mother and of the future babies. As it is immensely difficult for a woman to carry four or more embryos and dangerous for her health, and inevitably dangerous for the fetuses because they are bound to be born prematurely with ill-developed organ systems, he may very well in certain well-defined circumstances agree to fetal reduction. This is because Maimonides said about abortion 'the life of the mother takes precedence over that of the unborn child'. Under that ruling when labour became 'hard' so that the life of the mother was endangered, an embryotomy could be performed in order to save her life. This is quite the opposite teaching from that of the Catholic Church, as they say that the life of the fetus is at least equal to that of the mother. In Jewish tradition the child under certain circumstances may be considered as an aggressor, engaged in 'pursuing the life of the mother'. So abortion can be considered where the aggressor pursuing the mother is liable to the death sentence if it is threatening its mother's life. If the life of the mother is not threatened however, abortion is a

form of (non-capital) homicide. In 1974 the Chief Rabbinate of Israel declared the performance of an abortion to be an act of murder, but other authorities have said that it is not. The Israeli Chief Rabbi's view is similar to that of the Roman Catholic Church.

According to Biblical tradition the first commandment was 'to increase and multiply' and therefore a procedure such as *in vitro* fertilization, so long as it is carried out on a woman married to a man, with his semen, is certainly allowable. Although the rabbis have long said that artificial insemination from a donor is repugnant, the offspring of such an induced pregnancy are not considered according to longstanding tradition, to be 'bastards', whereas the offspring of an adulterous union where the adultery was a sexual act, is considered to be a bastard.

Jewish and Christian ethical tradition has always been against intercourse outside marriage, and particularly adulterous intercourse. Whereas some Christian sects, and particularly the Roman Catholics, view chastity throughout life as a virtue, others hold that this negates the command to increase and multiply. There are no Jewish monks or nuns. Both religions are against polygamy but the Moslem religion which is also derived from Judaism, allows polygamy for men, but not for women (Stewart McKay, 1901).

MODERN MEDICAL ETHICS AND DIFFERENT PHILOSOPHIES

It became clear at a conference on *in vitro* fertilization in 1983 that the attitude of Buddhists was entirely permissive and that infertility as a condition in Buddhists can be treated by *in vitro* fertilization, where both parties of the couple have a sincere desire to have a child. Buddhists also accept freezing embryos to reduce the hazards to patients of multiple attempts to retrieve oocytes and avoid the risk of failure of fertilization. 'Spare embryos' can be used for experimentation, but a Buddhist priest at the conference was opposed to surrogate motherhood because the mother–child relationship, he felt, was the most important. He was also opposed to gamete donation because of difficulty in bringing up the child, especially if it is deformed. It is quite possible then that the parents will not accept the child. He was very emphatic that infertility should not be accepted passively as is recommended by some Roman Catholic priests.

A Catholic priest at the same conference stated that it was a fundamental right for a couple to have children but he felt that freedom to abort was one of the big causes of infertility and therefore that was a problem to be tackled first. The motto, he said should be 'I am free', not 'I have freedom to do what I like'.

On the other hand, a Moslem priest stated that he was opposed to surrogacy because of the dilemma of whose child the infant really was.

THE ORIGINS OF MEDICAL JURISPRUDENCE

Ancient scriptures do deal with gynaecology and its relationship to the law. For instance, it says in the Old Testament that if two men are quarrelling with one another and they happen to knock into a pregnant woman who loses her pregnancy as a result, she is entitled to claim compensation. This is probably one of the earliest mentions of damages for a gynaecological misfortune. If it is unintentional the damages are in the nature of compensation for the woman and her husband and not to punish the person or persons responsible.

Medical jurisprudence really started with the use of doctors to give medical evidence. Apparently there are references in classical antiquity to this, but it took until the thirteenth century before medical experts were first appointed to advise law courts. About the same time, police surgeons were appointed in northern Italy, and occasionally post-mortems were carried out to determine the cause of death. In Germany medical evidence was used at the beginning of the sixteenth century, and the elector of Brandenberg in 1516 made provisions for the calling of medical evidence in criminal cases. It took until the middle of the seventeenth century before coroners could call on medical witnesses in their courts in England. Medical law was not taught in the UK until the beginning of the nineteenth century, when the first courses were held at Edinburgh University and just about this time the beginnings of medical jurisprudence were being taught in the USA at Columbia College in New York.

One of the first recorded cases of a medico-legal nature in gynaecology was that of Melchior Sebiz who wrote about the signs of virginity in 1630 (Sebiz, 1630). In 1666 Gottfried Welsh was writing on premature births (Welsh, 1667). Swammerdam discovered that newborn infants' lungs float in water if they have breathed, but sink if they have not breathed. When in 1681 a 15-year-old peasant girl was accused of infanticide, the

fact that the infant's lungs sank and it had therefore not breathed, helped to have her acquitted of the murder of the child (Swammerdam, 1667; Schreyer, 1690). Swammerdam's discovery was a very important one.

Nicolas de Blegny (1652–1722) founded the first French medical journal in 1679 and wrote an important work on the medico-legal relations of surgery (De Blegny, 1684).

The first book on medical jurisprudence was by Fortunato Fedeli in 1602 and in it he mentions the proof of virginity, the time of delivery and the formation of the fetus. So, the subject was debated throughout the ages, though not very thoroughly in England (Garrison, 1929).

HOW ENGLISH LAW DEVELOPED, PARTICULARLY IN RELATION TO OBSTETRICS AND GYNAECOLOGY

The 'law of England' as it exists to this day, has been derived from two sources, the first being *case law* in which the trial of somebody or an action, has resulted in a judgement (Figure 1). The legal principle or the *ratio decidendi* sustaining the judgement gave rise to the doctrine of judicial precedent and such precedents were quoted in subsequent trials or used as the basic standards on which to proceed further. The second is *statute law*. Statute law enunciates the law as enacted by Parliaments in the various Acts that they pass. The preliminary to an Act is the Bill which Members of Parliament or the Government present to the Houses of Parliament to debate before an Act is finally drawn up, after discussions in Committees and on the floors of both Houses of Parliament. The Alec Bourne (1939, ref. 1) case was a very good example of *case law* helping to formulate the 'Law of the Land' and adherence to the judgement in this case was the basis of the effective law until The Abortion Act of 1967 was passed. Because of the Alec Bourne case doctors felt slightly more free to perform abortions if they genuinely believed that the life of a mother was at risk. The Bourne case clarified the law as it was in 1939. It did not make new law but was immensely influential.

The judge held that it was not unlawful for Mr Alec Bourne, a consultant gynaecologist from St Mary's Hospital, London, to terminate the pregnancy of a 15-year-old girl, pregnant as a result of rape by several soldiers, because her life in the sense of her mental well-being, was at risk if the abortion had not been done.

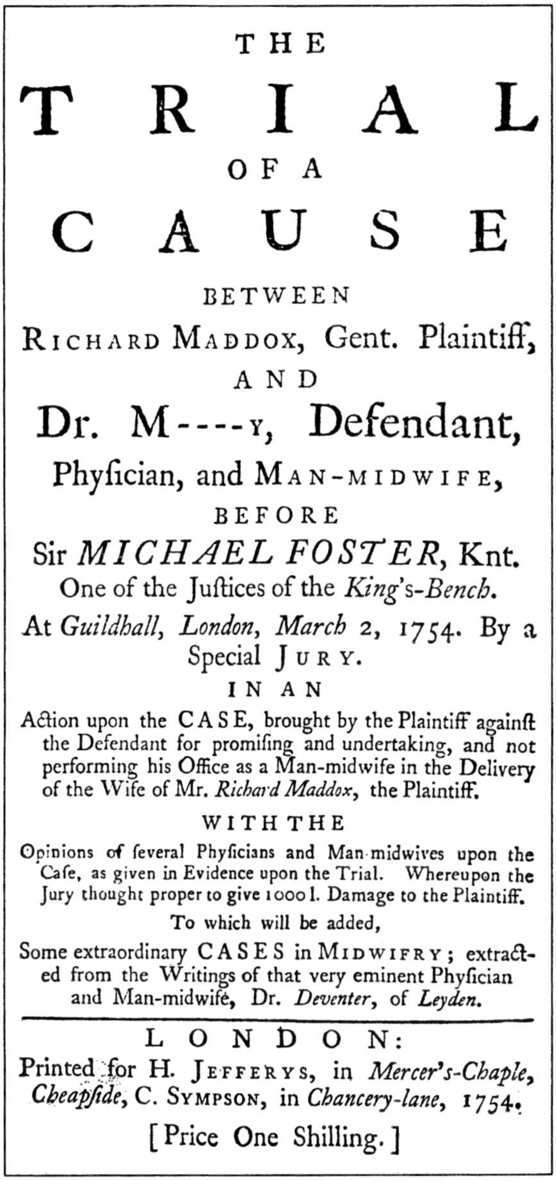

THE

T R I A L

O F A

C A U S E

BETWEEN

RICHARD MADDOX, Gent. Plaintiff,

AND

Dr. M ---- Y, Defendant,

Phyſician, and MAN-MIDWIFE,

BEFORE

Sir *MICHAEL FOSTER*, Knt.

One of the Juſtices of the *King's-Bench*.

At *Guildhall*, *London*, *March* 2, 1754. By a Special JURY.

IN AN

Action upon the CASE, brought by the Plaintiff againſt the Defendant for promiſing and undertaking, and not performing his Office as a Man-midwife in the Delivery of the Wife of Mr. *Richard Maddox*, the Plaintiff.

WITH THE

Opinions of ſeveral Phyſicians and Man-midwives upon the Caſe, as given in Evidence upon the Trial. Whereupon the Jury thought proper to give 1000 l. Damage to the Plaintiff.

To which will be added,

Some extraordinary CASES in MIDWIFRY; extracted from the Writings of that very eminent Phyſician and Man-midwife, Dr. *Deventer*, of *Leyden*.

──────────────

L O N D O N :

Printed for H. JEFFERYS, in *Mercer's-Chaple*, *Cheapſide*, C. SYMPSON, in *Chancery-lane*, 1754.

[Price One Shilling.]

Figure 1 The report of a trial before Sir Michael Foster with a special jury in 1754, of a man-midwife in a case of medical negligence

The passing of the Abortion Act in 1967 is a very good example of the way the law of England is formulated by *statute law*. The Abortion Act of 1967 was introduced by Mr (later Sir) David Steel, a Member of Parliament, because of great disquiet at the deaths occurring from so-called 'back-street abortions'. It legalized abortions carried out in National Health Service Hospitals and licensed Private Clinics providing that the abortions were done under certain clear-cut regulations. There is no doubt that the very high numbers of so-called therapeutic abortions carried out safely each year as a result of the Act, as well as the great spread of contraception and contraception knowledge have contributed to a marked lowering of the birth rate in the UK. There has also been a very marked lowering in the maternal mortality rate, some of which was due to septic abortions. The Abortion Act in the UK (1967) states that abortions should be performed only as a therapeutic measure. According to the Act, which was slightly modified in 1990, the decision to terminate pregnancy should be approved in writing by at least two doctors and the procedure should be performed by a doctor in premises approved by the appropriate authority. A doctor may opt out of performing or assisting at an abortion if his conscience so sways him. Until the Act of 1967 the performance of abortion otherwise than in accordance with the ruling in R. vs. Bourne (1939, ref. 1) was illegal because it contravened The Offences Against The Persons Act 1861. The Abortion Act has been slightly modified by the Human Fertilization and Embryology Act 1990.

This very important legal doctrine passed on a free (no political party pressures) vote, is concerned with the licensing and supervision of units that carry out *in vitro* fertilization (but not Gamete IntraFallopian Tube Transfer – GIFT). The clause that was debated most in the Bill before it became an act, concerned experimentation on human embryos. By clear majorities in both Houses of Parliament, it became legal to experiment on human embryos up to 14 days after conception, providing the experiments were carried out in units supervised by the statutory licensing authority, established under the Act.

The 1967 Abortion Act was passed after introduction by a private member of the House of Commons. The Human Fertilization and Embryology Act 1990 followed a Government Bill.

The Government and the formulation of the law

When policy with regard to an important subject such as abortion or *in vitro* fertilization is being formulated the Government often sets up a committee to take evidence from interested parties. For instance, the Lane Committee set up under a lady judge, the Hon. Mrs Justice Lane, DBE, to investigate the working of the 1967 Abortion Act, deliberated for 2 or 3 years and finally submitted a report in 1974, which recommended slight alterations in abortion procedures (Lane, 1974). Its deliberations are of great value whenever the abortion issue is debated in the Houses of Parliament (as it repeatedly is).

Assisted reproduction and the law

When it became obvious that 'assisted reproduction procedures' should be regulated the Warnock Committee was set up under the chairmanship of Dame, later Lady, Mary Warnock, a University Don and philosopher. It took evidence over 2–3 years about the running of *in vitro* fertilization and other fertility clinics. The Committee published a lengthy report in 1984 (Warnock, 1984) and the Parliamentary debates that took place in 1990 did so on the basis of that Warnock Report. The Warnock Committee that enquired into human fertilization and embryology, consisted of 15 members as well as the chairman. It took evidence from many interested parties including leaders of religion; and the subjects that were discussed by the committee included such controversial matters as surrogacy, semen and oocyte (egg) donation and the donation of embryos. Such difficult matters as cloning, biopsy of embryos and substitution of nuclei were also discussed. It was the Warnock Report's recommendations that formed the basis of all the arguments in Parliament which finally resulted in the passage of the Human Fertilization and Embryology Act in 1990. The interval of time between the publication of the Report and the debates allowed for prolonged discussion by interested parties to take place on the Report so that when the debates were held Members of Parliament were far better informed than they would have been if the Bill had been debated more quickly. 'Warnock' undoubtedly received much of its information from reports by ethical committees in various clinics operating at the time of Warnock's enquiry. In this way statute law was made; but it seems quite possible that many of the clauses of the 1990 Bill will have to be discussed in the courts when doubts arise, so that case law will be added to statute law to clarify the issues as the years go by.

Obstetricians are concerned with the rights of the fetus. In general the fetus has a right not to be injured by the wrongful act of a third party. The Congenital Disabilities (Civil Liability) Act in 1976 gave the fetus this protection, but only partially. This is not a good place to turn to the limitations of the Act; but partly because of these limitations historically a child can bring a claim in respect of 'wrongful life'. This arises when a child is born with disabilities because of the failure of an obstetrician to terminate the pregnancy, as for instance if the mother has been infected with rubella in early pregnancy and not been given the choice of having an abortion, and the child is born with multiple disabilities. The authority in an English court is that of the Court of Appeal's decision in 'McKay vs. Essex Area Health Authority 1982' (ref. 2).There is one difficulty about this case in that it was decided just before the Congenital Disabilities Act came into effect. In the McKay case the child was born with multiple defects as a result of rubella although the mother had been tested for the presence of rubella. The first blood sample was mislaid and the second one misinterpreted.

Another field in which law is involved is in the old historic principle of *consent*. It is not sufficient for a patient to consent to treatment, especially if such treatment would cause damage. The consent should be given only after full information. The situation is therefore known as *informed consent* . English law has no doctrine of 'informed' consent in the sense that full information must be given. Consent that has not been 'informed', i.e. where the consequences of the treatment have not been fully explained,can lead to legal actions against the doctors who have given the treatment. There are several such cases of which perhaps the most important is the case known as 'Bolam vs. Friern Hospital Management Committee 1957' (ref. 3). This case concerned a patient who was given electroconvulsive therapy and was damaged by the therapy. The doctor felt that the patient was mentally too ill to understand the explanation and therefore did not give any. So, already in the 1950s questions of consent arose, to be decided in the law courts. Another such case is that of Sidaway vs. Bethlem Royal Hospital Governors (1984; ref. 4) which is about the duty of a doctor to advise about the risk of treatments.

Surrogacy has entered the law courts when surrogate mothers have refused to give up a child to the genetic parents. A case was decided in the Californian courts in October 1990 where the dispute was between the genetic parents and the surrogate mother who was acting as a host for their offspring. The decision was in the first instance in favour of the genetic parents but it is understood that the case will go to appeal. Doctors were marginally, and only marginally involved in this case.

Gynaecologists, general practitioners and obstetricians do have to know a certain amount of law, because it is held that ignorance of the law is no excuse for breaking it. The law controls the professional behaviour of obstetricians and gynaecologists. It grows slowly; but since the 1980s there has been a proliferation of legislation to govern medical behaviour; some of it formulated by the Government.

Professional confidentiality

Subject to well-defined exceptions doctors have to keep secret what they hear in confidence from their patients. According to the modern law of England, doctors may find themselves legally in a difficult position in regard to professional secrecy which they are enjoined to keep. In English law, a judge may rule that some confidential medical information must on occasion be divulged in open court; and there is nothing whatever that any doctor can do to stop this ruling by a judge in a particular case. If a doctor still refuses to answer questions in open court he risks going to prison for contempt of court. Subject to two exceptions, a doctor however, does not have to give information to the police, although it may be his duty occasionally to let the police know if he thinks a criminal act is going to take place. This is justifiable only if the whole purpose of giving such information to the police is to protect the public from danger and sometimes to prevent repeated non-accidental injury to children.

INTERNATIONAL CODES AND HUMAN EXPERIMENTATION

Medicine can only advance by experimentation and both obstetrics and gynaecology as branches of medicine and surgery have benefited from trying out new techniques and treatments on human beings after animal experimentation. Hence the need for codes governing the ethics of human experimentation. Doctors, bound as they are by the spirit, if not the wording of the Hippocratic Oath, are also bound by several more recent series of DECLARATIONS. The first most important of these was the *Nuremberg Code* set out in 1947 by the World Medical Association. On 19 August 1947 23 Germans, most of whom were doctors, had

judgment passed on them. They had been accused of crimes involving experiments on human subjects including sterilization of women. In short the ethical and legal concepts of the 1947 Nuremberg Code are:

(1) The human subject must consent voluntarily to the experiment.

(2) The experiment should be such as to yield fruitful results for the good of society.

(3) The experiment should be based on the result of animal experimentation and the knowledge of the natural history of the disease, or the experiments should be so conducted so as to avoid all unnecessary physical and mental suffering and injury.

(4) No experiment should be conducted where there is good reason to believe that death or disabling injury will occur.

(5) The degree of risk to be taken should never exceed that determined by the humanitarian importance of the problem to be solved.

(6) Proper preparation should be made to protect the experimental subject against even the remote possibilities of injury or death.

(7) The experiment should be undertaken only by scientifically qualified persons using the highest degree of skill.

(8) In the course of the experiment the subject should be at liberty to bring the experiment to an end if he has reached the physical or mental state where continuation of the experiment seems to him to be impossible.

(9) The scientist in charge must also be prepared to terminate the experiment at any stage.

In the *Declaration of Geneva* 1948 which was amended in 1968, doctors were expected to pledge themselves on admission to the profession that they would behave according to the Hippocratic principles as modified in the light of modern conditions. A physician agrees to 'solemnly pledge myself to consecrate my life to the service of humanity; my teachers respect and gratitude which they are due; practice of my profession with consciousness and dignity; and have the health of my patient as my first consideration'. It goes on to state, as does the Hippocratic Oath, that the doctor will respect the secrets confided in him even after the patient has died, and that he will maintain the overall traditions of the medical profession. From the obstetrician's point of view he will maintain the utmost respect for human life from the time of conception; he will not permit considerations of religion, nationality, race, party politics or social standing to intervene between his duty and his patient.

In 1964 the *Declaration of Helsinki*, was formulated. It was revised in 1975. It gave recommendations guiding medical doctors in biomedical research involving human subjects. The declaration of Helsinki acknowledges that medical progress is based on research which ultimately must rest, in part, on experimentation involving human subjects. The purpose is to improve diagnostic, therapeutic and prophylactic procedures and the understanding of the aetiology and pathogenesis of diseases including gynaecological and obstetric illnesses. There were 12 basic principles involved. These stated that the research should conform to the following:

(1) It should conform to generally accepted scientific principles;

(2) It should follow an experimental protocol;

(3) It should be conducted only by scientifically qualified persons and under the supervision of a clinically competent medical person;

(4) The importance of the objective must be in proportion to the inherent risk to the subject;

(5) Predictable risks should be carefully assessed before the experiment is started;

(6) Every care should be taken to safeguard the rights of the research subject, his integrity, privacy and personality;

(7) Doctors engaged in the research must be satisfied that the hazards involved are believed to be predictable, and must stop the research if the hazards are found to outweigh the potential benefits;

(8) The research results have to be published accurately.

(9) The research when published must make readers aware of the aims, methods and anticipated benefits and all potential hazards.

(10) A doctor carrying out research should be particularly careful if the subject is in a dependent relationship to him or may consent under duress. This sort of situation would arise where an assistant in a medical department depended for promotion on his chief's recommendations and his chief wished to use him as an experimental object;

(11) Informed consent should be obtained either from the subject or his or her legal guardian; and

(12) The research protocol should always contain a statement of the ethical considerations involved.

There are six principles which govern medical research combined with professional care. Four principles govern non-therapeutic biomedical research involving human subjects.

The *Declaration of Sydney* 1968 deals with the determination of the time of death. This is particularly important since cadaver organs such as heart, lungs and kidneys have become used for transplantation and gynaecologists are now increasingly being asked for fetal tissues obtained at abortion for use in transplantation techniques, e.g. for treatment of Parkinson's disease. Transplantation of ovaries is a distinct possibility. It is obviously essential to know that the donor is dead before taking organs which are essential for the continuation of the donor's life.

The *Declaration of Tokyo* in 1975 was concerned with torture and other cruel inhuman or degrading treatments or punishments. This affects the conduct of doctors working for oppressive regimes. The Nazi doctors experimentally sterilized hundreds of women in the death camps; in Turkey in 1990 doctors were still involved in human torture on women as well as men.

The *Declaration of Hawaii* 1977 regulated to a great extent psychiatric treatments. The *Declaration of Oslo*, 1970 gives a statement on so called 'therapeutic' abortion. Important matters here concern:

(1) Respect for human life from the time of conception (a clause in the Declaration of Geneva 1948);

(2) The circumstances which bring the vital interests of the mother into conflict with the vital interests of her unborn child; and

(3) The diversity of response which results from the diversity of attitudes towards the life of the unborn child, and the Declaration states 'this is a matter for individual conviction and conscience which must be respected'. It is not the role for the medical profession to determine the attitudes and rules of any particular state or community in this matter.

610

There have been attempts to formulate the ethics of the patient–doctor relationship and there is for instance a patients' Bill of Rights drawn up by the American Hospital Association in 1973. This starts with 'the patient has the right to considerate and respectful care', and goes on to point out what information the patient should be receiving from the doctor, and what care he can expect.

Specifically in relation to obstetrics and gynaecology the Declaration of Oslo, 1970 confirmed the respect for human life whereas in the Declaration of Geneva it went on to show that there were circumstances which brought the vital interests of the mother into conflict with the vital interests of her unborn child, thus creating a dilemma. The response to this dilemma depended as 'a matter of individual conviction and conscience which must be respected'. The 1970 Declaration went on to discuss the circumstances in which an abortion could be performed. While these Declarations are binding world-wide, they are basically creations of the Western world.

MATTERS OF ETHICAL CONCERN IN INFERTILITY INVESTIGATION, TREATMENT AND RESEARCH (ASSISTED REPRODUCTION)

The birth of Louise Brown, the first baby born following *in vitro* fertilization , gave an impetus to much more research of a very sophisticated nature (Edwards and Steptoe, 1980). There was so much concern in society that the English Government set up a commission under the chairmanship of Dame Mary Warnock. The findings were published under the auspices of the Department of Health and Social Security in July 1984 (Warnock, 1984). The Government allowed plenty of time for the findings of the Warnock Report to be debated by the public and by politicians. The whole matter came before parliament first in the House of Lords and then in the House of Commons (Parliamentary Debates, 1989). It was finally enacted in the Human Fertilization and Embryology Act 1990 which came into effect in July 1991. The French also debated the matter of assisted reproduction or 'Les Procreations Artificielles'.

Research continues into the physiology and pathology of human embryos (Singer and Wells, 1984). Of the utmost ethical concern is the possibility of cloning of human beings. Concern is also expressed on the differentiation of cell lines which may give clues for cancer research, and also for the treatment of such conditions as Parkinson's disease and Huntington's chorea, which may be treated by inserting cells from abortuses into the brains of sufferers or potential sufferers from these diseases (Dawson, 1988).

Material from one embryo of one species can be incorporated into the material of an embryo of another species to produce what are called transgenic animals. Transgenic sheep can provide human blood-clotting protein to treat human haemophiliacs. The sex of an embryo can be predetermined by removing one cell from a six- or eight-cell embryo which is then frozen until the one cell has multiplied a few times and its chromosomal content has been studied. In 1990 the position of the gene for maleness in the Y chromosome was identified and experiments continued to try to remove this gene and replace it with a gene for femininity in the Y chromosome (Handyside, 1989). Animals can be cloned so that, in theory at any rate, identical male cattle can be born to produce good meat, or identical female cattle to produce good milk.

The problems of human surrogate motherhood raise ethical issues as do the problems of oocyte donation, of embryo flushing and embryo division. In the 1990s genetic engineering is just starting, bringing its own problems, of science, of ethics and of law which vary from community to community.

MEDICAL NEGLIGENCE

The growth in the 1970s and 1980s of patients actions against doctors was very large indeed especially against gynaecologists (Symonds, 1985). In the eighteenth century medicine had been described as 'a liberal profession . . . to be exercised by gentlemen of honour and ingenious manners' (Gregory, 1772). In the nineteenth century and the first half of the twentieth century medical men were recruited from the upper middle class but gradually the profession became more classless, and coincidentally patients began to question the decisions of doctors where they had not done so previously. There are three ways that patients can 'seek redress' from doctors if they think that they have not been handled correctly by them. The first is by complaints to representatives of the doctors' employing authority. The vast majority of doctors in the UK are employed by the National Health Service, i.e. by the State. If patients feel that the doctors have

611

been either cavalier to them or lacking in assiduousness in attending to their duties, they can complain to the various employing authorities. They may then have the satisfaction of seeing doctors censored; but they will not get any financial recompense in this way. The second way is to report the doctor to the General Medical Council for serious professional misconduct. The third way is to sue in the common courts. Alec Bourne was prosecuted in the criminal court by the Director of Public Prosecutions, as was Dr Leonard Arthur, a physician of great integrity who allowed a Down's syndrome baby to die through failure of adequate treatment when he considered that the baby's life was not worth living. He was accused of attempted murder, and acquitted after a lengthy trial.

The function of the civil courts in negligence claims is to act as a mediator to decide whether the doctor was negligent, and if so what compensation the patient should receive for such negligence. A good case illustrative of an obstetrician being sued for possible negligence is the famous case in 1980 of a senior registrar, Dr Jordan, was called to Birmingham hospital to attempt to deliver by forceps an infant whose mother's labour was prolonged. He applied the forceps, pulled but probably not excessively half a dozen times, and then abandoned the procedure and carried out a Caesarean operation. When the child was born it was appreciated that his mental functions were less than perfect. The mother sought compensation; and indeed the expenses to which she was put in bringing up such a mentally defective child were great. The procedure that had been attempted was called a 'trial of forceps'. It was conducted in such a way that if the baby was not delivered easily the senior registrar would resort to a Caesarean operation, which is in fact what he did, Whitehouse vs. Jordan, 1980 (see reference 5).

The trial judge in the first instance (the first High Court Judge) found that the senior registrar had pulled too hard and was therefore negligent. This finding of negligence was reversed in the Court of Appeal where Lord Denning stated that an error of judgment was not negligence. Mrs Whitehouse took the case on to the House of Lords who held that there had been insufficient evidence to justify the trial judge's finding of negligence, but the House of Lords disagreed with Lord Denning by stating that an error of judgment was not necessarily negligent. They said it could be negligent but it was not so in this case.

Thus in 1980 a memorable case was decided after the fullest possible hearings, in the High Court, the Court of Appeal and the House of Lords. Proven or admitted gross negligence will nearly always lead to damages being awarded. The fear in the UK is that these damages will reach astronomical proportions as they have done in the USA.

There have been historical developments in the law in negligence and in several other subjects of interest to obstetricians and gynaecologists. There is, for instance, the right of a woman to have an abortion. English law has looked fairly carefully at the decisions made in the supreme court in the USA in 1973 and the famous cases of Rowe vs. Wade and Doe vs. Bolton (ref. 6). The effect of the decisions in these two cases was that it was an invasion of a woman's constitutional right to privacy to limit her access to abortion by statute. This also applied to schoolchildren although their parents may still be informed of the circumstances.

From 1983 onwards the *Medical Defence Union*, which with the *Medical Protection Society* insures the vast majority of doctors practising not only in the UK but also in other countries such as Australia and Israel, started to report a very large increase in the number of claims for negligence in the case of brain damage in infants. In 1983 there were 50 cases a year and by 1989 the figure had gone up to 157 per year. The worrying thing for obstetricians about this was that the full extent of brain damage or presumed brain damage might not show up for up to 18 years after the birth of the child (the age of majority). Therefore doctors might be involved in actions for a delivery that had occurred 20 or more years previously.

By 1989 the situation had become so serious that almost 30% of all the costs and damages paid out for the entire medical profession were for actions against obstetricians and gynaecologists, and by 1987 the American College of Obstetricians and Gynecologists showed that 71% of their members had been sued for negligence at least once and 26% had experienced three or more claims.

Brain damage does not necessarily result from the way that a delivery is carried out. In fact in most cases it does not result from it at all, nor from birth asphyxia attributable to anything the obstetrician has done or not done. Unfortunately, continuous monitoring does not necessarily protect all babies at risk. In 1989 the American College of Obstetricians and Gynecologists decided it was not necessary to use the cardiotocograph monitoring instrument in labour because some of the readings it gave were completely false. For instance, a normal trace was obtained where it was known that the baby had definitely perished 24 hours previously. In any case cardiotocographs can be unreliable, so that the advent of this form of monitoring while it may be helpful to save babies' lives, does not help to prove or disprove anything in some legal cases. Medical negligence had become such a 'growth industry' that at the end of 1990 a large book was produced by Format Publishing written by Rodney Nelson-Jones and Frank Burton and entitled *Medical Negligence Case Law*. It has become a specialist form of law for solicitors and barristers (Lord Chancellor's Department, 1987).

THE LEGAL PROTECTION OF DOCTORS AND PATIENTS

The Medical Defence Union was founded in 1885 to counteract the attacks on medical practitioners animated by malice or on frivolous pretext. The original founder of the Union was Dr C.F. Rideal, who became its secretary. Its original objects now seem to have been slightly woolly in nature. It seemed to spend quite a lot of its earlier years supporting libel actions between doctors such as the famous case of Denholm vs. Tait. This was a libel action between two of the founder members of the Medical Defence Union. Ten years earlier, a Medical Defence Association had been formed to prosecute unqualified practitioners and to assist medical practitioners in their disputes, but by 1885 when two doctors defended themselves against charges of negligence they had to meet the costs of their successful defence out of their own pockets. The object of the Medical Defence Union from its beginning was to help other doctors in similar positions. There seems to have been a merger between the Medical Defence Association and the Medical Defence Union by 1889. But not all agreed with all the objects nor with all the personalities under Lawson Tait's presidency and the breakaway Medical Protection Society was formed in 1892. It was originally known as the London and Counties Medical Protection Society Limited. Some members of the Medical Defence Union left to join the Medical Protection Society, under the presidency of Mr, later Sir, Jonathan Hutchinson.

One of the first cases the Medical Defence Union had to deal with was an action for libel against Lawson Tait who had been rash in criticizing a colleague – a Dr Denholm. After that case a resolution was passed 'that this society being a Medical Defence Union, it is undesirable that finances should be used to defend or support any action made against another member of the profession and that this be a recommendation to Council'. Only if a matter of medical principle arises in a dispute between doctors, and the case goes to arbitration (and not to Law Courts) does the Medical Defence Union pay any costs. It is important to emphasize that the Medical Defence bodies are not insurance companies because if they were they would come under the Insurance Companies Act of 1974 and be controlled under that act by the Secretary of State.

Lest it be thought that the role of the Medical Defence Union is to protect the doctor solely against the patient, this is far from true. Dr S. Cochrane Shanks, a former president of the Medical Defence Union has said 'the Medical Defence Union has two functions equally important: one is to protect the doctor, the other is to compensate the patient'. Very large sums of money are often paid out by the defence societies if there is no likelihood of successfully contesting a case against a doctor because he has been negligent or ignorant.

Occasionally even when the union has defended doctors, large sums have been awarded against them; and these sums are paid by the medical defence societies together with legal expenses.

As far as gynaecology is concerned, among the most common accusations against doctors are those following a failure of sterilization. Sometimes the baby is eventually wanted in a pregnancy that results because of such a failure, but at other times the baby is not wanted and if the diagnosis of the pregnancy is made in time the woman may submit to its termination. At other times however, she may continue with the pregnancy as the information about her being pregnant is delivered too late. The awards made in these cases may include sums of money to help bring up the child. Dr Clifford Hawkins who has written a history of the Medical Defence Union lists in his book (Hawkins, 1985), many of the most interesting cases that the Medical Defence Union has had to defend.

Litigation becomes more and more common, partly as a result of examples set in the USA, particularly in California and New York State.

ETHICAL COMMITTEES FOR *IN VITRO* FERTILIZATION AND IN OBSTETRICS AND GYNAECOLOGY

Every large hospital where any medical research whatsoever is carried out should have an ethics committee. It is now recognized that no research on human beings should be carried out without the protocol for each piece of research being approved by an ethics committee. The ethics committee which rules on a piece of research must not include any member of the research team; although members of the research team can, and in fact should, be called in to present their research projects.

The ethics committees in gynaecological units usually consist of a chairman, who may or may not be a doctor but preferably is not; a lawyer; a lady who is often a Justice of the Peace or a schoolmistress; and in the sort of ethics committees that deal with obstetric and gynaecological matters, usually a woman general practitioner as well as other people. To illustrate the constitution of a good ethics committee, here is a list of the members' occupations of one of the most important *in vitro* fertilization treatment and research units in the country in 1989 (Bourn Hall, Cambridge).

The Chairman was a lady who had been involved with adoption societies and the supervision of schools in East Anglia.

The secretary was a parson, who was also a counsellor in infertility matters.

The scientist was a specialist in animal reproduction who was a Fellow of the Royal Society.

The University Regius Professor of Roman (Civil) Law was the lawyer.

A woman general practitioner, a teacher of biology, as well as a gynaecologist from a different city, constituted the rest of the ethics committee, with powers to vote; although a vote was never needed.

In attendance, moreover, at all meetings was the director of the clinic or his deputy, and the director of research. These did not have a vote but helped with the very technical information sometimes required by members of the committee. The leader of every team wanting to do research had to submit each protocol in writing, to be circulated to all members of the committee a few days before the meeting at which the protocol was to be discussed. Somebody from the research team had to be available to be questioned when the project was being discussed.

Naturally all the proceedings were highly confidential, and minutes were not circulated to anyone except members of the ethics committee.

SEX IN RELATIONSHIP TO OBSTETRICS AND GYNAECOLOGY (THE LEGAL POSITION)

The gynaecological organs are used for sexual intercourse as well as development of the fetus. Until the advent of artificial insemination as practised on a woman by John Hunter, intercourse was the sole method of reproduction. There were however, cases quoted in literature of women becoming pregnant accidentally by insemination from bath water into which semen had been passed, or by the discharge of semen near the genital organs, but not into them. Whether this left the woman as a virgin or whether she had already had intercourse is legally important, but not as important as the legal position of children conceived without intercourse.

The history of attempts to record the natural results of intercourse, pregnancy and childbirth and unnatural results of intercourse such as sexually transmitted diseases and sexual trauma, goes back millennia rather than centuries. All the same, the teaching of sexual behaviour in a moral and legal way, has only relatively recently become a matter for public discussion. The recognition by the law of the relationship between sex and reproduction has throughout history been, to put it mildly, somewhat controversial.

Sex, marriage and reproduction have throughout the ages been bound up with property rights, with religious injunctions and religious taboos, and later with the recognition of the advantages of contraception and birth control. This last had to wait for the approval of the law. The law in England made it difficult to teach anything about contraception so that Charles Bradlaugh in 1877, a Member of Parliament, together with Annie Besant were imprisoned because of a breach of the English Obscene Publications Act in 1857. The conviction was quashed because of a failure of the indictment to specify in which way the book they were advocating was obscene (Norray, 1991). The change was gradual from the end of the nineteenth century to the beginning of the twentieth, when writing about birth control was considered to be obscene and Dr Marie Stopes (not a medical doctor) was sued for obscenity in a famous or notorious case (ref. 7). Suddenly in the year 1967 attitudes and the law changed with the passage of the National Health Service Family Planning Act, which allowed local health authorities in England and Wales to provide contraceptive advice and treatment on the National Health Service. The Abortion Act of 1967 provided some defences to the crime of abortion, and the Sexual Offences Act 1967 legalized some homosexual acts.

Even in 1954 there was some doubt as to the legality of sterilization operations following Lord Denning's minority judgment in the case of Bravery vs. Bravery (1954; ref. 8) in that year. He then stated that if a sterilization operation is to be done to enable the person to have the pleasure of sexual intercourse without shouldering the reponsibilities attached to it . . . it would be illegal. By 1967 the view had changed and the Medical Defence Union confidentially advised its members that sterilization carried out merely as a convenient method of birth control was legitimate. The matter was put beyond doubt by the National Health Service Act 1967 mentioned above.

REFERENCES

Law cases listed separately by number.

Clifford, H. (1985). *History of the Medical Defence Union.*

Dawson, K. (1988). Bio-ethics, **2**, 1–14

De Blegny, N. (1684). *La Doctrine des Rapports de Chirurgie*, published in Lyons

Duncan, A.S., Dunstan, G.R. and Welbourn, B. (1981). *Dictionary of Medical Ethics*, p. xxviii. (London: Darton, Longman and Todd)

Edwards, R. and Steptoe, P. (1980). *A Matter of Life*, pp. 77 and 113. (London: Hutchinson)

Garrison, F.H. (1929). *An Introduction to the History of Medicine*, 4th edn. p. 272. (Philadelphia, London: W.B. Saunders & Co.)

Gregory, J. (1772). *Lectures on the Duties and Qualifications of the Physician.* Manuscript in the Royal Society of Medicine

Handyside, A.H. *et al.* (1989). Biopsy of human pre-implantation embryos and sexing by DNA amplification. *Lancet*, **1**, 347–9

Hawkins, C. (1985). *Mishap or Malpractice.* (Oxford: Blackwell Scientific Publications)

Lane, The Hon. Mrs Justice, (1974). *Report on the Working of the Abortion Act*, (3 vols.) (London: HMSO)

Lord Chancellor's Department (1987). Civil Justice Review: personal injuries litigation. *Br. Med. J.*, **294**, 1600

Mahoney, J. (1990). In Bromham, D.R., Dalton, M.E. and Jackson, J.C. (eds.) *Philosophical Ethics in Reproductive Medicine*, p. 85. (Manchester: The Manchester University Press)

Nelson-Jones, R. and Burton, F. (1990). *Medical Negligence Case Law.* (Format Publishing)

Norray, McK. (1991). *Family Planning Practice and the Law*, p. 9. (Aldershot: Dartmouth)

Parliamentary Debates, Thursday 7th December 1989, House of Lords Official Report. Hansard Volume 513, No 11, pages 1002–1114

Schreyer, J. (1690). Erorterung und oerlauterung der Frag: Ob es ein gewiss zeichen (etc.) Zeitz

Sebiz, M. (1630). *De Notis Virginitatis.*

Singer, P. and Wells, A. (1984). *The Reproduction Revolution.* (Oxford: Oxford University Press)

Swammerdam, J. (1667). *Tractatus phys-anat-med de respiratione usque pulmonum.* (Leiden)

Symonds, E.M. (1985). Litigation in obstetrics and gynaecology. *Br. J. Obstet. Gynaecol.*, **92**, 433–6

Warnock, Dame Mary (1984). *Report of the Committee of Inquiry into Human Fertilisation and Embryology.* (London: HMSO)

Welsh, G. (1667). *De gemellis et partu numerori.*

LAW CASES CITED

1. R. vs. Bourne (1939). 1KB 68, 1938, 3 All ER 615., 1938, 3 All ER 619

2. McKay vs. Essex Area Health Authority (1982). 2 All ER 771 2 WLR 890 CA

3. Bolam vs. Friern Hospital Management Committee (1957). 2 All ER 118 and (1957) 1 WLR 582

4. Sidaway vs. Bethlem Royal Hospital Governors (1984). 1 All ER 1018 and AC 8714

5. Whitehouse vs. Jordan (1980). 1 All ER Page 1650 onwards

6. Rowe vs. Wade; Doe vs. Bolton 93 S Ct 705 (1973), and 35 L Ed 2d 201 (1973) and HL vs. Matheson 101 S Ct 1164 (1981)

7. Stopes vs. Sutherland, (1924). 39 TLR 677CA

8. Bravery vs. Bravery (1954). 3 All ER 59 CA

BOOKS REFERRED TO

Brazier, M. (1987). Medicine, Patients and the Law, pp. 8–210. (Harmondsworth, Middlesex: Penguin Books Ltd.)

Forbes, R. (1945). *The Medical Defence Union Ltd.*, pp. 1–30. (London: Medical Defence Union)

Leonardo, R.A. (1944). *History of Gynecology.* (New York: Froben Press)

Mason, J.K. and McCall Smith, R.A. (1983). *Law and Medical Ethics*, p. 40. (London: Butterworths)

The Medical Defence Union Annual Report (1985). (London: Medical Defence Union Ltd.)

Stewart McKay, W.J. (1901). *The History of Ancient Gynaecology.* (London: Baillière Tindall and Cox)

Biographies

There is properly no history – only biography
Emerson

AETIUS (502–575)

Aetius of Amida in Mesopotamia was the Royal Physician to Justinian I (527–565) and lived in the Byzantine period (476–732). He said 'the [gynaecological] patient should fast, take sitzbaths, use wine soap tampons, and be bled; if necessary she should use pessaries of Iris, gallanum, turpentine, etc'. Aetius also wrote about carcinoma of the breast as well as about vaginal haemorrhages and he seems to have described fibroids.

It is believed that he may have used a vaginal speculum and carried out vaginal examinations as well as bimanual examinations, two fingers of the left hand being in the vagina while the right hand palpated the lower abdomen. Aetius differentiated between ulcerated cancers of the breast and of the womb and non-ulcerated ones – the ulcerated growths often causing bloody discharges or haemorrhages.

His book is called the *Tetrabiblion of Aetius*. In this book there is a chapter with directions for causing an abortion. The method he advocated was 'on the 13th day after the date of missed menstruation the patient is to be jerked about by several people, or she must lift heavy burdens, use high douches of strong herbs, take hot sitz baths, drink a tea of roux, artemisia, oxgall, eletrium, absinthe and violet roots. She must have poultices on the abdomen. On the 4th month the child will be dead and labour will commence. After labour the patient is to be bled profusely'.

It would appear that Aetius was taught by a woman doctor named *Aspasia*, and he in turn is quoted by *Paul of Aegina* (in about AD 660). Paul described the inclined position which we now call the Trendelenburg position of placing the woman with her shoulders lower than her pelvis in order to treat serious abdominal wounds, when the intestines were eviscerated. This is well illustrated in Caspars Stromayr's manuscript of 1559, the position first advocated by Aetius then being used to repair hernias. Stromayr's book is profusely illustrated with colour plates.

ALBUCASIS (936–1013)

Abul-Qasim Albucasis wrote important treatises on medicine and surgery and probably gave the earliest description of haemophilia in a book describing many operations and surgical instruments (Norman, 1991).

Norman, J.M. (ed.) (1991). *Morton's Medical Bibliography*, 5th edn. 3048; 3666. 82; and 5550. (Aldershot: Scolar Press)

ASCLEPIUS

Aesculapius (Latin) or Asclepius (Greek) was the Greek god of medicine; and his staff with *one* serpent coiled around it is the only true symbol of medicine. The Aesculapian staff must not be confused with a caduceus, which in classical mythology was a staff entwined by *two* serpents and which bore a pair of wings at the top. That staff was meant to be carried by Hermes (Mercury) as a messenger of the gods. That is not the true insignia for the medical profession (although it is used by the medical branch of the Royal Air Force).

Epidaurus, believed to be the mountain on which Asclepius was born, is opposite the mountain where a shrine to the god Apollo is situated (Charitonidou, 1978). Asclepius is reputed to have had a sanctuary in the plain beneath the mountain. His sanctuary was called an Asklepieion, where people paid for cures.

Homer referred to Asclepius in the Iliad as

'the blameless physician', a mortal who lived in Thessaly and who had infallible medical knowledge which he taught to his two soldier sons, Machaon and Podaleirios, who were also doctors, probably in the Army. Asclepius was considered to be a semi-god, born of a mortal woman and of the god Apollo. The Epidaurians may have altered the myth to place the birthplace of Asclepius in their region in opposition to the claims of the Thessalian city of Trikke (its present day name is Trikala), that it was Asclepius' birth place.

The sanctuary of Asclepius at Epidaurus is worth a visit. Parts of it were built in Roman times, over 5 years from 380 to 375 BC. In the Roman building there were warm baths. The architect was Theodotos. The sole purpose was to house the statue of the god, whose faithful worshipped outside the temple at an altar. Asclepius had a large family, the names of whose members are very familiar. They include: Hypnos, who gave sleep, Oneiros, who gave dreams, Hygeia, who gave health, and Panaceia and Aegle.

There is also a statue of gold and ivory fashioned by Thrasymedes in Epidaurus. This shows Asclepius seated on a throne, holding in one hand a staff with a snake coiled around it, while his other hand rests on the head of another snake. At his feet is a dog – the emblem of watchfulness.

The Asclepiades were the followers of Asclepius and Hippocrates is himself said to have been descended from the Asclepiades of Cos (Haggard, 1929).

Charitonidou, A. (1978). *Epidaurus, The Sanctuary of Asclepios and the Museum*, pp. 7–58. (Clio Editions)
Haggard, H.W. (1929). *Devils, Drugs and Doctors*, p. 15. (London: William Heinemann)

ASTRUC, JEAN (1684–1766)

Astruc qualified as a doctor at the age of 18 in 1702 in Montpellier. He first practised in Toulouse and then back in Montpellier before finally becoming Professor of Anatomy in Paris, and Physician to the King of France as well as to the King of Poland. There is a portrait of him by the French artist Vigée.

This remarkable physician is famous for his six-volume gynaecological thesis on the diseases of women, published by Cavelier in French in 1761 and translated into Latin in 1762. There had previously been a shorter edition, published in

1738. In that book it was stated that the first observation of an ovarian pregnancy had been in 1682 by St Maurice, a physician of Perigord, France (Astruc, 1767).

His book on obstetrics *L'art d'accoucher reduit a ses Principes* appeared in 1771. In it he advocated using Levret's forceps to extract a dead child; he quoted Levret as being the accoucheur of Madame La Dauphine, and said that Levret had written about Caesarean operations carried out 'D'une Maniere tres-judicieuse'. In the same book he also praised M.Soumain, a clever surgeon of Paris, for carrying out a Caesarean operation in Paris in 1740. It was successful and performed in the presence of many well-known surgeons, saving the lives, according to Astruc, of both mother and child.

Jean Astruc was a man of many parts, a very important anatomist, a physician and gynaecologist and also surprisingly the founder of modern biblical criticism. He had an authoritative knowledge of theology and Hebrew. His father was a Huguenot, who became a Catholic. His first biblical work was a publication that explained the character and mutual relations of various documents in the Pentateuch.

Astruc, J. (1767). *Treatise on all the diseases incident to women*, translated by J. R___n. *The art of midwifery reduced to principles* with a summary history of the art and an appendix by the translator on conception and pregnancy, translated by J. R___n. (London)

AVELING, JAMES HOBSON (1828–1892)

Aveling was 'this rather neglected British Historian of midwifery'. He was born on 25 January 1828 in Cambridgeshire, studied medicine at Aberdeen, and first practised near Sheffield after being Sir James Y. Simpson's pupil. He, in 1864, together with Jessop, Jackson and Keeling, founded the Sheffield Hospital for Women (The Jessop). He later practised in Upper Wimpole Street, London. Together with Thomas James, because he was too old for a junior position and because he found it difficult to secure a senior one, he founded a new hospital, The Chelsea Hospital for Women, in King's Road, Chelsea in 1871. He also founded the *Obstetrical Journal of Great Britain and Ireland* which started publication on 1 April 1873, the date chosen being the anniversary of William Harvey's birth.

Aveling designed several gynaecological and obstetrical instruments. He became interested in the operation for excision of the clitoris, which had been advocated by Baker Brown and others.

He was involved in 1876 in a case of ovariotomy and a discussion ensued between him, Spencer Wells and Marion Sims.

Most of what we know about the early midwives, such as Margaret Cobbe, Alice Massy, Elizabeth Gaynsford, Johane Hammulden (who was notorious for making remarks about the conjugal proceedings of Henry VIII and saying that Queen Anne was a harlot!), and Jane Carisbrycke, all from the sixteenth century comes from his book of 1872. He also wrote about Jane Sharp another famous midwife. His writing about William Harvey also states how much Percival Willughby (q.v.) was indebted to Harvey.

Aveling wrote a paper in 1879 on the curves of midwifery forceps, their origins and their usage and this appeared in the *Transactions of the Obstetrical Society of London*, volume 20, pages 130–151. He also in 1882 wrote a critical essay on the invention of the midwifery forceps which appeared in London, published by Churchill in that year (Thornton, 1967).

Aveling died on 12 December 1892 of typhoid fever. He had published a great deal during his life time, including writings on the use of chloroform in obstetrics, and two history books, one of which *'The English Midwives'* (1872) described the lives and characters of several midwives and the other about the development of obstetric forceps.

Aveling, J.H. (1872). *English Midwives, Their History and Prospects.* (London: J. & H. Churchill)
Thornton, J.L. (1967). *English Midwives* (as above) *together with a biographical sketch of the Author.* (London: Hugh K. Elliott Ltd.)

BALLANTYNE, JOHN WILLIAM (1861–1923)

John Ballantyne was the son of a seedsman and great-grandson of the botanist who re-afforested Scotland with Canadian trees, and the great-great-grandson of the man who introduced Himalayan Azaleas to Britain (Oakley, 1984). He was a dapper little man who was 'curteous and fastidious'. He opened the first venereal disease clinic in Edinburgh. Ballantyne was very cultured and a prolific writer of books. He was the first to advocate systematic antenatal care and wrote 'The first step . . . in the successful treatment of the unborn infant must be the successful treatment of the

pregnant mother'. He pointed out that the profession did not understand the physiological changes of pregnancy. In 1901 he was in favour of an annexe of his maternity hospital being used 'for the reception of women who are pregnant but who are not yet in labour'. Until this time there were no hospital antenatal beds. His ideas were not necessarily new, but he was the first to suggest that admission should be entirely on medical grounds and not on social grounds, such as being unmarried. He also wrote science fiction and an interesting article on Rösslin's *Birth of Mankynde.*

Oakley, A. (1984). *The Captured Womb – A History of the Medical Care of Pregnant Women*, p. 46. (Oxford: Blackwell Scientific Publications)
(Also see chapter on Antenatal Care, pp. 83–86.).

BECLERE, ANTOINE (1856–1939)

Beclere was the man who introduced medical radiology into France. Radiotherapy followed quickly on Roentgen's discovery that radiography could be used for diagnosis. In 1896 three Viennese doctors, Freund, Schiff and Kienbock demonstrated the effects of Roentgen therapy on skin diseases. Beclere had become a medical student in 1873. In 1897 he started a radiodiagnostic centre at the Hôpital Tenon which he later moved to the Hôpital St Antoine. He worked out some of the physical elements of radiology and designed new instruments for fluoroscopy. It was he who introduced X-rays into insurance examinations. He also started a radiotherapy department at the Hôpital St Antoine. It was the first radiotherapeutic clinic in Europe. His great contribution was to work out exact radiation dosages for treating various kinds of cancers between 1902 and 1934. Moreover, in 1934 and 1935 he found two hormones Prolan A and Prolan B, in different types of seminoma of the testis and in acromegaly. It was he who realized that treatment of fibroids of the uterus by radiotherapy depended on suppression of ovarian function. He published 17 papers on this subject between 1913 and 1929. He also wrote in 1934 a work comparing the hot flushes of the spontaneous menopause with those of the X-ray-induced menopause (Beclere, 1972).

Beclere, Antionette. (1972). *Antoine Beclere: Pioneer of Endocrinology: One of the founders of Radiology and Immunology, and Founder of French Radiology.* (Paris: J.B. Baillière)

BECQUEREL, ANTOINE HENRI (1852–1908)

Becquerel discovered radioactivity and thus was the father of atomic and nuclear physics. He was educated at the Ecole Polytechnique in France and obtained his training in engineering at the Ecole des Ponts et Chaussées. He became Professor of Physics in 1892 as successor to his father and his grandfather at the Musée National d'Histoire Naturelle.

Becquerel heard of Roentgen's discovery of X-rays. He initially thought that X-rays could be produced by stimulating crystals with ultraviolet light; but when he started investigating uranium salts he discovered the emissions of radioactive substances which were different from X-rays. He and Marie Curie (1867–1934, born in Warsaw, died in France), together with Pierre Curie (1859–1906) shared the Nobel Prize for their investigation of radioactivity. Becquerel carried out further research into the polarization of light, into magnetism and into the passage of light through crystals.

Becquerel's discovery of radioactivity in uranium was accidental, when he found that photographic plates in his dark-room were fogged by traces of the uranium ore in the room. It was Becquerel who suggested to the Curies that pitchblende should be investigated and it was that suggestion that led the Curies to discover radium.

BILLROTH, (CHRISTIAN ALBERT) THEODOR (1829–1894)

Billroth was born on the Island of Rugen, now in Germany, of Swedish parents. His father was a Pastor. He studied in Berlin and became assistant to Professor Bernhard von Langenbeck. From 1860 (when he was 31) to 1867, he was Professor in the University of Zurich, Switzerland; then he was appointed by the Emperor Franz Josef to the Chair of Surgery in Vienna. It is said that he and Lawson Tait (q.v.) 'led the way into abdominal surgery'. He experimented on animals before performing his operations on human beings.

Billroth performed the first gastrectomy for cancer of the pylorus of the stomach, and also the first total laryngectomy. He was the founder of the modern concept of reporting total departmental clinical experience. According to Harold Ellis in his book *Famous Operations*, Billroth warned 'statistics are like women, mirrors of virtue and truth, or like whores, to use as one pleases'.

In 1872 he performed the first partial oesophagectomy. He soon adopted antiseptic techniques, thus lowering his operative morbidity and mortality and setting an example to abdominal surgeons, including gynaecologists, everywhere.

Billroth was an intimate friend of Johannes Brahms, and was himself a good musician. He was also prominent in Austrian politics and was a member of the Upper House of Parliament. He was a leader among surgeons and an example for all time in that he was a fully rounded man who based his surgical techniques on Hunterian-like principals of 'try the experiment'.

Ellis, H. (1984). *Famous Operations*, pp. 29–36. (Media, PA: Harwal Publishing Co.)

BLAIR-BELL, WILLIAM (1861–1936) (Figure 1)

Blair-Bell did not make any particularly original contributions to obstetrics and gynaecology but he was a near genius in his own way. He founded what was at first the College of Obstetricians and Gynaecologists; which later became the Royal College of Obstetricians and Gynaecologists. Although he was involved with both research and clinical work as the senior surgeon of the Royal Infirmary Liverpool and later Professor of Obstetrics and Gynaecology at Liverpool University, it is as administrator and founder of this very important College, that has members and fellows in at least 85 different countries with world-wide influence, that he will always be remembered.

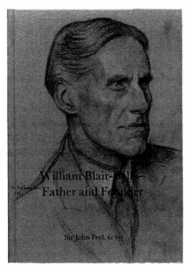

Figure 1 Frontispiece from the biography of William Blair-Bell, Father and Founder, by Sir John Peel

In 1911 Blair-Bell had founded the Gynaecological Visiting Society of Great Britain, whose
purpose was for chosen research workers to meet
together to discuss their different scientific problems, and also to visit clinics in the UK and abroad.
It was out of this Gynaecological Visiting Society
that the original idea came to found a College of
Obstetricians and Gynaecologists. Blair-Bell was
very keen that the College should be a Commonwealth college. He found and paid for the first
home for the College; and the money obtained
after the College's original building was sold was
invested so that the interest could be used for the
maintenance of the new building and College.
The College opened its doors in 1929 in Queen
Anne Street, London, in the house that Blair-Bell
gave, and Blair-Bell became its first president.

He managed to quarrel with too many of his
colleagues in the profession at that time to have
been a very popular man; but his contribution to
gynaecology with the founding of the College as
well as his work on hormones makes the description of him as a genius somewhere near the truth.
His Visiting Society still exists.

The function of the College is totally different
from that of a society. The sole purpose of societies is to meet and exchange ideas. This does
happen in specialist colleges, but the meetings
are nearly always much more formal than in societies. The lectures are held in front of large audiences and there is relatively little room for spontaneous discussion (Peel, 1976).

Peel, J. (1976). *Lives of the Fellows of the Royal College
of Obstetricians and Gynaecologists 1929–1969*, pp.
73–7. (London: William Heinemann Medical
Books)
Peel, J.H. (1980). *William Blair-Bell, Father and
Founder.* (London: RCOG)

BONNEY, WILLIAM FRANCES VICTOR
(1872–1953)

Bonney was the greatest operative gynaecological
technician of the twentieth century and possibly
of all time. He was a dapper, handsome man,
cultured and with widespread interests. His father
was a doctor in Chelsea who qualified at the
Middlesex Hospital in 1866, and both his grandfa-
thers were doctors. His mother was the daughter
of a French doctor; and he was a great Francophile.
Bonney trained the highest quality registrars in
the best possible manner. At one time it was said
that there was no teaching hospital in London

that did not have a trainee of Victor Bonney on its
consultant staff. His main claim to fame lies in his
publications, particularly his book on gynaecological surgery of which the ninth edition, much
modified and updated, is still in print. The first
edition appeared in 1911, when he wrote it together with Sir Comyns Berkeley, his senior gynaecological colleague at the Middlesex Hospital.

Although he carried out more than 500
Wertheim's operations, the most extended form
of gynaecological surgery known in his day, with a
low mortality in spite of poor anaesthesia, no
antibiotics, no relaxation for operation and no
blood transfusion, Bonney also practised conservative surgery. His book on *Extended Myomectomy and
Ovarian Cystectomy* was published in 1946. In it he
expounded how to remove fibroids and conserve
and reconstitute the uterus so that it was available
for childbearing. His last major operation in fact
was in the Middlesex Hospital in 1947 when at the
age of 75 he removed a large number of fibroids
and reconstructed the uterus.

He removed innocent cysts from ovaries and
rebuilt the ovaries so that they too could maintain
ovulation.

Between the years 1910 and 1945 he designed
many of the instruments used in gynaecological
surgery, in particular clamps to place around the
cervix when the extended myomectomy operation was being done.

He held that Wertheim's operation should be
performed only for cancer of the cervix, but as
radiotherapy developed he acknowledged that
radium and later caesium should replace some
Wertheim's operations.

Initially Bonney opposed the founding of the
Royal College of Obstetricians and Gynaecologists
because he felt that gynaecology should be a
branch of surgery and that every gynaecologist
should be able to cope with any organ that he
might come up against during operations. Thus
he himself was able to remove parts of bowel and
reconstruct continuity, similarly with the ureter.

Inevitably Bonney designed and modified obstetric forceps. In 1902 he modified Milne Murray
forceps, having them contructed slightly lighter
and with a simpler design. The detachable rods
fitted by a pin into a slot *inside* the blade unlike
the Milne Murray forceps where the slots fitted
outside.

Not only was Bonney a great surgeon but also
a self-taught artist; he drew most of the illustrations for his books himself. His great hobby was
dancing with his wife. They had no children. His

other hobbies were fly fishing, listening to good music and reading Milton and other poets.

Bonney, V. (1946). *The Technical Minutiae of Extended Myomectomy and Ovarian Cystectomy.* (London: Cassell)
Bonney, V. (1947). *A Textbook of Gynaecological Surgery.* (London: Cassell, 1st edn.: 8 subsequent editions by different publishers and editors)

CHAMBERLEN FAMILY

A beautiful book has been written by Dr Walter Radcliffe about this family and their 'invention' of the obstetric forceps. The book is entitled *The Secret Instrument* and was published by William Heinemann Medical Books Ltd. in 1947. On page 72 of this classic Dr Radcliffe has constructed a family tree of the Chamberlen family. The father of the family, one William Chamberlen, married Genevieve Vignon; he died before 1596. He had come as a Huguenot refugee from religious persecution in France to England, landing in Southampton in 1569. He had five children and somewhat unimaginatively named two of his sons Peter. They must have been alive at the same time because Peter 2nd died before Peter 1st in 1628. Peter 2nd was married to Sarah de Laune whose father Gideon de Laune is celebrated for having founded the Worshipful Society of Apothecaries of London. The Apothecaries is the only City Company of London which still has an undamaged hall, built in 1667 after the first hall was destroyed in the Great Fire of London in 1666. Peter 2nd (1575–1628) lived in London. His older brother Peter had stayed in Southampton. The London Peter soon got into trouble with the Barber-Surgeons' Company, for failing to attend lectures. He was also in trouble with the Royal College of Physicians as he did not want to obey the rules set up by William Harvey, who was immensely powerful although he had refused the Presidency of the College. (William Harvey, the famous discoverer of the circulation of the blood, had also written on the organs of generation.)

So bad was the trouble between Peter the Elder and his professional colleagues that he was arrested in 1612 and put in prison in spite of the fact that he had connections in the highest places and at that time had become surgeon to Queen Anne, the wife of James I and VI through the recommendation of the Archbishop of Canterbury. It is just possible that it was Peter 2nd who

had conceived the idea of the forceps. This latter Peter had eight children of whom the eldest was a doctor, also named Peter (1601–1683). By his first marriage that Peter had nine children of whom one was again inevitably called Peter. His oldest son Hugh was the man who carried on the family tradition. *His* eldest son was also called Hugh and his second son Peter. Elizabeth the first of the girls of the Dr Peter of 1601–1683, had four sons, one of whom became an Admiral. The second one Sir Chamberlen Walker (whose father was a Colonel William Walker of Ireland) was an obstetrician. He died in Dublin in 1780.

The time that interests us, however, is the beginning of the seventeenth century because Peter – the son of the William who had emigrated to England – tended the wives of both James I and Charles I in childbirth in the first half of the seventeenth century. It may well be that he invented the forceps in about 1630. His grandson Hugh, who was born in 1630 and may have lived until the age of 90, was the one who exploited the forceps more than anybody else, both in England and in France. In 1670 he offered the secret to the French government. He translated Francois Mauriceau's book on midwifery into English and made a reference to the forceps in his preface to that book. Peter Chamberlen the elder's patient Henrietta Maria was the wife of Charles I and the mother of the future Charles II.

The cause of the emigration of the Chamberlen family into England was the decree of Catherine De Medici (1519–1589), who ordered the slaughter of the Huguenots in France during the Wars of Religion (1562–1598). Her decree resulted from connivance with her son Charles IX at a period when she was attempting to make peace between the Catholics and Protestants and it was followed by the Massacre of the Huguenots on St Bartholomew's Day in August 1572.

Radcliffe, W. (1947). *The Secret Instrument.* (London: William Heinemann Medical Books Ltd.)

CHARAKA AND SUSRATA

Charaka was one of the great Indian doctors. He lived in the first century AD and was succeeded by Susrata who wrote the *Ayur Veda*, an old Indian obstetric text which talks about diseases, among them 24 diseases of the generative organs which were mostly concerned with disorders of menstruation. Charaka, however, described operations for vaginal tumours, and also for stone in the bladder. There was quite a marked similarity between Susrata's work and the Hippocratic collection, particularly in the sections relating to the ethics of medical practice. Susrata's description of lithotomy agrees almost exactly with the account given by Celsus. There seems to be some confusion between the authorities because according to Harvey Graham the *Ayur Veda* was one of the sacred books of Brahma of which there are four *Vedas*. These are all more recent than the Egyptian papyri and are known as the *Upavedas*. Charaka was supposed to be the court physician of King Kaniska of Peshawar. Peshawar is now in Pakistan but was a major city of the old Hindu empire.

As in Greek mythology (see Asclepius) there is some confusion between the healers who were human and those who were god-like in Hindu mythology. There is a legend of one Dadhyanchi who communicated the sounds of Brahmaveda which he had learned from Indra. For communicating it he had with his consent apparently, his head chopped off, and replaced by the head of a horse which Indra in turn chopped off; but everything was fine because there were other skilled surgeons around who could sew his original head back on! The sacred horses of Indra were called on in cases of difficult labour. It is very difficult for a Westerner to appreciate all the nuances of Indian mythology.

CROFT, SIR RICHARD B. (1762–1818)

This obstetrician, who was descended from a very ancient and distinguished family in Herefordshire, is given a place in this series of short biographies not because of what he taught or achieved, or discovered, but because of his one desperately tragic obstetric failure, which has been called by Sir Eardley Holland, co-founder of the Royal College of Obstetricians and Gynaecologists, 'a triple tragedy'.

He became quite early in his career, physician-accoucheur to 'the lying-in charity for delivering poor married women in their own habitations'. He was a member of the Medical and Chirurgical Society of London, and was appointed Surgeon in Ordinary to Princess Charlotte and her husband Prince Leopold on 3 November 1817. What happened at the delivery is not absolutely certain, but what is clear is that after receiving such antenatal care as was carried out in those days, the Princess Charlotte went into labour at 7 o'clock in the evening of Monday 3rd November. She was 42

weeks and 2 days from the first day of her last period, i.e. somewhat postmature. She had very sharp, acute and distressing pains for 20 hours. Her abdomen was noted to be remarkably large for a first pregnancy. After 20 hours it was thought that there may be a need for some assistance. Richard Croft called a Dr Sims along to assist him, but Dr Sims apparently never went into the room where the Princess was labouring. After a labour lasting 50 hours, the Princess delivered a stillborn male child. Forceps which were kept in readiness were never used. It is noted that the Princess during the first 20 hours or so of her labour was up and about and frequently walking about the rooms. Apparently the placenta was removed with some difficulty, probably because of an inert uterus. Manual removal was probably not undertaken. The Princess died after difficulty in breathing, five and a half hours after the delivery of the child. It is not certain whether application of forceps would have made any difference, but Richard Croft was blamed for not using them. The child weighed 9 lb (4.1 kg) and at post-mortem was found to be 'well-formed'. At Princess Charlotte's post-mortem, there was apparently an 'hour-glass contraction of the uterus. Had the baby been born alive and survived to adult life, he would have become King and Queen Victoria would never have come to the throne.

Sir Richard Croft committed suicide by shooting himself after there had been many letters calling for a public enquiry into the cause of Princess Charlotte's death. Croft is buried near William Hunter in St James's Church, Piccadilly, London.

Crainz, F. (1977). *An Obstetric Tragedy*. (London: Heinemann Medical Books Ltd.)

DALE, SIR HENRY HALLETT (1875–1968)

A splendid raconteur, a great admirer of Paul Ehrlich (q.v.) and a wonderful research worker, Dale establishes yet another example of how a scientist with no clinical input into obstetrics and gynaecology brought great changes in the subject.

He was a complete Cambridge man having been to school at the Leys school in Cambridge and having been an undergraduate and later a postgraduate at Trinity College, Cambridge. It was there too that he first started to research into neuroanatomy. Dale qualified as a doctor with a Cambridge degree having studied clinical medicine at St Bartholomew's Hospital, where he also worked in the laboratories. In 1904 he became director of the Wellcome Physiological Research Laboratories, and in 1914 he became a member of the staff of what was later the Medical Research Council. From 1928 to 1942 he was Director of the National Institute for Medical Research, and he was President of the Royal Sociey of which he had become a Fellow while at the Wellcome.

In 1938 he and O. Loewe shared the Nobel Prize for their discovery of the combined electrical and chemical transmission of nerve impulses. The stimulus for movement of an impulse down the nerve itself was electrical, but at nerve endings it became a chemical process and substances such as acetylcholine and noradrenaline were involved. He subdivided the actions of acetylcholine. From this was later developed the clinical use of tubocurarine, a powerful muscle relaxant. Derivatives of these are used daily in anaesthesia.

It was the work he did on ergot, the oxytocic used to contract the uterus during the third stage of labour, that was of the greatest possible importance, because from it and his great chemical research into the substance found on infected rye, many other developments occurred. Dale collaborated closely with W.C.W. Nixon on the use of oxytocics to speed up early labour and in the third stage of labour to deliver the placenta. Moreover, the isolation of various chemicals in ergot lead to later work on the α and β actions of adrenaline, and thus to the introduction of β-blockers, used for the treatment of heart conditions including angina. He also worked on the development of antihistamine drugs, now used in the treatment of hay fever and other allergic conditions. Even if it were only for his contributions to obstetrics he would have a place in the literature, but his total contributions to medicine were far, far greater.

Medvei, V.C. (1982). *A History of Clinical Endocrinology.* pp. 722–3. (Lancaster: MTP) 2nd edn. (1993) *The History of Clinical Endocrinology.* (Carnforth: Parthenon Publishing)

DENMAN, THOMAS (1733–1815) (Figure 2)

Denman published an atlas entitled *A Collection of Engravings Tending to Illustrate the Generation and Parturition of Animals and of the Human Species,* in London in 1787. He employed, as William Hunter had, Jan van Rymsdyk as one of his illustrators. His major textbook *Introduction to the Practice of*

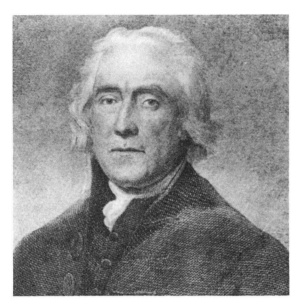

Figure 2 Thomas Denman, MD

Midwifery was first published in London in 1782. Like John Hunter, he initially worked at St George's Hospital and then joined the Navy where he stayed for 9 years as a ship's surgeon. His first training in midwifery was under William Smellie. In 1770 he was elected one of the man-midwives to the Middlesex Hospital, becoming in 1783 after William Hunter had died, 'the number one accoucheur' in London.

On 27 December 1783 he became the first licentiate in midwifery to be admitted by the College of Physicians. His connection with William Hunter and his passing on of the influence of William Hunter's conservatism may have led to his son-in-law Sir Richard Croft's (q.v.) extreme conservatism when looking after Princess Charlotte of Wales who died in childbirth in 1817.

DEVENTER, HENDRIK VAN (1651–1727)

Deventer was born in the Hague and died in Voorburg, both in The Netherlands. He first trained to be a goldsmith, though at the age of 20 he became articled to a chemist and pharmacist. Five years later he became a surgeon, and at the age of 28 started in practice as a man-midwife. In 1688 he journeyed to Copenhagen to see orthopaedic instruments being demonstrated, and while there was asked to treat the orthopaedic conditions of two of the King of Denmark's children.

Later he combined orthopaedics with obstetrics. Like Mauriceau, and like Celsus long before, he described the differences between male and female pelves, pointing out that the female pelvis is wider to allow the birth of a child through it. It is probable that it was his original training in orthopaedics that made him concentrate on the bony pelvis, as he was the first of the great obstetricians to do this. Previously most anatomical descriptions and discoveries were of the soft tissues, but Deventer wrote about the shape and position of the coccyx as well as of the sacrum. He realized, possibly before others, that a small-sized bony pelvis could cause delay, difficulty and failure to deliver a large baby. While he did not think that separation of the pubic bones was important to increase the diameters of the pelvis he did think the space between the ischial tuberosities and the coccyx was very important. He was one of the first, if not the first, to talk about the 'mechanisms' and to use a mechanistic approach to labour, although rotation of the head did not seem to figure much in his description (Fasbender, 1906).

He was the first to use the term 'placenta praevia'. His book, published in Leiden in 1701 was translated into many languages, and was considered to be the most lucid, useful and practical book for midwives. Even in the most obstructed labours he did not resort to Caesarean section. His senior contemporary in The Netherlands was Hendrik Van Roonhuyze, who became involved with the Chamberlens and their forceps. Roonhuyze was much more surgically minded than Deventer and he did perform Caesarean operations on living women. He also designed and carried out an operation for removal of a malignant breast.

An English edition of Deventer's book printed with smaller print and on smaller pages than the later French edition is entitled at length *The Art of Midwifery Improve'd – laying down whatever instructions are requisite to make a compleat midwife and the many errors of all the books hitherto written upon this subject clearly refute it, illustrated with 38 cuts curiously engraven on copper plates representing in their due proportion the several positions of a fetus. Also a new method demonstrating how infants still situated in the womb, whether obliquely or in a straight posture, may, by the hand only without the use of any instrument, be turned into their right position without hazarding either the life of the mother or of the child, written in Latin by Henry Deventer made English, to which is added a preface giving some account of his work by an eminent physician!* This book was printed in London by E. Curll at the Dial and Bible in 1716.

There is a beautiful description on page 74 of the first English edition, of his first wife's labour, who was like one of his patients whom 'I used to compare to a good Pye, out of which, if you take off the Top, and turn up the Bottom, the Pieces fall out of their own accord; and these almost with the same ease, were delivered of their Children'. His own wife 'because she was troubled a little in the Night with the Gripes, which she doubted were the genuine Pains of Labour, about Morning she desired me that I would try her by the Touch; which as soon as I had done, I said there was Work, except she would spoil the Bed; upon which my cloaths being cast about me, I was scarce out of the Chamber, but whilst I was knocking she called me back to help her in Labour; and placing herself upon the next Seat that was at hand, pouring as it were a Daughter into my Bosom, she made me a Father, before any Woman Could come to her help; I when this little infant was brought forth, thinking the swelling of the Mother's Belly was not sufficiently fallen, passing my Hand into her Womb, I perceived another just ready to come forth, which made us that were their parents fall a laughing; and since the Midwife was just ready, my Wife being committed to her Care, I went to the fire with my little One, where presently another Woman running to us, stirred up the Fire, and presently she was delivered of another Daughter . . .'

Hendrik van Deventer's book was written in Latin and translated into French by Jacques-Jean Bruier d'Ablaincourt and published in Paris by Cavelier in 1733 and again in 1739 under the title *Observations Importantes Sur Le Manuel des Accouchements.* This book is heavily illustrated with figures of the female pelvis both from above and laterally, as well as of the soft tissues. In particular there is a beautiful picture of a twin placenta showing two amnions. As important are the illustrations of fetuses presenting by the breech and in other ways and with compound presentations. Figure 13 shows a delivery chair with sides that can be removed and the back laid flat. There are also illustrations of transverse lies, of internal version as well as of breech delivery and descent into the pelvis – an altogether beautifully illustrated text.

Deventer wrote a text book for midwives containing anatomy, internal 'touching' and internal manoeuvres, birth of the baby, delivery of the afterbirth and the qualities of a surgeon who practises midwifery.

He said that men may undervalue the office of

midwife. Although his book for midwives is illustrated he does not illustrate the external 'secret parts' of a woman believing that such figures 'rather serve to excite impure thoughts and give occasion to obscene discourse'. He was an advocate of sitting rather than lying for the delivery, and in labour women should certainly walk or stand, being held up by somebody so the infant is brought forward for birth.

Deventer, H.A. van (1716). *The Art of Midwifery.* (London: Curll at the Dial and Bible)
Deventer, H.A. van (1733). *Observations Importantes sur le Manuel des Accouchements,* translated into French from the Latin by J.-J. Bruier d'Ablaincourt. (Paris: Cavelier)
Fasbender, H. (1906). *Geschichte der Geburtshülfe.* (Jena: Fischer)

DONALD, IAN (1910–1987)
(photographs pp. 403 and 517)

This gynaecologist, together with his contemporary Patrick Steptoe (q.v.), changed the face of obstetrics and gynaecology in the middle of the twentieth century more than any others did – he by the invention of ultrasound, and Steptoe by the development of laparoscopy. There are now few if any major obstetric, gynaecological or surgical departments in the developed world that do not use ultrasound.

Donald was born in Cornwall on 27 December 1910. He went to school in England but when he was 14 years of age his family moved to South Africa because of his father's ill health. His early education was in Edinburgh, and then in South Africa where he graduated in Arts in Cape Town. His father had been a doctor in Paisley and his grandfather was also a doctor.

His initial research after qualifying in medicine from St Thomas's Medical School in London in 1937 was in developing a respirator triggered by the respiratory efforts of the infant suffering from respiratory distress.

He was a brilliant teacher and his text book *Practical Obstetric Problems* went to five editions. He was later Professor of Obstetrics and Gynaecology in Glasgow at the Queen Mother's Hospital, where the maternity unit was built entirely to his design.

His fame, however, rests on his having adapted ultrasound for use in medicine. He preferred to call it 'sonar', which stands for Sound Navigation and Ranging. Sonar had first been developed for the Navy by Paul Langevin, a colleague of Marie

Curie's, who used the principle to locate submarines in the ocean by beams of sound waves of such high frequency as to be non-divergent and thus to be under directional control.

Donald fortunately had served in the Second World War from 1942 onwards with an Air Squadron of Coastal Command, whose task was to seek out and destroy German U-boats. They did this using a very primitive form of sonar. Donald, who was a yachtsman, also used echo sounders on his boat.

After the war Professor Donald was one day entertained to lunch by the research directors of Messrs. Babcock and Wilcox who at that time used an A-scanner to detect flaws in metals. He had with foresight taken with him to the lunch ovarian cysts and uterine fibroids removed by operations in the previous few days. He was able to demonstrate that they had different appearances when ultrasound was directed at them. From this beginning with metal-flaw detectors, he slowly evolved, with the help of engineers at Kelvin Hughes, apparatus for use in detecting abnormal masses in women's abdomens. Later, he was able to diagnose with fair assurance whether they were cystic or solid. He worked very hard at improving the apparatus with assistance from his University and various trust funds.

By 1960 he was able to develop a B-scanner, and later was able to identify and still later measure the fetal biparietal diameter. He recruited a physicist to his team and received the great help of his colleagues and assistants, particularly Dr James Willocks and Dr Stuart Campbell, later Professor of Obstetrics at King's College Hospital in London. Donald wrote an account of the first 25 years of medical sonar which was published in a volume edited by A. Kurjak (Kurjak, 1980).

Donald's opposition to the Abortion Act of 1967 was not admired by everybody. Possibly because of it some of the honours he might have received were withheld from him. He died on 19 June 1987 in his retirement home in Essex to which he and his wife Alix had gone in order to be able to indulge his hobbies of water colour painting and small boat sailing. In his last years he suffered very precarious health after three successive cardiac operations.

Kurjak, A. (ed.) (1980). *Recent Advances of Ultrasound Diagnoses, Proceedings of the International Symposium in Ultrasound Diagnosis,* Dubrovnik, 1–5 October 1979. (Amsterdam: Excerpta Medica)

EDWARDS, ROBERT (1925–)

Robert Edwards, born in 1925, came from a totally different background than his colleague Patrick Steptoe (q.v.). He, the second son in a working class family, was at the end of his professional life, a Professor at Cambridge University and a Don of Churchill College Cambridge. Trained as a biologist, he initially undertook postgraduate studies in agriculture. While working for his Ph.D. in Edinburgh University he learned that Alan Beaty, an expert on fertilization and the development of embryos in mice, had taken a fertilized egg from the uterus of one mouse and injected it into the uterus of another mouse. This had been successful in that a healthy baby mouse was born. He also learnt that the chromosomes of mouse embryos could be modified, and in Edinburgh, how he could modify the chromosome contents of mouse eggs that normally have 20 chromosomes in each gamete cell and 40 chromosomes in each adult cell.

Edwards married Ruth Fowler who was a granddaughter of Lord Rutherford the great physicist. Together they studied the biochemistry of mice eggs and embryos. They worked on stimulating mouse ovaries to produce more eggs for fertilization, and in fact they managed to induce mice to produce so many eggs at one time that the embryos resulting burst out of their wombs into the peritoneal cavities. One mouse produced 37 baby mice! Within a few years Edwards had become one of the most skilled embryologists in the world.

Edwards was one of the first people to superovulate mammals. Some of his original research work was done in California and later at the National Institute for Medical Research at Mill Hill, London. In California he obtained large quantities of human ovarian tissue in which he could ripen the eggs, particularly in cultures of the secretions of the female genital tract.

Before he even met Steptoe he was the first to fertilize a human egg outside the body. The egg had been taken from the ovary of a patient who was undergoing hysterectomy, and it was fertilized by human semen. There was no intention at that stage of putting the fertilized egg back into any woman. Edwards was the first to work out the 36-hour interval that the egg took to ripen after the luteinizing hormone surge in the human ovary; in 1965 he first published a paper in the Lancet about ripening ova and their fertilization, possibly outside the human body. He foresaw that certain inherited human diseases, particularly those that were sex-linked, could be eliminated.

The story of his work with Steptoe from 1968 onwards is well known and has been documented in *A Matter of Life* by Robert Edwards and Patrick Steptoe.

Edwards, R. and Steptoe, P. (1980). *A Matter of Life*. (London: Hutchison)

PAUL EHRLICH (1854–1915)

Paul Ehrlich, who first worked as a clinical assistant in the University of Berlin, was assistant to Robert Koch's Institute in Berlin until he became director of the Institute for the Investigation of Serum in Berlin, and later founded a new institute for experimental treatment in Frankfurt am Main. Most of his experimental work was on dye stuffs and stains. He was involved in the formulation of new biochemical theories and was the first to have the idea that diseases caused by protozoa could be treated by chemicals if such chemicals could be developed to kill the parasite without injuring the body. He discovered that if the doses given were too small the organisms would become resistant and that correct dosage was all important. It had to be strong enough to kill the parasite and not too strong to injure the normal tissues. His first tentatively successful experiments were on treating malaria with Methylene Blue and then he went on to other forms of 'chemotherapy' which was a term developed by Ehrlich himself. His work in developing arsenical drugs for the treatment of syphilis are described in the appropriate chapter in this book.

Ehrlich's work led to the development by Domagk, after an interval of some 25 years from the discovery of the arsenicals, of Prontosil Red. Prontosil was the first sulphanilamide drug. The initial work of Ehrlich then was of benefit in the treatment of syphilis rather than for purely gynaecological purposes, but it led gradually to the much larger development of chemotherapy and antibiotic therapy, now an enormous industry.

Ehrlich received the Nobel Prize in 1908 and Domagk in 1939.

FALLOPPIO, GABRIELE (1523–1562)
(portrait, p. 463)

Falloppio (or Fallopius) of Modena was a pupil and a successor of Vesalius in Padua. His book *Observationes Anatomicae,* published in Venice in

1561, contains his description of the Fallopian tubes. He also described the cochlea and labyrinth of the ear. He was among the first critics of Galen's teachings.

GALEN

Claudius Galenus (AD 131–201) was born at Pergamum in Mysia where he first studied in the medical school of the Shrine of Asclepius (q.v.), later moving to study at Smyrna, Corinth and Alexandria and still later going to Rome. He served the rulers of Venice and of Rome and tended Mark Aurelius and his two sons. He died in Sicily (Figure 3, p.631).

He was a prolific writer; but many now consider that Galen, (because of his huge reputation, and his poor understanding of physiology dominated by the Hippocratic four elements of heat, cold, wetness and dryness, and following these the humours, of blood, phlegm, choler, yellow bile and melancholy (black bile)) managed to hold back medicine for over 1000 years. Nobody dared contradict what he had written and thought (Mann, 1984).

Although his physiology was poor, his anatomy was not too obviously bad, but it was overturned when Andreas Vesalius in the sixteenth century produced his marvellous atlas and challenged and changed Galen's anatomy. Vesalius (q.v.) was the first to do so effectively. The work of William Harvey (q.v.) on the circulation of the blood was perhaps one of the most important discoveries that upset Galen's teachings.

It is at present the fashion to diminish the stature of Galen, who at this distance seems to have been hectoring, conceited, dogmatic and even guilty of distortion of the anatomical findings that he had made not only on the dead, but also on living animals; for he practised vivisection widely. Yet, the influence of his now discredited writings was so great that it lasted for 1500 years.

There is an interesting reference in Galen's writings to gynaecology in the 14th book of his 17-volume *De Usu Partium Corporis Humani*. In this Galen tried to establish an analogy between male and female parts of the genital organs. This was faulty both physiologically and anatomically. The fifth chapter of the sixth book of his work, entitled *De Locis Affectis*, is devoted to infections of the genital organs of women, and is mainly taken up with the subject of hysteria. Not unlike many other gynaecologists even into the twentieth century, Galen associated displacements of the uterus

with troubles of menstruation. He also wrote about haemorrhage in pregnancy. He wrote a whole book on the anatomy of the uterus *De Uteri Dissectione*. From this it seems quite clear that Galen had not dissected a human uterus although he had dissected animals. It does appear, however, that he was the first to point out that there are tubes to convey ova to the uterus, long before Fallopius, so that the modern tendency to decry him utterly seems unfair.

Mann, R.D. (1984). *Modern Drug Use – An Enquiry on Historical Principles*, pp. 123–9 and many others. (Lancaster: MTP)

Medvei, V.C. (1982). *A History of Endocrinology*, p. 735 and several other short references. (Lancaster: MTP)

Nuland, S.B. (1988). *Doctors*, pp. 31–60. (New York: Alfred A. Knopf)

Stuart McKay, W. J. (1901). *The History of Ancient Gynaecology*, pp. 133–48. (London: Bailliere, Tindal and Cox)

DE GRAAF, REGNIER (1641–1673)
(portrait, p. 62)

This Dutch physician, who was born in Schoonhoven on 30 July 1641, lived for only 32 years. He practised in Delft having obtained his M.D. at the University of Angers, France, in 1665. During his life he carried out an enormous amount of work and in 1668 published his remarkable book entitled *De Virorum Organis Generationi Inservientibus, De Clysteribus Et De Usu Siphonis In Anatomia*. This book gave the first exact and detailed account of the male reproductive system. It also contains his essay on the use of clysters which were becoming popular in the seventeenth century to give enemas. He not only described the male and female genital organs and gave the first description of the follicles of the ovaries, but he also studied the pancreas and its secretions. He demonstrated ovulation anatomically, pathologically and experimentally. He described for the first time the corpus luteum and gave the first account of the testis that showed that it was made up of tubes folded into lobules. The book was an immediate success. Reissued in 1672, it went into a second edition in 1677. The book was written in beautiful Latin. Apparently de Graaf was not only a very elegant man, as can be seen from his portraits to be found on the front pages of both his books (different portraits), but he was also said to be humorous. The illustrations in his book are accurate, artistic and delicate.

De Graaf produced a new syringe; and he used

mercury to inject blood vessels. This was a procedure that had also been used by Jan Swammerdam (1637–1680). Swammerdam disputed de Graaf's claim that he had made original observations on the gonads and it was possibly the row between them that hastened de Graaf's early death.

The anatomy of the female genital organs de Graaf described, included sections on the pudenda, clitoris, mons, the urethra, the vagina and the uterus as well as the ligaments and blood supply. It described also the arteries to the uterus and how much more vascular the pregnant uterus was than the non-pregnant one. It was Haller who named the Graafian follicles after de Graaf. Both de Graaf and Swammerdam had been pupils of Johannes van Horne, who was the first to attempt to show the difference between a corpus luteum and a simple ovarian cyst.

Following his magnum opus in 1668 de Graaf in the revised printing in 1672 described the lymphatic system of the uterus. We now know that this system is of immense importance for understanding the spread of cancer of the uterus. De Graaf had performed much of his work on a large fibroid uterus.

Among the interesting illustrations in the books are those of a ruptured Fallopian tube with a fairly advanced pregnancy in it (page 361, table XXI) and of Fallopian tubes with pus in them and with closed fimbrial ends. He also stated 'that a gonorrhoea has its source from the glandular body of the prostate (sic) and breaks out through the lacunae situated at the termination of the urinary passage; the dissection of a woman who died of this disease plainly demonstrated, for I found only the glandular body, or prostatas which embraced the urethra diseased while the uterus and vagina were perfectly sound'. De Graaf described the structure of the male prostate gland and of the seminal vesicles and in considerable detail in the 1677 edition which appeared posthumously, the structure of the pancreas and its ducts which are beautifully illustrated.

GUILLEMEAU, JACQUES (1550–1612)

Guillemeau was born in Orleans and died in Paris. He was Ambroise Paré's pupil and son-in-law, and it was he who translated Paré's work into Latin. He published a book on obstetrics entitled *De l'heureux accouchement des femmes* which appeared in 1609. He seems to have been a somewhat conservative obstetrician and prided himself on not using crotchets or other iron instruments. His book was translated into English, probably about 1612 (Fasbender, 1906).

Although Guillemeau claimed that he was conservative, chapter 28 of his second book speaks about Caesarean sections. He also wrote about adherent placentae and about the treatment of impotence.

He practised podalic version which he had learned from Ambroise Paré. He was probably the first to describe the technique now known as the Mauriceau–Smellie–Veit manoeuvre for delivery of the aftercoming head in breech deliveries.

Fasbender, H. (1906). *Geschichte der Geburtshülfe*, pp. 129–34. (Jena: Gustav Fischer)

HAMMURABIS

Hammurabis (also known as Hammurapi or Khammurabi) was the sixth ruler in the First Babylonian Dynasty and he lived according to different authorities at any time between 2300 BC and 1750 BC.

He was a great warrior who drove his enemies out of Babylon and created a large empire. His fame, however, rests more on his codification of the law, so that the Code of Hammurabis is considered the earliest legal code of all time. The medical parts that are of interest to us consist of the *Lex talionis* probably the original law of 'an eye for an eye and a tooth for a tooth'. In Judaic law, developed at about the same time, the penalties were not taken literally, but in the form of cash compensation.

At that time there was much trading, and among the commodities were slaves. Marriage itself was a form of contract. Although monogamy was the rule, a childless wife might give her husband a maid (who was not a wife), to bear him children and these were reckoned as the wife's children. The concubine was a wife, though not of the same rank. A slave could have children by her master, but these children were free and the mother could not be sold. So, childless wives might well give their slaves as concubines or mistresses to the husband so that he could have children.

If a wet-nurse substituted a changeling for the child that was entrusted to her to feed, her breasts would be cut off. If a surgeon operated and as a result his patient lost his life or a limb, the result was that the surgeon would have his hand cut off.

The Louvre in Paris has a stone pillar on which the code of Hammurabis is inscribed, including the laws relating to medical practice.

HARVEY, WILLIAM (1578–1657)

Harvey was one of the greatest men in the history of gynaecology. He not only elucidated the circulation of the blood, probably whilst in Padua, where he went after being a student at Gonville and Caius College Cambridge, but also turned his considerable intellect and knowledge of anatomy to researching reproduction. His investigations led him to write the very important book *Exercitationes de Generatione Animalium* (experiments concerning animal generation). This book, published in 1651, was written in Latin, and published originally in Amsterdam. On the title page he gives as his degrees Professor of Anatomy and Surgery in the London College of Medicine. Harvey's book not only criticized the work of Fabricius, under whom he studied in Padua, but also in an *additamenta* (pp. 353–82) there is a chapter on midwifery. However, Harvey's greatest contribution to medicine was contained in his book on the circulation of the blood *De Modu Cordis et Sanguinis in Animalibus* (on the motion of the heart and blood in animals) which was published in 1628.

Harvey practised as a physician rather than an obstetrician. He was admitted as a fellow of the Royal College of Physicians in 1607 and in 1609 became a physician at St Bartholomew's Hospital of London where he stayed until 1643. He was present when James I and VI died in 1625; and he became personal physician to Charles I. It is of passing interest that all the modern techniques of monitoring the fetal heart must originally derive from Harvey's work; although it required the discovery in 1775 of the nature of oxygen by Antoine Laurent Lavoisier for the sophisticated development of modern methods.

Harvey was originally somewhat loathe to publish his work on the generative organs, but after much persuasion, he gave the manuscript of his work to Dr Ent, who visited him at Christmas 1650 in the house of one of his brothers with whom Harvey was staying for the last years of his life. It was Dr Ent who arranged the 1651 publication of the book which was translated into English and published in 1653.

In 1654 Harvey was elected President of the Royal College of Physicians of London, but declined the honour because of his age and gouty infirmity. Harvey's master work on the circulation and the heart was first published in Frankfurt in 1628; and there is an almost perfect copy of it in the medical school of the Department of Obstetrics and Gynaecology in Kansas City, Kansas, USA.

HEAPE, WALTER (1855–1929)

Walter Heape was first a business man, but at the age of 25 he went to Cambridge to study reproductive science. In 1885 he started to work at the Marine Biology Institute in Plymouth. He is notable because on the 21 April 1890 he carried out the first embryo transfer from one rabbit to another, and this was the first embryo ever to be transferred from one mammal to another. His paper on the subject was presented to the Royal Society on 14 October 1890. This therefore was the forerunner of all embryo transfers which are the last stages, of all *in vitro* fertilization (IVF) and embryo transfer (ET) procedures.

Later the science of reproductive physiology was put on a proper basis by F.H.A. Marshall (Marshall, 1922) who founded the science of reproductive physiology within the physiology department of Cambridge University. It was Raoul Palmer in Paris however, who was the first to aspirate a human oocyte laparoscopically.

Marshall, F.H.A. (1922). *The Physiology of Reproduction*, with contributions by William Cramer, James Lochhead and Cresswell Scherer (London: Longmans)

HIPPOCRATES (460–377 BC) (sculpture, p. 46)

Hippocrates the great has been regarded from ages back as the Father of medicine. Although he was human he was given, as were so many eminent doctors, enormous god-like status, and was said to have been descended from Asclepius (q.v.). He was probably born on the Island of Cos, travelled widely throughout Greece and Asia Minor, and died in Larissa in Thessaly (Greece) (Figure 3). He probably lived to a very great age. He ran the medical school at Cos and helped to give it its very great fame. The Hippocratic collection of more than 60 works includes the famous Aphorisms; and his even more famous oath (which he may well not have composed himself) appears in *Jusjurandum*, which is another of his works. It was he who classified diseases, dividing them into two

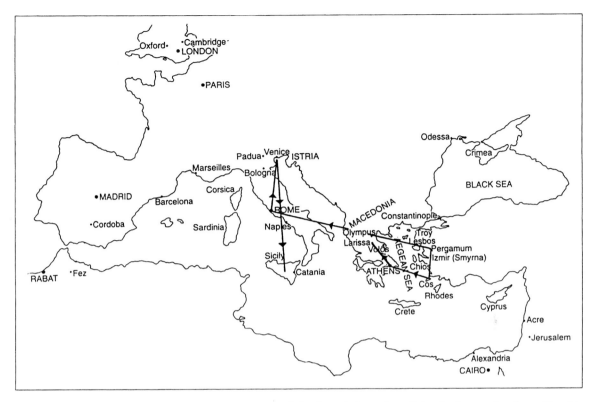

Figure 3 This map to shows how Hippocrates spread the knowledge of medicine by journeying from Cos, his birthplace, to Athens, then through Greece and Asia Minor, and finally to Larissa in Thessaly, where he died. Later, Galen travelled from Pergamum, his birthplace, to Smyrna, Rome, Venice and Sicily

classes; the first consisted of those caused by the influence of seasons, climates, water, geographical situations and so on, and the second class by more individual causes such as the food and exercise taken by the patient. He regarded the four humours of the body – blood, phlegm, yellow bile and black bile – as the primary seats of disease. (q.v. Galen.) If the combinations were right the man was healthy, if they were not right he was diseased. He believed that a baby had to fight its way out of the womb.

The first language into which Hippocrates' works were translated was Arabic; and the first time they were translated into a Western language was a Latin translation published in 1525 in Rome. The so-called writings of Hippocrates can be divided into genuine works of Hippocrates (Adams, 1849) and those that may or may not have been written by Hippocrates himself.

It does seem that Hippocrates knew the shape of the uterus; but he believed that it acted so as to suck and draw juices from various parts of the body. He also believed that 'dropsy' of the uterus

was due to the drinking of unwholesome water. Nobody knows whether his 'hydropsy of the uterus' has anything to do with hydatidiform changes occurring in the placental tissue in pregnancy, or to hydatid disease, which must have been fairly prevalent in Hippocrates' practice. Hippocrates believed that stones were less likely to form in the female bladder than the male because of the relative shortness of the female urethra; and he wrote about gynaecological matters in short in the *Works, Airs, Epidemics, Aphorisms*.

In his oath he says 'I will not give to any woman a pessary to produce abortion'. It does not seem likely that Hippocrates himself practised much gynaecology, but in the Hippocratic collection (that is not considered to be genuine) there is a mention of inspection and palpation of the abdomen and of the organs of generation. It is clear from those writings that vaginal examinations were made by medical men and also midwives and the patients were advised to practise self-examination in cases of sterility. Sounds to open the mouth of the womb 'previous to fumigation'; seem also to have existed. It also seems likely that there were pinewood uterine dilators, and possibly some made of lead and of tin. There were also catheters to wash out the cavity of the uterus. These were polished like a sound and made of silver, with the perforation at the side, slightly behind the tip of the catheter. Recent publications pour scorn on these descriptions by Adams, so it is difficult to know whether Hippocrates did describe various diseases that are mentioned in Stuart-Mackay's *History of Gynaecology* (1901). Hippocrates' writings were almost certainly brought together by the Alexandrian scholars of the third century (Stuart-Mackay, 1901).

Adams, F. (1849). *The Genuine Work of Hippocrates.* (London: Sydenham Society)
Stuart-Mackay, W.J. (1901). *The History of Gynaecology*, pp. 31–6. (London: Ballière, Tindall and Cox)

HOLMES, OLIVER WENDELL (1809–1894)

Holmes had a remarkable career. He started by reading law at Harvard University but then studied medicine and practised it. He also taught anatomy for 2 years at Dartmouth College in Hanover, New Hampshire. He became Professor of Anatomy and Physiology at Harvard in 1847 and later Dean of the Medical School. In 1843 he had written that he thought that puerperal fever was a contagious disease. His fame was mainly achieved as a humorist, writer and poet; and also as the father of his son with the same name, who became an eminent judge, legal historian and philosopher in Washington D.C. (Holmes, 1855).

When Holmes published his views, in great opposition to the orthodox physicians in Philadelphia, that students should not go from the post-mortem room or other sources of infection including other cases of puerperal fever, to healthy women and also that their hands should be washed in a solution of calcium chloride and that their clothes should be changed after attending a case of the disease, he mentioned that similar precautions were being taken by Semmelweis (q.v.). Holmes had already in 1840, tried to institute these precautions.

It is very likely that Holmes was the man who originally proposed the terms 'anaesthetic' and 'anaesthesia'. It was Sir James Young Simpson (q.v.) however, who on 19 January 1847 was the first man to use ether in midwifery and later in November 1847 was the first to use chloroform. The great Lord Lister recognized the contribu-

tions that both Oliver Wendell Holmes and Ignas Philipp Semmelweis had made in preventing the spread of infection.

One of the earliest contributions Holmes made was in 1843 when he lectured at the Boston Society for Medical Improvement on 'the contagiousness of puerperal fever'. This lecture was afterwards published in the *English Journal of Medicine and Surgery* and later enlarged and published in book form as *Puerperal Fever, as a private pestilence*, in Boston, in 1855 (Holmes, 1842; 1855).

Holmes, O.W. (1842). The contagiousness of puerperal fever. *N. Engl. Q. J. Med. Surg.*, **1**, 503–30
Holmes, O.W. (1855). *Puerperal Fever as a Private Pestilence.* (Boston: Ticknor & Fields)

HUNTER, WILLIAM (1718–1783)

William Hunter, the older brother of the even more famous John Hunter, was born in Long Calderwood, East Kilbride on 28 May 1718. He enrolled in Glasgow University at the age of 14, and spent 4 years there reading Humanity, Greek Logic and Natural Philosophy. This gave breadth to his education. In 1736 he went to William Cullen a local teacher of medicine and was apprenticed to him for 2 years until the age of 20 when he went to Edinburgh to attend anatomy lectures at the University. At the age of 22 he came to London to work with William Smellie, whom he had known in Hamilton and who was 21 years his senior. At the age of 30 William Hunter was elected Surgeon Accoucheur to the Middlesex Hospital which was then in Great Windmill Street, London. He was joined that year by his brother John. When he was 44 years of age he was made consultant to Queen Charlotte. At the age of 50 he was made a Fellow of the Royal Society and Professor of Anatomy at the Royal Academy and 2 years later he completed a building in Great Windmill Street into which he moved his Anatomy School from its original site in Covent Garden. He died at the age of 65 in 1783.

Hunter is most famous for his *Atlas of the Human Gravid Uterus*. He is also famous because he was one of the first obstetricians (men-midwives) to invade the field of childbirth which had been the prerogative of midwives for thousands of years. He was unlike other obstetricians of his day, because he was in no way meddlesome. In other words he was not prone to use the obstetric forceps and was even proud of the fact that his had rust on them.

His greatness lay in his ability to teach anatomy, some surgery and above all midwifery. His classes were attended by the most eminent as well as by young students, and there is a notable portrait of him teaching anatomy, painted by Zoffany, a well-known court painter of the day. He built up an enormous practice among the aristocracy and he literally cashed in on the cachet of being the royal doctor.

He was perhaps not as great a teacher as his older contemporary Smellie (q.v.), but his philosophy, that of conservatism, is illustrated by his phrase 'if his patient is a lady of eminence he must learn like Agag, to tread delicately lest he stray between the twin dangers of presumption and servility. But in return for his attention through months of waiting and his care on the night of agony he can expect gratitude and confidence beyond estimation'. Smellie was apparently unable to tread delicately between presumption and servility. Not all of Hunter's patients were aristocratic. For instance there were two who advertised 'Peg and Meg, comely with taking ways, two shillings each or three and six for the pair. Gentlemen welcome'.

Whereas the royal accoucheur of today does deliver babies, especially royal ones, it was not so in the case of Queen Charlotte who was delivered on 12 August 1762 of the Prince who was later to become George IV. Mrs Draper the midwife was inside the room and Hunter was kept outside, in case there was any emergency. His note book of the occasion is very interesting (Philipp, 1987). In it he described his care of the Queen. By the delivery of the third infant, having been kept out of the room for the first two, he got impatient and managed to persuade the Queen to be rid of Mrs Draper so that he himself could conduct the delivery. Hunter's other claims to fame after his marvellous Atlas are his wonderful collections of paintings, thousands of books, coins, anatomical specimens and particularly wax models of women who had died in different stages of pregnancy and labour. He died 12 days after collapsing whilst starting his last lecture in 1783, and was buried in St James' Piccadilly, as was poor Sir Richard Croft (q.v.) who had learnt the lessons of non-interference only too well. Just before his last lecture he had said 'I have now finished 20 years of lectures. However, as I presume I am still approved of I propose 20 years more, to begin next October, and after this is over I propose to settle in the world and take me a wife'. He never did.

Philipp, E.E. (1987). William Hunter; anatomist and obstetrician supreme. *Hunterian Soc. Trans.*, XLIV/XLV, 122–48

KIELLAND, CHRISTIAN CASPAR GABRIEL (1871–1941)

Kielland was born in Zululand, South Africa, where his father was a missionary. When Kielland was 3 years old his parents brought him back to Norway where, after leaving school, he became a Cadet in the Officers Training Corp, but switched to medicine and became a doctor, qualifying in 1899. He seems to have had a mixed private practice and University practice in Copenhagen, but he journeyed often to Germany and in 1915 demonstrated his forceps at the University Clinic in Munich, Germany, at a meeting of the Munich Gynaecological Society under the auspices of Professor Doederlein (Kielland, 1915). A year later he published a paper in the *German Journal of Obstetrics* pointing out that the application of the forceps was particularly indicated for the presenting head that needed rotation.

Kielland, C. (1915). Eine Neuen Form und Einfuhrungsweise der Geburtszange, Stets Biparietal an den Kindlichlen Schadel gelegt. *Munch. med. Wchnschr.*, 62, 923
(Further details in the Chapter 9, Labour & Delivery, under Forceps)

KRANTZ, KERMIT EDWARD (1923–)
(photograph, p. 412)

Krantz was born in Oak Park, Illinois in 1923. This extraordinarily productive gynaecologist who after being Assistant Professor in Arkansas became Gynaecologist in Chief at the University of Kansas School of Medicine, Bell Memorial Hospital, Kansas City in 1959, has produced hundreds of original papers on the anatomy of the pelvic organs and surgical techniques as well as eight films on operations.

His main claim to fame is the operation named after him and two of his collaborators Marshall and Marchetti, the Marshall–Marchetti–Krantz operation. He had performed over 4000 of these procedures before becoming the University Distinguished Professor at the Kansas School of Medicine, on his retirement from active teaching in 1990. He was able to evolve his operation because of his very detailed study of the anatomy of the supports of the uterus and bladder. The great contribution he made was to realize that the chances of curing stress incontinence were likely to be better if the operation was performed from above rather than below (Marshall, 1950).

It was as a result of the physiological work by Marshall and Marchetti and the anatomical work by Krantz that it was possible to appreciate that results might be better if the uterus and bladder were lifted up rather than held up by vaginal support.

Krantz declared his intention to continue to operate until 5000 of his operations had been completed.

Krantz was a pioneer in the use of microscopic surgery, and of laser for cervical intraepithelial neoplasia.

Marshall, V.F., Marchetti, A.A. and Krantz, K.E. (1949). The correction of stress incontinence by simple vesico-urethral suspension. *Surg. Gynecol. Obstet.*, **88**, 509

Krantz, K.E. (1980). Marshall–Marchetti–Krantz procedure for stress incontinence. *Perspectives in Gynecology*. (Pfizer Laboratories Division, Pfizer Inc.)

LANDSTEINER, CARL (1868–1943)

This immunologist and pathologist who received the 1930 Nobel Prize for physiology or medicine, discovered the major blood groups while working as a reseach assistant at the Vienna Pathological Institute in 1900. Had he not discovered and developed the ABO system of blood typing, it would not be possible to carry out blood transfusions. Forty years after his original discovery he with Wiener discovered the Rhesus Factor. The differences in human blood, are due to antigens which are sugar-containing substances attached to the outer envelope of red blood cells. He labelled them A and B. Later it was realized that there were four major types of human blood, A, B, AB and O. AB has no antibodies to the antigens of the other two blood groups and O no antigens. Therefore AB group people can be universal recipients of blood and O group people universal donors. However, reactions were still occurring. After Landsteiner had left his post as Professor of Pathology in the University of Vienna, he continued research until in 1940 he found together with Wiener the further blood groups containing anti-

gens (later named rhesus antigens). There were also rhesus antibodies. Landsteiner also found the MN groups in 1927. His is a great example of an outstanding pathologist continuing productive laboratory research over a period of more than 40 years.

LEVRET, ANDRÉ (1703–1780)

Levret was helped by Samuel Bernard, a rich man who gave him money so that he could become an obstetrician. He reached the acme of his profession by becoming the Royal Accoucheur. Among his patients was Maria Josepha of Saxony, consort of the Dauphin Louis whose third child became Louis XVI of France on the death of his grandfather Louis XV. Louis XVI was born in 1754 and died in 1793 under the guillotine. There is a story that when Levret was delivering the Dauphiness, her ladies-in-waiting said 'You must be pleased, Monsieur Levret, to be delivering the Dauphine, that will make your reputation', he replied 'If my reputation were not already made I should not be here'.

André Levret's great claim to fame was that he invented the long forceps, after having worked out in detail methods of estimating the size of the female pelvis. His forceps might quite possibly have been the first or one of the first pairs of forceps made with a screw to hold the two halves together.

Levret's forceps were an improvement on older forceps in that he modified Palfyn's Tire-Tete three ways. First by making a shallow groove on the internal edge of the forceps allowing them to come into better contact with the fetal head and ensuring a stronger hold than previously designed forceps had. The second modification consisted of covering the external part of the forceps on both sides by a very thin plate so that the two branches of the forceps were joined together by means of a groove and thirdly, and perhaps most important of all, the introduction of the pelvic curve in 1760.

During his time as an eminent obstetrician he was asked to examine a 'machine' invented by Madame Le Boursier du Coudray, a very popular and successful midwife of Paris. The machine really was a phantom pelvis with a doll used for teaching obstetric manoeuvres to midwives. Levret, together with another obstetrician Verdier, approved of Madame du Coudray's machine on a certificate dated 13 May 1756.

MAGNUS, ALBERTUS (?1193–1280)

One of the earliest printed anatomy books was prepared by a Dominican monk known as Albertus Magnus. He had been born Albert Volstadt, and probably lived from 1193 to 1280. He wrote his book in manuscript and it was only in the third quarter of the fifteenth century that somebody had the great idea of printing it. A section of it was devoted to gynaecology and that part is entitled *The comment on the secrets of women.* This incidentally contains one of the first printed endocrinological prescriptions; for Albertus Magnus advocated using the powdered testis of a hog in wine, for men of poor sexual power, and the powder from the womb of a hare in wine to make women fertile. A very similar prescription is to be found in an early fifteenth century manuscript which is in the British Library and has recently been printed in the Middle English text and translated into modern English by Beryl Rowland.

Rowland, B. (1981). *Trotula. Medieval Woman's Guide to Health.* The first English gynaecological handbook, Middle English text with introduction and Modern English translation by Rowland, B. (London: Croom Helm)

MAIMONIDES, MOSES (1135–1204)

This great Jewish intellectual figure of the early Middle Ages was born in Cordoba, Spain. His father who taught him was named Maimon and was a learned man. In 1148 when Maimonides was 13, the revolutionary Islamic Fundamentalist Faction captured Cordoba and gave the Jews of the city the alternatives of converting to Islam or leaving. The family finally left in 1159 and moved to Fez in Morocco where Moses studied rabbinics, Greek philosophy and, above all, medicine. When his teacher was executed in Fez the family had to move again and went to Palestine and from there to Egypt, settling near Cairo (Figure 4). His father

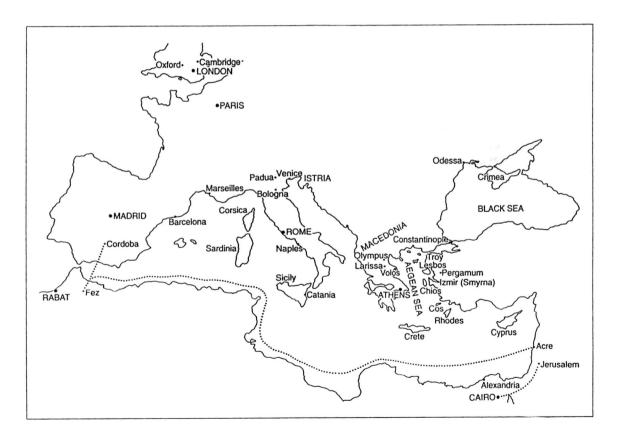

Figure 4 How the travels of *Maimonides* helped to spread the knowledge from the Iberian peninsula to North Africa and then by sea to the Eastern Mediterranean countries as indicated on the map

died soon after they arrived and his brother was drowned so Moses had to earn a living and this he did as a practising physician, becoming very soon Court Physician to the Sultan Saladin, the famous Muslim military leader. His medical writing (added to his enormous contribution to rabbinical writing) was in two parts. He dedicated to a nephew of Saladin his work on sexual intercourse *Fi al-Jamaah* which he wrote in Arabic as he did most of his writing.

He wrote an imitation of the aphorisms of Hippocrates and also a quite lengthy description of the anatomy of the uterus. It is unlikely that Maimonides ever practised dissection, so his descriptions must have been copied from other writers.

Another native of Cordoba was Albucasis who wrote widely on medical matters, including the use of the cautery which Maimonides also described in one of his writings. There was another important Jewish physician contemporary with Maimonides in Cordoba. His name was Avenzoar, who died in 1162. He was one of the first to question Galen's teachings.

Medicine in the twelfth and thirteenth centuries was dominated by the Mohammedan and Arabic influences. Among their principles were not to dissect because it was against their religion, for men not to deal with gynaecological or obstetrical matters because these were for midwives to deal with, for operations to be carried out by wandering specialists and to argue about fees! Yet there were great teaching hospitals in Baghdad, Damascus and Cairo of which the Hall of Wisdom in Cairo was the most famous.

Dissection of the human body had to wait for Mundinus (Mondino de'Luzzi) whose *Anothomia* was completed in 1316, but not published until 1487 in Padua. Of interest for gynaecology is that he carried out post-mortems on two female bodies in January and March 1315 to try to ascertain the relative size of the uterus in virgins and in those who had given birth.

Garrison, F. (1921). *History of Medicine,* p. 151. (London, Philadelphia: W. B. Saunders Co.)

MAURICEAU, FRANCOIS (1637–1709)

Mauriceau was born under very strange circumstances. His mother had smallpox while she was pregnant with him. He thought that he had been affected in the uterus while his mother hardly reacted. His older brother died of the illness (Witkowski, 1887.) Later he lost his sister from antepartum haemorrhage due to placenta praevia. Mauriceau's unfortunate sister was abandoned by all the doctors who were called to attend her because none of them wished to attempt an internal version which would have been the only way of saving her life at that time, and Mauriceau himself had to deliver her; but she died.

Mauriceau, apparently, could be easily angered and could be quite violent. He tended to quarrel with many of his colleagues including Viardel, de la Motte, and Peu who were audacious enough to criticize the apparatuses he had designed to pull dead babies out of their mothers. One of the disputes was on the significance of meconium in labour. In cephalic presentations it is of great significance, but of less with breech presentations which Mauriceau well understood, but the others did not. Many of the books of Mauriceau's era in the seventeenth century had beautiful illustrations, but Mauriceau's book on *Pregnancy and Delivery of Women* which appeared in Paris in 1715 is an exception. There is a nice portrait of him, however, on the front of this work.

Mauriceau was undoubtedly one of the greatest teachers of obstetrics of all time. He was the first fully trained French surgeon to take up obstetrics. The first edition of his great work appeared in Paris in 1668. It was called *Traité des Maladies des Femmes Grosses et Celles qui sont Accouchées.*

It was translated into Latin, German, Italian, Dutch (by Deventer) and English, the English version being by Hugh Chamberlen (q.v.). Hugh Chamberlen's translation of Mauriceau's book was printed in London in 1673 and went into many editions. In English it was entitled *The Accomplisht Midwife, Treating of the Diseases of Women and in Childbearing.*

Mauriceau was one of the first to point out the differences between male and female pelves; but thought wrongly that the fetus was fully formed from the earliest stages, and merely grew in the womb. He said 'the centre is made of menstrual blood from the mother which floats in the uterus and from this accumulation the parenchyma is formed'. He wrote about the circulation of blood in the fetus and said that there was a natural transfusion of blood from the umbilical vein which entered the liver of the fetus and from there it went to the vena cava and he described in considerable detail, even though falsely, the placental circulation. He described difficult labours due to short cords or to the cord becoming entangled with a limb making it difficult for the infant to descend into the pelvis. He also described for the first time several intrauterine manoeuvres. His authority was enormous.

The 1668 edition was the first of many publications. It was initially based on 700 deliveries, but finally on 3000 that Mauriceau conducted or supervised in the last 25 years of his practice. Even today this would be a very large number for any obstetrician to supervise personally. The Hotel Dieu in Paris, in which many great masters worked, must have had an enormous amount of clinical material. Mauriceau tried to work out the formation of the placenta from the maternal blood, and thought that blood that would otherwise flow at menstruation was in part responsible for the formation of the placenta. He also believed that blood circulating in the mother transfused not only to the fetus but back from the fetus to the mother. He wrote about the umbilical arteries and vein and postulated that amniotic fluid was made by the fetus passing urine.

In 1660 Mauriceau treated a young girl of about 20 who had lost her first child of 'the pox' (syphilis) with mercury ointment which he rubbed in five or six times. He had not been aware that she had been pregnant as she had concealed the pregnancy, four other surgeons having refused to treat her when they found out that she was pregnant. Mauriceau did treat her and she delivered a healthy baby.

Mauriceau sewed up tears in the perineum after cleaning them with red wine. He used three or four stitches or more. He covered the wound with liniment covered by linen to prevent the urine soiling it, and thus causing pain.

Mauriceau was the first to describe craniotomy and extraction of a dead child.

Mauriceau, F. (1715). *Observations Sur La Grossesse et L'Accouchement des Femmes et sur leurs Maladies et celles des Enfants nouveau-nez.* (Paris: La Compagnie des Librairies Associez)
Witkowski, G-J. (1887). (The book has no date in it) *Accoucheurs et Sages-Femmes Celebres*, p. 94. (Paris: Steinheil)

MERCURIO, GERONIMO SCIPIONE (1550–1616)

It is likely that Geronimo Scipione Mercurio was the first person to carry out Caesarean sections in Italy. Mercurio's book *La Comare o Riccoglitrice,* printed in Venice in 1596, was probably the first Italian book devoted to obstetrics.

MESNARD, JACQUES (18th C.; exact dates unknown)

Jacques Mesnard was a contemporary of André Levret. Unlike Levret, who worked in Paris, he worked in the provinces in Rouen, France. He also invented a forceps with a screw to hold the two sides together. These forceps, like Levret's, cross over and are based on Palfyn's design. Mesnard's book, published in Paris in 1743 entitled *Le Guide Des Accoucheurs, ou le Maistre dans l'art D'Accoucher les Femmes et de les Soulager . . .*, not only has illustrations of the three or four forceps designed by Mesnard, but also 12 plates of which the most interesting probably is the bed he invented for delivery of women. The interesting thing about this bed is that it had a basic mattress over the frame covering the whole length of the bed and in the top half it had a double mattress on top of this to raise the buttocks and trunk of the woman several inches. Above that was a large firm bolster to raise her head and shoulders. This was a worthy predecessor to the modern beds found in birthing rooms. Several of the illustrations in the book are similar to the far less elaborate ones produced by Smellie and Hunter. Jacques Mesnard's *Guide* posed several questions including those of the qualities needed in an accoucheur. He held there were six:

(1) He had to be intelligent, not alcoholic and calm;

(2) He had to be modest and discrete;

(3) He had to look nice and be gentle with patients, especially when he was operating on them;

(4) He had to be skilful;

(5) He had to be charitable to the poor; and

(6) He should know the theory of his profession.

Not bad qualities to be found in any obstetrician – still today!

Mesnard gives the explanations as to why an accoucheur should have all these qualities, on pages 3–7 of his book. On pages 299 and 300 he talks about Caesarean operations and on page 306 he describes his operative technique. On the next page there are illustrations not only of the site of the incision and how it should be sutured, but also of the instruments and the bandages to be used. Although there is no description of the 'machine' which appears in Boivin, Mesnard mentions Du Coudrey's book in which there appears a certificate for approval of the machine signed by him and Levret. This illustration slightly resembles the description of a demonstration model in Elisabeth Bennion's beautiful book (1979) as follows: 'Again from Italy is a stuffed leather and canvas semi-torso of a woman with foetus *in utero* and fully dilated cervix on which the various obstetrical forceps and hooks were demonstrated and practised' (Bennion, 1979).

Bennion, E. (1979). *Antique Medical Instruments*, pp. 286–8. (Berkeley and Los Angeles: Sotheby Parke Bernet Publications, University of California Press)

Mesnard, J. (1743). *Le Guide Des Accoucheurs, ou le Maistre dans l'art D'Accoucher les Femmes*. (Paris: De Bure, Le Breton Durand)

MILNE MURRAY, ROBERT (1855–1904)

Milne Murray designed a modification of the forceps previously invented by Tarnier. The idea had originated with Professor L.J. Humbert of Louvain who in 1860 had pointed out the dangers of traction on the handles of the forceps in the wrong direction. In the principle that he enunciated 'the direction of traction must coincide with the line that constitutes the axis of the blades of the forceps'. His son E. Humbert Jr. invented forceps which did not cross over but which it was claimed could follow the principle enunciated by his father. His forceps had a very marked pelvic curve.

Milne Murray pointed out that there were two important circumstances: first, the pelvic canal is curved; and second the fetal head is not a sphere, but must be regarded as an irregular ovoid or asymmetrical wedge.

In a very important contribution published in 1891 Milne Murray drew illustrations of the pelvis and of the fetal head and the relationship that the forceps had to have to the fetal head. He also illustrated Pajot's manoeuvre and the forceps designed by Herman to try to follow mechanically Pajot's principle. Milne Murray claimed that Humbert of Louvain was the man to whom the credit had to be given for the first practical suggestion of the solution of the axis–traction difficulty by simply adding a rigid bar to the handle. Milne Murray gave great attention to designing an instrument with the correct curves and to placing traction rods in the correct positions letting them hinge in the correct place; and in truth his forceps have stood the test of time because they can still be found in obstetric units.

McDOWELL, EPHRAIM (1771–1830)

Ephraim McDowell, who was born on 11 November 1771 in Rockbridge County, Virginia, was the ninth of 11 children and the sixth son. His family emigrated from Scotland to Northern Ireland in the mid-seventeenth century during the Protectorate of Cromwell and his Protestant great-grandfather, Ephraim McDowell, arrived in Pennsylvania on 4 September 1729. The family moved to Danville, Kentucky when he was 13. When he was 22, in 1793, he became a medical student at Edinburgh University, studying chemistry under the great Joseph Black and surgery under the equally great John Bell, whose younger brother later became Sir Charles Bell. The Bells were instrumental in emphasizing the importance of anatomy for surgeons. (John Bell died in Rome on 15 April 1820. In 1869 Sir James Y. Simpson (q.v.) visited the cemetery and had his gravestone repaired.)

McDowell returned to Danville after about two and a half years in Edinburgh. He had not taken a medical degree so far as the records tell but was allowed to practise in Danville, which at that time had fewer than 1000 inhabitants. All the same, it was an important town in Kentucky and patients came to Danville from all over the state.

After operating on Mrs Crawford (see account of McDowell's surgery under Operative Surgery in Chapter 29) McDowell continued as a surgeon in Danville until he died on 25 June 1830, having made an enormous contribution to surgery and having really placed the operation of opening the abdomen on the surgical map, for he performed a total of 13 operations to remove ovaries with eight recoveries, but this figure is disputed.

Ricci, J.V. (1945). *One Hundred Years of Gynaecology*, p. 59. (Philadelphia: Blakiston Co.)

NIHELL, ELIZABETH (1723–?)

Nihell was an eighteenth century midwife who, uniquely for an English midwife, trained for 2 years in Paris in the Hotel Dieu. In 1760 she wrote a book entitled *Treatise on the Art of Midwifery, setting forth various abuses therein, especially as to the practice with instruments.* 'The whole serving to put all National Enquiries in a fair Way, forming their own Judgement upon the question, which is best to employ in cases of Pregnancy and lying-in, a man-midwife or a Midwife. Against all male practitioners and particularly Smellie'. She mocked the disciples of Dr Smellie 'those self-constituted men-midwives made out of broken barbours, tailors or even pork butchers, I know myself one of this last trade, who, after passing half his life stuffing sausages has turned an intrepid physician and a man-midwife'. (Mowbray, 1724; Donnison, 1988; Towler, 1986).

Donnison, J. (1988). *Midwives and Medical Men,* pp. 43, 46–47, 52, 59 and 60. (New Barnet, London: Historical Publications)

Mowbray, J. (1724). *The Female Physician.* (London: J. Holland)

Towler, J. and Brammall, J. (1986). *Midwives in History and Society,* p. 102. (London: Croom Helm)

OULD, FIELDING (1710–1789)

Fielding Ould was a man-midwife in Dublin in the eighteenth century. He was notable for writing a treatise of midwifery in three parts (Ould, 1742). Fielding Ould worked in the College of Physicians and dedicated his treatise to the President, Censors and Fellows of the College of Physicians in Dublin. In his amusing preface he pointed out 'it is a common thing for some authors to calumnate all those who wrote before them, on the same subject, thereby to enhance the value of their own works'; but Ould said he was not going to do that, although he had previously he said, differed from others.

In the same preface he talks about the texture of the vagina, which is said to be 'as though it were knit like a stocking'; the great variety of shape that it is capable of, 'making it a probable conjecture, and besides', then he went on to say that he had looked at it through a magnifying glass as he had also examined the womb, and in his description of the way the womb dilates he disagreed with Mauriceau. He pointed out that whereas the bladder distended when filled with urine without gaining any weight, the uterus at the time of delivery of a child weighed 100 times more than before the pregnancy.

One of the interesting things in Ould's book is that he states 'though we be greatly indebted to our predecessors as Paré, Guillemeau, Liebuat, Bienassis, Portal, Peu, Mauriceau, Vierdel, Amand, Dionis, Lamotte, Chamberlen, Deventer and others; yet there is scarce one of their works that may not admit improvement as shall be remarked hereafter'. Indeed, in almost every one of the following chapters Ould criticizes adversely the writings of his predecessors, reserving special scorn from time to time for Deventer as well as for Mauriceau. He seemed to be against the use of instruments and also says 'yet it is not to be denied, but that such operations are very useful and necessary, when undertaken with caution, skill and prudence; and that, even when the child is alive'. Dublin, not only in Ould's day but for very many years before and after, was and still is, a great centre for the teaching of midwifery, the Rotunda Hospital being one of the three important teaching hospitals in that city.

Fielding Ould designed an instrument 'being a Piercer, to perforate the head of an infant, in order to lessen the size of it, by evacuating part of the brain; this Piercer is concealed in a sheath for the preservation of the mother, to be conducted to the part where it is to operate'. There are illustrations in his book of the Piercer which he named *terebra occulta.* He thought his instrument superior to that designed by Mauriceau which could damage not only the mother but the medical attendant as well.

Ould, F. (1742). A *Treatise on Midwifery.* (Dublin: Nelson and Connor)

PALFYNE, JEAN (1650–1730)

Jean Palfyne (also spelt Palfyn) who lived in Ghent, Flanders, Belgium, probably heard about the secret instrument made by the Chamberlen family when he visited London. He then constructed an instrument, consisting of two large iron spoons set in round wooden handles one to be applied on each side of the head of the fetus in difficult labours (the illustration for this is on page 135 of Witkowski's *Accoucheurs et Sages-Femmes Celebres).* Palfyne seems to have invented his 'Mains de Fer' (hands of iron), as he called his forceps, in 1713. He made several designs. The handles could be held together either by bandages, by leather, by metal strips or by chains. There was however no cross-over mechanism, but a screw lock was fitted to one of them. Once he had invented them, Jean Palfyne came back to London to demonstrate them, but by that time the Chamberlens had already invented their forceps and these are definitely the forerunners of those we know and use today. (See section on Forceps delivery in Chapter 9.)

PALMER, RAOUL (1906–1986)

In his day Palmer was the greatest figure in infertility. He was a Frenchman who had an enormous international practice in Paris which he conducted with the help of his wife Elisabeth, a Dutch doctor, who was also his operating theatre assistant. He was a surgical gynaecologist and she a medical gynaecologist.

He taught at the Hospital Broca in Paris, where he was head of the department; but surprisingly, was never made professor. His early work was on cancer and precancerous conditions of the cervix. He was one of the first in France to have a colposcope which he used routinely on all patients coming to his clinic both in the public and the private sector. He was one of the first to adopt the Papanicolaou smear technique. He was certainly the first to film laparoscopic examinations and explorations of the abdomen. He was one of the first to use carbon dioxide to insufflate the peritoneal cavity. He designed many of the instruments originally used in laparoscopic surgery. He was one of the first to try out external forms of illumination with a laparoscope, removing the bulb from the intraperitoneal end to a light source outside the body. His conservative operations on the Fallopian tubes and his myomectomy techniques were copied by countless gynaecologists who flocked to his operating sessions from all corners of the world. He wrote several textbooks.

Among his pupils who came to learn from him in Paris was Patrick Steptoe (q.v.) who was introduced to the laparoscope by Raoul Palmer in 1957. Palmer, together with Hans Frangenheim, changed from the French laparoscopes made by Drapier to the newer German ones made by Wolf and Storz. Palmer started the French Fertility Society and later was one of the founding fathers of the International Federation of Fertility Societies. Because of the esteem in which he was held throughout the world, he was probably more responsible than anyone for making the investigation and treatment of infertility a truly respectable art and science, taking it away from the doctors and lay-charlatans who had not treated the subject seriously nor scientifically.

PAPANICOLAOU, GEORGE NICHOLAS (1883–1962) (photograph, p. 547)

George Papanicolaou's great contribution to obstetrics and gynaecology was his discovery of recognizable cancer cells in secretions he was examining for other purposes.

He was born in the picturesque sea port of Kymi on the eastern slopes of the Greek island of Euboea. This is a wine-producing district and quite prosperous. His father was a medical practitioner and his family were not poor, but rather of the upper middle class. He received a broad education at Athens University where he not only obtained A grades in all his examinations, but also became a competent violinist. His father wished him to settle in Kymi as a family doctor but he had other ideas and went to Germany for postgraduate studies in several universities. In Munich, Hertwig, the head of the Zoological Institute gave him work on sex differentiation and determination of *Daphnia*, a genus of tiny, fresh water fleas with a transparent body that is much used in biological research. He completed a thesis in 1910 on the sexual differentiation of *Daphnia* and married in the same year. In 1911 he travelled with Prince Albert I of Monaco on the Prince's yacht as a physiologist studying the marine forms of 'the intermediary depth of the sea'. During the trip he dissected a false killer whale. In 1913 he emigrated to the USA and worked in the Department of Pathology and Bacteriology in the New York Hospital, a famous hospital founded by Sims (q.v.) which Sims left because it refused to accept cancer patients. There he worked on sex determination and sex control in guinea-pigs. Because he found it difficult to determine when ovulation occurred in these animals he bought a small nasal speculum to take smears from the guinea-pigs' vaginal discharges and found it possible to recognize different types of cells at different times in the oestrus cycle of the guinea-pig, and in 1917 published in the journals *Science* and the *American Journal of Anatomy*, with his senior C.R. Stockard (1917).

The observation of these cell changes led to the discovery of the corpus luteum hormones and to work done by other physiologists and biochemists.

He did not think it worthwhile at first to examine human vaginal secretions because menstruation furnished an external sign of the cyclical changes; but he did examine regularly vaginal secretions from a 'special patient', believed to be his wife, whose cycles were absolutely regular. He later examined the vaginal secretions of many other women. A newspaper reported on 5 January 1928 that he had made an announcement to the Race Betterment Conference in Battlecreek, Michigan, that he had found cancer cells in vaginal secretions. His technique was to observe cyclical changes in secretions obtained using a small pipette from normal women whose smears he examined daily. In 1933 he described the cytological appearances throughout the sexual cycle in the human female in the *American Journal of Anatomy*, and just about this time he and others developed a special cell-staining technique. He worked then with Dr H.F. Traut, aspirating cells from the posterior fornix of women's vaginas. He discovered cancer cells unexpectedly in an unsuspected case. In March 1941 together with Traut, they read a paper entitled *The Diagnostic Value of Vaginal Smears in Cancer of the Uterus* to the New York Obstetrical Society, and at the conclusion of that meeting I.C. Rubin (q.v.) said 'we have made a great advance in the armamentarium in this field'. Cytology is different from tissue pathology; and Papanicolaou was always at pains to point this out. A Mr Murayama, a meticulous artist, joined the team as an illustrator. In 1943 Papanicolaou, aided by the Empire Commonwealth Fund, published his famous and classic monograph *Diagnosis of Uterine Cancer by the Vaginal Smear* and in 1954 his *Atlas of Exfoliative Cytology*. As his biographer says, echoing the words of Pasteur 'chance favours the prepared mind' (Carmichael, 1973). George Papanicolaou had a mind prepared by an unlimited capacity for work, by strict mental and physical self-discipline and by a rare humility as well as by having a most supportive wife who was his partner in his work. He had luck or rather serendipity on his side in that his discovery was accidental, but only a man like he was would have recognized what he was seeing.

Carmichael, E. (1973). *The Pap Smear, Life of George N. Papanicolaou.* (Springfield, Illinois: Charles C. Thomas)
Stockard, C.R. and Papanicolaou, G.N. (1917). The existence of a typical oestrus cycle in the guinea-pig: with a study of its histological and physiological changes. *Am. J. Anat.*, **22**, 225–83

PARÉ, AMBROISE (1510–1590)

Paré, known as the father of French surgery and of modern surgical techniques, was born in Laval, France and, like so many great doctors trained in the Hotel Dieu, Paris. Paré was a very great military surgeon and was the first of his kind. He was a Huguenot, good and gentle, famous for his motto 'Je le pansay, Dieu le guairit' (I dressed his wounds, God healed him). He published a book

on anatomy and surgery of which the second half is entitled *Brieve Collection de l'administration Anatomique; Avec la maniere de conioindre les os: et de extraire les enfans tant mors que vivans dans le ventre de la mere lors que nature de soy ne peult venir a sons effect.* Paré wrote this book as a master barber-surgeon. It was published in Paris in 1550. It obviously was concerned with Caesarean sections, but it is not certain whether it is from the living mother or from the dead woman. In his writings Paré often referred to Galen, Hippocrates, Aristotle and the Arab medical teachers, as well as to the books by Rösslin and Rueff. He described the hymen and discussed pregnancy and sterility. For male infertility he suggested using the testicles of a cock as well as the genital organs of a bull (Malgaigne, 1840; Fasbender, 1906).

According to Malgaigne, Paré described the separation of the bones of the hips and pubis. Paré also seems to have described breech extraction and possibly also podalic version of the infant lying in an abnormal position which he taught to Guillemeau (q.v.). According to Fasbender, Paré undertook Caesarean section on two living women or else supervised his pupil Jacques Guillemeau doing them.

He taught Loyse Bourgeois dit Boursier (1563–1636) who practised midwifery among the poor of Paris as well as attending the French court and the Royal family. She delivered Marie de Medici of her sixth child Henrietta Maria in the Louvre in Paris on 25 November 1609. Henrietta Maria became Queen of England by her marriage to Charles I in 1625.

Paré's treatise and catalogue 'of monsters and prodigies' was illustrated by many woodcuts.

There is a full account of Paré's method of podalic version in Harvey Graham's *Eternal Eve* (1950) and in Malgaigne's writings (1840).

Fasbender, H. (1906). *Geschichte der Geburtshulfe*, pp. 124–9. (Jena: Gustav Fischer)
Graham, H. (1950). *Eternal Eve*, pp. 149–56. (London: Heinemann)
Malgaigne, J.F. (1840). *Histoire de la chirugie en Occident depuis du VIᵉᵐᵉ jusqu'au XVIᵉᵐᵉ siècle et histoire de la vie et des travaux d'Ambroise Paré.* (Paris: J.B. Baillière)

PASTEUR, LOUIS (1822–1895) (Figure 5)

The contributions of this great man to obstetrics and gynaecology can hardly be exaggerated. In 1879 (after he had already done remarkable work

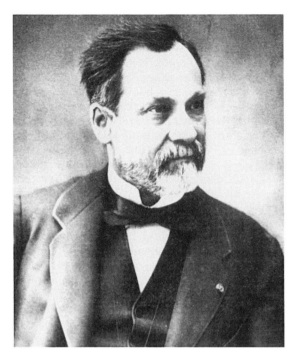

Figure 5 Louis Pasteur. Reproduced with kind permission from the Wellcome Institute Library, London

on fermentation of wines, on his discovery of bacteria in sour milk and on various infectious diseases as well as on silk worms), Pasteur interrupted a lecture being given by Professor Roux, to reveal how with his pupils Joubert, Chamberland, and Doleris he could demonstrate on a blackboard the chain of small circles representing bacterial colonies which they had found in patients suffering from puerperal fever.

Pasteur said that it was the nursing and medical staff who carried microbes from an infected to a healthy woman. Roux had said he thought the microbe would never be found. The very next day Pasteur had the opportunity to prove that the peritoneum of a woman who had died of puerperal fever had 'the organism with spherical grains associated by twos or fours, or forming strings (chains)' as he had described at the previous session of the Academy of Medicine. He had managed to take blood from the patient while she was still alive. Later, at 7 hours and 24 hours after her death he found the organisms in a pure state. Shortly afterwards another obstetrician, a Maurice Raynaud, sent in other samples of blood and discharges from a patient with puerperal fever in which the organism was also found. Pasteur was the first to culture these streptococci.

Pasteur and Lister met on a notable occasion organized to honour Pasteur. There is a famous picture of their meeting painted by M. Rixens. This was at a ceremony at the Sorbonne on 27 December 1892 when 2500 people filled the large theatre at the University. The audience included all the Ministers of State and members of the Pasteur Institute together with many delegates from French and foreign scientific bodies. Pasteur entered the hall leaning on the arm of the President of the Republic, and then Lister who represented both the Royal Society of London and the Royal Society of Edinburgh gave a fine address in French with Latin quotations. In his talk he explained how Pasteur had unravelled the cause of many infectious diseases. He particularly singled out rabies and said 'is it possible that a man who is neither a doctor nor a biologist could instruct us on an illness and exercise the best intelligences in medicine'. He praised Pasteur's scientific honesty and pointed out that infectious diseases at that time constituted the great majority of serious diseases to afflict the human being. Pasteur and Lister embraced one another after the end of Lister's oration which itself received a standing ovation. A contemporary said 'Pasteur rises to embrace Lister. The embrace of these two men was like a living picture of the brotherly unity of science in the relief of humanity'.

It is instructive to be able to follow first the observations made by Semmelweis and the measures he took to prevent the spread of puerperal fever, without knowing its cause, then on to the discovery of the organisms by Pasteur, and later on to the avoidance of their transmission and that of other bacteria by the antiseptic and aseptic work started by Lister. Pasteur's letters are distributed around the world because Pasteur's grandson, Pasteur Valery-Radot, quarrelled with the Institute Pasteur in Paris, and left the collection of letters that he had inherited and some of which he had annotated to be distributed via the Bibliotheque National in Paris. There are three letters about cholera vaccination, dated 1885, in the Barcelona Museum for the History of Medicine. These are from Pasteur to Jaume Ferran (1852-1929) head of the Institute of Immunology in Barcelona.

POMEROY, RALPH HAYWARD (1867–1925)

Pomeroy was an American obstetrician and gynaecologist whose main claim to fame is that he first described a method of sterilizing women by ligating the Fallopian tubes, which was only published by his associates Bishop and Nelmes 4 years after his death. He also described an obstetric manipulation to correct the posterior position of the occiput.

Pomeroy's sterilization consists of making a loop in the loose middle portion of the Fallopian tube, ligating it with absorbable suture material and excising the loop. By using absorbable material the ligated ends of the tube draw apart and avoid most of the risk of recanalization or of fistula formation because peritoneum grows over the ligated ends. It was important not to crush the tubes as was done in the older Madlener procedure.

READ, GRANTLY DICK (1890–1959) (Figure 6)

Read was an obstetrician who initially practised in Woking, UK, but after he published his book *Natural Childbirth* in 1933 he became an internationally known man. The 'Establishment' did not take kindly to his teachings which were that if women were informed adequately about the processes of pregnancy and labour and were

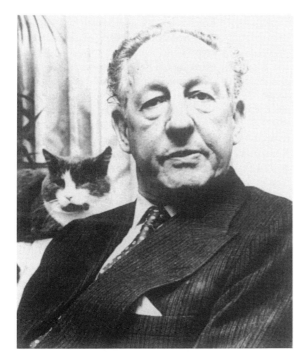

Figure 6 Grantly Dick Read. Reproduced with kind permission from the Wellcome Institute Library, London

encouraged to breathe rhythmically and in accordance with the type of contractions being suffered, labour could be if not painless, at least relatively so. He held that fear was one of the main causes of pain and that fear was partly engendered by the dissemination by the lay-press of information about abnormalities that were published in medical journals.

He aimed with his books and lectures to teach women that childbirth was and could be a physiological process, that it need not be painful, that it could even be joyful, and that forceps did not need to be applied except when labour was really prolonged.

Grantly Dick Read started the movement towards more instruction for labouring women. Adaptations of his breathing techniques were propounded by teachers such as Lamaze in France, and Lamaze's disciple Vellay. They held however that their methods of pain relief in childbirth were different from those of Grantly Dick Read and were based on Russian teachings which derived from Pavlovian theory. There are elements in both methods which invoke different stimuli passing into the brain and causing some form of distraction from pain sensations.

RECAMIER, J.C.A. (1774–1852)

A French gynaecologist; whilst certainly not the inventor of the speculum, Recamier did devise improved versions of it. He was probably the first regularly to use a uterine sound and a curette. He probably invented in 1843 a small scoop or spoon attached to a long blade, and he gave it the name *curette*. He used it to scrape small growths off the mucous membrane of the uterus. He had modified the uterine sound which had been advocated for some time by introducing a curve into it and to this very day, all curettes and uterine sounds do have curves to them. Not only speculae and curettes were used at the beginning of the nineteenth century but also special examination couches upholstered in such a way they would have been an adornment in any drawing room. The great Marion Sims modified Recamier's spoon curette which was made of soft metal, by introducing an instrument made of hard steel but shaped more to conform to the passage into the body of the uterus through the cervix. The worry with sounds and curettes then, and still today, is perforation of the uterus and Recamier himself reported three cases of such perforation followed by death. Perforation itself is not so dangerous where asepsis is used before passing instruments into the uterus. Its main danger however is the damage that can be caused to bowel or bladder after the instrument has been passed through the wall of the uterus.

VON ROKITANSKY, CARL FREIHERR (1804–1878)

This great pathologist who in his lifetime supervised 100 000 autopsies and performed 30 000 of them, is very important in obstetrics and gynaecology. He was born in Koniggratz, in what is now Czechoslovakia, and died in Vienna, where he was Professor of Pathology and Anatomy at the Vienna General Hospital. It was his encouragement to his pupil Semmelweis together with the encouragement given by Skoda, Hebra and Michaelis that enabled Semmelweis to do his very great work. Rokitansky stood by Semmelweis in opposition to some of the great names among the orthodox obstetricians such as Scanzoni and Karl Braun.

Rokitansky was the first to find bacteria in the lesions of malignant endocarditis. He also made a basis for differentiating lobar pneumonia from lobular pneumonia or bronchial pneumonia. His study of acute yellow atrophy of the liver is a classic. He was the first to describe spondylolisthesis, in 1839.

From the gynaecological point of view Rokitansky is important because by 1882 he had collected 95 cases of total removal of the malignant uterus. This was only 18 years before E. Wertheim described the technique for really radical removal of the uterus and the other tissues in the pelvis in cases of uterine malignancy. His name together with two others, Kuster and Hauser, has been given to the condition of congenital absence of the uterus and its replacement by a thin band of fibrous tissue.

Rokitansky's son followed his father as a pathologist and anatomist in Vienna.

RÖSSLIN, EUCHARIUS (d.1526)

Rösslin was the first man to have a textbook for midwives of the Renaissance printed; and in German instead of Latin so that the midwives could understand it. In its first edition in 1513 it was known as *Der Swangern Frawen an Hebammen Roszgarten*, which loosely translated would be called *The Garden of Roses for Pregnant Women and for Midwives*. It is known to antiquarians as *The Rose Garden*.

Two books by Ortollf of Bavaria (1477) had appeared a few years earlier. They were *A German Text of Popular Medicine* (1477) and *Frauenbuchlein* (1500). This latter was a popular handbook for lying-in women.

Rösslin's book which had been commissioned by Catherine, Duchess of Brunswick, was a very important work; though it was mainly a re-recital of the work of Soranus (q.v.). It revived podalic version. The illustrations were rather strange woodcuts executed by Martin Caldenbach, a pupil of the great Albrecht Dürer (1471–1528). In one of the editions there is an illustration showing the author presenting the book to the Duchess, his patroness (Haggard, 1929). *The Rose Garden* was translated into Dutch, Czech, French and Latin. The English translation printed in 1540 is known as *The Byrth of Mankynde – newly translated out of Latin into Englysshe by Richard Jonas*. The Latin translation had been by Rösslin's son. The English edition was produced by William Raynalde, published in 1545 with a lengthy prologue by Thomas Reynalde or Raynolde (the printer or editor who enlarged the Jonas-version) (Hibbott, 1990).

Rösslin's book was extremely influential in directing the practice of midwifery, especially that carried out by midwives for many centuries. It was the forerunner of Jacob Rueff's book *De Conceptu et Generatione Hominis*, which was published in Zurich in 1554. Rueff (1500–1558), who practised as a surgeon in Zurich, had also trained as a midwife. Rueff had emphasized that it was essential to know anatomy in order to practise midwifery. Rösslin's book became famous in many countries because of its many translations. It has been said that it brought midwifery out of the Dark Ages and into the Renaissance (Garrison, 1921).

Haggard, H. W. (1929). *Devils, Drugs and Doctors*, (London: William Heinemann (Medical Books) Ltd.)

Hibbott, Y. (1990). Medical books of the sixteenth century. In Besson, A. (ed.) *Thornton's Medical Books, Libraries and Collections*, 3rd edn. pp. 43–82. (Aldershot: Gower Publishing Co.)

RUBIN, ISIDOR CLINTON (1883–1958)

Rubin was a founder of the modern scientific investigation of infertility. He went to the College of Physicians and Surgeons and to Columbia

University, New York, and graduated at the age of 22. After 3 years' residency at the Mount Sinai Hospital in the same city he went to Austria and Germany and started a particular interest in gynaecological pathology, working with Schottlaender in Vienna and Ludwig Pick in Berlin.

Although he was recognized as the father figure in the field of women's infertility, his interests in gynaecology were much broader, and he improved on Wertheim's operation (q.v.) as well as on the surgery of fibroids. In 1910 he published his first paper on 'the pathological diagnosis of incipient carcinoma of the cervix'. In it he described in detail the microscopic appearance of biopsy specimens of the cervix, and paid particular attention to the structure of individual cells, thus presaging the work of Papanicolaou (q.v.). In 1913 he wrote about what is now known as carcinoma *in situ*, 'it is possible to recognize small cancer foci owing to a well-marked morphological cell-aberration even though the deep penetration of epithelial sprouts is barely present or altogether absent'. In 1914 both he and W.H. Cary independently demonstrated patency of the Fallopian tubes using a radio-opaque dye. His interest in using X-rays for gynaecological diagnosis declared itself with his epoch-making papers first on imaging the uterus (hysterography) and later the uterus and the tubes (hysterosalpingography).

He invented the Rubin test for tubal patency by insufflation, first with oxygen and then, because he realized that carbon dioxide was much more soluble in blood than oxygen and therefore had less danger of causing a gas embolus, with carbon dioxide. He watched pressure changes on a kymograph and found the sign of tubal patency which was fullness of the upper abdomen as the gases reached it, followed later by referred shoulder pain from accumulation of gas under the diaphragm.

By 1954 he had already published over 130 scientific papers, mostly dealing with infertility, but some also with other pathologies.

He was immensely popular throughout the world and received many honorary degrees including being made an Honorary Fellow of the Royal College of Obstetricians and Gynaecologists in 1957, having been President of the American Gynaecological Society in 1955. He was a kindly, friendly gentleman. He died suddenly in London from a heart attack, a few weeks after he had received a standing ovation in Mexico City where he had given an oration.

SEMMELWEIS, IGNAZ PHILIPP (1818–1865)

Most biographies and medical history books say that this very great man was born on 1 July 1818 in Buda, now part of Budapest. However, Dr Heinrich Fasbender, the compiler of the classical *Geschichte der Geburtshülfe* (Fasbender, 1906) gives the date of Semmelweis's birth as 17 July 1818 and the place as Ofen. It is of no consequence, but is quoted here only to show how difficult accurate research into history may be, especially since another biographer spells his first name with a 'c' instead of a 'z' and Philip with a single 'p'.

What is accepted by all is that Semmelweis studied as a student in the University of Vienna and qualified with a doctor's degree in 1844. He seems almost immediately to have been appointed Assistant in the first obstetric clinic in Vienna in July 1844, but he had to resign his clinical responsibilities when his predecessor, a Dr Breit, was unexpectedly given a 2-year extension of his position. This left Semmelweis in the clinic but without any clinical responsibility. So, he started to dissect the bodies of women who had died from puerperal fever. He tried very hard to work out an effective method of preventing this terrible disease.

At the same time there were in Vienna, two very famous men, the pathologist Rokitansky (q.v.) and Skoda, an imposing clinician. Rokitansky helped Semmelweis greatly with his post-mortem examinations, giving him any materials he needed. Semmelweis realized before long that puerperal fever killed women who were delivered by medical students and by doctors, but not those who were admitted to hospital, either having delivered outside or who were delivered in hospital by pupil midwives. So obvious was the difference between the mortality rates in the first clinic of the maternity unit, which had a death rate of 9.9% and the second unit where the midwives worked, which had a death rate of 3.9% that the women themselves were terrified of going into the first clinic and tried everything to be delivered in the second clinic.

All sorts of explanations were given for the very high toll in the first clinic and the relatively low toll (high enough in all conscience) in the second clinic. They were really all guesses without foundation. Doctors looked for such excuses as that the women who died were prostitutes or abandoned women; but there was the same number of those in the second clinic as in the first clinic. It was recognized that there was some resemblance between puerperal fever and erysipelas. Both, we now know, are caused by streptococci. Both give rise to an acute feverish illness. Erysipelas is an acute inflammation of the skin and the tissues beneath it. A doctor handling a case of erysipelas and going from that to a labouring woman and examining her without gloves would almost certainly infect the latter so that she would die of puerperal fever.

But it was not a case of erysipelas that suggested to Semmelweis the all important connection between doctors and students who worked in the post-mortem room and went straight from there to the labour wards, and carried the puerperal fever. It was the death of Jacob Kolletschka, a professor of medical jurisprudence in Vienna, who had formerly been Rokitansky's assistant, and whom Semmelweis worshipped. Kolletschka had had a small puncture wound on his finger, which was contaminated with material from a post-mortem body. He developed septicaemia and died. Semmelweis realized that the course of his illness was very much like the course and development of the fever that killed so many of the women. Furthermore the findings at Kolletschka's post-mortem closely resembled those in the women who died. Semmelweis wrote that the death of his friend 'revealed to my mind an identity' with the fatal cases of puerperal fever. Semmelweis reasoned that Kolletschka's finger that had been cut, had been contaminated with material from a dead body he had dissected. Both had open wounds, Kolletschka's on his finger and the woman in her uterus from where the afterbirth had been delivered. Both were infected by material taken from the post-mortem or dissecting room.

In May 1847 Semmelweis instructed his students to wash their hands after scrubbing them in a solution of chloride of lime. Dramatically, the death rate in his wards fell from 11.4% in 1846, to 3.8% by the end of 1847 and only 1.2% in 1848. This was even a little better than the very best maternal mortality rate of 1.33% in the wards where midwives conducted the deliveries. So, Semmelweis argued that 'puerperal fever is caused by conveyance to the pregnant woman of putrid particles derived from living organisms, through the agency of the examining fingers'. Semmelweis's effective order to his students to wash their hands meant that the chloride of lime washed away the particles carried on the students' hands from the dead bodies. There was nothing else with which to infect the labouring women.

This fitted in with other observations that Semmelweis had made. The previous professor in the Vienna Lying-in Hospital, Professor Lucas Johann Boer, had conducted his clinic and labour wards in the way that he had been taught by Charles White of Manchester (q.v.). Charles White was a very fine English obstetrician who had campaigned for women to be kept, if possible, each in a separate room which was well ventilated, and they were to be kept cool. This was in absolute contradistinction to the normal conduct of the day which was to have women wrapped up and kept in bed for 2 weeks after delivery. He had his patients walking around within 24 hours or so. He also insisted that the attendants should be clean. Boer was succeeded by Johann Klein who taught in the dissecting room and then went straight to labouring women. Boer's clinic's death rate which had been under 1% in his last year of office rose to as high as nearly 30% within some months of Klein's reign. It was during Klein's professorship that the obstetric work of the hospital was divided into the first clinic and the second clinic.

Semmelweis published his book *Die Aetiologie, der Begriff und die Prophylaxis des Kindbettfiebers* (the Aetiology, the Understanding and Prophylaxis of Childbirth Fever) in 1861. By this time he had been Professor in Pest since 1855. Pest is on the other side of the Danube from Buda, and there in his St Rochus Hospital, his mortality figures were down to 0.39%. In December 1847 his theories had been published in the *Journal of the Medical Society of Vienna*. In fact he had not mentioned them at all! The paper was written by Hebra, the editor of the journal. It was an editorial which drew attention to Semmelweis's observations that the condition which infected puerperal women could be taken from the cadaver of a woman who had died of cancer of the womb or from another with a foul ulcer of the leg. At that time there were not all that many post-mortems being carried out in the UK and USA. When Semmelweis first went back to Pest from Vienna he insisted that students who came in from the post-mortem room must wash their hands, but he still had high incidences of puerperal fever in some of his patients. He then discovered that in the obstetric clinic there, women were either delivered or nursed on sheets that were dirty and foul smelling from decomposed blood and lochia because the superintendent of midwives who was responsible for laundering the sheets had taken the money but had not laundered them! The stale blood and lochia had become infected between cases.

The manner of Semmelweis's death as recorded at the time, was particularly tragic. He suffered alternate manic depressive attacks possibly partly because of the way his book of 1861 had been received. Even the great pathologist Rudolf Virchow (1821–1902) (q.v.), refused to accept his teaching. By July 1865 he needed admission to a private asylum in Vienna, which was achieved because of the help of his friend Hebra, who had responded to a call from Semmelweis's wife. The myth is that just before admission Semmelweis had performed a gynaecological operation and cut his hand. The wound was said to have become infected and he died on 13 August 1865 from it, with, it was said, the very condition of generalized sepsis that was so like that which infected puerperal women.

However, according to Sherwin B. Nuland (1988), the story of the cut finger is a myth. Nuland thinks it more likely that he had a form of presenile Alzheimer's disease which of course at that time had not been described. What is certain is that Semmelweis was not accepted properly at the time of his death, nor were his theories.

Fasbender, H. (1906). *Geschichte der Geburtshülfe*, pp. 817–24. (Jena: Fisher)
Nuland, S.B. (1988). *Doctors*, pp. 238–62. (New York: Alfred A. Knopf)
Semmelweis, I. P. (1861). *Die Aetiologie der Begriff und die Prophylaxis des Kindbettfiebers*. (Pest, Liepzig: Hartleiben)

A report on confidential enquiries into maternal deaths in the United Kingdom 1985–87, (London: Department of Health, HMSO; 1991, pp. 64–7) shows that puerperal sepsis does still occur.

SHARP(E), JANE (17th C.)

Jane Sharp (e) lived during the reigns of Charles I and Charles II and the intervening Commonwealth. Her book initially entitled *The Midwives Book or The Whole Art of Midwifery Discovered: directing child-bearing women how to behave themselves in their conception, breeding, and nursing of children*, first appeared in 1671. Several editions followed but by the third one the title was shortened to *The Compleat Midwife's Companion*.

Jane Sharp's book dealt with the role of the midwife and also with obstetric matters, but quite a lot of it is concerned with the relationship between midwives and men-midwives (see Chapter 2, Narrative).

Donnison, J. (1988). *Midwives and Medical Men*, pp. 29–30 and 34. (New Barnet, London: Historical Publications)

SHIRODKAR, PROFESSOR V.N. (d.1971)

Shirodkar who died in 1971, was pre-eminent among the gynaecologists of the world, and in his deceptively simple manner probably advanced the subject as much as any gynaecologist of his generation. In 1962 he was elected a Fellow of the Royal College of Obstetricians and Gynaecologists, one of the first Indians to be so honoured.

Shirodkar's operation for encircling the incompetent internal cervical os was designed at the same time as Raoul Palmer in Paris designed his encircling operation, and saved thousands of babies who would otherwise have been aborted or born too premature to survive. Less well-known were his brilliant modifications of standard tubal operations whereby the cornu of the uterus is preserved without being weakened by a coring out procedure; and in the case of hydrosalpinx he preserved any little piece of fimbria which he thought could be of value. He was persistent, modest, brilliantly lucid, highly original and with all simplicity, in his day the acknowledged leader of the obstetricians and gynaecologists of India, respected not only in his home country, but also on the international scene.

SIMS, JAMES MARION (1813–1883) (Figure 7)

Sims invented the operation that inspired all subsequent repairs of fistulae. The broad details of J. Marion Sims' life are set out in *The Story of My Life* which is his autobiography, and which was edited by his son, H. Marion Sims, and published in 1884, after his death, in New York by D. Appleton & Company.

Sims was born in Lancaster County, South Carolina, USA, on 25 January 1813, 10 miles south of the village of Lancaster. His father, John Sims, was a descendant of English colonists of Virginia, and his mother was the daughter of a family of Scottish/Irish origin. There are interesting pages about the Second War of Independence which he calls 'The Revolution'.

There is a very full description of his preparatory school with a master given to flogging his pupils, and of his years in college in South Carolina, then to Jefferson Medical College in Philadelphia, graduating on 1 March 1835.

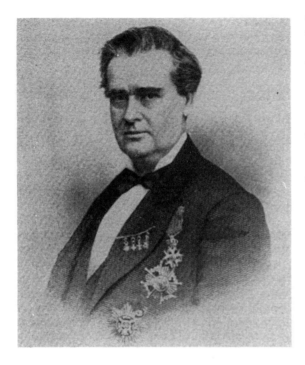

Figure 7 James Marion Sims (1813–1883)

Sims recounts movingly his romance with his future wife, Theresa Jones, the daughter of a doctor. He fell in love with her when he was 11 years old and she was 8. Nine years later on 23 July 1833 she gave him a rose-bud which he treasured for more than 50 years. That was when he was 20 and she was 17. She refused his original proposal of marriage but changed her mind 3 months later, and they married just about the time he graduated in medicine.

He started practising in his home village of Lancaster, and lost two patients rapidly, which demoralized him. He then moved to Mount Meigs in Alabama where he performed his first operation which was to open an abscess in a man's abdomen from which 2 quarts of pus were discharged.

He came to surgery 'after I had no particular interest in my profession at the beginning'. There is a splendid description of a very severe attack of malaria that he suffered, and how a local doctor gave him quinine which helped to cure him.

In Montgomery he started to do surgery and did a lot of it, including operating on a woman with an extremely bad hare-lip which he cured with the help of Dr Belangee, who made a plate for the roof of her mouth with four teeth on it.

This persuaded him to write up the case and that was his first publication, in the *Journal of Dental Surgery*. The first serious case of fistula that he saw was in a servant girl 'Betsey' about 17 or 18 years old, who had had the base of her bladder destroyed by a lengthy and difficult labour. The second one was a Negro girl 'Lucy' about 18 years old, who had given birth 2 months previously and who also had a bladder fistula.

By chance he happened to be called to an emergency – a stout fat woman, 46 years of age, who weighed nearly 200 pounds and who had been thrown from a pony that was frightened by a hog. He diagnosed that the woman may have had an acute retroversion of the uterus and remembered that one of his teachers in Charleston Medical College, a Dr Priolaeu said 'the patient must be placed in a genu-pectoral position', i.e. on her knees and elbows. He did this and introduced his middle and index fingers into her vagina and found the uterus and tried to push it back. Suddenly he realized that his manipulations had caused the vagina to fill with air, and incidentally had relieved the patient of her symptoms. From this he realized that he would be able to distend the vagina with air and see and perhaps cure the hitherto incurable cases of vesico-vaginal fistula. 'I jumped into my buggy and drove hurriedly home. Passing by the store of Hall, Mores and Roberts, I stopped and bought a pewter spoon. I went to my office where I had two medical students and said "Come boys, go to the hospital with me".' He placed Betsey into the genu-pectoral position supported by the two students and air rushed in even before he could get the bent spoon handle into the vagina. Once he had introduced the handle of the spoon 'I saw everything, as no man had ever seen before. The fistula was as plain as the nose on a man's face. The edges were clear and well-defined, and distinct, and the opening could be measured exactly, as if it had been cut out of a piece of plain paper. The walls of the vagina could be seen closing in every direction; the neck of the uterus was distinct and well-defined and even secretions from the neck could be seen as a tear glistening in the eye, clear even and distinct, and as plain as could be. I said at once "Why cannot these things be cured? It seems to me that there is nothing to do but to pare the edges of the fistula and bring it together nicely, introducing a catheter into the neck of the bladder, and drain the urine off continually, and the case will be cured"'. He felt sure that he was on the eve of one of the greatest discoveries of the day and started immediately to invent instruments necessary for performing the operation. He had not sent either Betsey or Lucy home, but asked another patient Anarcha, back to the hospital. He never dreamt that the operations could fail. The first patient he operated on was Lucy who had lost the base of her bladder and had a fistula at least 2 inches (5 cm) in diameter. At that time the self-containing catheter had not been invented. He tried to invent one but the patient became very ill because he had put a small sponge in the neck of the bladder to hold the catheter in. He realized that the sponge was becoming stone-like and removed it, but the fistula was much smaller than it had been. He operated on Betsey without using a sponge but keeping the catheter in some other way. He removed the catheter after 7 days which was too soon. Anarcha had a fistula into her rectum as well as into her bladder. He operated on the bladder fistula and again only partially cured her, but the fistula was smaller. He kept his three patients for up to 4 years, supervising them personally all the time. His brother-in-law tried to persuade him to give up. Suddenly in the middle of one night, the idea came to him as to how to secure the stitches because he had not been able to tie a suture situated high up in the vagina 'All at once an idea occurred to me to run a shot, a perforated shot, on the suture, and when it was drawn tight, to compress it with a pair of forceps which would make the knot perfectly secure'. He woke his wife up to tell her of what he had dreamt. The next day he performed the operation with the new suture on Lucy, but once more it failed, and he thought it was because he had been using silk. By chance he picked up a little brass wire in a yard, and that gave him an idea of asking his jeweller to make a little silver wire which he used on Anarcha. It was her 30th operation. It was the first time that cystitis had not resulted, as it had with the use of the previous sutures of silk. He then operated on Lucy and Betsey and after curing Anarcha, they too were cured. He realized that he had made an immensely important discovery.

He revelled in his very happy family life, and said that nothing could induce him to leave Montgomery, but in 1848 his second son, aged 3, died from diarrhoea which he himself contracted. A trip to New York did not do him any good. Then, emaciated he was persuaded to go to Cooper's Well via New Orleans where he drank the waters in 'this most God-forsaken looking place presided over by Mr Cooper a Methodist preacher'. In 27 days he gained 27 lb (12 kg) and his diarrhoea became controlled. He relapsed when he returned to Montgomery and then decided that the climate of New York with the pure water would be better for him as the diarrhoea continued. When lying in bed he wrote out his history of the operation of vesico-vaginal fistula.

Later in New York he set up a hospital after having demonstrated his operation to some New York surgeons. This was possibly the first woman's hospital opened specifically to deal with gynaecological surgery. When Sims arrived in New York in May 1853 the extreme conservatism of his profession was manifested. Once he had established his hospital he had to leave it because the board which administered it refused to allow him to have more than 15 onlookers at an operation, and his audiences were 30 or more. He could not see the difference in an anaesthetized patient's operation being observed by 30 people rather than 15. He sometimes had trouble with the anaesthetic which was nearly always chloroform, as some of the patients took it badly. One clause in the by-laws was that the assistant surgeon should be a woman. Later he appointed a man assistant surgeon, a Doctor Thomas Addis Emmet, the husband of a beautiful Southern young woman whom he had known since his childhood. The first hospital was at Clinton Hall in Astor place in New York and it opened in 1855 and flourished. In 1857 there were moves to have a bigger hospital and a larger staff of surgeons. Sims' diarrhoea, which he had had for 6 years, gradually got better, and he decided in 1861 to go to Europe. In Dublin he was 'dined and feted to satiety, particularly in the Rotunda hospital'. He operated on two cases of vesico-vaginal fistula there, and then he went to Edinburgh to see Simpson, Syme, Chrisleston and Mathews Duncan. He repeatedly saw Syme operate and considered him the best operator he had seen, although he had witnessed great surgeons in London, Paris and America.

He found that Simpson was not the prophet in his own country that he was abroad. He operated in the Samaritan Hospital in London, watched by Spencer Wells, Henry Savage, Routh, and other surgeons of that hospital. The patient unfortunately died 5 or 6 days afterwards. This was the first patient he had ever lost by the operation that he had now performed hundreds of times, and the reason for the death was that he had tied both the ureters. In Paris for the first time he wore glasses to operate in front of a host of French surgeons. He was invited to demonstrate his operation in Brussels, and did three in one morning. One patient died a week later because the nurse using the catheter had driven it through the posterior wall of the bladder into the peritoneal cavity. He was given a dinner and he did not understand a word of what was said! Later, he was made Chevalier of the Legion of Honour. He set up a hospital in Paris, determined not to return to New York until the war there was over. He was asked to settle in London. He was made a Knight of the Order of Leopold I 1862 in Brussels. He continued on his journeys and when he was not accompanied by his wife he wrote her the most loving letters. Sim's autobiography finished 20 years before he died. On 12 November 1883 he returned with his family to New York. He then operated on the wife of a prominent citizen highly successfully. He was jotting down memoranda until his wife urged him to sleep and put out the light. He died quickly with his wife beside him. 'His hand had not lost its skill or his eye its brightness. He had nearly rounded his 71st year and time had written scarce one wrinkle upon his brow'.

SIMPSON, JAMES YOUNG (1811–1870)

James Simpson was remarkable in every way. Because he was so brilliant he was made Professor of Obstetrics at Edinburgh University after marrying Jessie Grindlay of Liverpool at the age of 28. He knew an unmarried man would stand less chance, so because of 'the proprieties' of obtaining the post he became a married man. Simpson realized to get on one has not only to be good, but be seen to be so. He therefore spent £150.00 or more having testimonials printed and posted to everyone who had even the slightest influence at the town council.

Simpson naturally attracted a great deal of jealousy because of his large private practice, his prolific output in writing and his interest in operative gynaecology. It was Simpson who used a 'metallic uterine sound or bougie of nearly the size and shape of a small male catheter, which when introduced as it can easily be done into the interior of the uterus and manipulated there in different ways, proved to be a great service in rendering the diagnosis of the disease in question and more particularly those of the fundus, body, and cavity of the organ . . . much more precise (ly) than can be affected by any other means than which I am acquainted'.

This remarkable man produced a volume of essays on archaeology, published posthumously in 1872 after editing by John Stuart, an antiquary in Scotland, and several historical essays, some from as early as March 1841 on leprosy and continuing until 1862. One of the most interesting however, of all his essays was his inaugural address to the Medico-Chirurgical Society of Edinburgh when he was made their President in 1853. In this address he, in simple language, reviewed the progress of histological anatomy, pathological chemistry, medical diagnosis, materia-medica, medicine as a practical art and vaccination. He was a doughty opponent of homeopathy. In one of his obstetric essays 1844 he showed that statistically it was more dangerous to have a male than a female child. Simpson who died relatively young in 1870, packed so much into his life. One of the most remarkable of his discoveries was that of acupressure for stopping bleeding from large arteries. Needles were placed across the arteries before they were divided and then removed 42–78 hours later. It is difficult today to see how the pressure mechanism worked.

Simpson argued with Mauriceau's doctrine, which had misinterpreted Genesis 16:3 which says 'I will greatly multiply thy sorrow, and thy conception; in sorrow thou shall bring forth children; and thy desire shall be to thy husband, and he shall rule over thee'; Simpson countered that the Lord put Adam to sleep when he fashioned Eve out of one of his ribs!

Simpson was appointed physician to the Queen in Scotland in 1847, made a Baronet in 1866, and was responsible for Dr John Snow anaesthetizing Queen Victoria for two of her deliveries.

James Young Simpson was born in Bathgate, Linlithgowshire (now West Lothian) on 17 June 1811. He was the first to use both ether and chloroform in obstetrics, using ether soon after it was discovered by Morten on 19 January 1847. He started to experiment also with chloroform and the description of how he anaesthetized some of his friends after a long day's work, is a classic. There were three of them and they started to inhale from tumblers filled with chloroform, which incidentally Simpson had obtained from a chemist in Edinburgh, Messrs Duncan and Flockhart who are still important in the pharmaceutical industry. Simpson had been sent the substance and had put it away beneath a heap of wastepaper and empty bottles.

The three men almost immediately became amazingly talkative and were startled at first and delighted at the change, but then horrified as they crashed to the floor. Simpson who was the first to come round realized that the substance was better and stronger than ether. The other two, a Dr Duncan and a Dr Keith took longer to come round. It was very fortunate that they suffered no ill effects because they took part in the experiment several times in the same evening. Simpson himself was unconscious once for over 2 hours as the result of trying different substances. The first time he used chloroform on a patient was on a doctor's wife, and she christened the baby girl that was born 'Anaesthesia'. On 15 November 1847, Simpson was the anaesthetist for his friend Professor Miller when the latter removed one of the long bones in the forearm of a child, followed by another two operations which were watched by a huge crowd of doctors and students. Inevitably as with all modern advances, there were criticisms from other surgeons who were jealous and from religious authorities and moralists.

The long obstetric forceps Simpson designed are still occasionally used today. Simpson is almost as much revered in British obstetric circles as John Hunter is in surgical circles.

SMELLIE, WILLIAM (1697–1763)

Smellie, who was one of the most important obstetricians of all times and countries, was born in Lesmahagow, (Lanark), Scotland, in 1697. He was also married and finally buried in Lanarkshire. His tombstone bears the inscription 'this is Dr William Smellie's burial place, who died March 5th 1763, aged 66'. He first practised in Glaister in Lanarkshire, and then in London, where he was rather unhappy with what he was learning about obstetrics from teachings on the phantom of an artificial pelvis. He then went to Paris where he spent some time (nobody knows exactly how long) studying from the French masters.

Returning to London in about 1739–1740 he set up in practice, where he was soon joined by William Hunter (q.v.) in 1741. He set his mind to working out the mechanics of labour and was the first to measure the diagonal conjugate of the pelvis. He taught, using a real pelvis covered in leather; and he charged for allowing pupils to watch him conduct deliveries. He has been described as practical, logical and quickly able to pick up the meaning of signs and symptoms found in his patients.

His publications are very famous indeed. His treatise on the theory and practice of midwifery was published in 1752 and has been described as the first important textbook of obstetrics written by a Briton. Its success was so great that a second edition appeared in the same year. This was not a mere reprint of the first edition but heavily corrected; and 2 years later was followed by *A collection of cases and observations in midwifery* to illustrate 'his former treatise or first volume on that subject'.

The introduction to the treatise on the theory and practice of midwifery reviews some of the early writings, including those of Hippocrates and Plato. He quotes Plato thus: 'after affirming that there is implanted in the genitals of man, an imperious, headstrong, inobedient power that endeavours to subject everything to its furious lusts, he says the vulva and matrix of woman is also an animal ravenous after generation . . .'. Smellie quotes Celsus, Moschion, and many others including Galen; and he quotes from Linacre, Raynalde and other Arabic, Swiss, and Italian authors and lauds the writings of Francis Mauriceau. After his lengthy introduction to his treatise . . . Smellie described for the first time accurately, the bony pelvis and the different shapes and forms it could take.

He tried at first to use the French forceps, particularly Dussé's forceps, but found them wanting in some respects, so designed his own made with iron and covered with leather. Later he abandoned the leather cover on the blades. Before insertion into the vagina the blades were greased with hog's lard. He tried to use wooden forceps that he designed, thinking them likely to be less upsetting for patients, but found after three attempts that they did not really work well. His *Sett of Anatomical Tables, Explanations and Abridgements of the Practise of Midwifery, with a view to illustrate a treatise on that subject and a collection of cases*, was first printed in 1754 in London and a second edition of this masterly Atlas of 39 plates of which 26 were drawn by Rymsdyck (q.v. William Hunter) and 13 probably by Smellie himself, appeared in 1761. This is probably the most important anatomical obstetric atlas ever produced, but was followed fairly soon afterwards by William Hunter's *Atlas of the Gravid Uterus* and several others. Smellie was the first person to describe how to rotate the occipito-posterior positioned head with the forceps, and was the first to apply forceps to the aftercoming head in breech deliveries.

He did not have a smooth manner and managed to antagonize the midwives practising in

London, of whom one, Mrs Nihell (q.v.) a midwife practising in Haymarket with whom he quarrelled, called him 'a great horse God-mother of a he-midwife'.

His practice was much more among the poor of London than William Hunter's was, but he acquired immense experience. He had delivered over 1000 babies by 1752 and given hundreds of lectures. When he returned to Lanark in the summer of 1759 he devoted himself to updating his writings and in particular his collection of cases and his theories on the mechanisms of labour – many of which have stood the test of time. Although he was somewhat unpolished and dressed even in London in country clothes, the impression he made on the science of midwifery as well as the very sensible teachings he propounded, have made him, the acknowledged master of midwifery; not only because he introduced a new kind of lock into forceps which made them easier to use as well as a newly shaped curve and a double curve, but also because he wrote his extremely important books that indicated his great knowledge of the history of his subject, as well as having an immense practice.

Smellie, W. (1752). *Treatise on the Theory and Practice of Midwifery*, 2nd edn. corrected. (London: D. Wilson & T. Durhan)

SNOW, JOHN (1813–1858) (portrait, p. 437)

John Snow was the first to administer chloroform to Queen Victoria and he did so on two occasions. In fact he was the first full-time British anaesthetist. He published in the year of his death, his book *Chloroform and Other Anaesthetics* which has become a classic. He administered as many as 400 anaesthetics a year during the last 10 years of his short life.

John Snow was equally famous for tracing the source of the cholera epidemic which swept London in 1854. He found that it was due to contaminated water, and by suggesting taking away the handle of the pump from a well from which water was obtained for the City of London he stopped the cholera epidemic in 1854 from spreading.

SORANUS OF EPHESUS (AD 98–138)

Soranus was born in Ephesus, a city in Asia Minor, to Menandrus and his wife Phoebe. It seems that he studied in Alexandria, but eventually went to Rome where he practised medicine at the time of the Emperors Trajan (98–117) and Hadrian (117–138).

Soranus of Ephesus is the leading authority on the gynaecology and obstetrics of antiquity. He recognized atresia of the vagina as being congenital or acquired from inflammation. He packed the uterus for haemorrhage and performed hysterectomy for prolapse. He described podalic version. His book *Gynecology* in the original Greek was the most important work of the era and has been beautifully translated into English (in 1956) by Owsei Temkin. The *Gynecology* is probably the most important of Soranus' writings, but he also wrote about internal medicine, surgery, materia medica, and other subjects including embryology. Among those who praised him highly was Saint Augustine. Soranus was a member of the 'Methodist Sect', the third important sect in medicine, the other two being the 'Dogmatic Sect' and the 'Empirical Sect'.

Soranus discussed fertilization and embryology. In his remarkably complete book on gynaecology Soranus included, first the midwife and her subject, and then the physicians who were gynaecologists treating female illnesses. In difficult obstetric cases the male physician was called in and the physician was expected to include obstetrics and gynaecology in his field of knowledge. Soranus himself did.

Soranus described the female genitals, the hygiene of female sexual functions during pregnancy, normal labour and the puerperium, and finally some early paediatrics.

Soranus talked about positions of the fetus being longitudinal, the head or feet presenting first; transverse position with a side, back or abdomen presenting; and the doubled-up position where the head and legs or the abdomen or the hips were presenting. It was recognized that these were very bad presentations.

Soranus did not describe the management of the transverse position but Caelius Aurelianus suggested that Soranus did turn the fetus either to the head or feet presentation.

In his recital of the qualities necessary to become a midwife, he says 'she must be sound of limb and robust, endowed with long slim fingers and short nails at her finger tips . . . She must be literate, have a good memory, be able to impart information and be respectable'. Soranus divided midwives into faultless midwives (the average) and the best midwives. These are well versed not only in practice, but in theory as well, and are 'unafraid in danger'.

Talking about gynaecological hygiene he says this can be learnt from dissection, although he says this is useless! The term *uterus* or *metra* he also called *hysteria* and *delphys*. These terms are still all used today. The term metra comes from *meter*, the Greek word for 'mother' since the womb is the mother of all embryos. He gives fairly accurate descriptions of the anatomical position of the uterus and its relationship to the bladder and rectum.

There is a drawing on Plate I of a uterus that looks rather like the head of a small domesticated animal!

As for menstruation he uses the terms *katamenion* and *epimenion* (the food of the embryo), also the use of the word '*katharsis* . . . excreting blood from the body like excessive matter affects a purgation of the body'. He discusses whether the katharsis of the menses fulfils a helpful purpose and likens the salutary effect of menstruation to the way men rid themselves of surplus matter through athletics. He quotes Herophilius of Chalcedon who says that on occasion menstruation may be harmful. He discusses the value of virginity and of sexual intercourse for general health, and says there are two sides to the arguments. He discusses (on page 30) 'up to what time females should be kept virginal' and answers 'certainly till menstruation starts'.

The best time for fruitful intercourse 'is when menstruation is ending and abating, when urge and appetite for coitus are present, when the body is neither in want, nor too congested . . .'. He is an advocate of massage 'rub-down'. He does not seem to be certain whether conception is good for women's health or not, but he discusses the diagnosis of conception and the care that should be given to pregnant women. He points out that Hippocrates 'believed the male to be formed if the seed was conceived in the right part of the uterus, a female on the other hand if in the left part'. But in the physiological commentaries 'on generation we prove this untrue'. Antenatal care is discussed at some length. There are several pages on pica or *kissa* which is an upset stomach and dislike of certain foods together with an appetite for things not customary 'like earth, charcoal, tendons of the vine and ripeless fruit . . .'. There are several pages talking about 'what grows inside the uterus', impending abortions and abortive agents as well as contraceptives. The second of Soranus' four books deals with labour and childbirth and the selection of a wet-nurse as well as breastfeeding. The third book deals with

conditions familiar to women such as retention of menstruation, inflammation of the uterus, satyriasis – 'intense itching of the genitals together with pain, so that they continually bring their hands to this region. Because of this they develop an irresistible desire for sexual intercourse . . . which throws aside all sense of shame'. There is a disease called 'hysterical suffocation' a condition of air in the uterus, as well as moles, allergies, discharges (flux), atony and unusual positions of the uterus. The fourth book deals with difficult labours when the physician may well be called in. Plate II has an illustration of the different positions that the fetus (who looks incredibly adult) may occupy in the uterus.

Soranus (1956). *Gynecology* translated with an introduction by Owsei Temkin. (Baltimore: Johns Hopkins Press)

STEPTOE, PATRICK CHRISTOPHER (1913–1988)

Steptoe was born in Whitney, which is a small Oxfordshire market town near the Cotswold Hills in England, and he was one of eight children. He qualified as a doctor in 1939 and after one or two resident posts went into the Royal Navy. His ship was torpedoed, and he was a prisoner of war of the Italians for 2 years. In 1951 he obtained a consultant post in Oldham in Lancashire. This was somewhat of a disappointment as he had hoped to become a consultant in 'a centre of excellence' which Oldham certainly was not. In a way this was to stimulate him to become outstanding. In 1959 he saw Raoul Palmer (q.v.) the great French gynaecologist, demonstrate on film his laparoscope (see Chapter 27 laparoscopy). He wrote the first English book on the subject and went on developing the apparatus and techniques for operating using it. He was almost certainly the first in the English-speaking world to use it for diagnosis and later for operative treatment, and better still on many occasions, to avoid an open operation.

In 1968 there was a meeting of the Endocrinological and Gynaecological sections of the Royal Society of Medicine. At that meeting, Steptoe was the first in the English-speaking world to demonstrate beautifully illustrated slides of polycystic ovaries taken through the laparoscope. He had used a machine fitted with Hopkin's light system. From that meeting in 1968, which was also attended by Robert Edwards (q.v.), developed a research project that was to take 10 years until

Louise Brown, the first *in vitro* fertilization baby, was born at nearly midnight on 25 July 1978 by Caesarean section because of Mrs Brown's worsening toxaemia.

He and Edwards knew from the beginning that there would be heavy criticism and serious ethical problems to be solved (see Chapter 45 on Ethics). There were many firsts in their work. Before Louise Brown was born there was an ectopic pregnancy from which they were fortunately able to do chromosome studies which revealed a normal fetus. Later there was an unintentional abortion which showed triploidy. They were the first to describe these two cases following *in vitro* fertilization. There were serious unfounded worries that the incidence of abnormalities would be higher in *in vitro* fertilization babies than in others.

Steptoe had originally intended to be a musician and already at the age of 18 had been appointed Musical Director at Christ Church Oxford. He had been a pianist almost up to professional standard and had started by playing the piano for silent films at the local cinema in Oldham when he was 13 years of age. He had been shunned by the London Medical establishment, vilified by pro-life groups and starved of funds for research, particularly by the Medical Research Council. Yet, he with Robert Edwards a close friend and colleague, had been the first not only to produce a baby by *in vitro* fertilization but also a baby born from a frozen embryo and to start the donation of embryos. Because of his work the genetic structure of embryos can be analysed and perhaps later altered.

He died in March 1988. The last years of his life were clouded by his wife's paralysis following a brain haemorrhage and by his own cancer of the prostate. Yet he never wavered in his determination to go on leading the profession in the direction he knew it had to go.

SUSRATA see under *Charaka* and *Susrata*

TAIT, ROBERT LAWSON (1845–1899)

Lawson Tait was a 'real character'. He was, as are so many surgeons, aggressive, unusual, original and most dogmatic. People liked or disliked him; few were neutral about him. He operated brilliantly as he talked and as he wrote. Lawson Tait was trained in Edinburgh where he lived for a time with James Young Simpson.

In 1867 he was appointed resident surgeon at the Clayton Hosital, Wakefield, and a year later performed his first ovariotomy followed by four others in the following 3 years. He was one of the first abdominal surgeons and in 1880 one of the first to remove an inflamed appendix.

He did the first cholecystotomy in Europe in 1879, and in the same year a partial hepatectomy for hydatid cysts or tumours. He was appointed to the staff of the Women's Hospital in Birmingham when he was 26 years of age. He later became Professor of Gynaecology at Queen's College, Birmingham. By the age of 32 he had published 200 papers and books and before he was 40 he had carried out 1000 cases of laparotomy with a mortality rate of 9.3%. These included 307 appendicectomies, 54 hysterectomies and 13 cholecystotomies, 11 ectopics and the removal of a large number of ovaries. Many of these had nothing wrong with them (Tait, 1879).

Spaying ladies by removing their ovaries was not considered a mutilating operation (although doubtless Tait would not have liked his testes to be removed!). It was meant to improve women's health and perhaps make them more docile. In fact the results may well have been, or must have been, to induce an artificial menopause with all of its consequent ill effects. He was the first surgeon to carry out the operation of salpingectomy for tubal (ectopic) pregnancy in 1883, and he said that he thought that this was a life-saving and essential procedure.

Lawson Tait's part in the foundation in 1885 of the Medical Defence Union (Forbes, 1945), of which he became the first president, was of incalculable benefit to doctors, and especially surgeons, as well as to patients (Brazier, 1987) (see Chapter 45 on Ethics and the Law).

His rivalry with Spencer Wells (q.v.) was such that these two very great pioneers were not on speaking terms with one another. It was said that Lawson Tait and the great German Billroth (q.v.), 'led the way' into abdominal surgery (Clapesattle, 1941).

The following chronologically were the important achievements in Lawson Tait's life.

1873 He received the Hasting's Medal from the British Medical Association in Birmingham for his achievements in surgery.

1873 He used silk to close wounds.

1877 He published an essay on hospital mortality following bilateral salpingectomies.

1879 First cholecystotomy and first exploratory laparotomy for diagnosis.

1880 He had carried out 1000 cases of successful ovariotomy and attacked the ever spreading vogue for 'Listerism'.

1883 First salpingectomy for ruptured ectopic pregnancy.

1884 Thousandth laparotomy by Spencer Wells.

1885 President of the newly founded Medical Defence Union.

1886 Medical Defence Union considers a case of spaying (removal of both ovaries).

Brazier, M. (1987). *Medicine, Patients and the Law*, pp. 8–210. (Harmondsworth: Penguin Books Ltd.)
Clapesattle, H. (1941). *Doctors*. (Mayo, Minneapolis: University of Minnesota Press)
Forbes, R. (1945). *The Medical Defence Union Ltd.*, pp. 1–30. (London: Medical Defence Union)
Shepherd, J.A. (1965). *Spencer Wells*. (Edinburgh, London: E. & S. Livingstone)
Tait, R.L. (1879). Removal of normal ovaries. *Br. Med. J.*, 1, 813–14

VELPEAU, ALFRED ARMAND LOUIS MARIE (1795–1867)

He worked as a surgeon at the Hôpitals Sainte Antoine, la Pitie, and Charité Paris between the years 1828 and 1867. His chief written work was the *Traite Elementaire de l'art des Accouchements*. It was translated into English by Ch. D. Meigs in 1831 (Philadelphia: Grigg). He also in 1833 wrote one of the first authoritative works on embryology. He described, together with a colleague, hydatidiform moles. Velpeau also contributed to the debates on uterine retroversion, treatment of urinary fistulae and caesarean section.

VESALIUS, ANDREAS (1514–1564)

Vesalius (also known as Andreas Wesel) of Brussels was the son of an English mother. He was a student of the University of Louvain and later of Paris, and became a pupil of Sylvius. With his partner Jan Stephen van Calcar (1499–1546) he produced *De Humani Corporis Fabrica Libri Septem*, which Sir William Osler has called the greatest medical work ever printed. The first edition printed and published by Oporinus appeared in Basle in 1543. It was the first truly scientific anatomical work.

This marvellous atlas of human anatomy was the first to contradict the teachings of Galen and Aristotle. The atlas contains 663 folio pages and over 300 illustrations. There was a second edition in 1555. Only in this second edition did Vesalius express his doubts as to the character of Galen's physiology; and contradict its fundamental basis. It contains some beautiful woodcut illustrations including some of the female genital organs.

DA VINCI, LEONARDO (1452–1519) (Figure 8)

Although Leonardo da Vinci was certainly not a gynaecologist nor obstetrician no book of medical history would be complete without reference to this man, born at Vinci near Empoli, not far from Florence in Italy 'of unknown antecedents, left handed, unsexed' and considered by many to be the greatest genius of all time. He was a painter, sculptor, architect, engineer, musician, poet, philosopher, chemist, botanist and geologist. His painting of the Mona Lisa in the Louvre in Paris is

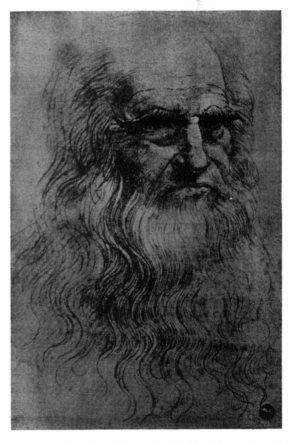

Figure 8 Portrait of Leonardo da Vinci. Reproduced with kind permission from the Royal Library, Windsor

probably the most visited painting in the world. His notebooks and drawings are remarkable. His engineering projects, helicopters, flying machines, aqueducts, were centuries ahead of his time, but for gynaecologists his first depiction of the uterus in a drawing in red crayon outlined with a pen, made from bodies he had dissected, was the nearest to anatomical accuracy that had been achieved up to his time. He probably dissected 30 male and female bodies. His depiction of the uterus as unilocular instead of making it look like a two-horned organ as in mammals, shows that he had almost certainly dissected a human uterus. He described the fetal membranes and even did a notable drawing of the human genitalia as they come together in sexual intercourse.

He was followed by Jacopo Berengario da Carpi (1470–1550) making anatomical drawings direct from nature. He was Professor of Anatomy in Padua. He described vaginal hysterectomy, an operation originally carried out by Soranus.

Leonardo, R.A. (1944). *A History of Gynecology*, pp. 185–7 and Plate 10. (New York: Froben Press)

VIRCHOW, RUDOLF LUDWIG KARL (1821–1902)

This nineteenth century German pathologist was known as 'The Master'. His specialty was pathological anatomy or histology. He became Professor first in the University in Wurzburg in 1849 and then in Berlin in 1856. He was a politician as well as one of the world's greatest histopathologists. He pioneered the idea of applying cell doctrine to the concept of disease. He discovered the neuroglia in the brain and spinal cord. His work on cell pathology, which was translated into English in 1868, is probably one of the most important books in the history of medicine because it laid the foundation stone for cellular pathology. He was the first to demonstrate that syphilis was a disease that involved all the organs and tissues of the body. The causal organism was transferred through the blood to various organs and tissues. While he was still young he founded the *Journal of Pathological Anatomy* and already at the age of 26 postulated that cancer might result from local irritation; but he was mistaken in thinking that carcinomas grow in connective tissues. He was the first to describe clearly thrombosis and embolism and was the first to name the condition of leukaemia. His contributions to gynaecological pathology were particularly important in descriptions of the cells in carcinomas.

This remarkable man wrote about town planning, anthropology and even craniology (the different shapes of the head according to ethnic origin). He also assisted in archeological excavations.

WELLS, THOMAS SPENCER (1818–1897)

Thomas Spencer Wells (Figure 9) was born in St Albans on 3 February 1818 and died at Cap d'Antibes on 31 January 1897 of apoplexy. His father was a builder. Thomas went to school first in St Albans, a school with a very long history dating back to 1100. He started training as a doctor at the age of 17 when he went as a pupil to Dr Michael Sadler of Barnsley where he stayed for a year and then went to Leeds to a Mr Marsden a para-surgeon where, before he was 19 years of age he had 'attended a great many poor women of Leeds in childbirth'. He then attended the Leeds Medical School, but in 1837 he spent a session at Trinity College Dublin during the summer months, returning to England and to St Thomas' Hospital where he qualified in 1841 with membership of the Royal College of Surgeons of London.

In 1841, he joined the Navy where he came under the influence of Sir William Burnett. He served in Malta where the hospital is beautifully built, well-ventilated and the wards are spacious, so that problems with infection did not militate against surgery. While in Malta he was made a Fellow of the Royal College of Surgeons, one of 300 elected without examination. He was later to become President of the Royal College of Surgeons. Not only did Spencer Wells look after Naval personnel, but also civilians on the island of Malta.

After his service in Malta, Spencer Wells visited Paris to study gunshot wounds. Later in Corfu, still as a Naval surgeon, Wells was able to operate with the assistance of medical officers of the Army in an Army hospital on a sailor of 24 with a tumour of the bones of the pelvis. In 1856 Wells was working in a civilian hospital in the Dardanelles.

After nearly 15 years in the Navy, part of which time he spent in private practice in London, and part working in an Army hospital during the Crimea, he left the Navy, mainly because of ill health. He did, in 1851, have pneumonia in the right lung. At the end of 1854 on New Year's Eve he was entertained by James Young Simpson in Edinburgh. Wells operated in Edinburgh and there is

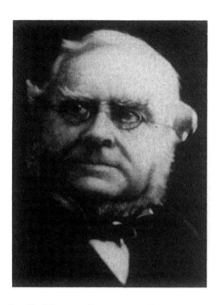

Figure 9 Sir Thomas Spencer Wells

no doubt that Simpson frequently watched him operate in London.

On 16 June 1854 when he had already tried to operate on a case of Simpson's for vesico-vaginal fistula, he was appointed to the staff of the Samaritan Hospital for Women and Children. It was in that hospital that he performed a large series of operations for ovarian disease.

The Samaritan Hospital is still today a very important gynaecological hospital. In 1886 it moved to its present site in Marylebone Road, having been established in Manchester Square in the West End of London in January 1847, as the 'gynae-pathic institute free hospital'.

He had not been at the Samaritan Hospital for long before he had to go the Crimean War, accompanied by his wife. Florence Nightingale was also out there at the time.

The first time Spencer Wells tried to remove an ovarian cyst was in December 1857. Although Robert Houston had already in 1701 opened an abdomen to extract the contents of an ovarian cyst and McDowell had in 1809 removed an ovarian tumour, not much surgery on ovaries had been carried out; although Lawson Tait (q.v.) of Birmingham was operating in that city.

In 1845 Spencer Wells was appointed a Surgeon to the Royal Household. By the age of 44 he had operated on 50 ovaries, and by 3 years later he had performed 100 ovariotomies. He retired from the Samaritan Hospital in 1877 20 years before he died in 1897 of a second stroke.

It is of historical interest that some time while Spencer Wells was working in it, the Samaritan Hospital was at 20 Orchard Street which is now Selfridges Store. Spencer Wells himself had his consulting rooms in Upper Grosvenor Street which is now the American Embassy. It is believed that by the time Spencer Wells died he had performed a total of 1200 ovariotomies. In his lifetime he benefited from the introduction of aseptic gynaecological surgery by Lawson Tait and by his own invention of the Spencer Wells clamp which he first used on the ovarian pedicle which initially he left exteriorized.

Shepherd, J.A. (1965). *Spencer Wells, The Life and Work of a Victorian Surgeon.* (Edinburgh, London: E. & S. Livingstone Ltd.)

WERTHEIM, ERNST (1864–1920)

Ernst Wertheim was born on 21 February 1864 in Graz, the ancient capital of Styria, a university town, an industrial centre, and the second city of Austria. He came from a distinguished scientific family. His father Theodore was a Professor of Chemistry and his mother, the sister of a Professor of Physics in the University. In 1988 he graduated M.D. at the University of Graz and worked with Kahler, Croback and the legendary Billroth (q.v.). By 1891 Wertheim was Schauta's first assistant and by October 1906, when he was invited to address the University Medical Society of Chicago, he had already published his description of 29 cases of carcinoma of the cervix, on whom he had carried out his radical operation. There was till then no really effective treatment for carcinoma of the cervix. Wertheim studied and understood quite a lot about its pathology and its modes of spread.

Although Wertheim realized that blood spread was possible he did not consider that there was any procedure that could effect a cure, or prevent this spread if it was going to happen. His operation was designed to prevent lymphatic spread. Wertheim felt that although carcinoma of the cervix was a local disease, it had to be treated by radical excision in order to obtain real cures.

Wertheim's operation was based on an operation designed in 1878 by William Alexander Freund of Breslau, who had carried out 66 radical operations, but with 50 deaths at operation! The vaginal approach had been tried, but until Schauta performed a radical operation vaginally the mortality rate was 96% within 5 years. Wertheim's operation included excision of the parametrium, which was only possible if the ureters were dissected throughout their length. To do this the operation had to be performed abdominally. The removal of the lymph nodes followed on Halstead's radical operation for removal of the breast together with the axillary and other lymph nodes.

Wertheim's first patient was a Madame Rudd, aged 39, and the operation was performed on 16 November 1898. There was no trained anaesthetist available. Intravenous blood transfusion was not available because it was only 2 years later in 1900 that Landsteiner (q.v.), also from Vienna, worked out the first four blood groups.

By the time he lectured in Chicago in 1906, 8 years after performing his first radical operation, Wertheim had operated on more than 300 cases of cancer of the cervix and was about to publish his classical work *De Erweiterte Abdominale Operation bei Carcinoma Colli Uteri* which recorded his first 500 cases. Wertheim spoke in Chicago to 360 surgeons and physicians. He pointed out 'the radical operation, can', he said, 'with justice, be described as the German–American operation'. German from Freund who originated the abdominal route and from Funke and Reis who advocated the systemic removal of regional nodes. American from Howard Kelly for his work on the ureter and Clark, Cullen and Prior (who were present with Kelly that night) for 'their persistence with the operation'. He pointed out how important it was to expose the ureter and to operate by the abdominal route and that only that way could infection be controlled.

Inevitably Wertheim was criticized in the Chicago meeting. One, Nicholas Sen, thought Wertheim's operation to be the most difficult a surgeon could undertake, and that it would never become routine. A Dr Xavier Oswald Wender, a Swiss who became President of the American Association of Obstetricians and Gynecologists in 1912 claimed that he had described Wertheim's operation 2 years before Wertheim himself had. (So often people claim to have done things when they could not have possibly done them, and even in our day, Steptoe and Edwards had to hear of claims that a 'test-tube baby' had been born in another provincial city in England as well as in a city in India, but neither of those claims could be substantiated.) In spite of his critics in Chicago, Wertheim continued to perform his operations so that by his death he had carried out 1300 radical operations.

When Madame Curie had isolated radium in 1911 and it was starting to be used in cancer therapy, Wertheim thought this affected his radical operation which 'has toppled and collapsed in an instance'. Radium bromide had been separated from Bohemium pitchblende, but had not yet been used in the treatment of carcinoma of the cervix. However, by 1990 it was obvious that radiotherapy did not supersede the operation, nor the radical operation exclude radiotherapy. Stallworthy has shown that the two can and often should be combined.

Wertheim died in 1920 aged 56, from pneumonia during the world-wide influenza epidemic.

As Sir Stanley Simmons, Past President of the Royal College of Obstetricians and Gynaecologists, who has contributed to the above biography of Wertheim, for which the authors of this book are immensely grateful, said at the end of his Presidential Address to the Section of Obstetrics and Gynaecology of the Royal Society of Medicine 'one notes with awe the astonishing explosion of talents in Vienna: Rokitansky, Semmelweis, Billroth, Freud, Landsteiner, Schauta and Wertheim, the city of Mozart, Haydn, Beethoven and Schubert.

WHITE, CHARLES (1728–1813) (portrait, p. 18)

This Manchester obstetrician played a very great role in the early history of prevention of puerperal fever. He was a general surgeon who also practised orthopaedic surgery.

His most important work is *A Treatise on the Management of Pregnant and Lying-in Women, and a means of curing, but more especially preventing the principal disorders to which they are liable*, which was printed in London in 1773. His practice of hand washing before attending labouring women was followed by Semmelweis (q.v.).

He wrote also *An enquiry into the nature and cause of that swelling in one or both of the lower extremities which sometimes happens to lying-in women*. This was published in Warrington in 1784 and contained the first accurate description of 'Phlegmasia Alba Dolens'.

White, C. (1773). *A Treatise on the Management of Pregnant and Lying-in Women*. (London: Diley)

WILLUGHBY, PERCIVALL (1596–1695)

Willughby was a friend and great admirer of Harvey (q.v.) and mentions him 16 times in his textbook. He practised in Derby, Stafford and London.

His book *The Country Midwives' Opusculum*, written in the seventeenth century, gave the case histories of 150 deliveries. It was however, only printed in 1863 under the general title of *Observations in Midwifery*. In it Willughby described many abnormalities of the mothers and their fetuses. His book was written to educate midwives; and he condemned some 'doctors' saying that bad medical practice was certainly as bad as ignorant midwives' practice. His daughter was a midwife. She called him in 1658 to help her deliver the wife of Sir Tennebs Evanks. His daughter had rightly diagnosed that the presentation was a breech presentation although Willughby at first thought it was a head presentation. He told his daughter to bring down a leg which she did, but then apparently lost her nerve. Willughby completed the delivery without, so it was said, the patient knowing that he was there as he had crawled into the room on hands and knees and delivered the baby under the cover of a sheet. (Men were not welcome at deliveries in the seventeenth century.)

Willughby believed all difficult deliveries could be undertaken by turning the fetus inside the uterus and extracting it by the feet. In spite of the fact that he did so many internal versions he did adjure midwives not to interfere unless it was absolutely necessary.

It seems that Willughby delivered his patients whenever possible 'kneeling at a convenient and fitting time, in a bending posture, holding her hands above another woman's neck, but sitteth before her . . .'. Willughby neither liked a midwives' stool nor delivering women on their backs.

He was visited in Derby by Harvey on several occasions and also in London. He said about midwives 'high and lofty conceited midwives, who will leave nothing unattempted to save their credits and cloak their ignorances'. He accused midwives of interfering and using instruments such as 'pot hooks, pack needles, silver spoons, thatcher's hooks and knives'. Midwives at that time according to Willughby were tossing patients about on blankets in order to try and hasten labour. Willughby was a great advocate of leaving things to nature. He adjured midwives to 'attend and wait on nature'. He advocated that sweet words be used to women in labour.

Graham, H. (1950). *Eternal Eve*, p. 256. (London: Heinemann)

Name index

Subject index

T - #1086 - 101024 - C0 - 254/190/31 - PB - 9781850700401 - Gloss Lamination